FOUNDATIONS OF CLINICAL RESEARCH

Applications to Evidence-Based Practice

Fourth Edition

Leslie G. Portney, DPT, PhD, FAPTA
Dean Emerita
MGH Institute of Health Professions
School of Health and Rehabilitation Sciences
Boston, Massachusetts

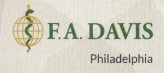

F.A. DAVIS

Philadelphia

F. A. Davis Company
1915 Arch Street
Philadelphia, PA 19103
www.fadavis.com

Printed in the United States of America

Last digit indicates print number: 10 9 8 7 6 5 4 3 2 1

Senior Sponsoring Editor: Jennifer Pine
Manager of Content Development: George W. Lang
Content Project Manager: Megan Suermann
Art and Design Manager: Carolyn O'Brien

As new scientific information becomes available through basic and clinical research, recommended treatments and drug therapies undergo changes. The author(s) and publisher have done everything possible to make this book accurate, up to date, and in accord with accepted standards at the time of publication. The author(s), editors, and publisher are not responsible for errors or omissions or for consequences from application of the book and make no warranty, expressed or implied, in regard to the contents of the book. Any practice described in this book should be applied by the reader in accordance with professional standards of care used in regard to the unique circumstances that may apply in each situation. The reader is advised always to check product information (package inserts) for changes and new information regarding dosage and contraindications before administering any drug. Caution is especially urged when using new or infrequently ordered drugs.

Library of Congress Cataloging-in-Publication Data
Names: Portney, Leslie Gross, author.
Title: Foundations of clinical research : applications to evidence-based
  practice / Leslie G. Portney.
Description: Fourth edition. | Philadelphia : F.A. Davis, [2020] | Includes
  bibliographical references and index. | Summary: "The text of this
  fourth edition has maintained its dual perspectives. It is designed for
  those who do research to generate new knowledge and examine theories and
  for those who want to be critical consumers of evidence to inform
  clinical decision-making. All of us need to be able to critically
  evaluate research reports to inform practice and further study. The
  scope of the text allows it to fulfill different needs at different
  times. This edition will continue to serve this wide audience. It
  incorporates several important contemporary themes, including the
  application of evidence-based practice (EBP) for clinical
  decision-making, the imperative of interprofessional collaboration, the
  implications of translational research, and the focus of healthcare on
  quality of life, meaningful outcomes, and patient values. These
  directions and priorities continue to define research philosophies that
  guide the conduct of clinical inquiry, the types of questions that are
  deemed important, and how they influence advances in measurement and
  analysis techniques"— Provided by publisher.
Identifiers: LCCN 2019044025 (print) | LCCN 2019044026 (ebook) | ISBN
  9780803661134 (hardcover) | ISBN 9780803661165 (ebook)
Subjects: MESH: Biomedical Research—methods | Evidence-Based
  Practice—methods | Clinical Decision-Making—methods | Statistics as
  Topic—methods | Research Design
Classification: LCC R853.C55 (print) | LCC R853.C55 (ebook) | NLM W 20.5
  | DDC 610.72/4—dc23
LC record available at https://lccn.loc.gov/2019044025
LC ebook record available at https://lccn.loc.gov/2019044026

To Hazel

. . . and joyful running hugs

Preface

It is now more than 25 years since this text was first published in 1993. It has become a classic reference, cited extensively in literature from researchers around the globe. It is gratifying to see its sustained and widespread use by clinicians, faculty, students, and researchers in a variety of fields including rehabilitation, medicine, public health, nursing, public policy, epidemiology, exercise physiology, and other disciplines concerned with healthcare. This edition will continue to serve this wide audience.

As I have approached each revision, I have been struck by how much the framework for research continues to evolve over time, and this edition is no different. It incorporates several important contemporary perspectives.

First, regardless of the role we play in healthcare, be it clinician, administrator, policy maker, or researcher, we all need to be critical consumers of evidence to inform decisions. This requires at least a basic understanding of principles of measurement, design, and analysis to enable reasonable and critical evaluation.

Second, the concept of evidence-based practice (EBP), although ubiquitous in healthcare discussion, must be understood in terms of its full purpose for clinical decision-making, relying not only on literature but also on clinical expertise, patient values, and environmental conditions. These considerations have influenced translational research and the need to address meaningful outcomes.

Third, today's healthcare enterprise mandates attention to interprofessional collaboration. I have included examples throughout the book to illustrate various concepts. These are drawn from many different fields, with the intent that all examples have wide application. I believe this is a distinct advantage of this book, to underscore the importance of appreciating research within and beyond one's own field.

And finally, the content will work for those who want to plan or implement research. Detailed examples are included for those who want more depth, both in the text as well as in online supplements.

These directions and priorities continue to define research philosophies that guide the conduct of clinical inquiry, the types of questions that are deemed important, and how they influence advances in measurement and analysis techniques.

The popular features of the book have not changed, such as its accessible tone, use of extensive clinical examples to illustrate applications of design and statistics, and careful logic in explanation of complex concepts. It remains a comprehensive text, meant to fulfill different needs at different times, serving as both an introduction and a reference as readers grow in their knowledge and experience. However, this fourth edition does represent a significant update in format, focus, and organization.

■ New and Updated

Perhaps most notable is the new design, intended to make the text more reader-friendly and engaging with full color. Tables and figures have a new look to facilitate interpretation. Starting with the book's title, the emphasis on EBP is clear, including the *Focus on Evidence* and *Case in Point* features in each chapter that illustrate the direct application of concepts in the literature. Additional information is included in boxes to clarify content, emphasize key points, offer interesting background and historical context—and a few fun facts along the way. Commentaries build on important concepts. Online resources have also been expanded, with chapter supplements, access to data files, and materials for instructors and students.

Five new chapters have been included in this edition, focusing on translational research (Chapter 2), evidence-based practice (Chapter 5), health measurement scales (Chapter 12), clinical trials (Chapter 14), and qualitative research (Chapter 21). All of these address content that was covered in previous editions but with greater depth and application.

Many chapters also include new or updated content to address current clinical research issues. For example,

- Examples provided throughout the book have been updated with more recent literature.
- The stronger emphasis on EBP includes use of the PICO strategy to answer clinical questions as well as to generate research questions. The EBP emphasis reflects a comprehensive model that includes research evidence, clinical expertise, patient values, and clinical circumstances.

- The chapter on searching the literature has been reorganized to provide stronger guidance in that process.
- The chapter on ethical principles has been updated to reflect recent changes in regulations and definitions.
- Measurement chapters provide a stronger emphasis on relative and absolute reliability, a broader context for construct validity, and extensive discussion on measuring change.
- The chapter on health measurement scales focuses on construct validity and reliability for questionnaires that are used to measure function, quality of life, and personal characteristics that impact health. It includes expanded coverage of Rasch analysis.
- Chapters on foundations of design cover contemporary issues related to clinical trials, such as translational research, efficacy and effectiveness, superiority and non-inferiority trials, pragmatic trials, N-of-1 trials, and implementation studies.
- Content related to observational designs has increased emphasis on use of these designs for diagnosis and prognosis, as well as for evaluating causal relationships.
- Qualitative research has a stronger presence throughout the book, including a new chapter that also addresses mixed methods. Although this coverage cannot substitute for a full reference on this topic, this content should facilitate reading and interpreting the literature, and will reinforce the relevance of qualitative research in a variety of contexts.
- The *International Classification of Functioning, Disability and Health (ICF)* is used as a framework for terminology as part of understanding patient-oriented research.
- Statistics chapters have added coverage of validity measures and regression and multivariate methods, such as exploratory and confirmatory factor analysis and structural equation modeling. Data files for all examples presented in tables can be accessed online.
- Information on power, effect size, and sample size calculations are integrated with statistical procedures and illustrated in detail in chapter supplements. Some analyses are done using SPSS and others using G*Power.
- The chapters on critical appraisal and dissemination include information on use of reporting guidelines for different types of studies.
- The chapter on systematic reviews has been expanded to include more detail related to meta-analyses and now includes information on scoping reviews.

■ Organization

Although the overall organization of the book remains the same with content in five parts, some chapters have been rearranged to better reflect their role in the research process. Each section focuses on a different phase of that process.

- **Part 1- Foundations of Research and Evidence** focuses on fundamental concepts that define the clinical research enterprise, such as types of research, frameworks of health, translational research, application of theory, ethical principles, how to frame clinical and research questions, literature search strategies, and the overarching structure of EBP for clinical decision-making. These chapters provide an overview of the research process that serves as a foundation for the rest of the text.
- **Part 2- Concepts of Measurement** includes the basic premises of measurement for all types of data collection, including validity and reliability. The chapter on surveys has been relocated to this section to emphasize their role as data collection tools rather than a design. Fundamental concepts in the design of health measurement scales are presented.
- **Part 3- Designing Clinical Research** includes content on descriptive, observational, and explanatory research, with extensive examples related to validity and application of these designs. These include a variety of clinical trial designs, single-subject designs, observational studies using cohort and case-control designs, and descriptive and qualitative studies.
- **Part 4- Analyzing Data** presents the full scope of statistical content, starting with descriptive statistics and developing concepts through multivariate procedures. Parametric and nonparametric statistics are described for comparative, predictive, and descriptive studies, validity and reliability, studies of diagnostic tests, and epidemiology related to risk assessments. Information is presented from an intuitive perspective without emphasis on mathematical derivation or statistical notation. These chapters include a review of output using SPSS to illustrate how statistical results can be interpreted. Data files can also be accessed online for all analyses.
- **Part 5- Putting It All Together** focuses on the aspects of research that incorporate all the principles of design and analysis that have been covered in preceding chapters. Chapter 35 describes guidelines for developing a research proposal. Chapter 36 addresses the process of critical appraisal for several types of studies. Chapter 37 provides an overview of methods for conducting and evaluating systematic reviews,

meta-analyses, and scoping reviews. Finally, Chapter 38 presents a format for preparing and disseminating research through publications and presentations.

Appendix A includes reference tables for major statistical tests and additional tables are provided in *Appendix A Online*. Appendix B includes an algorithm for choosing a statistical procedure based on design and measurement considerations. Appendix C covers content related to management of quantitative data, including data transformation. The glossary, also available online, provides a handy reference to define terms, symbols, and common abbreviations.

No matter how many years I have engaged in research, I continue to learn about advances in design and analysis that set new directions and priorities for clinical inquiry. This edition is intended to strengthen our collective commitment to new knowledge, discovery and innovation, and implementation of evidence, as we strive to provide the most effective care. The process remains a challenge to all of us engaged in healthcare, and this text will always be a work in progress. I look forward to continuing to hear from colleagues across disciplines regarding how to make this volume most useful.

Contributors

Jessica Bell, MS
Director of Library and Instructional Design
MGH Institute of Health Professions
Boston, Massachusetts

Marianne Beninato, DPT, PhD
Professor Emerita
MGH Institute of Health Professions
Boston, Massachusetts

Peter S. Cahn, PhD
Associate Provost for Academic Affairs
MGH Institute of Health Professions
Boston, Massachusetts

Heather Fritz, PhD, MSOT
Assistant Professor, Occupational Therapy Program
  and Institute of Gerontology
Eugene Applebaum College of Pharmacy and Health
  Sciences
Wayne State University
Detroit, Michigan

**K. Douglas Gross, MPT, DPT, ScD,
  FAAOMPT, CPed**
Associate Professor, Department of Physical Therapy
MGH Institute of Health Professions
School of Health and Rehabilitation Sciences
Boston, Massachusetts

Catherine Lysack, PhD, OT(C)
Associate Professor, Occupational Therapy
  and Gerontology
Eugene Applebaum College of Pharmacy and Health
  Sciences
Wayne State University
Detroit, Michigan

David A. Scalzitti, PT, PhD
Assistant Professor, Physical Therapy and Health
  Care Sciences
School of Medicine and Health Sciences
The George Washington University
Washington, DC

Reviewers

Jason Browning, OTR/L
Assistant Professor
Occupational Therapy
Jefferson College of Health Sciences
Roanoke, Virginia

Stephen Chao, PT, DPT, CSCS
Clinical Assistant Professor
Physical Therapy Department
School of Health Technology and Management
State University of New York at Stony Brook
Southampton, New York

Jennifer B. Christy, PT, PhD
Associate Professor
Physical Therapy
The University of Alabama at Birmingham
Birmingham, Alabama

Peter C. Douris, PT, EdD, DPT, OCS
Professor
Physical Therapy
New York Institute of Technology
Old Westbury, New York

Winnie Dunn, PhD, OTR, FAOTA
Distinguished Professor
Occupational Therapy
University of Missouri
Columbia, Missouri

Ashraf Elazzazi, PT, PhD
Associate Professor
Chair, Department of Physical Therapy
Utica College
Utica, New York

Simon French, BAppSc, MPH, PhD
Associate Professor
School of Rehabilitation Therapy
Queen's University
Kingston, Ontario, Canada

Joanne Gallagher Worthley, EdD, OTR/L, CAPS
Professor
Occupational Therapy
Worcester State University
Worcester, Massachusetts

Sean F. Griech, PT, DPT, OCS, COMT
Assistant Professor
Doctor of Physical Therapy Program
DeSales University
Center Valley, Pennsylvania

Emmanuel B. John, PT, DPT, PhD, MBA
Associate Professor & Chair
Department of Physical Therapy
Chapman University
Irvine, California

Steven G. Lesh, PhD, PT, SCS, ATC
Chair and Professor of Physical Therapy
Southwest Baptist University
Bolivar, Missouri

Jean MacLachlan, PhD, OTR/L
Associate Professor
Occupational Therapy
Salem State University
Salem, Massachusetts

Dennis McCarthy, PhD, OTR/L, FAOTA
Associate Professor
Occupational Therapy
Nova Southeastern University
Tampa, Florida

Raymond F. McKenna, PT, PhD, CSCS
Clinical Associate Professor
Physical Therapy
Stony Brook University
Stony Brook, New York

Saurabh Mehta, PT, PhD
Assistant Professor
School of Physical Therapy
Marshall University
Huntington, West Virginia

Tamara Mills, PhD, OTR/L, ATP
Assistant Professor
School of Occupational Therapy
Brenau University
Norcross, California

Pablo Mleziva, PT, OCS, CSCS
Physical Therapist-Assistant Professor
Physical Therapy
Loma Linda University
Loma Linda, California

Shannon Petersen, PT
Associate Professor
Physical Therapy
Des Moines University
Des Moines, Iowa

Lenny Ramsey, PhD
Assistant Professor
Physical Therapy
Carroll University
Waukesha, Wisconsin

David A. Scalzitti, PT, PhD
Assistant Professor, Physical Therapy and Health Care
    Sciences
School of Medicine and Health Sciences
The George Washington University
Washington, DC

Eric Schussler, PhD, PT, ATC
Assistant Professor
School of Physical Therapy and Athletic Training
Old Dominion University
Norfolk, Virginia

Mary P. Shotwell, PhD, OT/L, FAOTA
Professor
School of Occupational Therapy
Brenau University
Gainesville, Georgia

Matt S. Stock, PhD
Assistant Professor
Department of Health Professions
University of Central Florida
Orlando, Florida

Ying-Chih Wang, PhD
Associate Professor
Occupational Science & Technology
University of Wisconsin – Milwaukee
Milwaukee, Wisconsin

Jennifer B. Wasserman, DPT, MS, PhD
Associate Professor
Physical Therapy
Franklin Pierce University
Manchester, New Hampshire

Mark Patrick Wilhelm, PT, DPT
Assistant Professor
Physical Therapy
Walsh University
North Canton, Ohio

Acknowledgments

Taking on this edition as a solo effort has been an interesting challenge. I am so appreciative for the support of many friends and colleagues who have helped me through it. I am indebted to those who contributed to writing chapters—Jessica Bell, Marianne Beninato, Peter Cahn, Heather Fritz, Doug Gross, Cathy Lysack, and David Scalzitti. I am thankful to John Wong for many hours of invaluable guidance on statistics. I am also grateful to those who took the time to review sections of the book and provide valuable feedback—Marjorie Nicholas, Winnie Dunn, Lisa Connor and Saurabh Mehta among others. I also want to acknowledge the long-time support of colleagues at the MGH Institute of Health Professions, especially Alex Johnson, Mary Ellen Ferolito, Denis Stratford and the entire IT team, as well as the graduate assistants Jasmin Torres and Baothy Huynh, who will both be awesome Doctors of Occupational Therapy. I reserve a special note of deep appreciation for David Scalzitti who has reviewed every page of this book and who freely offered his advice along the way, in every instance providing important comments to make things more accurate, complete, and useful. Many of his "pearls" are included in the text. Additionally, I'd like to thank David for creating the online Test Bank questions and PowerPoint slides. Always a wonderful colleague, he has become a good friend.

The F. A. Davis team was remarkably patient with me over many years, providing incredible support. Special thanks to Jennifer Pine, Senior Sponsoring Editor, who held my hand and tolerated my missing every deadline. Megan Suermann, Content Project Manager, lived through every word, figure, and table, and all their changes. Thank you to everyone who helped with every aspect of the project—to Cassie Carey, Senior Production Editor at Graphic World Publishing Services; Kate Margeson, Illustration Coordinator; Nichole Liccio, Melissa Duffield, and especially to Margaret Biblis, Editor-in-Chief, who said "yes" so quickly.

I'd also like to acknowledge my dear friend and writing partner Mary Watkins, who retired several years ago and is happily ensconced in New Hampshire with her family. Our collaboration was a special part of our lives for more than 20 years, and I sorely missed her this time around.

Over the past 50 years of my professional life, of which 45 were spent in academia, I have had the good fortune to work with thousands of students, faculty colleagues, and teachers who have inspired and challenged me. Too numerous to mention by name, I thank them all for their friendship, mentorship, and dedication. I am also grateful to many people, some I know and many I have never met, from all over the world, who over the years have taken the time to stop me at conferences, or to call or send emails, telling me how much they appreciated the book— and pointing out the mistakes and where information needed updating. Those comments have been immensely rewarding and incredibly helpful. I hope these colleagues are pleased with the revisions they have inspired.

And of course, there is no way a project like this gets done without support and sacrifice from those closest to me. My parents, who were so proud of this work, have both passed away since the last edition was published, but they continue to inspire me every day. My husband Skip has given up so much of our together time, particularly once we were both supposed to be retired. He gave me the space and time I needed, and now I have a lot of dishes to wash to make up my share! My children, Devon and Jay and Lindsay and Dan, are always there to prop me up with love and understanding, and Lindsay was even able to help me through some of the more complex statistics—very cool. And finally, little Hazel, the ultimate joy that only a grandparent can understand. Her smile and hugs have lifted me up through many tough days. She confirms for me every day that the future is bright. What they say is so true—if I'd known grandchildren were so much fun, I would have had them first! With no pun intended, the next chapter awaits!

About the Author

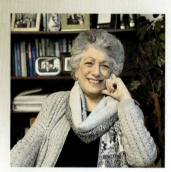

Dr. Leslie G. Portney is *Professor and Dean Emerita*, MGH Institute of Health Professions, having served as the inaugural Dean of the School of Health and Rehabilitation Sciences and Chair of the Department of Physical Therapy. She holds a PhD in Gerontology from the University Professors Program at Boston University, a Master of Science from Virginia Commonwealth University, a DPT from the MGH Institute of Health Professions, a certificate in Physical Therapy from the University of Pennsylvania, and a Bachelor of Arts from Queens College. Leslie has been an active researcher and educator for more than 50 years, with decades of teaching critical inquiry to graduate students from a variety of disciplines, which contributed to her being a staunch advocate of interprofessional education. She remains an active member of the American Physical Therapy Association, having served as chair of the Commission on Accreditation in Physical Therapy Education and inaugural president of the American Council of Academic Physical Therapy. She is the recipient of several awards, including receiving the 2014 Lifetime Achievement Award from the Department of Physical Therapy at Virginia Commonwealth University, being named the 2014 Pauline Cerasoli Lecturer for the Academy of Physical Therapy Education of the APTA, and being elected as a Catherine Worthingham Fellow of the American Physical Therapy Association in 2002. Leslie retired in 2018 but continues to contribute to professional projects and to consult with educational programs. She lives on Cape Cod with her husband, near to her children and granddaughter.

How to Use This Book

Since its first printing in 1993, this text has served several different audiences. Students may be assigned readings, using it as a class text. Clinicians may use it as a reference to explain material found in the literature. Researchers may use it to help generate questions, design studies, or develop analysis strategies. Some want only conceptual material while others want more in-depth coverage. I have tried to serve all these goals efficiently. Some material has been placed online to supplement content in the text as a way of providing in-depth material.

■ Examples

The extensive use of examples from literature has long been considered a strength of this text. Examples continue to be used throughout the book to illustrate how studies have incorporated specific designs or used various analysis techniques. The use of these examples does not necessarily advocate for the methodologic quality of the study.

- **Case in Point** features are used to clarify content through a description of a relevant study. The case is carried through discussion of a particular topic to illustrate applications. Some cases are from actual literature and others are hypothetical.
- Relevant examples are provided for certain designs using short descriptions that are highlighted in blue.
- **Focus on Evidence** features are included in each chapter to provide an example of how the material is relevant to evidence-based practice.
- **Numbered boxes** within chapters provide relevant information that will enhance understanding of content and will provide examples to illustrate material.

■ Clarifying Information

Clarifying information will also be presented in several small boxes throughout the text:

 Note boxes provide complementary content to enhance discussion of particular topics.

 Key Point boxes provide important information to emphasize concepts.

 Historical Notes offer interesting background that puts content into an historical context.

 Fun Facts illustrate concepts through a lighthearted look at relevant information.

 Statistics boxes are included with discussions of various designs to suggest relevant statistics that will be described fully in later chapters.

■ Statistical Material

Many statistical procedures are described in the text, some that will include calculations within tables or boxes. However, most procedures are presented conceptually, with the primary purpose of being able to apply principles to the literature. Formulas are included for some statistical measures where they are instructive. Some more detailed calculations are included in supplements.

- Many different statistical packages are available for data analysis, some proprietary and others free online. Their interfaces and formats are varied, and their output may look different, but most will generate comparable results. This text uses SPSS version 25, the most recent version at the time the book was published.
- In chapters 22-34, tables are included that illustrate SPSS statistical output. Tables and text will guide readers through interpretation of the results, including footnotes to identify relevant information. Some material is omitted from the output if it does not provide relevant information, but full output is included in online files. All data used for examples in tables are hypothetical unless otherwise specified.
- Appendix A includes tables of critical values that can be applied to statistical calculations. Additional

tables are also available in relevant chapter supplements as well as in *Appendix A Online*.

- The **Data Download** icon will indicate that the original data and full output for an example are available online in SPSS and CSV files. Full output will also be available as SPSS files or as PDF files for those who do not have access to SPSS. Data and output files will be named according to the number of the table that contains the relevant material. **Data Files** will be available online at www.fadavis.com.

- Hypothetical data are not intended to reflect any true physiological or theoretical relationships. They have been manipulated to illustrate certain statistical concepts—so please don't try to subject the results to a clinical rationale!

- Examples of how results can be presented in a research report are provided for each statistical procedure.

- This text is not a manual for using SPSS. Appendix C will introduce the basics of data management with SPSS, but please consult experts if you are unfamiliar with running statistical programs. Several texts are devoted to detailed instructions for applying SPSS.[1,2]

■ Supplements

Each chapter has supplemental material available online.

- **Chapter Overviews** include objectives, key terms, and a chapter summary.
- **Supplemental Materials** are included for many chapters with references highlighted in the text. Chapter material can be understood without referring to supplements, but the information in them may be important for teaching or for understanding the application of certain procedures. Where appropriate, supplements also provide links to relevant references or other resources related to the chapter's content.
- **Review Questions** are included for each chapter as a self-assessment to reinforce content for readers. Answers to these questions are also provided.

■ For Instructors

The order of chapters is based on the research process model introduced in Chapter 1. However, instructors may approach this order differently. The chapters will

work in any order that fits your needs. Material is cross-referenced throughout the book.

- It is not necessary to use all the chapters or all of the material in a given chapter, depending on the depth of interest in a particular topic. This book has always served as a teaching resource as well as a comprehensive reference for clinicians and researchers who run across unfamiliar content as they read through the literature. It will continue to be a useful reference for students following graduation.
- **Study Suggestions** are given for each chapter, providing activities and exercises that can be incorporated into teaching, assignments, or exams. Many include discussion topics that can be used for individual or small group work. Where relevant, answers are provided, or ideas are given for focusing discussions.
- A **Test Item Bank** includes multiple choice items for each chapter.
- **PowerPoint** slides outline chapter content, and can be incorporated into teaching or other presentations.
- An **Image Bank** offers access to all images within the text.

■ For Students

This book is intended to cover the concepts that will allow you to become a critical consumer of literature and to apply that knowledge within the context of evidence-based practice. It will also serve as a guide for planning and implementing research projects. Use the online resources to complement your readings.

It is unlikely that you will use the entire textbook within your courses but consider its usefulness as you move into your future role as an evidence-based practitioner. You may also find you are interested in doing some research once you have identified clinical questions. Don't be overwhelmed with the comprehensive content—the book will be a resource for you going forward, so keep it handy on the bookshelf!

■ Terminology

This text has a distinct and purposeful focus on inter-professional practice. However, many professions have particular jargon that may differ from terms used here. I have tried to define terms and abbreviations so that these words can be applied across disciplines.

- When statistical procedures and designs can be described using different terms, I have included these alternatives. Unfortunately, there are many such instances.

- The *International Classification of Functioning, Disability and Health (ICF)* is introduced in Chapter 1, defining the terms impairment, activity, and participation. These are used to reflect different types of outcome measures throughout the text.
- The pronouns "he" or "she" are used casually throughout the book to avoid using passive voice. There is no underlying intent with the choice of pronoun unless it is applied to a particular study.
- I have chosen to use the terms "subject," "participant," "patient," "person," "individual," or "case" interchangeably for two reasons. First, I recognize

that those we study may represent different roles in different types of research studies, and second, it is just an effort to vary language. Although the term "participant" has gained increasing favor, there is no consensus on which terms are preferable, and these terms continue to be used in federal regulations and research reports.

REFERENCES

1. Field A. *Discovering Statistics Using IBM SPSS Statistics*. 5th ed. Thousand Oaks, CA: Sage; 2018.
2. Green SB, Salkind NJ. *Using SPSS for Windows and Macintosh: Analyzing and Understanding Data*. 8th ed. New York: Pearson; 2017.

Contents

PART 1 Foundations of Research and Evidence

1 Frameworks for Generating and Applying Evidence, 2
The Research Imperative, 2
The Research Process, 4
Frameworks for Clinical Research, 5
Types of Research, 11

2 On the Road to Translational Research, 17
The Translation Gap, 17
The Translation Continuum, 18
Effectiveness Research, 21
Outcomes Research, 23
Implementation Studies, 25

3 Defining the Research Question, 29
Selecting a Topic, 29
The Research Problem, 29
The Research Rationale, 32
Types of Research, 34
Framing the Research Question, 34
Independent and Dependent Variables, 34
Research Objectives and Hypotheses, 38
What Makes a Good Research Question? 39

4 The Role of Theory in Research and Practice, 42
Defining Theory, 42
Purposes of Theories, 42
Components of Theories, 43
Models, 44
Theory Development and Testing, 45
Characteristics of Theories, 47
Theory, Research, and Practice, 48
Scope of Theories, 49

5 Understanding Evidence-Based Practice, 53
Why Is Evidence-Based Practice Important? 53
How Do We Know Things? 54
What Is Evidence-Based Practice? 56
The Process of Evidence-Based Practice, 57
Levels of Evidence, 62
Implementing Evidence-Based Practice, 65

6 Searching the Literature, 70
with Jessica Bell

Where We Find Evidence, 70
Databases, 71
The Search Process, 74
Keyword Searching, 74
Getting Results, 76
Medical Subject Headings, 77
Refining the Search, 80
Expanding Search Strategies, 83
Choosing What to Read, 83
Accessing Full Text, 84
Staying Current and Organized, 85
When Is the Search Done? 85

7 Ethical Issues in Clinical Research, 88
The Protection of Human Rights, 88
The Institutional Review Board, 91
Informed Consent, 92
Research Integrity, 98

PART 2 Concepts of Measurement

8 Principles of Measurement, 106
Why We Take Measurements, 106
Quantification and Measurement, 106
The Indirect Nature of Measurement, 107
Rules of Measurement, 108
Levels of Measurement, 109

9 Concepts of Measurement Reliability, 115
Concepts of Reliability, 115
Measuring Reliability, 117
Understanding Reliability, 118
Types of Reliability, 119
Reliability and Change, 122
Methodological Studies: Reliability, 124

10   Concepts of Measurement Validity, 127
with K. Douglas Gross

Defining Validity, 127
Types of Evidence for Validity, 128
Construct Validity, 132
Norm and Criterion Referencing, 135
Interpreting Change, 136
Methodological Studies: Validity, 138

11   Designing Surveys and Questionnaires, 141
Purposes of Surveys, 141
Survey Formats, 142
Planning the Survey, 143
Designing the Survey, 144
Types of Survey Questions, 145
Writing Good Questions, 148
Formatting the Survey, 150
Selecting a Sample, 150
Contacting Respondents, 152
Analysis of Questionnaire Data, 154
Ethics of Survey Administration, 155

12   Understanding Health Measurement Scales, 159
with Marianne Beninato

Understanding the Construct, 159
Summative Scales, 161
Visual Analog Scale, 164
Cumulative Scales, 167
Rasch Analysis, 168

PART 3   Designing Clinical Research

13   Choosing a Sample, 180
Populations and Samples, 180
Sampling, 183
Probability Sampling, 185
Nonprobability Sampling, 188

14   Principles of Clinical Trials, 192
Types of Clinical Trials, 192
Manipulation of Variables, 193
Random Assignment, 194
Control Groups, 198
Blinding, 199
Ideal Versus Pragmatic, 200
Phases of Clinical Trials, 201
Comparing Treatments: Better or No Worse? 204

15   Design Validity, 210
Validity Questions, 210
Statistical Conclusion Validity, 210
Internal Validity, 212
Construct Validity, 215
External Validity, 217
Strategies to Control for Subject Variability, 218
Non-compliance and Missing Data, 220
Handling Missing Data, 223

16   Experimental Designs, 227
Design Classifications, 227
Selecting a Design, 228
Pretest–Posttest Control Group Designs, 228
Posttest-Only Control Group Design, 230
Factorial Designs for Independent Groups, 231
Repeated Measures Designs, 233
Sequential Clinical Trials, 236

17   Quasi-Experimental Designs, 240
Validity Concerns, 240
Time Series Designs, 241
Nonequivalent Group Designs, 244

18   Single-Subject Designs, 249
Focus on the Individual, 249
Structure of Single-Subject Designs, 250
Defining the Research Question, 253
Measuring the Target Behavior, 253
Limitations of the A–B Design, 254
Withdrawal Designs, 254
Multiple Baseline Designs, 255
Designs With Multiple Treatments, 257
N-of-1 Trials, 259
Visual Data Analysis, 260
Statistical Analysis, 263
Generalization, 267

19   Exploratory Research: Observational Designs, 271
with K. Douglas Gross

Exploring Relationships, 272
Longitudinal Studies, 274
Cross-Sectional Studies, 276
Cohort Studies, 278
Case-Control Studies, 280

20   Descriptive Research, 285
Developmental Research, 286
Normative Studies, 287
Descriptive Surveys, 288
Case Reports, 289
Historical Research, 293

21 Qualitative Research, 297
with Heather Fritz and Cathy Lysack

Human Experience and Evidence, 297
The Research Question: Beyond "What" to "Why", 299
Perspectives in Qualitative Research, 302
Methods of Qualitative Data Collection, 305
Sampling, 308
Data Analysis and Interpretation, 309
Mixed Methods, 312

PART 4   Analyzing Data

22 Descriptive Statistics, 318
Frequency Distributions, 318
Shapes of Distributions, 322
Measures of Central Tendency, 322
Measures of Variability, 324
The Normal Distribution, 328

23 Foundations of Statistical Inference, 333
Probability, 333
Sampling Error, 334
Confidence Intervals, 336
Statistical Hypothesis Testing, 338
Errors in Hypothesis Testing, 340
Type I Error and Significance, 340
Type II Error and Power, 342
Concepts of Statistical Testing, 346
Parametric Versus Nonparametric Statistics, 348

24 Comparing Two Means: The *t*-Test, 351
The Conceptual Basis for Comparing Means, 351
The Independent Samples *t*-Test, 353
Paired Samples *t*-Test, 359
Power and Effect Size, 360
Inappropriate Use of Multiple *t*-Tests, 363

25 Comparing More Than Two Means: Analysis of Variance, 365
ANOVA Basics, 365
One-Way Analysis of Variance, 365
Two-Way Analysis of Variance, 370
Repeated Measures Analysis of Variance, 373
Mixed Designs, 378

26 Multiple Comparison Tests, 383
Corrections and Adjustments, 383
Post Hoc Multiple Comparisons, 384
Post Hoc Tests for Factorial Designs, 390
Post Hoc Tests for Repeated Measures, 392
Planned Comparisons, 394

27 Nonparametric Tests for Group Comparisons, 400
Criteria for Choosing Nonparametric Tests, 400
Procedure for Ranking Scores, 402
Tests for Independent Samples, 403
Tests for Related Samples, 407

28 Measuring Association for Categorical Variables: Chi-Square, 415
Testing Proportions, 415
Goodness of Fit, 416
Tests of Independence, 419
Power and Effect Size, 423
McNemar Test for Correlated Samples, 424

29 Correlation, 428
Concepts of Correlation, 428
Linear and Curvilinear Relationships, 430
Pearson Product–Moment Correlation Coefficient, 431
Correlation of Ranked Data, 432
Correlation of Dichotomies, 435
Interpreting Correlation Coefficients, 435
Partial Correlation, 437

30 Regression, 440
The Basics of Regression, 440
Simple Linear Regression, 441
Multiple Regression, 446
Power and Effect Size for Regression, 449
Stepwise Multiple Regression, 449
Dummy Variables, 453
Nonlinear Regression, 454
Logistic Regression, 456
Analysis of Covariance, 461

31 Multivariate Analysis, 468
Exploratory Factor Analysis, 468
Structural Equation Modeling, 474
Cluster Analysis, 477
Multivariate Analysis of Variance, 478
Survival Analysis, 481

32 Measurement Revisited: Reliability and Validity Statistics, 486
with K. Douglas Gross

Intraclass Correlation Coefficient, 486
Standard Error of Measurement, 492
Agreement, 494
Internal Consistency, 497
Limits of Agreement, 499
Measuring Change, 501

33 Diagnostic Accuracy, 509
Validity of Diagnostic Tests, 509
Pretest and Posttest Probabilities, 514
Receiver Operating Characteristic (ROC) Curves, 519
Clinical Prediction Rules, 523

34 Epidemiology: Measuring Risk, 529
The Scope of Epidemiology, 529
Descriptive Epidemiology, 530
Analytic Epidemiology: Measures of Risk, 533
Analytic Epidemiology: Measures of Treatment Effect, 539

PART 5 Putting It All Together

35 Writing a Research Proposal, 548
Purposes of the Research Proposal, 548
The Research Team, 548
Components of a Proposal, 549
Plan for Administrative Support, 552
Writing the Proposal, 554
Funding, 555
Submitting the Proposal, 555

36 Critical Appraisal: Evaluating Research Reports, 557
Levels of Evidence, 557
The Appraisal Process, 558
Core Questions, 558
Intervention Studies, 562

Studies of Diagnostic Accuracy, 564
Studies of Prognosis, 565
Qualitative Studies, 567
Critically Appraised Topics, 568

37 Synthesizing Literature: Systematic Reviews and Meta-Analyses, 574
with David Scalzitti

Purpose of Systematic Reviews, 575
The Research Question, 576
Methods, 578
Results, 581
Discussion and Conclusions, 586
Meta-Analysis, 587
Appraisal of Systematic Reviews and Meta-Analyses, 591
Scoping Reviews, 592

38 Disseminating Research, 597
with Peter S. Cahn

Choosing a Journal, 597
Authorship, 599
Standards for Reporting, 599
Structure of the Written Research Report, 602
Submitting the Manuscript, 605
Presentations, 607
Promoting Your Work, 610

Appendices

A   Statistical Tables, 613

B   Relating the Research Question to the Choice of Statistical Test, 622

C   Management of Quantitative Data, 629

Glossary, 637

Index, 659

Online Supplements

1 Frameworks for Generating and Applying Evidence
Evolving Models of Healthcare

2 On the Road to Translational Research
Ernest Codman: The "End Result Idea"

3 Defining the Research Question
Links to Study Examples

4 The Role of Theory in Research and Practice
No supplement

5 Understanding Evidence-Based Practice
Barriers and Facilitators of Evidence-Based Practice

6 Searching the Literature
Databases and Search Engines for Health Sciences

7 Ethical Issues in Clinical Research
2019 Changes to the Common Rule

8 Principles of Measurement
No supplement

9 Concepts of Measurement Reliability
No supplement

10 Concepts of Measurement Reliability
1. Content Validity Index
2. Sources of Evidence to Support Construct Validity

11 Designing Surveys and Questionnaires
1. Delphi Surveys
2. Q-Sort Methodology
3. Edwards et al: *Are People With Chronic Diseases Interested In Using Telehealth? A Cross-Sectional Postal Survey*

12 Understanding Health Measurement Scales
1. Likert Scales: The Multidimensional Health Locus of Control Scale
2. Further Understanding of Rasch Analysis

13 Choosing a Sample
1. Generating a Random Sample
2. Weightings for Disproportional Sampling

14 Principles of Clinical Trials
No supplement

15 Design Validity
No supplement

16 Experimental Designs
Sequential Clinical Trials

17 Quasi-Experimental Designs
No supplement

18 Single-Subject Designs
1. Variations of Single-Subject Designs
2. Drawing the Split Middle Line
3. Table of Probabilities Associated With the Binomial Test
4. Statistical Process Control
5. Calculating the C Statistics

19 Exploratory Research: Observational Designs
No supplement

20 Descriptive Research
Writing and Appraising Case Reports

21 Qualitative Research
No supplement

22 Descriptive Statistics
Calculating Variance and Standard Deviation

23 Foundations of Statistical Inference
Introduction to G*Power

24 Comparing Two Means: The *t*-Test
1. Calculation of the Unpaired *t*-Test With Unequal Variances
2. Estimating Power and Sample Size: *t*-Test

25 Comparing More Than Two Means: Analysis of Variance
1. Calculation of Sums of Squares
2. Estimating Power and Sample Size: Analysis of Variance

26 Multiple Comparison Tests
1. Critical Values of the Studentized Range Statistic, *q*
2. Calculating the Harmonic Mean
3. Choosing Multiple Comparison Tests

27 Nonparametric Tests for Group Comparisons
1. Multiple Comparisons for Nonparametric Tests
2. Tables of Critical Values for Nonparametric Tests
3. Estimating Power and Sample Size: Mann-Whitney *U* and Wilcoxon Signed-Ranks

28 Measuring Association for Categorical Variables: Chi-Square
Estimating Power and Sample Size: Chi-Square

29 Correlation
1. Calculation of the Pearson and Spearman Correlations
2. Correlation of Dichotomies
3. Eta Coefficient for Non-Linear Correlation
4. Estimating Power and Sample Size: Correlation

30 Regression
1. Calculating Linear Regression Coefficients
2. Probabilities in Logistic Regression
3. Estimating Power and Sample Size: Regression

31 Multivariate Statistics
1. Principal Components Analysis and Exploratory Factor Analysis
2. Direct, Indirect, and Total Effects in Sequential Equation Modeling

32 Measurement Revisited: Reliability and Validity Statistics
1. Calculating the Intraclass Correlation Coefficient
2. Generating ICCs With SPSS
3. Weighted Kappa
4. Response Stability: Method Error

33 Diagnostic Accuracy
Nomogram to Determine Posttest Probabilities

34 Epidemiology: Measuring Risk
Estimating Sample Size: Cohort and Case-Control Studies

35 Writing a Research Proposal
The NIH Biosketch Format

36 Critical Appraisal: Evaluating Research Reports
1. Appraisal Resources
2. Critical Appraisal Worksheets

37 Synthesizing Literature: Systematic Reviews and Meta-Analyses
1. Reporting Guidelines: PRISMA
2. Appraising Systematic Reviews: AMSTAR-2 Checklist
3. Resources for Systematic Reviews and Meta-Analyses
4. Data Extraction Forms
5. Lucas et al: *Interventions to Improve Gross Motor Performance in Children with Neurodevelopmental Disorders: A Meta-Analysis*
6. Olding et al: *Patient and Family Involvement in Adult Critical and Intensive Care Settings: A Scoping Review*

38 Disseminating Research
1. Links to Reporting Guidelines
2. Annotated Article: Travier et al: *Effects of an 18-Week Exercise Programme Started Early During Breast Cancer Treatment: A Randomised Controlled Trial*

PART 1

Foundations of Research and Evidence

CHAPTER 1 **Frameworks for Generating and Applying Evidence** 2

CHAPTER 2 **On the Road to Translational Research** 17

CHAPTER 3 **Defining the Research Question** 29

CHAPTER 4 **The Role of Theory in Research and Practice** 42

CHAPTER 5 **Understanding Evidence-Based Practice** 53

CHAPTER 6 **Searching the Literature** 70

CHAPTER 7 **Ethical Issues in Clinical Research** 88

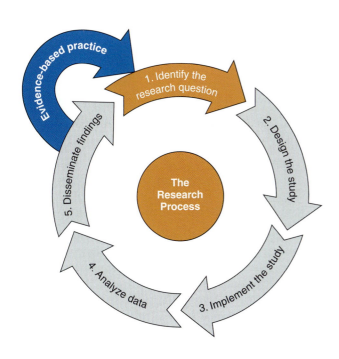

Frameworks for Generating and Applying Evidence

The ultimate goal of clinical research is to maximize the effectiveness of practice. To that end, health professionals have recognized the necessity for generating and applying evidence to clinical practice through rigorous and objective analysis and inquiry.

The purpose of this text is to provide a frame of reference that will bring together the comprehensive skills needed to promote critical inquiry as part of the clinical decision-making process for the varied and interdependent members of the healthcare team.

This chapter develops a concept of research that can be applied to clinical practice, as a method of generating new knowledge and providing evidence to inform healthcare decisions. We will also explore historic and contemporary healthcare frameworks and how they influence the different types of research that can be applied to translate research to practice.

■ The Research Imperative

The concept of research in health professions has evolved along with the development of techniques of practice and changes in the healthcare system. All stakeholders (including care providers and patients, policy analysts, administrators, and researchers) have an investment in knowing that intervention and healthcare services are effective, efficient, and safe.

Clinical research is essential to inform clinical judgments, as well as the organization and economics of practice. We must all exercise a commitment to scientific discovery that will lead to improvement in standards of care and patient outcomes. The task of addressing this need is one that falls on the shoulders of all those engaged in healthcare (whether we function as scientific investigators who collect meaningful data and analyze outcomes, or as consumers of professional literature who critically apply research findings to promote optimal care (see Box 1-1).

The importance of engaging in collaborative and interprofessional efforts cannot be overemphasized, as researchers and clinicians share the responsibility to explore complex theories and new approaches, as well as to contribute to balanced scientific thought and discovery.

Defining Clinical Research

Clinical research is a structured process of investigating facts and theories and of exploring connections, with the purpose of improving individual and public health. It proceeds in a systematic way to examine clinical or social conditions and outcomes, and to generate evidence for decision-making.

Although there is no one universal description of clinical research, the National Institutes of Health (NIH) has proposed the following three-part definition[1]:

1. **Patient-oriented research:** Studies conducted with human subjects to improve our understanding of the mechanisms of diseases and disorders, and of which therapeutic interventions will be most effective in treating them.
2. **Epidemiologic and behavioral studies:** Observational studies focused on describing patterns of disease and disability, as well as on identifying preventive and risk factors.

Box 1-1   Addressing the Triple Aim

Issues related to evidence-based practice (EBP) and population health are especially important in light of the economic, quality, and access challenges that continue to confront healthcare. In 2008, the Institute for Healthcare Improvement (*IHI*) proposed the *Triple Aim* framework to highlight the need to improve the patient experience and quality of care, to advance the health of populations, and to reduce the *per capita* cost of healthcare.[2] This goal will require extensive research efforts to collect data over time, understand population characteristics and barriers to access, and identify the dimensions of health and outcomes that are meaningful to providers and patients.

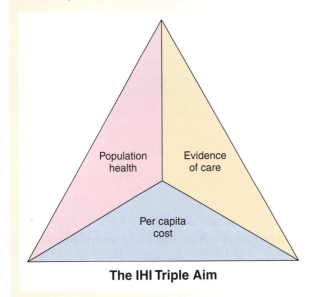

The IHI Triple Aim

Several organizations have proposed a *Quadruple Aim*, adding the clinician experience (avoiding burnout),[3] as well as other priorities, such as health equity.[4]

3. **Outcomes research and health services research:** Studies to determine the impact of research on population health and utilization of evidence-based therapeutic interventions.

All of these approaches are essential to establishing an evidence base for clinical practice and the provision of quality health services.

Qualitative and Quantitative Methods

The objective nature of research is a dynamic and creative activity, performed in many different settings, using a variety of measurement tools, and focusing on the application of clinical theory and interventions. In categorizing clinical inquiry, researchers often describe studies by distinguishing between qualitative and quantitative methods. Quantitative research is sometimes viewed as more accurate than qualitative study because it lends itself to objective statistical analysis, but this is an unfortunate and mistaken assumption because approaches to inquiry must best match the context of the question being asked. Each approach has inherent value and each can inform the other.

Qualitative Approach

Qualitative research strives to capture naturally occurring phenomena, following a tradition of *social constructivism*. This philosophy is focused on the belief that all reality is fundamentally social, and therefore the only way to understand it is through an individual's experience. Researchers often immerse themselves within the participants' social environment to better understand how phenomena are manifested under natural circumstances.

In qualitative methodology, "measurement" is based on subjective, narrative information, which can be obtained using focus groups, interviews, or observation. Analysis of narrative data is based on "thick description" to identify themes. The purpose of the research may be to simply describe the state of conditions, or it may be to explore associations, formulate theory, or generate hypotheses.

Qualitative research will be explored in more depth in Chapter 21.

Quantitative Approach

In contrast, quantitative research is based on a philosophy of *logical positivism*, in which human experience is assumed to be based on logical and controlled relationships among defined variables. It involves measurement of outcomes using numerical data under standardized conditions.

The advantage of the quantitative approach is the ability to summarize scales and to subject data to statistical analysis. Quantitative information may be obtained using formal instruments that address physical, behavioral, or physiological parameters, or by putting subjective information into an objective numerical scale.

The Scientific Method

Within the quantitative model, researchers attempt to reduce bias by using principles of the scientific method, which is based on the positivist philosophy that scientific truths exist and can be studied.[5] This approach is founded on two assumptions related to the nature of reality.

First, we assume that nature is orderly and regular and that events are, to some extent, consistent and predictable. Second, we assume that events or conditions are not random or accidental and, therefore, have one or more causes that can be discovered. These assumptions allow us to direct clinical thinking toward establishing cause-and-effect relationships so that we can develop rational solutions to clinical problems.

The scientific method has been defined as:

A systematic, empirical, and controlled critical examination of hypothetical propositions about the associations among natural phenomena.[6]

The *systematic* nature of research implies a logical sequence that leads from identification of a problem, through the organized collection and objective analysis of data, to the interpretation of findings.

The *empirical* component of scientific research refers to the necessity for documenting objective data through direct observation, thereby minimizing bias.

The element of *control* is perhaps the most important characteristic that allows the researcher to understand how one phenomenon relates to another, controlling factors that are not directly related to the variables in question.

A commitment to *critical examination* means that the researcher must subject findings to empirical testing and to the scrutiny of others. Scientific investigation is thereby characterized by a capacity for self-correction based on objective validation of data from primary sources of information.

Although the scientific method is considered the most rigorous form of acquiring knowledge, the complexity and variability within nature and the unique psychosocial and physiological capacities of individuals will always introduce some uncertainty into the interpretation and generalization of data. This means that researchers and clinicians must be acutely aware of extraneous influences to interpret findings in a meaningful way. Qualitative research can serve an important function in helping to understand these types of variables that can later be studied using quantitative methods.

■ The Research Process

The process of clinical research involves sequential steps that guide thinking, planning, and analysis. Whether one is collecting quantitative or qualitative data, the research process assures that there is a reasonable and logical framework for a study's design and conclusions. This is illustrated in Figure 1-1, recognizing that the order of steps may vary or overlap in different research models. Each of these steps is further described in succeeding chapters.

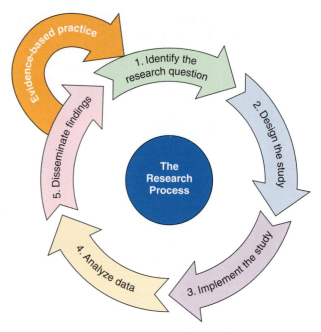

Figure 1–1 A model of the research process.

Step 1: Identify the Research Question

The first step of the research process involves delimiting the area of research and formulating a specific question that provides an opportunity for study (see Chapter 3). This requires a thorough review of scientific literature to provide a rationale for the study (see Chapters 6 and 37), justification of the need to investigate the problem, and a theoretical framework for interpreting results (see Chapter 4).

During this stage, the researcher must define the type of individual to whom the results will be generalized and the specific variables that will be studied. Research hypotheses are proposed to predict how these variables will be related and what clinically relevant outcomes can be expected. In descriptive or qualitative studies, guiding questions may be proposed that form the framework for the study.

Step 2: Design the Study

In step 2, the researcher designs the study and plans methods of implementation (see Chapters 14–21). The choice of research method reflects how the researcher conceptualizes the research question.

The first consideration is who will be studied and how subjects will be chosen (see Chapter 13). The researcher must carefully define all measurements and interventions so that outcomes will be reliable and valid (see Chapters 8–12), and the methods for data analysis are clear (see Chapters 22–34).

The completion of steps 1 and 2 leads to the development of a **research proposal** (see Chapter 35) that explains the research aims, sampling methods, and ethical considerations, including potential benefits and risks to participants. The proposal defines methods to show that the study can be carried out appropriately and that it should be able to deliver outcomes of some impact. It is submitted to an **Institutional Review Board (IRB)** for review and approval, to assure that ethical concerns are addressed (see Chapter 7).

Step 3: Implement the Study

In the third step, the researcher implements the plans designed in steps 1 and 2. Data collection is typically the most time-consuming part of the research process. Researchers may conduct pilot studies before beginning the full study to confirm that measurement methods and procedures work as expected, typically on a small sample.

Step 4: Analyze the Data

After data are collected, the researcher must reduce and collate the information into a useful form for analysis, often using tables or spreadsheets to compile "raw data." The fourth step of the research process involves analyzing, interpreting, and drawing valid conclusions about the obtained data.

Statistical procedures are applied to summarize and explore quantitative information in a meaningful way to address research hypotheses (see Chapters 22–34). In qualitative studies, the researcher organizes and categorizes data to identify themes and patterns that are guided by the research question and its underlying theoretical perspective (see Chapter 21).

Step 5: Disseminate Findings

In the fifth step of the research process, researchers have a responsibility to share their findings with the appropriate audience so that others can apply the information either to clinical practice or to further research. This step is the pulling together of all the materials relevant to the study, to apply them to a generalized or theoretical framework. Through the analysis of results, the researcher will interpret the impact on practice and where further study is needed.

Research reports can take many forms including journal articles, abstracts, oral presentations, poster presentations, and conference proceedings (see Chapter 38). Students may be required to report their work in the lengthier form of a thesis or dissertation.

Closing the Loop

Note that the research process is circular, as no study is a dead end. Results of one study invariably lead to new questions. Researchers contribute to the advancement of their own work by offering suggestions for further study, sometimes to address limitations in a study's design. Replication may be needed to confirm results with different samples in different settings.

The loop also includes application of evidence based on dissemination of research findings (see Chapter 5). This process will often lead to new questions, as we continue to deal with the uncertainties of practice.

■ Frameworks for Clinical Research

The context of clinical research is often seen within prevailing **paradigms**. A paradigm is a set of assumptions, concepts, or values that constitute a framework for viewing reality within an intellectual community.

Scientific paradigms have been described as ways of looking at the world that define what kinds of questions are important, which predictions and theories define a discipline, how the results of scientific studies should be interpreted, and the range of legitimate evidence that contributes to solutions. Quantitative and qualitative research approaches are based on different paradigms, for example, as they are founded on distinct assumptions and philosophies of science.

American physicist Thomas Kuhn[7] also defined **paradigm shifts** as fundamental transitions in the way disciplines think about priorities and relationships, stimulating change in perspectives, and fostering preferences for varied approaches to research.

We can appreciate changes in research standards and priorities in terms of four paradigm shifts that have emerged in healthcare, rehabilitation, and medicine in the United States as we have moved into the 21st century: evidence-based practice, a focus on translational research, the conceptualization of health and disability, and the importance of interprofessional collaboration.

Evidence-Based Practice

The concept of **evidence-based practice (EBP)** represents the fundamental principle that the provision of quality care will depend on our ability to make choices that are based on the best evidence currently available. As shown in Figure 1-1, the research process incorporates EBP as an important application of disseminated research.

When we look at the foundations of clinical practice, however, we are faced with the reality that often compels practitioners to make intelligent, logical, best-guess decisions when scientific evidence is either incomplete or unavailable. The Institute of Medicine (IOM) and other agencies have set a goal that, by 2020, "90% of clinical decisions will be supported by accurate, timely, and up-to-date clinical information, and will reflect the best available evidence."[8] As this date approaches, however, this goal continues to be elusive in light of barriers in education and healthcare resources.

Everyone engaged in healthcare must be able to utilize research as part of their practice. This means having a reasonable familiarity with research principles and being able to read literature critically. The concept of EBP is more than just reliance on published research, however, and must be put in perspective. Informed clinicians will make decisions based on available literature, as well as their own judgment and experience—all in the context of a clinical setting and patient encounter. Perhaps more aptly called *evidence-based decision-making*, this process requires considering all relevant information and then making choices that provide the best opportunity for a successful outcome given the patient-care environment and available resources.

The process of EBP will be covered in more detail in Chapter 5, and these concepts will be included throughout this text as we discuss research designs, analysis strategies, and the use of published research for clinical decision-making. Look for Focus on Evidence *examples in each chapter.*

Translational Research

The realization of EBP requires two major elements. The first is the availability of published research that has applicability to clinical care. Researchers must produce relevant data that can be used to support well-informed decisions about alternative strategies for treatment and diagnosis.[9] The second is the actual adoption of procedures that have been shown to be effective, so that the highest possible quality of care is provided. This is an implementation dilemma to be sure that research findings are in fact translated into practice and policy. Unfortunately, both of these elements can present a major challenge. The NIH has defined translational research as the application of basic scientific findings to clinically relevant issues and, simultaneously, the generation of scientific questions based on clinical dilemmas.[10]

Efficacy and Effectiveness

Researchers will often distinguish between efficacy and effectiveness in clinical studies. Efficacy is the benefit of an intervention as compared to a control, placebo, or standard program, tested in a carefully controlled environment, with the intent of establishing cause-and-effect relationships. Effectiveness refers to the benefits and use of procedures under "real-world" conditions in which circumstances cannot be controlled within an experimental setting.

Translation spans this continuum, often described as taking knowledge from "bench to bedside," or more practically from "bedside to bench and back to bedside."[11] The goal of translational research is to assure that basic discoveries are realized in practice, ultimately improving the health of populations.

The full scope of translational research will be covered in Chapter 2.

Models of Health and Disability

Cultural and professional views of health influence how illness and disability are perceived, how decisions are made in the delivery of healthcare, and the ensuing directions of research. An important concept in understanding the evolution of medical and rehabilitation research is related to the overriding framework for the delivery of healthcare, which continues to change over time.

Understanding Health

Historical measures of health were based on mortality rates, which were readily available. As medical care evolved, so did the view of health, moving from survival to freedom from disease, and more recently to concern for a person's ability to engage in activities of daily living and to achieve a reasonable quality of life.[12]

These changes led to important shifts in understanding disability over the past 50 years. Following World War II, disability research was largely focused on medical and vocational rehabilitation, based primarily on an economic model in which disability was associated with incapacity to work and the need for public benefits.[13] Today social and government policies recognize the impact of the individual and environment on one's ability to function. Subsequently, we have seen an important evolution in the way health and disability have been conceptualized and studied, from the medical model of disease to more recent models that incorporate social, psychological, and medical health as well as disability.[14–17]

The International Classification of Functioning, Disability and Health

In 2001, the World Health Organization (WHO) published the International Classification of Functioning, Disability and Health (ICF).[18] The ICF portrays health and function in a complex and multidimensional model, consisting of six components in two domains, illustrated in Figure 1-2. The relationships among these components are interactive, but importantly do not necessarily reflect causal links.

In practice, research, and policy arenas, the ICF can be used to reflect potentially needed health services, environmental adaptations, or guidelines that can maximize

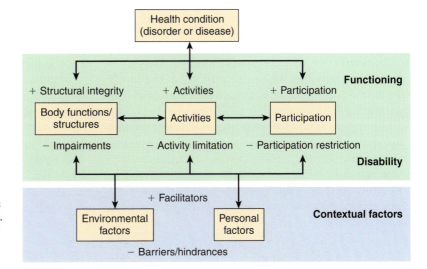

Figure 1–2 The International Classification of Functioning, Disability and Health (ICF). *Adapted from the World Health Organization. International Classification of Functioning, Disability and Health. Geneva, World Health Organization, 2001. Used with permission.*

function for individuals or create advantageous community services. Rather than focusing on the negative side of disability or simply mortality or disease, the intent of the ICF is to describe how people live with their health condition, shifting the focus to quality of life. This context makes the model useful for health promotion, prevention of illness and disability, and for the development of relevant research directions.

Functioning and Disability.
The first ICF domain, in the upper portion of the model, is *Functioning and Disability*, which reflects the relationship among health conditions, body functions and structures, activities, and participation. Each of these components can be described in positive or negative terms, as *facilitators* or *barriers*.

- **Body structures** refer to anatomical parts of the body, such as limbs and organs, such as the brain or heart. **Body functions** are physiological, such as movement or breathing, or psychological, such as cognition. Body systems or anatomical structures will be *intact* or *impaired*.
- **Activities** refer to the carrying out of tasks or actions, such as using a knife and fork, rising from a chair, or making complex decisions. Individuals will be able to perform specific activities or will demonstrate difficulties in executing tasks, described as *activity limitations*.
- **Participation** is involvement in life roles at home, work, or recreation, such as managing household finances, going to school, or taking care of a child. Individuals will either be able to participate in life roles or they may experience *participation restrictions*.

Contextual Factors.
The lower section of the model includes *Contextual Factors*, which consider the individual's health and function based on interaction with the environment and personal characteristics. Both of these contextual elements will either *facilitate* function or create *barriers*.

- **Environmental factors** include physical, social, and attitudinal aspects of the environment within which the individual functions. This may include architectural features such as stairs, furniture design, the availability of family or friends, or social policies that impact accessibility.
- **Personal factors** reflect the individual's own personality, abilities, preferences, and values. These may relate to characteristics such as age, gender, pain tolerance, education, family relationships, or physical strength and mobility. An individual will react to impairments or functional loss differently, depending on their previous experiences and attitudes.

The inclusion of contextual factors is a significant contribution of the ICF, as it allows us to put meaning to the term "disability." Think of our typical understanding of stroke, for example. The impairment of "brain infarct" is not the disabling component. The person's motor abilities may present some limitations, but the person's participation will also be influenced by financial support, home environment, availability of assistive devices or communication aids, as well as the complex interaction of factors such as societal attitudes, social policy, access to healthcare, education, community, and work.[19]

Capacity and Performance.   The activity and participation components of the ICF can be further conceptualized in terms of an individual's *capacity* to act versus actual *performance*; that is, what one is *able* to do versus what one actually *does*. These elements are defined with reference to the environment in which assessment is taking place.

The gap between capacity and performance reflects the impact of the environment on an individual's ability to perform.[18] In the activity/participation construct, there is a distinction made between a person's ability to perform a skill in the clinic or standardized setting and their ability to perform the same skill in their natural environment.

> Diwan et al[20] studied mobility patterns of children with cerebral palsy in India in three contexts—home, school, and community settings. Using a measure of motor capacity, they observed that 70% of the children were able to walk with or without support in the clinical setting, and 16% were able to crawl.

In the community, however, 52% were lifted by parents and only 6% used wheelchairs to get around; 22% of children who were able to walk with or without support were still lifted by parents in school and community settings. These results emphasize the importance of understanding environmental context, including culture, when evaluating a patient's performance and choosing measurements to investigate outcomes.

The ICF is the result of a multidisciplinary international effort to provide a common language for the classification and consequences of health conditions. In contrast to other models, the ICF recognizes functioning for its association with, but not necessarily as a consequence of, a health condition.

From a research and evidence standpoint, therefore, one cannot assume that measures of impairments or function always translate to understanding participation limitations. Much of the research on the ICF is focused on how these elements do or do not interact with specific types of health conditions (see Focus on Evidence 1-1).

📌 The ICF has been evaluated in a variety of patient populations, cultures, age groups, and diagnoses,[21–28] including a recent children's and youth version.[29] The model has been applied primarily within rehabilitation fields,[30–32] although medicine, nursing, and other professions have recognized its relevance.[19,33–35]

 An expanded discussion of models of health is included in the *Chapter 1 Supplement* with examples of studies that are based on the ICF. The evolution of these models has influenced priorities and methods in healthcare research.

Interprofessional and Interdisciplinary Research

A major challenge to translating new evidence into application is moving knowledge through the laboratory, academic, clinical, and public/private sectors—often a problem created by the existence of practical "silos."

Focus on Evidence 1–1
Health, Function, and Participation—Not Always a Straight Line

Three main consequences of chronic low back pain (LBP) are pain, functional limitations, and reduced productive capacity at work. A variety of outcome measures have been used to study the impact of LBP, mostly focusing on pain and function, with work status implied from the severity of functional limitation. Sivan et al[36] designed a cross-sectional study to analyze the correlation between work status and three standard functional outcome scales for LBP, to examine the extent to which they measure similar concepts.

The researchers looked at function and work status in 375 patients with chronic LBP who were receiving outpatient care. They considered two categories of outcomes:

1. Functional deficits related to pain, using the Oswestry Disability Index,[37] the Roland Morris Disability Questionnaire,[38] and the Orebro Musculoskeletal Pain Questionnaire[39]; and

2. Work status defined by the degree to which LBP interfered with participation in work activities, based on whether hours or duties had to be curtailed or changed.

Results showed only modest correlations between work status and the three LBP indices, even though some of the questionnaires include work-related questions. The authors concluded that vocational liability should not be implied from the severity of LBP because work status is influenced by other complex physical and psychosocial factors not necessarily related to LBP.

This study illustrates two central principles in applying the ICF—the importance of personal and environmental factors to understand participation, and the potential nonlinear relationship across impairments, function, and participation. The interaction of these factors, therefore, must be considered when setting treatment goals. This framework can also be used to direct research efforts, with a need to evaluate the ability of measurement tools to reflect the ICF components of body functions, activities, participation, environmental factors, and personal factors.

Translation can be slowed by limited communication across disciplines and settings, as well as substantial differences in scientific and social perspectives.

Just like the idea of interprofessional practice, the concept of collaboration across disciplines to address important research questions is not new, as many interdisciplinary fields have emerged over the decades to make significant contributions to health science, such as physical chemistry, bioinformatics, or astrophysics.

HISTORICAL NOTE
Interprofessional collaborations have led to many vital connections needed in the process of discovery.

- A fundamental observation by physicists in 1946 that nuclei can be oriented in a magnetic field eventually led to magnetic resonance imaging in collaboration with physical chemists and biologists.[40]
- The development of the cochlear implant required the integration of electrical engineering, physiology, and acoustics.[41]
- The sequencing of the human genome required techniques from physics, chemistry, biology, and computer science.[42]

Terminology

Discussions of interprofessional research are often hampered by a lack of consistency in terminology, starting with the difference between a discipline and a profession.

Disciplines represent fields of study or individual sciences, such as biology, chemistry, psychology, economics, or informatics. A *profession* has been defined as a disciplined group of individuals who are educated to apply a specialized knowledge base in the interest of society, and who adhere to ethical standards and hold themselves accountable for high standards of behavior.[43]

Therefore, occupational therapy, physical therapy, speech-language pathology, medicine, nursing, and pharmacy are examples of professions. Within a profession, different disciplines may be represented, such as neurology and orthopedics. Even within one profession, however, disciplinary norms may vary.

We can consider different levels of integration across disciplines or professions. The use of "discipline" or "profession" in these terms depends on the nature of the

individuals included and will often involve both. For the sake of simplicity, this discussion will continue to use the term "interprofessional," but "interdisciplinary" can be substituted appropriately.

Here are some useful distinctions related to how teams function to solve problems (see Fig. 1-3).[44] These definitions can be applied to interprofessional education, practice, or research.

- **Intraprofessional:** Members of one profession work together, sharing information through the lens of their own profession.
- **Multiprofessional:** An additive process whereby members of multiple professions work in parallel alongside each other to provide input, making complementary contributions, each staying within their own professional boundaries, working separately on distinct aspects of the problem.
- **Interprofessional:** Members of multiple professions work together, contributing their various skills in an integrative fashion, sharing perspectives to inform decision-making.
- **Transprofessional:** A high level of cooperation of professionals from multiple fields who understand each other's roles and perspectives sufficiently to blur boundaries, share skills and expertise, and use them to develop new ways of viewing a problem.

One comprehensive definition suggests that interprofessional research is:

. . . any study or group of studies undertaken by scholars from two or more distinct scientific disciplines. The research is based upon a conceptual model that links or integrates theoretical frameworks from those disciplines, uses study design and methodology that is not limited to any one field, and requires the use of perspectives and skills of the involved disciplines throughout multiple phases of the research process.[45]

This definition advocates that such scholars must develop skills and knowledge beyond their own core discipline. Interprofessional researchers should be open to perspectives of other professions, read journals outside

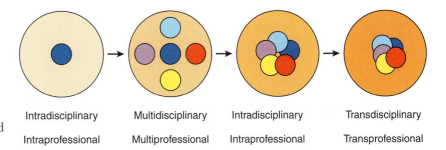

Figure 1–3 Levels of disciplinary and professional collaboration.

| Intradisciplinary | Multidisciplinary | Intradisciplinary | Transdisciplinary |
| Intraprofessional | Multiprofessional | Intraprofessional | Transprofessional |

of their own discipline, and be willing to consider theories that stretch their understanding of the problems at hand.[46] Just as professional education must give students collaborative tools that they can bring into practice, clinicians and investigators must be trained in the team science of interprofessional research.[47]

Supporting Translational Research

The entire concept of translational research, from basic science to effectiveness studies, makes the argument for interprofessional collaboration even stronger. Implementation of research requires strong teams to develop questions and study methodologies that go beyond any one discipline. This may include members who are not routinely part of most clinical trials, such as economists, sociologists and anthropologists, organizational scientists, quality-improvement (QI) experts and administrators, and patients and clinicians from various professions.[48]

 Contributing to translational research demands diversity of thinking that is best generated by collaborative teams.[49–51] Most importantly, we cannot ignore the importance of collaboration for evidence-based practice. Just as we need to consider interprofessional communication as an essential part of patient-centered care, we must look to research from many professions to inform our clinical decisions. Many funding agencies have set priorities for studies involving multiple disciplines.[52–54]

Barriers and Promoters in Interprofessional Research

Many barriers have been identified that limit the degree to which interprofessional research is carried out.[55] These include philosophical clashes, such as differences in professional cultures, perceived professional hierarchies, language and jargon disparities, preferences for different research methodologies, and conflicting theoretical or conceptual frameworks for prioritizing research questions.

Some barriers are more practical, such as insufficient funding, institutional constraints on time and space, difficulty identifying the right collaborators with expertise across disciplines, academic tenure requirements, concerns about authorship, and disagreements about where to publish the results. Many interdisciplinary and interprofessional journals have been developed, but these may not carry the same weight as publication within a discipline's flagship publication.

Successful collaborations have been described as those with strong cooperative teams and team leaders, flexibility and commitment of team members, physical proximity, and institutional support, clarity of roles, and a common vision and planning process involving the team members from the start.[55]

Making an Impact

The importance of collaboration in research cannot be overemphasized, as healthcare confronts the increasing complexity of health issues, technology, and social systems. Real-world problems seldom come in neat disciplinary packages. The progress of science and healthcare will depend on our ability to generate new ways of viewing those problems. In health education, service delivery, and policy implementation, the progress of healthcare will depend on contributions with different viewpoints as a way to offer innovative solutions when trying to solve multifaceted issues (see Focus on Evidence 1-2).[56]

The foundational healthcare frameworks that we have discussed in this chapter all demand interprofessional attention. In the *Triple Aim*, for example, the three concepts of population health, cost, and quality care, as well as the outcomes that would be the appropriate indicators of change, are almost by definition interprofessional and interdisciplinary.[57]

Focus on Evidence 1–2
Coming at a Question From Two Sides

Physical therapists identified a challenge in working with people with aphasia when administering the Berg Balance Scale, a commonly used tool to quantify dynamic sitting and standing balance to predict fall risk.[58] Although considered a valid test for older adults, the clinicians were concerned about the test's validity for those with aphasia because of its high demand for auditory comprehension and memory.

Collaborative work with speech-language pathologists resulted in a modified version of the scale, which included simplified verbal directions, visual and written cues, and modeling and repetition of instructions. The researchers compared performance on the standard and modified versions, finding that patients performed better with the modified test, which indicated that some portion of their performance difficulty was likely due to their communication deficit.

In this example, the clinicians from both professions brought important and different perspectives to the question and its research implementation that neither group could have done alone, adding to the understanding of the test's validity.

Examples throughout this text will illustrate the importance of interprofessional research topics that apply to healthcare researchers and clinicians across professions.

■ Types of Research

The research process delineates a general strategy for gathering, analyzing, and interpreting data to answer a question. A variety of classifications have been used to organize these strategies according to their purpose and objectives.

Basic research, also called *bench* or *preclinical research*, is directed toward the acquisition of new knowledge. This includes research in laboratories on animals, often focused on theory and understanding mechanisms of disease or therapies. The results of basic research may not have direct clinical application. In contrast, the purpose of **applied research**, also considered *clinical research*, is to advance the development of new diagnostic tests, drugs, therapies, and prevention strategies. It answers questions that have useful ends, testing theories that direct practice and evaluating the quality of healthcare services.

Research Classifications

Applied research can be viewed along a continuum that reflects the type of question the research is intended to answer, and whether the focus is on individuals, populations, or health systems. Within this continuum (see Fig. 1-4), research methods can be classified as descriptive, exploratory, or explanatory.

These classifications reflect different purposes of research, and within each one various types of research can be used. As a continuum suggests, however, different types of research can overlap in their purpose and may incorporate elements of more than one classification.

Importantly, this continuum is not a hierarchy. Each type of research fulfills a particular purpose and need. Each brings specific strengths to an investigation of clinical, social, or organizational phenomena. The appropriate use of various designs will depend on the research question and the available data, with questions related to intervention, diagnosis, and prognosis requiring different approaches. These will be described here and discussed in more detail in subsequent chapters.

Synthesis of Literature

As bodies of evidence continue to grow through publication of research, clinicians face the challenge of aggregating information to adequately answer a clinical question. **Systematic reviews** present a comprehensive analysis of the full range of literature on a particular topic, usually an intervention, diagnostic test, or prognostic factors. These studies look at methodological quality of studies to frame the state of knowledge on a topic.

Meta-analysis goes a step beyond systematic review, applying a process of statistically combining the findings from several studies to obtain a summary analysis. These analyses typically restrict the inclusion of studies based on design criteria to assure a rigorous analysis of the evidence.

Scoping reviews are a more recent contribution to this process, similar to systematic reviews, but incorporating a broader range of study designs and data-gathering methods to comprehensively synthesize evidence, often with the aims of informing practice, programs, and policy and of providing direction to future research.[59]

These synthesis methods are described in Chapter 37.

Explanatory Research

Explanatory research utilizes various types of **experimental designs** to compare two or more conditions or interventions. Different design approaches offer varied levels of control to establish cause and effect between interventions and outcomes (see Table 1-1). These trials address both efficacy and effectiveness.

Exploratory Research

In **exploratory research**, observational designs are used to examine a phenomenon of interest and explore its dimensions, often in populations or communities, and to examine how it relates to other factors (see Table 1-2). Using principles of **epidemiology**, health researchers examine associations to describe and predict risks or preventive strategies for certain conditions. Exploratory methods can also be used to establish associations between variables and to carry out **methodological research** to assess validity and reliability.

Descriptive Research

In **descriptive research** the researcher attempts to describe a group of individuals on a set of variables, to document their characteristics (see Table 1-3). Descriptive research may involve the use of questionnaires, interviews, direct observation, or the use of databases. Descriptive data allow researchers to classify and understand the scope of clinical or social phenomena, often providing the basis for further investigation. **Qualitative research** is considered descriptive in that it involves collection of data through interview and observation.

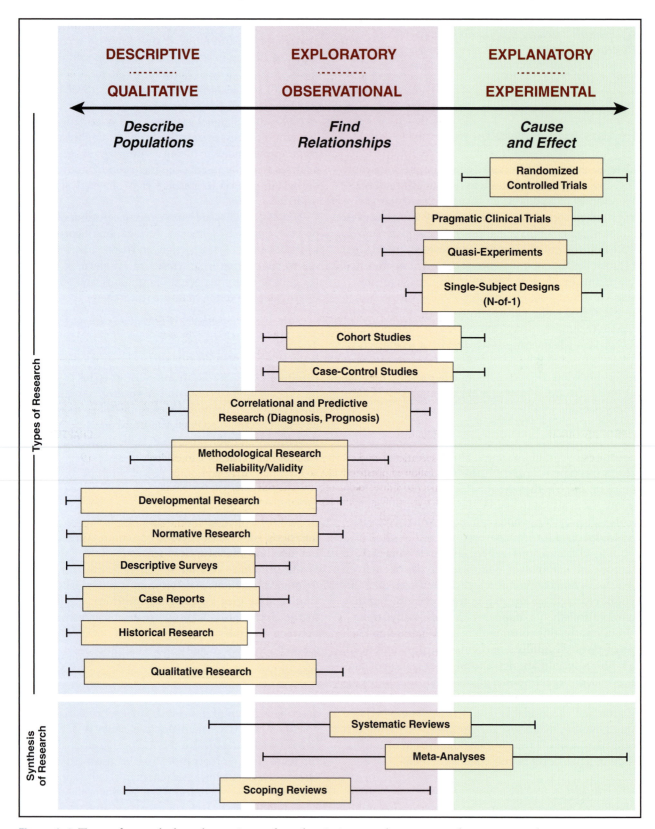

Figure 1–4 Types of research along the continuum from descriptive to exploratory to explanatory research.

Table 1-1 Types of Explanatory Research		
TYPE OF RESEARCH	**PURPOSE**	**CHAPTER**
Randomized Controlled Trial (RCT)	An efficacy trial involving the controlled comparison of an experimental intervention and a placebo, sham, or usual care condition. Through random assignment and restricted subject selection, the design controls for bias to allow cause-and-effect conclusions.	14,16
Pragmatic Clinical Trial (PCT)	An effectiveness trial with a focus on real-world outcomes. Participants represent the patients that would typically receive treatment, and testing takes place in clinical practice settings. Outcomes focus on issues of importance to patients and stakeholders, including quality of life, cost, and implementation.	2, 16
Quasi-Experimental Designs	Comparative designs that do not have a control group or randomization. Includes time-series designs that allow for repeated measurements over prolonged periods to document trends.	17
Single-Subject Designs (N-of-1 trials)	Systematic study of one or more subjects with repeated measurements under controlled and experimental conditions to show changes in responses with and without intervention, or comparing more than one intervention.	18

Table 1-2 Types of Exploratory/Observational Research		
TYPE OF RESEARCH	**PURPOSE**	**CHAPTER**
Cohort Studies	Observational studies where one or more cohorts of individuals are followed prospectively, to determine their status with respect to a disease or outcome and their exposure to certain risk factors. The design can be configured for retrospective analysis as well.	19
Case-Control Studies	Observational studies that compare patients with (cases) and without (controls) a disorder or outcome of interest. Cases and controls are compared on their exposure to a risk factor to determine the relationship between the risk factor and the disorder.	19
Correlational/Predictive Studies	Exploring relationships; can be used as a basis for decision-making, diagnosis, prognosis, and prevention.	19
Methodological Studies	Using correlational and comparative methods to demonstrate reliability and validity of measuring instruments, including interpretation of change and responsiveness.	9,10, 32, 33

Table 1-3 Types of Descriptive Research		
TYPE OF RESEARCH	**PURPOSE**	**CHAPTER**
Developmental Research	Investigation of patterns of growth and change over time; may chronicle natural history of a disease or disability.	20
Normative Research	Establishes normal values for specific variables; serves as guidelines for diagnosis and treatment planning.	20
Case Report/Case Series	Description of one or several patients or communities to document unusual conditions or the effect of innovative interventions.	20
Historical Research	Reconstructs the past to generate questions or suggest relationships of historical interest to inform contemporary perspectives.	20
Qualitative Research	Also called naturalistic research; observations or interviews explore the meaning of human experience as it occurs naturally, generating hypotheses about human behavior.	21
Mixed Methods Research	A combination of quantitative and qualitative research methods.	21

COMMENTARY

Research is to see what everyone else has seen, and to think what nobody else has thought.

—Albert Szent-Gyorgyi (1893–1986)

1937 Nobel Prize in Medicine

The focus of a text such as this one is naturally on the methods and procedures of conducting and interpreting research. By understanding definitions and analytic procedures, the clinician has the building blocks to structure an investigation or interpret the work of others.

Methodology is only part of the story, however. Research designs and statistical techniques cannot lead us to a research question, nor can they specify the technical procedures needed for studying that question. Designs cannot assign meaning to the way clinical phenomena behave. Our responsibility includes building the knowledge that will allow us to make sense of what is studied. This means that we also recognize the philosophy of a discipline, how subject matter is conceptualized, and which scientific approaches will contribute to an understanding of practice. As one scientist put it:

> *Questions are not settled; rather, they are given provisional answers for which it is contingent upon the imagination of followers to find more illuminating solutions.*[60]

How one conceives of a discipline's objectives and the scope of practice will influence the kinds of questions one will ask. We must appreciate the influence of professional values on these applications, reflecting what treatment alternatives will be considered viable. For instance, we might look at the slow adoption of qualitative research approaches in medicine, emphasizing the need to open ourselves to evidence that may hold important promise for our patients.[61] Some disciplines have embraced single-subject designs, whereas others have focused on randomized trials.[62] Research choices are often a matter of philosophical fit that can override issues of evidence, hindering knowledge translation.[63] This is especially relevant for interdisciplinary clinical associations and the shared research agenda that can emerge.

There is no right or wrong in these contrasts. As we explore the variety of research approaches and the context of EBP, clinicians and researchers will continually apply their own framework for applying these methods. The emphasis on clinical examples throughout the book is an attempt to demonstrate these connections.

REFERENCES

1. National Institutes of Health. Director's Panel on Clinical Research. Executive Summary, 1997. Available at http://grants.nih.gov/grants/NIH_Directors_Panel_Clinical_Research_Report_199712.pdf. Accessed December 25, 2015.
2. Stiefel M, Nolan K. A guide to measuring the triple aim: population health, experience of care, and per capita cost. IHI Innovation Series white paper. Cambridge, Massachusetts: Institute for Healthcare Improvement; 2012. Available at www.IHI.org. Accessed January 9, 2017.
3. Bodenheimer T, Sinsky C. From triple to quadruple aim: care of the patient requires care of the provider. *Ann Fam Med* 2014;12(6):573–576.
4. Feeley D. The triple aim or the quadruple aim? Four points to help set your strategy. Institute for Health Care Improvement. Available at http://www.ihi.org/communities/blogs/the-triple-aim-or-the-quadruple-aim-four-points-to-help-set-your-strategy. Accessed January 23, 2018.
5. Topping S. The quantitative-qualitative continuum. In: Gerrish K, Lacey A, eds. *The Research Process in Nursing*. 7 ed. Oxford: Wiley Blackwell, 2015:159–172.
6. Kerlinger FN. *Foundations of Behavioral Research*. New York: Holt, Rinehart & Winston, 1973.
7. Kuhn TS. *The Structure of Scientific Revolutions*. 3 ed. Chicago: University of Chicago Press, 1996.
8. Institute of Medicine. *Roundtable on Evidence-Based Medicine*. Washington, DC.: National Academies Press, 2009.
9. Tunis SR, Stryer DB, Clancy CM. Practical clinical trials: increasing the value of clinical research for decision making in clinical and health policy. *JAMA* 2003;290(12):1624–1632.
10. Rustgi AK. Translational research: what is it? *Gastroenterol* 1999;116(6):1285.
11. Fontanarosa PB, DeAngelis CD. Translational medical research. *JAMA* 2003;289(16):2133.
12. McDowell I. *Measuring Health: A Guide to Rating Scales and Questionnaires*. 3 ed. New York: Oxford University Press, 2006.
13. Scotch RK. Paradigms of American social research on disability. *Disability Studies Q* 2002;22(2):23–34.
14. Leimkuehler PE: Models of health and disability. American Academy of Orthotists and Prosthetists, Online Learning Center. Available at http://www.oandp.org/olc/lessons/html/SSC_09/module2.asp?frmCourseSectionId=7CC1D52A-9E9D-4A03-A2F0-78AE7DB64977. Accessed December 23, 2015.
15. Nagi SZ. Some conceptual issues in disability and rehabilitation. In: Sussman MB, ed. *Sociology and Rehabilitation*. Washington, DC: American Sociological Association, 1965.
16. Engel GL. The need for a new medical model: a challenge for biomedicine. *Science* 1977;196(4286):129–136.
17. Verbrugge LM, Jette AM. The disablement process. *Soc Sci Med* 1994;38:1–14.
18. World Health Organization. *International Classification of Functioning, Disability and Health*. Geneva: World Health Organization, 2001.
19. Kearney PM, Pryor J. The International Classification of Functioning, Disability and Health (ICF) and nursing. *J Adv Nurs* 2004;46(2):162–170.
20. Diwan S, Diwan J, Bansal AB, Patel PR. Changes in capacity and performance in mobility across different environmental settings in children with cerebral palsy: an exploratory study. *J Clin Diagn Res* 2015;9(8):YC01–YC03.
21. Bilbao A, Kennedy C, Chatterji S, Ustun B, Barquero JL, Barth JT. The ICF: applications of the WHO model of functioning, disability and health to brain injury rehabilitation. *NeuroRehabilitation* 2003;18(3):239–250.
22. Worral L, McCooey R, Davidson B, Larkins B, Hickson L. The validity of functional assessments of communication and the Activity/Participation components of the ICIDH-2: do they reflect what really happens in real-life? *J Commun Disord* 2002;35(2):107–137.
23. Geyh S, Kurt T, Brockow T, Cieza A, Ewert T, Omar Z, Resch KL. Identifying the concepts contained in outcome measures of clinical trials on stroke using the International Classification of Functioning, Disability and Health as a reference. *J Rehabil Med* 2004;(44 Suppl):56–62.
24. Brockow T, Duddeck K, Geyh S, Schwarzkopf S, Weigl M, Franke T, Brach M. Identifying the concepts contained in outcome measures of clinical trials on breast cancer using the International Classification of Functioning, Disability and Health as a reference. *J Rehabil Med* 2004;(44 Suppl):43–48.
25. Salih SA, Peel NM, Marshall W. Using the International Classification of Functioning, Disability and Health framework to categorise goals and assess goal attainment for transition care clients. *Australas J Ageing* 2015;34(4):E13–16.
26. Bruijning JE, van Rens G, Fick M, Knol DL, van Nispen R. Longitudinal observation, evaluation and interpretation of coping with mental (emotional) health in low vision rehabilitation using the Dutch ICF Activity Inventory. *Health Qual Life Outcomes* 2014;12:182.
27. Dur M, Coenen M, Stoffer MA, Fialka-Moser V, Kautzky-Willer A, Kjeken I, Dragoi RG, Mattsson M, Bostrom C, Smolen J, et al. Do patient-reported outcome measures cover personal factors important to people with rheumatoid arthritis? A mixed methods design using the International Classification of Functioning, Disability and Health as frame of reference. *Health Qual Life Outcomes* 2015;13:27.
28. Arvidsson P, Granlund M, Thyberg M. How are the activity and participation aspects of the ICF used? Examples from studies of people with intellectual disability. *NeuroRehabilitation* 2015;36(1):45–49.
29. World Health Organization. *International Classification of Functioning, Disability and Health: Children and Youth Version*. Geneva, Switzerland: World Health Organization, 2007.
30. Threats TT. The ICF and speech-language pathology: aspiring to a fuller realization of ethical and moral issues. *Int J Speech Lang Pathol* 2010;12(2):87–93.
31. Steiner WA, Ryser L, Huber E, Uebelhart D, Aeschlimann A, Stucki G. Use of the ICF model as a clinical problem-solving tool in physical therapy and rehabilitation medicine. *Phys Ther* 2002;82(11):1098–1107.
32. Haglund L, Henriksson C. Concepts in occupational therapy in relation to the ICF. *Occup Ther Int* 2003;10(4):253–268.
33. Stucki G, Grimby G. Applying the ICF in medicine. *J Rehabil Med* 2004;(44 Suppl):5–6.
34. Ankam N, Levinson M, Jerpbak C, Collins L, Umland E, Kern S, Egger S, Lucatorto K, Covelman K, Koeuth S.: A Common Language for Interprofessional Education: The World Health Organization's International Classification of Functioning, Disability and Health (ICF). MedEdPORTAL Publications; 2013. Available at https://www.mededportal.org/publication/9321. Accessed December 26, 2015.
35. Burger H. Can the International Classification of Functioning, Disability and Health (ICF) be used in a prosthetics and orthotics outpatient clinic? *Prosthet Orthot Int* 2011;35(3):302–309.
36. Sivan M, Sell B, Sell P. A comparison of functional assessment instruments and work status in chronic back pain. *Eur J Phys Rehabil Med* 2009;45(1):31–36.
37. Fairbank JC, Pynsent PB. The Oswestry Disability Index. *Spine* 2000;25(22):2940–2952.
38. Roland M, Morris R. A study of the natural history of back pain. Part I: development of a reliable and sensitive measure of disability in low-back pain. *Spine* 1983;8(2):141–144.
39. Linton SJ, Boersma K. Early identification of patients at risk of developing a persistent back problem: the predictive validity of the Orebro Musculoskeletal Pain Questionnaire. *Clin J Pain* 2003;19(2):80–86.
40. National Research Council (US) Committee for Monitoring the Nation's Changing Needs for Biomedical, Behavioral, and Clinical Personnel: Advancing the Nation's Health Needs: NIH

Research Training Programs. Washington (DC): National Academies Press, 2005. 8, Emerging Fields and Interdisciplinary Studies. Available at: http://www.ncbi.nlm.nih.gov/books/NBK22616/. Accessed December 26, 2015.

41. Luxford WM, Brackman DE. The history of cochlear implants. In: Gray R, ed. *Cochlear Implants*. San Diego, CA: College-Hill Press, 1985:1–26.

42. US Department of Energy OoSaTI: History of the DOE human genome program. Available at https://www.osti.gov/accomplishments/genomehistory.html. Accessed December 18, 2015.

43. Professions Australia: What is a profession? Available at http://www.professions.com.au/about-us/what-is-a-professional. Accessed January 23, 2017.

44. Choi BC, Pak AW. Multidisciplinarity, interdisciplinarity and transdisciplinarity in health research, services, education and policy: 1. definitions, objectives, and evidence of effectiveness. *Clin Invest Med* 2006;29(6):351–364.

45. Aboelela SW, Larson E, Bakken S, Carrasquillo O, Formicola A, Glied SA, Haas J, Gebbie KM.. Defining interdisciplinary research: conclusions from a critical review of the literature. *Health Serv Res* 2007;42(1 Pt 1):329–346.

46. Gebbie KM, Meier BM, Bakken S, Carrasquillo O, Formicola A, Aboelela SW, Glied S, Larson E. Training for interdisciplinary health research: defining the required competencies. *J Allied Health* 2008;37(2):65–70.

47. Little MM, St Hill CA, Ware KB, Swanoski MT, Chapman SA, Lutfiyya MN, Cerra FB. Team science as interprofessional collaborative research practice: a systematic review of the science of team science literature. *J Investig Med* 2017;65(1):15–22.

48. Bauer MS, Damschroder L, Hagedorn H, Smith J, Kilbourne AM. An introduction to implementation science for the non-specialist. *BMC Psychology* 2015;3(1):32.

49. Horn SD, DeJong G, Deutscher D. Practice-based evidence research in rehabilitation: an alternative to randomized controlled trials and traditional observational studies. *Arch Phys Med Rehabil* 2012;93(8 Suppl):S127–137.

50. Green LW. Making research relevant: if it is an evidence-based practice, where's the practice-based evidence? *Fam Pract* 2008;25 Suppl 1:i20–i24.

51. Westfall JM, Mold J, Fagnan L. Practice-based research—"Blue Highways" on the NIH roadmap. *JAMA* 2007;297(4):403–406.

52. Agency for Healthcare Research and Quality: US Department of Health and Human Services. Available at https://www.ahrq.gov. Accessed January 5, 2017.

53. Zerhouni E. Medicine. The NIH Roadmap. *Science* 2003; 302(5642):63–72.

54. Patient-Centered Outcomes Research Institute. Available at http://www.pcori.org/. Accessed January 5, 2017.

55. Choi BC, Pak AW. Multidisciplinarity, interdisciplinarity, and transdisciplinarity in health research, services, education and policy: 2. Promotors, barriers, and strategies of enhancement. *Clin Invest Med* 2007;30(6):E224–E232.

56. Committee on Facilitating Interdisciplinary Research: Facilitating Interdisciplinary Research. National Academy of Sciences, National Academy of Engineering, and the Institute of Medicine, 2004. Available at https://www.nap.edu/catalog/11153.html. Accessed January 24, 2017.

57. Berwick DM, Nolan TW, Whittington J. The triple aim: care, health, and cost. *Health Aff (Millwood)* 2008;27(3): 759–769.

58. Carter A, Nicholas M, Hunsaker E, Jacobson AM. Modified Berg Balance Scale: making assessment appropriate for people with aphasia. *Top Stroke Rehabil* 2015;22(2):83–93.

59. Arksey H, O'Malley L. Scoping studies: towards a methodological framework. *Int J Soc Res Methodol* 2005;8:19–32.

60. Baltimore D. Philosophical differences. *The New Yorker* January 27, 1997, p. 8.

61. Poses RM, Isen AM. Qualitative research in medicine and health care: questions and controversy. *J Gen Intern Med* 1998;13(1):32–38.

62. Welch CD, Polatajko HJ. Applied behavior analysis, autism, and occupational therapy: a search for understanding. *Am J Occup Ther* 2016;70(4):1–5.

63. Polatajko HJ, Welch C. Knowledge uptake and translation: a matter of evidence or of philosophy. *Can J Occup Ther* 2015;82(5):268–270.

On the Road to Translational Research

The imperative of evidence-based practice (EBP) must be supported by research that can be applied to clinical decisions. Unfortunately, many research efforts do not have clear relevance to every day practice, and many clinical questions remain unanswered. Our EBP efforts can be stymied by a lack of meaningful and useful research to support our clinical efforts.

The term translational research refers to the direct application of scientific discoveries into clinical practice. Often described as taking knowledge from "bench to bedside," this process is actually much broader in scope. Although certainly not a new concept, the healthcare community has experienced a renewed emphasis on the application of findings from laboratory and controlled studies to clinically important problems in real-world settings.

The purpose of this chapter is to describe the scope of translational research, including methods of efficacy and effectiveness research, and the importance of implementation research to make EBP a reality.

■ The Translation Gap

All too often, the successes of scientific breakthroughs in the laboratory or in animal models have not translated into major changes in medical or rehabilitative care for humans in a timely way. Of course, there are many notable success stories of research that has resulted in exceptionally important medical treatments, such as the discovery of penicillin in 1928[1] and the subsequent development of techniques to extract the antibiotic. Similarly, the discovery of insulin and its use in treating diabetes is a landmark achievement that has resulted in significant changes in medical care.[2]

There are many more examples, however, of lag times from 10 to 25 years or more for a discovery to reach publication, with several estimates of an average of 17 years for only 14% of new scientific discoveries to eventually reach clinical practice.[3] Given that these estimates are primarily based on publication records, it is likely that they are underestimates of true translation to health outcomes and impacts (see Focus on Evidence 2-1).[4] The *NIH Roadmap*, proposed in 2002, has called for a new paradigm of research to assure that "basic research discoveries are quickly transformed into drugs, treatments, or methods for prevention."[5]

Lag times are often due to sociocultural or scientific barriers, as well as systemic hurdles such as grant awards and institutional approvals, marketing and competition, policy and regulatory limitations, need for long-term follow-up in clinical trials, limited funding resources, guideline development, and dissemination. In the meantime, evidence-based clinicians who strive to adopt the

Focus on Evidence 2–1
A Translation Journey: The Lipid Hypothesis

It was more than 100 years ago, in 1913, that a young Russian experimental pathologist named Nikolai Anitschkow reported that feeding rabbits a high-cholesterol diet produced arterial plaques that resembled those in human atherosclerosis.[6] The disease had been well described in the medical literature by then, but was considered to be a predictable and nontreatable consequence of aging. At the time, one of the leading hypotheses as to its pathogenesis was that it was the result of excessive intake of animal proteins, and several scientists were attempting to provide evidence by feeding rabbits diets rich in milk, eggs, and meat, which did lead to vascular abnormalities. And although they found that egg yolks or whole eggs could also replicate the process, egg whites alone did not! Anitschkow showed that, by extracting cholesterol from egg yolks, he could duplicate the results without any added proteins.

Although some laboratories were able to confirm Anitschkow's findings using rabbits, most investigators were using other, more typical test animals, such as rats and dogs, and were not getting the same results. Reasons for these differences, understood today but not then, included different metabolic function in dogs and rabbits. So even though Anitschkow's work had been widely disseminated in German in 1913 and republished in English in 1933, there was no follow-up. Perhaps, too, the scientific community was indifferent to the findings because they ran contrary to the prevailing aging theory,

and it was considered implausible to mimic that outcome by feeding rabbits cholesterol![7] Steinberg,[8] a prominent researcher in this field, observed:

> Anitschkow's work should have galvanized the scientific community and encouraged innovative approaches to this major human disease problem. But nothing happened. Here was a classic example of how rigid, preconceived ideas sometimes stand in the way of scientific progress. Why did no one ask the (now) obvious questions?

Although Anitschkow's work did convincingly show that hypercholesterolemia in rabbits was sufficient to cause atherosclerosis, that did not necessarily mean that cholesterol in the human diet or blood had to be a factor in the disease. But basic questions about the pathogenesis of the disease were not being asked—how the cholesterol traveled in the rabbit's blood, how it became embedded in the arterial wall, or how a human diet might contribute to increased blood cholesterol. It wasn't until the 1950s that metabolic studies[10] and epidemiologic studies, such as the Framingham Heart Study,[9] sparked further investigation. Then, it took more than 30 years for the first clinical trial to be completed in 1984 to understand the relationship,[11] and the first statin was not approved until 1987. A century later, we have the benefit of basic laboratory studies, the development of medications, understanding genetic markers, and extensive clinical trials that have supported the century-old "lipid hypothesis."[12]

---

most effective treatment are at the mercy of the research enterprise—sometimes information on newer successful therapies is unavailable, or a study may support a new therapy, only to be disputed later with new information. This means that some patients may not get the best care, and others may unwittingly get unintentional harmful care.

 Another concept that is central to translational research is *knowledge translation (KT)*, a relatively new term that relates to underutilization of evidence. KT is a process of identifying clinical problems and accelerating the application of knowledge to improve outcomes and change the provision of care. It requires interprofessional support to close the gap between what we know and what we do. This concept will be covered in greater detail in Chapter 5.

■ The Translation Continuum

Many definitions have been proposed for translational research, and it can mean different things to different people.[13] Some view it as the development of new drugs, treatments, or devices, whereas others see its purpose to focus on getting research findings into practice. Whether driven by product, community, or policy interests, the importance of finding ways to ultimately influence clinical

decision-making and treatment effectiveness is paramount. One working definition is:

> *Translational research fosters the multidirectional integration of basic research, patient-oriented research, and population-based research, with the long-term aim of improving the health of the public.*[14]

Efficacy

Clinical trials are often distinguished by their design and purpose. The **randomized controlled trial (RCT)** is considered the "gold standard" design to study the **efficacy** of a new therapy by comparing it to a placebo or standard care. The design typically incorporates random allocation to groups and blinding to rule out sources of bias, allowing conclusions regarding the effect of the experimental treatment. This approach lets us examine theory and draw generalizations to large populations while controlling for unintended bias.

To provide sufficient control, however, RCTs must also carefully define and adhere to the treatment protocol, and will usually set strict inclusion and exclusion criteria for participants to eliminate possibly confounding factors such as comorbidities. The endpoints of such studies are usually directly related to the intervention's purpose, such as physiological responses, laboratory tests, or assessment of impairments that demonstrate the treatment's safety and biophysiological effect. These are necessary elements of the design process to assure that researchers can have confidence in observed outcomes.

Effectiveness

The major limitation of the efficacy approach is that it often eliminates the very patients who would likely be treated with the new therapy; that is, most of our patients come with comorbidities and other personal traits that cannot be controlled in practice. The testing environment will often be artificial, limiting the applicability of findings because they are not representative of the variable practice environment that cannot be controlled in the clinical community.

Therefore, effectiveness trials are needed to look at interventions under natural practice conditions, to make sure that the findings from RCTs translate to "real-world" clinical care. These trials are called pragmatic (practical) clinical trials (PCTs). PCTs will often incorporate measures of function or quality of life that are considered more relevant for patient satisfaction to understand if treatments have a meaningful effect on patient outcomes. Qualitative research, which highlights the human dimensions of health care, is especially useful in health services research to understand how patients' and providers' perceptions influence care delivery.

> Efficacy trials are sometimes referred to as *explanatory*, whereas effectiveness trials are called *pragmatic*. This distinction does not really clarify their differences, as both are seeking to discern the success of interventions. It is more appropriate to think of efficacy and effectiveness as ends of a continuum, with most trials somewhere in between.[15]

Chapters 14, 15, and 16 will cover the design and validity issues inherent in RCTs and PCTs. Chapter 21 will focus on the contributions of qualitative research.

Translation Blocks

Between 2000 and 2005, the *Institute of Medicine (IOM) Clinical Research Roundtable* identified two "translation blocks" that represented obstacles to realizing true health benefits from original research.[16] The first translation block, T1, reflected the challenge of transferring laboratory findings related to disease mechanisms into the development of new methods for diagnosis, treatment, and prevention. The second block, T2, reflected the need to translate results of clinical studies into everyday clinical practice and decision-making.

These blocks have since been expanded to reflect four stages in the translation of scientific knowledge to practice and health-care services. Although several models

have been proposed,[4,17–21] they all have a common trajectory for the translation process (see Fig. 2-1).

> ### ➤ CASE IN POINT #1
> The *botulinum* toxin, known to be a poisonous substance, is also now known to have important properties for relieving neurogenic disorders, including spasticity. Discoveries from basic mechanisms to clinical use illustrate the stages of translational research.

T0—Basic Research

The start of the translational continuum is characterized as basic research, representing investigations that focus on theory or biological inquiry, often utilizing animal models. These studies are typically necessary for the development of new drugs. The purpose is to define physiological mechanisms that will allow researchers to generate potential treatment options that can be tested.

> ➤ **T0:** The *Clostridium botulinum* bacterium was first identified in 1895 following the death of three people from food poisoning in a small Belgian town. Over time, laboratory studies were able to isolate the botulinum-A toxin (BTX) and researchers discovered that it blocked neuromuscular transmission by preventing the release of acetylcholine.[22]

T1—Translation to Humans:
DOES it work?

In this first translation stage, researchers must assess the potential for clinical application of basic science findings, testing new methods of diagnosis, treatment, and prevention. These studies are considered *Phase I* trials and case studies. They are usually small, focused studies, specifically looking at safety, accuracy, and dosage.

> ➤ **T1:** In 1977, the first human injections of BTX were given to relieve strabismus, with no systemic complications.[23] In 1985, injections were successful for 12 patients with torticollis.[24]
>
> Following these studies, in 1989 researchers demonstrated its effect on upper extremity spasticity in six patients post-stroke.[25] These studies also demonstrated the safety of this application.

T2—Translation to Patients:
CAN it work under ideal conditions?

Once clinical applications have been demonstrated, researchers must subject interventions and diagnostic procedures to rigorous testing using *Phase II* and *Phase III* trials, which are typically RCTs. These trials are larger efficacy studies, with specific controls and defined patient samples, comparing the intervention of interest with a placebo or usual care.

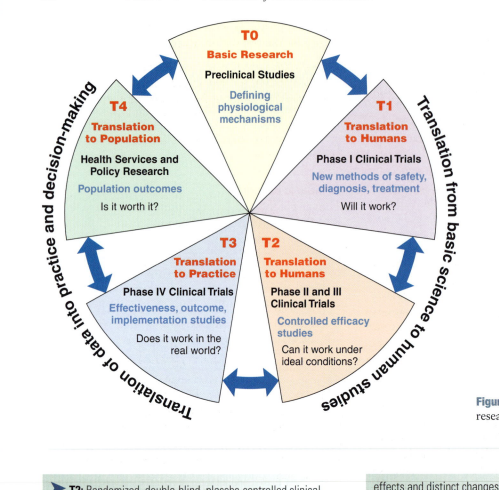

Figure 2–1 A model of translational research.

➤ **T2:** Randomized, double-blind, placebo-controlled clinical trials over 20 years demonstrated that BTX could safely reduce upper extremity spasticity over the long term.[26,27]

This phase of the translation process will often result in approval of a new drug or device by the Food and Drug Administration (FDA).

T3—Translation to Practice:

WILL it work in real-world conditions?

This is the practice-oriented stage, focusing on dissemination, to find out if treatments are as effective when applied in everyday practice as they were in controlled studies.

Phase IV clinical trials are typically implemented when devices or treatments have been approved and researchers continue to study them to learn about risk factors, benefits, and optimal use patterns. Outcomes are focused on issues that are relevant to patients, such as satisfaction and function, and studies are embedded into practice settings.

➤ **T3:** Effectiveness trials continue to demonstrate multiple uses of BTX. Spasticity studies have shown minimal adverse

effects and distinct changes in tone. Treatment aimed at prevention of contractures has had some success, although there is limited evidence regarding positive upper extremity functional outcomes.[28,29] Studies continue to look at dosage, dilutions, site of injections, and combination therapies.

T4—Translation to Populations:

Is it worth it?

This final translation stage is focused on health services and policy research to evaluate population outcomes and impact on population health, which can include attention to global health. It addresses how people get access to health-care services, the costs of care, and the system structures that control access. These are also considered Phase IV trials. They seek to inform stakeholders if the difference in treatment outcomes warrants the difference in cost for more expensive interventions, or if the "best" treatment gives the best "bang for the buck."[30]

The ultimate goal is to impact personal behaviors and quality of life for individuals and populations, and to provide information that will be used for clinical decision-making by patients, care providers, and policy makers. Although many therapies make their way through T1 to

T3 phases, they must still reach the communities that need them in cost-effective ways.

> ▶ **T4:** Researchers have been able to show improved quality of life in physical dimensions of function for patients with upper extremity spasticity,[31] and cost-effectiveness of using BTX based on a greater improvement in pretreatment functional targets that warrant continuation of therapy.[32] Guidelines for using BTX have also been established.[33]

Chapter 14 provides a fuller discussion of the four phases of clinical trials.

The Multidirectional Cycle

Although the translational continuum is presented as sequential stages, it is important to recognize that these stages truly represent an iterative and interactive pathway in multiple directions, not always starting with basic research questions. The bidirectional arrows reflect how new knowledge and hypotheses can be generated at each phase.

For example, many conditions, such as AIDS and fetal alcohol syndrome, were first described based on clinical observations presented in historical reports and case studies.[34,35] These were followed by decades of epidemiologic studies describing the syndromes, with later bench studies confirming physiological and developmental mechanisms through animal models and genetic investigation. Subsequent clinical trials focused on diagnostic tests, medications, and guidelines for treatment, often leading back to laboratory studies.

■ Effectiveness Research

Because the explicit goal of translational research is to bridge the gap between the controlled scientific environment and real-world practice settings, effectiveness trials specifically address generalizability and access. These varied study approaches have different names, with some overlap in their purposes, but they represent an important direction for clinical research to address T3 and T4 translation.

Federal and nonprofit agencies have created programs with significant funding to support effectiveness studies, most notably the Agency for Healthcare Research and Quality (AHRQ),[36] the Patient-Centered Outcomes Research Institute (PCORI),[37] and the National Institutes of Health (NIH) Clinical and Translational Science Awards (CTSA).[38]

Comparative Effectiveness Research

Comparative effectiveness research (CER) is designed to study the real-world application of research evidence to assist patients, providers, payers, and policy makers in making informed decisions about treatment choices. The IOM provides the following definition:

> *Comparative effectiveness research is the generation and synthesis of evidence that compares the benefits and harms of alternative methods to prevent, diagnose, treat and monitor or improve the delivery of care.*[39]

This purpose includes establishing a core of useful evidence that will address conditions that have a high impact on health care.

- For patients, this strategy means providing information about which approaches might work best, given their particular concerns, circumstances, and preferences.
- For clinicians, it means providing evidence-based information about questions they face daily in practice.
- For insurers and policy makers, it means producing evidence to help with decisions on how to improve health outcomes, costs, and access to services.[37]

CER may include studies on drugs, medical devices, surgeries, rehabilitation strategies, or methods of delivering care. These trials include studies done on patients who are typical of those seen in every day practice, with few exclusion criteria, and are typically embedded in routine care to improve generalizability of findings and to allow translation of findings into care for individuals and populations.

Study designs may include randomized trials as well as observational research, and CER may include original research or systematic reviews and meta-analyses that synthesize existing evidence.

> 🔑 An important distinction of CER is a focus on comparing alternative treatments, not comparing new treatments to a placebo or control. This "head-to-head" comparison is intended to compare at least two interventions that are effective enough to be the standard of care, to determine which one is "best." Because different patients may respond differently to treatments, CER will often focus on studying subgroups of populations.

Pragmatic Clinical Trials

Pragmatic trials have several important features that differ from RCTs (see Fig. 2-2).[40,41] In PCTs, the hypothesis and study design are formulated based on information needed to make a clinical decision.

Flexible Protocols

Pragmatic trials allow for a different level of flexibility in research design than an RCT. One such difference is in the specificity of the intervention.

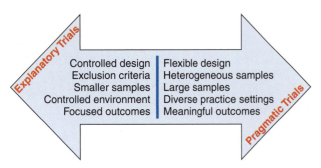

Controlled design | Flexible design
Exclusion criteria | Heterogeneous samples
Smaller samples | Large samples
Controlled environment | Diverse practice settings
Focused outcomes | Meaningful outcomes

Figure 2–2 The continuum from explanatory to pragmatic trials.

> ### ➤ CASE IN POINT #2
>
> Physical inactivity in elders can lead to functional decline and many physical and physiological disorders. Researchers designed a pragmatic trial to evaluate programs to promote physical activity and better functional outcomes among older people.[42] The study compared three treatments:
>
> - A group-based Falls Management Exercise (FaME) program held weekly for supervised exercise and unsupervised home exercises twice weekly.
> - A home-based exercise program involving unsupervised exercises to be done three times per week.
> - A usual care group that was not offered either program.
>
> Although a precise definition of the intervention is important in both types of studies, PCTs involve implementation as it would typically occur in practice. For example, in the FaME study, the way in which patients did home exercises would likely have variability that could not be controlled.

Patients may also receive modifications of treatment in a PCT to meet their specific needs, as long as they are based on a common management protocol or decision-making algorithm.[43] This is especially relevant to rehabilitation interventions, which may be based on the same approach, but have to be adapted to individual patient goals and conditions.

Diverse Settings and Samples

RCTs typically limit where the research is being done, whereas PCTs will try to embed the study in routine practice, such as primary care settings or communities.[44] The challenge with PCTs is balancing the need for sufficient control in the design to demonstrate cause and effect while being able to generalize findings to real-world practice.

One of the most important distinctions of a PCT is in the selection of participants and settings, both of which impact the generalization of findings. The PCT sample should reflect the variety of patients seen in practice for whom the interventions being studied would be

used. If you look at the method section of an RCT, you will often see a substantial list of exclusion criteria that restricts age or gender, and eliminates subjects with comorbidities, those at high risk, or those who take other medications. The purpose of these exclusions is to make the sample as homogeneous as possible to improve statistical estimates.

In clinical practice, however, we do not have the luxury of selecting patients with specific characteristics. Therefore, the PCT tries to include all those who fit the treatment population to better reflect the practical circumstances of patient care. A full description of demographics within a sample is important to this understanding.

> ➤ The FaME exercise study involved 43 general practices in three counties in the United Kingdom. All patients over 65 years of age were recruited. They had to be independently mobile so that they could participate in the exercise activities. The only exclusions were a history of at least three falls, not being able to follow instructions, or unstable clinical conditions precluding exercise.

Practice-Based Evidence

The term **practice-based evidence (PBE)** has also been used to describe an approach to research that is of high quality but developed and implemented in real-world settings. Developing PBE requires deriving research questions from real-world clinical problems. Applying evidence to practice is often difficult when studies do not fit well with practice needs. In a practice-based research model, the clinical setting becomes the "laboratory," involving front-line clinicians and "real" treatments and patients.[45]

> 📌 The ideas of EBP and PBE are often confused. EBP focuses on how the clinician uses research to inform clinical practice decisions. PBE refers to the type of evidence that is derived from real patient care problems, identifying gaps between recommended and actual practice.[46] EBP will be more meaningful when the available evidence has direct application to clinical situations—evidence that is practice based!

PBE studies often use observational cohorts, surveys, secondary analysis, or qualitative studies, with diverse samples from several clinical sites, with comprehensive data collection methods that include details on patient characteristics and their care (see Focus on Evidence 2-2). The studies are typically designed to create databases with many outcome variables and documentation standards.

Focus on Evidence 2–2
Patients and Providers: Understanding Perceptions

Nonadherence to drug regimens can lead to negative consequences, and patients often stop taking medications for various reasons. Having identified this problem in practice, researchers examined the differences between patient and physician perspectives related to drug adherence and drug importance in patients who were taking at least one long-term drug treatment.[47] The study recruited 128 patients, from both hospital and ambulatory settings, who were taking 498 drugs.

For each drug taken, they asked physicians to rate their knowledge of the patient's adherence and the importance of the drug to the patient's health. Patients were asked for the same two ratings, in addition to an open-ended question on why they were not adherent. Researchers found a weak agreement of both adherence and importance between patients and physicians. They found that the physicians considered 13% of the drugs being taken as unimportant, and that nearly 20% of the drugs that the physicians considered important were not being taken correctly by patients.

These findings have direct clinical implications for shared decision-making, including involving other professionals such as pharmacists. It points to the different perspectives of patients, who may see drugs primarily for symptom relief, whereas physicians may be focused on long-term prevention or changes in laboratory test values.

Outcomes Research

Effectiveness trials have also been distinguished from RCTs in terms of the endpoints that are typically used to determine if interventions are successful. Rather than using endpoints that focus on treatment response or impairment values, such as a change in blood pressure or range of motion, PCTs aim to incorporate measurements that reflect the values of various stakeholders, such as an improvement in function, quality of life, patient satisfaction, or cost.

Outcomes research is an umbrella term to describe studies that focus on the impact of results of healthcare practices and interventions. As part of health services research, outcome studies address both clinical and population-based questions with the intent of improving the benefits of health care to individual patients and communities.[48]

HISTORICAL NOTE
The need to document outcomes has not always been appreciated, but several historical influences have had important impacts. For example, in 1847, Ignaz Semmelweis, a Hungarian physician, was concerned about the high mortality rate among mothers and newborns due to "childbed fever," and was able to show a marked decline in the death rate after physicians began to wash their hands before delivering babies.[49] Florence Nightingale's efforts during the Crimean War in the 1850s were focused on better hygiene, nutrition, and less crowding, again resulting in significantly reduced mortality.[50]

Perhaps one of the most relevant influences was the work of Boston surgeon Ernest Codman in 1914, who advocated for the disclosure of hospital data to show the outcomes of medical and surgical intervention. His contributions are evident in many contemporary practices, such as keeping anesthesia records during surgery, holding mortality and morbidity rounds, creating patient registries, and establishing quality monitoring organizations.[51]

Codman's work had an important influence on how we record outcomes and how health care is evaluated. See the *Chapter 2 Supplement* for expanded discussion of his vital contributions. It is a story with many contemporary lessons.

Measuring What Matters

Historically, outcomes of health care were assessed in terms of morbidity, mortality, length of stay, and readmissions. Today, outcomes have a broader meaning, reflecting endpoints that matter to patients, which can be dramatically different from traditional measures of disease or impairment. Physiological measures and other objective assessments, such as symptoms or movement, are often not the primary focus for patients, although they give clinicians a sense of change.

Patients will typically be more interested in things that only they can perceive, such as pain, function, quality of life or satisfaction, and things that fall within activity and participation domains of the ICF (see Chapter 1). These are multidimensional constructs that require the development of a tool to gather relevant information. Understanding these various mechanisms and how they are reported in the literature can make a difference in treatment decisions.

In making the patient an important and explicit part of the EBP process, researchers and clinicians often seek **patient-oriented evidence that matters (POEM)**, referring to outcomes that measure things that a patient would care about, such as symptoms, quality of life, function, cost of care, length of stay, and so on.[52] This is in contrast to **disease-oriented evidence (DOE)**, which focuses more on changes in physiology and laboratory tests. DOE is important to understanding disease and diagnostic processes but may not be as informative in making choices for clinical management as POEM.

Patient-Reported Outcome Measures

The kinds of outcomes that are most important to patients are often assessed by using a **patient-reported outcome measure (PROM)**, which is:

. . . any report of the status of a patient's health condition that comes directly from the patient, without interpretation of the patient's response by a clinician or anyone else.[53,54]

These measures have been a mainstay in the design of pragmatic trials, but are becoming more common in RCTs in addition to more traditional outcomes. For example, research has shown that PROMs have a strong correlation to objective measures of movement and function.[55]

PROMs can be generic or condition specific. For measuring quality of life, for example, the *Short Form 36 Health Survey* provides a generic evaluation in domains related to physical, mental, emotional, and social functioning.[56] This tool has been tested across multiple populations. Similar tests are condition specific, such as the *Minnesota Living with Heart Failure Questionnaire*, which asks for patient perceptions relative to their heart condition.[57]

Other condition-specific measures include the Shoulder Pain and Disability Index (SPADI)[58] and the Stroke Impact Scale (SIS).[59] Clinicians need to understand a measure's theoretical foundation and the validity of these tools so they can select the one that will be appropriate to the condition and the information that will be relevant to decision-making (see Chapter 10).[60]

You may also see the term *patient-reported outcome (PRO)* used to refer to the outcome itself, such as satisfaction or health-related quality of life, as opposed to the PROM. For example. health-related quality of life is a PRO that can be measured using the Short Form 36 Health Survey, which is a PROM.

Patient-Centered Outcomes Research

Because patients and clinicians face a wide range of complex and often confusing choices in addressing health-care needs, they need reliable answers to their questions. Those answers may not exist, or they may not be available in ways that patients can understand.

As a form of CER, **patient-centered outcomes research (PCOR)** has the distinct goal of engaging patients and other stakeholders in the development of questions and outcome measures, encouraging them to become integral members of the research process (see Focus on Evidence 2-3). Funding for these studies is the primary mission of the *Patient-Centered Outcomes Research Institute (PCORI).*[37]

Focus on Evidence 2–3
Focusing on Patient Preferences

For research to be patient centered, assessments must be able to reflect what matters to patients, how they would judge the success of their treatment. In a study funded by PCORI, Allen et al[61] used a tool they developed called the Movement Abilities Measure (MAM), which evaluates movement in six dimensions: flexibility, strength, accuracy, speed, adaptability, and endurance. They wanted to know if there was a gap between what patients thought they could do and what movement ability they wanted to have. Patients completed questions at admission and discharge. Clinicians' notes on patient performance were analyzed for the same six dimensions, to see if there was agreement—did the physical therapists have the same perceptions as the patients in terms of their values for outcomes?

Responses were transformed to a six-point scale. For example, on the dimension of flexibility, patients were asked to rate their movement from 6 "I move so easily that I can stretch or reach . . ." to 0 "Stiffness or tightness keeps me from doing most of my daily

care." For each dimension, patients were asked what their current state was and what they would like it to be. The largest gap at admission was between the patients' current and preferred level of flexibility.

The gaps decreased following the episode of care, indicating that most patients perceived improvement, getting closer to where they wanted their movement to be. However, the clinicians did not rate the outcomes so highly and reported that 62% of patients did not meet all therapeutic goals. Interestingly, only 29% of the patients had their largest current–preferred gap in the same dimension as their therapist.

The important message in these results, which leads to many research opportunities, is that there appears to be considerable disagreement between clinicians and patients on the dimensions of movement that should be the goals of their care and how improvements are perceived. Such information would help clinicians understand what patients value most and how treatment can be focused on those preferences.

Primary and Secondary Outcomes

Trials will often study multiple endpoints, which will reflect outcomes at different levels. Researchers will typically designate one measure as a *primary outcome*, the one that will be used to arrive at a decision on the overall result of the study and that represents the greatest therapeutic benefit.[62] *Secondary outcomes* are other endpoint measures that may also be used to assess the effectiveness of the intervention, as well as side effects, costs, or other outcomes of interest.

> ➤ The primary outcome in the FaME exercise study was the proportion of patients reaching the recommended target of 150 minutes of moderate to vigorous physical activity per week at 12-months postintervention, based on a comprehensive self-report questionnaire. Secondary outcomes included number of falls, quality of life, balance and falls efficacy, and cost. A significantly higher proportion of the FaME participants achieved the physical activity target and showed better balance and decreased fall rate compared to the other two groups, but there were no differences in quality of life. The researchers also established that the FaME program was more expensive, averaging £1,740 (about $2,000 to us on the other side of the pond in 2017).

> 🔑 The decision regarding the primary outcome of a study is important for planning, as it will direct the estimate of the needed sample size, and thereby the power of a study (see Chapter 23). Because this estimate is determined by the expected size of the outcome effect, with multiple outcomes, researchers must base it on one value, usually the primary outcome.[63] However, alternatively, the one outcome variable that has the smallest effect, and thereby would require a larger sample, can be used.

■ Implementation Studies

As evidence mounts over time with efficacy and effectiveness studies, at some point "sufficient" evidence will be accumulated to warrant widespread implementation of a new practice, replacing standard care. This is the crux of the "translation gap."

For example, despite extraordinary global progress in immunizing children, in 2007, almost 20% of the children born each year (24 million children) did not get the complete routine immunizations scheduled for their first year of life. In most cases, this occurred in poorly served remote rural areas, deprived urban settings, and fragile and strife-torn regions.[64] This is not a problem of finding an effective intervention—it is a problem of *implementation*.

Implementation science is the next step beyond effectiveness research. It focuses on understanding the influence of environment and resources on whether research findings are actually translated to practice. Once trials have established that an intervention is effective, the question then turns to "how to make it happen."

> *Implementation science is the study of methods to promote the integration of research findings and evidence into health-care policy and practice. It seeks to understand the behavior of health-care professionals and other stakeholders as a key variable in the sustainable uptake, adoption, and implementation of evidence-based interventions.*[65]

This approach incorporates a broader scope than traditional clinical research, looking not only at the patient, but more so at the provider, organizational systems, and policy levels.

Implementation Science and Evidence-Based Practice

There is a key distinction between implementation studies and the evidence-based practices they seek to implement. An implementation study is focused on ways to change behavior, often incorporating education and training, team-based efforts, community engagement, or systemic infrastructure redesign. It is not intended to demonstrate the health benefits of a clinical intervention, but rather the rate and quality of the use of that intervention[66] and which adaptations are needed to achieve relevant outcomes.[67]

> ➤ **CASE IN POINT #3**
> Quanbeck et al[68] reported on the feasibility and effectiveness of an implementation program to improve adherence to clinical guidelines for opioid prescribing in primary care. They used a combination of quantitative and qualitative methods to determine the success of a 6-month intervention comparing four intervention clinics and four control clinics.

Types of Implementation Studies

Understanding implementation issues requires going beyond efficacy and effectiveness to recognize the geographic, cultural, socioeconomic, and regulatory contexts that influence utilization patterns.[69] The acceptance and adoption of interventions, no matter how significant clinical studies are, must be based on what works, for whom, under which circumstances, and whether the intervention can be scaled up sufficiently to enhance outcomes. There is an element of ethical urgency in this process, to find the mechanisms to assure that individuals and communities are getting the best care available.[70]

Implementation studies can address many types of intervention, including looking at clinical performance audits, the use of patient or provider alerts to remind them of guidelines, the influence of local leaders to adopt best practices, the investigation of consensus as a foundation for problem management, or patient education interventions.[71]

➤ The intervention in the opioid study consisted of a combination of monthly site visits and teleconferences, including consultations and facilitated discussions. Teams of six to eight staff members at each clinic included a combination of physician, nurse, medical assistant, and administrative personnel. Teams reviewed opioid prescribing guidelines and how to implement mental health screening and urine drug testing.

🔑 Implementation studies are closely related to quality improvement (QI) techniques. The difference lies in the focus of QI on a practical and specific system issue leading to local and immediate changes, usually with administrative or logistic concerns.[72] Implementation studies address utilization with the intent of generalizing beyond the individual system under study to populations, applying research principles, typically across multiple sites.

Implementation Outcomes

Implementation outcomes involve variables that describe the intentional activities to deliver services.[72] They typically focus on feasibility, acceptance, adoption, cost, and sustainability—all serving as indicators of success. These variables also provide insight into how the program contributes to health outcomes.

➤ The opioid study focused on attendance of clinic staff at monthly sessions and staff satisfaction with the meetings. At 6 and 12 months, they found significant improvement in the intervention clinics compared to controls. There was a reduction in prescribing rates, average daily dose for patients on long-term therapy, and the number of patients receiving mental health screens and urine tests. Costs were assessed and adjustments made as needed.

Data for implementation studies may be quantitative, based on structured surveys about attitudes or behaviors, or administrative data such as utilization rates. Qualitative data are also often collected to better understand the context of implementation, including semi-structured interviews, focus groups, and direct observation.

➤ The opioid study used qualitative data from focus groups, interviews, and ethnographic techniques to determine which types of adaptations were needed. They found that a personal touch was helpful to promote sustained engagement, with frequent communication at each stage being key. They also realized the need for clear expectations to team roles and responsibilities, as well as for linking the implementation process with the clinic's organizational workflows, policies, and values.

COMMENTARY

Knowing is not enough; we must apply. Willing is not enough; we must do.

—Johann Wolfgang von Goethe (1749–1832)

German writer and statesman

So much to think about. So much that still needs to be done. Which studies will tell us what we need to know—RCTs or PCTs? The answer may be less than satisfying—we need both.[15] They give us different information and we need to put each in perspective, use each for the right purpose.

Efficacy studies are often referred to as "proof of concept," to demonstrate if an intervention can work. If the answer is yes, the next step is to test it under "real-world" conditions. But real-world conditions are quite a conundrum in "research world," which tries to be orderly, logical, and consistent. Efficacy studies try to avoid confounding issues such as diverse patients or noncompliance that can interfere with therapeutic benefits. And effectiveness studies struggle with the lack of control that defines them, recognizing the potential for bias and the difficulty in demonstrating significant effects because of so much variability.

So we are left with the need to consider evidence across the continuum, with the onus on both practitioners and researchers to exchange ideas, understand priorities, and contribute to setting research agendas. It also means that both are responsible for creating information in a relevant format and using that information to make decisions. Collaboration is an essential approach to making translation a reality.

REFERENCES

1. Fleming A. Classics in infectious diseases: on the antibacterial action of cultures of a penicillium, with special reference to their use in the isolation of B. influenzae by Alexander Fleming, Reprinted from the *British Journal of Experimental Pathology* 10:226–236, 1929. *Rev Infect Dis* 1980;2(1):129–139.
2. Dunkley AJ, Bodicoat DH, Greaves CJ, Russell C, Yates T, Davies MJ, Khunti K. Diabetes prevention in the real world: effectiveness of pragmatic lifestyle interventions for the prevention of type 2 diabetes and of the impact of adherence to guideline recommendations: a systematic review and meta-analysis. *Diabetes Care* 2014;37(4):922–933.
3. Morris ZS, Wooding S, Grant J. The answer is 17 years, what is the question: understanding time lags in translational research. *J R Soc Med* 2011;104(12):510–520.
4. Trochim W, Kane C, Graham MJ, Pincus HA. Evaluating translational research: a process marker model. *Clin Transl Sci* 2011;4(3):153–162.
5. National Institutes of Health: Overview of the NIH Roadmap. Available at http://nihroadmap.nih.gov/overview.asp. Accessed January 30, 2005.
6. Anitschkow NN, Chalatow S. Üeber experimentelle Cholesterinsteatose und ihre Bedeutung für die Entstehung einiger pathologischer. *Prozesse Zentralbl Allg Pathol* 1913;24:1–9.
7. Steinberg D. *The Cholesterol Wars*. Amsterdam: Elsevier/Academic Press, 2007.
8. Steinberg D. In celebration of the 100th anniversary of the lipid hypothesis of atherosclerosis. *Journal of Lipid Research* 2013;54(11):2946–2949.
9. Dawber TR, Moore FE, Mann GV. Coronary heart disease in the Framingham study. *Am J Public Health Nations Health* 1957;47(4 Pt 2):4–24.
10. Gofman JW, Lindgren F. The role of lipids and lipoproteins in atherosclerosis. *Science* 1950;111(2877):166–171.
11. The Lipid Research Clinics Coronary Primary Prevention Trial results. II. The relationship of reduction in incidence of coronary heart disease to cholesterol lowering. *JAMA* 1984;251(3):365–374.
12. Goldstein JL, Brown MS. A century of cholesterol and coronaries: from plaques to genes to statins. *Cell* 2015;161(1):161–172.
13. Woolf SH. The meaning of translational research and why it matters. *JAMA* 2008;299(2):211–213.
14. Rubio DM, Schoenbaum EE, Lee LS, Schteingart DE, Marantz PR, Anderson KE, Platt LD, Baez A, Esposito K. Defining translational research: implications for training. *Acad Med* 2010;85(3):470–475.
15. Streiner DL. Statistics commentary series: Commentary #5—can it work or does it work? The difference between efficacy and effectiveness trials. *J Clin Psychopharmacol* 2014;34(6):672–674.
16. Institute of Medicine. *Roundtable on Evidence-Based Medicine*. Washington, DC.: National Academies Press, 2009.
17. Khoury MJ, Gwinn M, Yoon PW, Dowling N, Moore CA, Bradley L. The continuum of translation research in genomic medicine: how can we accelerate the appropriate integration of human genome discoveries into health care and disease prevention? *Genet Med* 2007;9(10):665–674.
18. Westfall JM, Mold J, Fagnan L. Practice-based research—"Blue Highways" on the NIH roadmap. *JAMA* 2007;297(4):403–406.
19. Dougherty D, Conway PH. The "3T's" road map to transform US health care: the "how" of high-quality care. *JAMA* 2008;299(19):2319–2321.
20. Sung NS, Crowley WF, Jr., Genel M, Salber P, Sandy L, Sherwood LM, Johnson SB, Catanese V, Tilson H, Getz K, et al. Central challenges facing the national clinical research enterprise. *JAMA* 2003;289(10):1278–1287.
21. Blumberg RS, Dittel B, Hafler D, von Herrath M, Nestle FO. Unraveling the autoimmune translational research process layer by layer. *Nat Med* 2012;18(1):35–41.
22. Devriese PP. On the discovery of Clostridium botulinum. *J Hist Neurosci* 1999;8(1):43–50.
23. Scott AB. Botulinum toxin injection into extraocular muscles as an alternative to strabismus surgery. *Ophthalmology* 1980;87(10):1044–1049.
24. Tsui JK, Eisen A, Mak E, Carruthers J, Scott A, Calne DB. A pilot study on the use of botulinum toxin in spasmodic torticollis. *Can J Neurol Sci* 1985;12(4):314–316.
25. Das TK, Park DM. Effect of treatment with botulinum toxin on spasticity. *Postgrad Med J* 1989;65(762):208–210.
26. Simpson DM, Alexander DN, O'Brien CF, Tagliati M, Aswad AS, Leon JM, Gibson J, Mordaunt JM, Monaghan EP. Botulinum toxin type A in the treatment of upper extremity spasticity: a randomized, double-blind, placebo-controlled trial. *Neurology* 1996;46(5):1306–1310.
27. Gordon MF, Brashear A, Elovic E, Kassicieh D, Marciniak C, Liu J, Turkel C. Repeated dosing of botulinum toxin type A for upper limb spasticity following stroke. *Neurology* 2004;63(10):1971–1973.
28. Ney JP, Joseph KR. Neurologic uses of botulinum neurotoxin type A. *Neuropsychiatri Dis Treat* 2007;3(6):785–798.
29. Intiso D, Simone V, Rienzo F, Santamato A, Russo M, Tolfa M, Basciani M. Does spasticity reduction by botulinum toxin type A improve upper limb functionality in adult post-stroke patients? A systematic review of relevant studies. *J Neurol Neurophysiol* 2013;4(4):167.
30. Woolf SH, Johnson RE. The break-even point: when medical advances are less important than improving the fidelity with which they are delivered. *Ann Fam Med* 2005;3(6):545–552.
31. Rychlik R, Kreimendahl F, Schnur N, Lambert-Baumann J, Dressler D. Quality of life and costs of spasticity treatment in German stroke patients. *Health Econ Rev* 2016;6:27.
32. Ward A, Roberts G, Warner J, Gillard S. Cost-effectiveness of botulinum toxin type A in the treatment of post-stroke spasticity. *J Rehabil Med* 2005;37(4):252–257.
33. Royal College of Physicians, British Society of Rehabilitation Medicine, Chartered Society of Physiotherapy, Association of Chartered Physiotherapists Interested in Neurology. Spasticity in adults: management using botulinum toxin. National guidelines. London: RCP, 2009. Available at http://www.bsrm.org.uk/downloads/spasticity-in-adults-management-botulinum-toxin.pdf. Accessed January 8, 2017.
34. Curran JW, Jaffe HW. AIDS: the early years and CDC's response. *MMWR Suppl* 2011;60(4):64–69.
35. Jones KL, Smith DW. Recognition of the fetal alcohol syndrome in early infancy. *Lancet* 1973;302(7836):999–1001.
36. Agency for Healthcare Research and Quality. US Department of Health and Human Services. Available at https://www.ahrq.gov. Accessed January 5, 2017.
37. Patient-Centered Outcomes Research Institute. Available at http://www.pcori.org/. Accessed January 5, 2017.
38. National Institutes of Health. National Center for Advancing Translational Sciences. Clinical and translational science awards (CTSA) program. Available at https://ncats.nih.gov/ctsa. Accessed January 6, 2017.
39. Institute of Medicine: Initial National Priorities for Comparative Effectiveness Research. Washington, DC, National Academies Press, 2009. Available at https://www.nap.edu/catalog/12648/initial-national-priorities-for-comparative-effectiveness-research. Accessed January 4, 2017.
40. Patsopoulos NA. A pragmatic view on pragmatic trials. *Dialogues Clin Neurosci* 2011;13(2):217–224.
41. Tunis SR, Stryer DB, Clancy CM. Practical clinical trials: increasing the value of clinical research for decision making in clinical and health policy. *JAMA* 2003;290(12):1624–1632.
42. Iliffe S, Kendrick D, Morris R, Griffin M, Haworth D, Carpenter H, Masud T, Skelton DA, Dinan-Young S, Bowling A, et al. Promoting physical activity in older people in general practice: ProAct65+ cluster randomised controlled trial. *Br J Gen Pract* 2015;65(640):e731–e738.

43. Roland M, Torgerson DJ. What are pragmatic trials? *BMJ* 1998;316(7127):285.

44. Godwin M, Ruhland L, Casson I, MacDonald S, Delva D, Birtwhistle R, Lam M, Seguin R. Pragmatic controlled clinical trials in primary care: the struggle between external and internal validity. *BMC Medical Research Methodology* 2003;3:28.

45. Horn SD, Gassaway J. Practice-based evidence study design for comparative effectiveness research. *Med Care* 2007;45 (10 Suppl 2):S50–S57.

46. Horn SD, DeJong G, Deutscher D. Practice-based evidence research in rehabilitation: an alternative to randomized controlled trials and traditional observational studies. *Arch Phys Med Rehabil* 2012;93(8 Suppl):S127–S137.

47. Sidorkiewicz S, Tran V-T, Cousyn C, Perrodeau E, Ravaud P. Discordance between drug adherence as reported by patients and drug importance as assessed by physicians. *Ann Fam Med* 2016;14(5):415–421.

48. Agency for Healthcare Research and Quality: Outcomes Research. Fact Sheet. Available at https://archive.ahrq.gov/research/findings/factsheets/outcomes/outfact/outcomes-and-research.html. Accessed January 12, 2017.

49. Semmelweis I. *The Etiology, Concept, and Prophylaxis of Childbed Fever*. Madison, WI: University of Wisconsin Press, 1983.

50. Nightingale F. *Introductory Notes on Lying-In Institutions, Together with a Proposal for Organising and Institution for Training Midwives and Midwifery Nurses*. London: Longmans Green & Co, 1871.

51. Mallon BE: Amory Codman: pioneer New England shoulder surgeon. New England Shoulder & Elbow Society. Available at http://neses.com/e-amory-codman-pioneer-new-england-shoulder-surgeon/. Accessed January 11, 2017.

52. Geyman JP. POEMs as a paradigm shift in teaching, learning, and clinical practice. Patient-oriented evidence that matters. *J Fam Pract* 1999;48(5):343–344.

53. Center for Evidence-based Physiotherapy: Physiotherapy Evidence Database. Available at http://www.pedro.fhs.usyd.edu.au/index.html. Accessed October 17, 2004

54. Food and Drug Administration: Guidance for industry: patient-reported outcome measures: use in medical product development to support labeling claims; 2009. Available at http://www.fda.gov/downloads/drugs/guidances/ucm193282.pdf. Accessed January 18, 2017.

55. Alcock L, O'Brien TD, Vanicek N. Age-related changes in physical functioning: correlates between objective and self-reported outcomes. *Physiother* 2015;101(2):204–213.

56. Hays RD, Morales LS. The RAND-36 measure of health-related quality of life. *Ann Med* 2001;33(5):350–357.

57. Bilbao A, Escobar A, García-Perez L, Navarro G, Quirós R. The Minnesota Living with Heart Failure Questionnaire: comparison of different factor structures. *Health Qual Life Outcomes* 2016;14(1):23.

58. Breckenridge JD, McAuley JH. Shoulder Pain and Disability Index (SPADI). *J Physiother* 2011;57(3):197.

59. Duncan PW, Bode RK, Min Lai S, Perera S. Rasch analysis of a new stroke-specific outcome scale: the Stroke Impact Scale. *Arch Phys Med Rehabil* 2003;84(7):950–963.

60. Perret-Guillaume C, Briancon S, Guillemin F, Wahl D, Empereur F, Nguyen Thi PL. Which generic health related Quality of Life questionnaire should be used in older inpatients: comparison of the Duke Health Profile and the MOS Short-Form SF-36? *J Nutr Health Aging* 2010;14(4):325–331.

61. Allen D, Talavera C, Baxter S, Topp K. Gaps between patients' reported current and preferred abilities versus clinicians' emphases during an episode of care: Any agreement? *Qual Life Res* 2015;24(5):1137–1143.

62. Sedgwick P. Primary and secondary outcome measures. *BMJ* 2010;340.

63. Choudhary D, Garg PK. Primary outcome in a randomized controlled trial: a critical issue. *Saudi J Gastroenterol* 2011;17(5):369–369.

64. World Health Organization, UNICER, World Bank. *State of the World's Vaccines and Immunization*. 3 ed. Geneva: World Health Organization, 2009.

65. NIH Fogarty International Center: Implementation Science Information and Resources. Available at https://www.fic.nih.gov/researchtopics/pages/implementationscience.aspx. Accessed January 10, 2017.

66. Bauer MS, Damschroder L, Hagedorn H, Smith J, Kilbourne AM. An introduction to implementation science for the non-specialist. *BMC Psychology* 2015;3(1):32.

67. Chambers DA, Glasgow RE, Stange KC. The dynamic sustainability framework: addressing the paradox of sustainment amid ongoing change. *Implement Sci* 2013;8:117.

68. Quanbeck A, Brown RT, Zgierska AE, Jacobson N, Robinson JM, Johnson RA, Deyo BM, Madden L, Tuan W, Alagoz E. A. A randomized matched-pairs study of feasibility, acceptability, and effectiveness of systems consultation: a novel implementation strategy for adopting clinical guidelines for opioid prescribing in primary care. *Implement Sci* 2018;13(1):21.

69. Edwards N, Barker PM. The importance of context in implementation research. *J Acquir Immune Defic Syndr* 2014;67 Suppl 2:S157–S162.

70. Solomon MZ. The ethical urgency of advancing implementation science. *Am J Bioeth* 2010;10(8):31–32.

71. Jette AM. Moving research from the bedside into practice. *Phys Ther* 2016;96(5):594–596.

72. Peters DH, Adam T, Alonge O, et al. Implementation research: what it is and how to do it. *BMJ* 2013;347:f6753.

Defining the Research Question

The start of any research effort is identification of the specific question that will be investigated. This is the most important and often most difficult part of the research process because it controls the direction of all subsequent planning and analysis.

The purpose of this chapter is to clarify the process for developing and refining a feasible research question, define the different types of variables that form the basis for a question, describe how research objectives guide a study, and discuss how the review of literature contributes to this process. Whether designing a study or appraising the work of others, we need to appreciate where research questions come from and how they direct study methods, analysis, and interpretation of outcomes.

■ Selecting a Topic

The research process begins when a researcher identifies a broad topic of interest. Questions grow out of a need to know something that is not already known, resolve a conflict, confirm previous findings, or clarify some piece of information that is not sufficiently documented. Researchers are usually able to identify interests in certain patient populations, specific types of interventions, clinical theory, or fundamental policy issues.

> ➤ **CASE IN POINT #1**
> To illustrate the process of identifying a research problem, let us start with an example. Assume a researcher is interested in exploring issues related to pressure ulcers, a common and serious health problem. Let us see how this interest can be developed.

■ The Research Problem

Once a topic is identified, the process of clarifying a research problem begins by sorting through ideas based on clinical experience and observation, theories, and professional literature to determine what we know and what we need to find out. The application of this information will lead to identification of a *research problem* that will eventually provide the foundation for delineating a specific question that can be answered in a single study.

Clarify the Problem

Typically, research problems start out broad, concerned with general clinical problems or theoretical issues. This is illustrated in the top portion of Figure 3-1, showing a process that will require many iterations of possible ideas that may go back and forth. These ideas must be manipulated and modified several times before they become narrowed sufficiently to propose a specific question. Beginning researchers are often unprepared for the amount of time and thought required to formulate and hone a precise question that is testable. It is sometimes frustrating to accept that only one small facet of a problem can be addressed in a single study. First, the topic has to be made more explicit, such as:

How can we effectively manage pressure ulcers?

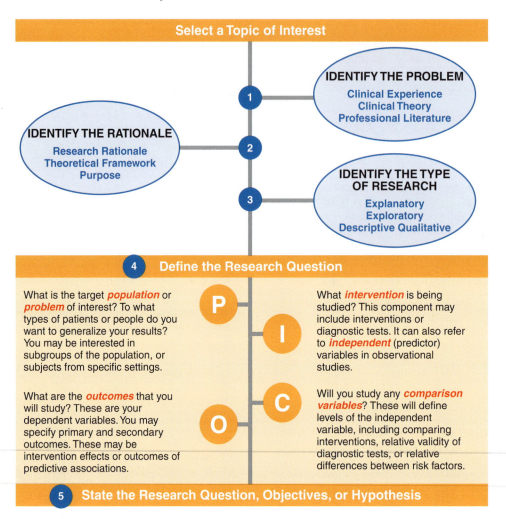

Figure 3–1 Five-step process for developing a research question. Portions of these steps may vary, depending on the type of research question being proposed.

This problem can be addressed in many ways, leading to several different types of studies. For example, one researcher might be interested in different interventions and their effect on healing time. Another might be concerned with identifying risk factors that can help to develop preventive strategies. Another might address the impact of pressure ulcers on patients' experience of care. Many other approaches could be taken to address the same general problem, and each one can contribute to the overall knowledge base in a different way.

🔑 The development of a question as the basis for a research study must be distinguished from the process for development of a clinical question for evidence-based practice (EBP). In the latter instance, the clinician formulates a question to guide a literature search that will address a particular decision regarding a patient's intervention, diagnosis,

or prognosis (see Chapter 5). In both instances, however, variables and outcome measures must be understood to support interpretation of findings.

Clinical Experience

Research problems often emerge from some aspect of practice that presents a dilemma. A clinician's knowledge, experience, and curiosity will influence the types of questions that are of interest. Discussing issues with other researchers or colleagues can often generate interesting ideas.

We may ask why a particular intervention is successful for some patients but not for others. Are new treatments more effective than established ones? Does one clinical problem consistently accompany others? What is the natural progression of a specific injury or disease? Often, through trial and error, clinicians find interesting solutions to clinical problems that need to be documented. For instance, would a particular treatment be more or less effective if we changed the technique of application or combined it with other treatments?

> ➤ Knowing that electrical stimulation and ultrasound have each been shown to have positive effects of healing in chronic wounds, researchers evaluated a novel device that combined the two modalities to study its effect on healing rates in severe pressure ulcers for patients in skilled nursing facilities.[1] Having seen the positive effects of the device on other types of wounds, they wanted to see if it held promise for chronic pressure ulcers as well.

Questions about methodology are also of interest. How can we measure change? Which tools are needed to document and diagnose patient problems? Many new instruments have been developed in recent years for measuring physical, physiological, and psychological performance. These need to be analyzed for reliability and validity under varied clinical conditions and on different patient groups.

> ➤ The Braden Scale is widely used to identify hospitalized patients at high risk for pressure ulcers.[2] Researchers found that the scale did not work as well, however, for critically ill patients and wanted to establish whether there were other clinical factors that needed to be considered to improve the scale's validity.[3] They modified the tool by adding eight clinical factors, including age, sex, diabetes, and other variables related to circulation and ventilation; they found that the revised scale significantly improved discrimination of risk.

> See the *Chapter 3 Supplement* for links to references used as examples throughout this chapter.

Clinical Theory

Clinicians will often examine the theories that govern their practice as a source of research questions. Theories allow us to explain relationships and to predict outcomes based on given information and observations. To formulate a specific research question, a clinician must first examine the principles behind a theory and then determine which clinical outcomes would support or not support the theory. The answers will be the basis for a research question.

> ➤ Several theories contribute to our understanding of patients' abilities to change health behaviors or take responsibility for their health. Guihan and Bombardier[4] recognized that clinicians

continue to educate patients regarding their self-care, and wanted to see if risk factors for pressure ulcers could be modified in patients with spinal cord injury to promote healing and prevention. They cited three behavioral models (transtheoretical change, health beliefs, and locus of control) as a foundation for their study of patient compliance and self-management.

See Chapter 4 for a full discussion of the role of theory in clinical research.

Professional Literature

Reference to professional literature plays the most essential role in the delineation of a research problem and ultimately in deriving the specific research question. In the initial phases, the literature will help the researcher determine the issues of importance. Using this information, an initially broad problem can begin to take a more structured and concise form. Professional literature provides the basis for developing a research problem in several important ways.

Finding Gaps and Conflicts in the Literature

Literature may point out holes in professional knowledge, areas where we do not have sufficient information for making clinical decisions.

> ➤ Cereda et al[5] noted that many studies had shown a relationship between poor nutrition and development of pressure ulcers, but that robust evidence from randomized controlled trials (RCTs) was still lacking and no high-level nutritional recommendations were available. This led them to a randomized investigation of the effect of a disease-specific nutritional treatment with specific enrichments compared to a standard protocol for improving the rate of pressure ulcer healing.

Another common source of ideas derives from conflicts in the literature, when studies present contradictory findings.

> ➤ A systematic review of risk factors for pressure ulcers revealed that studies identified many different factors as predictors, but with no consistency in frequency or significance.[6] These discrepancies make it difficult for clinicians to develop preventive strategies and can become the foundation for further research.

Identifying Methodological Limitations

Professional literature may also identify flaws or limitations in study design or measurement methods that suggest further research is needed.

> In a systematic review of behavioral and educational interventions to prevent pressure ulcers in adults with spinal cord injury, Cogan et al[7] found little evidence to support the success of these strategies, noting considerable methodological problems across studies with recruitment, intervention fidelity, participant adherence, and measurement of skin breakdown. These limitations make comparison of findings and clinical applications difficult.

Authors should address these limitations in discussion sections of publications and offer suggestions for further study.

Descriptive Research

Research questions arise out of data from descriptive studies, which document trends, patterns, or characteristics that can subsequently be examined more thoroughly using alternative research approaches.

> Spilsbury et al[8] provided qualitative data to characterize the impact of pressure ulcers on a patient's quality of life. Their findings emphasized the need to provide information to patients, understand the importance of comfort in positioning, and management of dressings, all of which contribute to the effectiveness of care.

Analysis of these elements can become the building blocks of other qualitative and quantitative research questions.

Replication

In many instances, replication of a study is a useful strategy to confirm previous findings, correct for design limitations, study different combinations of treatments, or examine outcomes with different populations or in different settings. A study may be repeated using the same variables and methods or slight variations of them.

> Researchers studied the effect of high-voltage electrical stimulation on healing in stage II and III pressure ulcers, and demonstrated that it improved the healing rate.[9] They also suggested, however, that their study needed replication to compare the effectiveness of using cathodal and anodal stimulation combined or alone and to determine the optimal duration of these two types of electrical stimulation.

Replication is an extremely important process in research because one study is never sufficient to confirm a theory or to verify the success or failure of a treatment. We are often unable to generalize findings of one study to a larger population because of the limitations of small sample size in clinical studies. Therefore, the more studies we find that support a particular outcome, the more confidence we can have in the validity of those findings (see Focus on Evidence 3-1).

■ The Research Rationale

Once the research problem has been identified, the next step is to dig deeper to develop a rationale for the research question to understand which variables are relevant, how they may be related, and which outcomes to expect. The rationale will guide decisions about the study design and, most importantly, provide the basis for interpreting results. It presents a logical argument that shows how and why the question makes sense, as well as provides a theoretical framework that offers a justification for the study (Fig. 3-1). A full review of the literature is essential to understand this foundation. For this example, we will consider a question

---

Focus on Evidence 3–1
The Sincerest Form of Flattery: But When Is It Time to Move On?

Although replication is important to confirm clinical findings, it is also important to consider its limits as a useful strategy. There will come a point when the question must move on to further knowledge, not just repeat it. Fergusson et al[10] provide an illustration of this point in their discussion of the use of the drug aprotinin to reduce perioperative blood loss. Through meta-analysis, they showed that 64 trials on the drug's effectiveness were published between 1987 and 2002, although the effectiveness had been thoroughly documented by 1992 after 12 trials. They suggested that the following 52 trials were unnecessary, wasteful, and even unethical, and that authors "were not adequately citing previous research, resulting in a large number of RCTs being

conducted to address efficacy questions that prior trials had already definitively answered." Replication is a reasonable approach, but only when prior research has not yet arrived at that threshold.

Many journals now require that authors have conducted a comprehensive review of literature, with justification for their question based on prior research. Authors need to provide a clear summary of previous research findings, preferably through use of a systematic review, and explain how their trial's findings contribute to the state of knowledge. When such reviews do not exist, authors are encouraged to do their own or describe in a structured way the qualitative association between their research and previous findings. Such practices will limit unnecessary clinical research, protect volunteers and patients, and guard against the abuse of resources.[11]

related to different types of dressings and their effect on the healing of pressure ulcers. Now let us see how we can refine this question based on a review of literature.

Review of Literature

Every research question can be considered an extension of all the thinking and investigation that has gone before it. The results of each study contribute to that accumulated knowledge and thereby stimulate further research. For this process to work, researchers must be able to identify prior relevant research and theory through a *review of literature*.

Start With a Systematic Review

The first strategy in this process should be reading recent **systematic reviews** or **meta-analyses** that synthesize the available literature on a particular topic, provide a critical appraisal of prior research, and help to summarize the state of knowledge on the topic (see Chapter 35). Importantly, systematic reviews can also establish the state of knowledge in an area of inquiry so that newer studies will build on that knowledge rather than repeat it (see Focus on Evidence 3-1).

> ➤ Reddy et al[12] did a systematic review of studies that looked at various therapies for pressure ulcers. Out of 103 RCTs, 54 directly evaluated different types of dressings. The studies were published from 1978 to 2008. They focused on patients of varied ages, in acute and long-term care, rehabilitation, and home settings, used varied outcome measures, and studied outcomes between 1 and 24 weeks. The authors concluded that the evidence did not show any one single dressing technique to be superior to others. However, most studies had low methodological quality (see Chapter 37) and they recognized the need for further research to better understand comparative effectiveness.

📌 Systematic reviews are an important first step but may not be sufficient, as they often restrict the kind of studies that are included; therefore, a more in-depth review will likely be necessary to include all relevant information.

Scope of the Review of Literature

Clinicians and students are often faced with a dilemma in starting a review of literature in terms of how extensive a review is necessary. How does a researcher know when a sufficient amount of material has been read? There is no magic formula to determine that 20, 50, or 100 articles will provide the necessary background for a project. The number of references needed depends first on the researcher's

familiarity with the topic. A beginning researcher may have limited knowledge and experience, and might have to cover a wider range of materials to feel comfortable with the information.

In addition, the scope of the review will depend on how much research has been done in the area and how many relevant references are available. Obviously, when a topic is new and has been studied only minimally, fewer materials will exist. In that situation, it is necessary to look at studies that support the theoretical framework for a question or related research questions.

Reviewing the literature occurs in two phases as part of the research process. The preliminary review is conducted as part of the identification of the research problem, intended to achieve a general understanding of the state of knowledge. Once the problem has been clearly formulated, however, the researcher begins a more comprehensive review to provide a complete understanding of the relevant background for the study.

 When a topic has been researched extensively, the researcher need only choose a representative sample of articles to provide sufficient background. After some review, it is common to reach a saturation point, when you will see the same articles appearing over and over in reference lists—and you will know you have hit the most relevant sources. The important consideration is the relevancy of the literature, not the quantity. Researchers will always read more than they will finally report in the written review of literature. The volume of literature reviewed may also depend on its purpose. For instance, a thesis or dissertation may require a fully comprehensive review of literature.

Strategies for carrying out a literature search are described in Chapter 6.

Establishing the Theoretical Framework

The review of literature should focus on several aspects of the study. As we have already discussed, the researcher tries to establish a theoretical rationale for the study based on generalizations from other studies (see Fig. 3-2). It is often necessary to review material on the patient population to understand the underlying pathology that is being studied. Researchers should also look for information on methods, including equipment used and operational definitions of variables. Often it is helpful to replicate procedures from previous studies so that results have a basis for comparison. It may be helpful to see which statistical techniques have been used by others for the same reason.

■ Types of Research

As the process moves toward defining the research question, the researcher must decide which approach to use. There are four general types of research objectives:

1. The study may be based on a *comparison* in an attempt to define a cause-and-effect relationship using an *explanatory* model. This includes the gold standard RCT as well as comparative effectiveness studies.
2. A second type of research objective is *exploratory*, looking for relationships to determine how clinical phenomena interact. These studies are considered observational because they do not involve manipulation of variables. By determining these relationships, studies can suggest risk factors that contribute to impaired function and provide ideas for prevention and treatment options. This approach is also used to study predictive patterns, such as in the use of diagnostic tests.
3. A third type of study is *descriptive*, seeking to characterize clinical phenomena or existing conditions in a particular population. Qualitative research is a unique type of descriptive research that focuses on systematic observation of behaviors and attitudes as they occur in natural settings.
4. A fourth type of study is *methodological*, stemming from the lack of appropriate measuring instruments to document outcomes. Studies may involve the investigation of reliability and validity in measuring tools to determine how different instruments can be used meaningfully for clinical decision-making. Sometimes, the problem will address different uses of a known tool, and other times it will suggest the need for a new instrument.

The choice of one of these approaches will frame the research design, the types of data collection that will be appropriate, and the applicable data analysis procedures. Each of these approaches is examined in detail in subsequent chapters.

📌 These concepts are focused on clinical research applications, and are not necessarily relevant to basic research designs.

■ Framing the Research Question

Now that the background work has been done, it is time to frame the research question. As shown in the lower portion of Figure 3-1, there are four essential components that must be specified, using a popular acronym, PICO:

- **Population** or **Problem.** The researcher must specify the **target population**, or the disease or condition of interest. This represents the characteristics of the group to which the results of the study will apply. It will also include eligibility criteria for participants (inclusion and exclusion).
- **Intervention.** This is the treatment of interest but may also include diagnostic tests and the predictive risk or prognostic factors.
- **Comparison** or **Control.** In explanatory studies, two or more treatment conditions will be compared. For studies of diagnostic or prognostic factors, or descriptive studies, this component may not be relevant.
- **Outcomes.** This component is the effect of intervention, measurement of the accuracy of a diagnostic test, or strength of an association between risk factors and clinical outcomes. Primary and secondary outcomes may be specified, as well as potential adverse effects that will be measured.

Figure 3-2 shows how these elements have been defined for a research question related to treatment of pressure ulcers.

📌 We will revisit the acronym PICO again in Chapters 5 and 6 when we discuss EBP and how these components help to develop a good question for searching the literature.

■ Independent and Dependent Variables

➤ CASE IN POINT #2

Let us use another example to look at the components of a research question. Chronic low back pain (LBP) is a common disorder resulting in pain and decreased physical function, as well as requiring substantial healthcare services. We can explore this problem using different types of research questions.

Now we must specify *what* we want to test. **Variables** are the building blocks of the research question. A variable is a property that can differentiate members of a group or set. It represents a concept, or **factor**, that can have more than one *value*. By definition, variables are characteristics that can vary. A factor becomes a variable by virtue of how it is used in a study.

Research variables are generally classified as independent or dependent, according to how they are used. A predictor variable is an **independent variable**. It is a condition, intervention, or characteristic that will predict or cause a

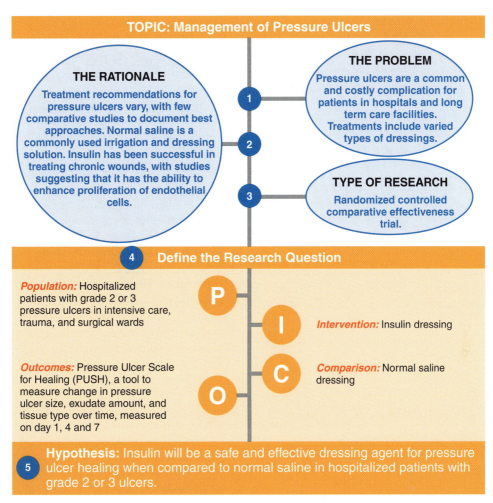

Figure 3–2 Development of a research question for an explanatory study of intervention for pressure ulcers. Based on Stephen S, Agnihotri M, Kaur S. A randomized controlled trial to assess the effect of topical insulin versus normal saline in pressure ulcer healing. *Ostomy Wound Manage* 2016;62(6):16–23.

given outcome. This is the **I** and **C** in PICO. The outcome variable is called the **dependent variable**, which is a response or effect that is presumed to vary depending on the independent variable. This is the **O** in PICO.

Explanatory Studies

Explanatory studies involve comparison of different conditions to investigate causal relationships, where the independent variable is controlled and the dependent variable is measured.

> ➤ Djavid et al[13] evaluated the effect of low-level laser therapy on chronic LBP. They studied 63 patients, randomly assigned to receive laser therapy and exercise, laser therapy alone, or placebo laser therapy plus exercise, with treatment performed twice a week for 6 weeks. The outcome measures were pain using a visual analog scale (VAS), lumbar range of motion (ROM), and disability.

The independent variable in this study is the treatment (intervention) and the dependent variables are pain level, ROM, and disability. A change in the dependent variables is presumed to be caused by the independent variable.

Comparative studies can be designed with more than one independent variable. We could look at the patients' sex in addition to intervention, for instance, to determine whether effectiveness of treatment is different for males and females. We would then have two independent variables: type of intervention and sex. A study can also have more than one dependent variable. In this example, the researchers included three dependent variables.

> 📌 The **I**ntervention and **C**omparison components of PICO are the levels of the independent variable in an explanatory study.

Levels of the Independent Variable

In comparative studies, independent variables are given "values" called **levels**. The levels represent groups or conditions that will be compared. Every independent variable will have at least two levels. Dependent variables are not described as having levels.

In the example of the study of laser therapy and LBP, the independent variable has three levels: laser therapy + exercise, laser therapy alone, and placebo + exercise (see Fig. 3-3).

 It is important to distinguish *levels* from *variables*. This study of laser therapy has one independent variable with three levels, not three independent variables. Dependent variables are not described as having levels.

Exploratory Studies

In exploratory studies, independent and dependent variables are usually measured together to determine whether they have a predictive relationship.

> ➤ Researchers were interested in predictors of chronic LBP in an office environment.[14] They studied 669 otherwise healthy office workers to assess individual, physical, and psychological variables such as body mass index, exercise and activity patterns, work habits, and job stress. They looked at the relationship among these variables and onset of LBP over 1 year (see Fig. 3-4).

The dependent outcome variable in this study was the onset of back pain (the **O** in PICO) and the independent predictor variables were the individual, physical, and psychological variables (the **I** in PICO). These types of studies often involve several independent variables, as the researcher tries to establish how different factors interrelate to explain the outcome variable. These studies are not concerned with cause and effect, and the comparison component of PICO would be ignored.

 Qualitative research studies do not incorporate comparisons or predictive relationships. They use a different process for development of a research question, which will be described in Chapter 21.

Operational Definitions

Once the variables of interest have been identified, the researcher still faces some major decisions. Exactly which procedures will be used? How will we measure a change in back pain? As the research question continues to be refined, we continually refer to the literature and our clinical experience to make these judgments. How often will subjects be treated and how often will they be tested? These questions must be answered before adequate definitions of variables are developed.

Variables must be defined in terms that explain how they will be used in the study. For research purposes, we distinguish between conceptual and operational definitions. A *conceptual definition* is the dictionary definition, one that describes the variable in general terms, without specific reference to its methodological use in a study. For instance, "back pain" can be defined as the degree of discomfort in the back. This definition is useless, however, for research purposes because it does not tell us what measure of discomfort is used or how we could interpret discomfort.

In contrast, an **operational definition** defines a variable according to its unique meaning within a study. The operational definition should be sufficiently detailed that another researcher could replicate the procedure or measurement. Independent variables are operationalized according to how they are manipulated by the investigator. Dependent variables are operationally defined by describing the method of measurement, including delineation of tools and procedures used to obtain measurements. For the study of laser therapy:

> ➤ ***Independent variable:*** The operational definition for laser therapy included the type of lamp, irradiation area, power, and dosage. The exercise activity was described as specific stretching and strengthening exercises, number of repetitions, and frequency.
> ***Dependent variables:*** The visual analogue scale was defined as a 10-cm line, with anchors at "0 = no pain" and "10 = severe pain." Lumbar ROM was measured using the Schober Test and disability using the Oswestry scale, a standardized 10-item self-report tool. Measurements were taken on admission and at 6 and 12 weeks.

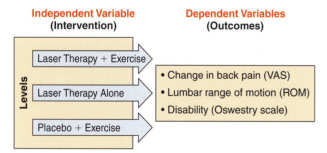

Independent Variable (Intervention)

Dependent Variables (Outcomes)

Levels:
- Laser Therapy + Exercise
- Laser Therapy Alone
- Placebo + Exercise

- Change in back pain (VAS)
- Lumbar range of motion (ROM)
- Disability (Oswestry scale)

Figure 3–3 Relationship between the independent and dependent variables in a study of low-level laser therapy for treatment of LBP. Based on Djavid GE, Mehrdad R, Ghasemi M, et al. In chronic low back pain, low level laser therapy combined with exercise is more beneficial than exercise alone in the long term: a randomised trial. *Aust J Physiother* 2007;53(3):155–60.

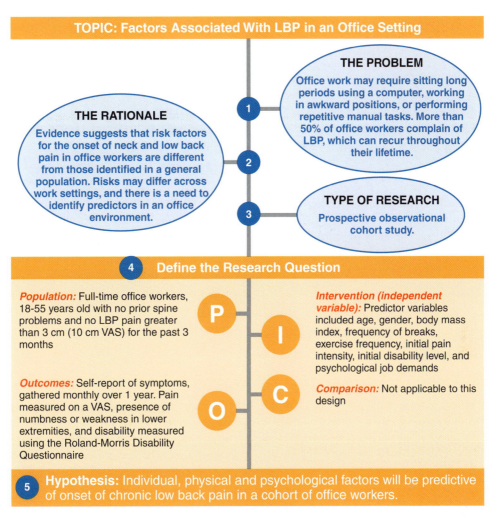

Figure 3–4 Process of developing a research question for an observational study to predict onset of LBP in an office environment. Based on Sihawong R, Sitthipornvorakul E, Paksaichol A, Janwantanakui P. Predictors for chronic neck and low back pain in office workers: a 1-year prospective cohort study. *J Occup Health* 2016;58(1):16–24.

Everything Needs to Be Defined!

There are a few variables that do not require substantial operational definitions, such as height and weight, which can be defined simply by specifying units of measurement and the type of measuring instrument. But most variables, even those whose definitions appear self-evident, still present sufficient possibilities for variation that they require explanation. Think about the debate over the interpretation of a "hanging chad" in the outcome of the 2000 presidential election! In a more relevant example, consider the concept of gender, which can require varied identities, or even strength, which can be measured in a variety of ways.

There are many examples of concepts for which multiple types of measurements may be acceptable. Researchers often find themselves faced with having to choose which method best represents the variable for purposes of a single study. For example, disability due to back pain can be measured using the Oswestry Disability Rating Scale or the Roland Morris Disability Questionnaire, among many others. Similarly, there are many different scales used to measure quality of life, depression, cognitive status, and so on. The results of studies using these different tools would be analyzed and interpreted quite differently because of the diverse information provided by each tool.[15] The measurement properties, feasibility of use, and sensitivity of an instrument should be considered in choosing the most appropriate dependent variable. A comparison of measurement methods can also become the basis for a research question.

■ Research Objectives and Hypotheses

The final step in delineating a researchable question is to clarify the objective of the study. This is the culmination of all the reasoning and reading that has gone before to determine the target population, describe the research rationale, and define the research variables. The objectives may be presented as hypotheses, specific aims, the purpose of the research, or they may be phrased as a research question.

The terms used will vary among researchers, journals, and disciplines. Most importantly, however, this statement must specifically and concisely delineate what the study is expected to accomplish. The research question is found in the introductory section of a research publication and should be framed in such a way that readers can easily understand the study's purpose.

Research and Statistical Hypotheses

For explanatory investigations and many exploratory studies involving the examination of relationships, the researcher must be more precise in setting expectations. This requires that the researcher propose an educated guess about the outcome of the study. This guess is presented as a **hypothesis**—a declarative statement that predicts the relationship between the independent and dependent variables.

The researcher generally formulates a **research hypothesis** following identification of the problem, a review of relevant literature, and final conceptualization of the research variables. The research hypothesis states the researcher's true expectation of results, guiding the interpretation of outcomes and conclusions. Hypotheses are developed at the outset to provide a definitive structure for the investigation by assisting the researcher in planning the design and methods, as well as in determining the data analysis procedures. The purpose of the study is to test the hypothesis and, ultimately, to provide evidence so that the researcher can accept or reject it.

Analysis of data is based on testing a **statistical hypothesis**, which differs from the research hypothesis in that it will always express no difference or no relationship between the independent and dependent variables. Therefore, the statistical hypothesis is called the **null hypothesis** (see Chapter 23).

 The statement of the research hypothesis must incorporate the PICO elements, including the target population, the independent variable and its levels, and the dependent outcome variables.

Explanatory Studies

Researchers use a great deal of flexibility in phrasing research hypotheses. The same research problem can be translated into a hypothesis in different ways. In the following examples, note how each one includes the PICO components.

Some research hypotheses predict *no difference* between variables:

1. *There is no difference in face-to-face interaction or perceived learning scores between students enrolled in on-line classes and those enrolled in on-campus courses.*[16]

More often, research hypotheses propose a relationship in terms of a difference:

2. *There will be a difference in expressive language scores at 6 and 12 months in preschool children with language delay who receive routine speech and language therapy as compared to those who are managed with a strategy of watchful waiting.*[17]

Hypotheses 1 and 2 are considered **nondirectional hypotheses** because they do not predict a direction of change.

In other cases, a researcher will have a definite idea about the expected direction of outcomes. Consider the following hypotheses:

3. *Children with cerebral palsy who receive botulinum toxin A (BTX) injections in combination with serial casting will have significantly faster resolution of contracture, greater reduction of spasticity, and greater improvement in gross motor function when compared with children who receive casting alone.*[18]
4. *Patients with chronic plantar fasciitis who are managed with a structure-specific plantar fascia–stretching program for 8 weeks have a better functional outcome than do patients managed with a standard Achilles tendon–stretching protocol.*[19]

These are examples of **directional hypotheses**. They not only describe the relationship between variables in terms of a difference, but they also assign a direction to that difference.

Exploratory Studies

Hypotheses can also be phrased to predict a *relationship* between variables, rather than a *difference*, as illustrated by the following:

5. *There is an association between decreased length of stay and reduced functional status at follow-up for patients receiving inpatient rehabilitation.*[20]
6. *Onset of LBP is related to individual, physical, and psychological factors in a cohort of office workers.*[14]

Hypothesis 5 is considered directional because the authors predict the presence of a relationship between two variables and the direction of that relationship. We can expect that patients with a shorter length of stay will tend to have poorer function. Hypothesis 6 does not tell us the expected direction of the proposed relationship (see Fig. 3-4).

Simple or Complex Hypotheses

Research hypotheses can be phrased in simple or complex forms. A *simple hypothesis* includes one independent variable and one dependent variable. For example, Hypotheses 1, 4, 5, and 6 are simple hypotheses. A *complex hypothesis* contains more than one independent or dependent variable. Hypotheses 2 and 3 contain several dependent variables. Complex hypotheses are often nondirectional because of the potential difficulty in clarifying multiple relationships. Complex hypotheses are efficient for expressing expected research outcomes in a research report, but they cannot be tested. Therefore, for analysis purposes, such statements must be broken down into several simple hypotheses. Several hypotheses can be addressed within a single study.

Guiding Questions

The purpose of descriptive studies will usually be based on *guiding questions* that describe the study's purpose. For instance, researchers may specify that they want to describe attitudes about a particular issue, the demographic profile of a given patient group, or the natural progression of a disease. Survey researchers will design a set of questions to organize a questionnaire (see Chapter 11). Because descriptive studies have no fixed design, it is important to put structure into place. Setting guiding questions allows the researcher to organize data and discuss findings in a meaningful way.

Specific Aims or Objectives

The *specific aims* of a study describe the purpose of a project, focusing on what the study seeks to accomplish. The statements reflect the relationships or comparisons that are intended and may reflect quantitative or qualitative goals. Aims may also expand on the study's hypothesis based on various analysis goals.

For example, consider again Hypothesis 6:

Onset of LBP is related to individual, physical, and psychological factors in a cohort of office workers.[14]

This was the overall goal of the study, but several approaches were incorporated as part of the study. The aims of this study were:

1. To document test-retest reliability of measures from questionnaire and physical examination outcomes.

2. To describe the demographic characteristics of workers who experience chronic neck and back pain.
3. To determine risk factors for chronic neck and back pain based on physical characteristics, work patterns, and psychological work demands.

A single study may have several aims, typically breaking down the hypothesis into analysis chunks. These define the scope of the study. Funding agencies often require statements of specific aims in the introduction to a grant proposal. The number of aims should be limited so that the scope of the study is clear and feasible.

■ What Makes a Good Research Question?

Throughout the process of identifying and refining a research question, four general criteria should be considered to determine that it is worth pursuing: the question should be important, answerable, ethical, and feasible for study.

Importance

Clinical research should have potential impact on treatment, understanding risk factors or theoretical foundations, or on policies related to practice. The time, effort, cost, and potential human risk associated with research must be "worth it." Researchers should look at trends in practice and health care to identify those problems that have clinical or professional significance for contributing to EBP. The research problem and rationale will generally support the importance of the study (see Figs. 3-2 and 3-3).

Statements that support the importance of the research question are often considered the *justification* for a study—every study should be able to pass the "*so what?*" test; that is, the results should be relevant, meaningful, and useful.

It may be relevant to ask how often this clinical problem occurs in practice. Will the findings provide useful information for clinical decision-making or be generalizable to other clinical situations? Will others be interested in the results? For example, in the earlier example of pressure ulcers, the prevalence and incidence of this health problem was cited to support the importance of the research.

New Information

Research studies should provide new information (see Focus on Evidence 3-1). Sometimes, the project addresses an innovation or novel idea, but more often the research will build on something that has already been studied in some way. Confirmation of previous findings may be important, as will variations in subjects or methods or clarification of inconsistencies.

Ethical Standards

A good research question must conform to ethical standards in terms of protection of human rights and researcher integrity (see Chapter 7). As part of the planning process, the researcher must be able to justify the demands that will be placed on the subjects during data collection in terms of the potential risks and benefits. The data must adhere to confidentiality standards. If the variables of interest pose an unacceptable physical, emotional, or psychological risk, the question should be reformulated. Questions about the ethical constraints in human studies research should be directed to an Institutional Review Board to assure compliance in the initial stages of study development.

Feasibility

Many factors influence the feasibility of a research study. Because of the commitment of time and resources required for research, a researcher should recognize the practicalities of carrying out a project and plan sufficiently to make the efforts successful.

Sample Size

Given the variables under study and the size of the projected outcomes, can a large enough sample be recruited to make the study worthwhile? This relates to the **power** of a study, or the likelihood that true differences can be demonstrated statistically (see Chapter 23). Preliminary estimates can be determined and researchers are often surprised by the number of subjects they will need. Recruitment strategies need to be considered, as well as the available pool of potential subjects (see Chapter 13). The choice of outcome variable can also make a difference and the researcher may look for measurements that will demonstrate larger effects.

Available Resources

Time, funding, space, personnel, equipment, and administrative support are all examples of resources that can make or break a study. Can a realistic timetable be developed? Pilot studies are helpful for estimating the time requirements of a study. What type of space or specialized equipment is needed to carry out the project, and will they be accessible? Will the necessary people be available to work on the project and can a realistic budget be developed? Resource needs should be assessed at the outset and modifications made as needed.

Scope of the Project

One of the most difficult parts of developing a good research question is the need to continue to hone the question into a reasonable chunk—not trying to measure too many variables or trying to answer too many questions at once. The enthusiasm generated by a project can make it difficult to sacrifice a side question, but judgment as to reasonable scope will make a successful outcome much more realistic.

Expertise

Those who are responsible for developing the question should have the relevant clinical, technical, and research expertise to understand the nuances of the variables being studied, as well as the ability to administer the study protocol. Consultants may need to be brought in for specific components of a study. This is often the case with statistical assistance, for example. Most importantly, anyone whose expertise is needed to carry out the project should be brought onto the team in the planning phases so that the study is designed to reach the desired goals.

COMMENTARY

You've got to be very careful if you don't know where you are going, because you might not get there.

—*Yogi Berra (1925–2015)*
Baseball catcher

Research is about answering questions. But before we can get to the answers, we must be able to ask the right question. Good questions do not necessarily lead to good outcomes, but a poorly conceived question will likely create problems that influence all further stages of a study.[21] It is no exaggeration to speak of the extreme importance of the development of the right question. Albert Einstein[22] once wrote:

> *The formation of a problem is far more often essential than its solution . . . to raise new questions, new possibilities, to regard old problems from a new angle,*

requires creative imagination and marks real advance in science.

A clear research question also allows those who read about the study to understand its intent. It is easy to report data on any response, but those data will be totally irrelevant if they do not form the context of a specific question. Those who read the literature will find themselves lost in a sea of results if a question has not been clearly articulated at the outset. The presentation of results and discussion in an article or presentation should focus on those data that address the question, thereby delimiting the theoretical framework within which the results of the study will be interpreted.

In the process of doing research, novice researchers will often jump to a methodology and design, eager to collect data and analyze it. It is an unfortunate situation that has occurred all too often, when a researcher has invested hours of work and has obtained reams of data but cannot figure out what to do with the information. There is nothing more frustrating than a statistical consultant trying to figure out what analysis to perform and asking the researcher, "What is the question you are trying to answer?" The frustrating part is when the researcher realizes that his question cannot be answered with the data that were collected. Beginning researchers often "spin their wheels" as they search for what to measure, rather than starting their search with the delineation of a specific and relevant question. It does not matter how complex or simple the design—when you are starting on the research road, it is not as important to know how to get the answer as it is to know how to ask the question![23]

REFERENCES

1. Rosenblum J, Papamichael M. Combined ultrasound and electric field stimulation aids the healing of chronic pressure ulcers. *J Gerontol Geriatr Res* 2016;5(319):2.
2. Agency for Healthcare Research and Quality. Preventing pressure ulcers in hospitals. Section 7. Tools and resources. Available at https://www.ahrq.gov/professionals/systems/hospital/pressureulcertoolkit/putool7b.html. Accessed May 22, 2018.
3. Ranzani OT, Simpson ES, Japiassu AM, Noritomi DT. The challenge of predicting pressure ulcers in critically ill patients. A multicenter cohort study. *Ann Am Thorac Soc* 2016;13(10):1775–1783.
4. Guihan M, Bombardier CH. Potentially modifiable risk factors among veterans with spinal cord injury hospitalized for severe pressure ulcers: a descriptive study. *J Spinal Cord Med* 2012;35(4):240–250.
5. Cereda E, Gini A, Pedrolli C, Vanotti A. Disease-specific, versus standard, nutritional support for the treatment of pressure ulcers in institutionalized older adults: a randomized controlled trial. *J Am Geriatr Soc* 2009;57(8):1395–1402.
6. Coleman S, Gorecki C, Nelson EA, Closs SJ, Defloor T, Halfens R, Farrin A, Brown J, Schoonhoven L, Nixon J. Patient risk factors for pressure ulcer development: systematic review. *Int J Nurs Stud* 2013;50(7):974–1003.
7. Cogan AM, Blanchard J, Garber SL, Vigen CLP, Carlson M, Clark FA. Systematic review of behavioral and educational interventions to prevent pressure ulcers in adults with spinal cord injury. *Clinical Rehabilitation* 2016:0269215516660855.
8. Spilsbury K, Nelson A, Cullum N, Iglesias C, Nixon J, Mason S. Pressure ulcers and their treatment and effects on quality of life: hospital inpatient perspectives. *J Adv Nurs* 2007;57(5):494–504.
9. Franek A, Kostur R, Polak A, Taradaj J, Szlachta Z, Blaszczak E, Dolibog P, Dolibog P, Koczy B, Kucio C. Using high-voltage electrical stimulation in the treatment of recalcitrant pressure ulcers: results of a randomized, controlled clinical study. *Ostomy Wound Manage* 2012;58(3):30–44.
10. Fergusson D, Glass KC, Hutton B, Shapiro S. Randomized controlled trials of aprotinin in cardiac surgery: could clinical equipoise have stopped the bleeding? *Clin Trials* 2005;2(3):218–229; discussion 29–32.
11. Young C, Horton R. Putting clinical trials into context. *Lancet* 2005;366(9480):107–108.
12. Reddy M, Gill SS, Kalkar SR, Wu W, Anderson PJ, Rochon PA. Treatment of pressure ulcers: A systematic review. *JAMA* 2008;300(22):2647–2662.
13. Djavid GE, Mehrdad R, Ghasemi M, Hasan-Zadeh H, Sotoodeh-Manesh A, Pouryaghoub G. In chronic low back pain, low level laser therapy combined with exercise is more beneficial than exercise alone in the long term: a randomised trial. *Aust J Physiother* 2007;53(3):155–160.
14. Sihawong R, Sitthipornvorakul E, Paksaichol A, Janwantanakul P. Predictors for chronic neck and low back pain in office workers: a 1-year prospective cohort study. *J Occup Health* 2016;58(1):16–24.
15. Chiarotto A, Maxwell LJ, Terwee CB, Wells GA, Tugwell P, Ostelo RW. Roland-Morris Disability Questionnaire and Oswestry Disability Index: which has better measurement properties for measuring physical functioning in nonspecific low back pain? Systematic review and meta-analysis. *Phys Ther* 2016;96(10):1620–1637.
16. Fortune MF, Shifflett B, Sibley RE. A comparison of online (high tech) and traditional (high touch) learning in business communication courses in Silicon Valley. *J Educ for Business* 2006;81(4):210–214.
17. Glogowska M, Roulstone S, Enderby P, Peters TJ. Randomised controlled trial of community based speech and language therapy in preschool children. *BMJ* 2000;321(7266):923–926.
18. Kay RM, Rethlefsen SA, Fern-Buneo A, Wren TA, Skaggs DL. Botulinum toxin as an adjunct to serial casting treatment in children with cerebral palsy. *J Bone Joint Surg Am* 2004;86-a(11):2377–2384.
19. DiGiovanni BF, Nawoczenski DA, Lintal ME, Moore EA, Murray JC, Wilding GE, Baumhauer JF. Tissue-specific plantar fascia-stretching exercise enhances outcomes in patients with chronic heel pain. A prospective, randomized study. *J Bone Joint Surg Am* 2003;85-a(7):1270–1277.
20. Ottenbacher KJ, Smith PM, Illig SB, Linn RT, Ostir GV, Granger CV. Trends in length of stay, living setting, functional outcome, and mortality following medical rehabilitation. *JAMA* 2004;292(14):1687–1695.
21. Agee J. Developing qualitative research questions: a reflective process. *Int J Qual Studies Educ* 2009;22(4):431-447.
22. Einstein A, Infield L. *The Evolution of Physics*. New York: Simon and Shuster, 1938.
23. Findley TW. Research in physical medicine and rehabilitation. I. How to ask the question. *Am J Phys Med Rehabil* 1991;70 (Suppl)(1):S11–S16.

The Role of Theory in Research and Practice

In the development of questions for research or the use of published studies for evidence-based practice (EBP), we must be able to establish logical foundations for questions so that we can interpret findings. This is the essential interplay between theory and research, each integral to the other for advancing knowledge. Theories are created out of a need to organize and give meaning to a complex collection of individual facts and observations. The purpose of this chapter is to discuss components of theories, mechanisms for developing and testing clinical theories, and how we apply theory to research and the application of evidence.

■ Defining Theory

Scientific theory today deals with the empirical world of observation and experience, and requires constant verification. We use theory to generalize beyond a specific situation and to make predictions about what *should* happen in other similar situations. Without such explanations, we risk having to reinvent the wheel each time we are faced with a clinical problem.

> *A theory is a set of interrelated concepts, definitions, or propositions that specifies relationships among variables and represents a systematic view of specific phenomena.*[1]

Research methods are the means by which we conduct investigations in a reliable and valid way so that we can observe clinical phenomena. But it is theory that lets us speculate on the questions of why and how things work, accounting for observed relationships. It allows us to name what we observe, provide potential explanations, and thereby figure out how we can change things in the future.

HISTORICAL NOTE

Theories have always been a part of human cultures, although not all have been scientific. Philosophy and religion have historically played a significant part in the acceptance of theory. The medieval view that the world was flat was born out of the theory that angels held up the four corners of the earth. Naturally, the men of the day were justified in believing that if one sailed toward the horizon, eventually one would fall off the edge of the earth. In healthcare we are aware of significant modifications to our understanding of the human body, as evidenced in the shift from Galen's view of "pores" in the heart to Harvey's theory of circulation. In the middle ages, medical theory was based on a balance among four "humours" (blood, black bile, yellow bile, and phlegm) and patients were bled and purged, made to vomit, and made to take snuff to correct imbalances. As theories change, so does our understanding of science and health.

■ Purposes of Theories

Theories can serve several purposes in science and clinical practice, depending on how we choose to use them.

- ***Theories summarize existing knowledge to explain observable events***—giving meaning to isolated empirical findings. They provide a framework for interpretation of observations. For example, a theory of motor learning would explain the relationship between feedback and feedforward mechanisms in the learning, performance, and refinement of a motor skill.

- *Theories allow us to predict what should occur*—even when they cannot be empirically verified. For instance, through deductions from mathematical theories, Newton was able to predict the motion of planets around the sun long before technology was available to confirm their orbits.

  The germ theory of disease allows us to predict how changes in the environment will affect the incidence of disease, which in turn suggests mechanisms for control, such as the use of drugs, vaccines, or attention to hygiene.

- *Theories stimulate development of new knowledge*—by providing motivation and guidance for asking significant clinical questions. On the basis of a theoretical premise, a clinician can formulate a hypothesis that can then be tested, providing evidence to support, reject, or modify the theory. For instance, based on the theory that reinforcement will facilitate learning, a clinician might propose that verbal encouragement will decrease the time required for a patient to learn a home program. This hypothesis can be tested by comparing patients who do and do not receive reinforcement. The results of hypothesis testing will provide additional affirmation of the theory or demonstrate specific situations where the theory is not substantiated.

- *Theories provide the basis for asking a question in applied research*. As discussed in Chapter 3, research questions are based on a theoretical rationale that provides the foundation for the design and interpretation of the study. Sometimes, there will be sufficient background in the literature to build this framework; other times, the researcher must build an argument based on what is known from basic science. In qualitative or exploratory research, the study's findings may contribute to the development of theory. This theoretical framework is usually discussed within the introduction and discussion sections of a paper.

■ Components of Theories

The role of theory in clinical practice and research is best described by examining the structure of a theory. Figure 4-1 shows the basic organization of scientific thought, building from observation of facts to laws of nature.

The essential building blocks of a theory are **concepts**. Concepts are abstractions that allow us to classify natural phenomena and empirical observations. From birth we begin to structure empirical impressions of the world around us in the form of concepts, such as "tall" or "far," each of which implies a complex set of recognitions and expectations. We supply labels to sets of behaviors, objects, or processes that allow us to identify them and discuss them. Therefore, concepts must be defined operationally. When concepts can be assigned values, they can be manipulated as **variables**, so that relationships can be examined. In this context, variables become the concepts used for building theories and planning research.

Constructs

Some physical concepts, such as height and distance, are observable and varying amounts are easily distinguishable. But other concepts are less tangible and can be defined only by inference. Concepts that represent nonobservable behaviors or events are called **constructs**. Constructs are invented names for abstract variables that cannot be seen directly, also called **latent variables**. Measurement of a construct can only be inferred by

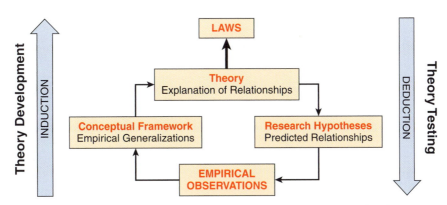

Figure 4–1 A model of scientific thought, showing the circular relationship between empirical observations and theory, and the integration of inductive and deductive reasoning.

assessing relevant or correlated behaviors that are observable. Many important variables in healthcare research are constructs, such as function, patient satisfaction, pain, even strength.

Most constructs must be defined as a function of many interrelated concepts or multiple dimensions. Consider the construct of disability as an example. We each have a conceptual understanding of the clinical term "disability," but researchers still struggle to develop meaningful ways to measure it. How might an occupational therapist look at disability as compared to a physical therapist, nurse, physician, psychologist, neurologist, social worker, or architect? Can we devise a scale so that one sum or average number is indicative of a patient's level of disability?

Many such scales exist. But can we make the inferential leap from this number to an assessment of the psychological, social, physical, or economic manifestations of disability? To do so we must be able to define disability in terms of specific and limited properties of behavior that are relevant to our own frame of reference. It is important to appreciate this difficulty in operationally defining construct measures as a basis for interpretation of clinical variables.

Issues related to measurement of constructs will be discussed further in Chapters 8, 10, and 12.

Propositions

Once the concepts that relate to a theory are delineated, they are formed into a generalized statement, or **proposition**. Propositions assert the theoretical linkages between concepts, which can then be tested. Hypotheses are derived from these statements to describe or predict presumed relationships. This will provide the foundation for testing the theory.

For example, the *transtheoretical model* is a theory that proposes a continuum of motivational readiness for health behavior change.[2] Rather than seeing change as a single act or decision, such as simply quitting smoking or starting to exercise all at once, this model suggests that individuals progress through a series of five stages in recognizing the need to change, eventually engaging in a new behavior (see Fig. 4-2). Starting with "thinking about it," they go through a planning stage to take action and finally maintain the new behavior. When behaviors relapse, the individual can enter the cycle again.

One proposition derived from this theory is that the "pros" of changing behavior will be higher in contemplation than precontemplation, and the "cons" will be decreased from contemplation to action.[3] From this proposition, many hypotheses can be derived.

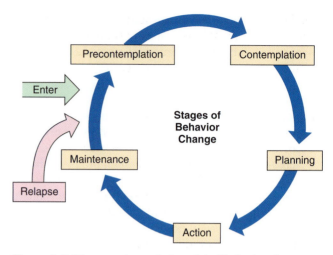

Figure 4–2 The transtheoretical model of behavior change, an example of a process model. Based on the work of Prochaska JO, Velicer WF. The transtheoretical model of health behavior change. *Am J Health Promot* 1997; 12(1):38–48.

In a study of smoking cessation among primary care clients, researchers hypothesized that they could develop educational material matched to the person's current stage in the transtheoretical model and that these targeted materials would be more effective than general educational materials.[4] Their findings, however, did not support their hypothesis and they found no differences in outcomes between those receiving targeted versus general intervention.

This example illustrates the situation where theory guides an approach but may not support it.

■ Models

Many of the concepts we deal with in professional practice are so complex that we use **models** to comprehend their real nature. In an effort to understand them, we try to simplify them using an analogy for the real phenomenon. To understand the concept of an "atom," for example, it was helpful for scientists to delineate a conceptual model that is likened to a solar system. The intricacies of genetic processes were clarified by the development of a helical model of DNA. Function of the neuromuscular system is often taught using a model of the muscle spindle.

Models are considered simplified approximations of reality. They leave out much of the detail but describe the conceptual structure closely enough to give us a better understanding of the phenomenon. Therefore, models are symbolic representations of the elements within a system. Where a theory is an explanation of phenomena, a model is a structural representation of the concepts that comprise that theory.

Types of Models

Physical models are used to demonstrate how the real behavior might occur. For example, engineers study models of bridges to examine how stresses on cables and different loading conditions affect the structure. The benefit of such models is that they obey the same laws as the original but can be controlled and manipulated to examine the effects of various conditions in ways that would not otherwise be possible and without risk. Computer simulations are the most recent contributions to the development of physical models.

A *process model* provides a guide for progressing through a course of action or thought process. The structural image of the transtheoretical model in Figure 4-2 is an example of this approach.

A *quantitative model* is used to describe the relationship among variables by using numerical representations. Such models usually contain some degree of error resulting from the variability of human behavior and physical characteristics. For instance, a clinician might want to set a goal for increasing the level of strength a patient could be expected to achieve following a period of training. A model that demonstrates the influence of a person's height, weight, and age on muscle strength would be useful in making this determination.[5–7] This type of quantitative model can serve as a guide for setting long-term goals and for predicting functional outcomes. Research studies provide the basis for testing these models and estimating their degree of accuracy for making such predictions.

■ Theory Development and Testing

As previous examples illustrate, theories are not discovered, they are created. A set of observable facts may exist, but they do not become a theory unless someone has the insight to understand the relevance of the observed information and pulls the facts together to make sense of them. Surely, many people observed apples falling from trees before Newton was stimulated to consider the force of gravity! Theories can be developed using inductive or deductive processes (see Fig. 4-3).

Deductive Reasoning

Deductive reasoning is characterized by the acceptance of a general proposition, or premise, and the subsequent

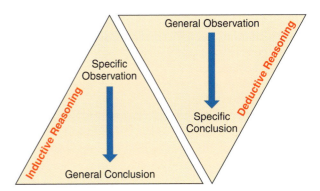

Figure 4–3 The relationship between deductive and inductive reasoning.

inferences that can be drawn in specific cases. The ancient Greek philosophers introduced this systematic method for drawing conclusions by using a series of three interrelated statements called a *syllogism*, containing (1) a major premise, (2) a minor premise, and (3) a conclusion. A classic syllogism will serve as an example:

1. All living things must die. [*major premise*]
2. Man is a living thing. [*minor premise*]
3. Therefore, all men must die. [*conclusion*]

In deductive reasoning, if the premises are true, then it follows that the conclusion must be true. Scientists use deductive logic to ask a research question by beginning with known principles or generalizations and deducing explicit assertions that are relevant to a specific question. The subsequent observations will confirm, reject, or modify the conclusion. Of course, the usefulness of this method is totally dependent on the truth of its premises (see Focus on Evidence 4-1).

✒ **HISTORICAL NOTE**

The following statement, attributed to the ancient Greek physician Galen of Pergamon (c. 130–210 A.D.), illustrates the potential abuse of logic and evidence:

All who drink of this remedy recover in a short time, except those whom it does not help, who all die. Therefore, it is obvious that it fails only in incurable cases.[8]

Deductive Theories

The deductive approach to theory building is the intuitive approach, whereby a theory is developed on the basis of great insight and understanding of an event and the variables most likely to impact that event. This type of theory, called a *hypothetical-deductive theory*, is

Focus on Evidence 4–1
The Deductive Road to a Research Question

Deductive reasoning is often the basis for development of a research question. It is also applied as part of the clinical decision-making process to support treatment options. For example, we might use previous research to reason that exercise will be an effective intervention to prevent falls in the elderly in the following way:

1. Impaired postural stability results in falls.
2. Exercise improves postural stability.
3. Therefore, exercise will decrease the risk of falls.

This system of deductive reasoning produces a testable hypothesis: If we develop an exercise program to improve impaired stability, we should see a decrease in the number of falls. Li et al[10] used this logic as the theoretical premise for their study comparing tai chi exercise, stretching, and resistance exercise to improve postural stability in patients with Parkinson's disease. Carter et al[11] designed an exercise program aimed at modifying risk factors for falls in elderly women with osteoporosis. Similarly, Mansfield et al[12] demonstrated the effect of a perturbation-based training program on balance reactions in older adults with a recent history of falls. All three studies found that stability exercise programs reduced the incidence of falls or improved balance behaviors, supporting the premise from which the treatment was deduced.

---

developed with few or no prior observations, and often requires the generation of new concepts to provide adequate explanation. Freud's theory of personality fits this definition.[9] It required that he create concepts such as "id," "ego," and "superego" to explain psychological interactions and motivations.

Because they are not developed from existing facts, hypothetical-deductive theories must be continually tested in the "real world" to develop a database that will support them. Einstein's theory of relativity is an excellent example of this type of theory; it was first advanced in 1905 and is still being tested and refined through research today.

Inductive Reasoning

Inductive reasoning reflects the reverse type of logic, developing generalizations from specific observations. It begins with experience and results in conclusions or generalizations that are probably true. Facts gathered on a sample of events could lead to inferences about the whole. This reasoning gave birth to the scientific method and often acts as the basis for common sense.

Inductive Theories

Inductive theories are data based and evolve through a process of inductive reasoning, beginning with empirically verifiable observations. Through multiple investigations and observations, researchers determine those variables that are related to a specific phenomenon and those that are not. The patterns that emerge from these studies are developed into a systematic conceptual framework, which forms the basis for generalizations. This process involves a degree of abstraction and imagination, as ideas are manipulated and concepts reorganized, until some structural pattern is evident in their relationship.

Glaser and Strauss used the term "grounded theory" to describe the development of theory by reflecting on individual experiences in qualitative research.[13] As an example, Resnik and Jensen used this method to describe characteristics of therapists who were classified as "expert" or "average" based on patient outcomes.[14] Building on their observations, they theorized that the meaning of "expert" was not based on years of experience, but on academic and work experience, utilization of colleagues, use of reflection, a patient-centered approach to care, and collaborative clinical reasoning.

Most theories are formulated using a combination of both inductive and hypothetical-deductive processes. Observations initiate the theoretical premise and then hypotheses derived from the theory are tested. As researchers go back and forth in the process of building and testing the theory, concepts are redefined and restructured.

Both deductive and inductive reasoning are used to design research studies and interpret research data. Introductory statements in an article often illustrate deductive logic, as the author explains how a research hypothesis was developed. Inductive reasoning is used in the discussion section, where generalizations or conclusions are proposed from the observed data. It is the clinical scientist's responsibility to evaluate the validity of the information and draw reasonable conclusions. This process occurs along a circular continuum between observation and theory, whereby a theory can be built on observations which must then be tested to confirm them (Fig. 4-1).

Theory Testing

Ultimately, a theory can never be "proven" or even completely confirmed or refuted. Hypotheses are tested to demonstrate whether the premises of the theory hold true in certain circumstances, always with some probability that the outcomes could be spurious. A replication study may show a different outcome or other logical explanations can be offered. EBP requires that we consider the latest research in the context of our own clinical judgment and experience. We cannot ignore the possibility that any theory will need to be modified or discarded at some point in the future.

When we speak of testing a theory, we should realize that a theory itself is not testable. The validity of a theory is derived through the empirical testing of hypotheses that are deduced from it and from observation of the phenomenon the theory describes. The hypotheses predict the relationships of variables included in the theory. The results of research will demonstrate certain facts, which will either support or not support the hypothesis. If the hypothesis is supported, then the theory from which it was deduced is also supported.

■ Characteristics of Theories

As we explore the many uses of theories in clinical research, we should also consider criteria that can be used to evaluate the utility of a theory.

- *A theory should be rational.* First and foremost, a theory should provide a reasonable explanation of observed facts that makes sense given current knowledge and beliefs (see Focus on Evidence 4-2).
- *A theory should be testable.* It should provide a basis for classifying relevant variables and predicting their relationships, thereby providing a means for its own verification; that is, it should be sufficiently developed and clear enough to permit deductions that form testable hypotheses.
- *A theory should be economical.* It should be an efficient explanation of the phenomenon, using only those concepts that are truly relevant and necessary to the explanation offered by the theory.
- *A theory should be relevant.* It should reflect that which is judged significant by those who will use it. In this sense, theories become the mirror of a profession's values and identity.
- *A theory should be adaptable.* Theories must be consistent with observed facts and the already established body of knowledge but must also be able to adapt to changes in that knowledge as technology and scientific evidence improve. Many theories that are accepted today will be discarded tomorrow (see Box 4-1). Some will be "disproved" by new evidence and others may be superseded by new theories that integrate the older ones.

Focus on Evidence 4–2
The Tomato Effect

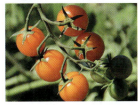

Did you know that up until the 19th century, tomatoes were not cultivated or eaten in North America? Although they were a staple in continental European diets, the tomato was shunned in America because it was "known" to be poisonous and so it would have been foolish to eat one. It seems that many European aristocrats would eat them, become ill, and die. What was actually happening was that they were eating off pewter plates, which interacted with the acid in the tomato, and they were dying from lead poisoning.[15] But at the time, the fact that tomatoes were poisonous was just that—a known fact.

It was not until June 20, 1820, when an American, Robert Gibbon, stood on the courthouse steps in Salem, New Jersey, and ate a juicy tomato without incident that the myth was finally dispelled and Americans began consuming and cultivating tomatoes.[16]

This little-known agricultural history provides the derivation of the "tomato effect," which occurs when an effective treatment is ignored or rejected because it does not "make sense" in light of contemporary theories of disease.[17]

One relevant example is the historic use of acetylsalicylic acid, marketed under the name "aspirin" by Bayer in 1899, a compound known to relieve pain, fever, and inflammation.[18] Among other disorders, this therapy was used successfully in the late 1800s to treat acute rheumatic fever, with several research reports also demonstrating its efficacy for rheumatoid arthritis (RA).

But from 1900 to 1950, medical textbooks barely mention this treatment for RA, coinciding with the acceptance of the "infectious theory of disease" in medicine, which saw bacteria as the prime culprit in disease.[19] Because aspirin was a medication for fever and pain, it did not "make sense" that it would have an effect on a chronic infectious process—and so the treatment approach was ignored.

By 1950, the infectious theory was discarded and RA was recognized as a chronic inflammatory disease that would respond to the anti-inflammatory properties of aspirin. Although many newer treatments for RA have since been adopted, this history is an important lesson in how theory can influence research and practice.

Photo courtesy of Rob Bertholf. Found at https://commons.wikimedia.org/

Box 4-1   Finding Meaning in Aging

The *disengagement theory of aging* was originally proposed to account for observations of age-related decreases in social interaction, explaining that older individuals withdrew from social involvements in anticipation of death.[21] The *activity theory* later countered this explanation by suggesting that remaining active and engaged with society is pivotal to satisfaction in old age, necessitating new interests and relationships to replace those lost in later life.[22] *Continuity theory* then built upon activity theory, suggesting that personality and values are consistent through the life span.[23] These theories continue to change and be challenged, as explanations of observed psychosocial behavior evolve and as our understanding and perceptions of aging and social interaction have grown.[24]

HISTORICAL NOTE

Karl Popper (1902–1994) was one of the most influential philosophers of the 20th century. He proffered a *falsificationist* methodology, suggesting that all theories are characterized by predictions that future observations may reveal to be false.[20] This process causes scientists to revise theory, reject it in favor of a different theory, or change the hypothesis that originally supported it.

■ Theory, Research, and Practice

Every theory serves, in part, as a research directive. The empirical outcomes of research can be organized and ordered to build theories using inductive reasoning. Conversely, theories must be tested by subjecting deductive hypotheses to scientific scrutiny. The processes of theory development and theory testing are represented in the model shown in Figure 4-1. The figure integrates the concepts of inductive and deductive reasoning as they relate to the elements of theory design.

Practical Applications of Theory

Clinicians are actually engaged in theory testing on a regular basis in practice. Theories guide us in making clinical decisions every day, although we often miss the connection because we are focused on the pragmatics of the situation. Specific therapeutic modalities are chosen for treatment because of expected outcomes that are based on theoretical assumptions about physiological effects. Treatments are modified according to the presence of risk factors, again based on theoretical relationships.

Therefore, theories are tested each time the clinician evaluates treatment outcomes.

These theoretical frameworks, used as rationale for intervention, may not rise to the level of a "named" theory, but that does not diminish their importance in setting the context for interpreting outcomes. Sometimes we anticipate a certain outcome based on this framework, and it does not work out as expected, indicating that something in our thought process needs to be re-examined. Are we using a theoretical rationale that is not valid? Did we not measure outcomes in a meaningful way? Are there intervening factors that could have influenced the outcome? These are questions that take us back to the theoretical frameworks that supported our initial decisions and our examination of the evidence that led us there (see Focus on Evidence 4-3).

HISTORICAL NOTE

For centuries, physicians believed that illnesses were caused by "humoral imbalances." This theory was the basis for diagnosis and treatment, and bloodletting was one of the most popular interventions to end the imbalances. Although patients suffered and died from this practice, it persisted into the end of the 19th century. In 1892, even William Osler, one of the most influential medical authorities, stated that "we have certainly bled too little."[25] Because research finally showed the harm it caused, bloodletting has been abandoned for more than a century—except that it is back for some modern applications. Leeches are used today to restore venous circulation and reduce engorgement in limb reattachments.[26]

Same practice, different theory.

Understanding of a clinical phenomenon cannot be achieved in a single study. It requires a process involving discussion, criticism, and intellectual exchange among a community of researchers and clinicians, to analyze the connection between new and previous findings and explanations. This type of exchange allows inconsistencies to surface, to identify findings that cannot be explained by current theories.

Theory and Research Questions

The importance of theory for understanding research findings is often misunderstood. Whenever a research question is formulated, there is an implicit theoretical rationale that suggests how the variables of interest should be related (see Chapter 3). Unfortunately, many authors do not make this foundation explicit. Empirical results are often described with only a general explanation or an admission that the author can

Focus on Evidence 4–3
Applying Theory to Guide Practice

Researchers have long lamented the difficulties in running clinical trials to study treatments that involve clinical judgment, patient interaction, and combinations of interventions for individualized care because of the challenge in providing consistent operational definitions.[27] For instance, in designing rehabilitation programs, therapists will often incorporate many activities which can vary greatly from one patient to another, even if they have the same diagnosis. One way to address this dilemma is to rely on theory to provide guidelines and rationale about mechanisms of action. Even if the specific intervention activities are not identical from patient to patient, the treatment decisions can all be directed by the same theoretical premise.

Whyte[28] provides a useful perspective by distinguishing theories related to treatment and enablement. *Treatment theory* specifies the mechanism of action for an intervention, or the "active ingredient" that is intended to produce change in an aspect of function or health.[29] For example, Mueller and Maluf[30] have described *physical stress theory*, which states that changes in stress to biological tissues (such as muscle) will cause a predictable adaptive response. Therefore, we can predict that, when muscle is challenged at high stresses (as through exercise), we should see increases in contractile strength. With a lack of stress (inactivity) we should see declines in strength. The treatment target is typically an impairment that can be measured as a direct result of the intervention,[28] in this case strength or force of movement. In contrast, *enablement theory* provides the link from theory to outcomes, reflecting the relative importance of clinical changes to activity and participation. In this example, it would be a link from increased strength to improved mobility and function.

To illustrate this application, Dibble et al[31] conducted a randomized controlled trial (RCT) to compare active exercise with resistance exercises for patients with Parkinson's disease (PD) in order to evaluate changes in muscle force production and mobility. They theorized that the more challenging resistive exercises would be more effective in improving muscular force (measured with a dynamometer), gait (measured by the Functional Gait Assessment),[32] and quality of life (measured using the Parkinson's Disease Questionnaire [PDQ-39]).[33] They found, however, that both groups showed similar improvement in muscle force and gait—suggesting that it was not the type of exercise that was relevant, but the presence of an exercise component. They also found that neither group improved in the quality of life measure. Their interpretation suggested that exercise may not be sufficient to impact health status in the PD population. The impairment and activity level treatment targets (strength and mobility) showed improvement, but this did not link to participation activities, at least as it was measured in this study.

The PDQ-39 focuses on difficulty of movement tasks as well as emotional consequences of PD. Enablement theory leads us to hypothesize that intervention may need to be designed to more directly influence these elements of quality of life and, therefore, this measure might not have been a relevant outcome based on the theoretical premise of the intervention, which focused on the neurological and musculoskeletal influence of exercise.

From an EBP perspective, this example illustrates the need to be wary of simple conclusions (resistive exercise does not improve function in PD). The theoretical basis for decision-making will affect how outcomes will be interpreted and applied to practice.

Concepts of impairment, activity, and participation are discussed within the framework of the International Classification of Functioning, Disability and Health in Chapter 1.

find no explanation. It is the author's responsibility, however, to consider what is known, to examine potential relationships, and help the reader understand the context within which the results can be understood. It is incumbent upon all researchers to project their expectations into the realm of theory, to offer an interpretation of findings, and thereby contribute to the growth of knowledge.

 We should be careful not to assign the rank of theory to an "approach" to treatment. For example, neurophysiological treatment approaches, often given imposing names such as neurodevelopmental treatment (NDT) or proprioceptive neuromuscular facilitation (PNF), are not theories, but are developed from theories of motor control and neurophysiology.

■ Scope of Theories

Theories can range in scope from simple to complex and may have specific applications versus broad relevance. Most of the theoretical frameworks that are applied to practice are built on clinical knowledge that supports a particular approach. Published research can provide evidence to help us identify what these frameworks are. Other theories build on observations to create broader perspectives that allow us to generate specific hypotheses.

Middle-Range Theories

Most theories relevant to clinical practice seek to explain a specific set of phenomena. **Middle-range theories** sit between the basic hypotheses that guide everyday practice and the systematic efforts to develop a unified theory to explain a set of social behaviors.[34] They form the bridge of theory with empirical observations. For example, the transtheoretical model of behavior change (shown in Figure 4-2) can be described as a middle-range theory, providing many opportunities for hypothesis testing and guiding clinical practice.

Grand Theories

A **grand theory** is a comprehensive idea that tries to explain phenomena at the societal level. As a highly abstract approach, this type of theory has broad application. Some of the "grandest" examples include Darwin's theory of evolution[35] and Einstein's theory of relativity.[36] Other more relevant examples include Piaget's theory of cognitive development, a comprehensive view of how humans acquire, construct, and use intelligence,[37] and Erikson's theory of human personality development, delineating stages of growth through the lifespan.[38]

Meta-Theory

The concept of **meta-theory** has been used to reflect theories that attempt to reconcile several theoretical perspectives in the explanation of sociological, psychological, and physiological phenomena.[39] For example, researchers examined the complex phenomenon of postpartum depression and constructed a meta-theory of *critical realism* that incorporated theoretical frames of stress, social isolation, social exclusion, and several other psychological theories.[40] Other meta-theories include adaptation to chronic illness[41] and compensatory phenomena observed in studies of early brain damage.[42]

Laws

When a theory reaches the level of absolute consistency in outcomes, it turns into a **law**. Laws allow precise predictions. For example, Newton made many mathematical observations that were used to describe the motion of the planets around the sun. These motions can be described with great precision, allowing great accuracy of prediction. What started as a theoretical observation eventually came to be accepted as a universal law.

Generally, laws are not established in the applied sciences as they are in the physical sciences. The nature of human beings and their interactions with the environment do not allow our theories to become so precise in their prediction. We are left, therefore, with the necessity of continuing the quest for affirmation of our theories.

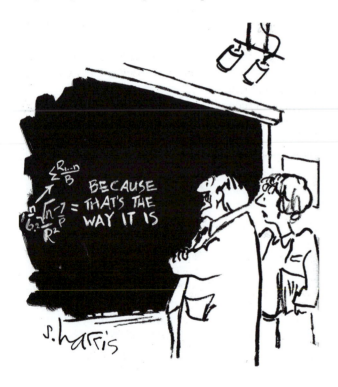

"IS THAT IT? IS THAT THE GRAND UNIFIED THEORY?"

Illustration courtesy of Sidney Harris. Used with permission from ScienceCartoons Plus.com.

COMMENTARY

Theory is knowledge that doesn't work. Practice is when everything works and you don't know why.

—Hermann Hesse (1877–1962)

German poet

Theories are approximations of reality, plausible explanations of observable events. This leaves us with much uncertainty in the continued search for understanding clinical behavior. Steven Hawking offered this caution:

Any physical theory is always provisional, in the sense that it is only a hypothesis; you can never prove it. No matter how many times the results of experiments agree with some theory, you can never be sure that the next time the result will not contradict the theory.[43]

In essence, the more that research does *not disconfirm* a theory, the more the theory is supported. This may sound backward, but in actuality we can only demonstrate that a theoretical premise *does not hold true* in a specific situation. Hawking also offered this proviso:

On the other hand, you can disprove a theory by finding even a single observation that disagrees with the predictions of the theory.[43]

Hawking's admonition is probably useful in physical sciences but has to be considered with less conviction in behavioral and health sciences. We do not always know which variables are relevant to a theory. If we choose one way to test it and the outcome does not support the theory, the theory may still have validity. It may mean we need to test it differently, choosing different variables or measuring instruments in different circumstances, or choosing subjects with different characteristics. Or the theory may need to be clarified as to its scope. This is where "making sense" is an important criterion and why operationally defining constructs is so important.

Conversely, we may find that certain treatments are continually successful, even though we cannot explain the theoretical underpinnings. This is often the case, for example, when working with neurological conditions. We may find that theoretical foundations change over time, but this does not mean that the treatment does not work. It simply means we do not yet fully understand the mechanisms at work. Eventually, we have to reformulate the theories to reflect more precisely what we actually observe in practice.

This is the constant challenge—finding how the pieces of the puzzle fit. Most importantly, researchers and evidence-based practitioners must consider how theory helps to balance uncertainty to allow for reasoned decisions and interpretations of outcomes, remembering that today's theoretical beliefs may be tomorrow's tomatoes!

REFERENCES

1. Kerlinger FN. *Foundations of Behavioral Research*. New York: Holt, Rinehart & Winston, 1973.
2. Prochaska JO, Velicer WF. The transtheoretical model of health behavior change. *Am J Health Promot* 1997;12(1):38–48.
3. Prochaska JO, Wright JA, Velicer WF. Evaluating theories of health behavior change: a hierarchy of criteria applied to the transtheoretical model. *Appl Psychol: An Internat Rev* 2008; 57(4):561–588.
4. Aveyard P, Massey L, Parsons A, Manaseki S, Griffin C. The effect of transtheoretical model based interventions on smoking cessation. *Soc Sci Med* 2009;68(3):397–403.
5. Hamzat TK. Physical characteristics as predictors of quadriceps muscle isometric strength: a pilot study. *Afr J Med Med Sci* 2001;30(3):179–181.
6. Neder JA, Nery LE, Shinzato GT, Andrade MS, Peres C, Silva AC. Reference values for concentric knee isokinetic strength and power in nonathletic men and women from 20 to 80 years old. *J Orthop Sports Phys Ther* 1999;29(2):116–126.
7. Hanten WP, Chen WY, Austin AA, Brooks RE, Carter HC, Law CA, Morgan MK, Sanders DJ, Swan CA, Vanderslice AL. Maximum grip strength in normal subjects from 20 to 64 years of age. *J Hand Ther* 1999;12(3):193–200.
8. Silverman WA. *Human Experimentation: A Guided Step into the Unknown*. New York: Oxford University Press, 1985.
9. Keutz Pv. The character concept of Sigmund Freud. *Schweiz Arch Neurol Neurochir Psychiatr* 1971;109(2):343–365.
10. Li F, Harmer P, Fitzgerald K, Eckstrom E, Stock R, Galver J, Maddalozzo G, Batya SS. Tai chi and postural stability in patients with Parkinson's disease. *N Engl J Med* 2012;366(6):511–519.
11. Carter ND, Khan KM, McKay HA, Petit MA, Waterman C, Heinonen A, Janssen PA, Donaldson MG, Mallinson A, Riddell L, et al. Community-based exercise program reduces risk factors for falls in 65- to 75-year-old women with osteoporosis: randomized controlled trial. *CMAJ* 2002;167(9):997–1004.
12. Mansfield A, Peters AL, Liu BA, Maki BE. Effect of a perturbation-based balance training program on compensatory stepping and grasping reactions in older adults: a randomized controlled trial. *Phys Ther* 2010;90(4):476–491.

13. Glaser BG, Strauss AI. *The Discovery of Grounded Theory: Strategies for Qualitative Research*. New York: Aldine, 1967.

14. Resnik L, Jensen GM. Using clinical outcomes to explore the theory of expert practice in physical therapy. *Phys Ther* 2003;83(12):1090–1106.

15. Smith KA. Why the tomato was feared in Europe for more than 200 years. Smithsonian.com. Available at http://www.smithsonianmag.com/arts-culture/why-the-tomato-was-feared-in-europe-for-more-than-200-years-863735/. Accessed February 10, 2017.

16. Belief that the tomato is poisonous is disproven. History Channel. Available at http://www.historychannel.com.au/this-day-in-history/belief-that-the-tomato-is-poisonous-is-disproven/. Accessed February 9, 2017.

17. Goodwin JS, Goodwin JM. The tomato effect. Rejection of highly efficacious therapies. *JAMA* 1984;251(18):2387–2390.

18. Ugurlucan M, Caglar IM, Caglar FN, Ziyade S, Karatepe O, Yildiz Y, Zencirci E, Ugurlucan FG, Arslan AH, Korkmaz S, et al. Aspirin: from a historical perspective. *Recent Pat Cardiovasc Drug Discov* 2012;7(1):71–76.

19. Goodwin JS, Goodwin JM. Failure to recognize efficacious treatments: a history of salicylate therapy in rheumatoid arthritis. *Perspect Biol Med* 1981;25(1):78–92.

20. Popper KR. *Conjectures and Refutations: The Growth of Scientific Knowledge*. 2 ed. London: Routledge Classics, 2002.

21. Cummings E, Henry WE. *Growing Old: The Process of Disengagement*. New York: Basic Books, 1961.

22. Havighurst RJ. Successful aging. In: Williams RH, Tibbits C, Donohue W, eds. *Process of Aging: Social and Pyschological Perspectives, Volume 1*. New Brunswick, NJ: Transaction Publishers, 1963:299–320.

23. Atchley RC. A continuity theory of normal aging. *Gerontologist* 1989;29(2):183–190.

24. Jewell AJ. Tornstam's notion of gerotranscendence: re-examining and questioning the theory. *J Aging Stud* 2014;30:112–120.

25. Osler W, McCrae T. *The Principles and Practice of Medicine*. New York: D. Appleton and Company, 1921.

26. Smoot EC, 3rd, Debs N, Banducci D, Poole M, Roth A. Leech therapy and bleeding wound techniques to relieve venous congestion. *J Reconstr Microsurg* 1990;6(3):245–250.

27. Johnston MV. Desiderata for clinical trials in medical rehabilitation. *Am J Phys Med Rehabil* 2003;82(10 Suppl):S3–S7.

28. Whyte J. Contributions of treatment theory and enablement theory to rehabilitation research and practice. *Arch Phys Med Rehabil* 2014;95(1 Suppl):S17–23.e2.

29. Whyte J, Barrett AM. Advancing the evidence base of rehabilitation treatments: a developmental approach. *Arch Phys Med Rehabil* 2012;93(8 Suppl):S101–S110.

30. Mueller MJ, Maluf KS. Tissue adaptation to physical stress: a proposed "Physical Stress Theory" to guide physical therapist practice, education, and research. *Phys Ther* 2002;82(4):383–403.

31. Dibble LE, Foreman KB, Addison O, Marcus RL, LaStayo PC. Exercise and medication effects on persons with Parkinson disease across the domains of disability: a randomized clinical trial. *J Neurol Phys Ther* 2015;39(2):85–92.

32. Wrisley DM, Marchetti GF, Kuharsky DK, Whitney SL. Reliability, internal consistency, and validity of data obtained with the functional gait assessment. *Phys Ther* 2004;84(10):906–918.

33. Fitzpatrick R, Jenkinson C, Peto V, Hyman N, Greenhall R. Desirable properties for instruments assessing quality of life: evidence from the PDQ-39. *J Neurol Neurosurg Psychiatry* 1997;62(1):104.

34. Merton RK. *Social Theory and Social Structure*. New York: The Free Press, 1968.

35. van Whye J. *Darwin: The Story of the Man and His Theories of Evolution*. London: Andre Deutsch Ltd, 2008.

36. Einstein A. *Relativity: The Special and General Theory*. New York: Holt and Company, 1916.

37. Wadsworth BJ. *Piaget's Theory of Cognitive and Affective Development: Foundations of Constructivism*. 5 ed. New York: Longman Publishing, 1996.

38. Erikson EH, Erikson JM. *The Life Cycle Completed-Extended Version*. New York: W.W. Norton, 1997.

39. Abrams D, Hogg MA. Metatheory: lessons from social identity research. *Pers Soc Psychol Rev* 2004;8(2):98–106.

40. Eastwood JG, Kemp LA, Jalaludin BB. Realist theory construction for a mixed method multilevel study of neighbourhood context and postnatal depression. *Springerplus* 2016;5(1):1081.

41. Paterson BL. The shifting perspectives model of chronic illness. *J Nurs Scholarsh* 2001;33(1):21–26.

42. Gottlieb G. The relevance of developmental-psychobiological metatheory to developmental neuropsychology. *Dev Neuropsychol* 2001;19(1):1–9.

43. Hawking S. *A Brief History of Time From the Big Bang to Black Holes*. New York: Bantam Dell Publishing Group, 1988.

Understanding Evidence-Based Practice

Evidence-based practice (EBP) is about clinical decision-making—how we find and use information and how we integrate knowledge, experience, and judgment to address clinical problems. EBP requires a mindset that values evidence as an important component of quality care and a skill set in searching the literature, critical appraisal, synthesis, and reasoning to determine the applicability of evidence to current issues. The ultimate goal is to create a culture of inquiry and rigorous evaluation that provides a basis for balancing quality with the uncertainty that is found in practice—all in the effort to improve patient care.

The purpose of this chapter is to clarify how evidence contributes to clinical decision-making, describe the process of EBP and the types of evidence that are meaningful, and discuss the barriers that often limit successful implementation. This discussion will continue throughout the text in relation to specific elements of research design and analysis.

■ Why Is Evidence-Based Practice Important?

In a landmark 2001 report, *Crossing the Quality Chasm*,[1] the Institute of Medicine (IOM) documented a significant gap between *what we know* and *what we do*, between the care people *should* receive and the care they *actually* receive, between published evidence and healthcare practice. The IOM estimates that one-third of healthcare spending is for therapies that do not improve health.[2] Another review suggests that 50% of healthcare practices are of unknown effectiveness and 15% are potentially harmful or unlikely to be beneficial.[3,4] Consider, for example, the change in recommendations for infant sleep position, for many years preferred on the stomach, to reduce the possibility of spitting up and choking. In 1992, this recommendation was changed to sleeping on the back, which improved breathing and drastically changed the incidence of sudden infant death syndrome (SIDS).[5]

Clinicians tackle questions every day in practice, constantly faced with the task of interpreting results of diagnostic tests, determining the efficacy of therapeutic and preventive regimens, the potential harm associated with different treatments, the course and prognosis of specific disorders, costs of tests or interventions, and whether guidelines are sound. Despite having these questions, however, and even with an emphasis on EBP across healthcare, practitioners in most professional disciplines do not seek answers or they express a lack of confidence in evidence, with a higher value placed on experience, collegial advice, or anecdotal evidence than on research to support clinical decisions.[6,7]

From an evidence-based standpoint, research has continued to document escalating healthcare costs, disparities in access to healthcare, and unwarranted variations in accepted practice—with geography, ethnicity, socioeconomic status, and clinical setting often cited as major determinants.[8–11] Addressing these issues requires understanding how evidence informs our choices to support quality care.

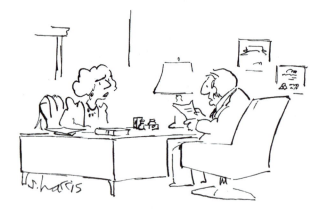

"I MUST TELL YOU THAT THE DRUG THAT CURED YOU HAS BEEN PROVEN COMPLETELY INEFFECTIVE."

Illustration courtesy of Sidney Harris. Used with permission from ScienceCartoons Plus.com.

Where Are the Gaps?

As discussed in Chapter 2, the focus on translational research has highlighted the need for research to provide practical solutions to clinical problems in a timely way, further fueling the urgency for a more evidence-based framework for healthcare.

Generalizing results from randomized controlled trials (RCTs) is often difficult because patients and circumstances in the real world do not match experimental conditions. Clinicians often contend with reimbursement policies that can interfere with decisions regarding effective treatment choices (see Focus on Evidence 5-1). They may also be faced with changes in recommendations, as research uncovers inconsistencies or errors in previous studies and recommendations are reversed.[12]

Three primary issues drive this discussion, all related to the quality of care: *overuse* of procedures without justification, *underuse* of established procedures, and *misuse* of available procedures.[13] Table 5-1 provides examples of each of these quality concerns. These issues are exacerbated by a lack of attention to research findings as well as difficulties in applying results to practice.

■ How Do We Know Things?

How do we decide which test to perform, which intervention to apply, or which patients have the best chance of responding positively to a given treatment? As far back as ancient times, healthcare providers have relied on three typical sources of knowledge (see Fig. 5-1).

- **Tradition**

"That's the way it has always been done."

Conventional wisdom in each era supports theories of the day as "given." We inherit knowledge and accept precedent without further validation. Something is thought to be true simply because people have always known it to be true.

- **Authority**

"That's what the experts say."

When an authority states that something is true, we often accept it. Influential leaders can set longtime standards. We may also find ourselves committed to one approach over others based on what we were taught, relying on that information even years later, without finding out if knowledge has expanded or changed.

🖋 HISTORICAL NOTE

Galen of Pergamon (130–200 A.D.), the ancient Greek physician, was the authority on medical practices for centuries. His authority held such weight that centuries later, when scientists performed autopsies and could not corroborate his teachings with their physical findings, his followers commented that, if the new findings did not agree with his teachings, *"the discrepancy should be attributed to the fact that nature had changed."*[29]

- **Experience**

"It's worked for me before."

Sometimes a product of trial and error, experience is a powerful teacher. Occasionally, it will be the experience of a colleague that is shared. The more experienced the clinician, the stronger the belief in that experience!

◎ FUN FACT

Although somewhat tongue-in-cheek, unyielding trust in authority has also been called *"eminence-based medicine,"* the persistent reliance on the experience of those considered the experts.[30] Such faith has been defined as *"making the same mistakes with increasing confidence over an impressive number of years."*[31]

These "ways of knowing" can be efficient and they may actually achieve positive outcomes. But over time they are more likely to result in a lack of progress, limited understanding of current knowledge, or resistance to change—even in the face of evidence. With a greater understanding of the scientific method, logic, and evidence, however, "knowing" has taken on a more stringent emphasis (see Chapter 4). Seeking evidence can substantiate or refute experience, authority, and tradition, and can thereby strengthen foundations to consider new, more valid methods.

Focus on Evidence 5–1
The Direct Line from Evidence to Practice

Treatment to improve healing of chronic wounds remains a serious healthcare challenge.[14] Standard care includes optimization of nutritional status, débridement, dressings to maintain granulation tissue, and treatment to resolve infections.[15] Electrical stimulation (ES) has been used as an alternative therapy since the 1960s, especially for chronic wounds, with numerous clinical reports showing accelerated healing.[16,17]

Despite several decades of successful use of the modality and Medicare coverage for such treatment since 1980, in May 1997, the Health Care Financing Administration (HCFA, now the Centers for Medicare and Medicaid Services, CMS) announced that it would no longer reimburse for the use of ES for wound healing. The agency claimed that a review of literature determined there was insufficient evidence to support such coverage and that ES did not appear to be superior to conventional therapies.[18]

In July 1997, the American Physical Therapy Association (APTA) filed a lawsuit along with six Medicare beneficiaries seeking a temporary injunction against HCFA from enforcing its decision.[15] The APTA included several supporting documents, including a CPG for pressure ulcers issued by the Agency for Health Care Policy and Research (now the Agency for Healthcare Research and Quality, AHRQ). Although several clinical trials were cited, supportive evidence was not considered strong. Therapists who opposed

HCFA's decision cited their experience and informal data, insisting that the treatment made an important difference for many patients.[18]

This prompted the gathering of more formal evidence and further analysis to show that ES was indeed effective for reducing healing time for chronic wounds.[15] Based on this information, in 2002 CMS reversed the decision and coverage was approved, but only for use with chronic ulcers, defined as ulcers that have not healed within 30 days of occurrence.

One of the continuing issues with research in this area is the lack of consistency across trials in parameters of ES application, including dosage, waveforms, duration of treatment, and the delivery system. Interpretations are further complicated by varied protocols, types of wounds studied, generally small samples, and different types of comparisons within the trials.[14,19] This type of variability in design still threatens the weight of evidence, in this and many other areas of clinical inquiry. This is not an isolated experience.

This story emphasizes why the use of evidence in practice is not optional. "Insisting" that a treatment works is not sufficient. Our ability to provide appropriate care, change policy, and be reimbursed for services rests on how we have justified interventions and diagnostic procedures through valid research—not just for our own decision-making, but for those who influence how our care is provided and paid for and, of course, ultimately for the benefit of our patients.

Table 5-1	Quality Issues That Can Be Addressed Through EBP		
QUALITY ISSUE	**DEFINITION**	**CONSEQUENCES**	**EXAMPLE**
Overuse	Occurs when treatment or tests are given without medical justification. At best, this can result in wasted resources; at worst, it can result in harm.	Overuse contributes to high costs, with some estimates attributing up to 30% of U.S. health spending to overuse.[20]	Even with evidence that 80% of childhood ear infections will resolve within 3 days without medication, antibiotics are still prescribed most of the time, despite potential risks of side effects and antibiotic resistance.[21]
Underuse	Occurs when clinicians fail to provide necessary care or tests, employ preventive strategies, or follow practice guidelines. Underuse may also be a factor of nonadherence on the part of patients, lack of referral to proper services, or implementation barriers.	It has been estimated that children and adults in the United States receive less than 50% of recommended healthcare and preventive services.[4,22,23]	Almost 200,000 people get pneumococcal pneumonia each year, from which 3% die, despite the availability of a vaccine.[24]
Misuse	Inappropriate use of interventions or tests, often resulting in medical errors that reduce the benefit of treatment or cause harm.	Updated estimates suggest that preventable harm in hospitals is responsible for over 200,000 deaths per year[25] and one-third of healthcare spending.[26]	Despite common use for deep heating therapy and potential risks, several systematic reviews have shown that ultrasound is not effective for that purpose.[27,28]

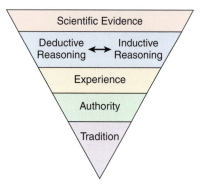

Figure 5–1 Ways of knowing.

■ What Is Evidence-Based Practice?

Evidence-based practice is an approach to decision-making that incorporates scientific information with other sources of knowledge. The widely accepted definition of EBP incorporates several important elements:

> *Evidence-based practice is the conscientious, explicit and judicious use of current best evidence in making decisions about the care of individual patients.*[32]

But it is also. . .

> *the integration of best research evidence with clinical expertise and the patient's unique values and circumstances.*[33]

This evidence may be related to accuracy of diagnostic tests, prognostic factors, or the effectiveness and safety of therapies and preventive strategies.

HISTORICAL NOTE

The idea of using evidence as a basis for clinical decision-making is not new. Healthcare providers have understood the importance of applying knowledge to practice since the time of Hippocrates, but their sources of knowledge were heavily reliant on ancient theory and observation. Gordon Guyatt and colleagues from McMaster University first coined the term "evidence-based medicine" (EBM) in 1991, promoting an approach to clinical decision-making that did not rely solely on authority, tradition, or experience.[34] They proposed that the medical community needed to stress the importance of using published research as the foundation for practice. Although their work was geared toward physicians, the relevance of this approach for all healthcare fields has now been widely adopted under the terminology of *evidence-based practice*.

Misconceptions

When the EBP concept was first introduced, there were many misconceptions about what it meant.[32] Proponents argued that this was an essential and responsible way to make clinical decisions, tying practice to scientific standards that would allow metrics of efficacy, greater consistency, and better-informed patients and clinicians. Detractors argued that it would lead to "cook book" medicine, requiring practitioners to follow certain procedures for all patients, taking away the "art" of providing care, and removing the ability to make judgments about individual cases. They also argued, with some validity, that there was not sufficient evidence to make the process viable. But these objections reflect a misunderstanding of the intent of EBP as part of a larger process that includes experience and judgment, beginning and ending with the patient. Let's look closely at the definition of EBP to clarify this process (see Fig. 5-2).

Components of EBP

. . . the integration of best research evidence

The bottom line of EBP is the use of published evidence to support clinical decisions whenever possible. This requires three primary things—the ability to search the literature to find the evidence, the skill to critically appraise the evidence to determine its quality and applicability, and the availability of such evidence to be found! Stipulating "current" best evidence implies that we understand that knowledge and acceptable treatment methods will change over time. The best we can do is keep up with today's knowledge—no small feat given the volume of information being added every day to professional literature.

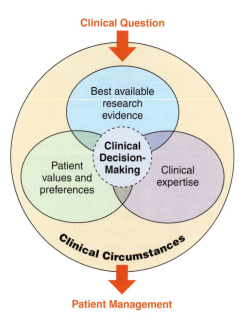

Figure 5–2 The components of EBP as a framework for clinical decision-making.

📌 There are estimates that more than 2,000 citations are being added to databases every day! In 2018, PubMed included over 28 million citations.

The concept of "best" evidence implies that it might not be a perfect fit to answer our questions. Sometimes we have to refer to basic science research to establish a theoretical premise, when no other direct evidence is available. It is also important to know that not everything that is published is of sufficient quality or relevance to warrant application. This means we have to be able to apply skills of critical appraisal to make those judgments.

. . . with clinical expertise

EBP makes no attempt to stifle the essential elements of judgment, experience, skill, and expertise in the identification of patient problems and the individual risks and benefits of particular therapies. Clinical skill and exposure to a variety of patients takes time to develop and plays an important role in building expertise and the application of published evidence to practice. As much as we know the scientific method is not perfect, clinical decisions are constantly being made under conditions of uncertainty and variability—that is the "art" of clinical practice. But we cannot dissociate the art from the science that supports it. Sackett[32] implores us to recognize that:

> . . . *without clinical expertise, practice risks being tyrannized by evidence, for even excellent external advice may be inapplicable to or inappropriate for an individual patient. Without current best evidence, practice risks becoming rapidly out of date, to the detriment of patients.*

. . . the patient's unique values

A key element of the EBP definition is the inclusion of the patient in decision-making. It is not just about finding evidence but finding evidence that matters to patients. Patients have personal values, cultural traits, belief systems, family norms and expectations, and preferences that influence choices; these must all be weighed against the evidence. Patients may opt for one treatment over another because of comfort, cost, convenience, or other beliefs. Patients understand the importance of evidence, but also see value in personalized choices and clinical judgment.[35] This is especially important when evidence is not conclusive and multiple options exist. This implies, however, that the clinician discusses the evidence with the patient in an understandable way so that decisions are considered collaboratively. Evidence supports better outcomes with patient participation in decision-making.[36-38]

. . . and circumstances

This last element of the EBP definition is a critical one. The final decisions about care must also take into account the organizational context within which care is delivered, including available resources in the community, costs, clinical culture and constraints, accessibility of the environment, and the nature of the healthcare system. All of these can have a direct influence on what is possible or preferable. For instance, evidence may clearly support a particular treatment approach, but your clinic may not be able to afford the necessary equipment, you may not have the skills to perform techniques adequately, an institutional policy may preclude a certain approach, or the patient's insurance coverage may be inadequate. Choices must always be made within pragmatic reality.

 It is essential to appreciate all the components of EBP and the fact that ***evidence does not make a decision***. The clinician and patient will do that together—with all the relevant and available evidence to inform them for optimal shared decision-making.

■ The Process of Evidence-Based Practice

The process of EBP is generally described in five phases—the 5 A's—all revolving around the patient's condition and care needs (see Fig. 5-3). This can best be illustrated with an example.

➤ CASE IN POINT

Mrs. H. is 67 years old with a 10-year history of type 2 diabetes, which she considers essentially asymptomatic. She has mild peripheral neuropathies in both feet and poor balance, which has resulted in two noninjurious falls. She is relatively sedentary and overweight, and although she knows she should be exercising more, she admits she "hates to exercise."

Her HbA1c has remained around 7.5 for the past 5 years, slightly above the recommended level of less than 7.0. She is on several oral medications and just began using a noninsulin injectable once daily. She claims to be "relatively compliant" with her medications and complains of periodic gastrointestinal problems, which she attributes to side effects.

Three months ago, Mrs. H started complaining of pain and limited range of motion (ROM) in her right shoulder. She had an MRI and was diagnosed with adhesive capsulitis (frozen shoulder), which has continued to get worse. She considers this her primary health concern right now and is asking about treatment options.

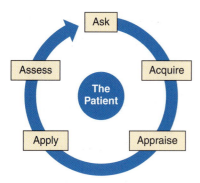

Figure 5–3 The five steps in the EBP process: 1) **Ask** a clinical question, 2) **Acquire** relevant literature, 3) **Appraise** the literature, 4) **Apply** findings to clinical decision-making, 5) **Assess** success of the process.

STEP 1: Ask a Clinical Question

The first step in EBP is asking a clear clinical question that is relevant to a patient's problem and structured to provide direction for searching for the answer. This can be a challenging task because it represents an uncertainty about a patient's care.

Being an evidence-based practitioner does not mean that every patient encounter requires asking a question. Often, clinicians will find themselves in familiar territory, being knowledgeable about the approaches that are appropriate for their patient's condition. But there will also be many instances in which questions arise out of uncertainty about new therapies or technologies or a patient's curiosity about a new treatment. Sometimes a new treatment is not as effective as expected and you need to consider alternatives. Perhaps the patient presents with a unique combination of problems, or has a condition that is rarely seen, or a standard treatment has not been effective. These are the uncertainties that occur in everyday practice and the reasons for needing to understand how to apply evidence.

There are two general types of questions that are asked as part of the search for evidence—questions that refer to background information and those that focus on patient management decisions.

Background Questions

A background question is related to etiology or general knowledge about a patient's condition, referring to the cause of a disease or condition, its natural history, its signs and symptoms, or the anatomical or physiological mechanisms that relate to pathophysiology. This type of question may also focus on the physiology of a treatment or test in order to understand how they work. These questions will generally have a "who, what, where, when, how, or why" root.

Background questions are commonly asked by patients in an effort to understand their own conditions. They may also be more frequent for clinicians who have less experience with a given condition. For Mrs. H, for example, we may ask:

Is frozen shoulder a common condition in patients with type 2 diabetes?

Basic research studies may help with this type of question, but they can often be answered easily using textbooks or Web-based resources—with the proviso that the clinician is wary of the degree to which that content is updated and valid. Over time, clinicians tend to ask fewer background questions, as they become more experienced with various types of patient conditions.

➤ Several studies have documented an increased risk of shoulder adhesive capsulitis in individuals with type 2 diabetes.[39] A meta-analysis has demonstrated that patients with diabetes are five times more likely to have the condition than individuals who do not have diabetes, with an estimated prevalence of diabetes in those with adhesive capsulitis of 30%.[40]

📌 Another source of questions is the need for continuous professional development, staying current in your area of practice. Clinicians who have specialized areas of practice, or who see certain types of patients more often, will find keeping up with the literature helpful in making everyday decisions.

Foreground Questions

The more common type of clinical question for EBP is one that focuses on specific knowledge to inform decisions about patient management, called a foreground question. Foreground questions are stated using four components:

- **P**opulation or **P**roblem
- **I**ntervention (*exposure or test*)
- **C**omparison (*if relevant*)
- **O**utcome

These components are described using the acronym **PICO** (see Fig. 5-4). The phrasing of a complete question with these four elements is most important for finding an answer—to identify search terms for the acquisition of literature and to interpret findings to determine whether they help with the problem under consideration.

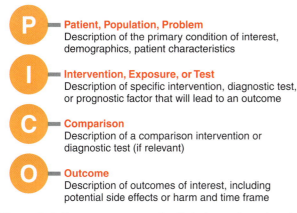

Figure 5–4 Four components of a clinical question using the PICO format.

Other formats have been proposed to structure EBP questions, including PICOT (adding **T**ime frame),[41] PICOTS (adding **T**ime frame and **S**etting),[42] PICOS (adding **S**tudy design),[43] and PESICO (adding **E**nvironment and **S**takeholders).[44] The term PIO has also been used for observational or descriptive studies that do not include comparisons.

A strategy for qualitative research has been proposed using SPIDER[45] (**S**ample, **P**henomenon of **I**nterest, **D**esign, **E**valuation, **R**esearch type).

The PICO structure was introduced in Chapter 3 as a basis for framing a research question—and as promised, here it is again!

Sources of Clinical Questions

Foreground questions can focus on four main areas of evidence:

- Diagnosis and measurement
- Prognosis
- Intervention
- Patient experiences

Questions may include outcomes related to changes in impairments, function, or participation, as well as cost and resource use. The questions may also incorporate qualitative outcomes, such as understanding the impact of health conditions on a patient's experience of care.

Applying PICO

Many different questions can arise for a single patient, depending on the clinician's and patient's concerns and preferences. Let's use one as an example.

> ➤ Mrs. H is very concerned about her shoulder, which is painful and severely limits her function. She has been told that she needs therapy but has also read that corticosteroid injections can be helpful and asks about that option.

How can we address this concern using PICO?

P: Type 2 diabetes, frozen shoulder (adhesive capsulitis), age 65, female
I: Physical therapy
C: Corticosteroid injection
O: Reduced shoulder disability, decreased pain, and increased ROM

We can then formulate a question to guide a search for evidence:

In a patient with type 2 diabetes who has adhesive capsulitis, is a corticosteroid injection more effective than physical therapy for reducing shoulder disability and pain and for increasing range of motion?

Table 5-2 shows how PICO components are used to phrase other questions related to Mrs. H.

STEP 2: Acquire Relevant Literature

The question leads to a search for the best evidence that can contribute to a decision about the patient's care, guided by the PICO terms. Searching is not always a straightforward process and finding relevant literature can be a challenge. How the question is phrased can make a huge difference in being able to find an answer.

The search process must be thorough yet focused to be effective and efficient. It is important to use a variety of resources and to consider literature across disciplines to improve the likelihood of finding relevant information (see Box 5-1). The help of a research librarian can be invaluable in creating a comprehensive search strategy.

Different types of studies will be explored, depending on the nature of the clinical question (see Table 5-2).

- **Diagnosis and measurement:** These questions will typically be answered using methodological studies for validity and reliability, epidemiologic methods to assess diagnostic accuracy, or RCTs to answer questions about comparison of diagnostic tests.
- **Prognosis:** These questions will usually involve observational cohort and case-control studies, exploring relationships to determine which factors are relevant to predicting outcomes.
- **Intervention:** The RCT is considered the standard but pragmatic trials may also be used. Single-subject and observational designs can also be applied, especially with conditions for which RCTs are less feasible.
- **Patient experiences:** Qualitative studies provide a rich source of information about patient preferences. Descriptive surveys may also be useful to gather this information.

Table 5-2   Sources of Foreground Clinical Questions

CLINICAL ISSUE	SAMPLE QUESTIONS (PICO)
Diagnosis and Measurement	
Diagnostic tests: Which diagnostic tests should be performed, considering their accuracy and expense? Are there clinical prediction rules that can be applied? **History and physical examination:** Which tools, assessments, or measurements should be used, and how should they be interpreted? Are measures reliable and valid?	Are measures of peripheral sensation valid for assessing peripheral neuropathies in patients with type 2 diabetes?[46,47] In patients with type 2 diabetes who have peripheral neuropathy, which measure of balance will provide the best assessment to predict falls?[48]
Prognosis	
What is the likely course of the condition over time or the potential complications? Which factors should help to understand risks and benefits of care?	Are patients with type 2 diabetes and an HbA1C of 7.5 likely to develop peripheral neuropathies?[49]
Intervention	
Therapy: Which treatments are likely to be most effective? Are they worth the efforts of using them? What is the balance between potential benefit and harm? **Prevention:** Which steps can be taken to reduce the chance of a condition developing or worsening? What are potential mediating risk factors and screening opportunities?	In patients with type 2 diabetes who experience a frozen shoulder, will a corticosteroid injection be more effective than physical therapy to improve shoulder function?[50] Can personal leisure activities be developed to encourage exercise in sedentary individuals with diabetes?[51]
Patient Experiences	
How do patient preferences, values, or goals influence choices and progress?	In patients with type 2 diabetes, which factors contribute to a lack of adherence to a medication regimen and exercise?[52]

Box 5-1   We Are in This Together

The mandates for interprofessional practice have become a central focus of healthcare today, touting the need to move out of our professional silos to support quality and safety in the provision of patient-centered care.[1,54] And yet, when it comes to EBP, the silos may be perpetuated with resources being developed for "evidence-based medicine,"[33] "evidence-based occupational therapy,"[55] "evidence-based physical therapy,"[56] "evidence-based nursing,"[57] and so on.

By thinking about "disciplinary evidence," we risk becoming short-sighted about how we ask questions, look for evidence, or use information to make clinical decisions. Although each discipline surely has its unique knowledge base (albeit with overlaps), we must be sure to think *interprofessionally* to phrase questions and gather evidence broadly enough to reflect the best care for a particular patient, including understanding how such evidence can inform our role as a member of the team responsible for the patient's total management.

Finding relevant literature requires knowledge of search parameters and access to appropriate databases. Sometimes searches are not successful in locating relevant resources to answer a particular question. This may be due to a lack of sophistication in searching or it may be because studies addressing a particular question have not been done!

Comprehensive information about searching the literature to answer this question will be presented in Chapter 6.

Evidence Reviews

One of most useful contributions to EBP has been the development of critical reviews of literature that summarize and appraise current literature on a particular topic. For clinicians who do not have the time or skill to read and assess large numbers of studies, these reviews provide a comprehensive summary of available evidence. Reviews are not necessarily available for every clinical question but, whenever possible, such reviews should be sought as a first source of information. Many excellent resources provide evidence-based reviews on particular topics (see Chapter 37).

Systematic reviews are studies in which the authors carry out an extensive and focused search for research on a clinical topic, followed by appraisal and summaries of findings, usually to answer a specific question.

> ➤ Blanchard et al[53] compiled a systematic review to look at the effectiveness of corticosteroid injections compared to physical therapy intervention for adhesive capsulitis. They evaluated six randomized trials, with varied quality and sample sizes. They found that the corticosteroid injections had a

greater effect on mobility in the short term (6–7 weeks) compared to physical therapy, but with no difference in pain. At 1 year, there was no difference in shoulder disability between the two groups, with a small benefit in terms of pain for those who got the injection.

Meta-analyses are systematic reviews that use quantitative methods to summarize the results from multiple studies. Summary reviews are also used to establish **clinical practice guidelines (CPGs)** for specific conditions, translating critical analysis of the literature into a set of recommendations.

Another type of knowledge synthesis is called a **scoping review**, which also includes a review of literature but with a broader focus on a topic of interest to provide direction for future research and policy considerations.[58]

STEP 3: Appraise the Literature

Once pertinent articles are found, they need to be critically appraised to determine whether they meet quality standards and whether the findings are important and relevant to the clinical question. Although different types of studies will have different criteria for determining validity, three major categories should be addressed for each article:

1. Is the study valid?
2. Are the results meaningful?
3. Are results relevant to my patient?

These criteria are described in Table 5-3. Each question will require evaluations that are specific to the type of study, with an understanding of the validity issues that are relevant to the design. Clinicians must be able to determine to what extent the results of a study inform their practice, especially when some studies will have "significant" findings and others will not (see Chapter 36). Having a working knowledge of research design and analysis approaches is essential for making these judgments.

Appraisal is also dependent on the extent to which authors present clear and complete descriptions of their research question, study design, analysis procedures, results, and conclusions. Checklists have been developed for various types of studies that list specific content that should be included in a written report to assure transparency (see Chapter 38).

STEP 4: Apply the Evidence

Once the literature is reviewed, analyzed, and interpreted, the clinician must then determine whether research results can be applied to a given clinical situation, with integration of expertise, patient values, and the context of the clinical setting. This is where the "rubber meets the road," so to speak—putting it all together to

Table 5-3	Outline of General Criteria for Critical Appraisal

1. Is the study valid?
This is the determination of the quality of the design and analysis, as well as the extent to which you can be confident in the study's findings. Various scales can be used to assess the methodological quality of a study.
- Is the research question important, and is it based on a theoretical rationale? Is the study design appropriate for the research question?
- Was the study sample selected appropriately? Was the sample size large enough to demonstrate meaningful effects? Were subjects followed for a long enough time to document outcomes?
- Was bias sufficiently controlled? For an intervention trial, was randomization and blinding used? For observational studies, was there control of potential confounders?
- Was the sample size large enough to demonstrate treatment effects?
- What were the outcome measures? Were they valid and reliable? Were they operationally defined? Were they appropriate to the research question?
- Were data analysis procedures applied and interpreted appropriately? Do data support conclusions?

2. Are the results meaningful?
Results must be interpreted in terms of their impact on patient responses and outcomes. They may be related to primary and secondary outcomes.
- Is the sample sufficiently representative of the target population so that results can be generalized?
- How large was the effect of intervention, the accuracy of the diagnostic test, or the degree of risk associated with prognostic factors?
- Is the effect large enough to be clinically meaningful?

3. Are the results relevant to my patient?
Finally, you must determine whether the findings will be applicable to your patient and clinical decisions.
- Were the subjects in the study sufficiently similar to my patient?
- Can I apply these results to my patient's problem? What are the potential benefits or harms?
- Is the approach feasible in my setting and will it be acceptable to my patient?
- Is this approach worth the effort to incorporate it into my treatment plan?

inform a clinical decision. This conclusion may not be simple, however. Research studies may not fit your patient's situation exactly. For instance, in the case of Mrs. H, many studies and systematic reviews have shown results for patients with adhesive capsulitis but did not focus specifically on people with diabetes.

And then there is the unhelpful situation where you could not find the evidence—because your search strategy was not sufficient, no one has studied the problem, or studies have shown no positive effects (see Box 5-2). This is where the decision-making process meets uncertainty and where judgment is needed to determine what constitutes best evidence for a specific clinical question. For Mrs. H, we can go through the thought process shown in Figure 5-5, resulting in a decision to explore corticosteroid injection as a supplement to physical therapy.

STEP 5: Assess the Effectiveness of the Evidence

The final step in the EBP process is to determine whether the application of the evidence resulted in a positive outcome. Did Mrs. H improve as expected? If she did not, the clinician must then reflect on why the evidence may not have been valid for the patient's situation, whether additional evidence is needed to answer the clinical question, or whether other factors need to be considered to find the best treatment approach for her.

This step is often ignored but in the end may be the most important, as we must continue to learn from the evidence—what works and what does not. The process shown in Figure 5-3 is circular because, through this assessment, we may generate further questions in the search of the "best evidence." These questions may facilitate a new search process or they may be the basis for a research study.

■ Levels of Evidence

As we search for evidence, we want to find the most accurate and valid information possible. Depending on the kind of question being asked, different types of studies will provide the strongest evidence. To assist in this effort, studies can be assigned to **levels of evidence**, which essentially reflect a rating system. These levels represent the expected rigor of the design and control of bias, thereby indicating the level of confidence that may be placed in the findings.

Levels of evidence are viewed as a hierarchy, with studies at the top representing stronger evidence and those at the bottom being weaker. This hierarchy can be used by clinicians, researchers, and patients as a guide to find the likely best evidence.[61] These levels are also used as a basis for selecting studies for incorporation into guidelines and systematic reviews.

Classification Schemes

Several classifications of evidence have been developed, with varying terminology and grading systems.[62,63] The most commonly cited system has been developed by the Oxford Centre for Evidence-Based Medicine (OCEBM), shown in Table 5-4. This system includes five study types:[61]

- **Diagnosis:** *Is this diagnostic or monitoring test accurate?*
  Questions about diagnostic tests or measurement reliability and validity are most effectively studied using cross-sectional studies applying a consistent reference standard and blinding.
- **Prognosis:** *What will happen if we do not add a therapy?*
  Studies of prognosis look for relationships among predictor and outcome variables using observational designs.
- **Intervention:** *Does this intervention help?*
  This question is most effectively studied using an RCT, although strong observational studies may also be used. The latest version of this classification includes the N-of-1 trial as an acceptable alternative to the standard RCT.
- **Harm:** *What are the common or rare harms?*
  RCTs and observational studies can identify adverse effects. Outcomes from N-of-1 trials can provide evidence specific to a particular patient.
- **Screening:** *Is this early detection test worthwhile?*
  RCTs are also the strongest design for this purpose to determine whether screening tests are effective by comparing outcomes for those who do and do not get the test.

The Hierarchy of Evidence

Hierarchies are delineated for each type of research question to distinguish the designs that provide the strongest form of evidence for that purpose. The OCEBM structure is based on five levels of evidence:

- **Level 1** evidence comes from systematic reviews or meta-analyses that critically summarize several studies. These reviews are the best first pass when searching for information on a specific question (see Chapter 37).
- **Level 2** includes individual RCTs or observational studies with strong design and outcomes (see Chapters 14 and 19).
  The studies included in levels 1 and 2 are intended to reflect the strongest designs, including RCTs for assessment of interventions, harms, and screening procedures, as well as prospective observational studies for diagnosis and prognosis.
- **Level 3** includes studies that do not have strong controls of bias, such as nonrandomized studies, retrospective cohorts, or diagnostic studies that do not have a consistent reference standard (see Chapters 17, 19).

Box 5-2   An invisible unicorn is grazing in my office. . . prove me wrong!

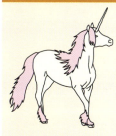

This fantastical challenge carries an important message about evidence.[59] Try to prove that the invisible unicorn does not exist. Come visit my office and you will probably find no evidence that it does, but perhaps you are not looking in the right places, or carefully enough, or for the right kind of evidence. Proving a negative is difficult, if not impossible.

Consider a hypothetical trial to investigate the effectiveness of a corticosteroid injection to improve shoulder function. Ten patients with adhesive capsulitis are randomly assigned to two groups, one group getting the active injection and the other a placebo, with subjects and experimenters all blinded to assignment. In the end, one person in each group improves. What is the conclusion?

The evidence shows that the drug does not work—OR—*The study provides no evidence that the drug works.*

This is no small distinction. The first conclusion is about the "*evidence of absence*," suggesting that there is evidence to show there is no effect. The second conclusion is about the "*absence of evidence*," indicating that we have not found evidence to show that it works—we just do not know yet.

There are many possible reasons why the study did not show an effect. Maybe if the sample were larger we would have seen more people respond positively; maybe we could have measured function more precisely to show a difference; maybe our sample was biased; maybe the effect is just too small to be meaningful—or maybe the injection just does not work! Evidence is not black and white. We have to consider many questions when we evaluate what we find. How big a difference is going to matter? What are the relevant costs, potential adverse outcomes, the patient's preferences? Was the analysis of data appropriate? Was the sample large enough to show a difference? Did the design control for potential biases? Are these results confirmed in more than one study? Can we have confidence in the outcomes? Conclusions of an absent effect can be misleading. It is always possible that the treatment is not effective, but it is also possible that the study simply was not powerful enough to show a difference. Beware of the invisible unicorn! *Absence of evidence is not evidence of absence.*[60]

We will revisit this issue from a statistical perspective in Chapter 23.

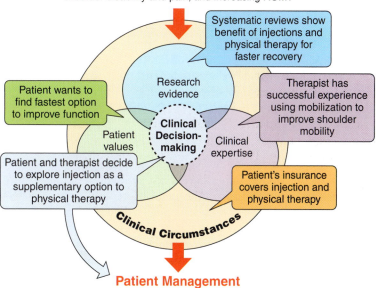

Figure 5–5 EBP framework, showing the process to decide on appropriate treatment for a patient with diabetes who has adhesive capsulitis. After considering all relevant information, a decision is made to pursue a particular treatment approach.

Table 5-4   Levels of Evidence

TYPE OF QUESTION	LEVEL 1 STRONGEST	LEVEL 2 →	LEVEL 3	LEVEL 4	LEVEL 5 WEAKEST
Diagnosis	• Systematic review of cross-sectional studies • Consistently applied reference standard • Blinding	• Cross-sectional study • Consistently applied reference standard • Blinding	• Nonconsecutive studies • Studies without consistent reference standard	• Case-control studies • Nonindependent reference standard	• Mechanistic reasoning
Prognosis	• Systematic review of inception cohort studies	• Inception cohort studies	• Cohort study • Control arm of RCT	• Case series or case-control studies • Poor-quality cohort study	• n/a
Intervention	• Systematic review of RCTs • N-of-1 trial*	• RCT • Observational study with dramatic effect	• Nonrandomized controlled cohort • Follow-up study	• Case series • Case-control studies • Historical controls	• Mechanistic reasoning
Harm†	• Systematic review of RCTs • Systematic review of nested case-control studies • N-of-1 trial* • Observational study with dramatic effect	• RCT • Observational study with dramatic effect	• Nonrandomized controlled cohort • Follow-up study‡	• Case series • Case-control study • Historical controls	• Mechanistic reasoning
Screening	• Systematic review of RCTs	• RCT	• Nonrandomized controlled cohort • Follow-up study	• Case series • Case control • Historical controls	• Mechanistic reasoning

Adapted from Oxford Centre for Evidence-Based Medicine (OCEBM): http://www.cebm.net/index.aspx?o=5653.

OCEBM Levels of Evidence Working Group: The Oxford 2011 Levels of Evidence. Used with permission.

*N-of-1 trial with a patient who has raised the question.

† Harm relates to adverse effects of treatment and can be described as rare or common.

‡ Numbers must be sufficient to rule out common harm; duration of follow-up must be sufficient to show long-term harm.

- **Level 4** is a relatively low level of evidence, primarily including descriptive studies such as case series or studies that use historical controls (see Chapter 20).
- **Level 5** is based on *mechanistic reasoning*, whereby evidence-based decisions are founded on logical connections, including pathophysiological rationale.[67] This may be based on biological plausibility or basic research. Case reports that focus on describing such mechanisms in one or more individuals can be informative at this level of evidence.

As the nature of EBP has matured, hierarchies of evidence have been modified over time. In previous versions of levels of evidence, the "bottom" level included case reports, expert opinion, anecdotal evidence, and basic research. With the most recent OCEBM modifications in 2011, these sources have been replaced by *mechanistic reasoning*, suggesting that such "opinions" must still be based on logical rationale. Also omitted are questions about economics for which there is less consensus on what counts as good evidence.[61]

Qualitative and Descriptive Research Evidence

The framework for levels of evidence has been based on designs used in quantitative studies. Studies that produce qualitative or descriptive data have been excluded from the hierarchy, and are sometimes not seen as true forms of evidence. These research approaches do, however, make significant contributions to our knowledge base and identification of mechanisms, and will often provide an important perspective for appreciating patients' concerns. Quantitative studies can tell us which treatment is better or the degree of correlation between variables, but qualitative inquiry can help us understand the context of care and how the patient experience impacts outcomes—factors that can have substantial influence on clinical decisions (see Chapter 21). Therefore, rather than thinking of qualitative study as a low level of evidence in a quantitative paradigm, a different set of criteria need to be applied that focus on the various approaches and kinds of questions relevant to qualitative research.[64,65]

Qualitative research stands apart from other forms of inquiry because of its deep-rooted intent to understand the personal and social experience of patients, families, and providers. Daly et al[66] have proposed a hierarchy with four levels of evidence, emphasizing the capacity for qualitative research to inform practice and policy.

- **Level 1**, at the top of the hierarchy, represents *generalizable studies.* These are qualitative studies that are guided by theory, and include sample selection that extends beyond one specific population to capture diversity of experiences. Findings are put into the context of previous research, demonstrating broad application. Data collection and analysis procedures are comprehensive and clear.
- **Level 2** includes *conceptual studies* that analyze data according to conceptual themes but have narrower application based on limited diversity in the sample. Further research is needed to confirm concepts.
- **Level 3** includes *descriptive studies* that are focused on describing participant views or experiences with narrative summaries and quotations, but with no detailed analysis.
- **Level 4** includes *case studies*, exploring insights that have not been addressed before, often leading to recognition of unusual phenomena.

Quality of Evidence

Levels of evidence are intended to serve as a guide to accessing and prioritizing the strongest possible research on a given topic. However, levels are based on design characteristics, not quality. An RCT may have serious flaws because of bias, restricted samples, inappropriate data analysis, or inappropriate interpretation of results. At the same time, level 4 studies may provide important relevant information that may influence decision-making for a particular patient.

Grading Evidence Up or Down

Hierarchies used to classify quality of published research should serve as a guide for searching and identifying higher quality studies, but are not absolute. By evaluating the quality of the evidence presented, we may find that a higher-quality study at a lower level of evidence may be more helpful than one at a higher level that has design or analysis flaws (see Chapter 37). For instance, a well-designed cohort study may be more applicable than a poorly designed RCT. The level of evidence for a strong observational study may be graded up if there is a substantial treatment effect. An RCT can be graded down based on poor study quality, lack of agreement between studied variables and the PICO question, inconsistency between studies, or because the absolute effect size is very small.

Levels of evidence are based on the assumption that systematic reviews and meta-analyses provide stronger evidence than individual trials in all categories. The content of reviews, however, is not always sufficiently detailed to provide applicable information for clinical decision-making. For example, reviews often lack specifics on patient characteristics, operational definitions about interventions, or adverse effects, which can vary across studies. Individual references may still need to be consulted to inform clinical decisions.

■ Implementing Evidence-Based Practice

Although the concepts and elements of EBP were introduced more than 20 years ago, the integration of EBP into everyday practice has continued to be a challenge in all healthcare disciplines. As we explore evidence, it is important to keep a perspective regarding its translation to practice. The ultimate purpose of EBP is to improve patient care, but this cannot happen by only using published research. The clinician must be able to make the connections between study results, sound judgment, patient needs, and clinical resources.

The literature is replete with studies that have examined the degree to which clinicians and administrators have been able to implement EBP as part of their practice. It is a concern that appears to affect all health professions and practice settings, as well as healthcare cultures across many countries. For the most part, research has shown that issues do not stem from devaluing evidence-based practice. Although healthcare providers appreciate their professional responsibility to work in an evidence-based way, they also recognize the difficulties in achieving that goal from personal and organizational perspectives, particularly related to availability of time and resources, as well as establishing an evidence-based clinical culture.[67]

Several strategies can be incorporated to build an EBP clinical environment. See the *Chapter 5 Supplement* for further discussion.

Knowledge Translation

As we come to better appreciate the importance of EBP, we must also appreciate the journey we face in getting from evidence to practice. Implementation studies can help us see how evidence can be integrated into practice. But then there is still one more hurdle—securing the knowledge that facilitates actual utilization of evidence.

Knowledge translation (KT) is a relatively new term that has been used to describe the longstanding problem of underutilization of evidence in healthcare.[68] It describes the process of accelerating the application of knowledge to improve outcomes and change behavior for all those involved in providing care. It is a process that needs interprofessional support, including disciplines such as informatics, public policy, organizational theory, and educational and social psychology to close the gap between what we know and what we do (see Chapter 2).[69]

Although the term KT has been widely used, its definition has been ambiguous, often used interchangeably with other terms such as knowledge transfer, knowledge exchange, research utilization, diffusion, implementation, dissemination, and evidence implementation.[70,71] The Canadian Institutes of Health Research (CIHR) have offered the following definition:

> *Knowledge translation is a dynamic and iterative process that includes synthesis, dissemination, exchange and ethically-sound application of knowledge to improve health, . . . provide more effective health services, and products and strengthen the health care system.*[72]

Knowledge-to-Action Framework

This definition characterizes KT as a multidimensional concept involving the adaptation of quality research into relevant priorities, recognizing that KT goes beyond dissemination and continuing education.[70] KT includes both creation and application of knowledge—what has been called the *knowledge-to-action framework*.[71]

Knowledge creation addresses specific needs and priorities, with three phases:

1. **Inquiry**—including completion of primary research.
2. **Synthesis**—bringing disparate findings together, typically in systematic reviews, to reflect the totality of evidence on a topic.
3. **Development of tools**—further distilling knowledge into creation of decision-making tools such as clinical guidelines.

The action cycle begins with identification of a problem, reflecting the current state of knowledge. It then leads to application and evaluation of the process for achieving stable outcomes. Integral to the framework is the input of stakeholders, including patients, clinicians, managers, and policy makers (see Focus on Evidence 5-2).[71]

Knowledge, Implementation, and Evidence

There is an obvious overlap of knowledge translation, implementation research, and EBP, all representing a process of moving research knowledge to application. Although the definitions appear to coincide, KT has a broader meaning, encompassing the full scope of knowledge development, starting with asking the right questions, conducting relevant research, disseminating findings that relate to a clinical context, applying that knowledge, and studying its impact.

KT is seen as a collaborative engagement between researchers and practitioners, reflecting together on practice needs and consequences of research choices, with mutual accountability.[75] It is an interactive, cyclical, and dynamic process that integrates an interprofessional approach to change. In contrast, implementation science focuses on testing how interventions work in real settings, and what solutions need to be introduced into a health system to promote sustainability.[76] KT is a complementary process with a stronger emphasis on the development, exchange, and synthesis of knowledge.

In further contrast, EBP is used more narrowly to refer to the specific part of that process involving the application of information to clinical decision making for a particular patient, including the influence of the patient's values and the practitioner's expertise. In a broader framework, KT formalizes the relationship between the researcher and the practitioner, including mechanisms to remove barriers to EBP.

Focus on Evidence 5–2
From Knowledge to Action

Although there is substantial evidence for the importance of physical activity for children, school and community programs often do not achieve their full potential, either because of poor quality of programming or lack of engaging activities. Based on a review of relevant data and several theories related to activity and goal achievement, a set of principles was designed to address documented limitations: Supportive, Active, Autonomous, Fair, Enjoyable (SAAFE).[75] The purpose of SAAFE was to guide planning, delivery, and evaluation of organized physical activity. The process involved teachers, students, community leaders, and after-school staff, and was tested in several different environments to document changes in behavior and programming, including adoption of teacher training strategies, development of research protocols for evaluation, and dissemination of findings across settings.

This is an example of the knowledge-to-action cycle, requiring multiple inputs, recognition of barriers, and iterations of contributions to understand how evidence can be implemented in real-world environments.

COMMENTARY

Don't accept your dog's admiration as conclusive evidence that you are wonderful.

— *Ann Landers (1918–2002)*

Advice columnist

The central message of EBP is the need to establish logical connections that will strengthen our ability to make sound decisions regarding patient care—but because we base research results on samples, we make lots of assumptions about how findings represent larger populations or individual patients. We also know that all patients do not respond in the same way and, therefore, the causal nature of treatments is not absolute. Several studies looking at the same questions can present different findings. Unique patient characteristics and circumstances can influence outcomes. Studies often try to examine subgroups to determine the basis for these differences, but even those data are subject to variance that cannot be explained or anticipated. This is why clinical decisions should be informed by multiple sources of knowledge, including theory and experience.

In his classic paper, *Things I Have Learned (So Far)*, Cohen[77] cautions us as researchers and practitioners:

Remember that throughout the process, . . . it is on your informed judgment as a scientist that you must rely, and this holds as much for the statistical aspects of the work as it does for all the others. . . . and that informed judgment also governs the conclusions you will draw.

So although the need for EBP seems uncontroversial, it has not yet achieved its full promise. As we shall see in upcoming chapters, uncertainty is ever-present in practice and clinical research. Even when evidence appears strong and convincing, clinical decisions can vary based on practitioner and patient values.[78] We need to apply good principles of design and statistics with sound clinical judgment to strengthen the likelihood that our conclusions, and therefore our actions, have merit.

REFERENCES

1. Institute of Medicine. *Crossing the Quality Chasm: A New Health System for the 21st Century*. Washington, DC: National Academy Press, 2001.
2. Institute of Medicine. *Best care at lower cost: The path to continuously learning health care in America*. Washington, DC: The National Academies Press, 2013.
3. BMJ Clinical Evidence: What conclusions has clinical evidence drawn about what works, what doesn't based on randomised controlled trial evidence? Available at http://clinicalevidence.bmj.com/x/set/static/cms/efficacy-categorisations.html. Accessed June 25, 2017.
4. Fox JB, Shaw FE. Relationship of income and health care coverage to receipt of recommended clinical preventive services by adults - United States, 2011–2012. *MMWR Morb Mortal Wkly Rep* 2014;63(31):666–670.
5. American Academy of Pediatrics Task Force on Infant Positioning and SIDS. Positioning and sudden infant death syndrome (SIDS): update. *Pediatrics* 1996;98(6 Pt 1):1216–1218.
6. Schreiber J, Stern P. A review of literature on evidence-based practice in physical therapy. *Internet J Allied Health Sci and Pract* 2005;3(4).
7. Ely JW, Osheroff JA, Maviglia SM, Rosenbaum ME. Patient-care questions that physicians are unable to answer. *J Am Med Inform Assoc* 2007;14(4):407–414.
8. Timmermans S, Mauck A. The promises and pitfalls of evidence-based medicine. *Health Aff (Millwood)* 2005;24(1):18–28.
9. Mercuri M, Gafni A. Medical practice variations: what the literature tells us (or does not) about what are warranted and unwarranted variations. *J Eval Clin Pract* 2011;17(4):671–677.
10. Lee HY, Ahn HS, Jang JA, Lee YM, Hann HJ, Park MS, Ahn DS. Comparison of evidence-based therapeutic intervention

between community- and hospital-based primary care clinics. *Int J Clin Pract* 2005;59(8):975–980.

11. Fiscella K, Sanders MR. Racial and ethnic disparities in the quality of health care. *Annu Rev Public Health* 2016;37:375–394.

12. Prasad V, Vandross A, Toomey C, Cheung M, Rho J, Quinn S, Chacko SJ, Borkar D, Gall V, Selvaraj S, et al. A decade of reversal: an analysis of 146 contradicted medical practices. *Mayo Clinic Proceedings* 2013;88(8):790–798.

13. National Partnership for Women and Families: Overuse, underuse and misuse of medical care. Fact Sheet. Available at http://go.nationalpartnership.org/site/DocServer/Three_Categories_of_Quality.pdf. Accessed February 17, 2017.

14. Isseroff RR, Dahle SE. Electrical stimulation therapy and wound healing: where are we now? *Advances in Wound Care* 2012;1(6):238–243.

15. Centers for Medicare and Medicaid Services: Decision Memo for Electrostimulation for Wounds (CAG-00068N). Available at https://www.cms.gov/medicare-coverage-database/details/nca-decision-memo.aspx?NCAId=27&fromdb=true. Accessed May 20, 2017.

16. Kloth LC. Electrical stimulation for wound healing: a review of evidence from in vitro studies, animal experiments, and clinical trials. *Int J Low Extrem Wounds* 2005;4(1):23–44.

17. Ennis WJ, Lee C, Gellada K, Corbiere TF, Koh TJ. Advanced technologies to improve wound healing: electrical stimulation, vibration therapy, and ultrasound—what is the evidence? *Plast Reconstr Surg* 2016;138(3 Suppl):94s–104s.

18. AHC Media: Association files suit over reimbursement change. Electrical stimulation funding at issue. Available at https://www.ahcmedia.com/articles/48484-association-files-suit-over-reimbursement-change. Accessed May 20, 2017.

19. Ashrafi M, Alonso-Rasgado T, Baguneid M, Bayat A. The efficacy of electrical stimulation in lower extremity cutaneous wound healing: a systematic review. *Exp Dermatol* 2017; 26(2):171–178.

20. Korenstein D, Falk R, Howell EA, Bishop T, Keyhani S. Overuse of health care services in the United States: an understudied problem. *Arch Intern Med* 2012;172(2):171–178.

21. Takata GS, Chan LS, Shekelle P, Morton SC, Mason W, Marcy SM. Evidence assessment of management of acute otitis media: I. The role of antibiotics in treatment of uncomplicated acute otitis media. *Pediatrics* 2001;108(2):239–247.

22. Mangione-Smith R, DeCristofaro AH, Setodji CM, Keesey J, Klein DJ, Adams JL, Schuster MA, McGlynn EA. The quality of ambulatory care delivered to children in the United States. *N Engl J Med* 2007;357(15):1515–1523.

23. McGlynn EA, Asch SM, Adams J, Keesey J, Hicks J, DeCristofaro A, Kerr EA. The quality of health care delivered to adults in the United States. *N Engl J Med* 2003;348(26):2635–2645.

24. National Foundation for Infectious Diseases: Pneumococcal disease fact sheet for the media. Available at http://www.nfid.org/idinfo/pneumococcal/media-factsheet.html. Accessed February 17, 2017.

25. James JT. A new, evidence-based estimate of patient harms associated with hospital care. *J Patient Saf* 2013;9(3):122–128.

26. Pronovost PJ, Bo-Linn GW. Preventing patient harms through systems of care. *JAMA* 2012;308(8):769–770.

27. Desmeules F, Boudreault J, Roy JS, Dionne C, Fremont P, MacDermid JC. The efficacy of therapeutic ultrasound for rotator cuff tendinopathy: a systematic review and meta-analysis. *Phys Ther Sport* 2015;16(3):276–284.

28. Ebadi S, Henschke N, Nakhostin Ansari N, Fallah E, van Tulder MW. Therapeutic ultrasound for chronic low-back pain. *Cochrane Database Syst Rev* 2014(3):Cd009169.

29. Silverman WA. *Human Experimentation: A Guided Step into the Unknown*. New York: Oxford University Press, 1985.

30. Isaacs D, Fitzgerald D. Seven alternatives to evidence based medicine. *BMJ* 1999;319:1618.

31. O'Donnell M. *A Sceptic's Medical Dictionary*. London: BMJ Books, 1997.

32. Sackett DL, Rosenberg WM, Gray JA, Haynes RB, Richardson WS. Evidence based medicine: what it is and what it isn't. *BMJ* 1996;312:71–72.

33. Straus SE, Glasziou P, Richardson WS, Haynes RB, Pattani R, Veroniki AA. *Evidence-Based Medicine: How to Practice and Teach It*. London: Elsevier, 2019.

34. Guyatt GH. Evidence-based medicine. *ACP J Club* 1991; 114(2):A16.

35. Carman KL, Maurer M, Mangrum R, Yang M, Ginsburg M, Sofaer S, Gold MR, Pathak-Sen E, Gilmore D, Richmond J, et al. Understanding an informed public's views on the role of evidence in making health care decisions. *Health Affairs* 2016;35(4):566–574.

36. Epstein RM, Alper BS, Quill TE. Communicating evidence for participatory decision making. *JAMA* 2004;291(19): 2359–2366.

37. Stewart M, Meredith L, Brown JB, Galajda J. The influence of older patient-physician communication on health and health-related outcomes. *Clin Geriatr Med* 2000;16(1):25–36, vii–viii.

38. Bastian H, Glasziou P, Chalmers I. Seventy-five trials and eleven systematic reviews a day: how will we ever keep up? *PLoS Med* 2010;7(9):e1000326.

39. Huang YP, Fann CY, Chiu YH, Yen MF, Chen LS, Chen HH, Pan SL. Association of diabetes mellitus with the risk of developing adhesive capsulitis of the shoulder: a longitudinal population-based followup study. *Arthritis Care Res* 2013;65(7): 1197–1202.

40. Zreik NH, Malik RA, Charalambous CP. Adhesive capsulitis of the shoulder and diabetes: a meta-analysis of prevalence. *Muscles Ligaments Tendons J* 2016;6(1):26–34.

41. Haynes RB, Sackett DL, Guyatt GH, Tugwell PS. *Clinical Epidemiology: How To Do Clinical Practice Research*. 3 ed. Philadelphia: Lippincott Willliams & Wilkins, 2006.

42. Samson D, Schoelles KM. Chapter 2: medical tests guidance (2) developing the topic and structuring systematic reviews of medical tests: utility of PICOTS, analytic frameworks, decision trees, and other frameworks. *J Gen Intern Med* 2012;27 Suppl 1:S11–S119.

43. Centre for Reviews and Dissemination. Systematic Reviews: CRD's Guidance for Undertaking Reviews in Health Care. York: University of York, 2006. Available at https://www.york.ac.uk/media/crd/Systematic_Reviews.pdf. Accessed February 3, 2017.

44. Schlosser RW, Koul R, Costello J. Asking well-built questions for evidence-based practice in augmentative and alternative communication. *J Commun Disord* 2007;40(3):225–238.

45. Cooke A, Smith D, Booth A. Beyond PICO: the SPIDER tool for qualitative evidence synthesis. *Qual Health Res* 2012;22(10): 1435–1443.

46. Perkins BA, Olaleye D, Zinman B, Bril V. Simple screening tests for peripheral neuropathy in the diabetes clinic. *Diabetes Care* 2001;24(2):250–256.

47. Donaghy A, DeMott T, Allet L, Kim H, Ashton-Miller J, Richardson JK. Accuracy of clinical techniques for evaluating lower limb sensorimotor functions associated with increased fall risk. *PM R* 2016;8(4):331–339.

48. Jernigan SD, Pohl PS, Mahnken JD, Kluding PM. Diagnostic accuracy of fall risk assessment tools in people with diabetic peripheral neuropathy. *Phys Ther* 2012;92(11):1461–1470.

49. Montori VM, Fernandez-Balsells M. Glycemic control in type 2 diabetes: time for an evidence-based about-face? *Ann Intern Med* 2009;150(11):803–808.

50. Roh YH, Yi SR, Noh JH, Lee SY, Oh JH, Gong HS, Baek GH. Intra-articular corticosteroid injection in diabetic patients with adhesive capsulitis: a randomized controlled trial. *Knee Surg Sports Traumatol Arthrosc* 2012;20(10):1947–1952.

51. Pai LW, Li TC, Hwu YJ, Chang SC, Chen LL, Chang PY. The effectiveness of regular leisure-time physical activities on long-term glycemic control in people with type 2 diabetes: A systematic review and meta-analysis. *Diabetes Res Clin Pract* 2016; 113:77–85.

52. Berenguera A, Mollo-Inesta A, Mata-Cases M, Franch-Nadal J, Bolibar B, Rubinat E, Mauricio D. Understanding the physical, social, and emotional experiences of people with uncontrolled type 2 diabetes: a qualitative study. *Patient Prefer Adherence* 2016;10:2323–2332.

53. Blanchard V, Barr S, Cerisola FL. The effectiveness of corticosteroid injections compared with physiotherapeutic interventions for adhesive capsulitis: a systematic review. *Physiother* 2010; 96(2):95–107.

54. Interprofessional Education Collaborative. *Core competencies for interprofessional collaborative practice: 2016 update.* Washington, DC: Interprofessional Education Collaborative, 2016.

55. Rappolt S. The role of professional expertise in evidence-based occupational therapy. *Am J Occup Ther* 2003;57(5):589–593.

56. Fetters L, Tilson J. *Evidence Based Physical Therapy*. Philadelphia: FA Davis, 2012.

57. Brown SJ. *Evidence-Based Nursing: The Research-Practice Connection*. Norwich, VT: Jones & Bartlett, 2018.

58. Arksey H, O'Malley L. Scoping studies: towards a methodological framework. *Int J Soc Res Methodol* 2005;8:19–32.

59. Burton M. An invisible unicorn has been grazing in my office for a month. . . Prove me wrong. Evidently Cochrane, October 7, 2016. Available at http://www.evidentlycochrane. net/invisible-unicorn-grazing-office/. Accessed June 16, 2017.

60. Alderson P. Absence of evidence is not evidence of absence. *BMJ* 2004;328(7438):476–477.

61. Centre for Evidence-Based Medicine: OCEBM Levels of Evidence. Available at http://www.cebm.net/ocebm-levels-of-evidence/. Accessed April 28, 2017.

62. Wright JG. A practical guide to assigning levels of evidence. *J Bone Joint Surg Am* 2007;89(5):1128-1130.

63. Guyatt G, Gutterman D, Baumann MH, Addrizzo-Harris D, Hylek EM, Phillips B, Raskob G, Lewis SZ, Schunemann H. Grading strength of recommendations and quality of evidence in clinical guidelines: report from an American College of Chest Physicians task force. *Chest* 2006;129(1):174-181.

64. Levin RF. Qualitative and quantitative evidence hierarchies: mixing oranges and apples. *Res Theory Nurs Pract* 2014;28(2): 110-112.

65. Giacomini MK. The rocky road: qualitative research as evidence. *ACP J Club* 2001;134(1):A11-13.

66. Daly J, Willis K, Small R, Green J, Welch N, Kealy M, Hughes E. A hierarchy of evidence for assessing qualitative health research. *J Clin Epidemiol* 2007;60(1):43-49.

67. Snöljung A, Mattsson K, Gustafsson LK. The diverging perception among physiotherapists of how to work with the concept of evidence: a phenomenographic analysis. *J Eval Clin Pract* 2014; 20(6):759–766.

68. Grol R, Grimshaw J. From best evidence to best practice: effective implementation of change in patients' care. *Lancet* 2003;362(9391):1225–1230.

69. Davis D, Evans M, Jadad A, Perrier L, Rath D, Ryan D, Sibbald G, Straus S, Rappolt S, Wowk M, et al. The case for knowledge translation: shortening the journey from evidence to effect. *BMJ* 2003;327(7405):33–35.

70. Graham ID, Logan J, Harrison MB, Straus SE, Tetroe J, Caswell W, Robinson N. Lost in knowledge translation: time for a map? *J Contin Educ Health Prof* 2006;26(1):13–24.

71. Straus SE, Tetroe J, Graham I. Defining knowledge translation. *CMAJ* 2009;181(3–4):165–168.

72. Candian Institutes of Health Research: Knowledge translation. Available at http://www.cihr-irsc.gc.ca/e/29418.html#2. Accessed July 14, 2017.

73. National Center for Dissemination of Disability Research: What is knowledge translation? *Focus: A Technical Brief from the National Center for the Dissemination of Disability Research.* Number 10. Available at http://ktdrr.org/ktlibrary/articles_pubs/ncddrwork/focus/focus10/Focus10.pdf. Accessed April 17, 2017.

74. Lubans DR, Lonsdale C, Cohen K, Eather N, Beauchamp MR, Morgan PJ, Sylvester BD, Smith JJ. Framework for the design and delivery of organized physical activity sessions for children and adolescents: rationale and description of the 'SAAFE' teaching principles. *Int J Behav Nutr Phys Act* 2017;14(1):24.

75. Oborn E, Barrett M, Racko G. *Knowledge Translation in Health Care: A Review of the Literature*. Cambridge, UK: Cambridge Judge Business School 2010.

76. Khalil H. Knowledge translation and implementation science: what is the difference? *Int J Evid Based Healthc* 2016;14(2):39-40.

77. Cohen J. Things I have learned (so far). *Am Pyschologist* 1990; 45(12):1304–1312.

78. Rubenfeld GD. Understanding why we agree on the evidence but disagree on the medicine. *Respir Care* 2001;46(12): 1442–1449.

Searching the Literature

—with Jessica Bell

Although most of us have had some experience obtaining references for term papers or assignments, technology has forever changed how we locate information, how quickly we want it, and the volume of data available. Clinicians often go to the literature to stay on top of scientific advances as part of professional development, or they may gather evidence specific to a patient for clinical decision-making. Researchers will review the literature to build the rationale for a study and to help interpret findings. This process, of course, assumes that we can locate and retrieve the relevant research literature. The purpose of this chapter is to describe strategies for successful literature searches that will serve the full range of information-seeking needs to support evidence-based practice (EBP).

■ Where We Find Evidence

We can think of "literature" broadly to include all scholarly products, including original research articles, editorials and position papers, reviews and meta-analyses, books and dissertations, conference proceedings and abstracts, and website materials.

Scientific Journals

When we think of searching for information in the health sciences, we typically will turn first to published journal articles. Thousands of journals are published by professional associations, societies or academies of practice, and other special interest groups, each with a specific disciplinary or content focus.

Most of these journals are **peer reviewed**, which means that manuscripts are scrutinized by experts before they are accepted for publication to assure a level of quality. It is important to appreciate this process, as it may have implications for the quality and validity of papers that we read.

Magazines

Scientific magazines are periodicals that include opinion pieces, news, information on policy, and reports of popular interest. These publications are often read by the public or by professionals from a particular field. Magazine pieces are not peer reviewed, do not generally contain primary research reports, and may present biased views. Most professional associations publish magazines that provide useful summaries of published studies or industry information that can give direction to further searching.

Government and Professional Websites

Government agencies, nongovernmental organizations, hospitals, advocacy organizations, and professional associations are eager to share the information and knowledge they have acquired, and frequently do so on their websites. Those sites are easily discoverable with a few well-worded searches in a Web search engine. A close examination of the source is always recommended to ensure its authority and accuracy of the information provided.

Grey Literature

Many useful sources of information can be found in what is called the **grey literature**, which is anything not produced by a commercial publisher. Government documents, reports, fact sheets, practice guidelines, conference proceedings, and theses or dissertations are some of the many nonjournal types of literature that fall under this category.[1] The grey literature can provide information such as demographic statistics, preliminary data on new interventions and professional recommendations, and results of experimental, observational, and qualitative inquiries that never made it to formal publication. Studies with null findings are particularly vulnerable to rejection by publishers. Regardless, these unpublished studies can be an important source of evidence.[2]

 Research reports have shown that journals are less likely to publish studies with negative findings or findings of no significant difference.[3] This **publication bias** must be considered when searching for relevant literature, clearly impacting what we can learn from published work (see Chapter 37). For instance, studies have shown that, by excluding grey literature, systematic reviews may overestimate intervention effects.[4,5]

Searching for grey literature does present a challenge. There are several databases, developed in the United States, Canada, and Europe (such as *Open Grey*,[6] *GreySource*,[7] and *Grey Net*[8]) that focus on grey literature. Unfortunately, many of these databases are not comprehensive and full references can be difficult to obtain. Internet strategies can be useful for locating grey literature. *Google* can locate websites related to your topic, and once identified, browsing through their pages can uncover many items of relevance.[9,10]

Any of the thousands of governmental and advocacy organizations, think tanks, and conference websites may have hidden gems that Google does not unearth. For instance, *ClinicalTrials.gov*, developed by the National Library of Medicine (NLM), is a database of ongoing and completed privately and publicly funded clinical studies conducted around the world.[10] You may also find that contacting researchers in a particular area of study will provide insight into ongoing studies.

Grey Matters is a comprehensive resource that provides guides to a variety of options for searching grey literature websites, including library websites that have created convenient databases.[11]

Primary and Secondary Sources

In the search for relevant literature, clinicians should be seeking primary data sources as much as possible. A **primary source** is a report provided directly by the investigator. Most research articles in professional journals are primary sources, as are dissertations or presentations of research results at conferences.

A **secondary source** is a description or review of one or more studies presented by someone other than the original authors. Review articles and textbooks are examples of secondary sources, as are reports of studies that often appear in newspapers, professional magazines, websites, or television news. Patients often receive their information about research through such methods.

Secondary sources may be convenient, but they can be incomplete, inaccurate, biased, or out-of-date, or they can present misleading information. Clinicians are frequently amazed, when they go back to the original reference, to discover how different their own interpretation of results may be from descriptions provided by others.

Systematic Reviews

Systematic reviews, meta-analyses, and clinical guidelines that include a critical analysis of published works may technically be secondary references, but they become primary sources as a form of research in generating new knowledge through rigorous selection criteria, evaluation of methodological quality, and conclusions drawn from the synthesis of previous research. Even then, however, when study details are relevant, evidence-based decisions will be better served by going back to the original reference. Reviews do not typically provide sufficient information on operational definitions, for example, for decisions to be based on a full understanding of an intervention or a measurement.

■ Databases

Regardless of the type of literature you seek, the most commonly used resources are literature databases. A **database** is an index of citations that is searchable by keywords, author, title, or journal. Some databases have been created by public agencies, others by private companies or publishers with varying levels of access (see Table 6-1). Many journals provide free full-text options as part of their listings within a database. The most commonly used databases in healthcare are MEDLINE, CINAHL, and the Cochrane Database of Systematic Reviews. Every health science clinician and researcher should be familiar with these databases at a minimum.

MEDLINE

MEDLINE is by far the most frequently used database in health-related sciences. Offered through the NLM, it indexes more than 5,200 journal titles and over 24 million

Table 6-1   Major Databases and Search Engines in Health and Social Sciences

DATABASE/SEARCH ENGINE	DESCRIPTION
ASHAWire *American Speech-Language- Hearing Association (ASHA)* pubs.asha.org	Catalogs articles from any ASHA publication. Searching is free but full text available by subscription or membership. *Free access.*
CINAHL *Cumulative Index to Nursing and Allied Health Literature* www.cinahl.com	Indexes published articles and other references relevant to nursing and the health professions. Coverage from 1937. *Requires subscription.*
ClinicalTrials.gov *National Institutes of Health* www.clinicaltrials.gov	The U.S. registry for clinical trials, which includes new, ongoing, and completed studies. *Free access.*
Cochrane Library of Systematic Reviews *The Cochrane Collaboration* www.cochranelibrary.com	Full-text systematic reviews of primary research in healthcare and health policy. Can be accessed through PubMed. *Free access, some full text.*
MEDLINE *National Library of Medicine* www.ncbi.nlm.nih.gov/pubmed/ www.pubmed.gov	Citations from life sciences and biomedical literature. Primary access through PubMed. *Free access, some full text.*
OT Search *American Occupational Therapy Association* www1.aota.org/otsearch/	Citations and abstracts from the occupational therapy literature and its related subject areas. *Fee-based subscription.*
PEDro *Center for Evidence-based Physiotherapy, University of Sydney, Australia* www.pedro.org.au/	Physiotherapy Evidence Database that includes abstracts of randomized clinical trials, systematic reviews, and practice guidelines. All trials include quality ratings using the PEDro scale. *Free access.*
PTNow Article Search *American Physical Therapy Association* www.ptnow.org	Full-text articles, clinical summaries synthesizing evidence for management of specific conditions, and resources on tests and measures. Provides access to other databases. *Requires APTA membership.*
SPORTDiscus *EBSCO* www.ebsco.com	Citations and full text for sports-related references, including nutrition, physical therapy, occupational health, exercise physiology, and kinesiology. *Requires subscription.*
UpToDate *Wolters Kluwer* www.uptodate.com	Point-of-care, clinical reference tool for EBP. Contains original entries written specifically for UpToDate that synthesize available evidence about clinically important topics. *Requires subscription.*

references in 40 languages.[12] A growing number of references include free full-text articles. Full references are available back to 1966. Earlier citations from 1946–1965 can be obtained through OLD MEDLINE, a limited data set available through PubMed and other platforms.[13]

PubMed

MEDLINE can be accessed through various platforms, but its primary access is obtained through PubMed, a platform developed and maintained by the National Center for Biotechnology Information (NCBI). It is undoubtedly the most-used health science application because it is free, readily available through the internet,

and comprehensive. PubMed includes the entirety of the MEDLINE database as well as supplemental content, including publications that are "ahead of print." It also includes information on studies that are funded through the National Institutes of Health (NIH), which are required to be freely accessible through the *PubMed Central (PMC)* repository.

CINAHL

The Cumulative Index to Nursing and Allied Health Literature (CINAHL) indexes references from nursing, biomedicine, health sciences, alternative/complementary medicine, consumer health, and 17 other health disciplines.[14] It is also a major point of access for citations from health sciences publications that do not appear in MEDLINE. Although there is substantial overlap with MEDLINE, its unique content is an important supplement. It is more likely to contain citations from smaller, specialty journals in the nursing, clinical, and rehabilitation fields.

CINAHL indexes more than 3.8 million records from more than 3,100 journals, with 70 full-text journals. It contains a mix of scholarly and other types of publications, including healthcare books, dissertations, conference proceedings, standards of practice, audiovisuals and book chapters, and trade publications that contain opinion and news items. Therefore, searchers need to be discerning when reviewing articles to be sure they know the validity of sources.

 To be included in MEDLINE, journal editors must submit an application.[12] They must be able to demonstrate that the journal records research progress in an area of life sciences and influences development and implementation of related policy. Many smaller or newer journals that do not yet qualify for MEDLINE will be accessible through CINAHL.

Cochrane Database of Systematic Reviews

As its the name implies, the **Cochrane Database of Systematic Reviews** contains citations of systematic reviews (see Chapter 37). It is managed by a global network of researchers and people interested in healthcare, involving more than 37,000 contributors from 130 countries.[15] Reviews are prepared and regularly updated by 53 Review Groups made up of individuals interested in particular topic areas. Cochrane systematic reviews are considered high quality with rigorous standards. References can be accessed directly through the Cochrane group or through other databases such as MEDLINE or Embase.

Evidence-Based Resources

Separate from literature reviews that are published as articles, there are databases devoted to helping clinicians with decision-making. These EBP databases come in a variety of types. Some provide single-article analyses such as the *Physiotherapy Evidence Database (PEDro)*, which includes quality assessments of randomized trials, listings of systematic reviews, and clinical practice guidelines. The *Cochrane Library* focuses on high-quality systematic reviews. Others, such as *UpToDate*, are "point of care" sources to provide clinicians with a quick overview of the research pertaining to all aspects of a diagnosis, treatment, or prognosis. Many journals include EBP reviews in specialized content.[16–18]

Search Engines

Search engines are platforms that access one or more databases. Some databases, such as MEDLINE, can be accessed from different search engines. In addition to PubMed, which is freely available, libraries will often provide access through OVID (an integrated system covering more than 100 databases[19]) or EBSCO,[14] both of which also offer access to e-books and other scholarly products. *Translating Research into Practice (Trip)* is a search engine geared primarily toward EBP and clinicians, searching multiple databases, and providing a search algorithm based on PICO.[20] *Google Scholar* provides free searching for a wide spectrum of references, including grey literature (see Focus on Evidence 6-1).[21]

Focus on Evidence 6–1
"'Google' is not a synonym for 'research.'"
— *Dan Brown, The Lost Symbol*

Everyone is familiar with Google and the ease of searching for just about anything. Google is not particularly useful in the search for research evidence, however. Although it may locate some sources, it does not focus on scientific literature and does not have the ability to designate search parameters to get relevant citations.

Google Scholar is a search engine that locates articles, books, and theses on a wide variety of topics and disciplines, generally from traditional academic publishers.[21] Although searches can be limited to specific authors or a certain time frame, it does not have search limits for research designs or languages, study subject characteristics, or many of the other features most databases have. Google Scholar can match PubMed in locating primary sources but will also find many more irrelevant citations.[22] It is best used in combination with other databases.

Google Scholar can be helpful at the beginning of your literature searching when you are struggling to find the right keywords, and will often provide full-text files for articles and reports that are not available from other sites.[23] It can also be helpful when searching for grey literature, but it requires thorough searching since these references will often be buried after 100 pages.[24]

Like its parent search engine, Google Scholar ranks results by popularity and filters results based on browser version, geographic location, and previously entered search strings.[25,26] Therefore, it is not recommended as a primary resource for systematic reviews or other searches because it cannot be replicated.

Many databases offer mobile apps as well as their full Web versions. PubMed and UpToDate are two that make it easy to keep the information you need right at your fingertips. PubMed's app even helps you set up a PICO search.

There are many additional resources available to broaden a search. See the *Chapter 6 Supplement* for an expanded table of available databases.

■ The Search Process

Whether you are asking a question for research or clinical purposes, the search process begins with identification of a question or topic of interest, which will lead to determination of appropriate search terms and databases (see Fig. 6-1). The PICO approach, introduced in Chapters 3 and 5, can be used to frame a search strategy. Implementing the search includes reviewing citations, reading abstracts, and choosing which references should be read.

Successful searches require several iterations, revising keyword strategies and using different databases. As you progress through a search, you will come to better understand the various terms that are used and thereby improve your search outcome. Do not be afraid to try different ways of entering keywords—you may discover useful alternatives.

Databases tend to have common approaches to the search process, although there will be some unique features and different interfaces. Given its widespread use, we will use PubMed to illustrate the major steps in searching. All databases have tutorials that will explain their specific use.

■ Keyword Searching

All electronic databases will utilize some form of algorithm to generate a list of citations based on the keywords you choose. For articles and books, citations will generally be brought up if a keyword is present in the title or abstract. Some databases will search the full contents of the reference, which leads to many more hits.

> ### ➤ CASE IN POINT
>
> Consider again the case presented in Chapter 5 of Mrs. H, a 67-year-old woman who has type 2 diabetes and was recently diagnosed with a frozen shoulder (adhesive capsulitis). It severely limits her function and her ability to do everyday chores. She has asked about the benefit of treatment options, including physical therapy and cortisone injection, to improve her recovery.

A clinician working with this patient may be interested in finding out the relative benefits of physical therapy or corticosteroid injections for someone with diabetes and frozen shoulder.

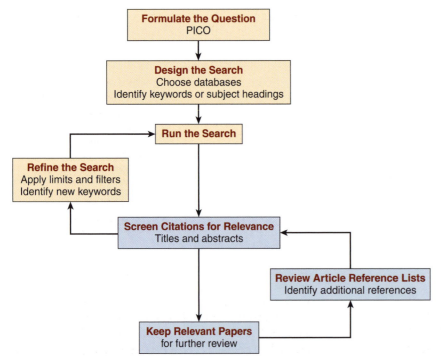

Figure 6–1 Overview of the search process.

> In patients with type 2 diabetes who have adhesive capsulitis, will physical therapy combined with corticosteroid injection be more effective than physical therapy alone to reduce pain, increase range of motion (ROM), and reduce shoulder disability?

We start by listing the elements of our question as they correspond to the PICO format (see Fig. 6-2). These words will help us generate search terms that will be entered into a database to find relevant references.

Finding the Right Words

We must determine how specific we need to be to identify the right references. At the start of a search, it is useful to brainstorm about the range of words that may apply to your topic, including synonyms and word variations.

P: Is "diabetes" sufficient or do we need to specify "type 2"? Is the patient's sex or age important for identifying relevant research? What terms best identify the patient's condition? For instance, "frozen shoulder" is more accurately termed "adhesive capsulitis."

I: Do we search for "physical therapy" or more specifically for a technique such as "exercise," "manual therapy," or "mobilization?"

C: Should the comparison treatment be called "cortisone" or "corticosteroid injection?"

O: Are pain and ROM the only variables of interest, or would we also want to look at measures of shoulder disability?

We must now choose the words we consider most relevant. We start our search at the PubMed homepage (see Fig. 6-3), entering keywords in the search window.

Keyword Phrases

When you are searching for phrases of two or more words, such as "adhesive capsulitis," some databases assume you always want those words next to each other and some do not. Enclosing a phrase in quotes will tell the database to consider the phrase a single term in the search.

Truncation and Wildcards

Truncation and **wildcards** are useful tools when a keyword has different forms, has alternate spellings, or could be pluralized. Truncation uses a symbol to replace endings on words and a wildcard uses a symbol to replace a letter in the middle of a word.

Typically, truncation uses an asterisk, but some databases may use $ or # instead. For example, the search term "mobiliz*" will bring back items with variations, such as "mobilize" or "mobilization."

A question mark is the typical symbol for wildcards. The most common use for wildcards is spelling variations between American and British English. For example, searching "mobili?ation" will bring back items that use "mobilization" as well as "mobilisation."

Boolean Logic

It is important to fine-tune the choice of keywords or reference terms to narrow the search. The PICO terms become possible keywords, but then we must consider how to combine them to generate citations that will relate to our question. Most databases and search engines use a system called **Boolean logic**, which uses three primary operators: AND, OR, and NOT.

Venn diagrams can be useful in helping to explain the way these operators function, as shown in Figure 6-4. The circles represent the citations resulting from a specific keyword search. Each time we combine keywords using one of the operators, our search returns those citations in the green sections.

🪶 HISTORICAL NOTE

George Boole (1815–1864), a British mathematician and philosopher, developed what came to be known as *Boolean algebra* in the mid-19th century. This new approach applied algebraic methods to logical reasoning and *Boolean logic* later became a foundational premise in computer sciences.

Several years later, John Venn (1834–1923), a British logician, introduced a new way to visualize this blend of algebra and logic using overlapping circles to represent common and unique elements in a system—a technique that would bear his name.

Boolean logic has become the basis for specifying sets of terms to focus searches and is typically represented by *Venn diagrams*.[4]

Boolean Operators

AND is used to combine two keywords, resulting in only citations that contain both. Figure 6-4A shows the combination of "adhesive capsulitis" and "physical therapy," represented by the blue overlapped section. Typically, AND

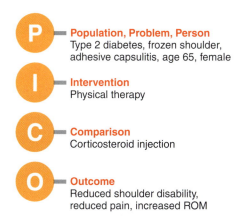

P — **Population, Problem, Person**
Type 2 diabetes, frozen shoulder, adhesive capsulitis, age 65, female

I — **Intervention**
Physical therapy

C — **Comparison**
Corticosteroid injection

O — **Outcome**
Reduced shoulder disability, reduced pain, increased ROM

Figure 6–2 Elements of a question using the PICO format.

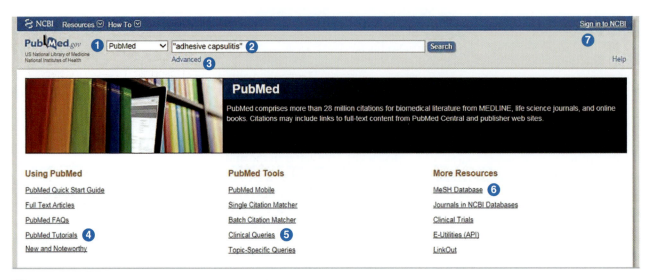

① This dropdown menu allows access to other databases provided by the National Library of Medicine, including *PubMed Central (PMC)*, and MeSH headings.

② We start the search by entering keywords or phrases into this search window.

③ Several advanced features can be accessed through this link, including combining and building complex searches (see Figure 6.8).

④ Tutorials and FAQs are useful for new and experienced users.

⑤ Clinical Queries allows searching specifically for references on therapy (intervention), diagnosis, prognosis, etiology, or clinical guidelines (see Figure 6.9).

⑥ MeSH terms can be accessed directly through this link.

⑦ *My NCBI* allows users to set up a free account, to personalize settings and save searches.

Figure 6–3 The search starts by entering keywords on the PubMed homepage. This page also lists several useful resources. *Accessed from The National Center for Biotechnology Information.*

is used to connect keywords representing different topics and will narrow the search only to references that include both. By adding a third term, "mobilization," we have further restricted our results to only those studies that use all three terms (see Fig. 6-4B).

OR broadens the search by combining two keywords, resulting in all citations that mention either word. Typically, OR is used to connect keywords that describe similar ideas that may be synonyms. Figure 6-4C shows the combination of "physical therapy" OR "mobilization," since both terms may be used for the intervention.

NOT excludes words from the search. For example, in this search we do not want to include studies that use "manipulation" for this condition. In Figure 6-4D, all references that include that term are omitted from the results. The NOT operator should be used judiciously, as it will often eliminate citations you might have found relevant. Other ways of narrowing the search should be tried first, such as strategies for refining the search, to be described shortly.

Nesting

Sometimes the focus of a search requires various combinations of keywords. Note, for example, the combination of **AND** and **OR** in Figure 6-4E. We have expanded the

search using OR to include articles that use either "physical therapy" or "mobilization," but we have put them in parentheses to connect them with "adhesive capsulitis" using AND. This is called **nesting** and is necessary for the database to interpret your search correctly. For example, if we had entered:

"adhesive capsulitis" AND "physical therapy" OR mobilization

without the parentheses, "OR mobilization" will be seen as an independent term, and all references to mobilization will be included, regardless of their connection to the first two terms.

■ Getting Results

Your search will result in a list of citations that match the keywords (see Fig. 6-5). As in this example, which shows 1,035 citations, initial searches often provide an overly long list that must be further refined. Looking through the titles can give you an idea of how closely the results match your intended search.

Clicking on any title will get you to the study abstract (see Fig. 6-6). All research papers, including systematic

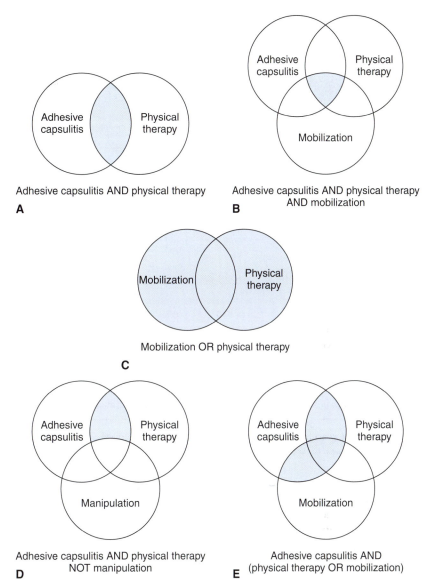

Figure 6–4 Venn diagrams illustrating the Boolean operators AND, OR, and NOT. The shaded areas reflect the results of the search.

reviews, are required to have an abstract, although the content can vary greatly depending on the journal. Most journals have a required format for abstracts, with specific categories of content, such as background, the study question or objective, population, study design, setting, methods, analysis, results, and conclusions. The abstract should give you a good idea of whether reading the full article will be worth your time.

■ Medical Subject Headings

The more traditional databases have added subject heading descriptors to help searchers find the most relevant content. These words are assigned to each article or book in the database and provide a consistent vocabulary

that can alleviate the need to brainstorm synonyms and word variations that arise when authors use different terminology for the same concepts. In the health sciences, the most well-known subject heading system has been developed by the NLM, called **Medical Subject Headings (MeSH)**. Although specifically developed for use with MEDLINE, many other databases have adopted the system.

MeSH consists of sets of terms in a hierarchical structure or "tree" that permits searching at various levels of specificity. The tree starts with broad categories and gradually narrows to more specific terms. In general, using both keywords and subject headings helps to ensure a more comprehensive list of results from your search, especially for systematic reviews. That said, there is not always a relevant subject heading for your needs.

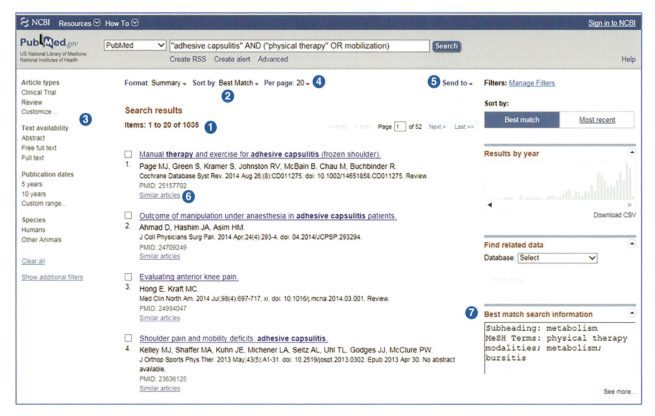

1 A total of 1,035 citations were returned. Only the first 20 are displayed.

2 The citations are sorted by "Best Match," based on an algorithm of the frequency of use of keywords. This dropdown menu includes other options such as "Most Recent," which lists citations in order of publication date, or alphabetical by author, journal, or title.

3 The left menu bar lists several limits that can be set for the search, including type of article, full-text options, and publication dates. The list of "Article Types" can be expanded using "Customize…" to specify RCTs, systematic reviews, or other formats. "Additional filters" include language, sex, age, and other descriptors. Clicking on these links will result in a revised display.

4 This dropdown menu allows you to set the number of citations viewed on the screen between 5 and 200.

5 The "Send to" dropdown menu allows you to save selected citations in several formats (see Figure 6.10).

6 Clicking on "Similar Articles" will generate a new list of citations with content similar to that article. Those citations will be listed in order of relevance to the original article.

7 MeSH terms are provided for the entered keywords. Note that "bursitis" is the heading under which "adhesive capsulitis" will be listed (see Figure 6.7).

Figure 6–5 Results of the initial search using "adhesive capsulitis" AND ("physical therapy" OR "mobilization") as keywords. This page offers several options for the display of results. *This search was run on April 5, 2018. Accessed from The National Center for Biotechnology Information.*

PubMed uses a feature called *automatic term mapping* to match your keywords to relevant MeSH terms and then automatically includes those headings in your search. These phrases do not need to be in quotes to be recognized. However, sometimes the keywords are matched to a heading that is not useful for your search. For example, by using *adhesive capsulitis* (without quotes), the MeSH term is *bursitis* (see Fig. 6-5 **7**). This will result in citations including studies of hip, knee, and shoulder joints, with many irrelevant results. If this happens, placing your phrase in quotation marks will force the search to limit results only to the exact phrase. You may want to try your search with and without quotation marks, just to see which works better for your particular topic.

Exploding and Focusing

When conducting subject heading searches, some databases give you features to help you broaden or narrow your search. **Exploding** the search means that the search will retrieve results using the selected term and all its narrower headings. For example, in our search related to Mrs. H., we may want to find articles related to diabetes. If our search includes the MeSH term "Diabetes

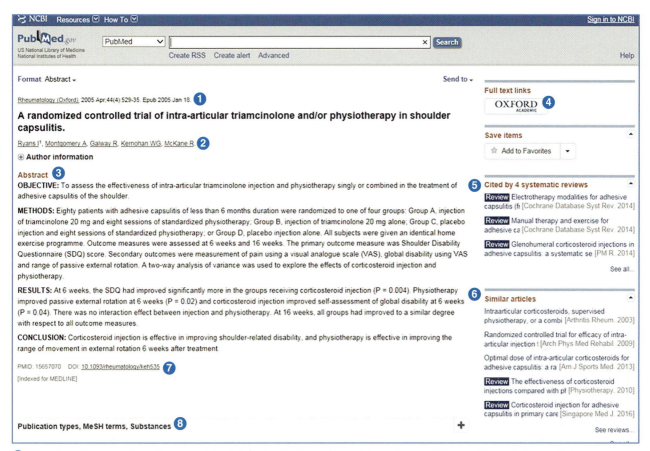

① The title and source information are provided, including the journal title, date, and pages. "Epub" indicates that this article was originally published electronically ahead of print.

② The authors' names are listed and clicking on an author's name will bring up a new list of citations by that author. "Author Information" can be expanded to reveal contact information.

③ The full abstract is provided. Formats will differ among journals.

④ This icon tells you that this article is available in full text. This may or may not be free. Click on the icon to get information on availability.

⑤ Systematic reviews that have referenced this study are listed here.

⑥ Articles with similar content are listed here. Clicking on these links will bring you to the abstract for that article.

⑦ "PMID" is the PubMed identifier. "DOI" is the digital object identifier, a unique number assigned to academic scholarly articles. These numbers are often included in reference lists and can be used to locate particular articles in a search.

⑧ Clicking on this link will provide a list of MeSH terms for the search keywords (see Figure 6.7).

Figure 6–6 The abstract display in PubMed, obtained by clicking on a citation link from the results page. *Accessed from The National Center for Biotechnology Information.*

Mellitus," the explode function allows that search to also include articles tagged with the narrower MeSH terms "diabetes mellitus, Type 1" and "Diabetes Mellitus, Type 2" along with several other subtypes of the disease. Some databases and search engines have the explode feature turned on automatically. This is true in PubMed.

Focusing the search means that it will be limited to documents for which the subject heading has been identified as a major point of the article. In Figure 6-7, you can tell which terms have been designated as major points because they are followed by asterisks. In PubMed, you can find the focus feature on the page for the MeSH term as a check box labeled "Restrict to MeSH Major Topic."

Subheadings

MEDLINE also uses a system of subheadings to further detail each MeSH term. In Figure 6-7, you can see the MeSH terms for one of the articles found in our PubMed search. You will notice that some of the terms are followed by a slash and a subheading, such as "Shoulder Joint/physiopathology." If you only want articles about the physiopathology of shoulder joints, this is one way to narrow your search.

Publication types, MeSH terms, Substances

Publication types
Clinical Trial
Comparative Study
Randomized Controlled Trial
Research Support, Non-U.S. Gov't

MeSH terms
Adult
Bursitis/drug therapy*
Bursitis/physiopathology
Bursitis/rehabilitation*
Double-Blind Method
Factor Analysis, Statistical
Female
Glucocorticoids/therapeutic use*
Humans
Injections, Intra-Articular
Male
Middle Aged
Pain Measurement/methods
Physical Therapy Modalities*
Range of Motion, Articular
Shoulder Joint/physiopathology
Single-Blind Method
Treatment Outcome
Triamcinolone/therapeutic use*

Substances
Glucocorticoids
Triamcinolone

Figure 6–7 MeSH terms listed by expanding the link at the bottom of the abstract in Figure 6-6 ❽. *Accessed from The National Center for Biotechnology Information.*

📌 The MeSH database can also be accessed from the PubMed homepage (see Fig. 6-3 ❻). Other databases have a mapping feature to help you find relevant headings. Look for a tutorial in the database you are using if you are not familiar with this process.

■ Refining the Search

Very rarely does a search hit the mark on the first try. Different combinations of words will provide different results; searching generally requires trying out those combinations to see which work best. As you read the

articles from your search, your familiarity with the topic increases, resulting in new terminology to use in your searching.

If your search provides too few articles, you may need to remove some of the specificity from your topic. Focus on the core ideas and remove any details that are not absolutely necessary. This is also a good time to brainstorm synonyms and spelling variations. For instance, including "OR frozen shoulder" or "OR exercise" may broaden the scope of results. MeSH terms may suggest alternate terminology.

If your search results in too many citations, you should be more specific in describing the population, intervention, or outcomes. Figure 6-8 shows how an iterative search using various combinations of terms has allowed us to narrow our results, including the use of some filters.

In search #7, the term "type 2 diabetes" yields a large number of items. However, when that term is combined with the previous comprehensive search (#6), we get only two results. This tells us that of the 66 citations in search #6, only 2 include "type 2 diabetes" in the title, abstract, or subject headings. That does not mean, however, that none of those other articles include "type 2 diabetes" in the body of the article. For example, that information could be a few pages into the article in the section describing the study participants. To be sure, we would have to return to the list of 66 and look through the full text of each article.

Limits and Filters

Search strategies can be refined by setting specific **limits** or **filters**, such as restricting results to studies of humans or animals, specific age groups or sexes, language, dates of publication, or studies that are provided as full text (see Fig. 6-5 ❸). Many databases also include limits relating to study design, such as case studies, randomized trials, or systematic reviews. In our search, we have used a filter to limit results to articles in English (Fig. 6-8 ❺). Clicking on these limits will result in a revised display of citations.

📌 The search described here was conducted using PubMed on April 5, 2018. Try running the same search to compare the results you get. You will likely find additional references since more information has undoubtedly been published since then! You may try to use some other search terms that might refine the search. You can also repeat the same search in another database, such as CINAHL, to see the difference in your results. Remember that CINAHL includes many publications that are not listed in MEDLINE, and may not index all of the references listed in PubMed.

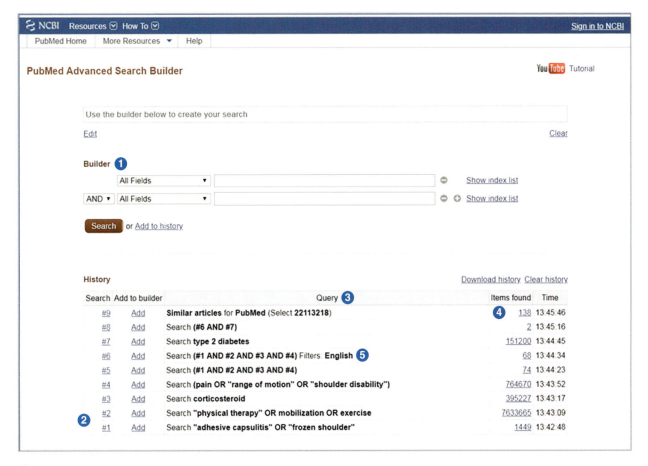

1 The search builder allows you to enter successive terms to create a comprehensive search.

2 Each successive search is numbered, with the most recent at the top.

3 The detailed terms for each search are provided. Searches can be combined by using keywords or using search numbers for prior searches.

4 The number of citations for each search is provided. By clicking on the number of items, the results of that search will be displayed.

5 If filters are applied (in this case for language), they will be indicated. There were six references from search #5 that were not published in English.

Figure 6–8 The Advanced Search page, obtained by clicking the link "Advanced" from the results or abstract page (see Figure 6-3 3). This page shows the details of a search history, allowing you to combine search components and to see the results of various keyword combinations. *Accessed from The National Center for Biotechnology Information.*

Clinical Queries

PubMed has developed predesigned strategies, called **Clinical Queries**, to target a search for studies on therapy (interventions), diagnosis, etiology, prognosis, or clinical prediction rules (see Fig. 6-9). It will generate references for clinical trials and systematic reviews.

Sensitivity and Specificity

Sensitivity is the proportion of relevant articles identified by a search out of all relevant articles that exist on that topic. It is a measure of the ability of the search strategy to identify all pertinent citations. A sensitive search casts a wide net to make sure that the search is comprehensive

and, therefore, may also retrieve may irrelevant references. In the PubMed Clinical Queries search, you can make the scope of your search more sensitive by using the drop-down menu to select "Broad" (see Fig. 6-9 3).

Specificity is the proportion of relevant citations that the search is able to retrieve, or a measure of the ability of the search strategy to exclude irrelevant articles. A specific search has more precision, trying to find only relevant documents. Therefore, while it is more likely to include only relevant studies, it might also exclude some relevant ones. In the Clinical Queries search, you can make the scope of your search more specific by using the drop-down menu to select "Narrow" (see Fig. 6-9 3).

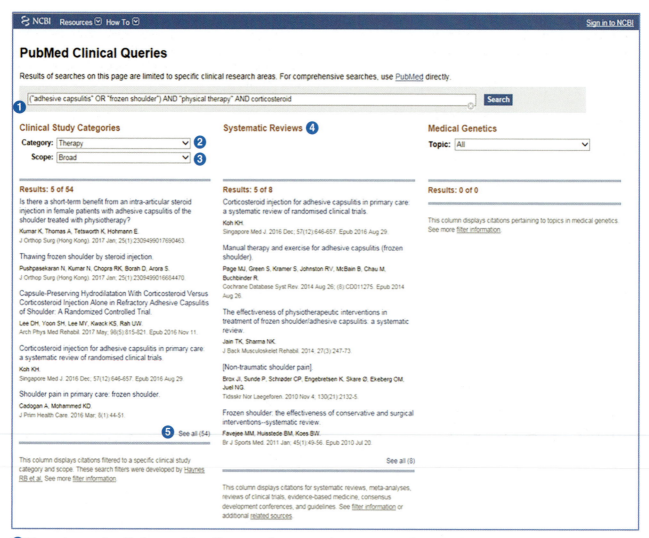

① Keywords are entered in the search box. Phrases are in quotes and terms are nested.

② Results are given for clinical study categories, with a dropdown menu that allows you to choose studies based on the type of clinical question: etiology, diagnosis, therapy (intervention), prognosis, or clinical prediction guides.

③ Dropdown menu for scope allows you to choose a narrow or broad focus, making the search more selective or more comprehensive. With a broad scope, we obtained 54 citations. If we had applied a narrow scope, the result would have only been 12 citations.

④ A separate category for systematic reviews is included.

⑤ The number of citations displayed can be expanded.

Figure 6–9 Screenshot of results of a search in "Clinical Queries," showing results for clinical trials and systematic reviews. A "Medical Genetics" search is a regular part of this feature, but does not result in any citations for this topic. This feature is accessed through a link on the PubMed homepage (see Figure 6-3 ⑤). *Accessed from The National Center for Biotechnology Information.*

📌 You will find analogous applications of the terms "sensitivity" and "specificity" in the use of diagnostic tests (see Chapter 33).

Find a Good Review

Clinicians and researchers will find systematic reviews to be a good place to start to identify gaps, understand the state of knowledge on a topic, and determine whether the question has already been answered in a valid way. Many databases have established specific search strategies to find these types of studies. For instance, in PubMed, reviews on a given topic can be obtained by checking "systematic reviews" under "Subsets" on the "Limits" tab (see Fig. 6-3 ③) or looking at the list of systematic reviews under "Clinical Queries" (see Fig. 6-9 ④).

To be sure that a systematic review encompasses the most recent findings, it is important to note the dates of the review, and if updates have been written.

Expanding Search Strategies

In many cases, database searching will not be sufficient to create a comprehensive literature review. Databases are not necessarily all-inclusive repositories and even expertly crafted searches will miss relevant materials. Therefore, researchers should employ techniques beyond keyword and subject heading searches.

Related References

Several databases offer an option to search "related articles" or "similar articles" once a relevant citation has been found (see Fig. 6-5 ❻ and 6-6 ❺). By using this function, one relevant article becomes the key to a list of useful references. These citations will usually be displayed in order of their relevance to the original reference.

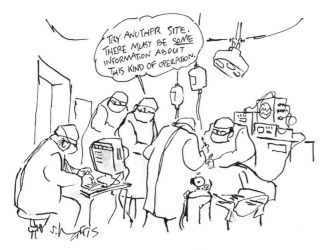

Illustration from Sidney Harris, courtesy of ScienceCartoonsPlus.com.

Reference Lists

The reference list at the end of published articles will provide a handy inventory of sources that were used by other authors in their review of literature. The obvious disadvantage of this approach is that you will only identify references that are older than the original article. But it is often a good place to start and to distinguish classic references that are used repeatedly. With electronic access, some journals provide direct links in their references using the PubMed ID or the DOI (see Fig. 6-6 ❼).

Cited Reference Searching

Many databases will allow you to discover whether an article has been cited by another (see Fig. 6-6 ❺). It is

similar to looking at an article's reference list but, instead of finding older articles, it finds articles published since the one in question. Look for links next to identified articles that say, "times cited in this database" or, "find citing articles."

> *Web of Science* is an entire database dedicated to helping track literature forward and backward. It can be an important component to any comprehensive search.

Journal and Author Searching

If an author is an expert on a subject, there is a good chance he or she has published more than one article on that topic. Most online databases make it easy to track down an author's other articles by making the name a link (see Fig. 6-6). Similarly, if you notice that a particular journal frequently publishes articles on your topic, browsing its tables of contents or doing general keyword searches limited to that journal may be advisable.

Choosing What to Read

As we have seen from our sample search, the number of references we locate may be daunting. To choose which articles to look at, the first pass is based on titles. Unfortunately, titles can sometimes be vague, and useful studies can be missed because authors did not provide an informative title. Therefore, a good strategy at this early stage is to be generous in your assessment and to choose all articles that seem potentially relevant.

The depth and scope of your search may depend on its purpose. When looking for references to inform a clinical decision, a good review or a few strong trials may be sufficient, especially if they are on point and the evidence is consistent. When trying to develop the rationale for a research question or do a systematic review, a more comprehensive literature review will be necessary. Always look for the highest level of evidence possible in choosing which references to consider (see Chapter 5).

Abstracts

The next step is to read the abstract (see Fig. 6-6). Remember, however, that abstracts are concise summaries of a study, usually with word limitations, and may not provide full details to understand the design, methods, or analysis. If the abstract suggests the study is relevant to your question, you will want to get the full text. Because abstracts can be incomplete in describing a study, it is not a substitute for reading the article.

📌 Opinion papers, commentaries, editorials, letters, and other nonresearch submissions do not have abstracts; you will generally have nothing but the title to inform you of the content.

■ Accessing Full Text

Many of us do not have access to large academic libraries and the impressive collections of journal subscriptions they offer, but reading the full text of articles is essential. Fortunately, there are several options available to obtain full-text articles.

Publishers

Many publishers will offer the full text of articles for a fee. When searching in PubMed, for example, you can click on the journal icon (see Fig. 6-6 ❹) to determine whether free text is available. If not, you will see information with rates for purchasing the article, which can be expensive. Some journals allow you to "rent" a copy for a limited time at less expense.

Some references will have a label under their citation that says, "Free Article." All articles published as part of *PMC* or the *Public Library of Science (PLOS)* will show icons for free full text.

Interlibrary Loan

If you have access to an academic library, it will generally offer free text from various journals through electronic subscriptions. If the article you need is not available, you can request a copy using **interlibrary loan**, whereby your home library will find another library with a subscription to the journal you need, request your article from that library, and send it to you electronically. Your library may charge for this service, but even when they do, the charge is generally far cheaper than the cost of purchasing directly from the publisher.

PubMed allows you to obtain articles by clicking on "Order" on the "Send to" menu (see Fig. 6-10) through a service called *Lonesome Doc*. You do this by agreement with an area library and it does incur a fee.

📌 Although you can limit a search to only articles that are available in full text (see Fig. 6-5 ❸), this can be counterproductive. You are likely to miss many important studies that will be essential to your search. Find citations for the articles that appear relevant and then consider the other ways to obtain the needed articles in full text if necessary.

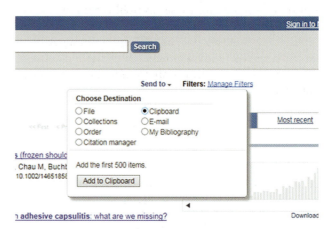

Figure 6–10 The "Send to" dropdown menu lists options to send selected citations from the results page to a saved file, collection, or clipboard (in My NCBI), a citation manager, an e-mail message, or a formatted bibliography. Articles can also be ordered in full text. This menu can be accessed from the results page or abstract page for a particular citation. *Accessed from The National Center for Biotechnology Information.*

Public Libraries

The electronic journal collections at most public libraries are better than you might think. Largely because of federal and state funding, most public libraries have been able to expand their online full-text databases to such an extent that it is worth a look if an academic library is not an option for you. You can usually access these resources from off-site.

Author Requests

Contact information for the first author of a paper is always provided with the publication, usually including mailing and e-mail addresses on the first page of the article. Electronic databases may include institutional information as a link with abstracts (see Fig. 6-6 ❷). Readers should take advantage of this information to communicate directly with authors to request copies of articles.

Open Access Journals

Open access is a term used to describe articles and journals that are free of restrictions on access. There are many journals that are entirely open access, meaning every article they publish is free. In addition, many traditional journals give authors an open access option for their articles, although that option often comes with a fee (See Chapter 38). Since 2005, the NIH has required that all funded articles be available as open access and made available through PMC.

Epub Ahead of Print

Articles often appear on publishers' websites prior to the release of a journal issue. Publishers also have the option of submitting these prepublication articles to PubMed, which will include the notation "Epub" followed by a date (see Fig. 6-6 ❶). Full-text availability of this type of article varies depending on the publisher, as many will limit access only to individuals or library subscribers.

■ Staying Current and Organized

The volume of literature that is available in healthcare can be truly overwhelming and the rates at which new information is produced is staggering. Many of us subscribe to a variety of journals that concentrate on our areas of clinical interest and just keeping up with that reading can be an overwhelming task. As one strives to stay up to date in an environment that is increasingly focused on evidence, taking advantage of tools and applications is a necessity.

My NCBI

Establishing an NCBI account through PubMed allows you to save records and searches, as well as customize your results display with filters and other personalized options (see Fig. 6-3 ❼). Registration with a password is required and access is free. Most databases have similar features. Look for links to log in or create an account.

Saving Searches

When proceeding through several iterations of a search, sometimes over more than 1 day, you do not want to lose your work. You can save your searches in a number of ways. In PubMed, you can save references by "sending" them to a *clipboard*, which will hold a list of selected references for up to 8 hours (see Fig. 6-10). For a more permanent option, you can save references to various *collections* that you specify so that you can refer to them later. If you have established a profile through *My NCBI*, you can refer selected references to a previously identified collection or name a new one.

E-mail Alerts

Many databases provide a way to let the literature come to you. E-mail alert services provide regular automatic updates delivered to your inbox. These services are usually free. They deliver current citations (with abstracts) or the table of contents of selected journals. Databases such as PubMed (through My NCBI), CINAHL, and many others let you set up alerts based on a saved search profile. Many journals allow individuals to register to receive free alerts for their tables of contents each month. Some journals will also send out alerts for early release of certain articles.

Social Media

Several online forums help researchers make connections and find out about colleagues' research activities. One popular site is *ResearchGate*, which is an international network of more than 14 million members, providing the opportunity for researchers to share papers, ask and answer questions, and find collaborators.[27] You can make direct requests for full text to authors through this site. By registering, authors can catalogue their publications, receive notifications of reprint requests, and obtain citation statistics for their articles.

Researchers frequently use *Twitter* to share early results or updates. Many conferences also encourage attendees to tweet with designated hash tags so that people who are not attending can follow along. Be warned that if you use any of these tools in your personal life, you may want to create a separate persona for your professional communication.

Citation Management Applications

With the amount of information available to researchers, it is easy to lose track of references. If you are working on a research study or gathering literature on a particular clinical topic, you will undoubtedly want to save your references. Many citation management tools are available to help you organize your searches, also called reference or bibliographic management applications. They help you store and organize references and full-text *pdf* files in a library, search for references, and, even more importantly, format your reference lists in a written paper. Citations can be saved using the "Send To" menu on the results or abstract page (see Fig. 6-10).

Two of the most commonly used tools are *RefWorks*,[28] which is Web based, and *EndNote*,[29] which is computer based. They both require purchase or subscription but may be free if you are affiliated with an academic library. Free reference tools are also available, such as *Mendeley*[30] and *Zotero*,[31] two of the most highly regarded. Whether free or through subscription, each tool has strengths and weaknesses; it is advisable to try one or more of them before launching into any project that requires a large amount of information gathering. Most of these programs will allow importing and exporting references between them.

■ When Is the Search Done?

Good question—but one that will probably depend on the purpose of your search. You need to be thorough, but at the same time exercise judgment to know when you have found the bulk of relevant literature so you can move on to the next phase of your decision-making or research. Do not let your literature search be a "forever" task!

Looking for Evidence

If you are looking for evidence to support a clinical decision, you may find yourself sufficiently informed by finding a few recent clinical trials or systematic reviews that provide a broad enough perspective for you to move forward. Meta-analyses provide additional information on the size of effects or the statistical significance of outcomes. You will want to see some consistency across these studies to help you feel confident in results. In addition, you will want to critically appraise the quality of the studies to determine whether they provide adequate validity for their findings (see Chapter 36).

Depending on the amount of literature that exists on your topic, you may need to think broadly about the pathophysiology and theoretical issues that pertain to your patient's problem. For example, you may not find references on adhesive capsulitis and corticosteroid injections specific to 67-year-old women and, as we have seen, perhaps not even specific to type 2 diabetes. You will need to connect the dots and may have to ask background questions to substantiate your decisions (see Chapter 5). Allow yourself to be satisfied once you have obtained relevant references that provide consistent, logical rationale.

Review of Literature

If your purpose is to establish a foundation for a research question, your approach will need to be more comprehensive. There are likely to be many different topics that need to be addressed, including theoretical underpinnings of your question, how variables have been defined, which design and analysis strategies have been used, and what results have been obtained in prior studies. It is essential to establish the state of knowledge on the topic of interest; therefore, a thorough review is necessary.

Starting with a recent systematic review is the best strategy, assuming one is available, but you will need to get full-text references to determine the actual study methods. As you review recent studies, you will find that reference lists contain the same citations and eventually you will be able to determine that you have obtained the most relevant information. You will also likely continue to search the literature as your study goes on, especially as you interpret your results, needing to compare your findings with other study outcomes. Setting e-mail alerts for related topics can be helpful as your study progresses.

Next Steps

Searching and retrieval of references is one early step in the process of reviewing literature. Whatever your purpose, you will now need to determine how useful the references are. Most importantly, you will need to assess their quality—how well the studies have been executed. You need to determine whether the results are valid and whether they provide sufficient information for you to incorporate into your clinical decisions or research plan. This requires an understanding of design and analysis concepts.

COMMENTARY

If at first you don't succeed, search, search again. That's why they call it research.
—*Unknown*

Information is essential to the health professions. Whatever the reason for your literature search, be it for research or clinical purposes, it can be a frustrating process if you are not knowledgeable and experienced in the use of resources available to you. Although we have reviewed some of the basic strategies for identifying relevant databases and putting searches together, we cannot begin to cover all the possible search strategies or variations a particular search may require. Take advantage of the tutorials and tips offered by most search engines and databases, or classes sponsored by many libraries.

Because of our unlimited access to the internet, many of us, at least the digital natives, feel very self-sufficient in searching for information. But searching for the right literature to inform practice or support research rationale is not always so simple. The lament we have heard all too often is, "I've spent 5 hours searching and haven't found anything!" This is not a good use of anyone's time! Whether you are just beginning to conceptualize your question, have hit a dead end in your search, or need advice about evaluating and organizing the information you have found, reference librarians can help. Do not hesitate to take advantage of these experts who understand how information is created, organized, stored, and retrieved, and who are experienced in working with researchers of all types. They will also be able to keep you apprised of changes in databases or search options, as these are often updated.

REFERENCES

1. Blackhall K. Finding studies for inclusion in systematic reviews of interventions for injury prevention: the importance of grey and unpublished literature. *Inj Prev* 2007;13(5):359.
2. Citrome L. Beyond PubMed: Searching the "Grey Literature" for clinical trial results. *Innov Clin Neurosci* 2014;11(7–8):42–46.
3. Joober R, Schmitz N, Annable L, Boksa P. Publication bias: what are the challenges and can they be overcome? *J Psychiatry Neurosci* 2012;37(3):149–152.
4. Hopewell S, McDonald S, Clarke M, Egger M. Grey literature in meta-analyses of randomized trials of health care interventions. *Cochrane Database Syst Rev* 2007(2):Mr000010.
5. McAuley L, Pham B, Tugwell P, Moher D. Does the inclusion of grey literature influence estimates of intervention effectiveness reported in meta-analyses? *Lancet* 2000;356(9237):1228–1231.
6. Open Grey. Available at http://www.opengrey.eu/. Accessed April 10, 2018.
7. GreySource. Available at http://www.greynet.org/greysourceindex.html. Accessed April 10, 2018.
8. GreyNet International 2018. Available at http://www.greynet.org/. Accessed April 10, 2018.
9. Godin K, Stapleton J, Kirkpatrick SI, Hanning RM, Leatherdale ST. Applying systematic review search methods to the grey literature: a case study examining guidelines for school-based breakfast programs in Canada. *Syst Rev* 2015;4:138.
10. ClinicalTrials.gov. Available at https://clinicaltrials.gov/ct2/home. Accessed April 21, 2018.
11. CADTH Information Services: Grey Matters: A Practical Tool for Searching Health-related Grey Literature. Canadian Agency for Drugs and Technologies in Health, 2015. Available at https://www.cadth.ca/resources/finding-evidence/grey-matters. Accessed April 10, 2018.
12. US National Library of Medicine: Fact Sheet: MEDLINE. Available at https://www.nlm.nih.gov/pubs/factsheets/medline.html. Accessed January 30, 2018.
13. US National Library of Medicine: OLDMEDLINE Data. Available at https://www.nlm.nih.gov/databases/databases_oldmedline.html. Accessed January 30, 2018.
14. EBSCO Health. CINAHL Database. Available at https://health.ebsco.com/products/the-cinahl-database. Accessed February 4, 2018.
15. Cochrane Collaboration. Available at http://www.cochrane.org/. Accessed March 25, 2018.
16. ACP Journal Club: *Annals of Internal Medicine*. Available at http://annals.org/aim/journal-club. Accessed April 21, 2018.
17. BMJ Evidence-Based Medicine: *BMJ Journals*. Available at http://ebm.bmj.com/. Accessed April 21, 2018.
18. Family Physicians Inquiries Network: Evidence-Based Practice. Available at http://fpin.org/page/EBPAbout. Accessed April 21, 2018.
19. Ovid Technologies: Databases on Ovid. Available at http://www.ovid.com/site/catalog/databases/index.jsp. Accessed February 5, 2018.
20. Translating Research into Practice. Available at https://www.tripdatabase.com/. Accessed March 31, 2018.
21. Google Scholar. Available at http://scholar.google.com. Accessed February 16, 2018.
22. Freeman MK, Lauderdale SA, Kendrach MG, Woolley TW. Google Scholar versus PubMed in locating primary literature to answer drug-related questions. *Ann Pharmacother* 2009;43(3):478–484.
23. Shariff SZ, Bejaimal SA, Sontrop JM, Iansavichus AV, Haynes RB, Weir MA, Garg AX. Retrieving clinical evidence: a comparison of PubMed and Google Scholar for quick clinical searches. *J Med Internet Res* 2013;15(8):e164.
24. Haddaway NR, Collins AM, Coughlin D, Kirk S. The role of Google Scholar in evidence reviews and its applicability to grey literature searching. *PLoS One* 2015;10(9):e0138237.
25. Bates ME. Is Google hiding my news? *Online* 2011;35(6):64.
26. Mahood Q, Van Eerd D, Irvin E. Searching for grey literature for systematic reviews: challenges and benefits. *Res Synth Methods* 2014;5(3):221–234.
27. ResearchGate. Available at https://www.researchgate.net. Accessed March 3, 2018.
28. RefWorks 2.0 Quick Start Guide. Available at https://www.refworks.com/refworks2/help/RefWorks_QSG_EN_Dec11.pdf. Accessed March 4, 2018.
29. EndNote. Available at http://www.endnote.com/. Accessed March 4, 2018.
30. Mendeley. Available at https://www.mendeley.com/. Accessed March 4, 2018.
31. Zotero. Available at https://www.zotero.org/. Accessed March 4, 2018.

Ethical Issues in Clinical Research

Ethical issues are of concern in all health professions, with principles delineated in codes of ethics that address all aspects of practice and professional behavior. Clinical research requires special considerations because it involves the participation of people for the purpose of gaining new knowledge that may or may not have a direct impact on their lives or health. We ask them to contribute to our efforts because we seek answers to questions that we believe will eventually be of benefit to society. Because their participation may put them at risk, or at least some inconvenience, it is our responsibility to ensure that they are treated with respect and that we look out for their safety and well-being. We also know that published findings may influence clinical decisions, potentially affecting the lives of patients or the operation of health systems. Therefore, we must be vigilant to ensure the integrity of data.

The purpose of this chapter is to present general principles and practices that have become standards in the planning, implementation, and reporting of research involving human subjects or scientific theory. These principles apply to quantitative and qualitative studies, and they elucidate the ethical obligation of researchers to ensure protection of the participants, to safeguard scientific truth, and to engage in meaningful research.

■ The Protection of Human Rights

In our society, we recognize a responsibility to research subjects for assuring their rights as individuals. It is unfortunate that our history is replete with examples of unconscionable research practices that have violated ethical and moral tenets.[1] One of the more well-known examples is the Tuskegee syphilis study, begun in the 1930s, in which treatment for syphilis was withheld from rural, black men to observe the natural course of the disease.[2] This study continued until the early 1970s, long after penicillin had been identified as an effective cure.

One would like to think that most examples of unethical healthcare research have occurred because of misguided intentions and not because of purposeful malice. Nonetheless, the number of instances in which such behavior has been perpetrated in both human and animal research mandates that we pay attention to both direct and indirect consequences of such choices (see Focus on Evidence 7-1).

Regulations for Conducting Human Subjects Research

Since the middle of the 20th century, the rules of conducting research have been and continue to be discussed, legislated, and codified. Establishment of formal guidelines delineating rights of research subjects and obligations of professional investigators became a societal necessity as clear abuses of experimentation came to light.

Nuremberg Code

The first formal document to address ethical human research practices was the 1949 *Nuremberg Code*.[3] These

Focus on Evidence 7–1
The Failings of Research—Two Important Examples

Willowbrook Hospital Hepatitis Study

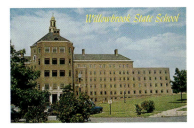

Courtesy of The New York Public Library Digital Collections.

The Remarkable Cells of Henrietta Lacks

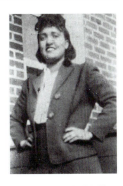

Photo courtesy of https://en.wikipedia.org/wiki/File:Henrietta_Lacks_(1920-1951).jpg

In 1965, the Willowbrook State School in Staten Island, NY, housed 6,000 children with severe intellectual disabilities, with major overcrowding and understaffing. With a 90% rate of infection with hepatitis in the school, Dr. Saul Krugman was brought in to study the natural history of the disease. Through the 1960s, children were deliberately exposed to live hepatitis virus and observed for changes in skin, eyes, and eating habits.[9] Krugman[10] reasoned that the process was ethical because most of the children would get hepatitis anyway, they would be isolated to avoid exposure to other diseases, and their infections would eventually lead to immunity. Although they obtained informed consent from parents following group information sessions, and approvals through New York University (prior to IRBs),[11] the ethical dimensions of these studies raise serious concerns by today's standards. The abuses and deplorable conditions at Willowbrook were uncovered in a shattering television exposé by Geraldo Rivera in 1972,[12] and the school was eventually closed in 1987.

Henrietta Lacks was a patient at Johns Hopkins Hospital in 1951, where she was assessed for a lump in her cervix.[13] A small tissue sample was obtained and she was subsequently diagnosed with cancer. In the process of testing the sample, however, scientists discovered something unusual. One of the difficulties in cancer research was that human cells would not stay alive long enough for long-range study—but Henrietta's cancer cells not only survived, they continued to grow. The line of cells obtained from her, named HeLa, has now been used in labs around the world for decades, and has fostered large-scale commercial research initiatives.

Neither Henrietta nor her family ever gave permission for the cells to be used, nor were they even aware of their use until 1973, long after her death in 1951. And of course, they accrued no benefit from the financial gains that were based on her genetic material. The family sued, but was denied rights to the cell line, as it was considered "discarded material."[14] The DNA of the cell line has also been published, without permission of the family. There have since been negotiations, assuring that the family would have some involvement in further applications of the cell line. The Henrietta Lacks Foundation was established in 2010 to "help individuals who have made important contributions to scientific research without personally benefiting from those contributions, particularly those used in research without their knowledge or consent."[15] This compelling story has been chronicled in *The Immortal Life of Henrietta Lacks*,[13] which has been turned into a movie.

guidelines were developed in concert with the Nuremberg trials of Nazi physicians who conducted criminal experimentation on captive victims during World War II. The most common defense in that trial was that there were no laws defining the legality of such actions.[4]

The *Nuremberg Code* clearly emphasized that every individual should voluntarily consent to participate as a research subject. Consent should be given only after the subject has sufficient knowledge of the purposes, procedures, inconveniences, and potential hazards of the experiment. This principle underlies the current practice

of obtaining informed consent prior to initiation of clinical research or therapeutic intervention. The Nuremberg Code also addresses the competence of the investigator, stating that research "should be conducted only by scientifically qualified persons."

Declaration of Helsinki

The World Medical Association adopted the *Declaration of Helsinki* in 1964.[5] It has been amended and reaffirmed several times, most recently in 2013. This document addresses the concept of independent review of research protocols by a committee of individuals who are not associated with the proposed project. It also declares that reports of research that has not been conducted according to stated principles should not be accepted for publication. This led to an editorial challenge to professional journals to obtain assurance that submitted reports of human studies do indeed reflect proper attention to ethical conduct. Most journals now require acknowledgment that informed consent was obtained from subjects and that studies received approval from a review board prior to initiating the research.

National Research Act

In 1974, the National Research Act was signed into law by Richard Nixon, largely in response to public recognition of misconduct in the Tuskegee syphilis study.[6] This law requires the development of a full research proposal that identifies the importance of the study, obtaining informed consent, and review by an **Institutional Review Board (IRB)**. These essential principles have been incorporated into federal regulations for the protection of human subjects.[7]

Belmont Report

The National Research Act established the National Commission for the Protection of Human Subjects of Biomedical and Behavioral Research. The deliberations and recommendations of this Commission resulted in the *Belmont Report* in 1979, which delineates the guiding ethical principles for human research studies.[8] The Belmont Report also established the rules and regulations that govern research efforts of the Department of Health and Human Services (DHHS) and the Food and Drug Administration (FDA). The Office for Human Research Protection (OHPR) is the administrative arm of the DHHS that is responsible for implementing the regulations and providing guidance to those who conduct human studies.

> The *Belmont Report* established boundaries between research and practice.[8] Although both often take place in similar settings and may be implemented by the same people, practice is considered routine intervention for the benefit of an individual that has reasonable expectation of success. In contrast, research is an activity designed to test a hypothesis, draw conclusions, and contribute to generalizable knowledge, which may or may not benefit the individual being studied. Research is also typically described in a formal protocol that sets objectives and procedures.

The Common Rule

Based on tenets in the Belmont Report, the Federal Policy for the Protection of Human Subjects, known as the *Common Rule*, outlines the basic provisions for ethical research. Originally published in 1991, revised in 2011 and again in 2019, this rule codifies regulations adopted by many federal departments and agencies, with a focus on institutional guidelines, informed consent, and review of proposals for the protection of participants. Researchers should become familiar with the substantial changes in the 2019 revision, as these will also require changes to institutional guidelines.[16] Technically, studies that are not federally funded are not required to follow these regulations, although most institutions use the Common Rule as a guide nonetheless.

> See the *Chapter 7 Supplement* for a description of the major 2019 revisions to the Common Rule.

> The *Health Insurance Portability and Accountability Act (HIPAA)* of 1996 and the resultant regulations (the *Privacy Rule*) issued by the DHHS have added a new dimension to the process of protecting research subjects related specifically to the protection of private health information.[17]

Guiding Ethical Principles

The Belmont Report established three basic ethical principles that have become the foundation for research efforts, serving as justification for human actions: respect for persons, beneficence, and justice.[8]

Respect for Persons

Respecting human dignity is essential to ethical behavior. This principle incorporates two considerations. The first is personal **autonomy**, referring to self-determination and the capacity of individuals to make decisions affecting their lives and to act on those decisions. This principle also recognizes that those with diminished autonomy must be protected. Some individuals who may be appropriate subjects for research, such as children or patients with cognitive problems, may be unable to deliberate about personal goals. In these cases, the researcher is obliged to ensure that an authorized surrogate decision-maker is available, has the ability to make a reasoned decision, and is committed to the well-being of the compromised individual.

Beneficence

Beneficence refers to the obligation to attend to the well-being of individuals. This extends to research projects and the entire research enterprise to ensure that all who engage in clinical research are bound to maximize possible benefits and minimize possible harm. Risks may be physical, psychological, social, or economic harm that goes beyond expected experiences in daily life. Research benefits may include new knowledge that can be applied to future subjects or patients, or that may have a direct impact on study participants, such as improved health status. The analysis of the *risk-benefit* relationship measures the probability and magnitude of benefit against the probability of anticipated harm or discomfort. Beneficence requires that an investigation be justified when studying a treatment to determine its benefits despite known risks, especially if these risks are substantial.[8] The attempted justification for the Willowbrook hepatitis study, for example, would challenge this principle.

Justice

Justice refers to fairness in the research process, or the equitable distribution of the benefits and burdens.[8] This principle speaks to the fair selection of subjects who are appropriate for a given study, drawn from a defined population that is most likely to benefit from the research findings. The selection of subjects should not be discriminatory based on an irrelevant criterion, but on reasons directly related to the problem being studied. Studies supported by public funds must demonstrate that they are including a full range of subjects who might benefit from the research applications. Questions of justice also apply to the burden of research, especially if subjects are drawn from less fortunate populations. For example, patients with fewer resources may be targeted, even though benefits will favor those who can afford better care. The Tuskegee study is an example, as syphilis was by no means confined to that population.[8]

■ The Institutional Review Board

According to federal regulations, an IRB must review research proposals prior to implementation to ensure that the rights of research subjects are protected.[7] The IRB must have at least five members with diverse backgrounds that facilitate complete and adequate reviews of the scientific and ethical details of proposed research. At least one member must be concerned primarily with nonscientific issues and may be a lawyer, clergyman, or ethicist.

Federal regulations require that all those involved in the design and conduct of research undergo training in safety and ethics of research. This includes all personnel who will be involved with subjects or handling of data. One of most widely used services is the Collaborative Institutional Training Initiative (CITI) Program,[18] which provides several courses in biomedical and social-behavioral-educational research. Certification by CITI is required for all individuals engaged in research at any institutions that have funding through the National Institutes of Health (NIH).

Review of Proposals

The responsibility of the IRB is to review research proposals at convened meetings. The decision to approve, require modifications in, defer approval, or deny approval of a proposal must be that of a majority. In arriving at a decision, the IRB considers the scientific merit of the project, the competence of the investigators, the risk to subjects, and the feasibility based on identified resources. The IRB also has the authority to terminate approval if research is not being conducted in accordance with requirements, or if participants are being subjected to unexpected harms.

If a project is not scientifically sound or practical, there can be no benefit; therefore, no risk to subjects is justified. Reviewers will consider the risk-benefit ratio, based on evidence that the risks and discomforts to the subject are reasonable, have been minimized, and are sufficiently outweighed by the potential benefits of the proposed study. The IRB also looks at the procedures for selecting subjects, ensuring that they are equitable, and that voluntary informed consent is based on complete and understandable descriptions and conforming to the applicable elements of privacy. The majority of proposals submitted to an IRB are reviewed in this detailed manner.

Expedited or Exempt Review

Some categories of research activity may qualify for an expedited review or may be exempted from the review process. A project may qualify for *expedited review* in circumstances such as "recording data from subjects 18 years of age or older using noninvasive procedures routinely employed in clinical practice," or "moderate exercise by healthy volunteers."[7] IRBs may expedite review of projects involving retrospective studies, when data are used from medical records, and all subjects are de-identified. The advantage of expedited review is that it is usually completed in less time than that required for a full IRB review.

Exempt reviews may be allowed for surveys, interviews, or studies of existing records, provided that the data are collected in such a way that subjects cannot be identified. The revisions to the Common Rule have established several exempt categories, including research in educational settings that involve normal learning situations, studies involving benign behavioral interventions, secondary research, and demonstration projects focused on public benefits.[16]

All proposals for studies involving human subjects must be submitted to the IRB, which then determines whether a project qualifies for full review, expedited review, or is exempt (see Fig. 7-1). The researcher does not make that determination.

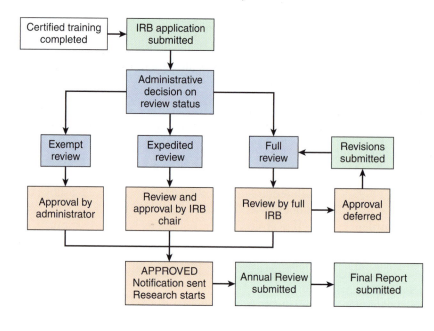

Figure 7–1 Progress of a proposal through the IRB process with different levels of review.

 Under the revised Common Rule, *broad consent* is a new standard that can be applied to the storage, maintenance, and secondary use of identifiable data or biospecimens in future, yet-to-be specified research. This does require identification of the types of research that may be conducted with the data.[19]

Institutional Guidelines

Each institution establishes its own guidelines for review in accordance with federal and state regulations. Researchers should, therefore, become familiar with the requirements in their own institutions, especially as the new Common Rule is being implemented. For instance, one useful change is a new provision that studies conducted at multiple sites only need to obtain approval from one IRB that will oversee the study. The approval process can take several weeks, depending on the IRB's schedule and whether the proposal needs revision. This review process should be included in the timetable for any research project. Research on human subjects should not be started without prior review and approval of a designated review committee.

IRBs require regular reporting of ongoing studies, typically on an annual basis. Researchers must be able to document the current status of the project. Any changes to the protocol must also be filed for approval before they take effect. Researchers are also responsible for notifying the IRB promptly of any critical incidents associated with the project. A final notification must be submitted when the study is completed, which will include information on subjects and study outcomes. Under the new Common Rule, studies involving minimal risk may no longer be required to submit annual reports, but will still need to keep the IRB updated regarding any changes or problems that arise.[16]

■ Informed Consent

Perhaps the most important ethical tenet in human studies is the individual's ability to agree to participate with full understanding of what will happen to him. The **informed consent** process and all its elements address the basic principles of respect, beneficence, and justice.

> **➤ CASE IN POINT**
> A trial was conducted to evaluate the effects of accelerated or delayed rehabilitation protocols on recovery of range of motion (ROM) following arthroscopic rotator cuff repair.[20] Patients were randomly assigned to begin exercises 2 weeks or 4 weeks following surgery. Both groups received the same protocol. Active ROM was assessed at postoperative weeks 3, 5, 8, 12, and 24. Written informed consent was obtained from all patients.

The components of the informed consent process include two important elements: information and consent (see Table 7-1).[8] Each of these elements must be incorporated into an informed consent form. Many institutions have created templates that require consistent

Table 7-1   Elements of Informed Consent

Informed consent forms should be on institutional letterhead and should identify relevant personnel. Sections should include the following elements. The initial summary may include information that would otherwise be included in later sections, and they do not have to be repeated if there is no additional relevant information:

1. **Concise introductory summary**
   - Invitation to participate and explanation of voluntary nature of study. This section must include a concise presentation of key information that would allow an individual to determine if they want to participate, including the purpose of the study, duration of commitment, procedures to be followed, foreseeable risks, potential benefits, and appropriate alternative treatments that may be beneficial to the individual.
2. **Purpose of the research**
   - A clear explanation of the purpose of the study and why it is important.
   - Why this individual is included and how they were selected.
3. **Procedures**
   - A clear, detailed explanation of what will be done to or by the individual.
   - Expectations for subject performance, including time commitment.
4. **Potential risks and discomforts**
   - Truthful and inclusive statements of foreseeable risks that may result and discomforts that can be expected.
5. **Potential benefits**
   - A description of potential benefits to the individual participant, to general knowledge, or to future administration of healthcare.
6. **Information on study outcomes**
   - A statement about whether the clinical results, including individual research results, will be available to the subject, and if so, under what circumstances.
7. **Alternatives to participation**
   - A description of reasonable alternative procedures that might be used in the treatment of this individual when a treatment intervention is being studied.
8. **Confidentiality**
   - Statements of the procedures used to ensure the anonymity of the individual in collecting, storing, and reporting information, as well as who (persons or agencies) will have access to the information.
9. **Compensation**
   - Compensation may be in the form of reimbursement, stipends, or other incentives.
   - Full description of arrangements for compensation, if being offered.
   - Description of any costs to the subject that may occur from participation.
10. **Contact information and request for more information**
    - A statement that the individual may ask questions about or discuss participation in the study at any time, naming an individual to contact.
    - Contact information for participants who may have questions or complaints.
11. **Consent statement**
    - A confirmation that the individual voluntarily consents to participate in the research project.
    - A statement that the individual may refuse to participate or discontinue participation at any time without prejudice.
12. **Signatures**
    - Participant, parent, or guardian (for the care of minors).
    - Assent of minors over age 7.
    - Person explaining the research, indicating they have answered all questions.

inclusion of content and some boilerplate language. The sample in Figure 7-2 offers a generic format for informed consent to demonstrate how various elements can be included.

Information Elements

Information elements include disclosure of information and the subject's comprehension of that information.

Subjects Must Be Fully Informed

The informed consent process begins with an invitation to participate. A statement of the purpose of the study permits potential subjects to decide whether they believe in or agree with the worth and importance of the research. The process then requires that the researcher provide, in writing, a fair explanation of the procedures to be used and how they will be applied. This explanation must

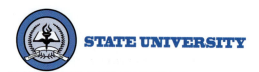

INFORMED CONSENT FORM

Title: The Effect of Accelerated or Delayed Rehabilitation Following Rotator Cuff Repair
Principle Investigator: John Smith, PT, DPT, PhD
Additional Investigators: Alice Jones, MD; Jennifer Ames, OTD

1   Brief Summary

You are being asked to participate in a research study that will evaluate the effect of starting exercises 2 or 4 weeks following rotator cuff repair. This informed consent document will provide important information about the study, to make clear that your participation is voluntary, explain potential risks and benefits, and allow you to make an informed decision if you want to participate. This summary will be followed by more detailed information.

Your participation in this study will go across 14 weeks, as you participate in exercise sessions three times per week. These exercises will be supervised by a physical therapist, who will also take measurements of your progress in shoulder movement. You may experience pain in your shoulder, and we will limit the activity in your shoulder to minimize pain. The range of motion of your shoulder may improve as you continue this exercise program, which may be accompanied by less pain. If you decide not to participate in the study, you may choose to work with another therapist who will be able to provide standard care for rotator cuff repair. You may also choose to contact your surgeon, primary care provider, or other health provider to discuss the best approach to regain movement in your shoulder following surgery.

2   What is the purpose of this research?

You are being asked to take part in this research because you recently underwent arthroscopic surgery for a rotator cuff tear, and you were referred to our clinic by your surgeon. We want to find out if movement recovery will be better if exercises are started within 2 weeks or 4 weeks after your surgery. We do not know which schedule is most beneficial for improving active range of motion.

3   What will happen if I take part in this study?

If you agree to participate, you will be randomly assigned to begin your physical therapy exercises either 2 weeks or 4 weeks after your surgery. All patients in both groups will receive the same exercises, starting with gentle movements in the first week, followed by more active movements the second week, and moving to exercises with resistance in the third week. You will be asked to attend exercise sessions three times a week for 14 weeks. Each session will take up to 1 hour.

Before your program begins, at your initial visit, you will be asked to provide descriptive information about you, including your age, height, weight and other health information regarding other conditions you might have. You are free to decline to provide any information. This information will be used to describe the group of people who are part of this study.

A physical therapist will measure several movements in your shoulder by asking you to raise your arm in different directions. This measurement will happen 4 times during the study, at the 3rd, 5th, 8th, and 12th week. You will also be asked to return at the 24th week following your surgery for a final measurement. Measurements will be taken by a different therapist than the one who works with you at each exercise session. These tests should take approximately 20 minutes.

Therapists who will gather your personal information and who will perform your testing will not know which group you are part of. We ask that you do not tell them.

4   What risks or discomfort may result from this study?

During the testing and your exercise activities, you may experience pain in your shoulder. You should report this immediately to the therapist working with you. Should you be injured while taking part in this study, we will obtain medical help for you as soon as possible. If this happens, you should refrain from any further movement of your arm.

5   What are the benefits from participating in this study?

Participating in the this study may allow you to improve the range of motion of your shoulder and experience less pain over time. The results of this research may guide future exercise programs for individuals with rotator cuff repair, helping us understand the most beneficial timing for rehabilitation.

6   How will outcomes be shared?

You are entitled to learn about results of your participation. We will provide a summary of results to all participants at the end of the study. You will also be able to monitor your own progress during the study to understand how much the movement in your shoulder has changed.

Figure 7–2 Sample informed consent form. Numbers in the left margin correspond to required elements listed in Table 7-1. Content in the form is based on the protocol described by Düzgün I, Baltaci G, Turgut E, Atay OA. Effects of slow and accelerated rehabilitation protocols on range of motion after arthroscopic rotator cuff repair. *Acta Orthop Traumatol Turc* 2014;48(6):642–648.

7 **Are there alternatives to participation?**
If you choose not to participate, you have the option of working with a therapist who is not involved in this study and who will work with you providing standard care for rotator cuff repair. You may also choose to contact your surgeon, primary care provider, or other health provider to discuss the best approach to regain movement in your shoulder following surgery.

8 **How will my information be protected?**
All information obtained as part of your participation in this study will remain completely confidential. Information will be stored in password-protected computer files. You will be given a code number to represent your information, and you will not be identified by name. Your name will be tied to your code number in a file that will be stored in a separate file. When the study is over, your information will be kept on file for future use, but it will not contain information that could directly identify you.

9 **What are costs related to my participation in this research?**
You will not be directly compensated for your participation in this research. However, we will cover your costs of parking in our university garage or fare for a taxi or other transportation to our facility. You will need to provide receipts for reimbursement.

Should you be injured during your participation, treatment costs will be charged to your insurance carrier. If for any reason these costs are not covered, they will be your responsibility. You will also be responsible for any deductible or co-pay costs.

10 **Where can I get additional information?**
You have the right to ask questions you may have about this research. If you have questions, concerns or complaints, or believe you have developed an injury related to this research, please contact the primary investigator, John Smith, at 866-555-5465 as soon as possible, or your health care provider.

If you have questions about your rights as a research participant, or you wish to ask questions about this study of someone other than the researchers, please contact the State University Institutional Review Board at 617-555-4343, Email: irb@su.edu.

11 **Your participation is voluntary.**
It is completely up to you to decide if you want to participate in this study. You do not have to answer any questions you do not want to answer. If you choose to participate, you are free to withdraw your permission for use of your information at any time by contacting the primary investigator. You may also choose to end your participation at any time without any effect on your health care or your rights as a patient. If you choose to withdraw, we may continue to use the information that we have already collected as part of your participation in our analysis of the data for the entire group, to maintain the soundness of our overall research. Your information will remain confidential.

12 **Your consent**
By signing this document, you are agreeing to participate in this study. Please make sure you understand what the study is about and what will be expected of you before you sign. You will be given a copy of this document for your records. We will keep the signed copy with our study records. If you have questions after you sign the document, you can contact the study team using the information provided above.

I understand what the study is about and my questions so far have been answered. I agree to take part in this study.

Participant signature	Date	Printed name
Parent/legally authorized representative/relationship	Date	Printed name
Investigator signature	Date	Printed name

Figure 7–2—cont'd

be complete, with no deception by virtue of commission or omission. Subjects should know what will be done to them, how long it will take, what they will feel, which side effects can be expected, and what types of questions they may be asked. An important revision to the Common Rule includes the requirement that informed consent forms must begin with a concise presentation of the "key information" that a reasonable person would want to have in order to make an informed decision about whether to participate.[16] This means that participants do not have to wade through a long, detailed form to find crucial information.

▶ For the rotator cuff study, subjects should be told what kinds of exercises they will be doing. They should be informed about the schedule of assessments, how often they have to visit the clinic for measurement, and how long each visit will last.

If subjects cannot read the informed consent document, it should be read to them. Children should be informed to whatever extent is reasonable for their age. Subjects should also know why they have been selected to participate in terms of inclusion criteria for the study, such as clinical condition or age. If the subjects are patients, they should understand the distinction between procedures that are experimental and procedures, if any, that are proposed to serve their personal needs.

 New common rule regulations also require statements in informed consent forms regarding use of identifiable information or biospecimens, commercialization, and results of whole genome sequencing.[16] These changes would have addressed the concerns in the case of Henrietta Lacks.

Control Groups

The researcher is obliged to inform the potential participants when a study is planned that includes a control group. Experimental subjects receive the studied intervention, whereas control subjects may receive an alternative treatment, usual care, a placebo, or no treatment at all. When the study involves random assignment, subjects should know that there is a chance they will be assigned to either group (see Box 7-1).

▶ In the rotator cuff study, subjects were randomly assigned to receive intervention on different timelines. They should be told that there are varied time periods and how they differ.

According to the *Declaration of Helsinki*, as a form of compensation, the experimental treatment may be offered to the control participants after data collection is complete, if results indicate that treatment is beneficial.[5] As clinician-researchers, we are obliged to discuss alternative treatments that would be appropriate for each patient/subject if such alternatives are employed in clinical practice.

See Chapter 14 for a description of various strategies for random assignment of subjects, including wait-list controls.

Disclosure

An ethical dilemma occurs when complete disclosure of procedures might hinder the outcomes of a study by biasing the subjects so that they do not respond in a typical way. When the risks are not great, review boards may allow researchers to pursue a deceptive course, but subjects must be told that information is being withheld and that they will be informed of all procedures after completion of data collection. For example, when the research design includes a control or placebo group,

---

Box 7-1   Uncertainty and Placebos

There is an ethical concept in the design of clinical trials called **equipoise**, which means that we should only conduct trials under conditions of uncertainty when we do not already have sufficient evidence of the benefit of a treatment.[21] The *Declaration of Helsinki* addresses this issue, stating that: "The benefits, risks, burdens and effectiveness of a new method should be tested against those of the best current prophylactic, diagnostic, and therapeutic methods."[5]

This concept also means that placebos must be used judiciously. There may be some clinical conditions for which no treatments have been effective. In that case, it is necessary to compare a new treatment with a no-treatment condition. It is also necessary to make such a comparison when the purpose of the research is to determine whether a particular treatment approach is not effective. In situations where the efficacy of a treatment is being questioned because current knowledge is inadequate, it may actually be more ethical to take the time to make appropriate controlled comparisons than to continue clinical practice using potentially ineffective techniques. The *Declaration of Helsinki* specifically states that placebos are permissible "when no proven intervention exists" or when a compelling scientific rationale for a placebo can be provided, with the assurance that control subjects will not be at risk.[22]

Based on this principle, trials should include a comparison with standard care or other recognized interventions as one of the treatment arms, as long as such treatment is available.[23] It is also considered unethical to include an alternative therapy that is known to be inferior to any other treatment.[21]

---

subjects may not know which treatment they are receiving to preserve blinding. They should know that they will be told their group assignment at the completion of the study.

Potential Risks

An important aspect of informed consent is the description of all reasonable foreseeable risks or discomforts to which the patient will be subjected, directly or indirectly, as part of the study. The researcher should detail the steps that will be taken to protect against these risks and the treatments that are available for potential side effects. The informed consent form is not binding on subjects and subjects never waive their rights to redress if their participation should cause them harm. The form should not contain language that appears to release the researcher from liability.

▶ The subjects in the rotator cuff study needed to be informed about the potential for pain or fatigue from exercises. ROM measurement could also result in some pain as the joint is stretched. The subjects should know what kind of pain is potentially expected and how long it should last.

If the research involves more than minimal risk, a statement should be included concerning the availability of medical care and whether compensation will be provided. Subjects should also be informed of new information, such as the identification of previously unknown risks that becomes available during the course of the study. This may affect their willingness to continue participation.

Potential Benefits

The informed consent form must also delineate the potential benefits of participation. Some studies may result in a reduction of symptoms, improvement in function, or a cure. The subject should be advised that such a benefit is possible but is not guaranteed. When a study involves a form of therapeutic intervention, subjects must be informed that alternative treatments are available and that they have the right to choose among them instead of accepting the experimental intervention. Patients must also be told whether "standard" treatments to which they are entitled are being withheld as part of the study. Studies that are geared more toward theory testing may provide no direct benefits. The researcher should explain the potential application of theoretical findings and how the findings will contribute to future research or patient care. New regulations also require that informed consent indicates if outcomes of the study will be shared with subjects.

> ➤ Subjects in the rotator cuff study may benefit from the exercise program for pain relief as well as improved movement and function.

Subject Information Should Be Confidential and Anonymous

Research subjects should be told that steps are being taken to ensure confidentiality of all information, including descriptive and experimental data. Whenever possible, a subject's anonymity should be protected. This becomes an issue with surveys, for example, when respondents wish to remain unidentified. In experimental situations, anonymity is often not feasible, but the researcher can *de-identify* the data by using subject codes without names. The key to names and codes must be kept separate from the rest of the data. All hard copy data should be stored in locked cabinets, and digital data should be secured within encrypted files or drives. Researchers should be aware of this responsibility when disseminating results. They also have a responsibility to know the requirements of the Privacy Rule and the procedures established by their Institutional Review Boards.

 The methods used to de-identify data must be specified in a research protocol and will be reviewed by the IRB.[24] Information that could identify a person (such as medical record number, date of birth, or zip code) should not be included in the analyzed dataset.

If video or photographs are going to be used during the study, this should be disclosed in the consent form. The subject should know who will have access to recordings or photographs, who will keep them, and how they will be used. Subjects retain the right to review such material and to withdraw permission for its use at any time. Subjects should also be informed if one-way windows will be used and who the observers will be.

The Informed Consent Form Must Be Written in Lay Language

Informed consent is more than telling subjects about the research. The process implies that they understand what they are being told or reading. The language must be clear and basic so that the average reasonable individual can follow it. Professional jargon is unacceptable. As a rule of thumb, language should be written for the lowest educational level that would be expected for subjects, typically considered 6th- or 8th-grade level.[25]

The Researcher Must Offer to Answer Questions at Any Time

The researcher is responsible for ensuring that the subject understands all relevant information. Even with a written form, a verbal description is almost always a part of the process so that the researcher can "personalize" the information for each subject. The subjects should have sufficient time to assimilate the details of the proposed project, prior to making their decision to participate. They should feel free to question the procedures at any time during the course of the study, and should be provided with the name and telephone number of an appropriate contact person.

Consent Elements

Consent Must Be Voluntary

Subjects should participate in a research project of their own free will. Patients are often quite motivated to help, but they must be informed that there is no penalty to them if they refuse. Some studies may involve monetary compensation for participation. It should be clear if such compensation will be received whether or not the subject completes the study.

Special Consideration for "Vulnerable" Participants

The IRB will be particularly concerned with research that involves subjects who are vulnerable to coercion or undue influence, such as children, prisoners, those with impaired decision-making capacity, or those who are educationally or economically disadvantaged. More subtle circumstances exist with the involvement of hospitalized patients, nursing home residents, or students. In these cases, the sense of pleasing those in authority may affect the subject's decisions. Importantly, consent implies that there is no intimidation. Researchers must be able to demonstrate how safeguards are included in the protocol to protect the rights and welfare of such subjects. If a subject is not competent, consent must be obtained from a legally authorized representative.[7]

The regulations regarding children as research subjects require that parents or guardians give permission for participation. Furthermore, if a child is considered competent to understand, regardless of age, his or her *assent* should be expressed as affirmative agreement to participate.

Subjects Must Be Free to Withdraw Consent at Any Time

The informed consent document must indicate that the subject is free to discontinue participation for any reason at any time without prejudice; that is, the subject should be assured that no steps will be taken against them, and, if they are a patient, that the quality of their care will not be affected. This can occur before or during an experiment, or even after data collection when a subject might request that their data be discarded. The informed consent form should include a statement that subjects will be informed about important new findings arising during the course of the study that may be relevant to their continued participation. It should also provide information about anticipated circumstances under which the subject's participation may be terminated by the investigator for the subject's safety or comfort.

Format of the Informed Consent Form

All subjects must give informed consent prior to participating in a project. The written form should be signed and dated by the subject and researcher. Subjects should receive a copy of this form and the researcher must retain the signed copy.

Required formats for consent forms may vary at different institutions. The format of the sample provided in Figure 7-1 follows recommendations from the NIH and is similar to those used in many institutions. It specifically identifies and acknowledges all the elements of informed consent.[26] Of special note, signatures should not be on a separate page, but should appear with some of the text to show that the signatures are applied in the context of the larger document. Although written consent is preferable, some agencies allow oral consent in selected circumstances. In this case, a written "short form" can be used that describes the information presented orally to the subject or their legally authorized representative.[7] This short form is submitted to the IRB for approval.

> 📌 The example that is provided in Figure 7-1 is just one possible version of an informed consent form in a concise format. It is only presented as a sample, and may require expanded explanations, depending on the nature of the research. It does not include sample language, for instance, for the use of biospecimens, genome sequencing, educational or psychological research, use of secondary data, or data that contain private information and identifiers. Institutions often have different policies, templates, or boilerplate language that must be incorporated into these forms. Guidelines are usually available through IRBs as well as through the Department of Health and Human Services.[27] Given the changes to the Common Rule it is important for researchers to review relevant information. The new rule also requires that consent forms for federally funded studies be posted on a public website.[27]

Informed Consent and Usual Care

Clinical research studies are often designed to test specific treatment protocols that are accepted as standard care, and subjects are recruited from those who would receive such treatments. Clinicians often ask whether informed consent is necessary for a research study when the procedures would have been used anyway. The answer is yes! Even where treatment is viewed as usual care, patients are entitled to understand alternatives that are available to them. Patients must always be informed of the use of the data that are collected during their treatments, and they should have sufficient information to decide to participate or not, regardless of whether treatment is viewed as experimental or accepted clinical practice.

■ Research Integrity

Although truth and objectivity are hallmarks of science, there are unfortunate instances in which researchers have misrepresented data. As we strive to build our evidence base for practice, all researchers and clinicians must be vigilant in their evaluation of the integrity of clinical inquiry.

Research Misconduct

According to the U.S. Office of Research Integrity:

Research misconduct means fabrication, falsification, or plagiarism in proposing, performing, or reviewing research, or in reporting research results.[28]

Fabrication

Fabrication is making up data or results and recording or reporting them. This includes presenting observations that never occurred or describing experiments that were never performed.

From 1996 to 2008, Dr. Scott Reuben, from Baystate Medical Center in Massachusetts, published a series of placebo-controlled studies that examined the role of COX-2 inhibitors in controlling postoperative pain following orthopedic surgery.[29] In 2008 an investigation determined that he had fabricated his data and that he had never enrolled patients in some of his studies. He was required to pay significant restitution to drug companies and served 6 months in prison.

Although this work has been retracted, it had already influenced the management of millions of patients and led to the sale of billions of dollars of drugs like Celebrex and Vioxx.[30]

Falsification

Falsification is manipulating research materials, equipment, or processes, or changing or omitting data or results such that the data are not accurately represented in the research record (see Focus on Evidence 7-2).

Dr. Jan Hendrick Schön, a physicist at Bell Laboratories, was considered a pioneer in research on transistors.[31] In 2002, evidence was presented that figures in 13 articles published over 2 years were suspiciously similar, some with identical data. An investigative report found that Schön had manipulated data, and independent efforts to replicate his findings had all failed.

Prior to retractions of these papers, this work had already impacted the discipline of field effect transistors, with estimates that more than 100 groups worldwide were working on related projects.[32]

Plagiarism

Plagiarism is the appropriation of another person's ideas, processes, results, or words without giving appropriate credit or attribution, and representing the work as one's own.

In 2011, a reviewer examining studies related to osteoarthritis (OA) found an article that was published in 2006 in the *Journal of Orthopaedic Research* under the title "Chondrocyte Gene Expression in Osteoarthritis: Correlation with Disease Severity."[33] In 2011, the exact same article, word for word, was published in the

---

Focus on Evidence 7–2
Fraudulent Science: A Detriment to Public Health

In 1998, Dr. Andrew Wakefield and 12 colleagues[46] published a study in *The Lancet* that implied a link between the measles, mumps, and rubella (MMR) vaccine and a "new syndrome" of autism and gastrointestinal disease. The paper was based on a case series of 12 children whose parents described the children's history of normal development followed by loss of acquired skills and an onset of behavioral symptoms following MMR vaccination. Although the authors did state that their study could not "prove" this connection, they asserted that the MMR vaccination was the "apparent precipitating event."

The report received significant media attention and triggered a notable decline in immunizations and a rise in measles outbreaks.[47] *The Lancet* received a barrage of letters objecting to the study's implications and prospective impact. Critics pointed out several limitations of the study, including no controls, children with multiple disorders, and data based on parental recall and beliefs.[48] Most importantly, however, over the following two decades, dozens of epidemiologic studies consistently demonstrated no evidence of this link.[49–52]

In 2004, *The Lancet* editors were made aware that Wakefield failed to disclose that he had received significant compensation prior to the study as a consultant to attorneys representing parents of children allegedly harmed by the MMR vaccine.[53] Soon after, 11 of the

contributing authors to the original paper published a retraction of the interpretation that there was a causal link between MMR vaccine and autism.[54]

These events triggered a formal investigation by the British General Medical Council in 2010, which found that the study had not been approved by a bioethics committee, that the researchers had exposed children to invasive colonoscopies and lumbar punctures that were not germane to the study, that the children were not drawn at random but were from families already reporting an association between autism and MMR vaccine, and that the coauthors of the paper all claimed to be unaware of these lapses despite their authorship.[55] Further investigation revealed that facts about the children's histories had been altered and that none of their medical records could be reconciled with the descriptions in the published paper.[56] Based on these findings, Wakefield's license to practice medicine in England was revoked.

The Lancet retracted the paper,[57] and in 2011 the *British Medical Journal* declared it a fraud.[56] However, despite the fact that the study has been widely discredited for both scientific and ethical reasons, and even with the overwhelming scientific evidence to the contrary, popular opinion and the internet seem to perpetuate the vaccine scare.[58–61] The tremendous harm caused by this fraud is evident in the increasing numbers of outbreaks of measles—a disease that had been declared eradicated in 2000—with the majority of those infected being unvaccinated.[62,63]

Romanian *Journal of Morphology and Embryology* under a different title with different authors.[33] The editor of the Romanian journal withdrew the article, banned the authors from further publication, and notified the dean of medicine and the ethics review board at their institution.

Both articles are still listed in PubMed.

 Research misconduct does not include honest error or differences of opinion. Mistakes in data entry or forgetting to report a value, for example, are considered honest errors.

As these examples show, many instances of misconduct have been documented over the past 50 years, some quite notorious. Such violations can have serious external effects, including damaging careers, delaying scientific progress, damaging public perception of clinical trials, and, most egregiously, providing misinformation about treatment efficacy that can influence healthcare decisions to the detriment of patients.[35]

It is important to note that because many of these studies attract public attention, the frequency of such violations may be incorrectly perceived. The actual incidence of such fraud is assumed to be quite low, although hard to estimate.[36] For those who would like to know more about interesting and significant examples of research misconduct, several informative reviews have been written.[35–38]

HISTORICAL NOTE

Throughout history, there have been many claims that scientists have fudged data in ways that would be considered misconduct today. Ptolemy is purported to have obtained his astronomical results by plagiarizing 200-year-old data or making up numbers to fit his theory of the Earth being the center of the universe.[39] Sir Isaac Newton may have adjusted calculations to fit his observations,[40] and Gregor Mendel is suspected of selectively reporting data on his pea plants to show patterns that are cleaner than might be expected experimentally.[41]

Although none of these can be proven, the suspicions arise from statistical evidence that observed results are just a little too close to expected values to be compatible with the chance that affects experimental data.[36]

Conflicts of Interest

A **conflict of interest (COI)** occurs when an individual's connections present a risk that professional judgment will be influenced. It can be defined as:

. . . a set of conditions in which professional judgment concerning a primary interest (such as patients' welfare

or the validity of research) tends to be unduly influenced by a secondary interest (such as financial gain).[42]

Such conflicts can undermine the objectivity and integrity of research endeavors, whether real or perceived. Conflicts can occur if an investigator has a relationship with a pharmaceutical company or manufacturer, for example, in which the outcome of a clinical trial may result in commercial benefits and there may be pressure to draw favorable conclusions.[43] Researchers may sit on agency boards or be involved with government, industry, or academic sponsors that can compromise judgment. Conflicts of interest can also apply to reputational benefits or simply conflicting commitments of time.[44] Patients and research participants present a particular source of concern, especially when they are solicited as subjects. Their welfare can be compromised if researchers are provided incentives, if they have intellectual property interests, or if subjects are students or employees, especially if they are led to believe that the study will be of specific benefit to them.[45]

Most professional codes of ethics include language warning against COIs, and universities or research laboratories usually require that investigators declare potential conflicts as part of ethics committee approval. Many journals and professional organizations now require formal declarations of COI for research publications or presentations.

Peer Review

One hallmark of a reputable scientific journal is its process for vetting articles, known as **peer review**. The purpose of peer review is to provide feedback to an editor who will make decisions about whether a manuscript should be accepted, revised, or rejected. Peer review requires the expertise of colleagues who offer their time to read and critique the paper, and provide an assessment of the study's validity, the data reporting, and the author's conclusions. Journals and researchers recognize the necessity of this process to support the quality of scholarship.

In recent years, many journals have asked authors to recommend or solicit reviewers to facilitate finding people who are willing to give the necessary time. Because reviews are now done electronically, contacts are typically made through e-mail. This has allowed some deceitful practices, where authors have made up identities and have reviewed their own articles, or groups have reviewed each other's papers.[64–66] Hundreds of articles have been retracted over the past few years because of this practice and many journals are now taking steps to properly identify reviewers to avoid such situations.

Retractions

An important characteristic of science is its commitment to self-correction in the pursuit of knowledge. A major mechanism for this process is *retraction* of published studies that are found to be fraudulent or containing error.

The first article retraction was in 1977, for a paper published in 1973. Since then there have been well over 2,000 articles retracted, 21% attributable to error and 67% attributable to misconduct, including fraud or suspected fraud (43%), duplicate publication (14%), and plagiarism (10%).[67] The percentage of scientific articles retracted because of fraud has increased approximately 10-fold since 1975, but this may be an underestimate.[36,68]

For some researchers, the evidence of misconduct extends over many years and several studies. For instance, in 2012, the University of Connecticut found the director of their Cardiovascular Research Center guilty of 145 counts of fabrication and falsification of data in his studies on the benefits of red wine for cardiovascular health.[69] At least 20 of his articles in 11 journals, published over a 7-year span, have now been retracted.

It can take an average of 4 years for an article to be retracted, although some can take more than 10 years. This is especially true in cases of fraud, depending on when the fraud is first suspected and when an investigative panel presents its findings. Many articles are cited hundreds of times in that interim, compounding the detrimental effect of the inaccurate research. For example, the Wakefield article on autism and MMR vaccine, described earlier, was cited 758 times before its retraction, which occurred 12 years after its publication![70]

Although the increase in number of retractions and the underlying reasons are concerning, it is important to emphasize that these represent a very small percentage of the total number of papers published each year. However, given the high profile of many of these cases, the funding involved, and the damage they do to the public trust, the data underscore the importance of vigilance by reviewers, editors, and readers, as well as of investigations by institutions and government agencies in identifying and exposing research misconduct.[67]

The Ultimate Goal: Scientific Truth

The scientific process is not only affected by deliberate misconduct of investigators. Many other concerns are relevant to understanding how the integrity of the research enterprise can be compromised. Some practices are intentional, some may be systemic issues, and some occur because of a lack of understanding of good research principles. Any of them can present ethical concerns, however, by interfering with solid evidence-based practice (EBP).

Replication

Research study results are based on data from samples, and through statistical analysis investigators determine the likelihood that their hypotheses have been supported by their data—always knowing that there is some probability, however small, that their conclusions may be due to chance. This recognition of uncertainty is why replication studies are so important. One study cannot be the final word, and results need to be reproduced on other samples to lend credence to conclusions. Finding disagreement in replication does not mean that the first study was wrong and the second was right. Many explanations can be put forth to explain differences, and these must be considered critically. The study described earlier on autism and the MMR vaccine exemplifies this point and its importance.[46]

To illustrate the extent of this issue, an ambitious 2015 study in *Science* described replications of 100 experimental and correlational studies published in three psychology journals.[71] The authors found that replication effects were half the magnitude of original effects. Although 97% of the original studies had statistically significant results, this was true in only 36% of replications.

Replication does not carry the same weight of innovation or recognition that original studies have, and funding opportunities may be slim, which is why many investigators do not go down that path. However, it is a vital opportunity to confirm outcomes in support of evidence. Reproducing results can increase certainty when findings confirm the original data, or it can promote progress and change when they do not.

Citations for retracted articles are maintained in literature databases, but notification of the retraction is prominently featured in the citation along with a link to a retraction notice in the relevant journal. The publication type is listed as "retracted publication" in PubMed.

Focus on Evidence 3-1 (Chapter 3) highlights the opposite argument—that researchers must realize when replication goes too far, when further corroboration is no longer needed to support an intervention, creating a potentially unethical use of human and financial resources.

Underpowered Clinical Trials

In the statistical analysis of clinical trials, the ability to document significant effects is dependent on two main elements: the size of the effect of the intervention or test, and the sample size included in the study. These two elements relate to the statistical concept of power. A study that does not have sufficient power is unlikely to find significant effects (see Chapter 23). Researchers are generally expected to do a power analysis as part of the planning process to determine the appropriate sample size that will provide the best opportunity for successful outcomes.

When a research study results in a nonsignificant finding, it may be because the treatment did not work, or it could be because the study did not have sufficient power. In the latter case, studies may present an undue risk to subjects with little expectation of benefit. Underpowered studies can contribute, however, as part of meta-analyses that take into account several studies of the same intervention, and may therefore still provide useful data (see Chapter 37). From an ethical standpoint, however, subjects should be informed that the study, as designed, may only indirectly contribute to future health benefits.[72]

Validity in Study Design and Analysis

The application of research evidence depends on the reliability and transparency of data. We rely on authors to honestly share their methods, operational definitions, and analytic procedures so that we can be critical consumers and make judgments about the utility of their findings. We also understand that research is based on data drawn from samples, with the intent of generalizing findings to others. Researchers draw inferences from these samples, knowing that their data will have some degree of inaccuracy, but doing so within probability guidelines.

Starting in the planning stages, researchers must engage in the process with commitment to established principles of design and statistical testing.[71] This means following the "rules":

- Formulating hypotheses and developing analysis plans before data are collected.
- Adhering to the research protocol.
- Taking responsibility to ensure a large enough sample to secure reasonable power.
- Choosing the appropriate statistical procedures and interpreting them without manipulation, even when outcomes are not as expected.[74]
- Not being selective in choosing relevant findings after the fact but analyzing and reporting all data.

COMMENTARY

Science cannot stop while ethics catches up . . .

—Elvin Charles Stakman (1885–1979)

American plant pathologist

The last century has seen remarkable changes in technology that have influenced the landscape of research and clinical practice. Guidelines continue to be evaluated and revised to address regulatory gaps that continue to widen as legal and ethical standards try to keep up with advances. The development of copyright laws, for example, originally followed the invention of the printing press in the 1400s, an advance that severely challenged the political and religious norms of the day and changed forever how information could be disseminated.[75] Our recent history has had to deal with changes in electronic distribution of intellectual property in ways that could never have been anticipated even 20 years ago.

Many scientific and technological advances bring with them ethical and legal questions that also challenge research endeavors. The use of social media creates many concerns regarding accessibility of information, spreading of misinformation, and processes for recruiting research participants. Personal profiles and digital footprints may allow personal information to become available, violating privacy rules. The human genome project and wide availability of genetic information bring concerns about confidentiality while providing important opportunities for personalized healthcare. Electronic medical records must adhere to HIPAA provisions, but also provide access to patient information for research purposes. And how do we deal with three-dimensional printing to create models for human organs,[76] developing surgical and mechanical human enhancements to substitute for human function,[77] or cloning of primates?[78]

It was only after blatant examples of unethical conduct were uncovered in the last century that regulations began to address the necessary precautions. Surely today's advances will uncover new concerns that will require continued vigilance regarding their implications for practice and research. But without individuals who volunteer to participate in studies, the research enterprise would be stymied. All the while, we must maintain the cornerstones of ethical standards—adhering to ethical and professional principles in reporting, providing adequate information to participants, maintaining privacy and confidentiality, and, above all, attending to the well-being of those we study and those to whom our research findings will apply.

REFERENCES

1. Beecher HK. Ethics and clinical research. *N Engl J Med* 1966;274(24):1354–1360.
2. Reverby SM. *Examining Tuskegee: The Infamous Syphilis Study and Its Legacy.* Chapel Hill, NC: The University of North Carolina Press, 2009.
3. Office of Human Research Protections: Ethical codes and research standards. Available at https://www.hhs.gov/ohrp/international/ethical-codes-and-research-standards/index.html. Accessed January 20, 2018.
4. United States Holocaust Museum: Holocaust Encyclopedia. Nazi medical experiments. Available at https://www.ushmm.org/wlc/en/article.php?ModuleId=10005168. Accessed January 20, 2018.
5. World Medical Association. Declaration of Helsinki-Ethical Principles for Medical Research Involving Human Subjects. Available at https://www.wma.net/policies-post/wma-declaration-of-helsinki-ethical-principles-for-medical-research-involving-human-subjects/. Accessed January 20, 2018.
6. Centers for Disease Control and Prevention (CDC): US Public Health Service Syphilis Study at Tuskegee. Research implications: How Tuskegee changed research practices. Available at https://www.cdc.gov/tuskegee/after.htm. Accessed January 20, 2018.
7. Office of Human Research Protections: Code of Federal Regulations, Title 45, Public Welfare. Department of Health and Human Services. Part 46: Protection of Human Subjects. Effective July 14, 2009. Available at https://www.hhs.gov/ohrp/regulations-and-policy/regulations/45-cfr-46/index.html. Accessed January 20, 2018.
8. Office of Human Research Protections: *The Belmont Report: Ethical Principles and Guidelines for the Protection of Human Subjects of Research.* National Commission for the Protection of Human Subjects of Biomedical and Behavioral Research. Available at https://www.hhs.gov/ohrp/regulations-and-policy/belmont-report/read-the-belmont-report/index.html. Accessed January 20, 2018.
9. Offit PA. *Vaccinated: One Man's Quest to Defeat the World's Deadliest Diseases.* New York: Smithsonian Books, 2007.
10. Krugman S. Experiments at the Willowbrook State School. *Lancet* 1971;297(7706):927–980.
11. Krugman S. The Willowbrook hepatitis studies revisited: ethical aspects. *Rev Infect Dis* 1986;8(1):157–162.
12. Rivera G. *Willowbrook: A Report on How It Is and Why It Doesn't Have to Be That Way.* New York: Random House, 1972.
13. Skloot R. *The Immortal Life of Henrietta Lacks.* New York: Crown, 2010.
14. Callaway E. Deal done over HeLa cell line. *Nature* 2013; 500(7461):132–133.
15. The Henrietta Lacks Foundation. Available at http://henriettalacksfoundation.org/. Accessed January 20, 2018.
16. Office of Human Research Protections: Federal policy for the protection of human subjects ('Common Rule'). Available at https://www.hhs.gov/ohrp/regulations-and-policy/regulations/common-rule/index.html. Accessed January 27, 2018.
17. National Institutes of Health: HIPAA Resources. Available at https://privacyruleandresearch.nih.gov/. Accessed January 30, 2018.
18. Collaborative Institutional Training Initiative (CITI Program). Available at https://about.citiprogram.org/en/series/human-subjects-research-hsr/. Accessed January 21, 2018.
19. National Institutes of Health: Clinical research and the HIPAA privacy rule. Available at https://privacyruleandresearch.nih.gov/clin_research.asp. Accessed January 21, 2018.
20. Düzgün I, Baltaci G, Turgut E, Atay OA. Effects of slow and accelerated rehabilitation protocols on range of motion after arthroscopic rotator cuff repair. *Acta Orthop Traumatol Turc* 2014;48(6):642–648.
21. Stanley K. Design of randomized controlled trials. *Circulation* 2007;115(9):1164–1169.
22. WMA Declaration of Helsinki-Ethical Principles for Medical Research Involving Human Subjects. Amended October, 2013. Available at http://www.wma.net/en/30publications/10policies/b3/. Accessed March 27, 2017.
23. D'Agostino RB, Sr., Massaro JM, Sullivan LM. Non-inferiority trials: design concepts and issues - the encounters of academic consultants in statistics. *Stat Med* 2003;22(2): 169–186.
24. US Department of Health and Human Services. Guidance regarding methods for de-identification of protected health information in accordance with the Health Insurance Portability and Accountability act (HIPAA) Privacy Rule. Available at https://www.hhs.gov/hipaa/for-professionals/privacy/special-topics/de-identification/index.html#rationale. Accessed May 25, 2018.
25. Plain Language Action and Information Network. Plain language makes it easier for the public to read, understand, and use government communications. Available at https://www.plainlanguage.gov/. Accessed February 25, 2019.
26. National Institute on Aging: Informed consent. Available at https://www.nia.nih.gov/research/dgcg/clinical-research-study-investigators-toolbox/informed-consent. Accessed January 30, 2018.
27. Office of Human Research Protections. Federal policy for the protection of human subjects ('Common Rule'). Available at https://www.hhs.gov/ohrp/regulations-and-policy/regulations/common-rule/index.html. Accessed January 27, 2019.
28. Office of Research Integrity: Definition of research misconduct. Available at https://ori.hhs.gov/definition-misconduct. Accessed March 11, 2017.
29. Reuben SS, Buvanendran A. Preventing the development of chronic pain after orthopaedic surgery with preventive multimodal analgesic techniques. *J Bone Joint Surg Am* 2007; 89(6):1343–1358 [Paper officially retracted in: Heckman, JD. Retractions. *J Bone Joint Surg Am* 2009;91(4):965].
30. White PF, Rosow CE, Shafer SL. The Scott Reuben saga: one last retraction. *Anesth Analg* 2011;112(3):512–515.
31. Schon JH, Meng H, Bao Z. Self-assembled monolayer organic field-effect transistors. *Nature* 2001;413(6857):713–716 (Retraction in *Nature* 2003;422(6927):92).
32. Service RF. Bell Labs inquiry. Physicists question safeguards, ponder their next moves. *Science* 2002;296(5573):1584–1585.

33. Eid K, Thornhill TS, Glowacki J. Chondrocyte gene expression in osteoarthritis: correlation with disease severity. *J Orthop Res* 2006;24(5):1062–1068.

34. Jalbă BA, Jalbă CS, Vlădoi AD, Gherghina F, Stefan E, Cruce M. Alterations in expression of cartilage-specific genes for aggrecan and collagen type II in osteoarthritis. *Rom J Morphol Embryol* 2011;52(2):587–591.

35. Stroebe W, Postmes T, Spears R. Scientific misconduct and the myth of self-correction in science. *Perspect Psycholog Sci* 2012; 7(6):670–688.

36. George SL, Buyse M. Data fraud in clinical trials. *Clin Investig (Lond)* 2015;5(2):161–173.

37. Buckwalter JA, Tolo VT, O'Keefe RJ. How do you know it is true? Integrity in research and publications: AOA critical issues. *J Bone Joint Surg Am* 2015;97(1):e2.

38. Sovacool BK. Exploring scientific misconduct: misconduct, isolated individuals, impure institutions, or an inevitable idiom of modern science? *Biothical Inq* 2008;5:271–582.

39. Newton RR. *The Crime of Claudius Ptolemy.* Baltimore: Johns Hopkins University Press, 1977.

40. Judson HF. *The Great Betrayal: Fraud in Science.* Orlando, FL: Harcourt Books, 2004.

41. Galton DJ. Did Mendel falsify his data? *Qjm* 2012;105(2): 215–216.

42. Thompson DF. Understanding financial conflicts of interest. *N Engl J Med* 1993;329(8):573-576.

43. Bekelman JE, Li Y, Gross CP. Scope and impact of financial conflicts of interest in biomedical research: a systematic review. *JAMA* 2003;298(4):454-465.

44. Horner J, Minifie FD. Research ethics III: publication practices and authorship, conflicts of interest, and research misconduct. *J Speech Lang Hear Res* 2011;54(1):S346–S362.

45. Williams JR. The physician's role in the protection of human research subjects. *Sci Eng Ethics* 2006;12(1):5-12.

46. Wakefield AJ, Murch SH, Anthony A, Linnell J, Casson DM, Malik M, Berelowitz M, Dhillon AP, Thomson MA, Harvey P, et al. Ileal-lymphoid-nodular hyperplasia, non-specific colitis, and pervasive developmental disorder in children. *Lancet* 1998;351(9103):637–641.

47. Flaherty DK. The vaccine-autism connection: a public health crisis caused by unethical medical practices and fraudulent science. *Ann Pharmacother* 2011;45(10):1302–1304.

48. Payne C, Mason B. Autism, inflammatory bowel disease, and MMR vaccine. *Lancet* 1998;351(9106):907; author reply 908–909.

49. Jain A, Marshall J, Buikema A, Bancroft T, Kelly JP, Newschaffer CJ. Autism occurrence by MMR vaccine status among US children with older siblings with and without autism. *JAMA* 2015;313(15):1534–1540.

50. Uno Y, Uchiyama T, Kurosawa M, Aleksic B, Ozaki N. Early exposure to the combined measles-mumps-rubella vaccine and thimerosal-containing vaccines and risk of autism spectrum disorder. *Vaccine* 2015;33(21):2511–2516.

51. Taylor LE, Swerdfeger AL, Eslick GD. Vaccines are not associated with autism: an evidence-based meta-analysis of case-control and cohort studies. *Vaccine* 2014;32(29):3623–3629.

52. DeStefano F. Vaccines and autism: evidence does not support a causal association. *Clin Pharmacol Ther* 2007;82(6):756–759.

53. Deer B. How the case against the MMR vaccine was fixed. *BMJ* 2011;342:c5347.

54. Murch SH, Anthony A, Casson DH, Malik M, Berelowitz M, Dhillon AP, Thomson MA, Valentine A, Davies SE, Walker-Smith JA. Retraction of an interpretation. *Lancet* 2004;363(9411):750.

55. General Medical Council: Fitness to practise panel hearing, 28 January 2010. Available at http://www.casewatch.org/foreign/wakefield/gmc_findings.pdf. Accessed March 10, 2017.

56. Godlee F, Smith J, Marcovitch H. Wakefield's article linking MMR vaccine and autism was fraudulent. *BMJ* 2011;342:c7452.

57. Retraction—Ileal-lymphoid-nodular hyperplasia, non-specific colitis, and pervasive developmental disorder in children. *Lancet* 2010;375(9713):445.

58. Basch CH, Zybert P, Reeves R, Basch CE. What do popular YouTube™ videos say about vaccines? *Child Care Health Dev* 2017;43(4):499–503.

59. Fischbach RL, Harris MJ, Ballan MS, Fischbach GD, Link BG. Is there concordance in attitudes and beliefs between parents and scientists about autism spectrum disorder? *Autism* 2016; 20(3):353–363.

60. Venkatraman A, Garg N, Kumar N. Greater freedom of speech on Web 2.0 correlates with dominance of views linking vaccines to autism. *Vaccine* 2015;33(12):1422–1425.

61. Bazzano A, Zeldin A, Schuster E, Barrett C, Lehrer D. Vaccine-related beliefs and practices of parents of children with autism spectrum disorders. *Am J Intellect Dev Disabil* 2012;117(3):233–242.

62. Centers for Disease Control and Prevention (CDC): Measles (Rubeola). Available at https://www.cdc.gov/measles/index.html. Accessed April 29, 2019.

63. Vera A. Washington is under a state of emergency as measles cases rise. CNN, January 16, 2019. Available at https://www.cnn.com/2019/01/26/health/washington-state-measles-state-of-emergency/index.html. Accessed February 25, 2019.

64. Ferguson C. The peer-review scam. *Nature* 2014;515: 480–482.

65. Kaplan S. Major publisher retracts 64 scientific papers in fake peer review outbreak. Washington Post, August 18, 015. Available at http://www.washingtonpost.com/news/morning-mix/wp/2015/08/18/outbreak-of-fake-peer-reviews-widens-as-major-publisher-retracts-64-scientific-papers/. Accessed August 20, 2015.

66. Stigbrand T. Retraction note to multiple articles in Tumor Biology. *Tumor Biology* 2017:1–6.

67. Fang FC, Steen RG, Casadevall A. Misconduct accounts for the majority of retracted scientific publications. *Proc Natl Acad Sci U S A* 2012;109(42):17028–17033.

68. Kakuk P. The legacy of the Hwang case: research misconduct in biosciences. *Sci Eng Ethics* 2009;15(4):545–562.

69. Bartlett T. UConn investigation finds that health researcher fabricated data. *The Chronicle of Higher Education*. January 11, 2012. Available at http://www.chronicle.com/blogs/percolator/uconn-investigation-finds-that-health-researcher-fabricated-data/28291. Accessed March 12, 2017.

70. Steen RG, Casadevall A, Fang FC. Why has the number of scientific retractions increased? *PLoS One* 2013;8(7):e68397.

71. Estimating the reproducibility of psychological science. *Science* 2015;349(6251):aac4716.

72. Halpern SD, Karlawish JH, Berlin JA. The continuing unethical conduct of underpowered clinical trials. *JAMA* 2002;288(3):358–362.

73. Bailar IJC. Science, statistics, and deception. *Annals of Internal Medicine* 1986;104(2):259–260.

74. Altman DG. Statistics and ethics in medical research. Misuse of statistics is unethical. *Br Med J* 1980;281(6249):1182–1184.

75. Wadhwa V. Laws and ethics can't keep pace with technology. *MIT Technology Review*, April 15, 2014. Available at https://www.technologyreview.com/s/526401/laws-and-ethics-cant-keep-pace-with-technology/. Accessed January 20, 2018.

76. Griggs B. The next frontier in 3-D printing: human organs. CNN, April 5, 2014. Available at https://www.cnn.com/2014/04/03/tech/innovation/3-d-printing-human-organs/index.html. Accessed January 28, 2018.

77. Human enhancements. John J. Reilly Center, University of Notre Dame. Available at https://reilly.nd.edu/outreach/emerging-ethical-dilemmas-and-policy-issues-in-science-and-technology/human-enhancements/. Accessed January 28, 2018.

78. Katz B. Scientists successfully clone monkeys, breaking new ground in a controversial field. Smithsonian.com, January 25, 2018. Available at https://www.smithsonianmag.com/smart-news/two-cloned-monkeys-scientists-break-new-ground-controversial-field-180967950/. Accessed January 28, 2018.

PART 2

Concepts of Measurement

CHAPTER 8 **Principles of Measurement** 106

CHAPTER 9 **Concepts of Measurement Reliability** 115

CHAPTER 10 **Concepts of Measurement Validity** 127

CHAPTER 11 **Designing Surveys and Questionnaires** 141

CHAPTER 12 **Understanding Health Measurement Scales** 159

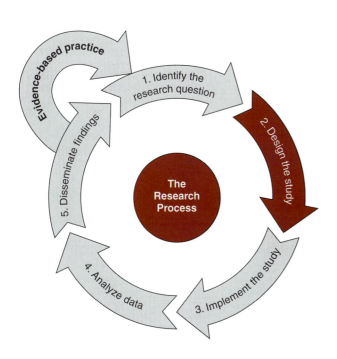

Principles of Measurement

Scientists and clinicians use measurement as a way of understanding, evaluating, and differentiating characteristics of people, objects, and systems. Measurement provides a mechanism for achieving a degree of precision in this understanding so that we can describe physical or behavioral characteristics according to their quantity, degree, capacity, or quality. This allows us to communicate in objective terms, giving us a common sense of "how much" or "how little" without ambiguous interpretation. There are virtually no clinical decisions or actions that are independent of some type of measurement.

The purpose of this chapter is to explore principles of measurement as they are applied to clinical research and evidence-based practice (EBP). Discussion will focus on several aspects of measurement theory and how these relate to quantitative assessment, analysis, and interpretation of clinical variables.

■ Why We Take Measurements

We use measurement as a basis for making decisions or drawing conclusions in several ways:

- Describing quantity of an existing variable to determine its value.

- Making decisions based on a criterion or standard of performance.
- Drawing comparisons to choose between courses of action.
- Evaluating responses to assess a patient's condition by documenting change or progress.
- Discriminating among individuals who present different profiles related to their conditions or characteristics.
- Predicting outcomes to draw conclusions about relationships and consider expected responses.
- "Measurement" has been defined as:

The process of assigning numerals to variables to represent quantities of characteristics according to certain rules.[1]

Let us explore the three essential elements of this definition.

■ Quantification and Measurement

The first part of the definition of measurement emphasizes the *process of assigning numerals to variables*. A variable is a property that can differentiate individuals or objects. It represents an attribute that can have more than one value. Value can denote quantity (such as age or blood pressure) or an attribute (such as sex or geographic region).

Numerals and Numbers

Numerals are used as labels, with no quantitative meaning, such as coding data on an opinion scale from "1" Strongly Disagree to "5" Strongly Agree. When the variable can take on only two values, such as using "0" to represent "No" and a "1" to represent "Yes" on a survey question, the measure is considered **dichotomous**. Variables that can have multiple values, such as a five-point opinion scale, are called **polytomous**.

A *number* represents a known quantity of a variable. Accordingly, quantitative variables can be operationalized and assigned values, independent of historical, cultural, or social contexts within which performance is observed. Numbers can take on different kinds of values.

Continuous Variables

A continuous variable can theoretically take on any value along a continuum within a defined range. Between any two integer values, an indefinitely large number of fractional values can occur. In reality, continuous values can never be measured exactly but are limited by the precision of the measuring instrument.

For instance, weight could be measured as 50 pounds, 50.4 pounds, or even 50.4352 pounds, depending on the calibration of the scale. Strength, distance, weight, and chronological time are other examples of continuous variables.

Discrete Variables

Some variables can be described only in whole integer units and are considered discrete variables. Heart rate, for example, is measured in beats per minute, not in fractions of a beat. Variables such as the number of trials needed to learn a motor task or the number of children in a family are also examples of discrete variables.

Precision

Precision refers to the exactness of a measure. For statistical purposes, this term is usually used to indicate the number of decimal places to which a number is taken. Therefore, 1.47382 is a number of greater precision than 1.47. The degree of precision is a function of the sensitivity of the measuring instrument and data analysis system as well as the variable itself (see Focus on Evidence 8-1).

It is not useful, for example, to record blood pressure in anything less than integer units (whole numbers with no decimal places). It may be important, however, to record strength to a tenth or hundredth of a kilogram. Computer programs will often record values with three or more decimal places by default. It is generally not informative, however, to report results to so many places. How important is it to know that a mean age is 84.5 years as opposed to 84.528 years? Such precision has been characterized as statistical "clutter" and is generally not meaningful.[2] In clinical research, greater precision may be used in analysis, but numbers will usually be reported to one or two decimal places.

■ The Indirect Nature of Measurement

The definition of measurement also indicates that measured values *represent quantities of characteristics*. Most measurement is a form of abstraction or conceptualization; that is, very few variables are measured directly. Range of motion in degrees and length in centimeters are among the few examples of measures that involve direct observation of a physical property. We can actually see how far a limb rotates or measure the size of a wound, and we can compare angles and size between people.

Most characteristics are not directly observable, however, and we can measure only a proxy of the actual property. For example, we do not observe temperature, but only the height of a column of mercury in a thermometer. We are not capable of visualizing the electrical activity of a heartbeat or muscle contraction, although

Focus on Evidence 8–1
Units of Measurement and Medication Dosing Errors

Parents often make dosing errors when administering oral liquid medications to children, with potentially serious consequences. Confusion is common because there is no standard unit, with measurements prescribed in milliliters, teaspoons, tablespoons, dropperfuls, and cubic centimeters, among the many variations. The actual instrument used to administer the liquid can also vary, including the use of household teaspoons and tablespoons, which can vary greatly in size and shape. Parents with low health literacy or language fluency challenges may be particularly vulnerable.

Yin et al[4] performed a cross-sectional analysis of data from a larger study of provider communication and medication errors, looking at 287 parents whose children were prescribed liquid medications.

Errors were defined in terms of knowledge of prescribed dose and actual observed dose. After adjusting for factors such as parent age, language, socioeconomic status, and education, they found that 40% of parents made an error in measurement of the intended dose and 17% used a nonstandard instrument. Compared to those who used milliliters only, those who used teaspoons or tablespoons were twice as likely to make an error. The authors recommended that a move to a milliliter-only standard may promote the safe use of pediatric liquid medications among groups at particular risk for misunderstanding medication instructions.

The importance of measurement precision will depend on how the measurement is applied and the seriousness of small errors. In this case, for example, confusion related to units of measurement contribute to more than 10,000 calls to poison control centers every year.[5]

we can evaluate the associated recording of an electro-cardiogram or electromyogram. For most variables, then, we use some form of direct observation to *infer* a value for a phenomenon.

Constructs

The ability to measure a variable, no matter how indirectly, is dependent on one's ability to define it. Unless we know what a term means, we cannot show that it exists. This is not difficult for variables such as temperature and heart rate which are based on physical and physiological properties, but is much harder for abstract terms such as intelligence, health, strength, mobility, depression, or pain. Any explanation of what these variables mean will undoubtedly involve descriptions of behaviors or outcomes that indicate whether someone is more or less "intelligent," "healthy," "strong," "mobile," "depressed," or "in pain." However, there is no logical, unidimensional definition that will satisfy these terms.

> Although some variables, such as strength, represent physical behaviors that are readily understood, they can still be abstract. For example, strength can be assessed in many different ways, yielding very different values. These include strain gauges, dynamometers, lifting weights, or manual resistance, with specific reference to type of contraction, joint position, speed of movement, and type of resistance. No one measurement can be interpreted as the absolute measure of a person's "strength."

These types of abstract variables, or **constructs**, are measured according to expectations of how a person who possesses the specified trait would behave, look, or feel in certain situations (see Chapter 4). Therefore, a construct is associated with some value that is *assumed* to represent the underlying variable. This presents a special challenge for measurement because there is no direct way to assign values or estimate the "amount" of a construct. Therefore, it must be defined by how we choose to measure it. Because the true nature of a construct only reflects something within a person and does not exist as an externally observable event, it is also called a **latent trait**.

We may think of mobility, for instance, in terms of how quickly someone can walk across a room or street. But the counting of seconds does not necessarily provide a linear measure of mobility.[3] It can be described in many ways other than simply time, including a reflection of capacity and intent of movement. Measuring a construct means understanding the fundamental meaning of a variable and finding ways to characterize it.

■ Rules of Measurement

The last element of the definition of measurement concerns the need for assigning values to objects *according to certain rules*. These rules reflect both amount and units of measurement. In some cases, the rules are obvious and easily learned, as in the use of a yardstick (inches), scale (pounds), thermometer (degrees), or dynamometer (newtons of force). Physiological and laboratory measures have carefully defined procedures to assign values.

The criteria for assigning values and units must be systematically defined so that levels of the behavior can be objectively differentiated; that is, rules of assignment stipulate certain relationships among numbers or numerals. For example, we assume that relationships are consistent within a specific measurement system so that objects or attributes can be equated or differentiated. We assume that either A equals B, or A does not equal B, but both cannot be true. We also assume that if A equals B, and B equals C, then A should also equal C (see Box 8-1).

Relative Order

Numbers are also used to denote relative order among variables. If A is greater than B, and B is greater than C, it should also be true that A is greater than C. We can readily see how this rule can be applied to a direct variable such as height or heart rate.

As logical as this may seem, however, there are measurement scales that do not fit within this structure. For example, we could ask two patients to rate their level of pain using a numerical rating scale from 0 to 10. Even if they both indicated their pain was a "6," there is no way to establish that their perceived levels of pain are equal. Another patient might indicate a pain level of 4, but their actual pain level might be the same as the first two patients' levels. However, if a patient rates their pain at 6 before intervention and at 2 afterward, we can assume the second measure is less than the first. The "rules" for this measurement define a system of order that is valid *within* an individual, but not *across* individuals. Therefore, clinicians must understand the conceptual basis of a particular measurement to appreciate how the rules for that measurement can logically be applied.

> Researchers and clinicians must recognize that any mathematical manipulation can be performed on any set of numbers, although they may not contribute to an understanding of the data. In his classic paper on football jersey numbers, Lord[6] cautions that numbers don't know where they come from and they will respond the same way every time! We can multiply 2×4 and get the same answer each time, whether

If you ever doubt the "far-reaching" consequences of not specifying well-defined terms, consider this. On December 11, 1998, the National Aeronautics and Space Administration (NASA) launched the Mars Climate Orbiter, designed to be the world's first complete weather satellite orbiting another planet, with a price tag of $125 million.

On September 23, 1999, the orbiter crashed into the red planet, disintegrating on contact. After a journey of 415 million miles over 9 months, the orbiter came within 36 miles of the planet's surface, lower than the lowest orbit the craft was designed to survive.

After several days of investigation, NASA officials admitted to an embarrassingly simple mistake.[9] The project team of engineers at Lockheed Martin in Colorado, who had built the spacecraft, transmitted the orbiter's final course and velocity to Mission Control in Pasadena using units of *pounds per second* of force. The navigation team at Mission Control, however, used the metric system in their calculations, which is generally the accepted practice in science and engineering. Their computers sent final commands to the spacecraft in *grams per second* of force (a measure of newtons). As a result, the ship just flew too close to the planet's surface and was destroyed by atmospheric stresses. Oops!

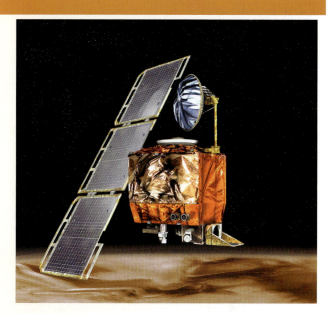

Photo courtesy of NASA/JPL/Corby Waste.

the numbers represent football jerseys, manual muscle test (MMT) grades, or inches on a ruler—but what will the answer mean? The numbers may not know but we must understand their origin to make reasonable interpretations.

■ Levels of Measurement

In 1946, Stanley Stevens,[7] a noted experimental psychologist, wondered about how different types of variables were measured and classified. He proposed a scheme to classify variables on their characteristics, rather than the number assigned to them. To clarify this process, Stevens identified four **levels of measurement**—nominal, ordinal, interval, and ratio—each with a special set of rules for manipulating and interpreting numerical data.[8] The characteristics of these four scales are summarized in Figure 8-1.

> ➤ **CASE IN POINT**
>
> Researchers studied the effects of participation in an early intervention (EI) program for low-birth-weight premature infants.[10] They collected data on several baseline measures, including sex of the child, mother's ethnicity, mother's level of education, child's birth order, the neonatal health index, the mother's age, and the child's birth weight.

These variables can be classified by different levels of measurement.

Nominal Scale

The lowest level of measurement is the **nominal scale**, also referred to as the *classificatory scale*. Objects or people are assigned to categories according to some criterion. Categories may be coded by name, number, letter, or symbol, although these are purely labels and have no quantitative value or relative order. Blood type and handedness are examples of nominal variables. A researcher might decide, for example, to assign the value of 0 to identify right-handed individuals, 1 to identify left-handed individuals, and 2 to identify ambidextrous individuals.

> ➤ In the EI study, variables of sex and ethnicity are nominal measurements. In this case, sex is male/female (a dichotomous variable), and ethnicity was defined as Black, Hispanic, or White/Other.

Based on the assumption that relationships are consistent within a measurement system, nominal categories are *mutually exclusive* so that no object or person can logically be assigned to more than one. This means that the members within a category must be equivalent on the property being scaled, but different from those in other

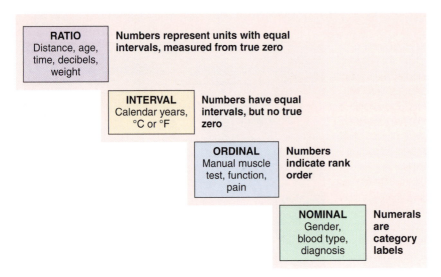

Figure 8–1 Four levels of measurement.

categories. We also assume that the rules for classifying a set of attributes are *exhaustive*; that is, every subject can be accurately assigned to one category. One can argue, for instance, that using a dichotomous classification of sex does not reflect a full range of classification according to contemporary mores.

Arithmetic Properties of Nominal Scales

The numbers or symbols used to designate groups on a nominal scale cannot be ordered based on their assigned numerals; that is, there is no inherent rank. The only permissible mathematical operation is *counting* the number of subjects within each category. Statements can then be made concerning the frequency of occurrence of a particular characteristic or the proportions of a total group that fall within each category.

> ➤ In the EI study, there were 562 girls and 520 boys. For mothers' ethnicity, 573 were Black, 119 were Hispanic, and 390 were classified as White/Other.

Ordinal Scale

More information can be obtained if countable events are ordered into successive categories that increase or decrease along an underlying continuum. Measurement on an **ordinal scale** requires that categories be rank-ordered based on an operationally defined characteristic, creating a "greater than–less than" relationship. Many clinical measurements are based on this scale, such as sensation (rated normal > impaired > absent). Tests of constructs such as function, strength, pain, and quality of life are also based on ranked scores. Surveys often create ordinal scales to describe attitudes or preferences (strongly agree > agree).

> ➤ In the EI study, level of mother's education was ranked as 1 = "some high school," 2 = "completed high school," 3 = "some college," or 4 = "completed college." Birth order also represents a rank.

Even though a measure is scored in ordinal categories, it still can represent an underlying continuous variable. To be useful, the ordinal scale should cover the full range of values for that characteristic. For example, in the EI study, the education rankings did not cover those who did not go to high school or those who had advanced education.

Importantly, the intervals between ranks on an ordinal scale may not be consistent and, indeed, may not be known. This means that although the objects assigned to one rank are considered equivalent on the rank criterion, they may not actually be of equal value along the continuum that underlies the scale (see Focus on Evidence 8-2). Therefore, ordinal scales often record ties even when true values are unequal. For example, the category of "some college" can represent any number of years. Therefore, the interval between those ranks is not really known and two individuals within one rank may not have equal education.

Arithmetic Properties of Ordinal Scales

Ordinal scales present several limitations for interpretation. Perhaps most important is the lack of arithmetic properties for ordinal "numbers." Because ranks are assigned according to discrete categories, ordinal scores are essentially labels, similar to nominal values; that is, an ordinal value does not represent quantity, but only relative *position* within a distribution. Therefore, if researchers coded education levels from 1 through 4, an individual with a score of 4 does not have twice as much

Focus on Evidence 8–2
Misleading Intervals

Using precise and accurate measurements is important in documenting therapeutic efficacy, especially when defining progression of disease. Andres et al[11] illustrated this point in a study that examined changes in strength in patients with amyotrophic lateral sclerosis, a disease that results in progressive decline in motor function. MMT has typically been used to grade strength according the patient's ability to move against gravity and hold against an examiner's resistance. Using a 12-point ordinal scale (from 0 = "no contraction" to 12 = "normal strength"), the researchers questioned the sensitivity of MMT grades to change.

They collected strength data for 20 subjects over multiple trials using MMT grades and percent of maximal voluntary isometric contraction (MVIC) using a strain gauge (ratio scale). The graph presents results for shoulder flexion, showing that there was a substantial range of strength within a single MMT grade. For example, MVIC ranged from 10% to 52% for an MMT score of 7. An MVIC of 30% could be graded between 4 and 9 on the MMT scale. These methods provide varying sensitivity, which will affect determination of progress and change over time. The choice of tool, therefore, could make a distinct difference in evaluative decisions.

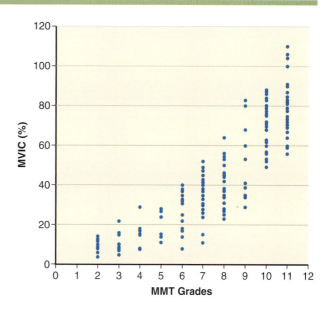

Adapted from Andres PL, Skerry LM, Thornell B, Portney LG, Finison LJ, Munsat TL. A comparison of three measures of disease progression in ALS. *J Neurol Sci* 1996;139 Suppl:64–70, Figure 2, p. 67. Used with permission.

---

education as one with a score of 2. Therefore, ordinal scores cannot meaningfully be added, subtracted, multiplied or divided, which has implications for statistical analysis, such as taking means and assessing variance.

Ordinal scores, therefore, are often described according to counts or percentages. In the EI study, 37% had some high school, 27% completed high school, 22% had some college, and 13% completed college. The median score within a distribution can also be useful (see Chapter 22).

Ordinal scales can be distinguished based on whether or not they contain a true zero point. In some cases, an ordinal scale can incorporate an artificial origin within the series of categories so that ranked scores can occur in either direction away from the origin (+ and -). This type of scale is often constructed to assess attitude or opinion, such as agree–neutral–disagree. For some construct variables, it may be reasonable to define a true zero, such as having no pain. For others it may be impossible to locate a true zero. For example, what is zero function? A category labeled "zero" may simply refer to performance below a certain criterion rather than the total absence of function.

Interval Scale

An **interval scale** possesses the rank-order characteristics of an ordinal scale, but also demonstrates known and equal intervals between consecutive values. Therefore,

relative difference and equivalence within a scale can be determined. What is not supplied by an interval scale is the absolute magnitude of an attribute because interval measures are not anchored to a true zero point (similar to an ordinal scale without a natural origin). Since the value of zero on an interval scale is not indicative of the complete absence of the measured trait, negative values are also possible and may simply represent lesser amounts of the attribute rather than a substantive deficit.

> ➤ In the EI study, the neonatal health index was defined as the length of stay in the neonatal nursery adjusted for birth weight and standardized to a mean of 100. A higher score is indicative of better health. This is an interval scale because it has no true zero and the scores are standardized based on an underlying continuum rather than representing a true quantity.

The standard numbering of years on the Gregorian calendar (B.C. and A.D.) is an interval scale. The year 1 was an arbitrary historical designation, not the beginning of time, which is why we have different years, for example, for the Chinese and Hebrew calendars. Measures of temperature using Fahrenheit and Celsius scales are also at the interval level. Both have artificial zero points that do not represent a total absence of heat and can indicate temperature in negative degrees. Within each temperature scale, we can identify that the numerical difference between 10° and 20° is equal to the numerical difference between 70° and 80°, but the actual difference in amount of heat or molecular motion generated between each 10° interval is not necessarily the same (see Fig. 8-2).

Arithmetic Properties of Interval Scales

Because of the nature of the interval scale, we must consider the practical implications for interpreting measured differences. Interval values can be added and subtracted, but these operations cannot be used to interpret actual quantities. The interval scale of temperature best illustrates this point. We know that the freezing point on the Celsius scale is 0°, whereas on the Fahrenheit scale it is 32°. This is so because the zero point on each scale is arbitrary. Therefore, although each scale maintains the integrity of its intervals and relative position of each quantity, measurement of the same quantities will yield different values. Therefore, it is not reasonable to develop a ratio based on interval data because the numbers cannot be logically measured against true zero. For example, 10°C is half of 20°C, a ratio of 1:2. The equivalent temperatures on the Fahrenheit scale are 50°F and 68°F, a ratio of 1:1.36.

The actual values within any two interval scales are not equivalent and, therefore, one interval scale cannot be directly transformed to another. Because the actual values are irrelevant, it is the ordinal positions of points or the equality of intervals that must be maintained in any mathematical operation. Consequently, we can transform scales by multiplying or adding a constant, which will not change the relative position of any single value within the scale. After the transformation is made, intervals separating units will be in the same proportion as they were in the original scale. This is classically illustrated by the transformation of Celsius to Fahrenheit by multiplying by 9/5 and adding 32.

 Measurement properties of many ordinal scales have been studied using an approach called Rasch analysis that provides a reasonable model for handling ordinal data as interval.[12-14] This is especially important in scales in which ordinal values are summed across multiple items and a total score is used to reflect an individual's performance. This issue is addressed fully in Chapter 12.

Ratio Scale

The highest level of measurement is achieved by the **ratio scale**, which is an interval scale with an absolute zero point that has empirical, rather than arbitrary, meaning. A score of zero at the ratio level represents a total absence of whatever property is being measured. Therefore, negative values are not possible. Height, weight, and force are all examples of ratio scales. Although a zero on such scales is actually theoretical (it could not be measured), it is nonetheless unambiguous.

➤ In the EI study, mother's age (years) and child's birth weight (grams) are examples of ratio level measures.

Arithmetic Properties of Ratio Scales

Numbers on the ratio scale reflect actual amounts of the variable being measured. It makes sense, then, to say that one baby is twice as heavy as another or that one mother is half the age of another. Ratio data can also be directly transformed from one scale to another. All mathematical and statistical operations are permissible with ratio level data.

Identifying Levels of Measurement

As shown in Figure 8-1, the four levels of measurement constitute a hierarchy based on the relative precision of assigned values, with nominal measurement at the bottom and ratio measurement at the top. Although variables will be optimally measured at the highest possible level of measurement, we can always operationally define a variable at lower levels.

Suppose we were interested in measuring step length in a sample of four children. We could use a tape measure with graduated centimeter markings to measure the distance from heel strike to heel strike. This would constitute a ratio scale. Our measurements would allow us to determine the actual length of each child's step, as well as which children took longer steps than others and by how much. Hypothetical data for such measures are presented in Table 8-1.

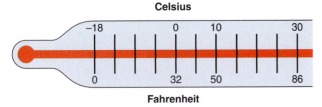

Celsius

| −18 | 0 | 10 | 30 |

| 0 | 32 | 50 | 86 |

Fahrenheit

Figure 8–2 Temperature as an interval scale, showing degrees expressed with two different zero points on Celsius and Fahrenheit scales.

Table 8-1	Hypothetical Data for Step Length Measured on Different Scales			
SUBJECT	RATIO (cm)	INTERVAL	ORDINAL	NOMINAL
A	23	4	2	Long
B	24	5	3	Long
C	19	0	1	Short
D	28	9	4	Long

We could convert these ratio measures to an interval scale by arbitrarily assigning a score of zero to the lowest value and adjusting the intervals accordingly. We would still know which children took longer steps, and we would have a relative idea of how much longer they were, but we would no longer know what the actual step length was. We would also no longer be able to determine that Subject D takes a step 1.5 times as great as Subject C. In fact, using interval data, it erroneously appears as if Subject D takes a step nine times the length of Subject C.

An ordinal measure can be achieved by simply ranking the children's step lengths. With this scale we no longer have any indication of the magnitude of the differences. Based on ordinal data, we could not establish that Subjects A and B were more alike than any others.

We can eventually reduce our measurement to a nominal scale by setting a criterion for "long" versus "short" steps and classifying each child accordingly. With this measurement, we have no way of distinguishing any differences in performance between Subjects A, B, and D.

Clearly, we have lost significant amounts of information with each successive reduction in scale. It will always be an advantage, therefore, to achieve the highest possible level of measurement. Data can always be manipulated to use a lower scale, but not vice versa. In reality, clinical researchers usually have access to a limited variety of measurement tools, and the choice is often dictated by the instrumentation available and the clinician's preference or skill. Even though step length was assessed using four different scales, the true nature of the variable remains unchanged. Therefore, we must distinguish between the underlying nature of a variable and the scale used to measure it.

Statistics and Levels of Measurement

An understanding of the levels of measurement is more than an academic exercise. The importance of determining the measurement scale for a variable lies in the determination of which mathematical operations are appropriate and which interpretations are meaningful. All statistical tests have been designed around certain assumptions about data, including the level of measurement. **Parametric tests** apply arithmetic manipulations, requiring interval or ratio data. **Nonparametric tests** do not make the same assumptions and are designed to be used with ordinal and nominal data (see Chapter 27).

In many cases, using parametric or nonparametric procedures can make a difference as to how data will be interpreted (see Chapter 23). Therefore, distinctions about levels of measurement are not trivial. However, identifying the level of measurement may not be simple. The underlying properties of many behavioral variables do not fit neatly into one scale or another. For example, behavioral scientists continue to question the classification of intelligence quotient (IQ) scores as either ordinal or interval measures.[15] Can we assume that intervals are equal so that the difference between scores of 50 and 100 is the same as the difference between 100 and 150, or are these scores only reflective of relative order? Can we say that someone with an IQ of 200 is twice as intelligent as someone with a score of 100? Is everyone with a score of 100 equally intelligent? Is there a "unit" of intelligence? Most likely the true scale is somewhere between ordinal and interval. The importance of this issue will be relevant in how data are analyzed and interpreted.

COMMENTARY

It is really just as bad technique to make a measurement more accurately than is necessary as it is to make it not accurately enough.

—Arthur David Ritchie (1891–1967)

British philosopher

Although there are clear differentiations among statistical tests regarding data assumptions, we find innumerable instances throughout the clinical and behavioral science literature in which parametric statistical operations are used with ordinal data. The question is, how serious are the consequences of misassumptions about scale properties to the interpretation of statistical research results? Some say quite serious,[16,17] whereas others indicate that the answer is "not very."[18,19] Many researchers are comfortable constructing ordinal scales using categories that are assumed to logically represent equal intervals of the test variable and treating the scores as interval data,[18,20] especially when the scale incorporates some type of natural origin. Questions using a five-point Likert scale ("Strongly Agree" to "Strongly Disagree") would be considered ordinal, but if several item responses are summed, the total is typically treated as an interval measurement.[21]

Because ordinal measures occur frequently in the behavioral and social sciences, this issue is of significant import to the reasonable interpretation of clinical data. Kerlinger[22] suggests that most psychological and educational scales approximate equal intervals fairly well, and that the results of statistical analyses using these measures provide satisfactory and useful information.

McDowell[23] suggests that the classification of a measurement as ordinal or interval in a health scale is less about inherent numerical properties than it is about how scores will be interpreted. Therefore, this issue will take on varied importance depending on the nature of the variables being measured and the precision needed to use them meaningfully. For the most part, it would seem appropriate to continue treating ordinal measurements as ranked rather than interval data; however, if the interval approach is defensible, the degree of error associated with this practice may be quite tolerable in the long run.[15] Even Stevens,[7] in his landmark paper, makes a practical concession:

> *In the strictest propriety the ordinary statistics involving means and standard deviations ought not to be used with these [ordinal] scales, for these statistics imply a knowledge of something more than the relative rank-order of data. On the other hand, for this "illegal" statisticizing there can be invoked a kind of pragmatic sanction: In numerous instances it leads to fruitful results.*

As researchers and evidence-based practitioners, we must scrutinize the underlying theoretical construct that defines a scale and remain responsible for justifying the application of statistical procedures and the subsequent interpretations of the data.

REFERENCES

1. Nunnally J, Bernstein IH. *Psychometric Theory*. 3 ed. New York: McGraw-Hill, 1994.
2. Cohen J. Things I have learned (so far). *Am Psychologist* 1990; 45(12):1304–1312.
3. Wright BD, Linacre JM. Observations are always ordinal; measurements, however, must be interval. *Arch Phys Med Rehabil* 1989;70(12):857–860.
4. Yin HS, Dreyer BP, Ugboaja DC, Sanchez DC, Paul IM, Moreira HA, Rodriguez L, Mendelsohn AL. Unit of measurement used and parent medication dosing errors. *Pediatrics* 2014;134(2):e354–e361.
5. Bronstein AC, Spyker DA, Cantilena LR, Jr., Rumack BH, Dart RC. 2011 Annual report of the American Association of Poison Control Centers' National Poison Data System (NPDS): 29th annual report. *Clin Toxicol* 2012;50(10):911–1164.
6. Lord FM. On the statistical treatment of football numbers. *Am Psychologist* 1953;8(12):750–751.
7. Stevens SS. On the Theory of Scales of Measurement. *Science* 1946;103(2684):677–680.
8. Stevens SS. Mathematics, measurement and psychophysics. In: Stevens SS, ed. *Handbook of Experimental Psychology*. New York: Wiley, 1951.
9. Metric mishap caused loss of NASA orbiter. CNN.com. September 30, 1999. Available at https://edition.cnn.com/TECH/space/9909/30/mars.metric.02/. Accessed January 25, 2018.
10. Hill JL, Brooks-Gunn J, Waldfogel J. Sustained effects of high participation in an early intervention for low-birth-weight premature infants. *Dev Psychol* 2003;39(4):730–744.
11. Andres PL, Skerry LM, Thornell B, Portney LG, Finison LJ, Munsat TL. A comparison of three measures of disease progression in ALS. *J Neurol Sci* 1996;139 Suppl:64–70.
12. White LJ, Velozo CA. The use of Rasch measurement to improve the Oswestry classification scheme. *Arch Phys Med Rehabil* 2002;83(6):822–831.
13. Decruynaere C, Thonnard JL, Plaghki L. Measure of experimental pain using Rasch analysis. *Eur J Pain* 2007;11(4):469–474.
14. Jacobusse G, van Buuren S, Verkerk PH. An interval scale for development of children aged 0–2 years. *Stat Med* 2006;25(13): 2272–2283.
15. Knapp TR. Treating ordinal scales as interval scales: an attempt to resolve the controversy. *Nurs Res* 1990;39(2):121–123.
16. Jakobsson U. Statistical presentation and analysis of ordinal data in nursing research. *Scand J Caring Sci* 2004;18(4):437–440.
17. Merbitz C, Morris J, Grip JC. Ordinal scales and foundations of misinference. *Arch Phys Med Rehabil* 1989;70:308–312.
18. Wang ST, Yu ML, Wang CJ, Huang CC. Bridging the gap between the pros and cons in treating ordinal scales as interval scales from an analysis point of view. *Nurs Res* 1999;48(4):226–229.
19. Cohen ME. Analysis of ordinal dental data: evaluation of conflicting recommendations. *J Dent Res* 2001;80(1):309–313.
20. Gaito J. Measurement scales and statistics: resurgence of an old misconception. *Psychol Bull* 1980;87:564–567.
21. Wigley CJ. Dispelling three myths about Likert scales in communication trait research. *Commun Res Reports* 2013;30(4):366–372.
22. Kerlinger FN. *Foundations of Behavioral Research*. 3 ed. New York: Holt, Rinehart & Winston, 1985.
23. McDowell I. *Measuring Health: A Guide to Rating Scales and Questionnaires*. 3 ed. New York: Oxford University Press, 2006.

Concepts of Measurement Reliability

The usefulness of measurement in clinical decision-making depends on the extent to which clinicians can rely on data as accurate and meaningful indicators of a behavior or attribute. The first prerequisite, at the heart of accurate measurement, is reliability, or the extent to which a measured value can be obtained consistently during repeated assessment of unchanging behavior. Without sufficient reliability, we cannot have confidence in the data we collect nor can we draw rational conclusions about stable or changing performance.

The purpose of this chapter is to present the conceptual basis of reliability and describe different approaches to testing the reliability of clinical measurements. Further discussion of reliability statistics is found in Chapter 32.

■ Concepts of Reliability

Reliability is fundamental to all aspects of measurement. If a patient's behavior is reliable, we can expect consistent responses under given conditions. A reliable examiner is one who assigns consistent scores to a patient's unchanging behavior. A reliable instrument is one that will perform with predictable accuracy under steady conditions. The nature of reality is such that measurements are rarely perfectly reliable. All instruments are fallible to some extent and all humans respond with some level of inconsistency.

Measurement Error

Consider the simple process of measuring an individual's height with a tape measure. First, assume that the individual's height is stable—it is not changing, and therefore, there is a theoretical *true value* for the person's actual height. Now let us take measurements, recorded to the nearest 1/16 inch, on three separate occasions, either by one examiner or by three different examiners. Given the fallibility of our methods, we can expect some differences in the values recorded from each trial. Assuming that all measurements were acquired using similar procedures and with equal concern for accuracy, it may not be possible to determine which of the three measured values was the truer representation of the subject's actual height. Indeed, we would have no way of knowing exactly how much error was included in each of the measured values.

According to classical measurement theory, any *observed score* (X_O) consists of two components: a *true score* (X_T) that is a fixed value, and an unknown *error component* (E) that may be large or small depending on the accuracy and precision of our measurement procedures. This relationship is summarized by the equation:

$$X_O = X_T \pm E$$

Any difference between the true value and the observed value is regarded as *measurement error*, or "noise," that gets in the way of our finding the true score. Although it is theoretically possible that a single measured value is right on the money (with no error), it is far more likely that an observed score will either overestimate or underestimate the true value to some degree. Reliability can be conceptually defined as an estimate of the extent to which an observed test score is free from error; that is, how well observed scores reflect true scores.

Whereas reliability is all about the consistency or replicability of measured values, validity describes the extent to which a measurement serves its intended purpose by quantifying the target construct (see Chapter 10). Both reliability and validity are essential considerations for how measurement accuracy is evaluated in research, as well as for how measured data are used as evidence to inform clinical practice.

Types of Measurement Error

To understand reliability, we must distinguish between two basic types of measurement errors: systematic and random. Figure 9-1 illustrates this relationship, using a target analogy in which the center represents the true score.

Systematic Error

Systematic errors are predictable errors of measurement. They occur in one direction, consistently overestimating or underestimating the true score. If a systematic error is detected, it is usually a simple matter to correct it either by recalibrating the instrument or by adding or subtracting the appropriate constant from each observed value. For example, if the end of a tape measure is incorrectly marked, such that markings actually begin 0.25 inch from the end of the tape, measurements of height will consistently record values that are too short by 0.25 inch. We can correct this error by cutting off the extra length at the end of the tape (thereby recalibrating the instrument) or by adding the appropriate constant (0.25 inch) to each observed value.

By definition, systematic errors are consistent. Consequently, systematic errors are not a threat to reliability. Instead, systematic errors only threaten the validity of a measure because, despite highly replicable values over repeated assessments, none of the observed values will succeed in accurately quantifying the target construct.

Random Error

Presuming that an instrument is well calibrated and there is no other source of systematic bias, measurement errors can be considered "random" since their effect on the observed score is not predictable. **Random errors** are just as likely to result in an overestimate of the true score as an underestimate. These errors are a matter of chance, possibly arising from factors such as examiner or subject inattention, instrument imprecision, or unanticipated environmental fluctuation.

For example, if a patient is fidgeting while their height is being measured, random errors may cause the observed scores to vary in unpredictable ways from trial to trial. The examiner may be inconsistently positioning herself when observing the tape, or the tape may be stretched out to a greater or lesser extent during some trials, resulting in unpredictable errors. We can think of any single measurement as one of an infinite number of possible measures that could have been taken at that point in time.

If we assume random errors are a matter of chance with erroneous overestimates and underestimates occurring with equal frequency, recording the average across several trials should allow the positive and negative random errors to cancel each other out, bringing us closer to the true score. For example, if we were to take the average of scores shown as random error in Figure 9-1, we would end up with a score closer to the true score at the center of the target. One possible strategy for reducing random error and improving reliability is to record the average across several repetitions of a measurement rather than just the results of a single trial.

Sources of Measurement Error

In the development or testing of a measuring instrument, a protocol should be specified to maximize reliability, detailing procedures and instructions for using the instrument in the same way each time. When designing the protocol, researchers should anticipate sources of error which, once identified, can often be controlled.

> ➤ **CASE IN POINT #1**
> The Timed "Up & Go" (TUG) test is a commonly used functional assessment to measure balance and gait speed, as well as to estimate risk for falls.[1] Using a stopwatch, a clinician measures in seconds the time it takes for a subject to rise from a chair, walk a distance of 3 meters, turn, walk back to the chair, and sit. Faster times indicate better balance and less fall risk. The reliability and validity of the TUG have been studied under a variety of circumstances and in several populations.[2]

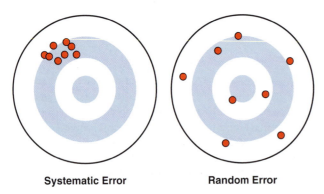

Systematic Error   **Random Error**

Figure 9–1 Depiction of systematic and random errors.

The simplicity and efficiency of the TUG make it a useful example to illustrate reliability concepts.

Measurement errors can generally be attributed to three sources:

1. **The individual taking the measurements (the rater):** Errors can result from a lack of skill, not following the protocol, distraction, inaccurately recording or transcribing values, or an unconscious bias.

> ➤ The rater for the TUG is the clinician who observes the test and times it with a stopwatch. The rater must be able to follow the protocol to be consistent from trial to trial. For example, the rater must determine criteria for the exact moment the patient rises from the chair and sits back down. Instructions to the subject should be the same each time.

2. **The measuring instrument itself:** Imprecise instruments or environmental changes affecting instrument performance can also contribute to random error. Many instruments, especially mechanical ones, are subject to some level of background noise or fluctuating performance.

> ➤ The stopwatch must be working properly to record TUG time accurately. For instance, the battery could be weak or the stem of the stopwatch could occasionally stick. If the stopwatch were calibrated to measure time to the nearest second rather than fractions of a second, random measurement errors could result.

3. **Variability of the characteristic being measured:** Errors often occur from variations in physiological response or changes in subject performance. Blood pressure is an example of a response that can vary from moment to moment. Responses can be influenced by personal characteristics such as changes in motivation, cooperation, or fatigue, or by environmental factors such as transient noise or ambient temperature fluctuations. If the targeted response variable is inherently unstable, it may be difficult or impossible to quantify reliably (see Focus on Evidence 9-1).

> ➤ A patient's TUG performance in rising, walking, and turning quickly can vary from moment to moment depending on their physical or emotional status. For example, multiple trials can cause some patients to fatigue. A patient with Parkinson's disease (PD) may experience physiological changes in response to recent medication. If a patient is feeling anxious, they may walk cautiously, but move more quickly during periods of lessened anxiety.

Where errors result solely from the inherent instability of a response variable, they may be difficult to avoid. In other instances, however, measurement error can be substantially reduced through improved training of the rater or careful standardization of the protocol. It is important for clinicians and researchers to understand the theoretical and practical nature of the response variable so that sources of error affecting reliability can be anticipated and properly interpreted or controlled.

■ Measuring Reliability

As it is not possible to know a true score with certainty, the actual reliability of a test can never be directly calculated. Instead, we estimate the reliability of a test based on the statistical concept of **variance**, which is a measure of the variability among scores in a sample (see Chapter 22). The greater the dispersion of scores, the larger the variance; the more homogeneous the scores, the smaller the variance. Within any sample, the total variance in scores will be due to two primary sources.

To illustrate, suppose we ask two clinicians to score five patients performing the TUG. Let us also assume that the true scores remain constant. Across the 10 scores that are recorded, we would undoubtedly find that scores differed from one another. One source of variance comes

---

Focus on Evidence 9–1
Real Differences or Random Error?

Kluge et al[3] wanted to establish the reliability of a mobile gait analysis system to measure several parameters, including timing of stride, stance and swing phases, and walking velocity. They studied 15 patients, 11 healthy and 4 with Parkinson's disease. The participants were asked to walk at three self-selected speeds: fast, normal, and slow.

Researchers found excellent reliability for all parameters—except for gait velocity during slow walking. Although the lower reliability could have resulted from other unidentified sources of measurement error that are unique to slow-paced walking, the researchers suggested that a more likely explanation was that slow walking velocities were inherently less stable than parameters of fast or normal speed gait. They speculated that people do not use a consistent pattern for walking at a slow pace, making it difficult to measure with high reliability.

from differences among true scores for different patients. This is expected when testing unique individuals, as some will walk faster than others. However, the second source of variance is a function of measurement error, which is reflected in discrepancies in the clinicians' ratings of any individual patient.

Reliability can be estimated by comparing the relative contributions of true variance versus random measurement error to the total variability observed in a set of test scores. Reliability increases when the error component is only a small proportion of the total variance, with true variance across individuals making up a larger proportion of the total variance observed. This relationship can be expressed statistically as a **reliability coefficient**. There are several different forms of reliability coefficients, each appropriate to different study designs and types of data.

Several examples of reliability coefficients will be described briefly here, with related statistical concepts presented in detail in Chapter 32.

Relative Reliability

Relative reliability coefficients reflect true variance as a proportion of the total variance in a set of scores. With maximum reliability (no error), this ratio will produce a coefficient of 1.00, indicating that all the observed variance was due to true differences among individual subjects with no measurement error. As error increases, the value of the coefficient approaches zero. As a ratio, this type of coefficient results in "unitless" values between 0.00 and 1.00.

 Because reliability is hardly ever perfect and chance is always operating, reliability coefficients of 1.00 or 0.00 are rare.

Because they are unitless, these relative values allow us to compare the reliability of different tests. For instance, if we studied reliability for the TUG, recorded in seconds, and the Berg Balance Test, a 14-item summative scale, we could determine which was more reliable using a relative index. The most reliable test would be the one whose relative reliability coefficient was closest to 1.00.

The most commonly used relative reliability indices are the **intraclass correlation coefficient (ICC)** for quantitative data and the **kappa (κ)** coefficient for categorical data.

> Studies have shown that the TUG has strong rater reliability in patients with lumbar disc disease (ICC = 0.97),[4] and stroke (ICC >0.95).[5]

> Although the Pearson correlation coefficient (r) is sometimes reported as a relative reliability coefficient, its usefulness for capturing reliability is limited and other statistics are generally preferred.

Absolute Reliability

Relative reliability indices are useful for estimating reliability for groups and for comparing the reliability of different tests, but they do not help us understand the actual degree to which measured values are expected to vary for any individual. Therefore, although conceptually helpful, they are less useful for interpreting clinical measurements obtained from an individual patient.

In contrast, **absolute reliability** statistics do indicate something about how much of a measured value, expressed in the original units, is likely to be due to error. The most commonly used absolute reliability index is the **standard error of measurement (SEM)**. The SEM provides a range of scores within which the true score for a given test is likely to lie.

> A study has shown that the SEM for the TUG is 10.2 seconds for patients who have had knee or hip replacement surgery.[6] This means that if a patient records a TUG score of 30.0 seconds, the true score for that patient, accounting for likely measurement error, is probably within the range of 19.8 to 40.2 seconds (i.e., 30.0 ± 10.2 seconds).

■ Understanding Reliability

Two considerations are important when interpreting results of a reliability study or making judgments about clinical instruments.

Reliability Exists in a Context

Reliability is not an inherent or immutable trait of a measurement tool. It can only be understood within the context of a tool's application, including the characteristics of the subjects, the training and skill of the examiners, the setting, and the number and timing of test trials.[7,8] Studies have also evaluated the unique reliability of various questionnaire tools when translated into different languages or administered to people of different cultures.[9–11] Without consideration of contextual factors, the reliability of an instrument cannot be fairly judged (see Box 9-1).

Reliability Is Not All-or-None

Reliability is not an all-or-none trait but exists to some extent in any instrument. References made to an instrument as either "reliable" or "unreliable" should be

Box 9-1   Generalizing Reliability: It's Not All Random

When we consider methods to improve reliability, we must be able to identify which factors contribute to error, recognizing that many of these factors can be controlled. Where classical measurement theory sees all error as random, the concept of **generalizability theory** has been proposed to account for specific sources of error.[14] If we can identify relevant testing conditions that influence scores, then we should be able to explain more of the variance in a set of scores, effectively leaving less variance unexplained as random error.

For example, a single TUG score of 15 seconds would be one of a universe of possible scores that might be obtained by the same examiner with the same test–retest interval. In classical measurement theory, all error would be considered random. However, by accounting for variance of rater performance and test intervals, less error variance will be unexplained, improving our understanding of reliability.

The concept of generalizability is especially relevant for development and standardization of measurement tools, because it provides a frame of reference for interpretation of reliability coefficients and suggests areas for improvement of protocols. When adopting a tool, a clinician can determine the conditions under which a reliability coefficient is applicable. If the use of a tool requires extensive training, then the results of a reliability study would only be generalizable to raters who had that training. If the

study incorporated test intervals of 1 hour, then results would apply only to that time frame. A questionnaire in English may not be reliable when translated into a different language or used with patients from different backgrounds. Therefore, generalizability theory provides a strong basis for clinical interpretation of reliability.

---

avoided since these labels fail to recognize this distinction. Reliability coefficients provide values that can help us estimate the degree of reliability present in a measurement system, but we must always exercise judgment in deciding whether a measurement is sufficiently reliable for its intended application. Application of reliability measures from published studies must be based on the generalizability of the study to clinical circumstances. A test's reliability is not necessarily the same in all situations.

🔑 Just how large does a relative reliability coefficient have to be to be considered acceptable? The short answer is, "it depends." The amount of error that is tolerable depends on the type of reliability being studied, the specific coefficient used, and the intended purpose of the measurement. Various cutoff values have been proposed for interpreting a coefficient as indicating poor, moderate, or high reliability. Generally, clinical measures should have reliability coefficient above 0.80,[12,13] but this could be higher or lower depending on the precision needed for clinical assessment.

There are no similar guidelines to judge whether absolute measures of reliability are strong or weak. These measures can be interpreted only in relation to the units of measurement, the variables being assessed, and how much error is tolerable for clinical decision-making.

This important issue of magnitude of reliability will be addressed again in Chapter 32.

■ Types of Reliability

Estimates of relative reliability vary depending on the type of reliability being analyzed. This section will introduce design considerations for four general approaches to reliability testing: test–retest reliability, rater reliability, alternate forms reliability, and internal consistency.

Test–Retest Reliability

Reliable measurement is impossible without a stable measuring instrument—one that obtains the same results over repeated administrations, assuming that no real change in performance has occurred. **Test–retest reliability** assessments determine the ability of an instrument to measure subject performance consistently.

➤ CASE IN POINT #2

The Falls Efficacy Scale-International (FES-I) is a 16-item self-report questionnaire that assesses fear of falling.[15] Using a 4-point Likert scale ("Strongly Disagree" to "Strongly Agree"), patients are asked to rate their concerns about the possibility of falling when performing specific activities, with higher summative scores indicating greater fear.

To perform a test–retest study, a sample of individuals is subjected to the identical test on two separate occasions, keeping all testing conditions as constant as possible. The coefficient derived from this type of analysis is called a *test–retest reliability coefficient*. It estimates reliability in situations in which raters are minimally involved, such as patient self-report questionnaires or instrumented physiological tests that provide automated digital readouts.

> The FES-I is a self-report inventory completed by an individual using pencil and paper. It has been evaluated for test–retest reliability by asking subjects to repeat the inventory on two separate occasions one week apart.[15]

> 🔑 Because the FES-I is a questionnaire completed by the patient, error cannot be attributed to a rater, and therefore test–retest reliability is a measure of the instrument's consistency. With a performance-based test such as the TUG, however, where the rater is a central part of the measurement system, consistent scoring will depend on adequate rater reliability and test–retest reliability cannot be logically measured.

Test–Retest Intervals

Because the stability of a response variable is such a significant factor, the time interval between tests must be considered. Intervals should be far enough apart to avoid fatigue, learning, or memory effects, but close enough to avoid genuine changes in the targeted variable.

> In the study of the FES-I, a 1-week interval was considered reasonable to ensure that significant changes in balance or fear of falling were unlikely but sufficient for subjects to no longer be influenced by recollection of their initial answers.[15]

Other measures may require different intervals. For instance, measurements of blood pressure need to be repeated in rapid succession to avoid changes in this labile response variable. Tests of infant development might need to be taken within several days to avoid the natural developmental changes that occur at early ages. If, however, we are interested in establishing the ability of an intelligence quotient (IQ) test to provide a stable assessment of intelligence over time, it might be more meaningful to test a child using intervals of a year or more. A researcher must be able to anticipate the inherent stability of the targeted response variable prior to making test–retest assessments.

Carryover

When a test is administered on two or more occasions, reliability can be influenced by carryover effects, wherein practice or learning during the initial trial alters performance on subsequent trials. A test of dexterity may improve due to motor learning. Strength measurements can improve following warm-up trials. Sometimes subjects are given a series of pretest trials to neutralize this effect and data are collected only after performance has stabilized. Because a retest score can be influenced by a subject's effort to improve, some researchers will conceal scores from the subjects between trials.

Testing Effects

When the test itself is responsible for observed changes in a measured variable, the change is considered a **testing effect**. For example, range of motion testing can stretch soft tissue structures around a joint, thereby increasing the arc of motion on subsequent testing. The initial trial of a strength test could provoke joint pain, thereby weakening responses on the second trial.

Oftentimes, testing and carryover effects will manifest as systematic error, creating unidirectional changes across all subjects. Such an effect will not necessarily affect reliability coefficients, for reasons we have already discussed.

📈 **Coefficients for Test–Retest Reliability**
Test–retest reliability of quantitative measurements is most often assessed using the ICC. With categorical data, percent agreement can be calculated and the kappa statistic applied. In clinical situations, the SEM, being an absolute reliability measure, provides a more useful estimate for interpreting how much error is likely to be present in a single measurement.

Rater Reliability

Many clinical measurements require that a human observer, or *rater*, is part of the measurement system. In some cases, the rater constitutes the only measuring instrument, such as in observation of gait, or palpation of lymph nodes or joint mobility. Other times, a test involves physical manipulation of a tool by the rater, as in the taking of blood pressure using a sphygmomanometer.

Rater reliability is important whether one or several testers are involved. Training and standardization may be necessary, especially when measuring devices are new or unfamiliar, or when subjective observations are used. Even when raters are experienced, however, rater reliability should be documented.

To establish rater reliability, the instrument and the response variable are assumed to be stable so that any differences between scores on repeated tests can be attributed solely to rater error. In many situations, this may be a large assumption and varied contributions to reliability should be considered (see Box 9-1).

Intra-Rater Reliability

Intra-rater reliability refers to the stability of data recorded by one tester across two or more trials. When carryover effects are not an issue, intra-rater reliability is usually assessed using trials that follow each other with short intervals. The number of trials needed is dependent on the expected variability in the response.

In a test–retest situation, when a rater's skill is relevant to the accuracy of the test, intra-rater reliability and test–retest reliability are essentially the same. In measuring blood pressure, for instance, it is not possible to distinguish the skill of the examiner versus the consistency of the sphygmomanometer.

> ➤ A single rater can observe and record scores from the TUG on successive trials. Part of the skill is being able to determine the exact time to click the stopwatch to start and stop the trial, as the patient rises from and sits in the chair.

We must also consider the possibility of bias when one rater takes two measurements. Raters can be influenced by their memory of the first score. This is most relevant in cases in which human observers use subjective criteria to rate responses. The most effective way to control for this type of error is to blind the tester in some way so that the first score remains unknown until after the second trial is completed.

> ➤ When a tester is administering the TUG, a second person could read the stopwatch and record scores so that the tester remains unaware of current or previous scores.

Because many clinical measurements are observational, such a technique is often unreasonable. For instance, we could not blind a clinician to measures of balance, function, muscle testing, or gait, where the tester is an integral part of the measurement system. The major protections against tester bias are to develop grading criteria that are as objective as possible to train the testers in the use of the instrument and to document reliability across raters.

Inter-Rater Reliability

Inter-rater reliability concerns variation between two or more raters who measure the same subjects. Even with detailed operational definitions and equal skill, different raters are not always in agreement about the quality or quantity of the variable being assessed.

> 🔑 Intra-rater reliability should be established for each individual rater before comparing raters to each other.

Inter-rater reliability is best assessed when all raters are able to measure a response during a single trial, in which they can observe a subject simultaneously yet independently of one another. This eliminates true differences in scores as a possible source of measurement error. Videotapes of patients performing activities have proved useful for allowing multiple raters to observe the exact same performance.[16–18]

> ➤ Two testers can observe a patient performing the TUG simultaneously, each with their own stopwatch, independently recording their times.

Simultaneous scoring is not possible, however, for many variables that require interaction of the tester and subject. For example, range of motion and manual muscle testing could not be tested simultaneously by two clinicians. With these types of measures, rater reliability may be affected if there is a testing effect or if, for some other reason, the actual performance changes from trial to trial.

Researchers will often decide to use one rater in a study to avoid the necessity of establishing inter-rater reliability. Although this may be useful for improving consistency within the study, it limits generalizability of the research outcomes to other people or clinics. If inter-rater reliability has not been established, we cannot assume that other raters would have obtained similar results.

📈 Coefficients for Rater Reliability

With quantitative data, the ICC should be used to evaluate rater reliability. Different models of this statistic are applied for intra- and inter-rater reliability, depending on the intent to generalize results. With categorical data, the kappa statistic is used.

Alternate Forms

Some variables can be assessed using alternative versions of the same tool. This is common in standardized educational testing, for example, to ensure that answers are not shared among test-takers. Alternate forms can also be applied in clinical situations in which two versions of an instrument are compared to see if they obtain similar scores. For example, studies have looked at the agreement between human counting of heart rate and automated monitors,[19] the agreement of paper and pencil or electronic versions of a pain visual analog scale (VAS),[20] and comparison of a pocket-sized ultrasound machine with standard equipment for routine prenatal scans.[21] These different versions are considered reliable alternatives based on their statistical equivalence.

Alternate forms reliability, also called *equivalent* or *parallel forms*, assesses the differences between scores on the different forms to determine whether they agree. It is also used as an alternative to test–retest reliability when the intention is to derive comparable versions of a test to minimize the threat posed when subjects recall their responses.

Coefficients for Alternate Forms Reliability

Correlation coefficients have been used to examine alternate forms reliability. Comparative tests, such as the *t*-test, can be used to compare mean scores on the different test versions, but this will not be a true measure of reliability. A test of *limits of agreement* can be used to estimate the range of error expected when using two different versions of an instrument. This estimate is based on how performance on the two versions of the test differs across a range of mean scores.

Internal Consistency

Instruments such as surveys, questionnaires, written examinations, and interviews are composed of a set of questions or items intended to measure the various aspects of a coherent area of knowledge or the different attributes of a multifaceted construct. **internal consistency**, or *homogeneity*, reflects the extent to which the items that comprise a multi-item test succeed in measuring the various aspects of the same characteristic and nothing else. For example, if we assess a patient's ability to perform daily tasks using a multi-item physical function inventory, then the items on the inventory should relate to aspects of physical function only. If some items evaluate psychological or social characteristics, then the items would not be considered internally consistent.

The most common approach to assessing internal consistency involves looking at correlations among each of the items comprising a scale, as well as correlations between each item and a summative test score. For most instruments, it is desirable to see some relationship among items to reflect measurement of the same attribute, especially if the scale score is summed. Therefore, for inventories that are intended to be multidimensional, researchers generally establish subscales that are homogenous on a particular trait.

Internal consistency, a measure of reliability, is sometimes confused with assessment of construct validity, which is also concerned with the ability of an instrument to measure a single characteristic (see Chapter 10). The difference is that internal consistency looks at the homogeneity of items in inventory, but does not assess whether it is the construct of interest that is being addressed.

Split-Half Reliability

If we wanted to establish the reliability of a questionnaire or educational test, it would be necessary to administer the instrument on two separate occasions, but recall can then become a potential threat. This concern is usually handled by combining two sets of items testing the same content into one longer instrument, with half the items being redundant of the other half. One group of subjects takes the combined test at a single session. The items are then divided into two comparable halves for scoring, creating two separate scores for each subject. Reliability is assessed by correlating results of two halves of the test. This is called **split-half reliability**. In essence, the two halves can be considered alternate forms of the same test.

Coefficients for Internal Consistency

The statistic most often used for internal consistency is Cronbach's coefficient alpha (α). As a relative measure of reliability, this index can take on values from 0.00 to 1.00, with higher scores indicating greater correlation among items and between each item and the summative inventory score. Values between 0.70 and 0.90 are considered strong. For example, for the FES-I, $\alpha = 0.96$.[15] For split-half reliability assessments, the *Spearman-Brown prophecy* statistic is used to estimate the correlation of the two halves of the test.

■ Reliability and Change

Reliability is of special interest in the assessment of change. When we take two measurements of the same variable at different times, we are usually doing so to determine whether there is a difference or improvement, perhaps due to a specific intervention or the passage of time. Therefore, we need to have confidence that the instrument is reliable so we can assume that the observed difference represents true change and not just measurement error.

Change Scores

When we want to show improvement following an intervention, we use a **change score**, obtained by measuring the difference between a pretest and posttest. Reliability will greatly influence the interpretation of this score. Suppose we use an intervention that has no effect, and the true score really does not change from pretest to posttest. We do not know this, however, and we find a difference when we take our imperfect measurements, which we want to attribute to the intervention. Measurement theory suggests that when we subtract pretest from posttest scores, the true value will cancel out and we will be left with only error. Clearly, reliability in our measurements is a necessary precondition for being able to interpret change scores.

Regression Toward the Mean

One concern in measuring change is related to the extremeness of observed scores; that is, very high scores may reflect substantial positive error and very low scores may reflect substantial negative error. When extreme scores are used in the calculation of measured change, they can contribute to a phenomenon called **regression toward the mean (RTM)**. According to this statistical phenomenon, extreme scores on an initial test are expected to move closer, or *regress*, toward the group average (the mean) on a second test; that is, the error component of an extreme pretest score is likely to be less extreme on a second test. If we think of measurement error as a random effect, then we might expect that performance might be "lucky" on one occasion and not so lucky on a subsequent test.

This phenomenon is potentially most serious in situations in which subjects are specifically assigned to groups on the basis of their extreme initial scores. With RTM, higher or lower baseline scores tend to move closer to the mean on a second trial. Therefore, even in situations in which treatment has no effect, we may see some change on follow-up among those with extreme pretest scores because high scores on the first test may have included substantial positive error, whereas low scores may have included substantial negative error. Measures with strong reliability, since they are less susceptible to measurement error, are less likely to exhibit regression.

◎ FUN FACT

The *Sports Illustrated (SI)* "cover jinx" may be an example of RTM. The story goes that appearing on the *SI* cover jinxes future performance. One of the earliest examples was in 1957. The Oklahoma Sooners football team was on a 47 consecutive-game winning streak, when their star player appeared on the *SI* cover, with the headline, "Why Oklahoma Is Unbeatable." They lost the next game to Notre Dame 7 to 0.

In 1978, Pete Rose was on the cover, with a 44-game hitting streak in progress (going after DiMaggio's 56-game record), only to see the streak broken the following week. In 2003, the Kansas City Chiefs were off to a 9–0 record when their quarterback, Trent Green, was featured on the cover. After that, they went 4–3 and lost in the first round of play-offs. There are many more examples that support the "jinx," making fans and players very nervous about being featured on the cover!

In 2002, *SI* ran a story about the jinx, with the picture of a black cat on the cover, with the caption, "The Cover No One Would Pose For." Although all players and teams will have good and bad streaks, they generally only get on the *SI* cover because of a winning streak. So, based on regression theory, the good streak is statistically likely to be followed by falling back to average performance!

Bad luck, or just unfortunate statistics?

Minimal Detectable Change

In any test–retest situation, we can appreciate that some portion of change may be error and some portion may be real. The concept of **minimal detectable change (MDC)** has been used to define that amount of change in a variable that must be achieved before we can be confident that error does not account for the entire measured difference and that some true change must have occurred.[22] The greater the reliability of an instrument, the smaller the MDC. The MDC is based on the SEM.

🔑 The MDC may also be called the *minimal detectable difference (MDD)*,[23] the *smallest real difference (SRD)*,[24] the *smallest detectable change (SDC)*,[25] the *coefficient of repeatability (CR)*,[12,26] or the *reliability change index (RCI)*.[22] Sorry, they all mean the same thing. Do not count on statisticians for consistent terminology!

➤ Several studies have looked at the MDC for the TUG test in different populations. For example, in a study of patients with PD, the MDC was 3.5 seconds, with an ICC of 0.80.[27] In a study of patients with knee osteoarthritis (OA), the MDC was 1.1 seconds with an ICC of 0.97.[28]

These data underscore the important relationship between reliability and the MDC. With lower reliability (lower ICC) in the PD study, we see a larger MDC, indicating that with greater error in the measurement, greater change scores are needed before we are able to rule out measurement error as being solely responsible (see Fig. 9-2). If we wanted to establish the effect of an

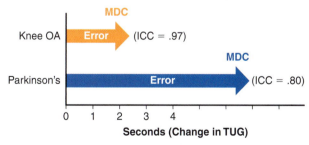

Figure 9–2 Depiction of MDC for the TUG test for patients with knee OA and PD, illustrating the relationship between MDC and reliability (ICC). Based on data from: 1) Huang SL, Hsieh CL, Wu RM, Tai CH, Lin CH, Lu WS. Minimal detectable change of the timed "up & go" test and the dynamic gait index in people with Parkinson disease. *Phys Ther* 2011;91(1):114–21; and 2) Alghadir A, Anwer S, Brismée JM. The reliability and minimal detectable change of Timed Up and Go test in individuals with grade 1–3 knee osteoarthritis. *BMC Musculoskelet Disord* 2015;16:174.

intervention for the group with PD, we would need to see a change of at least 3.5 seconds in the TUG to conclude that some true change had occurred. In a population with knee OA, we would only need to see a difference of at least 1.1 seconds to conclude that some of the change was real.

Procedures for calculating and interpreting the MDC will be presented in Chapter 32.

■ Methodological Studies: Reliability

Methodological research involves the development and testing of measuring instruments for use in research or clinical practice. These studies emphasize the use of outcome instruments as a way of indicating quality of care and effectiveness of intervention. Establishing reliability often requires multiple approaches, looking at different components with several indices to fully understand a tool's accuracy. The implications of the results of these studies are far-reaching, as we decide which tools will serve us best to demonstrate the efficacy of our services. It is essential, therefore, that we understand the designs and analyses of methodological study so we can choose appropriate instruments and defend the decisions that we make.

Obviously, we want to develop tools that have the best chance of assessing patients accurately. There are many strategies that can be incorporated into studies and clinical practice to maximize reliability.

- **Standardize measurement protocols.** By creating clear operational definitions and instructions for performing a test, observers, raters, and patients will have a better chance of being consistent. This includes creating a standard environment and timeline to ensure that everyone is performing in the same way.

- **Train raters.** Depending on the complexity of the task, training raters is important to ensure that all measurements are taken in the same way. Reliability analyses can be done during training to determine its effectiveness. For some scales, formal training procedures are required for certification.

- **Calibrate and improve the instrument.** For new instruments, continued efforts to refine and improve a tool are warranted for both reliability and validity. For mechanical instruments, a defined calibration procedure should be documented.

- **Take multiple measurements.** Using the mean of two or more trials may be effective in reducing overall error, especially for less stable measurements (see Commentary).

- **Choose a sample with a range of scores.** Testing for reliability requires that the sample has some variance; that is, subjects must have a range of scores. Even if scores are consistent from trial 1 to trial 2, if they are all similar to each other, it is not possible to establish whether they contain error. Samples for reliability studies must include subjects with scores across the continuum to show reliability.

- **Pilot testing.** Even when an instrument has been tested for reliability before, researchers should document reliability for their own studies. Pilot studies are "try outs" to make sure procedures work and to establish reliability prior to the start of actual data collection.

COMMENTARY

Measure twice, cut once.

—English proverb

It's hard to imagine any measurement system that is free from error. What strategies can we apply in data collection procedures to ensure the most reliable outcome? One approach is to take more than one measurement of a behavior or characteristic whenever possible. You have probably experienced this in your own healthcare, as clinicians often take more than one blood pressure measurement, for example. But then we must ask, out of several trials, which value best represents the individual's true score?

Investigators may not want to use the first score alone as the test value. The initial trial is often confounded by a warm-up or learning effect that will be evident as performance improves on subsequent trials. Therefore, warm-up or practice trials are often incorporated into a design.

Some researchers use the final score in a series. They rationalize that the last repetition in a set of trials will be stabilized following warm-up or practice. However, depending on the number of trials, the final score may also be influenced by fatigue or a practice effect, and therefore will not necessarily represent the subject's true effort.

Other researchers may use the subject's "best" effort of several trials as a reflection of what the subject is maximally capable of doing. If we consider reliability theory, however, this is not necessarily the most accurate representation because random error can contribute both positive and negative error to an observed score.

Theoretically, then, the most representative score is obtained by acquiring several measurements and calculating the mean or average. In the "long run," calculating the average will cancel out the error components of each overestimate and underestimate. Of course, there is room for argument in this rationale because this theory is based on a large number of trials. With only a few trials, this may be an unrealistic assumption. However, studies have shown that taking a mean value provides a more reliable measurement than any single value in a series of trials.[29,30]

So, bottom line? There is no simple answer to which score should be used. Generally, reliability of measurements that are less stable can be improved if averages are used. This is an important issue for statistical inference, as greater error (low reliability) will reduce the chances of finding statistically significant differences when comparing groups or looking for change. Clinicians should understand how reliability was determined to generalize findings to clinical situations.

REFERENCES

1. Podsiadlo D, Richardson S. The timed "Up & Go": a test of basic functional mobility for frail elderly persons. *J Am Geriatr Soc* 1991;39(2):142–148.
2. Beauchet O, Fantino B, Allali G, Muir SW, Montero-Odasso M, Annweiler C. Timed Up and Go test and risk of falls in older adults: a systematic review. *J Nutr Health Aging* 2011;15(10):933–938.
3. Kluge F, Gaßner H, Hannink J, Pasluosta C, Klucken J, Eskofier BM. Towards mobile gait analysis: concurrent validity and test-retest reliability of an inertial measurement system for the assessment of spatio-temporal gait parameters. *Sensors* 2017;17(7):1522.
4. Gautschi OP, Smoll NR, Corniola MV, Joswig H, Chau I, Hildebrandt G, Schaller K, Stienen MN. Validity and reliability of a measurement of objective functional impairment in lumbar degenerative disc disease: the Timed Up and Go (TUG) test. *Neurosurgery* 2016;79(2):270–278.
5. Hafsteinsdóttir TB, Rensink M, Schuurmans M. Clinimetric properties of the Timed Up and Go Test for patients with stroke: a systematic review. *Top Stroke Rehabil* 2014;21(3):197–210.
6. Yeung TS, Wessel J, Stratford PW, MacDermid JC. The timed up and go test for use on an inpatient orthopaedic rehabilitation ward. *J Orthop Sports Phys Ther* 2008;38(7):410–417.
7. Messick S. Validity. In: Linn RI, ed. *Educational Measurement.* 3 ed. Phoenix, AZ: ORYZ Press, 1993:13–104.
8. Riddle DL, Stratford PW. *Is This a Real Change? Interpreting Patient Outcomes in Physical Therapy.* Philadelphia: F.A. Davis, 2013.
9. Klassen AF, Riff KWW, Longmire NM, Albert A, Allen GC, Aydin MA, Baker SB, Cano SJ, Chan AJ, Courtemanche DJ, et al. Psychometric findings and normative values for the CLEFT-Q based on 2434 children and young adult patients with cleft lip and/or palate from 12 countries. *CMAJ* 2018;190(15):E455–E462.
10. Choi JT, Seo JH, Ko MH, Park SH, Kim GW, Won YH. Validation of Korean version of the London Chest Activity of Daily Living scale in patients with chronic obstructive pulmonary disease. *Ann Rehabil Med* 2018;42(2):329–335.
11. Paddick SM, Gray WK, Ogunjimi L, Lwezuala B, Olakehinde O, Kisoli A, Kissima J, Mbowe G, Mkenda S, Dotchin CL, et al. Validation of the Identification and Intervention for Dementia in Elderly Africans (IDEA) cognitive screen in Nigeria and Tanzania. *BMC Geriatr* 2015;15:53.
12. Dimitrov D, Rumrill P, Fitzgerald S, Hennessey M. Reliability in rehabilitation measurement. *Work* 2001;16(2):159–164.
13. Nunnally J, Bernstein IH. *Psychometric Theory.* 3 ed. New York: McGraw-Hill, 1994.
14. Cronbach LJ, Gleser GC, Nanda H, Rajaratnam N. *The Dependability of Behavioral Measurements: Theory of Generalizability for Scores and Profiles.* New York: Wiley, 1972.
15. Yardley L, Beyer N, Hauer K, Kempen G, Piot-Ziegler C, Todd C. Development and initial validation of the Falls Efficacy Scale-International (FES-I). *Age Ageing* 2005;34(6):614–619.
16. Cusick A, Vasquez M, Knowles L, Wallen M. Effect of rater training on reliability of Melbourne Assessment of Unilateral Upper Limb Function scores. *Dev Med Child Neurol* 2005;47(1):39–45.
17. McConvey J, Bennett SE. Reliability of the Dynamic Gait Index in individuals with multiple sclerosis. *Arch Phys Med Rehabil* 2005;86(1):130–133.
18. Baer GD, Smith MT, Rowe PJ, Masterton L. Establishing the reliability of Mobility Milestones as an outcome measure for stroke. *Arch Phys Med Rehabil* 2003;84(7):977–981.
19. Lin T, Wang C, Liao M, Lai C. Agreement between automated and human measurements of heart rate in patients with atrial fibrillation. *J Cardiovasc Nurs* 2018;33(5):492–499.
20. Bird ML, Callisaya ML, Cannell J, Gibbons T, Smith ST, Ahuja KD. Accuracy, validity, and reliability of an electronic visual analog scale for pain on a touch screen tablet in healthy older adults: a clinical trial. *Interact J Med Res* 2016;5(1):e3.
21. Galjaard S, Baeck S, Ameye L, Bourne T, Timmerman D, Devlieger R. Use of a pocket-sized ultrasound machine (PUM) for routine examinations in the third trimester of pregnancy. *Ultrasound Obstet Gynecol* 2014;44(1):64–68.
22. Beaton DE, Bombardier C, Katz JN, Wright JG. A taxonomy for responsiveness. *J Clin Epidemiol* 2001;54(12):1204–1217.
23. Stratford PW, Binkley J, Solomon P, Finch E, Gill C, Moreland J. Defining the minimum level of detectable change for the Roland-Morris questionnaire. *Phys Ther* 1996;76(4):359–365.
24. Schuck P, Zwingmann C. The 'smallest real difference' as a measure of sensitivity to change: a critical analysis. *Int J Rehabil Res* 2003;26(2):85–91.
25. Mokkink LB, Terwee CB, Patrick DL, Alonso J, Stratford P, Knol DL, Bouter LM, de Vet HC. *COSMIN Checklist Manual.* Amsterdam, Netherlands: EMGO Institute for Health and Care Research. Available at http://www.cosmin.nl/the_cosmin_checklist.html. Accessed March 9, 2018.

26. Vaz S, Falkmer T, Passmore AE, Parsons R, Andreou P. The case for using the repeatability coefficient when calculating test-retest reliability. *PLoS One* 2013;8(9):e73990.

27. Huang SL, Hsieh CL, Wu RM, Tai CH, Lin CH, Lu WS. Minimal detectable change of the timed "up & go" test and the dynamic gait index in people with Parkinson disease. *Phys Ther* 2011;91(1):114–121.

28. Alghadir A, Anwer S, Brismée JM. The reliability and minimal detectable change of Timed Up and Go test in individuals with grade 1–3 knee osteoarthritis. *BMC Musculoskelet Disord* 2015;16:174.

29. Beattie P, Isaacson K, Riddle DL, Rothstein JM. Validity of derived measurements of leg-length differences obtained by use of a tape measure. *Phys Ther* 1990;70(3):150–157.

30. Mathiowetz V, Weber K, Volland G, Kashman N. Reliability and validity of grip and pinch strength evaluations. *J Hand Surg [Am]* 1984;9(2):222–226.

Concepts of Measurement Validity

—with K. Douglas Gross

Clinical decision-making is dependent on the accuracy and appropriate application of measurements. Whether for diagnosis, prognosis, or treatment purposes, without meaningful assessment of a patient's condition, we have no basis for choosing the right interventions or making reasoned judgments. **Validity** relates to the confidence we have that our measurement tools are giving us accurate information about a relevant construct so that we can apply results in a meaningful way.

The purpose of this chapter is to describe the types of evidence needed to support validity and the application of this evidence to the interpretation of clinical measurements. Statistical procedures related to validity will be identified, with full coverage in Chapter 32.

■ Defining Validity

Validity concerns the meaning or interpretation that we give to a measurement.[1] A longstanding definition characterizes validity as the *extent to which a test measures what it is intended to measure*. Therefore, a test for depression should be able to identify someone who is depressed and not merely tired. Similarly, an assessment of learning disabilities should be able to identify children with difficulties processing information rather than difficulties with physical performance.

Validity also addresses the interpretation and application of measured values.[2] Beyond the tool itself, validity reflects the meaning ascribed to a score, recognizing the relevance of measurements to clinical decisions, as well as to the person being assessed.[3,4]

We draw inferences from measurements that go beyond just the obtained scores. For example, in clinical applications, when we measure variables such as muscle strength or blood pressure, it is not the muscle grade or blood pressure value that is of interest for its own sake, but what those values mean in terms of the integrity of the patient's physical and physiological health.

Validity addresses three types of questions:

- Is a test capable of *discriminating* among individuals with and without certain traits, diagnoses, or conditions?
- Can the test *evaluate* the magnitude or quality of a variable or the degree of change from one time to another?
- Can we make useful and accurate *predictions* about a patient's future status based on the outcome of a test?

We use those values to infer something about the cause of symptoms or presence of disease, to set goals, and to determine which interventions are appropriate. They may indicate how much assistance will be required and if there has been improvement following treatment. Such scores may also have policy implications, influencing the continuation of therapy, discharge disposition, or reimbursement for services. Measurements, therefore, have consequences for actions and decisions.[5] A valid measure is one that offers sound footing to support the inferences and decisions that are made.

Validity and Reliability

A ruler is considered a valid instrument for calibrating length because we can judge how long an object is by measuring linear inches or centimeters. We would, however, question any attempt to assess the severity of low back pain using measurements of leg length because we cannot make reasonable inferences about back pain based on that measurement.

Although validity and reliability are both needed to buttress confidence in our ability to accurately capture a target construct, it is important to distinguish between these two measurement properties. Reliability describes the extent to which a test is free of random error. With high reliability, a test will deliver consistent results over repeated trials. A reliable test may still suffer from systematic error, however. Such a test would deliver results that are consistently "off the mark." For example, although a precise ruler may deliver highly reproducible measurements of leg length, these values would continue to "miss the mark" as indicators of back pain severity.

Hitting the Target

Validity concerns the extent to which measurements align with the targeted construct. Validity can be likened to hitting the center of a target, as shown in Figure 10-1. In (A), the hits are consistent, but missing the center each time. This is a reliable measure, but one that is systematically measuring the wrong thing and is therefore invalid. In (B), the hits are randomly distributed around the center with an equal number of over-estimates and underestimates, reflecting both the poor reliability of the measure and the absence of any systematic error. However, by calculating an average score for the group, the overestimates and underestimates should cancel each other out, providing us with a valid score that is close to the center of the target.

In (C), the error reflects both poor reliability and poor validity. There is an inconsistent scatter, but there is also a pattern of being systematically off the mark in one direction. Even a calculated average score would still miss the intended target. Finally, in (D), the hits all cluster tightly around the center of the target and are therefore both highly reliable and highly valid.

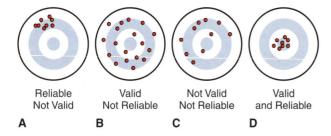

Figure 10–1 Illustration of the distinction between validity and reliability. The center of the target represents the true score. A) Scores are reliable, but not valid, showing systematic error. B) Scores demonstrate random error but will provide a valid score on average. C) Scores are neither reliable nor valid. D) Scores hit the center of the target, indicating high reliability and validity.

What Validity Is and Is Not

Because inferences are difficult to verify, establishing validity is not as straightforward as establishing reliability. For many variables, there are no obvious rules for judging whether a test is measuring the critical property of interest. As with reliability, we do not think of validity in an all-or-none sense, but rather as a characteristic that may be present to a greater or lesser degree.

Also as with reliability, validity is not an immutable characteristic of an instrument itself. Instead, validity can be evaluated only within the context of an instrument's intended use, including the population and setting to which it will be applied. There are no valid or invalid instruments per se. The extent of validity is specific to the instrument's intended application, including its ability to assess change or quantify outcomes.[6] Rather than asking, "*Is an instrument valid or invalid?*," it is more appropriate to ask, "*How valid are the results of a test for a given purpose within this setting?*"

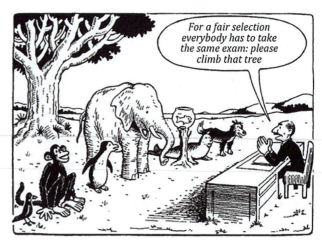

Source unknown.

For some physical variables, such as distance or speed, measurements can be acquired by direct observation. However, for variables that represent abstract constructs (such as anxiety, depression, intelligence, or pain), direct observation may not be possible and we are required to take measurements of a correlate or proxy of the actual property under consideration. Therefore, we make inferences about the magnitude of a latent trait (such as anxiety) based on observations of related discernible behaviors (such as restlessness and agitation). In this way, abstract constructs are in large part defined by the methods or instruments used to measure them.[7]

■ Types of Evidence for Validity

Validity is established by constructing an "evidentiary chain" that links the actual methods of measurement to the intended application.[8] By way of theory, hypothesis, logic, and data, evidence-based practitioners seek to establish that an instrument's output is related and proportional to the target construct and that it can provide a sound basis upon which to make clinical decisions. A measurement may only represent a highly abstruse construct to a degree, but perhaps not perfectly.[9] As we have emphasized, validity is never an "all-or-none" characteristic, and choices are often necessary when determining whether the validity of a measure is sufficient for the current task.

Several types of evidence can be used to support a tool's use, depending on specific conditions. Often referred to as the "3 Cs," the most common forms of evidence reflect content validity, criterion-related validity, and construct validity (see Fig. 10-2 and Table 10-1).

> ▶ **CASE IN POINT #1**
>
> The Harris Infant Neuromotor Test (HINT) is a screening tool that can be used for early identification of neuromotor, cognitive, and behavioral disorders during the first year of life.[10] The test is intended to identify difficulties that are often missed until they become more obvious in preschool years.[11] It consists of three parts, including background information, a parent questionnaire, and an infant examination. A lower score indicates greater maturity and a higher score indicates greater risk for developmental delay. The test has demonstrated strong rater and test–retest reliability (ICC = 0.99).[12] Instructions for administration have been formalized in a training manual.[13]

Content Validity

Many behavioral variables have a wide theoretical domain or *universe of content* that consists of all the traits

Table 10-1   Evidence to Support Measurement Validity: The 3 Cs

TYPE OF VALIDITY	PURPOSE
Content Validity	Establishes that the multiple items that make up a questionnaire, inventory, or scale adequately sample the universe of content that defines the construct being measured.
Criterion-Related Validity	Establishes the correspondence between a target test and a reference or gold standard measure of the same construct.
Concurrent Validity	The extent to which the target test correlates with a reference standard taken at relatively the same time.
Predictive Validity	The extent to which the target test can predict a future reference standard.
Construct Validity	Establishes the ability of an instrument to measure the dimensions and theoretical foundation of an abstract construct.
Convergent Validity	The extent to which a test correlates with other tests of closely related constructs.
Discriminant Validity	The extent to which a test is uncorrelated with tests of distinct or contrasting constructs.

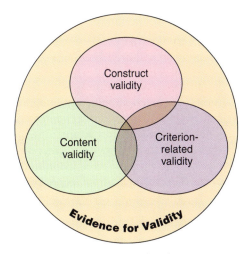

Figure 10–2 The "3 Cs": Types of evidence to support validity include evidence from content, criterion-related, and construct validation. These forms of evidence may provide complementary information to reflect different components of a construct.

or behaviors that are thought to characterize that variable. Questionnaires attempting to evaluate these multifaceted variables will assess a range of information using multiple test items or questions. Examples include educational tests, attitude scales, and clinical measures of function or quality of life. The multiple items that comprise these tests help to define the facets of the construct being measured. **Content validity** refers to the adequacy with which the complete universe of content is sampled by a test's items. Because the content universe cannot be covered in totality, the items must be representative of the whole.

Content validity demands three things of the items in a test:[3]

- The items must adequately represent the full scope of the construct being studied.
- The number of items that address each component should reflect the relative importance of that component.
- The test should not contain irrelevant items.

The Universe of Content

Some content domains are obvious—the questions on an exam can easily be based on assigned readings and lectures. But for many clinical constructs, this is not so obvious. Consider the range of activities that might be scored to determine a patient's overall "function." Should a functional status questionnaire include items related to the physical, cognitive, social, or emotional domains of function? How important are each of these domains when assessing a patient who has suffered a stroke or a spinal cord injury, or assessing a well elderly person? Will occupational therapists define the relevant content universe differently from nurses or physical therapists?

These types of questions must be answered before other issues of validity can be addressed. A review of the literature is important to provide a thorough context and to consider how relevant content has been incorporated into other instruments. The content universe should be described in sufficient detail so that the construct of interest is clearly identified for all who will use the instrument.

> ➤ Content for the HINT was based on reviewing the literature to develop a definition for the constructs of "neuromotor function" and "cognitive delay," with a focus on early identification of high-risk infants.[14] Items were developed to represent locomotion, posture, and movement, based on previous predictive validity studies.[10]

Judging Content Validity

The typical approach for judging content validity is essentially a subjective process using a panel of experts, which may include patients, providers, and other stakeholders. The experts review draft versions of the instrument to determine whether the items appropriately represent the relevant content domain. Panelists may provide independent ratings of the relevance of each item, and agreement between them can be determined (see Chapter 32). Opinions may also be obtained through focus groups, interviews, or Delphi panels (see Chapter 11 Supplement). Items that generate significant disagreement are assessed for ambiguity before they are modified or deleted. This process often requires several revisions of the instrument. When reviewers reach consensus that the content domain has been adequately sampled, content validity is supported.

> ➤ Harris and Daniels[14] assessed content validity of the HINT using a panel of 26 researchers and clinicians from several disciplines who reviewed all three sections of the tool. They were asked to rate items based on ability to reflect important neurodevelopmental characteristics, likelihood to discriminate between infants with and without neuromotor developmental problems, clarity of wording, and not being culturally biased. Their percent agreement was evaluated and, based on their feedback, the researchers added some questions, revised wording, and expanded grading criteria for the infant assessment portion.

Although most techniques for analyzing content validity focus on expert analysis and consensus, a quantitative method called the **content validity index (CVI)** can be used to reflect the extent of agreement among reviewers regarding relevance and clarity of individual items and a total scale.

> See the *Chapter 10 Supplement* for a description of the content validity index.

Face Validity

Another way to assess the usefulness of a test is by its **face validity**, which is actually not validity in its true sense. Face validity simply implies that an instrument *appears* to test what it is intended to and may be a plausible method for doing so. Although lacking in rigor, face validity is still an important property of many tests. An instrument lacking in face validity may not be well received or have its relevance understood by those who administer it, those who are tested by it, or those who will apply the results.

Content and face validation may seem like similar concepts, as both are based on subjective judgments, but there is an important distinction between them. Face validity is a judgment made after an instrument is constructed, generally by those who use it, whereas content validity evolves out of the process of planning and constructing a test, derived through evaluation by content experts of a test's objectives, theoretical context, and multi-item composition.

Criterion-Related Validity

Criterion-related validity is based on the ability of the test to align with results obtained on an external criterion. The test to be validated, called the *target test*, is compared to a **gold standard**, or *criterion measure*, that is already established and assumed to be valid. If results from the two tests are correlated or in agreement, the target test is considered a valid indicator of the criterion score.

Finding the Gold Standard

A crucial element of criterion validation is identification of an acceptable criterion measure. The relationship between the target test and the criterion measure should make theoretical sense in terms of the construct that both tests represent.[3] We must feel confident in assuming that the criterion itself is a valid measure of that construct. In many areas of physical and physiological science, standard criteria are readily available for validating clinical tools. For instance, heart rate (the target test) has been established as a valid indicator of energy cost during exercise by correlating it with standardized oxygen consumption values (the gold standard).[15] Unfortunately, the choice of a gold standard for more abstract constructs is not always as obvious. For instance, if we want to establish the validity of a new quality of life questionnaire, with which referent should it be compared?

Sometimes, the best one can do is use another instrument that has already achieved some degree of acceptance. In these instances, criterion-related validation may be based on comparison to a **reference standard** that, although not considered a true gold standard, is still regarded as an acceptable criterion.

Criterion-related validity can be separated into two basic approaches: concurrent validation and predictive validation, differentiated by the time frame within which measurements are acquired.

Concurrent Validity

Concurrent validity is studied when target and criterion test scores are obtained at approximately the same time so that they both reflect the same incident of behavior. This approach is often used to establish the validity of diagnostic or screening tests to determine the presence or absence of diseases or other health conditions (see Box 10-1).

> ➤ Concurrent validity for the HINT was established by correlating HINT scores to contemporaneous scores on the Ages and States Questionnaire ($r = .84$),[17] the Bayley Scale of Infant Development Mental Scale ($r = -.73$) and Motor Scale ($r = -.89$),[12] and the Alberta Infant Motor Scale ($r = -.93$ for at-risk infants at 10 to 12 months).[18]

The reference standards used to evaluate the concurrent validity of the HINT represent similar constructs, although none could be considered a true gold standard for the construct of "developmental delay." We risk becoming mired in circular reasoning if we are not

---

Box 10-1 Diagnostic and Screening Accuracy

Criterion measures are often applied to validate diagnostic or screening tools. They may require concurrent or predictive approaches depending on when the condition is manifested. A comparison of findings on the criterion and target tests generates data to indicate **sensitivity**, or the extent to which the target test can accurately identify those with the condition (*true-positive* findings), and **specificity**, which is the ability of the target test to identify those whom the criterion has determined are without the condition (*true-negative* findings). These are presented as percentages, with values closer to 100% indicating better accuracy.

These analyses also provide information about *false positive* and *false negative* findings, which can impact the appropriate use of a test. For example, the HINT parent questionnaire was shown to have high sensitivity (80%) and specificity (90.9%) for identifying infants with development concerns, using the Bayley Motor Scale of Infant Development as the criterion.[16] The high specificity indicates that there is a low risk of a false positive; that is, a low risk of identifying a normally developing child as having developmental delay. The 80% sensitivity also suggests that there is minimal risk of a false negative result, wherein a child with developmental delay remains undetected.

See Chapter 33 for a full description of procedures for diagnostic accuracy.

---

convinced that the reference standard itself has sufficient validity. Concurrent validation is useful in situations in which a new or untested tool is potentially more efficient, easier to administer, more practical, or safer than the current method, and when it is being proposed as an alternative.

Predictive Validity

Predictive validity assessments determine whether a measure will be a valid predictor of some future criterion score or behavior. To assess predictive validity, a target test is administered at a baseline session, followed by a period of time before the criterion score is obtained. The interval between these two tests is dependent on the time needed to achieve the criterion and may be as long as several years.

> ➤ Researchers evaluated the predictive validity of the HINT by administering the test to a sample of children at 3 to 12 months of age and then performing the Bayley Scale of Infant Development-II at 17 to 22 months. They found that there was a weak correlation for the HINT and Bayley-II Mental Scale ($r = -.11$), but a moderate correlation with the Motor Scale ($r = -.49$).[12]

Predictive validation can be used for several purposes, such as validating screening procedures used to identify risk factors for future disease or to determine the validity of prognostic indicators used to predict treatment outcomes.

 Analysis of Criterion Validity

Criterion validity, both concurrent and predictive, is typically assessed using a correlation coefficient or regression procedure (see Chapters 29 and 30). With two tools using the same units, the ICC can be used. *Limits of agreement* can also be applied to show how scores from two tools agree or disagree (see Chapter 32).

■ Construct Validity

Construct validity reflects the ability of an instrument to measure the theoretical dimensions of a construct. Because abstract constructs do not directly manifest as physical events, we often make inferences through observable behaviors, measurable performance, or patient self-report.

Constructs and Content

For measurements that use questionnaires, part of construct validity is based on content validity; that is, one must be able to define the content universe that represents a construct to develop a test that measures it. Thus, one can generate hypotheses regarding the overt behaviors of individuals with high and low scores on the test. An instrument is said to be a valid measure of a construct when its measurements support these theoretical assumptions (see Focus on Evidence 10-1).

Methods of Construct Validation

Because of the abstract and complex nature of constructs, construct validation is never fully realized. Each attempt to validate an instrument provides evidence to support or refute the theoretical framework behind the construct. This evidence can be gathered by a variety of methods (see Box 10-2). The more commonly used procedures include the known groups method, methods of convergence or discrimination, and factor analysis.

Known Groups Method

The most general type of evidence in support of construct validity is provided when a test can discriminate between individuals who are known to have the trait and those who do not. Using the **known groups method**, a criterion is chosen to identify the presence or absence of a particular characteristic and hypotheses are constructed to predict how these different groups are expected to behave. The validity of a target test is supported if the test's results document these anticipated differences.

> ➤ Megens et al[19] evaluated construct validity of the HINT by looking at both low- and high-risk infants. They recruited the low-risk group from well-baby clinics and day-care centers. The high-risk infants were recruited from neonatal follow-up programs and were considered at high risk for developmental delay because of premature birth, low birth weight, prenatal exposure to alcohol or drugs, or other major medical concerns. They found significantly different scores for the two groups, confirming that the HINT was effective in discriminating between high- and low-risk infants at 4, 5, 7, and 8 months of age.

Focus on Evidence 10–1
Constructing Pain

Pain is a difficult construct to define because of its subjective and unobservable nature. Perceptions of pain and pain relief may be subject to cognitive and behavioral influences that are specific to individuals and to cultural, sociological, or religious beliefs.[21] Many different assessment tools have been developed to measure acute and chronic pain, some with a disease-specific focus, others based on patient-specific function. In the development of scales or the choice of a clinical tool, the theoretical context of the measurement must be determined.

For instance, it is possible that acute pain is a more unidimensional construct, and its presence and intensity during a particular time period can be defined using a numerical rating scale or VAS. Grilo et al[22] used this method to demonstrate changes in patients with acute pain from rheumatic conditions, showing a correlated linear decline in score with a VAS and perceived level of pain.

Chronic pain, however, will have a very different context, with multiple dimensions related to physical, emotional, cognitive, and social functions, including quality of life.[23] For example, in a systematic review of measures for cancer pain, Abahussin et al[24] reviewed eight tools, each with different scoring rubrics and subscales, reflecting traits such as severity, impact on function, stoicism, quality of life, sensory, and affective components. They concluded that most studies of these tools had poor methodological quality and that further study was needed to determine validity characteristics for use with that population.

How one chooses to measure pain will greatly affect how the outcome will be interpreted. Different elements may be important, depending on the nature of the underlying cause of or intervention for the pain.

Box 10-2 It's All About the Construct

As we explore different forms of evidence to establish validity, it is clear that the underlying construct is a common thread.[3] Even with content or criterion validity, we still have to refer to the theoretical domain of the construct. The overlap among these elements is reflected in the widespread use of all three in many studies to support the full scope of validity of an instrument. This was well illustrated in the comprehensive and extensive validity testing of the HINT.

Standards for evaluating validity have been expanded based on a revised definition that considers construct validity the overarching concept that reflects:

. . . the degree to which evidence and theory support the interpretation of test scores for proposed uses of tests.[2,9]

This definition has been adopted in education and psychology, and more recently in health applications.[5,20] It supports five types of evidence, capturing and expanding on the traditional "3 Cs." These are not considered different types of validity, but rather they form a framework for gathering cumulative evidence to support construct validity. The first three of these correspond to traditional definitions of content, criterion, and construct validity:

1. **Test Content:** The process of analysis of items, including identification of the construct and the process for developing the scale.
2. **Relationship to Other Variables:** Including all the processes described under criterion-related and construct validity, demonstrating how the interpretation of scores can be generalized across groups, settings, and behaviors.
3. **Internal Structure:** Focusing on how the components of the scale fit the construct, including typical approaches to

construct validation, such as factor analysis and known groups analysis.

In the new framework, two additional types of evidence present a contemporary perspective that adds to a comprehensive understanding of construct validity:

4. **Response Process:** This evidence focuses on how response choices are worded and how patients or raters respond to items, recognizing the importance of reliability, data collection methods, adequacy of instructions, rater training, how scores are reported and summarized, and establishing a lack of bias in the process.
5. **Consequences of Testing:** Evidence should reflect intended or unintended consequences of a measure and may contribute to quality improvement efforts. For instance, a major premise of the HINT is the need to determine whether a child needs early intervention services, standardized assessment, follow-up screening, or no action. Therefore, depending on the score, some children who could use services might not be recommended for them. Validity ultimately relates to how a test's score can influence treatment decisions and patient outcomes.

Importantly, these evidence strategies put an emphasis on the use of assessment, rather than on the tool itself, to establish validity for both quantitative and qualitative applications.[3]

 See the *Chapter 10 Supplement* for examples of indicators for the five types of evidence to support construct validity.

Convergence and Discrimination

Construct validity of a test can be evaluated in terms of how its measures compare to other tests of closely related or contrasting constructs.[25] In other words, it is important to demonstrate what a test *does* measure as well as what it *does not* measure. This determination is based on the concepts of convergence and discrimination.

➤ CASE IN POINT #2

Children diagnosed with autism spectrum disorder (ASD) often experience anxiety. It is important to determine, however, whether measures of ASD can distinguish between anxiety and ASD symptoms as separate constructs, or whether these two traits are part of a common neurological process. This information is essential to determine appropriate diagnostic and intervention strategies.

Convergent validity indicates that two measures believed to reflect similar underlying phenomena will yield comparable results or scores that are correlated. Convergence also implies that the theoretical context behind the construct will be supported by these related tests. **Discriminant validity**, also called *divergent validity*, indicates that different results, or low correlations, are expected from measures that assess distinct or contrasting characteristics.

To document these types of relationships, Campbell and Fiske[25] suggested that validity should be evaluated in terms of both the characteristic being measured and the method used to measure it, using a technique called the **multitrait–multimethod matrix (MTMM)**. In this approach, two or more traits are measured by two or more methods. The correlations among variables within and between methods should show that different tests measuring overlapping traits produce high correlations, demonstrating convergent validity, whereas those that measure distinct traits produce low correlations, demonstrating discriminant validity.

> ➤ Renno and Wood[26] studied 88 children with ASD, aged 7 to 11 years, who were referred for concerns about anxiety. They used two methods—standardized interviews and questionnaires—to assess both ASD severity and anxiety, which included:
>
> - The Autism Diagnostic Interview (ADI)
> - The Social Responsiveness Scale (SRS)
> - The Anxiety Disorders Interview Schedule (ADIS)
> - The Multidimensional Anxiety Scale for Children (MASC)

This study used these two methods (questionnaire and interview) to assess two traits (autism and anxiety). Using an MTMM, they were able to document that the two measures of autism had correlated scores, as did the two measures of anxiety—indicating convergence. They were also able to show that the scores of autism and anxiety did not have high correlations—indicating discrimination.

Factor Analysis

Another common approach to construct validation is the use of a statistical procedure called **factor analysis** to evaluate whether a scale is unidimensional or whether it is comprised of several underlying dimensions. For example, we often think of intelligence as consisting of several theoretical components, related to mathematical, verbal, motoric, memory, and emotional skills. Similarly, health and function are often conceptualized as multidimensional constructs including physical, social, and emotional aspects. Factor analysis can help to identify subscales that represent distinct components of an overall construct.

Factor analysis can be run as an exploratory or confirmatory technique. It looks at the structure within a large number of items in a scale and tries to explain interrelationships by grouping highly correlated items into *factors*. A factor represents a subset of test items that are closely related to each other but are not closely related to items in other factors; that is, each factor represents a combination of items that reflects a different theoretical component of the overall construct (see Chapter 31).

> ### ➤ CASE IN POINT #3
> The Arthritis Impact Measurement Scale (AIMS) is a self-report health status questionnaire that assesses well-being in individuals with rheumatic diseases.[27] The scale has been widely used, with items rated on a 5-point Likert scale. The items are grouped into nine subscales.

Exploratory factor analysis (EFA) is used to study a set of items when the purpose is to determine how the variables cluster or to establish which concepts may be

present in the construct. The final model characterizes the target construct based on an analysis of how the items correlate without substantial limitations placed on the model at the outset.

> ➤ The AIMS is composed of 45 items. Through an EFA, the items were grouped into three components of health status, identifying distinct areas of physical disability, psychological disability, and pain.[28]
>
> Over time, researchers considered the need to expand the theoretical framework of the AIMS. They ran an EFA on a larger sample and identified five factors: lower extremity function, upper extremity function, affect, symptom, and social interaction.[29]

The breakdown of these analyses is shown in Figure 10-3. For instance, we can see that social interaction did not fit with any groupings in the three-factor outcome but did load as its own factor when five factors were identified. In this case, the authors believed the five-factor structure provided a clearer picture of the components of health status operationalized by the nine subscales, particularly differentiating upper and lower extremity function.[29] Because of the exploratory nature of factor analysis, results must be interpreted based on statistical criteria, which sometimes requires judgments on the part of the researcher. Therefore, different outcomes can be presented, as illustrated here. The full AIMS can be accessed online.[30]

Confirmatory factor analysis (CFA) is used to support the theoretical structure of an instrument to determine whether it fits with current empirical understanding of a construct. In this process, the researcher specifies in advance which factors are expected and runs the CFA to see if data support those expectations.

> ➤ Researchers examined the structure of the AIMS by running a CFA to confirm that each of the nine subscales represented a single factor.[31] They found that each set of items did load highly on one factor, which means that the items included in that factor all related clearly to that subscale. The exception was "Household Activities," which appeared to contain items that related to both physical and intellectual components.

> ### 📈 Analysis of Construct Validity
> Known groups can be compared using *t*-tests, analysis of variance, or regression procedures. Convergent and discriminant validity are analyzed using correlation procedures and factor analysis. Construct validity can also be examined using Rasch analysis to evaluate the linearity of a summative scale (see Chapter 12).

Arthritis Impact Measurement Scale (AIMS) Factor Analysis

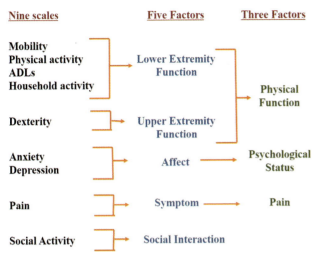

Figure 10–3 Factor analysis of the AIMS, showing breakdown of subscales in a three-factor and five-factor solution. Adapted from Mason JH, Anderson JJ, Meenan RF. A model of health status for rheumatoid arthritis. A factor analysis of the Arthritis Impact Measurement Scales. *Arthritis Rheum* 1988;31(6):714–20, Figure 2, p. 718. Used with permission.

■ Norm and Criterion Referencing

The validity of a test depends on evidence supporting its use for a specified purpose. Tests can be designed to document performance in relation to an external standard, indicating an individual's actual abilities, or to document ability in relation to a representative group.

> ### ▶ CASE IN POINT #4
> Rikli and Jones[32] have developed standards for fitness testing in older adults, predicting the level of capacity needed for maintaining physical independence in later life. The Senior Fitness Test (SFT) consists of a battery of tasks. One task is the chair stand test, which is a test of lower body strength, recording the number of times an individual can fully stand from sitting over 30 seconds with arms folded across the chest.[33]

Criterion Referencing

A **criterion-referenced test** is interpreted according to a fixed standard that represents an acceptable level of performance. In educational programs, for example, a minimum grade on a test might be used to specify competence for the material being tested. Criterion scores have been established for laboratory tests, based on medically established standards. These standards indicate acceptable performance irrespective of how others perform. It is possible that everyone could "pass" or everyone could "fail."

The validity of a criterion-referenced score depends on the validity of the criterion itself. Consequently, if we were to establish a score of 70 as the minimal passing score for an exam, it would be important to know that a score of 70 can distinguish those who truly are competent with the material from those who were not. Criterion scores may also change over time, such as the lowering of standard blood sugar levels to diagnose diabetes or lowering blood pressure standards for a diagnosis of hypertension.

> ▶ The predictive validity of the SFT was analyzed using the Composite Physical Function (CPF) scale as the reference criterion.[34] This is a 12-item self-report scale that assesses physical function as high, moderate, or low. Based on this criterion, physical independence was defined as having the ability to perform at least seven of the CPF activities without assistance.

Based on this criterion, Rikli and Jones[32] were able to establish a cutoff point for the chair stand test to indicate fitness level that would support future physical independence.

> ▶ For women, the standard for the chair stand test is:
>
> | | |
> |---|---|
> | 60–64 years: 15 reps | 80–84 years: 12 reps |
> | 65–69 years: 15 reps | 85–89 years: 11 reps |
> | 70–74 years: 14 reps | 90–94 years: 9 reps |
> | 75–79 years: 13 reps | |

These standards can be used to determine which patients are likely or unlikely to maintain physical independence and to set goals for intervention. Criterion-based scores are useful for establishing treatment goals, planning intervention, and measuring change, as they are based on an analysis of scores that are required for successful performance.

Norm Referencing

Norm-referenced tests are standardized assessments designed to compare and rank individuals within a defined population. Such a measure indicates how individuals perform relative to one another. Often scaled from 0 to 100, the norm-referenced score is obtained by taking raw scores and converting them to a standardized score based on the distribution of test-takers. This means that a judgment is not made based on how large or small a measurement is, but rather on how the measured value relates to a representative distribution of the population.

For example, you are probably familiar with standardized tests such as the SAT or GRE. If you recall, your scores were provided as percentiles, indicating how you did relative to others who took the test at the same time. On a different day, your friend might get the same score as you but be in a different percentile. If a professor decides to "curve" test scores so that the grades of the majority of the class are considered a "C," regardless of a student's absolute score, then the test would be norm-referenced.

Norm-referenced scores are often based on a distribution of "normal" values obtained through testing a large group that meets a certain profile (see Chapter 20). The mean of the distribution of scores for the reference group, along with standard deviations, is used as the standard to determine how an individual performs. For example, we can look at charts to determine whether we fit the profile for average weight for our height. These "norms" can be converted to norm-referenced values. Norm-referenced scores are typically reported as ranks or percentiles, indicating an individual's position within a set of scores (see Chapter 22).

> Normative values for the SFT were established on data from over 7,000 individuals aged 60 to 94 from 20 states.[33] These norms were converted to percentiles as a way of judging how individuals performed relative to their age group. For example, among men, percentile scores for the chair stand for those aged 60 to 64 years were:
>
> | 25th: 14 stands | 75th: 19 stands |
> |---|---|
> | 50th: 16 stands | 90th: 22 stands |

These values allow us to interpret an individual's score by determining whether they scored better or worse than their peers. These values do not, however, provide a basis for determining whether a person's demonstrated fitness level is sufficient to maintain functional independence in later years, nor will they help to design intervention or allow measurement of actual change. Such a determination would require a criterion-referenced comparison. Tests may provide both norm- and criterion-referenced methods (see Focus on Evidence 10-2).

■ Interpreting Change

One of the most important purposes of clinical measurement is to accurately capture change, whether improvement or decline. Change scores can serve the purpose of demonstrating the effectiveness of intervention, tracking the course of a disorder over time, or providing a context for evidence-based clinical decision-making. To be useful, an instrument should be able to detect small but meaningful change in a patient's performance. This aspect of validity is the **responsiveness** of an instrument.

This section offers a brief discussion of concepts of change. Further discussion of MDC and MCID, including methods for calculating and interpreting them, are provided in Chapter 32.

Minimal Clinically Important Difference

In Chapter 9, we introduced the concept of **minimal detectable change (MDC)**, which is the minimum amount of measured change needed before we can rule out measurement error as being solely responsible. When change scores exceed the MDC, we can be confident that some real change in status has occurred. This is a matter of reliability. Beyond this, however, the MDC is not helpful in determining whether the changes that have been measured are sufficient to impact the patient or their care in meaningful ways.

The **minimal clinically important difference (MCID)** is the smallest difference in a measured variable that signifies an *important* difference in the patient's condition.[39] It acts as an indicator of the instrument's ability to reflect impactful changes when they have occurred. The MCID is a reflection of the test's validity and can be helpful when choosing an instrument, setting goals for treatment, and determining whether treatment is successful.

The MCID is based on a criterion that establishes when sufficient change has taken place to be considered "important."[40] This criterion is a subjective determination, typically by the patient, who is asked to indicate whether they feel "better" or "worse" to varying levels. The average score that matches those who have indicated at least "somewhat better" or "somewhat worse" is usually used to demarcate the MCID.

📌 The MCID may also be called the *minimal clinically important change (MCIC)*,[41] *minimal important difference (MID)*,[42] or *minimal important change (MIC)*.[43,44] The term *minimal clinically important improvement (MCII)* has been used when the change is only measured as improvement.[45,46]

➤ CASE IN POINT #5

The ability to detect changes in patient-perceived pain is critical to patient management. Danoff et al[47] studied the MCID for visual analog scale (VAS) scores in patients with total knee arthroplasty (TKA) and total hip arthroplasty (THA). Data were collected on 304 patients during their period of postoperative hospitalization. Patients indicated their perception of change using a 5-point Likert scale: "much worse," "somewhat worse," "no change,"

Focus on Evidence 10–2
Defining Normal

The Pediatric Evaluation of Disability Inventory (PEDI) was developed to evaluate age-related capabilities of children with disabilities, aged 0 to 8 years. The test is organized in three domains, including self-care, mobility, and social function.[35] It is scored by summing raw scores within each domain based on ability to perform tasks and the amount of assistance needed. The raw scores are then converted to a normed value ranging from 0 to 100. Higher scores indicate lesser degree of disability. The normal values were standardized based on a sample of 412 children within the appropriate age groups who did not exhibit any functional disabilities.

Haley et al[36] generated reference curves that provide raw scores and percentiles for different age groups. For example, data for the motor subscale is shown here. Scale scores can serve as a criterion reference for evaluative purposes, such as determining the actual amount of change that occurred following intervention. The norm-referenced percentile scores can be used to distinguish children with high or low function as a basis for determining eligibility for disability-related services.[37] These two approaches can provide useful normative and clinical profiles of patients.[38]

From Haley SM, Fragala-Pinkham MA, Ni PS, et al. Pediatric physical functioning reference curves. *Pediatr Neurol* 2004;31(5):333–41, Figure 1, p. 337. Used with permission.

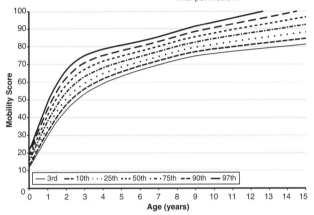

"somewhat better," and "much better." Scores on the VAS were measured as change in distance (in millimeters) along the scale. Negative change scores indicate improvement (less pain). The MCID was based on the mean VAS score for those who indicated a change of at least "somewhat better" or "somewhat worse."

See Chapter 12 for a full discussion of VAS and Likert scales.

The investigators found that some patients improved and some got worse. Therefore, they calculated an MCID to interpret change in both directions (see Fig. 10-4).

> The MCID for improvement was −18.6 mm in patients with THA and −22.6 mm for TKA. For those who exhibited worse pain, the MCID was 23.6 mm for THA and 29.1 mm for TKA.
> The MDC for the VAS scores in the arthroplasty study was 14.9 mm for THA and 16.1 mm for TKA. Therefore, the amount of measured change needed before error could be ruled out was greater for the patients with TKA than for those with THA.

Interpretation of the MCID must be made within the context of a given study, with specific reference to

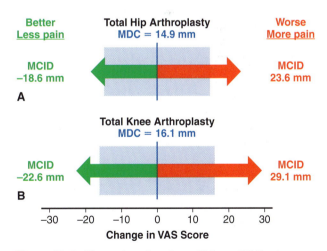

Figure 10–4 Change in pain using a 100 mm VAS pain score for patients following A) THA and B) TKA. The center line indicates initial pain level. A negative score indicates improvement (less pain); a positive score indicates worsening. The MDC is represented by the blue shaded area. Based on data from Danoff JR, Goel R, Sutton R, Maltenfort MG, Austin MS. How much pain is significant? Defining the minimal clinically important difference for the visual analog scale for pain after total joint arthroplasty. *J Arthroplasty* 2018;33(7S):S71–S75.e2.

the outcome measures used, the population and setting, and the design of the study. It is not a fixed value for a given test. In this case, we can see that the results are not the same for patients with different surgical interventions and that they depend on whether they saw improvement or got worse. Those who had TKA needed to show greater improvement to be clinically meaningful. Many studies do not make this important distinction regarding generalization of the MCID, which may lead to misleading conclusions, depending on the direction of change.[46,48]

Ceiling and Floor Effects

One concern in the interpretation of improvement or decline is the ability of an instrument to reflect changes at extremes of a scale. Some instruments exhibit a **floor effect**, which is not being able to show small differences when patients are near the bottom of the scale. For instance, a developmental assessment with a floor effect might not be able to distinguish small improvements in children who are low functioning. Conversely, a patient who is functioning at a high level may show no improvement if a scale is not able to distinguish small changes at the top, called a **ceiling effect**.

> ### ▶ CASE IN POINT #6
> Elbers et al[49] studied the measurement properties of the Multidimensional Fatigue Inventory (MFI) to assess elements of fatigue in patients with Parkinson's disease. The MFI is a self-report questionnaire with items in five subscales. Each subscale contains four items, scored 1 to 5 on a Likert scale. Scores are determined for the total test (maximum 100) as well as for each subscale (range 4 to 20).

The determination of ceiling and floor effects has been based on finding more than 15% of scores clustering at the lower or higher end of a scale.[50,51]

> ▶ Researchers in the fatigue study found no floor or ceiling effects when analyzing the total score, but did see a floor effect with the mental fatigue subscale (18.3% of patients at lowest end) and a ceiling effect for the physical fatigue subscale (16.3% at high end).

These findings suggest that these subscales should be examined to determine whether they can adequately convey the degree of improvement or decline in these dimensions of fatigue in this population. For instance, floor effects would attenuate the ability to capture improvement in patients who were "worse off" at baseline, potentially underestimating the effect of an intervention.[52]

■ Methodological Studies: Validity

Methodological research incorporates testing of both reliability and validity to determine their application and interpretation in a variety of clinical situations. Several important strategies are important as one approaches validity studies.

- **Fully understand the construct.** Validity studies require substantial background to understand the theoretical dimensions of the construct of interest. Through a thorough review of literature, it is important to know which other tools have been used for the same or similar constructs and how they have been analyzed.
- **Consider the clinical context.** Tools that have already gone through validity testing may not be applicable to all clinical circumstances or patient populations and may need further testing if applied for different purposes than used in original validity studies.
- **Consider several approaches.** Validity testing requires looking at all aspects of validity and will benefit from multiple analysis approaches. The broader the testing methods, the more the test's validity can be generalized.
- **Consider validity issues if adapting existing tools.** Many clinicians find that existing tools do not fit their applications exactly, and thus will adapt sections or definitions to fit their needs. Although it is useful to start with existing tools, changing a tool's properties can alter validity, and testing should be done to ensure that validity is maintained.
- **Cross-validate outcomes.** Validity properties that are documented on one sample may not be the same if tested on a different sample. This issue is especially important when cutoff scores or predictive values are being generated for application to a larger population. Cross-validation allows us to demonstrate the consistency of outcomes on a second sample to determine whether the test criteria can be generalized across samples.

COMMENTARY

In our lust for measurement, we frequently measure that which we can rather than that which we wish to measure . . . and forget that there is a difference.

—*George Yule (1871-1951)*

British statistician

The importance of validity for evidence-based practice cannot be overemphasized. All measurements have a purpose, which must be understood if we are to apply them appropriately and obtain meaningful data. For example, fitness standards for elderly individuals may influence whether a patient is referred for therapy and whether insurance coverage will be recommended. The application of MCID scores can impact whether a patient is considered improved and whether payers will reimburse for continued care. Diagnostic criteria must be accurate if we are to determine whether an intervention is warranted, especially if that intervention has associated risks. From an evidence perspective, we must be able to determine whether outcomes of clinical trials are applicable to practice, understanding the consequences of using measurements for clinical decisions. Because validity is context-driven, we must have confidence in the choice of instrument and validity of the data that are generated.

REFERENCES

1. McDowell I. *Measuring Health: A Guide to Rating Scales and Questionnaires.* 3 ed. New York: Oxford University Press, 2006.
2. American Educational Research Association, American Psychological Association, National Council on Measurement in Education, et al. *Standards for Educational and Psychological Testing.* Washington, DC: American Educational Research Association, 2014.
3. Messick S. Validity of psychological assessment: validation of inferences from persons' responses and performances as scientific inquiry into score meaning. *Am Psychol* 1995;50(9):741–749.
4. Streiner DL. Statistics commentary series: commentary no. 17-validity. *J Clin Psychopharmacol* 2016;36(6):542–544.
5. Brown T. Construct validity: a unitary concept for occupational therapy assessment and measurement. *Hong Kong J Occup Ther* 2010;20(1):30–42.
6. Patrick DL, Chiang YP. Measurement of health outcomes in treatment effectiveness evaluations: conceptual and methodological challenges. *Med Care* 2000;38(9 Suppl):II14–25.
7. Whelton PK, Carey RM, Aronow WS, Casey DE, Jr., Collins KJ, Dennison Himmelfarb C, DePalma SM, Gidding S, Jamerson KA, Jones DW, et al. 2017 ACC/AHA/AAPA/ABC/ACPM/AGS/APhA/ASH/ASPC/NMA/PCNA guideline for the prevention, detection, evaluation, and management of high blood pressure in adults: a report of the American College of Cardiology/American Heart Association Task Force on Clinical Practice Guidelines. *Hypertension* 2018; 71(6):e13–e115.
8. Downing SM. Validity: on meaningful interpretation of assessment data. *Med Educ* 2003;37(9):830–837.
9. Cook DA, Beckman TJ. Current concepts in validity and reliability for psychometric instruments: theory and application. *Am J Med* 2006;119(2):166.e7–e16.
10. Harris SR, Megens AM, Backman CL, Hayes V. Development and standardization of the Harris Infant Neuromotor Test. *Intants & Young Children* 2003;16(2):143–151.
11. Harris SR. Early identification of motor delay: family-centered screening tool. *Can Fam Physician* 2016;62(8):629–632.
12. Harris SR, Daniels LE. Reliability and validity of the Harris Infant Neuromotor Test. *J Pediatr* 2001;139(2):249–253.
13. Harris SR, Megens AM, Daniels LE: *Harris Infant Neuromotor Infant Test (HINT). Test User's Manual Version 1.0. Clinical Edition.* Chicago, IL: Infant Motor Performance Scales, 2010. Available at http://thetimp.com/store/large/382h6/TIMP_Products/HINT_Test_Manual.html. Accessed June 14, 2017.
14. Harris SR, Daniels LE. Content validity of the Harris Infant Neuromotor Test. *Phys Ther* 1996;76(7):727–737.
15. Buckley JP, Sim J, Eston RG, Hession R, Fox R. Reliability and validity of measures taken during the Chester step test to predict aerobic power and to prescribe aerobic exercise. *Br J Sports Med* 2004;38(2):197–205.
16. Harris SR. Parents' and caregivers' perceptions of their children's development. *Dev Med Child Neurol* 1994;36(10): 918–923.
17. Westcott McCoy S, Bowman A, Smith-Blockley J, Sanders K, Megens AM, Harris SR. Harris Infant Neuromotor Test: comparison of US and Canadian normative data and examination of concurrent validity with the Ages and Stages Questionnaire. *Phys Ther* 2009;89(2):173–180.
18. Tse L, Mayson TA, Leo S, Lee LL, Harris SR, Hayes VE, Backman CL, Cameron D, Tardif M. Concurrent validity of the Harris Infant Neuromotor Test and the Alberta Infant Motor Scale. *J Pediatr Nurs* 2008;23(1):28–36.
19. Megens AM, Harris SR, Backman CL, Hayes VE. Known-groups analysis of the Harris Infant Neuromotor Test. *Phys Ther* 2007;87(2):164–169.
20. Waltz CF, Strickland O, Lenz ER. *Measurement in Nursing and Health Research.* 4 ed. New York: Springer Publishing, 2010.
21. Melzack R, Katz J. The McGill Pain Questionnnaire: appraisal and current status. In: Turk DC, Melzack R, eds. *Handbook of Pain Assessment.* New York: Guilford Press, 1992.
22. Grilo RM, Treves R, Preux PM, Vergne-Salle P, Bertin P. Clinically relevant VAS pain score change in patients with acute rheumatic conditions. *Joint Bone Spine* 2007;74(4): 358–361.
23. Breivik H, Borchgrevink PC, Allen SM, Rosseland LA, Romundstad L, Hals EK, Kvarstein G, Stubhaug A. Assessment of pain. *Br J Anaesth* 2008;101(1):17–24.
24. Abahussin AA, West RM, Wong DC, Ziegler LE. PROMs for pain in adult cancer patients: a systematic review of measurement properties. *Pain Pract* 2019;19(1):93–117.

25. Campbell DT, Fiske DW. Convergent and discriminant validation by the multitrait-multimethod matrix. *Psychol Bull* 1959;56:81.

26. Renno P, Wood JJ. Discriminant and convergent validity of the anxiety construct in children with autism spectrum disorders. *J Autism Dev Disord* 2013;43(9):2135–2146.

27. Meenan RF, Mason JH, Anderson JJ, Guccione AA, Kazis LE. AIMS2. The content and properties of a revised and expanded Arthritis Impact Measurement Scales Health Status Questionnaire. *Arthritis Rheum* 1992;35(1):1–10.

28. Brown JH, Kazis LE, Spitz PW, Gertman P, Fries JF, Meenan RF. The dimensions of health outcomes: a cross-validated examination of health status measurement. *Am J Public Health* 1984;74(2):159–161.

29. Mason JH, Anderson JJ, Meenan RF. A model of health status for rheumatoid arthritis. A factor analysis of the Arthritis Impact Measurement Scales. *Arthritis Rheum* 1988;31(6):714–720.

30. Arthritis Impact Measurement Scales 2 (AIMS2). Available at http://geriatrictoolkit.missouri.edu/aims2/AIMS2-ORIGINAL.pdf. Accessed September 3, 2018.

31. Meenan RF, Gertman PM, Mason JH, Dunaif R. The arthritis impact measurement scales. Further investigations of a health status measure. *Arthritis Rheum* 1982;25(9):1048–1053.

32. Rikli RE, Jones CJ. *Senior Fitness Test Manual*. 2 ed. Champaign, IL: Human Kinetics, 2013.

33. Rikli RE, Jones CJ. Functional fitness normative scores for community-residing older adults, ages 60–94. *J Aging Phys Act* 1999;7(2):162–181.

34. Rikli RE, Jones CJ. Development and validation of criterion-referenced clinically relevant fitness standards for maintaining physical independence in later years. *Gerontologist* 2013; 53(2):255–267.

35. Feldman AB, Haley SM, Coryell J. Concurrent and construct validity of the Pediatric Evaluation of Disability Inventory. *Phys Ther* 1990;70(10):602–610.

36. Haley SM, Fragala-Pinkham MA, Ni PS, Skrinar AM, Kaye EM. Pediatric physical functioning reference curves. *Pediatr Neurol* 2004;31(5):333–341.

37. Haley SM, Coster WI, Kao YC, Dumas HM, Fragala-Pinkham MA, Kramer JM, Ludlow LH, Moed R. Lessons from use of the Pediatric Evaluation of Disability Inventory: where do we go from here? *Pediatr Phys Ther* 2010;22(1):69–75.

38. Kothari DH, Haley SM, Gill-Body KM, Dumas HM. Measuring functional change in children with acquired brain injury (ABI): comparison of generic and ABI-specific scales using the Pediatric Evaluation of Disability Inventory (PEDI). *Phys Ther* 2003;83(9):776–785.

39. Redelmeier DA, Guyatt GH, Goldstein RS. Assessing the minimal important difference in symptoms: a comparison of two techniques. *J Clin Epidemiol* 1996;49(11):1215–1219.

40. Wright JG. The minimal important difference: who's to say what is important? *J Clin Epidemiol* 1996;49(11):1221–1222.

41. Soer R, Reneman MF, Vroomen PC, Stegeman P, Coppes MH. Responsiveness and minimal clinically important change of the Pain Disability Index in patients with chronic back pain. *Spine* 2012;37(8):711–715.

42. Khair RM, Nwaneri C, Damico RL, Kolb T, Hassoun PM, Mathai SC. The minimal important difference in Borg Dyspnea Score in pulmonary arterial hypertension. *Ann Am Thorac Soc* 2016;13(6):842–849.

43. Rodrigues JN, Mabvuure NT, Nikkhah D, Shariff Z, Davis TR. Minimal important changes and differences in elective hand surgery. *J Hand Surg Eur Vol* 2015;40(9):900–912.

44. Terwee CB, Roorda LD, Dekker J, Bierma-Zeinstra SM, Peat G, Jordan KP, Croft P, de Vet HC. Mind the MIC: large variation among populations and methods. *J Clin Epidemiol* 2010;63(5):524–534.

45. Tubach F, Ravaud P, Baron G, Falissard B, Logeart I, Bellamy N, Bombardier C, Felson D, Hochberg M, van der Heijde D, et al. Evaluation of clinically relevant changes in patient reported outcomes in knee and hip osteoarthritis: the minimal clinically important improvement. *Ann Rheum Dis* 2005; 64(1):29–33.

46. Wang YC, Hart DL, Stratford PW, Mioduski JE. Baseline dependency of minimal clinically important improvement. *Phys Ther* 2011;91(5):675–688.

47. Danoff JR, Goel R, Sutton R, Maltenfort MG, Austin MS. How much pain is significant? Defining the minimal clinically important difference for the visual analog scale for pain after total joint arthroplasty. *J Arthroplasty* 2018;33(7S):S71–S75.e2.

48. de Vet HC, Terwee CB, Ostelo RW, Beckerman H, Knol DL, Bouter LM. Minimal changes in health status questionnaires: distinction between minimally detectable change and minimally important change. *Health Qual Life Outcomes* 2006;4:54.

49. Elbers RG, van Wegen EE, Verhoef J, Kwakkel G. Reliability and structural validity of the Multidimensional Fatigue Inventory (MFI) in patients with idiopathic Parkinson's disease. *Parkinsonism Relat Disord* 2012;18(5):532–536.

50. McHorney CA, Tarlov AR. Individual-patient monitoring in clinical practice: are available health status surveys adequate? *Qual Life Res* 1995;4(4):293–307.

51. Terwee CB, Bot SD, de Boer MR, van der Windt DA, Knol DL, Dekker J, Bouter LM, de Vet HC. Quality criteria were proposed for measurement properties of health status questionnaires. *J Clin Epidemiol* 2007;60(1):34–42.

52. Feeny DH, Eckstrom E, Whitlock EP, Perdue LA. *A Primer for Systematic Reviewers on the Measurement of Functional Status and Health-Related Quality of Life in Older Adults.* (Prepared by the Kaiser Permanente Research Affiliates Evidence-based Practice Center under Contract No. 290-2007-10057-I.) AHRQ Publication No. 13-EHC128-EF. Rockville, MD: Agency for Healthcare Research and Quality. September 2013. Available at https://www.ncbi.nlm.nih.gov/pubmedhealth/PMH0076940/. Accessed July 5, 2018.

Designing Surveys and Questionnaires

One of the most popular methods for collecting information is the survey approach. A **survey** consists of a set of questions that elicits quantitative or qualitative responses. Surveys can be conducted for a variety of purposes using different formats and delivery methods, including **questionnaires** in hard copy or online, and face-to-face or telephone interviews.

Surveys can be used as a data gathering technique in descriptive, exploratory, or explanatory studies. Data may be intended for generalization to a larger population or as a description of a smaller defined group. The purpose of this chapter is to present an overview of the structure of survey instruments, with a focus on essential elements of survey design, construction, question writing, and delivery methods.

■ Purposes of Surveys

Surveys can be used for descriptive purposes or to generate data to test specific hypotheses.

Descriptive Surveys

Descriptive surveys are intended to characterize knowledge, behaviors, patterns, attitudes, or demographics of individuals within a given population. Such surveys are often used to inform marketing decisions, public policy, or quality improvement. For instance, many healthcare institutions use surveys to determine patient satisfaction[1] and to describe patient demographics.[2]

Data can be accessed for many federal and state surveys.[3] For example, large national surveys such as the U.S. Census, the National Health Interview Survey,[4] and the National Nursing Home Survey[5] provide important population data that can be used for many varied purposes, including documenting the incidence of disease, estimating research needs, describing the quality of life of different groups, and generating policy recommendations.

Testing Hypotheses

Surveys may also involve testing hypotheses about the nature of relationships within a population. Data can be used to establish outcomes following intervention, explore relationships among clinical variables, or examine risk factors for disease or disability. Surveys can be used for data collection in experimental studies to compare outcomes across groups when studying variables such as attitudes and perceptions.

For example, questionnaires have been used to compare quality of life following bilateral or unilateral cochlear implants,[6] to establish the relationship between medical adherence and health literacy,[7] and to study the influence of life-style preferences and comorbidities on type 2 diabetes.[8]

Standardized questionnaires are also used extensively as self-report instruments for assessing outcomes related to broad clinical constructs such as function, pain, health status, and quality of life. These instruments are designed to generate scores that can be used to evaluate patient improvement and to support clinical decision making, requiring extensive validation procedures. We will discuss these types of scales in Chapter 12, but the concepts presented here related to designing surveys will apply to those instruments as well.

Other types of survey instruments will be discussed in the *Chapter 11 Supplement*, including the Delphi survey and Q-sort.

internet or email. Depending on the nature of the target population, this can provide a bias, especially based on age, education, or socioeconomic status.[9]

■ Survey Formats

The two main formats for surveys are questionnaires and interviews. The appropriate method will depend on the nature of the research question and the study variables.

Questionnaires

Most of us are familiar with questionnaires, a type of structured survey that is usually self-administered, asking individuals to respond to a series of questions. The advantages of using questionnaires are many. They are generally efficient, allowing respondents to complete them on their own time. Data can be gathered from a large sample in a wide geographical distribution in a relatively short period of time at minimal expense. Questionnaires are standardized so that everyone is exposed to the same questions in the same way. Respondents can take time to think about their answers and to consult records for specific information when needed. Questionnaires also provide anonymity, encouraging honest and candid responses.

Questionnaires are particularly useful as a research method for examining phenomena that can be best assessed through self-observation, such as attitudes, values, and perceptions. The primary disadvantages of the written questionnaire are the potential for misunderstanding or misinterpreting questions or response choices, and unknown accuracy or motivation of the respondent.

Surveys can be used for retrospective or prospective studies. Most often, surveys are based on a cross-sectional sample, meaning that a large group of respondents are tested at relatively the same point in time. Surveys can, however, be used in longitudinal studies by giving follow-up interviews or questionnaires to document changes in attitudes or behaviors over time.

Questionnaires are usually distributed through the mail or by electronic means, although many research situations do allow for in-person distribution.

Electronic distribution of questionnaires is less expensive, faster to send and return, and generally easier to complete and submit than written mail questionnaires. Many free electronic platforms are available online, and many provide automatic downloading of data, eliminating data entry and associated time or errors.

Electronic surveys do require, however, that respondents have the appropriate technological skill and access to the

Interviews

In an interview, the researcher asks respondents specific questions and records their answers for later analysis. Interviews can take a few minutes or several hours, depending on the nature of the questions and the respondent's willingness to share information. Interviews can be conducted face-to-face or over the telephone.

Face-to-Face Interviews

Interviews conducted in person tend to be most effective for establishing rapport between the interviewer and the respondent. This interaction can be important for eliciting forthright responses to questions that are of a personal nature.

The advantage of this approach is the opportunity for in-depth analysis of respondents' behaviors and opinions because the researcher can follow up responses with probes to clarify answers and directly observe respondents' reactions. Therefore, interviews are a common approach to obtain qualitative information. To avoid errors of interpretation of replies, many researchers will record interview sessions (with the participant's consent). The major disadvantages of face-to-face interviews include cost and time, need for trained personnel to carry out the interviews, scheduling, and the lack of anonymity of the respondents.

Structure of Interviews

Interviews can be *structured*, consisting of a standardized set of questions that will be asked of all participants. In this way, all respondents are exposed to the same questions, in the same order, and are given the same choices for responses.

Qualitative studies often use interviews with a less strict format. In a *semi-structured* interview, the interviewer follows a list of questions and topics that need to be covered but is able to follow lines of discussion that may stray from the guide when appropriate. In an *unstructured* interview, the interviewer does not have a fixed agenda, and can proceed informally to question and discuss issues of concern. This format is typically conversational and is often carried out in the respondent's natural setting. Data are analyzed based on themes of narrative data.

If a study involves the use of interviewers, a formal training process should be incorporated. Interviewers must be consistent in how questions are asked and how probing follow-up questions are used (if they are to be allowed). The interviewers must understand the process of recording responses, an important skill when open-ended questions are used.

Further discussion of interviewing techniques for qualitative research is included in Chapter 21.

Telephone Interviews

Telephone interviews have been shown to be an effective alternative to in-person discussions and have the advantage of being less expensive, especially if respondents are geographically diverse. Disadvantages include not being able to establish the same level of rapport as personal interviews without a visual connection, more limited time as people become fatigued when on the phone too long, and the "annoyance factor" that we have all experienced when contacted over the phone (typically at dinner time!). [10,11] Prior contact to set up an appointment can help with this. There are also issues with availability depending on what kinds of phone listings are available.

An important use of telephone interviews is gathering follow-up data in research studies.

> *Data were analyzed from a 17-center, prospective cohort study of infants (age <1 year) who were hospitalized with bronchiolitis during three consecutive fall/winter seasons.[12] Parents were called at 6-month intervals after discharge to assess respiratory problems. The primary outcome was status at 12 months. They were able to follow up with 87% of the families and were able to document differences in response rate among socioeconomic and ethnic subgroups.*

📌 Survey researchers often utilize more than one mode of data collection to improve response rates.[13] Using a mixed methods approach, offering written or online questionnaires and interviews or telephone surveys, researchers attempt to appeal to respondent preferences, reduce costs, and obtain greater coverage. Data are typically a combination of qualitative and quantitative information.

Self-Report

Survey data that are collected using either an interview or questionnaire are based on **self-report**. The researcher does not directly observe the respondent's behavior or attitudes, but only records the respondent's report of them. There is always some potential for bias or inaccuracy in self-reports, particularly if the questions concern personal or controversial issues. The phenomenon of **recall bias** can be a problem when respondents are asked to remember past events, especially if these events were of a sensitive nature or if they occurred a long time ago.

Research has shown, however, that self-report measures are generally valid. For instance, variables such as mobility have been reported accurately. [14,15] However, some studies have shown a poorer correlation between performance, healthcare utilization, and self-report measures. [16,17] These differences point out the need to understand the target population and the respondents' abilities to answer the questions posed.

For many variables, self-report is the only direct way to obtain information. Data obtained from standardized questionnaires that evaluate health and quality of life must be interpreted as the respondent's perception of those characteristics, rather than performance measures.

Although surveys can be administered through several methods, we will focus primarily on written questionnaires for the remainder of this chapter. Most of the principles in designing questionnaires can be applied to interviews as well.

■ Planning the Survey

The process of developing a survey instrument is perhaps more time consuming than people realize. Most problems that arise with survey research go back to the original design process, requiring well-defined goals and a full understanding of how the information gathered will be used.

Creating a survey involves several stages, within which the instrument is planned, written, and revised, until it is finally ready for use as a research tool (see Fig. 11-1).

Always Start with a Question

The first consideration in every research effort is delineation of the overall research question. The purpose of the research must be identified with reference to a target population and the specific type of information that will be sought. These decisions will form the structure for deciding the appropriate research design. A survey is appropriate when the question requires obtaining information from respondents, rather than measuring performance.

> ➤ **CASE IN POINT**
>
> For many older adults, access to healthcare is a challenge. Healthcare systems have begun to explore the efficacy of tele-health technologies for the delivery of education, monitoring of health status, and supplementing personal visits. However, before such efforts can be implemented effectively, attitudes toward such technology must be evaluated. Edwards et al[18] used a questionnaire to study acceptance of a telehealth approach for patients with chronic disease to determine which factors could influence successful outcomes.

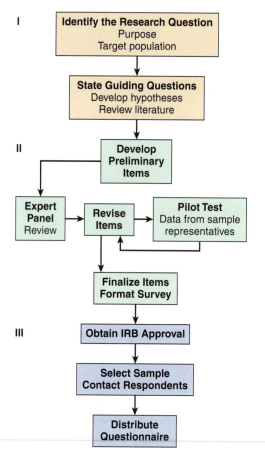

I

Identify the Research Question
Purpose
Target population

State Guiding Questions
Develop hypotheses
Review literature

II

Develop Preliminary Items

Expert Panel
Review

Revise Items

Pilot Test
Data from sample representatives

Finalize Items Format Survey

III

Obtain IRB Approval

Select Sample Contact Respondents

Distribute Questionnaire

Figure 11–1 Process for development of a questionnaire in three stages. In stage I, planning includes delineation of the research question, the target population, and hypotheses. In stage II, development includes designing the survey, as well as creating and testing items to finalize the format. Stage III includes IRB approval, selection of a sample, and distribution of the survey.

Review of Literature

Once the purpose of the research and the target population are identified, a review of literature is important to understand what is known and to inform the survey's focus and content. Previous research will inform defining constructs and the development of questions, as well as provide background for a rationale to support expected outcomes.

> ➤ Edwards et al[18] were able to find several studies that had looked at effectiveness and costs related to telehealth, with mixed results. Although some studies were able to document reduced mortality and admission rates, the researchers identified a lack of evidence focused on chronic diseases.

Guiding Questions and Hypotheses

The next step is to clarify the survey's purpose through a series of guiding questions, aims, or hypotheses that delineate what the researcher is trying to find out. This allows the researcher to describe the group to be studied and to examine specific relationships. This process will help to frame the content and questions included in the questionnaire.

> ➤ The aim of the telehealth study was to explore the key factors that influence interest in using telehealth in two exemplar chronic diseases: depression and cardiovascular disease (CVD) risk.

Stating useful hypotheses that support an overall research question requires that the researcher have a clear conceptualization of the phenomenon or characteristics being studied. If the phenomenon is poorly understood, it will be hard to construct questions that explore its component behaviors.

> ➤ The researchers hypothesized that interest in telehealth would be predicted by sociodemographic factors, health needs, difficulties and confidence in accessing technology, and prior use of telehealth.

By delineating the specific variables and expected outcomes, the authors were able to clearly structure the analysis and discussion of their findings.

> 📌 Depending on the nature of the research question, as a preliminary technique, researchers will often hold *focus groups* to explore people's attitudes and interests. Results can be informative in terms of how questions should be conceptualized and which issues would be most important to the target population.

■ Designing the Survey

Once hypotheses are formulated, investigators must develop a detailed outline, listing each item of information that will be needed to answer the research question. Each item should relate back to at least one of the study's objectives and should add to a larger informational context that will contribute to conclusions.

As with any other measurement approach, validity is a major concern in the design of a survey instrument; that is, the questionnaire or interview must provide data that are meaningful. Questions are not asked out of casual interest or curiosity, but because they reflect essential pieces of information that, taken as a whole, will address the proposed research question.

Developing Content

The researcher begins by writing a series of questions that address each behavior, knowledge, skill, or attitude reflected in the guiding questions.

> The telehealth study was organized around six categories of questions:
>
> 1. Sociodemographics
> 2. Current access to healthcare
> 3. Technology-related factors
>   - Availability of technology
>   - Confidence in using technology
>   - Perceived advantages or disadvantages of technology
> 4. Past telehealth satisfaction
> 5. Interest in using telehealth
> 6. Current health status

Questions should be grouped and organized to reflect each category or topic. The first draft of a questionnaire should include several questions for each topic so that these can eventually be compared and weeded out.

Using Existing Instruments

Depending on the nature of the research question, it is always helpful to review existing instruments to determine if they are applicable or adaptable for your study. Many investigators have developed and validated instruments for a variety of purposes, and these instruments can often be borrowed directly or in part, or they can be modified to fit new research situations, saving a great deal of time.[19] Tools like the Beck Depression Inventory,[20] the Mini-Mental State Examination (MMSE),[21] and the Short Form (SF)-36 or SF-12 health status questionnaires[22] are often applied as part of studies.

> To assess generic health status, researchers in the telehealth study used the SF-12 health survey, which has been validated across populations. This survey derives summary scores for physical and mental health components.

A benefit of using an existing tool is that your data can then be compared with outcomes of prior studies. It is not wise, however, to adopt previously used surveys blindly, without considering differences in populations being studied, the specific objectives of the instrument, and its established validity. This is an important part of the review of literature. But whenever possible, don't reinvent the wheel!

Expert Review

The preliminary draft of the survey should be distributed to a panel of colleagues who can review the document, identify problems with questions, including wording and organization. Using the guiding questions as a reference, these experts should be asked to make suggestions for constructive change. No matter how carefully the survey has been designed, the researcher is often too close to it to see its flaws.

Based on the panel's comments, the survey should be revised and then presented to the panel again for further comment. The revision process should continue with additional feedback until the researcher is satisfied that the instrument is concise and clear, as well as serves its intended purpose. This process is indeed time consuming but necessary, and helps to establish the content validity of the instrument.

Pilot Testing and Revisions

The revised questionnaire should then be pilot tested on a small representative sample, perhaps 5 to 10 individuals from the target population. The researcher should interview these respondents to determine where questions were unclear or misleading. If the researcher is unsure about the appropriateness of specific wording, several versions of a question can be asked to elicit the same information in different ways, and responses can be compared for their reliability.

It is also useful to monitor the time it takes for respondents to complete the questionnaire and to examine missing answers and inconsistencies. It may be helpful to administer the survey to this group on two occasions, perhaps separated by several days, to see if the responses are consistent, as a way of estimating test–retest reliability. Based on the results of pilot testing, the questionnaire will again be revised and retested until the final instrument attains an acceptable level of validity.

■ Types of Survey Questions

Using our example of surveying patients regarding the use of telehealth, let's look at various types of questions that can be asked. There are essentially two kinds of questions: open-ended and closed-ended questions.

Open-Ended Questions

Open-ended questions ask respondents to answer in their own words. This approach is useful for probing respondents' feelings and opinions without biases or limits imposed by the researcher. For example:

How do you use technology, such as phones, computers, and social media?

This would require the respondent to provide specific examples of using devices or the internet. This format is useful when the researcher is not sure of all possible responses to a question. Therefore, respondents are given the opportunity to provide answers from their own perspective. Sometimes researchers will use open-ended questions in a pilot study to determine a range of responses that can then be converted to a multiple-choice item.

Open-ended questions are, however, difficult to code and analyze because so many different responses can be obtained. If open-ended questions are misunderstood, they may elicit answers that are essentially irrelevant to the researcher's goal. Respondents may not want to take the time to write a full answer, or they may answer in a way that is clear to them but uninterpretable, vague, or incomplete to the researcher. For instance, the question about technology use could elicit a long list of specific devices and apps, or it could result in a general description of technology use. If the purpose of the question is to find out if the respondent uses specific types of technology, it would be better to provide a list of options.

Some open-ended questions request a numerical response, such as exact age, annual income, height, or weight. The question must specify exactly how it should be answered, such as to the nearest year, gross annual income, or to the nearest inch or pound.

 Open-ended questions can be most effective in interviews because the interviewer can clarify the respondent's answers using follow-up questions.

Closed-Ended Questions

Closed-ended questions ask respondents to select an answer from among several fixed choices. There are several formats that can be used for closed-ended questions, depending on the nature of the information being requested.

🌐 Questions used as examples in this section are taken or adapted from the telehealth study by Edwards at al.[18] See the *Chapter 11 Supplement* for the full survey.

Multiple Choice Questions

One of the most common formats is the use of multiple choice options. This type of question is easily coded and provides greater uniformity across responses. Its

disadvantage is that it does not allow respondents to express their own personal viewpoints and, therefore, may provide a biased response set.

There are two basic considerations in constructing multiple choice questions. First, the responses should be *exhaustive*, including all possible responses that can be expected. Second, the response categories should be *mutually exclusive* so that each choice clearly represents a unique answer with no overlap. In Question 1, for instance, it is possible that respondents could be in school and work at the same time, or taking care of a household could be interpreted as unemployed. As a protection, it is often advisable to include a category for "not applicable" (NA), "don't know," or "other (please specify ____)."

Question 1
Which one of these best describes your current situation? *Please check only one.*

- ◯ Full-time paid work (≥30 hrs/wk)
- ◯ Part-time paid work (<30 hrs/wk)
- ◯ Full-time school
- ◯ Unemployed
- ◯ Unable to work due to illness or disability
- ◯ Fully retired
- ◯ Taking care of household
- ◯ Doing something else (*please describe*)
  _____

Where only one response is desired, it may be useful to add an instruction to the question asking respondents to select the *one best answer* or the answer that is most important. However, this technique does not substitute for carefully worded questions and choices.

Dichotomous Questions

The simplest form of closed-ended question is one that presents two choices, or *dichotomous* responses, as shown in Question 2a. Even this seemingly simple question, however, can be ambiguous, as definitions of gender identity are no longer obvious using this dichotomous description. To be sensitive to social issues, Question 2b is an alternative.[23]

Question 2a
What is your gender?
- ◯ Male   ◯ Female

Question 2b
What is your gender identity?

- ◯ Man
- ◯ Woman
- ◯ Another identity, please specify_____
- ◯ I would prefer not to answer

Check All That Apply

Sometimes the researcher is interested in more than one answer to a question, as in Question 3a. However, coding multiple responses in a single question can be difficult. When multiple responses are of interest, it is better to ask respondents to mark each choice separately, as in Question 3b.

Question 3a

Do you have any of the following easily available for your use at home, at work, or at the home of friends or family? *Please check all that apply.*

- O   A telephone (land line)
- O   A mobile phone
- O   Internet access
- O   Personal email

Question 3b

Please indicate if you have each of the following easily available for your use at home, at work, or at the home of friends or family.

	Not Available	Available
1. A telephone	O	O
2. A mobile phone	O	O
3. Internet access	O	O
4. Personal email	O	O

Measuring Intensity

When questions address a characteristic that is on a continuum, such as attitudes or quality of performance, it is useful to provide a range of choices so that the respondent can represent the appropriate intensity of response. Usually, three to five multiple-choice options are provided, as shown in Question 4. An option for "Don't know" or "Unsure" may be included.

Checklists

When a series of questions use the same format, a checklist can provide a more efficient presentation, as illustrated in Question 4. With this approach, instructions for using the response choices need only be given once, and the respondent can quickly go through many questions without reading a new set of choices. Question 5 shows a checklist using a **Likert scale** (see Chapter 12).

Measurement Scales

Questions may be formatted as a scale to create a summative outcome related to a construct such as function or quality of life. Instruments such as the Barthel Index[24] and the Functional Independence Measure (FIM)[25] are examples of health questionnaires that use total scores to summarize functional levels.

See Chapter 12 for a robust discussion of measurement scales.

Visual Analog Scales

A commonly used approach incorporates **visual analog scales (VAS)**. This format is usually based on a 10-cm line with anchors on each side that reflect extremes of the variable being measured. Subjects are asked to place a mark along the scale that reflects the intensity of their response. Although mostly used to assess pain, the VAS can be used for any variable that has a relative intensity (see Chapter 12).

Question 4

Sometimes people find it hard to get the health support and advice they would like. Have you had any difficulty with the following:

	No Difficulty	Some Difficulty	Lots of Difficulty
a. Getting to appointments outside of your home due to your physical health?	O	O	O
b. Getting to appointments outside of your home due to psychologic or emotional difficulties?	O	O	O
c. Getting to appointments outside of your home due to difficulties with transportation or travel?	O	O	O
d. Cost of transportation and travel to get to appointments?	O	O	O

Question 5

How confident do you feel about doing the following:

	Not at all confident	Quite confident	Extremely confident	I have never tried this	I don't know what this is
1. Using a mobile phone for phone calls	O	O	O	O	O
2. Using a mobile phone for text messages	O	O	O	O	O
3. Using a computer	O	O	O	O	O
4. Sending and receiving emails	O	O	O	O	O
5. Finding information on the internet	O	O	O	O	O
6. Using social media sites like Facebook	O	O	O	O	O

Rank-Order Questions

An alternative question format is the *rank-order* question, shown in Question 6, where the respondent is presented with a series of responses and is asked to rank them on an ordinal scale. This format can be difficult, however, as respondents have to constantly adjust their opinion to determine relative importance as they sort through the list. It is also easy to misunderstand which rank is highest or lowest. It may be clearer to present each option on a Likert scale asking respondents to rate their level of interest from none to high.

Question 6

People have different interests in using technology for support of healthcare. Please rank the following items in terms of interest to you, ranking from 1 (MOST INTEREST) to 5 (LEAST INTEREST).

__ Using a landline
__ Using a mobile phone
__ Using text messages on a mobile phone
__ Using a computer to view websites
__ Sending and receiving emails

Branching

Some question sequences try to follow up on specific answers with more detailed questions, using a technique called *branching*. Depending on the response to an initial question, the respondent will be directed to answer additional questions or to skip ahead to a later question. This process saves time by avoiding questions that are irrelevant to a specific respondent. Branching can be confusing, however, and can be avoided by different phrasing, such as simply adding a choice of "none of the above." It can also present a challenge to data analysis, as the number of answered items will differ among respondents.

■ Writing Good Questions

The validity of surveys is highly dependent on the quality of the questions, how well they are understood, and how easily respondents can determine their answers. Survey questions must be clear and purposeful if they are going to provide useful information to answer the research question. Some useful considerations include:[26]

- *Every question should be answerable by every respondent.* Even if that response is "not applicable,"

every question must be relevant for all respondents. You want to avoid leaving blank answers. Having a choice for "Other" (with a space to indicate the other option) can also help. It is often useful to add a choice for "Don't know," but this should only be used for factual questions, not for questions about attitudes or opinions.

- *Respondents should be able to answer questions easily.* If they have to ponder the answer, they may not want to take the time to give a thoughtful response. Questions that require respondents to look up information can be burdensome and may be left blank.

- *Can respondents recall information accurately?* It can be difficult to remember details, especially over a long time period.

- *Will respondents be honest in their answers?* If the response is potentially embarrassing, they may not want to answer accurately. Sensitive topics need to be addressed carefully.

- *Try to use a variety of question types.* Just to give the survey some interest, and to prevent rote answers, try to incorporate different question formats. However, it is helpful to group question types so respondents can move quickly from one response to the next.

- *Questions should generate varied responses.* It is not useful to include questions that all respondents will agree with. If they are answered the same way by everyone, results will not help to distinguish outcomes.

Wording Questions

Simplicity is a key to good questionnaires. Sentences should be succinct and grammatically correct. The author of the questionnaire should assume that respondents will read and answer questions quickly and should provide choices that will be understood at a glance.

Purposeful Language

Questions should be written in common language for the lowest educational level that might be encountered. Generally, shorter questions and responses are more likely to be understood and to keep the respondent's attention. The length of the question is not, however, the determining factor in the clarity of the question. Sometimes, longer questions are needed to provide sufficient information to elicit the appropriate response.

Language may be an issue if respondents do not speak English or English is a second language. Idioms or subtle cultural expressions should be carefully avoided. The researcher may have the questionnaire translated into another language for specific sample groups. The translation must account for cultural biases.

Avoid Bias

Questions should not imply a "right" or "preferred" response. Similarly, response options should also be neutral. Words that suggest a bias should also be avoided. For example:

Do you often go to your physician with trivial problems?

This implies an undesirable behavior.

Clarity

It goes without saying that survey questions must be clear and unambiguous. Questions that require subtle distinctions to interpret responses are more likely to be misunderstood. For example, consider the question:

Do you use technology devices in your daily life?

There are two ambiguous terms here. First, there may be different ways to define technology devices. Do they include phones, computers, tablets, watches? Second, what constitutes use? Does it mean a simple phone call, accessing the internet, just telling time? This type of ambiguity can be corrected by providing the respondent with appropriate definitions.

Clarity also requires avoiding the use of jargon, abbreviations, or unnecessarily complex sentences. Generally, wording should be at the 8th grade reading level. Don't use words that can be ambiguous, like "most people" or "several." Phrase questions in the positive direction when using disagree–agree options. Avoid using "not," "rarely," "never," and negative prefixes.

Double-Barreled Questions

Each question should be confined to a single idea. Surveys should avoid the use of *double-barreled questions*, using "or" or "and" to assess two things within a single question. For instance:

"Do you have difficulty using mobile phones or computers to access information?"

It is obviously possible to experience these technologies differently, making it impossible to answer the question. It is better to ask two separate questions to assess each activity separately.

Frequency and Time Measures

Researchers are often interested in quantifying behavior in terms of frequency and time. For example, it might be of interest to ask:

How often do you use a mobile phone each day?

These types of questions may be difficult to answer, however, because the frequency of the behavior may vary greatly from day to day, month to month, or even season to season.

The researcher should determine exactly which aspect of the behavior is most relevant to the study and provide an appropriate time frame for interpreting the question (Question 7). For instance, the question could ask about a particular period, such as use of a phone within the last week, or the respondent can be asked to calculate an average daily time. This assumes, of course, that this time period is adequately representative for purposes of the study.

Question 7
Do you do any of the following at least once a day?

	Yes	No
Phone call on mobile phone	○	○
Access email	○	○
Access the internet	○	○

Alternatively, the question could ask for an estimate of "typical" or "usual" behaviors. This approach makes an assumption about the respondent's ability to form such an estimate. Some behaviors are much more erratic than others. For example, it may be relatively easy to estimate the number of times someone uses a computer each day, but harder to estimate typical phone use because that can vary so much.

Questions related to time should also be specific. For instance, Question 8a may be difficult to answer if it is not a consistent problem. It is better to provide a time frame for reference, as in Question 8b. Many function, pain, and health status questionnaires specify time periods such as within the last month, last week, or last 24 hours. Avoid ambiguous terms like "recently" or "often."

Question 8a
Have you had difficulty obtaining transportation to attend visits to your healthcare provider?

Question 8b
Have you had difficulty obtaining transportation to attend visits to your healthcare provider within the past month?

Sensitive Questions

Questionnaires often deal with sensitive or personal issues that can cause some discomfort on the part of the respondent. Although some people are only too willing to express personal views, others are hesitant, even when they know their responses are anonymous. Some questions may address social issues or behaviors that have negative associations, such as smoking, sexual practices, or drug use. Question 2b is an example where social issues should be addressed thoughtfully.

Questions may inquire about behaviors that respondents are not anxious to admit to, such as ignorance of facts they feel they should know, or compliance with medications or exercise programs. It may be useful to preface such questions with a statement to put them at ease so they feel okay if they fit into that category, as in Question 9.

Question 9

Many people have different levels of familiarity with newer technology and electronic communication. Which of these do you feel comfortable using?

O Mobile phone
O Computer
O Social media (like Facebook)

Sensitive questions may also be subject to recall bias. For example, respondents may be selective in their memory of risk factors for disease or disability. Respondents should be reminded in the introduction to the survey that they may refuse to answer any questions.

Personal information can also be sensitive. For example, respondents may not want to share income information, even when this is important to the research question. Asking an open-ended question for annual salary may not feel comfortable but putting responses in ranges can make this response more palatable.

■ Formatting the Survey

The format of a survey is an essential consideration, as it can easily impact a respondent's desire to fill it out. The layout should be visually appealing and language should be easy to read. The survey should begin with a short introduction that provides general instructions for answering questions. Researchers will often give the survey a title that provides an overview of its purpose.

Question Order

Content should flow so that the respondent's thought processes will follow a logical sequence, with smooth transitions from topic to topic. This allows the respondent to continue with relevant thoughts as the survey progresses and requires that questions be organized by topic.

Questions should proceed from the general to the specific. The initial questions should pique the respondent's

interest, or at least be "neutral." Sensitive questions should come later. Leaving a space for comments at the end of a survey or after specific questions can allow respondents to provide clarification of their answers.

Length of the Survey

The length of the survey should be considered. More often than not, the initial versions will be too long. Long questionnaires are less likely to maintain the respondent's attention and motivation, resulting in potentially invalid or unreliable responses or, more significantly, nonresponses. The importance of each item for the interpretation of the study should be examined, and only those questions that make direct and meaningful contributions should be retained. Best advice—keep it as short as possible.

Demographics

Typically, researchers include questions about important demographic information in a survey.

➤ The telehealth survey started with questions on gender, ethnic group, and age. These were followed by questions regarding current work status, level of education, and home status (own, rent).

Depending on the nature of the research question, other factors may be relevant such as employment setting, length of employment, marital status, and income.

Demographic information is needed to describe the characteristics of the respondents to compare the characteristics of the sample with those of the population to which the results will be generalized, and to interpret how personal characteristics are related to the participant's responses on other questions. Some researchers put demographic questions at the beginning, but many prefer to keep these less interesting questions for the end.

■ Selecting a Sample

Surveys are used to describe characteristics of a **population**, the entire group to which the results will be generalized. Most often, a smaller **sample** of the population will be asked to complete the survey as a representative group. Therefore, it is vitally important that the sample adequately represents the qualities of that population.

There are many strategies for choosing samples, with some important considerations for survey research. A **probability sample** is one that is chosen at random from a population, where every individual has the same chance of being chosen. A **nonprobability sample** is one that is not chosen at random.

Because we draw inferences from a sample, a probability sample provides the highest confidence that the sample represents all the varied characteristics and opinions of that group. Depending on the nature of the research question, this can be a vital concern when results are intended to provide strong generalization.

> ➤ In the telehealth study, participants were drawn from 32 practices from two geographical areas of the U.K., representing a wide mix of socioeconomic characteristics. The researchers randomly selected 54 patients from each practice, providing approximately 1,700 patients across both disease groups. Males and females were sampled in proportion to the number of eligible patients in each practice and the sample was stratified by age.

When generalizing the results of this study, it will be important to consider that it was performed in the U.K. with patients who participated in the National Health Service. Therefore, issues around accessibility could be influenced by the setting and applicability to other health systems may be limited.

Sampling Errors

Errors from sampling processes can impact results. **Sampling error** refers to the difference between collected data and the true scores in the population, potentially occurring when the sample is too small or not randomly drawn.

In survey research, *coverage error* occurs when all the members of a population are not included in the sampling process and, therefore, some will have no chance of being selected. This relates to the validity of lists that are obtained from which respondents will be chosen. Mailing lists can be purchased from professional associations or organizations. Published lists of schools or hospitals can usually be obtained from libraries or professional organizations. Depending on the source of lists, they may be incomplete or outdated.

> ➤ Patients in the telehealth study were identified by health records at each practice based on having been prescribed antidepressant medication or being identified as at increased risk for CVD.

Nonresponse error occurs when the people who respond to the survey are different from those who do not respond in a way that is relevant to the study. When possible, researchers try to compare demographics of respondents and nonrespondents to clarify these differences, but such data may not be available.

> ➤ Researchers in the telehealth study were able to compare the proportion of invited participants who did and did not respond to the survey by gender and location, finding no significant differences.

 Sometimes the population of interest is a defined group that will make sampling easier. For example, you may be interested in opinions of occupational therapist educators on interprofessional education. You could conceivably contact all faculty members of academic programs in the U.S. Or you may want to sample all occupational therapists who work in nursing homes within a certain community. When the population is much larger or diffuse, however, defining the sample becomes an important process to be sure you will be able to generalize your findings.

Chapter 13 includes a comprehensive discussion of various probability and nonprobability sampling methods that can be applied to survey research.

Response Rate

Response rate is the percentage of people who receive the survey who actually complete it. This is a constant threat to validity in survey research, as response rates tend to be disappointingly low. There is no consensus on what a "good" response rate is, but generally responses of 30% or more are considered high.[27,28]

> ➤ Of the 3,329 patients who were sent the telehealth questionnaire, 1,478 (44.4%) returned it. The response rate was higher for patients with CVD (50.1%) than for those with depression (38.1%). Response rates in both groups were higher in older people.

Response rates can indicate an important source of potential bias. The researcher might question why patients with CVD or older patients were more likely to respond to the telehealth survey. This differential could affect conclusions drawn from the study.

Response rates can vary by the delivery method and by the nature of the group being sampled. Research has shown that respondents are more likely to return surveys if:[29–31]

- They know and value the sponsoring organization
- The purpose and focus of the survey are clear
- The invitation to participate is personalized
- They understand why they are being asked and feel that they are a stakeholder
- The topic is important to them
- The questionnaire is clearly designed with a simple layout

Response rates can also be affected by the length of the survey, how long it takes to complete, and its complexity. With Web-based surveys, technical difficulties can interfere with return, as well as the computer literacy of the respondent. Respondents may not be comfortable sharing certain types of information online for safety purposes.

Incentives

Many researchers will use a form of incentive to inspire respondents to return a survey.[32] These are often small monetary tokens, such as gift cards. This does require a budget for the survey and can be prohibitive with a large sample. The amount really depends on the audience.

Many include this token with the initial request and mention it in a cover letter. Others will indicate that it will be available for all those who respond or that respondents will be put into a lottery, but these post-awards tend to be less effective. Estimates are variable as to whether monetary incentives do increase participation. Some data suggest that monetary incentives may produce biased differential responses by being more attractive to those with lower economic resources.[33]

Sample Size

Because response rates for surveys are generally low, sample size becomes an important consideration to adequately represent the population. Survey sample size determinations are based on three projections regarding the sample and expected responses:

- The size of the population from which respondents will be recruited
- The acceptable margin of error
- The confidence level desired, typically 95%

You are probably familiar with the concept of margin of error from political polls that always report this range, which is especially important when poll numbers are close. Most often they use a margin of ±5% or ±3%. The confidence level is based on the statistical concept of probability, which will be covered fully in Chapter 23. The most commonly used confidence level is 95%.

Determining Sample Size

Generally, as a population gets larger, a smaller proportion needs to be sampled to get a representative list. Table 11-1 shows some estimates based on ±5% and ±3% margins of error. Most importantly, these sample sizes represent the *actual number of completed surveys* that are needed, not the number of respondents originally invited to participate.

> ➤ Assuming a response rate of 60%, researchers in the telehealth study wanted approximately 960 responses for each chronic disease group, or a total of 1,920. Therefore, they needed to initially invite at least 3,200 patients.

Table 11-1   Survey Sample Size Estimates*

POPULATION SIZE	MARGIN OF ERROR	
	±5%	±3%
100	80	92
500	218	341
1,000	278	517
1,500	306	624
5,000	357	880
10,000	370	965

*Based on 95% confidence level.
Data obtained using sample size calculator from Survey Monkey.[34]

Other considerations in the determination of sample size will be addressed in Chapter 23.

Once the population exceeds 5,000, sample sizes of around 400 or 1,000 are generally sufficient for a ±5% or ±3% margin of error, respectively.[10,26] While larger samples are generally better, they do not necessarily make a sample more representative. Although these numbers probably appear quite large, the ease of contacting people may vary with the population and their availability.

Other considerations in the determination of sample size will be addressed in Chapter 23.

> 📌 You can figure out your own sample size estimates and margin of error preferences using convenient online calculators.[34,35] Actual recruitment needs are based on projected return rates. With an expected response rate of 30%, for instance, with a population of 5,000 and a ±5% margin of error, it would be necessary to send out 1,200 questionnaires to expect a return of 360 (divide 360 by 30%). With smaller populations, it may be necessary to contact the entire population to get a reasonable return.

■ Contacting Respondents

Recruitment is an important part of survey research. Because response rates are of concern, multiple contacts should be planned.[26] If possible, these communications should be personalized. The researcher needs to get buy-in to encourage respondents to take the time to fill out and return a survey.

Prior Communication

Shortly before sending out the survey, potential respondents should be contacted by mail or email to let them know they will be getting the survey. In a brief communication, they should be told the purpose of the survey, its importance, and why they are being asked to participate. It should identify the sponsor of the research. This will help to legitimize the survey.

For interviews, respondents will typically be within a local geographic area and may be recruited from agencies or clinics. Before an interview is administered, the potential respondents should be contacted to elicit their cooperation. For telephone interviews, it is appropriate to send advance notice in the mail that the phone call will be coming as a means of introduction and as a way of establishing the legitimacy of the phone call.

The Cover Letter

The questionnaire should be sent to respondents, whether by mail or electronic means, with a cover letter explaining why their response is important. Because a questionnaire can easily be tossed away, the cover letter becomes vitally important to encourage a return. The letter should include the following elements (illustrated in Figure 11-2):

1. Start with the purpose of the study. Be concise and on message. Provide brief background that will emphasize the importance of the study. This should be

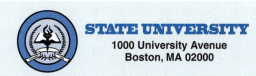

STATE UNIVERSITY
1000 University Avenue
Boston, MA 02000

June 10, 2019

Dear Mrs. Jones,

1   I am part of a research group that is trying to find the best ways to assure access to health care for older adults. Two weeks ago you received a letter from your primary care provider, introducing our research team, and letting you know that we would be contacting you regarding an important survey on the use of electronic devices and technology by older adults.

     I am writing now to ask for your help in this study. The purpose of the study is to explore whether technology can be used to contribute to your health care, and whether individuals like yourself would be comfortable with such use. Only by understanding how patients feel about different ways of communicating with providers can we learn how to be most effective in providing care.

2   We would appreciate your completing the enclosed questionnaire. Your name was selected at random from a list of patients from your health center because you gave your permission to be contacted for research purposes. Patients in this study are over 65 years old and have been diagnosed with either depression or risk for cardiovascular disease.

3   The questionnaire is completely confidential and your name will not be attached to any responses. All data will be presented in summary form only. Your health care will not be affected, whether or not you choose to participate. Your returning the questionnaire will indicate your consent to use your data for this research. This study has been approved by the Institutional Review Board at State University.

4   The questionnaire should take approximately 15 minutes to complete. We are interested in your honest opinions. If you prefer not to answer a question, please leave it blank. A stamped envelope is included for your convenience in returning the questionnaire. We would appreciate your returning the completed form within the next two weeks, by June 24, 2019.

5   If you have any questions or comments about this study, please feel free to contact me by mail at the address on the letterhead, or by phone or email at the bottom of this letter.

6,7   Thank you in advance for your cooperation with this important effort. Although there is no direct compensation for your participation, your answers will make a significant contribution to our understanding of contemporary issues that affect all of us involved in health care.

8   If you would like a summary of our findings, please fill in your name and address on the enclosed request form, and we will be happy to forward our findings to you when the study is completed.

9   Sincerely,

Jane Smith

Jane Smith, PhD
Professor and Director of Health Service Research at State University
Phone: (800) 555-9000, Email: jsmith@xsu.edu

Figure 11–2 Sample cover letter. Numbers in the left margin match the list of elements in the text.

done in a way that appeals to the participant and presents no bias in its impact. If the research is sponsored by an agency or is a student project, this information should be included.

2. Indicate why the respondent has been chosen for the survey.

3. Assure the respondents that answers will be confidential and, if appropriate, that they will remain anonymous. Encourage them to be honest in their answers and assure them that they can refuse to answer any questions that make them uncomfortable.

4. Some electronic survey platforms allow for a respondent to enter a personal identification number (PIN) so that their results can be tied to other information or a follow-up survey. If this is an important part of the study, it should be explained in the cover letter as a way of maintaining anonymity.

5. Give instructions for completing the survey, including how long it should take to fill out. Provide a deadline date with instructions for sending back the survey. It is reasonable to give 2 to 3 weeks for a response. A shorter time is an imposition, and longer may result in the questionnaire being put aside. Paper surveys should always include a stamped self-addressed envelope. Electronic surveys, of course, are automatically "returned" once submitted online.

6. Provide contact information if they have any questions.

7. Thank respondents for their cooperation.

8. If you are providing incentives, indicate what they are and how they will be offered.

9. Offer an opportunity for them to receive a summary of the report.

10. Sign the letter, including your name, degrees, and affiliation. If there are several investigators, it is appropriate to include all signatures. Use real signatures rather than fancy font.

The cover letter should be concise. If the research is being conducted as part of a professional activity, the organizational letterhead should be used. If possible, the letter should be personally addressed to each individual respondent. This is easily accomplished through mail merge programs.

Follow-Up Communication

Although the majority of surveys will be returned within the first 2 weeks, a reasonable improvement can usually be obtained through follow-up.

- **Follow-up:** A week or two after sending the questionnaire, a postcard or email can be sent out to thank respondents for their response or, if they have not yet returned the survey, to ask them to respond soon. Some people may have just forgotten about it.

- **Replacement:** A replacement questionnaire or the link can be resent to nonrespondents 2 to 4 weeks later, encouraging them to respond and emphasizing the importance of their response to the success of your study.

- **Final contact:** A final contact may be made by phone or email if needed to bolster the return rate.

■ Analysis of Questionnaire Data

The first step in the analysis of data is to collate responses and enter them into a computer. Each item on the survey is a data point and must be given a variable name, often an item number.

The researcher must sort through each questionnaire as it is returned, or through all responses from an interview, to determine if responses are valid.

In many instances, the respondent will have incorrectly filled out the survey and that respondent may have to be eliminated from the analysis. The researcher must keep track of all unusable questionnaires to report this percentage in the final report. Some questions may have to be eliminated from individual questionnaires because they were answered incorrectly, such as putting two answers in for a question that asked for a single response. There may be instances where a question is not answered correctly across most respondents and the question may be eliminated from the study.

Coding

Analyzing survey data requires summarizing responses. This in turn requires a form of coding, which allows counting how many respondents answered a certain way.

Multiple Choice Responses

Responses to closed-ended questions are given numeric codes that provide labels for data entry. For instance, sex can be coded 0 = male, 1 = female. We could code hospital size as 1 = less than 50 beds, 2 = 50 to 100 beds, and 3 = over 100 beds. These codes are entered into the computer to identify responses. Using codes, the researcher can easily obtain frequency counts and percentages for each question to determine how many participants checked each response.

When responses allow for more than one choice ("check all that apply"), analysis requires that each item in the list be coded as checked or unchecked. Coding does not allow for multiple answers to a single item. For example, referring back to Question 3a, each choice option would be considered an item in the final analysis. Question 3b provides an alternative format that makes this type of question easier to code.

> Codes should be determined at the time the survey is written so that there is no confusion later about how to account for each response. See codes imbedded in the telehealth survey in the *Chapter 11 Supplement.*

Open-Ended Responses

Coding open-ended responses is a bit more challenging. One approach is to use qualitative analysis to describe responses (see Chapter 21). If a more concise summary is desired, the researcher must sort through responses to identify themes and assign codes to reflect these themes. This requires interpretation of the answer to determine similar responses. The challenge comes when individual respondents provide unique answers, which must often be coded as "Other."

Summarizing Survey Data

The analysis of survey data may take many forms. Most often, descriptive statistics are used to summarize responses (see Chapter 22). When quantitative data such as age are collected, the researcher will usually present averages. With categorical data, the researcher reports the frequency of responses to specific questions. These frequencies are typically converted to a percentage of the total sample. For example, a researcher might report that 30% of the sample was male and 70% was female, or in a question about opinions, that 31% strongly agree, 20% agree, 5% disagree, and so on. Descriptive data are usually presented in tabular or graphic form. Percentages should always be accompanied by reference to the total sample size so that the reader can determine the actual number of responses in each category. Percentages are usually more meaningful than actual frequencies because sample sizes may differ greatly among studies.

Looking for Significant Associations

Another common approach to data analysis involves the description of relationships between two or more sets of responses (see Focus on Evidence 11-1). For instance, the telehealth survey asked questions about interest in various technologies and compared them across the two chronic disease groups.

Cross-tabulations are often used to analyze the relationship between two categorical variables. For instance, we can look at the number of males and females who indicate they do or do not use particular devices. Statistical tests can then be used to examine this association to determine if there is a significant relationship between gender and device use (see Chapter 28). Other statistical analyses can also be used to compare group scores or to establish predictive relationships. Correlational and regression statistics are often used for this purpose (see Chapters 29 and 30).

Missing Data

A common problem in surveys is handling of missing data, when respondents leave questions blank. It may be difficult to know why they have refused to answer. It could be because they didn't understand the question, their preferred choice was not there, they found the question offensive, they didn't know the answer—or they just missed it. The reason for leaving it blank, however, can be important and can create bias in the results. Providing a response choice of "Don't Know" or "I prefer not to answer" may allow some reasons to be clarified. For interviews, a code can be used to indicate a participant's refusal to answer a question.

When a response is not valid, the researcher will also record the response as "missing," but can code it to reflect the fact that it was an invalid answer. Chapter 15 includes discussion of strategies for handling missing data.

■ Ethics of Survey Administration

Like all forms of research, studies that involve interviews or questionnaires must go through a formal process of review and approval by an Institutional Review Board (IRB). Even though there may not be any direct physical risk, researchers must be able to demonstrate the protection of subjects from psychological or emotional risk or invasion of privacy. Researchers should also be vigilant about securing the confidentiality of data, even if surveys are de-identified (see Chapter 7).

The IRB will want assurances that all relevant individuals have been notified and are in support of the project. This may include healthcare providers, the rest of the research team, and administrators. Surveys will often receive expedited reviews.

Informed Consent

Consent for mail or electronic questionnaires is implied by the return of the questionnaire. The cover letter provides the information needed, serving the function of an

Focus on Evidence 11–1
Presenting Lots of Information

In their study of telehealth, Edwards et al[18] used a variety of presentations for results to look at interest in using phone-based, email/internet-based, and social media-based telehealth.

In a table, demographics of age, sex, and location were presented for responders and nonresponders to show differences for patients with CVD risk and those with depression. They were able to show that there were no significant differences between those who returned the questionnaire and those who did not. This provided confidence that the sample was not biased.

The researchers looked at the proportion of respondents interested in individual telehealth technologies by patient group and provided a bar chart to show these relationships, as shown. The responses were dichotomized to reflect some versus no interest. The data showed that patients with depression were more interested than those with CVD risk in most forms of technology. Landlines were clearly preferred, followed by finding information on the internet, with little interest in social media.

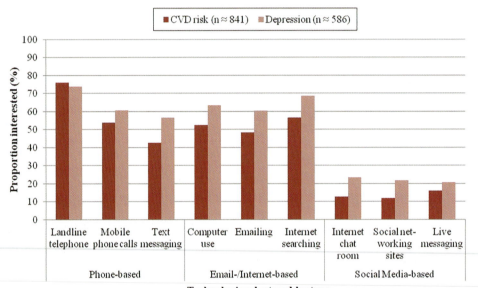

To address which factors influenced interest in telehealth, they used regression models to determine various relationships (see Chapter 30). They found several important outcomes:

- Those who had greater confidence in using technology showed more interest in telehealth.
- For patients with depression only, greater difficulties with getting convenient care were related to more interest in phone and internet technologies.
- Both groups showed greater interest if they had satisfactory experiences in the past using such technologies.
- Health needs, access difficulties, technology availability, and sociodemographic factors did not consistently have an effect on interest in telehealth across either patient group. Respondents with good or poor health, with more or less difficulty accessing care, and older and younger patients had the similar levels of interest. Interestingly, availability of technology was high, but this also did not relate to interest in telehealth.

These findings provide important information for policy makers and health professionals seeking to expand health services using different formats.

Source: Edwards L, Thomas C, Gregory A, et al. Are people with chronic disease interested in using telehealth? A cross-sectional postal survey. *J Med Internet Res* 2014;16(5):e123, Figure 2 (http://jmir.org/). Used under Creative Commons license (BY/2.0) (http://creativecommons.org/licenses/by/2.0/).

informed consent form (see Fig. 11-2). Individuals who participate in face-to-face interviews can be given an informed consent form to sign in the presence of the interviewer. For telephone interviews, the researcher is obliged to give respondents full information at the beginning of the call so that they can decide whether they want to continue with the interview. Consent to participate is obtained verbally up front in the conversation, letting respondents know that they can refuse to continue.

COMMENTARY

Surveys show that the #1 fear of Americans is public speaking. #2 is death. That means that at a funeral, the average American would rather be in the casket than doing the eulogy.

—Jerry Seinfeld (1954–)

American comedian

The term "survey research" is often interpreted as a research design, but it is more accurate to think of surveys as a form of data collection. Like any other data collection method, survey development requires an understanding of theory, content and construct validity, and basic principles of measurement. Surveys must be used for appropriate purposes and analyzed to ascribe valid meaning to results.

Because of the nature of clinical variables, and the emphasis on patient perceptions and values in evidence-based practice, surveys are an important methodology, providing information that cannot be ascertained through observational techniques. Many questionnaires have been developed as instruments for assessing constructs that are relevant to patient care. Such instruments are applicable to explanatory, exploratory, and descriptive research designs.

Those interested in pursuing the survey approach are encouraged to consult researchers who have had experience with questionnaires, as well as several informative texts listed at the end of this chapter.[26,36–38]

REFERENCES

1. Jenkinson C, Coulter A, Bruster S, Richards N, Chandola T. Patients' experiences and satisfaction with health care: results of a questionnaire study of specific aspects of care. *Qual Saf Health Care* 2002;11(4):335–339.
2. Calancie B, Molano MR, Broton JG. Epidemiology and demography of acute spinal cord injury in a large urban setting. *J Spinal Cord Med* 2005;28(2):92–96.
3. Freburger JK, Konrad TR. The use of federal and state databases to conduct health services research related to physical and occupational therapy. *Arch Phys Med Rehabil* 2002;83(6): 837-845.
4. Centers for Disease Control and Prevention (CDC). National Health Interview Survey: National Center for Health Statistics. Available at https://www.cdc.gov/nchs/nhis/data-questionnaires-documentation.htm. Accessed June 30, 2017.
5. National Center for Health Statistics: National Nursing Home Survey. Survey methodology, documentation, and data files survey. Available at https://www.cdc.gov/nchs/nnhs/nnhs_questionnaires.htm. Accessed February 7, 2018.
6. van Zon A, Smulders YE, Stegeman I, Ramakers GG, Kraaijenga VJ, Koenraads SP, Zanten GA, Rinia AB, et al. Stable benefits of bilateral over unilateral cochlear implantation after two years: A randomized controlled trial. *Laryngoscope* 2017;127(5):1161–1668.
7. Owen-Smith AA, Smith DH, Rand CS, Tom JO, Laws R, Waterbury A, et al. Difference in effectiveness of medication adherence intervention by health literacy level. *Perm J* 2016; 20(3):38–44.
8. Adjemian MK, Volpe RJ, Adjemian J. Relationships between diet, alcohol preference, and heart disease and type 2 diabetes among Americans. *PLoS One* 2015;10(5):e0124351.
9. Mandal A, Eaden J, Mayberry MK, Mayberry JF. Questionnaire surveys in medical research. *J Eval Clin Pract* 2000;6(4): 395–403.
10. Leedy PD, Ormrod JE. *Practical Research: Planning and Design.* Upper Saddle River, NJ: Prentice Hall, 2001.
11. Carr EC, Worth A. The use of the telephone interview for research. *J Res Nursing* 2001;6(1):511–524.
12. Wu V, Abo-Sido N, Espinola JA, Tierney CN, Tedesco KT, Sullivan AF, et al. Predictors of successful telephone follow-up in a multicenter study of infants with severe bronchiolitis. *Ann Epidemiol* 2017;27(7):454–458.e1.
13. Insights Association: Mixed-Mode Surveys. May 24, 2016. Available at http://www.insightsassociation.org/issues-policies/best-practice/mixed-mode-surveys. Accessed July 3, 2017.
14. Shumway-Cook A, Patla A, Stewart AL, Ferrucci L, Ciol MA, Guralnik JM. Assessing environmentally determined mobility disability: self-report versus observed community mobility. *J Am Geriatr Soc* 2005;53(4):700–704.
15. Stepan JG, London DA, Boyer MI, Calfee RP. Accuracy of patient recall of hand and elbow disability on the QuickDASH questionnaire over a two-year period. *J Bone Joint Surg Am* 2013;95(22):e176.
16. Brusco NK, Watts JJ. Empirical evidence of recall bias for primary health care visits. *BMC Health Serv Res* 2015;15:381.
17. Reneman MF, Jorritsma W, Schellekens JM, Goeken LN. Concurrent validity of questionnaire and performance-based disability measurements in patients with chronic nonspecific low back pain. *J Occup Rehabil* 2002;12(3):119–129.
18. Edwards L, Thomas C, Gregory A, Yardley L, O'Cathain A, Montgomery AA, et al. Are people with chronic diseases interested in using telehealth? A cross-sectional postal survey. *J Med Internet Res* 2014;16(5):e123.
19. McDowell I. *Measuring Health: A Guide to Rating Scales and Questionnaires.* 3 ed. New York: Oxford University Press, 2006.
20. Beck AT, Steer RA, Carbin MG. Psychometric properties of the Beck Depression Inventory: Twenty-five years of evaluation. *Clin Psychol Rev* 1988;8(1):77–100.

21. Creavin ST, Wisniewski S, Noel-Storr AH, Trevelyan CM, Hampton T, Rayment D, et al. Mini-Mental State Examination (MMSE) for the detection of dementia in clinically unevaluated people aged 65 and over in community and primary care populations. *Cochrane Database Syst Rev* 2016(1):Cd011145.

22. Ware J Jr, Kosinski M, Keller SD. A 12-Item Short-Form Health Survey: construction of scales and preliminary tests of reliability and validity. *Med Care* 1996;34(3):220–233.

23. National Survey of Student Engagement: Gender identify and sexual orientation: survey challenges and lessons learned. Available at http://nsse.indiana.edu/pdf/presentations/2016/AIR_2016_Gender_ID_handout.pdf. Accessed February 9, 2018.

24. Quinn TJ, Langhorne P, Stott DJ. Barthel index for stroke trials: development, properties, and application. *Stroke* 2011; 42(4):1146–1151.

25. Brown AW, Therneau TM, Schultz BA, Niewczyk PM, Granger CV. Measure of functional independence dominates discharge outcome prediction after inpatient rehabilitation for stroke. *Stroke* 2015;46(4):1038–1044.

26. Dillman DA, Smyth JD, Christian LM. *Internet, Phone, Mail, and Mixed-Mode Surveys: The Tailored Design Method*. 3 ed. Hoboken, NJ: John Wiley & Sons, 2014.

27. Survey Monkey: Survey sample size. Available at https://www.surveymonkey.com/mp/sample-size/. Accessed July 1, 2017.

28. Burgess TF: A general introduction to the design of questionnaires for survey research. University of Leeds, May, 2001. Available at http://iss.leeds.ac.uk/downloads/top2.pdf. Accessed June 29, 2017.

29. Fan W, Yan Z. Factors affecting response rates of the web survey: a systematic review. *Computers Hum Behav* 2010;26: 132–139.

30. Boynton PM, Greenhalgh T. Selecting, designing, and developing your questionnaire. *BMJ* 2004;328(7451):1312–1315.

31. Shih TH, Fan X. Comparing response rates from web and mail surveys: a meta-analysis. *Field Methods* 2008;20:249–271.

32. Millar MM, Dillman DA. Improving response to web and mixed mode surveys. *Public Opin Q* 2011;75(2):249–269.

33. Galea S, Tracy M. Participation rates in epidemiologic studies. *Ann Epidemiol* 2007;17(9):643–653.

34. Survey Monkey: Sample Size Calculator. Available at https://www.surveymonkey.com/mp/sample-size-calculator/. Accessed June 30, 2017.

35. CheckMarket: Sample Size Calculator. Available at https://www.checkmarket.com/sample-size-calculator/. Accessed June 30, 2017.

36. Oppenheim AN. *Questionnaire Design, Interviewing and Attitude Measurement*. 2 ed. London: Bloomsbury Academic, 2000.

37. Converse JM, Presser S. *Survey Questions: Handcrafting the Standardized Questionnaire*. Thousand Oaks, CA: Sage, 1986.

38. Saris WE, Gallhofer IN. *Design, Evaluation, and Analysis of Questionnaires for Survey Research*. 2 ed. Hoboken, NJ: John Wiley & Sons, 2014.

Understanding Health Measurement Scales

—with Marianne Beninato

The foundational measurement concepts described in preceding chapters create a context for understanding how we can use evidence to interpret scores from appropriate measurement tools. Because many aspects of health reflect intangible constructs, they require data that must be converted to a scale that will indicate "how much" of a health factor is present in an individual.

The purpose of this chapter is to describe different types of scales used in questionnaires to assess health. These may be self-report inventories or performance-based instruments. This discussion will focus on validity of four types of scales, including summative, visual analog, and cumulative scales, and the Rasch measurement model. Whether you are trying to use or modify established instruments or construct a new tool, an understanding of scale properties is essential for interpretation of scores and application to clinical decision-making.

■ Understanding the Construct

The first essential step in choosing or developing a health scale is understanding the construct being measured. The items in a scale must reflect the underlying latent trait and the dimensions that define it (see Chapter 10). Scales require substantial measurement scrutiny to establish their reliability and validity, as we strive to confirm utility with different populations and under different clinical conditions.

Theoretical Foundations

An important characteristic of a scale's validity is its focus on a common dimension of the trait being measured. This requires a clear theoretical foundation, including behavioral expectations when the trait is present to different degrees, and an understanding of distinct components of the construct.

Consider the study of pain, which can be manifested in several dimensions, including differences between acute and chronic pain, and potential biopsychosocial impacts related to symptoms, how it affects movement, or its impact on quality of life.[1] For example, the McGill Pain Questionnaire incorporates pain ratings as well qualitative descriptors, based on Melzack's theory of pain reflecting sensory, affective, and evaluative dimensions of pain.[2] It focuses on various aspects of pain, such as intensity, type of pain, and duration. In contrast, the Roland Morris Disability Questionnaire (RMDQ) was designed to assess physical disability due to low back pain.[3] Therefore, the framework for the RMDQ is based on how back pain influences daily life, not on a description of the pain itself.

Measuring Health

For many clinical variables, a single indicator, such as blood pressure or hematocrit, can provide relevant information regarding a specific aspect of health. These tests are typically interpreted with reference to a criterion that defines a normal range. These values play an important role in identifying disease or indicating appropriate treatment.

As the concept of health has broadened, however, single indicators are not sufficient to reflect the dimensions of important clinical traits. Assessing health requires the use of subjective measures that involve judgment on the part of a patient, caregiver, clinician, or researcher.[4] These judgments may reflect different perceptions, which will influence which indicators are appropriate. Therefore, to measure variables such as depression, function, or balance, it is necessary to develop a set of items that address multiple aspects of health. For function, for example, questions should address physical, social, and emotional considerations as they affect daily activities.

Health Scales

A **scale** is an ordered system based on a series of questions or items, resulting in a score that represents the degree to which a respondent possesses a particular attitude, value, or characteristic. The items used will usually be in the same format so that responses can be summed. The purpose of a scale is to distinguish among people who demonstrate different intensities of the characteristic and to document change in individuals over time.

Typically designed as questionnaires, health scales are often composed of self-report items that probe the latent trait being studied according to the individual's own perceptions. Scales may also include tasks that are observed by another. For example, instruments like the Beck Depression Inventory ask respondents to indicate the intensity of emotional, behavioral, and somatic symptoms they are experiencing related to depression.[5] Tests of function, such as the Barthel Index[6] or Functional Independence Measure (FIM),[7] rely on a clinician's judgment regarding a patient's performance in completing basic activities of daily living (ADLs). To characterize balance, clinicians usually observe patients performing several tasks using tests such as the Berg Balance Scale (BBS).[8]

Creating a scale requires establishing a scoring process that will yield a total score. Therefore, numbers have to be assigned to subjective judgments on a scale that can indicate high or low levels of the variable.[4] Because most health scales use ordinal response categories, we must be cognizant of the limitations in interpretation of ordinal scores (see Chapter 8).

Unidemensionality

For a scale to be meaningful, it should be unidimensional, representing a singular overall construct. When different dimensions exist, subscales can be created for each one. Content validity should be evaluated to establish that items represent the full scope of the construct. Statistical techniques, such as factor analysis, are useful to determine the construct validity, indicating how items cluster into different components (see Chapter 31).

For instance, the Short Form-36 (SF-36) health status questionnaire is based on eight subscales, including vitality, physical functioning, bodily pain, general health perceptions, physical role functioning, emotional role functioning, social role functioning, and mental health.[9] Each of these represent a different element of health that is assessed with different items. Users must be aware of the differences among subscales, understanding why a total score would be uninterpretable.

Short Forms

Health questionnaires are often lengthy and short forms have been developed for many scales. For example, the original 116-item Medical Outcomes Study was first reduced to the SF-36 health questionnaire[9] and was then condensed to the SF-12[10] and the SF-8.[11] The numbers in these scale names refer to the number of items in the scale. Because fewer representative items are used in the short form, the subscales have been truncated to two summary subscales of physical and mental health functioning.

Validation of these short forms follows full validation of the original scale. Typically, researchers use factor analysis and other construct validity approaches to demonstrate that the shorter version can generate a meaningful score that correlates with the longer scale and is consistent with the target construct. The obvious benefit of a short form test is efficiency of time and effort.

The Target Population

Scales may be generic or they may be geared toward specific patient groups, age ranges, or care settings. Therefore, a target population must be specified. For instance, the SF-36 is considered a generic measure of health status,[12] whereas the Arthritis Impact Measurement Scale (AIMS),[13] the Functional Living Index-Cancer,[14] and the Spinal Cord Injury–Quality of Life measurement system[15] were all created to address issues specific to those conditions. The Pediatric Quality of Life Inventory[16] and the Older Peoples Quality of Life Questionnaire[17] focus on those age-related populations, and the COOP Charts are specifically designed to measure quality of life in primary care settings.[18]

Cultural validity of an instrument also requires consideration of how language and other societal norms vary across populations. Many instruments have been validated in different languages and countries, often requiring nuanced changes in questions or wording.

The words used to reflect ordered grades in a scale must have a common meaning for respondents. In an interesting study of nine world regions, Szabo[19] found that "quite often" in England was equivalent to "often" in India, "from time to time" in Zambia, "sometimes" in Melbourne and Seattle, "now and then" in the Netherlands, and "usually" in Zagreb.

■ Summative Scales

A **summative scale** is one that presents a total score by adding values across a set of items.

Quantifying Health

Summative scales include several items scored on an ordinal scale. These items represent a unidimensional construct, and therefore the sum of the item scores is intended to indicate the "amount" of the latent trait that is present in an individual. By summing the items, this type of scale is based on an assumption that all items contribute equally to the total and does not account for items that are more or less difficult.

> ➤ **CASE IN POINT #1**
> The Functional Gait Assessment (FGA) is a 10-item scale that assesses a person's stability and balance while performing 10 walking tasks of differing difficulty.[20] It has been used with community-dwelling elderly individuals, as well as patients who have had a stroke, Parkinson disease (PD), and vestibular disorders. Clinicians observe performance and score each item from 0 to 3, with lower scores indicating greater impairment.

This type of ordinal scoring is typical of health scales, with numerals assigned to label ordinal categories. Although these numbers are arbitrary labels and do not represent actual quantity, they must represent increasing or decreasing function in a logical way for a summary score to be interpretable.

➤ The items on the FGA require the patient to walk a distance of 6 meters on a level surface under different conditions. Each item is scored as:

3 = *Normal*
2 = *Mild impairment*
1 = *Moderate impairment*
0 = *Severe impairment*
    Detailed definitions are provided for each grade.[20]

Even though these levels are operationally defined for each task, we are not able to determine if intervals are equal between steps. For example, we cannot assume that the threshold to move from *normal* to *mild impairment* is the same as the threshold from *moderate* to *severe impairment* within any one item. This pattern of thresholds may differ within an item or from item to item. This has important implications for analysis, especially when statistics such as means are generated for group data. For instance, we cannot consider the average of *moderate* and *mild* to be "mild-and-a-half," regardless of what integers have been used to represent each grade.[21]

We also do not know if two individuals with the same score of *mild impairment* will look exactly alike. We do know that *moderate impairment* is worse than *mild impairment*, but we do not know by "how much." We cannot, therefore, establish the linearity of the scale. Because we do not know if intervals across ordinal grades are consistent, a summative score presents a challenge for analysis. This challenge can be addressed using Rasch analysis, to be discussed later in this chapter.

> See the *Chapter 12 Supplement* for a link to the full Functional Gait Assessment, with descriptions of grading criteria for each item.

Putting Questions in Context

The items included in a health scale will place the underlying construct in a behavioral context. For example, an instrument that evaluates ADLs according to an individual's perception of the *difficulty* of performing given tasks will produce a measurement that is interpreted differently than one that focuses on the level of *pain* associated with specific tasks. For tests of function, questions may relate to observations of the *time* needed to perform, the amount of *assistance* required, or the *quality* of performance of varied tasks.

> ➤ The response categories in the FGA are based on the degree of impairment in performing the tasks, such as needing an assistive device, reducing speed, or making adjustments from normal gait patterns.

Questions may draw a distinction between what a person actually does versus his *capacity* (see Chapter 1), such as the difference between, "I do not shop for groceries" and, "I cannot shop for groceries."

Cut-off Scores

When scales are used as screening tools, a cut-off score can be used to demarcate a positive or negative test. Cut-off scores are determined using statistical procedures that examine how well varied scores predict the true positive and true negative outcomes (see Chapter 33).

➤ Using the Timed "Up & Go" (TUG) as the reference standard, an FGA score of ≤22 correctly identified 91% of those considered at risk for falls (true positives) and 87% of those who were not at risk (true negatives).[20] Based on this score, those with a score of ≤22 were 6 times more likely to be classified as having an increased risk of falling than those who scored >22.

Likert Scales

A commonly used format for summative scales is the **Likert scale**, in which individuals choose among answer options that range from one extreme to another to reflect attitudes, beliefs, perceptions, or values. Likert scales typically include five categories, such as: strongly disagree (SD), disagree (D), neutral (N), agree (A), and strongly agree (SA).[22] Likert scales can be used to assess a wide variety of traits, as shown in Figure 12-1.[23]

⊘ FUN FACT
The name Likert is widely mispronounced as "*lie-kert.*" The scale is named for Rensis Likert (1903–1981), an American psychologist who developed the five-point scale—but most people don't know that he pronounced his name "*lick'-ert.*" Spread the word!

Categories

Many modifications to Likert scales have been used, sometimes extending to seven categories (including "somewhat disagree" and "somewhat agree"). There is no consensus regarding the number of response categories that should be used, although data suggest a smaller number of categories will yield better reliability.[24,25] Using more categories does not necessarily translate into more information if respondents are unable to make fine distinctions.

➤ CASE IN POINT #2
The *Multidimensional Health Locus of Control (MHLC) Scale* was developed to assess an individual's beliefs about the source of reinforcements for health-related behaviors.[26] The MHLC is composed of three subscales, indicating if the individual believes controlling health is primarily *internal*, a matter of *chance*, or under the control of *powerful others*. The scale includes 18 statements, 6 in each subscale. The individual is asked to indicate level of agreement with each of the statements.

Some scales eliminate the neutral choice with an even number of categories, although the most common approach allows for an odd number of choices. Likert[22] argued that if we believe the attribute being measured exists on a bipolar continuum, we should offer a midpoint choice. When a "neutral" choice is not given, the scale presents a "forced choice," requiring that the respondent commit to agree or disagree.

➤ The MHLC scale uses six categories, as shown in Figure 12-2, ranging from 1 for "Strongly Disagree" to 6 for "Strongly Agree." The developers of the scale chose an even rather than an odd number of response alternatives because they wanted to "force" subjects to agree or disagree with each item.[27]

Subscales

Subscales are created when unique dimensions form a construct. For instance, in the process of defining health

	1	2	3	4	5
Agreement	Strongly Disagree	Disagree	Neither Agree nor Disagree	Agree	Strongly Agree
Difficulty	Very Difficult	Difficult	Neutral	Easy	Very Easy
Frequency	Never	Rarely	Sometimes	Often	Always
Importance	Not at all Important	Low Importance	Neutral	Important	Very Important
Likelihood	Extremely Unlikely	Unlikely	Equally Likely as Unlikely	Likely	Extremely Likely
Satisfaction	Very Dissatisfied	Dissatisfied	Unsure	Satisfied	Very Satisfied

Figure 12–1 Variety of Likert scales for different contexts.

Form A

Instructions: Each item below is a belief statement about your medical condition with which you may agree or disagree. Beside each statement is a scale which ranges from strongly disagree (1) to strongly agree (6). For each item we would like you to circle the number that represents the extent to which you agree or disagree with that statement. The more you agree with a statement, the higher will be the number you circle. The more you disagree with a statement, the lower will be the number you circle. Please make sure that you answer **EVERY ITEM** and that you circle **ONLY ONE** number per item. This is a measure of your personal beliefs; obviously, there are no right or wrong answers.

1 = STRONGLY DISAGREE (**SD**)   4 = SLIGHTLY AGREE (**A**)
2 = MODERATELY DISAGREE (**MD**)   5 = MODERATELY AGREE (**MA**)
3 = SLIGHTLY DISAGREE (**D**)   6 = STRONGLY AGREE (**SA**)

	No. Question	SD	MD	D	A	MA	SA
I	1. If I get sick, it is my own behavior that determines how soon I get well again.	1	2	3	4	5	6
C	2. No matter what I do, if I am going to get sick, I will get sick.	1	2	3	4	5	6
P	3. Having regular contact with my physician is the best way for me to avoid illness.	1	2	3	4	5	6
C	4. Most things that affect my health happen to me by accident.	1	2	3	4	5	6
P	5. Whenever I don't feel well, I should consult a medically trained professional.	1	2	3	4	5	6
I	6. I am in control of my health.	1	2	3	4	5	6
P	7. My family has a lot to do with my becoming sick or staying healthy.	1	2	3	4	5	6
I	8. When I get sick, I am to blame.	1	2	3	4	5	6
C	9. Luck plays a big part in determining how soon I will recover from an illness.	1	2	3	4	5	6
P	10. Health professionals control my health.	1	2	3	4	5	6
C	11. My good health is largely a matter of good fortune.	1	2	3	4	5	6
I	12. The main thing that affects my health is what I myself do.	1	2	3	4	5	6
I	13. If I take care of myself, I can avoid illness.	1	2	3	4	5	6
P	14. When I recover from an illness, it's usually because other people (like doctors, nurses, family, friends) have been taking good care of me.	1	2	3	4	5	6
C	15. No matter what I do, I am likely to get sick.	1	2	3	4	5	6
C	16. If it's meant to be, I will stay healthy.	1	2	3	4	5	6
I	17. If I take the right actions, I can stay healthy.	1	2	3	4	5	6
P	18. Regarding my health, I can only do what my doctor tells me to do.	1	2	3	4	5	6

Figure 12–2 The Multidimensional Health Locus of Control Scale (Form A), illustrating a six-point Likert scale. Subscales are shown on the left: I = Internal, C = Chance, P = Powerful others. (These codes are not included when the test is administered.) Adapted from Wallston KA. Multidimensional Health Locus of Control Scales. Available at https://nursing.vanderbilt.edu/projects/wallstonk/. Accessed September 16, 2018.

locus of control, three dimensions were identified, each one represented by its own total score.

▶ The three MHLC subscales of "internal," "chance," and "powerful others" each result in a total from 6 to 36. The items are interspersed when presenting the scale to prevent bias, but scoring requires reorganizing and summing the items within each subscale. Studies have demonstrated good convergent and divergent validity to support these dimensions.[26]

Constructing a Likert Scale

Constructing a Likert scale requires more than just listing a group of statements. A large pool of items should be developed that reflect an equal number of both favorable and unfavorable attitudes. It is generally not necessary to include items that are intended to elicit neutral responses because these will not help to distinguish respondents.

A Likert scale should be validated by performing item analyses that will indicate which items are truly discriminating between those with positive and negative attitudes. These items are then retained as the final version of the scale and others are eliminated. The basis of the item analysis is that there should be correlation between an individual's total score and each item response (see Chapter 32). Those who score highest should also agree with positively worded statements and those who obtain the lowest total scores should disagree. Those items that generate agreement from both those with high and low scores are probably irrelevant to the characteristic being studied and should be omitted.

Many of the principles of survey design described in Chapter 11 will also apply to the design of a health status questionnaire, such as organization, wording, clarity, and so on. However, as opposed to a descriptive survey, the construction of a scale that is intended to generate a total score that reflects a health trait must establish its construct validity to support its psychometric properties.

Alternative Forms

Depending on the nature of a scale, alternative forms may be developed to prevent bias from those who take the inventory on more than one occasion.

> The MHLC scale has three forms. Forms A and B contain items on the same three subscales, but with slightly different wording and in different order (the items in Figure 12-1 are from Form A). Form C is designed to be condition specific and can be used in place of Form A/B when studying people with an existing health/medical condition. Form C also has 18 items, but the "Powerful Others" subscale is further divided to consider doctors and other people separately.[28]

Forms A and B have been shown to be comparable using a split-half reliability test (see Chapter 9).[29] The development of Form C was based on a different conceptualization of health perceptions when one has a health condition, as opposed to when one is currently healthy.[28]

 See the *Chapter 12 Supplement* for full versions of Forms A, B, and C of the MHLC scale.

■ Visual Analog Scale

A **visual analog scale (VAS)** is one of the simplest methods to assess the intensity or magnitude of a subjective perception. A line is drawn, usually fixed at 100 mm in length, with word anchors on either end that represent extremes of the characteristic being measured. The left anchor represents the absence of the trait, such as "no pain," and the right anchor represents the most extreme condition, such as the "worst pain imaginable."

Intermediate points along the line are not defined. Respondents are asked to place a mark along the line corresponding to their perceived level for that characteristic (see Fig. 12-3). The VAS is scored by measuring the distance of the mark, usually in millimeters, from the left-hand anchor. The higher the score, the more severe the condition.

The VAS is considered an easy and quick self-report measure that can be applied in any setting. Although it has been used most extensively to measure pain, it has also been used to assess a variety of other characteristics (see Table 12-1).[30] The VAS can be used to evaluate a variable at a given point in time, or it can be used before and after intervention to reflect degree of change over time.

Constructing the VAS

Creating a VAS requires that the trait being measured is well understood in a single dimension (see Focus on Evidence 12-1). Pain, for example, can be evaluated in terms of its intensity, duration, or impact on quality of life. Each VAS must refer to only one dimension so that the individual completing the scale understands the nature of the perception that is being assessed. This definition will also provide guidance for the anchors of the VAS. When administering the VAS, the patient should be provided clear instructions about how to mark the line and what the anchors mean. A time frame should be included, such as, "your perception of pain right now" or, "pain over the past week."

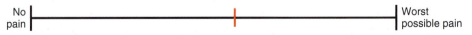

Figure 12–3 Visual analogue pain scale, showing a patient's mark (in red).

Table 12-1 Examples of VAS Anchors Used for Different Traits

TRAIT	LEFT ANCHOR		RIGHT ANCHOR
Pain[39]	No pain	I————————I	Worse pain imaginable
Stress[40]	Not at all stressed	I————————I	Extremely stressed
Anxiety[41]	Not anxious at all	I————————I	Extremely anxious
Fear of falling[34]	No fear of falling	I————————I	Extreme fear of falling
Disability[36]	No disability	I————————I	Very severe disability
Fatigue[42]	No fatigue	I————————I	Worst possible fatigue
Health-related quality of life[43,44]	Best imaginable health	I————————I	Worst imaginable health
Dyspnea[45]	Not breathless at all	I————————I	Most breathless I have ever been
Burden of care[46]	Giving care is very easy	I————————I	Giving care is very difficult
Readiness to change behavior[42,47]	Not at all	I————————I	Very much

Focus on Evidence 12–1
It's Not Really That Simple

The VAS is widely used to reflect many different types of subjective assessments because of its great convenience and apparent simplicity. Appropriately, reliability and validity of the VAS have been the subject of substantial research, which has generally found strong measurement properties for this scale.[31-35] However, while it may seem like a straightforward measure, we should be vigilant in deciding when to use it. Because of its unidimensional approach, the VAS may be limited in its use to evaluate complex clinical phenomena.

To illustrate this caveat, Boonstra et al[36] conducted a study to determine the validity of a VAS to measure disability in patients with chronic musculoskeletal pain. Their aim was to determine if a single-item measure could be used to measure the overall construct of disability, in place of established multi-item instruments that are lengthy and time consuming to use.

They developed a VAS with a left anchor of "no disability" and a right anchor of "very severe disability." Validity testing was based on comparisons with two tools that have long been considered valid measures of disability for this population: the SF-36[9] and the RMDQ.[37] They also included a standard VAS for pain.

They found weak correlations of the disability VAS with the SF-36 and RMDQ, but a strong correlation with the pain VAS. Their interpretation was that pain was likely a clearer concept than disability, and its impact on function was probably better understood than "disability." Therefore, they concluded that their VAS was not a valid measure of self-reported disability.

Their findings provide important general and specific lessons in the use of visual analog scales, as we seek to find more efficient ways to measure clinical variables. It is tempting to create measures with an easy format like the VAS, but this can be deceptive when dealing with multidimensional concepts, especially with variables like disability or pain that are less well understood. It is essential to appreciate the necessity for validation to assure that a construct is being adequately evaluated.

Choosing Anchors

There are no standards for choosing anchors for a VAS. As Table 12-1 illustrates, there is great variation in defining the extremes. The left anchor is usually easy to understand, as it represents the absence of the trait—no pain, no anxiety, no fatigue. The right anchor presents a greater challenge, as the extreme may not have a common context. For example, depending on our experience, we may not all have the same sense of the "worst possible pain," "extreme stress," or "difficulty in providing care." The expectation, however, is that the individual's perception of these endpoints will stay consistent for repeated measurement.

Variations of the VAS

Numerical Rating Scale

The *numerical rating scale (NRS)* is a variation on the VAS, as shown in Figure 12-4. In panel A, the NRS creates a distinct ordinal scale. This format may be easier for some individuals to understand, essentially providing steps in intensity of the trait being measured. Some researchers have added verbal descriptors to a NRS to

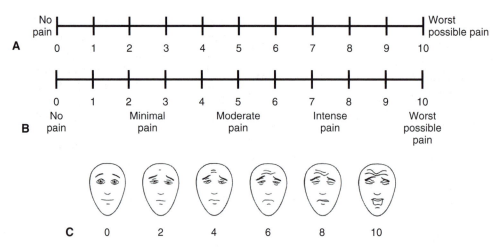

Figure 12–4 Variations of VAS scales. **A.** A 0-to-10 numerical pain rating scale; **B.** NRS with interim descriptors; **C.** The Faces Pain Scale-Revised (Part C used with permission of the International Association for the Study of Pain. Available at www.iasp-pain.org/FPSR. Accessed December 13, 2018.)

enhance understanding of the range of scores, as shown in panel B.[38] The NRS is often administered verbally, such as asking a patient to rate their pain on a scale from 0 to 10, defining the anchors. This approach differs from the VAS in that the increments of measurement are limited to 11 points, potentially providing less sensitivity. Although research has shown that the two versions are highly correlated,[48] the VAS may be more sensitive to small changes over time.[49]

Faces Rating Scale

The *faces rating scale*, in panel C, is considered useful when working with individuals who may have difficulty conceptualizing how a line represents subjective feelings. Several variations have been developed, primarily for use with children but this format has also been validated with mature populations in varied settings.[50-53] Versions of the faces scale have included up to 11 facial variations, but children may not be able to distinguish as many levels as adults.[54]

Visual analog scales can be presented horizontally or vertically. Although the horizontal configuration is used most often, both orientations have been found to show similar results.[55] For example, a vertical numerical scale has been incorporated into the Stroke Impact Scale to assess the patient's perception of recovery, with anchors from "no recovery" to "full recovery."[56] The vertical orientation was used to account for the potential impact of neglect on one side, which could impact a patient's ability to visualize the full scale.

Mechanical and computerized versions of the VAS have also been developed that allow for automatic measurement of marks.[57,58]

Multiple-Item VAS Measures

Because many clinical measures reflect complex constructs, one VAS may not be able to capture the full breadth of a multidimensional trait. Multiple VAS lines can be incorporated into an instrument, each with different anchors, to assess related aspects of the characteristic being measured.

► CASE IN POINT #3

Altenburg et al[59] studied quality of life in patients with bronchiectasis. As part of their study, they devised a five-item questionnaire that focused on dyspnea, fatigue, cough, sputum color, and pain.

The researchers based these five items on a review of literature that indicated these five symptoms of respiratory infection were the most frequently reported by patients, and had impact on quality of life in this population.

► Each symptom was presented as a VAS with unique anchors:
- No shortness of breath → Worst possible shortness of breath
- No tiredness → Worst possible tiredness
- I do not cough → Worst possible cough
- White phlegm → Dark green phlegm
- No pain → Worst possible pain

Each VAS was measured individually and a total score obtained for all five symptoms.

The design of the scale suggests that each symptom has equal weight in describing these traits for this population.

Analyzing VAS Scores

Because VAS scores are recorded in millimeters, the measurement is often interpreted as a ratio measure. However, the underlying scale is more accurately ordinal. Figure 12-5 illustrates hypothetical scores from three individuals rating their pain on two occasions. Even though they started at different points and ended at the same point, we don't know if actual pain levels are different at the first mark, the same at the second mark, or if the amount of change is different among patients. We only know that all three improved. This type of scale is consistent within a patient, but not across patients. This concept is important whether using a traditional VAS, a NRS, or a faces rating scale.

One argument suggests that the individual marking the line is not truly able to appreciate the nuances of a full continuum and, therefore, the mark does not represent a specific ratio score but more of a general estimate. Therefore, even though the actual readings from the scale are obviously at the ratio level, the true measurement properties are less precise.

> The issue of level of measurement is relevant for the choice of statistical procedures in data analysis. Although truly ordinal, VAS scores are often analyzed as ratio scores using parametric statistics (see Chapter 8).

■ Cumulative Scales

The dilemma with a summative scale, where several item responses are added to create a total score, is that the total score can be interpreted in more than one way.

Suppose we have a scale, scored from 0 to 100, that measures physical function, including elements related to locomotion, personal hygiene, dressing, and feeding. Individuals who achieve the same score of 50 may have obtained this score for very different reasons. One may be able to walk but is unable to perform the necessary upper extremity movements for self-care. Another may be in a wheelchair but is able to take care of his personal needs. Or a third individual may do all tasks, but poorly. Therefore, people with the same score will not necessarily have the same profile. This potential outcome reflects the fact that the items within the scale actually reflect different components of the latent trait being measured, in this case physical function, which are not all equal.

Cumulative scales (also called *Guttman scales*) provide an alternative approach, wherein a set of statements is presented that reflects increasing severity of the characteristic being measured. This technique is designed to ensure that there is only one dimension within a set of responses—only one unique combination of responses that can achieve a particular score. Each item in the scale is dichotomous.

> ➤ **CASE IN POINT #4**
>
> Gothwal et al[60] evaluated the Distance Vision Scale (DVS), an assessment of visual acuity in which letter reading becomes progressively difficult, to determine if the scale's properties held up in patients with cataracts.

The DVS asks individuals to respond to five statements, each scored "1" for yes and "0" for no. A total is computed, with a maximum score of 5.

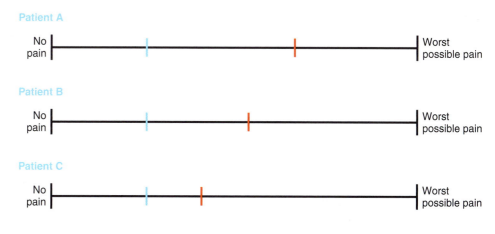

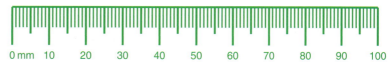

Figure 12–5 VAS measures of pain for three patients. ❘ represents the initial mark and ❘ represents pain at follow-up.

> When wearing glasses:
1. Can you see well enough to recognize a friend if you get close to his face?
2. Can you see well enough to recognize a friend who is an arm's length away?
3. Can you see well enough to recognize a friend across the room?
4. Can you see well enough to recognize a friend across a street?
5. Do you have any problems seeing distant objects?

In a cumulative scale, a respondent who agrees with an item must also agree with all items before it. For the DVS, all those who can recognize a friend across the room (item 3) should also be able to recognize them at arm's length (item 2) and face to face (item 1). Although there may be several combinations of responses that will result in a total score for a summative scale, there is only one way to achieve that score on a cumulative scale. Therefore, subjects who get the same score should have the same level of ability. The development of the scale is based on a theoretical premise that there is a hierarchy to this distance dimension of vision. This means we can predict a patient's visual acuity by knowing the total score.

 When an individual indicates scores for the items on a cumulative scale, the item order is rearranged so that the hierarchy is not obvious.

Validating a Cumulative Scale

To construct a cumulative scale, a set of items is developed that should reflect incremental degrees of the trait being measured. A statistical technique, called *scalogram analysis*, has been used to determine whether a unidimensional scale structure exists among the set of items.[61] This involves administration of the proposed scale to a sample of respondents, and the creation of a matrix that shows their responses. The analysis sorts the statements based on those that have more or less frequent agreement. Items that do not fit the hierarchical structure may be removed from the scale.

In reality, such scales are not free of error, and some of the subjects can be expected to present inconsistent patterns of response. In the analysis of the items for the DVS, for example, two subjects did have inconsistent responses, but all other responses maintained the expected order. A scalogram analysis will provide an analysis of the error rate within the scale. Scalogram analysis is used less often today in favor of the Rasch model, which will be discussed next.

■ Rasch Analysis

The scales described thus far are based on **classical measurement theory**, whereby a trait is assessed by getting a total numerical score that represents a person's overall performance. Most scales include dichotomous or ordinal values that are summed, and this "summary" score is treated as a continuous measure for purposes of assessing the degree to which an individual exhibits a certain trait.

Whether used in an educational test as the total number of correct answers, or as a quantitative representation of a functional score, we have already established that individuals with the same score may not have "passed" the same items, and therefore may not have the same "amount" of the trait being measured. Two students with the same exam grade may not have equal knowledge of the subject. Patients with the same functional score may not have the same abilities in all functional tasks. Because items are typically based on ordinal scoring, we also cannot know that intervals between grades are equal. Therefore, moving from one level of ability to another does not necessarily occur in a linear fashion.

Another limitation in the use of classical measurement approaches is that the observed score is dependent on the items used and the sample on which they are tested. Therefore, different measures of the same construct are not comparable. Consider, for example, the measurement of a physical attribute such as length. Regardless of whether you use a ruler, tape measure, caliper, or a laser, the "amount" of length should be the same. This is not the case, however, for latent traits. For instance, there are several different instruments that have been developed to measure balance, but their scoring systems do not reflect the "amount" of balance in the same way, and therefore cannot be compared.

Item Response Theory

Item response theory (IRT) is a different measurement approach that addresses these shortcomings based on two important premises.[62] First, scores should represent the amount of a unidimensional trait so that all persons with the same level of ability should get the same score. Therefore, regardless of the instrument used, items should be measuring the same thing and the person's ability level should be invariant across populations.

Second, the probability that an individual will "pass" an item should increase as an individual's ability increases. Therefore, individuals with less ability should do well only on easier items, and those with more ability should achieve higher scores on more difficult items.

The unidimensionality of a scale can be confirmed using factor analysis (see Chapter 31) and a measure of internal consistency (see Chapter 32).

The Rasch Model

Although there are several IRT models, the one most commonly used is a statistical technique called **Rasch analysis**, named for Georg Rasch (1901–1980), a Danish psychometrician. Using data from a patient sample and specialized computer programs, a model is generated that plots a linear metric on an interval scale that locates items in order of difficulty and persons in order of ability. In an approach similar to Guttman scaling, the Rasch model is based on the assumption that there is a relationship between an item's difficulty and an individual's ability level.

This discussion will focus on a conceptual understanding of Rasch analysis and how reported data can be interpreted. There are many good references for those who want to delve further into this approach.[63-69]

The Person-Item Map

The conceptual structure of a Rasch analysis is illustrated in Figure 12-6. The vertical line represents the continuum of the construct being measured. Using a common metric, items are plotted on the right, indicating their level of difficulty. On the left, people are positioned according to their ability level, based on "how much" or "how little" of the trait they have. This presentation is called a **person-item map**.

The scale is a linear measure in natural log units called **logits**. Logit scores are assigned to items and person ability, with a central zero point at the mean of item distribution, allowing items to be scaled as positive or negative. A logit scale is considered an equal-interval measure, thereby creating an interval scale that has linear, additive properties.

This transformation of ordinal data into interval values is an important feature of Rasch analysis. It allows us to not only rank items, but to determine how much more or less difficult each item is than another. Likewise, given a specific trait, we can determine how much more or less able one person is than another.

The items are ordered on the map according to the probability that an individual with a specific ability level will score high on that item. Therefore, persons 1 and 2 have lower ability levels and can only achieve item 1. Person 3 can achieve items 1 and 3, and person 4 can achieve all three items, including item 2, which is the most difficult item. People are located on the person-item map

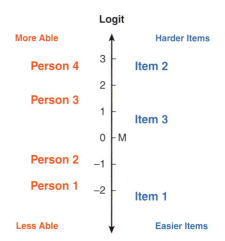

Figure 12–6 Person-item map, showing the relative position of items and persons along a linear scale in a Rasch model. The scale increases vertically from less able/easier items to more able/harder items. M = mean logit of item distribution.

according to the highest item on which they have a 50% probability of succeeding.[70,71]

A good fitting scale should reflect the full range of difficulty of items. Ideally, the scale items should not be redundant of each other, but should be distributed across the continuum of the trait being measured. Therefore, there should be no gaps where items are missing along the continuum, and no floor or ceiling effects. We should also find that the rank order of difficulty does not change from person to person. The analysis examines the extent to which an instrument's responses fit the predicted hierarchical model.[65,70,72,73]

Establishing the Hierarchy

> ► **CASE IN POINT #1: REVISITED**
> Recall the description of the Functional Gait Assessment (FGA), presented earlier. The FGA is a 10-item scale that assesses a person's ability to balance while walking.[20] Each item is scored 0 to 3, with lower scores indicating greater impairment. Beninato and Ludlow[74] studied the FGA with 179 older adults to determine if items mapped along a meaningful continuum, determine if the spread of tasks was sufficient to measure patients with varying functional abilities, and describe psychometric properties of individual items.

The 10 items in the FGA are listed in Table 12-2. Figure 12-7 illustrates the full person-item map obtained in this study, showing the distribution of these 10 items and the patients.

The person-item map shows that item 2 (gait speed) was the easiest, and item 7 (narrow base) was the most

Table 12-2   Items on the FGA (in Order of Administration)[75]

1. Gait on level surface
2. Change in gait speed
3. Gait with horizontal head turn
4. Gait with vertical head turn
5. Gait and pivot turn
6. Step over obstacle
7. Gait with narrow base of support
8. Gait with eyes closed
9. Walking backwards
10. Steps

difficult. There was a good spread of patients across the continuum, with a cluster around a logit of +1.

📌 Several specialized software options are available to run Rasch analysis.[76] The two most commonly used packages are WINSTEPS[77] and RUMM2030.[78] Both are available for purchase. The person-item map in Figure 12-7 was generated using WINSTEPS.[74]

Thresholds

The Rasch model was originally proposed for *dichotomous* items (yes/no), where grading is based on "passing" or "failing" an item. It has been further developed to accommodate *polytomous* items with multiple choice categories.[68] Grading for these items is based on thresholds of moving from one category to another.

For a good fitting item, 50% of the sample at that functional level should succeed on that item.[79] Similarly, person ability is determined by the probability of successful performance on each item. Persons with less ability should have a high probability of reporting difficulty performing tasks, and those with more ability should have a low probability of reporting difficulty performing the same tasks.

The category choices for each item should clearly identify people of different abilities, with minimal overlap of adjacent categories. Rasch analysis can indicate where the structure of category choices for a given item does not work as intended. When category choices are *disordered*, it may be necessary to collapse categories into fewer options.[80]

🔑 The logit for a given polytomous item is defined as the mean of the natural logarithm of the odds that a person with average ability will transition from one category to the next higher one (such as going from a rating of 1 to 2, 2 to 3).

Item Distribution

The determination of the item hierarchy can indicate if there are redundant items or gaps along the difficulty continuum.[71]

➤ In the distribution of FGA scores, items 10 (steps), 3 (horizontal head turns), and 9 (walking backwards) all locate at the same level of difficulty, at logit −0.25.

This redundancy suggests that it might be possible to eliminate one or two of these items without adversely affecting the scale's psychometric properties. Patients who attain this level of function should get the same score.

➤ We can also see that there is a large gap between item 8 (eyes closed, at +1.41) and the most difficult item 7 (narrow base of support, at +2.98).

A good scale will allow distinction of difficulty and ability throughout the continuum of the construct being measured. A large gap indicates that the scale is not sensitive to variations among those with higher ability. An additional item at a higher level of difficulty could improve the scale's capacity to distinguish individuals who have higher levels of ability.

We can also use this map to identify floor and ceiling effects, which would be evident if many patients were clustered at the extremes, especially if they exceed the difficulty levels of the scale in either direction (see Chapter 10).

➤ The FGA data showed a good distribution of patients across the full scale, with few patients scoring beyond the least and most difficult items, indicating no floor or ceiling effects.

 See the *Chapter 12 Supplement* for additional resources related to Rasch analysis of person-item thresholds and item characteristic curves.

Item and Person Separation

Item separation refers to the spread of items and *person separation* represents the spread of individuals. Ideally, the analysis will show that items can be separated into at least three *strata* that represent low, medium, and high difficulty,[81] although a good scale may actually delineate many strata to clarify the construct. Statistically, this spread is related to measurement error or reliability. The more reliable the scale, the more likely the item or person score represents the true score. This property can be assessed using a reliability coefficient.[70]

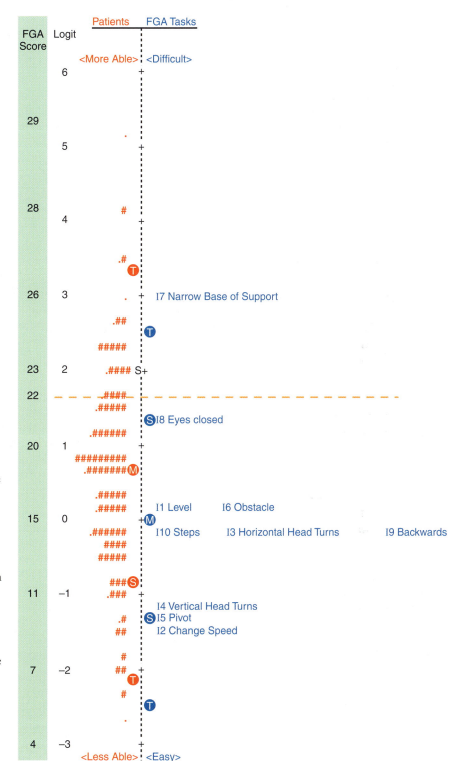

Figure 12–7 Person-item map for a Rasch analysis of the Functional Gait Assessment (FGA). Scores to the left (green bar) are the actual FGA scores. Logit scores are evenly spaced. The numbered test items are listed in blue (for example, item 7 is numbered I7). The number of patients who were able to achieve different ability levels is indicated in red (. = one person; # = 2 people). The gold dashed horizontal line indicates a cutoff score of ≤22, which indicates risk for falls on the FGA. Circled letters: M = mean ability or mean difficulty; S = 1 standard deviation from the mean; T = 2 standard deviations from the mean. From Beninato M, Ludlow LH. The Functional Gait Assessment in older adults: validation through Rasch modeling. *Phys Ther* 2016;96(4): 456–468. Adapted from Figure 1, p. 459. Used with permission of the American Physical Therapy Association.

> The FGA scale demonstrated internal consistency ($\alpha = 0.83$) and item separation reliability ($r = 0.99$), supporting overall consistency of scores and spread of task difficulty.[70]

Fit to the Rasch Model

Fit statistics indicate how well the data conform to the predicted Rasch measurement model.[66,71,82] They tell us how well each individual item contributes to the measurement of the unidimensional construct. To demonstrate goodness of fit, high ratings on more difficult items should be accomplished by people of greater ability, and people should have a higher probability of attaining higher scores on easier items than on more difficult ones.

Mean Square Estimate

Fit statistics are reported using two values. The *mean square (MSQ)* statistic is used to identify person or item ratings that deviate from Rasch model predictions. It is the ratio of the variance of observed scores to the expected variance based on the model.

Standardized residuals (ZSTD) are also generated, which represent the difference between the score the patient achieved and the model's predicted score for a particular item. A positive residual means that the obtained score is higher than predicted, and a negative residual means that the obtained score is lower than predicted.

Higher MSQ values or residuals indicate greater discrepancy from the model, where an item is not consistent in its level of difficulty across patients. Ideally, the MSQ will equal 1 and residuals will equal zero, indicating that the data fit the predicted distribution perfectly. If the MSQ is greater than 1, there is more variation in the data than would be predicted by the model—in other words, too unpredictable. When the ratio is less than 1, there is less variance in the data than the model would predict—or too predictable.

Infit and Outfit

Fit is expressed in two ways. *Infit* is sensitive to erratic or unexpected response patterns for items that are close to a patient's level of ability, such as a person of high ability performing poorly on a difficult item that is near their predicted ability level. A large infit value would indicate a problem with the item's fit with the unidimensional model.

Outfit reflects the occurrence of extremely unexpected or rare responses, such as a person of low ability scoring high on a difficult item. A large outfit value suggests that some patients have unique patterns of impairment and may reflect a different population.

Fit statistics for the FGA study are shown in Table 12-3 for four of the scale's items. There are no hard and fast rules about the upper and lower limits of acceptable fit

		INFIT		OUTFIT	
ITEM	LOGIT	MSQ	ZSTD	MSQ	ZSTD
7. Gait with narrow base of support	2.98	1.94	6.8	1.53	3.3
9. Ambulating backwards	−0.25	0.67	−3.6	0.68	−3.4
10. Climbing steps	−0.25	0.63	−4.2	0.77	−2.4
5. Gait and pivot turn	−1.32	1.01	0.1	1.18	1.4

Table 12-3 Fit Statistics for Selected FGA Items (in Order of Decreasing Difficulty)[74]

MSQ = mean square; ZSTD = standardized residual

statistics, in part because they are dependent on sample size. For a sample of 100 subjects, for example, MSQ values in the range of 0.7 to 1.3 are considered acceptable.[68] Others have suggested more flexible criteria.[66,74] ZSTD provide a significance test for the MSQ, and typically values greater than 2 are flagged as misfitting.[66]

> In the FGA study, we can see that item 7 is at a high level of difficulty (logit = 2.98), but also has a large MSQ for both infit and outfit. This suggests unexpected performance on this item. In contrast, item 5 is much easier (logit = −1.32) and MSQ scores are close to 1. This item is consistent with the predicted model.

Items that do not fit are those that deviate from the expected difficulty/ability hierarchy that the Rasch model generates. The poorly fitting items should trigger further investigation. It might be reasonable to consider revising the scale, either by eliminating the item, rewording it to remove ambiguity, or reducing the number of response categories.

Person Fit

Fit statistics are also generated for subjects. *Misfitting* subjects perform in an unexpected manner compared to that predicted by the Rasch model. The researcher must examine these patients' characteristics, potentially identifying subgroups in the population or to further investigate unexpected difficulties with specific activities that may direct intervention for specific individuals.[83]

Conversion Scores

The Rasch approach is complex and its clinical usefulness may be less than obvious to the clinician. As Rasch modelling is conducted on more and more clinical measures, however, it is important for the clinician to appreciate how these analyses can inform their practice. For example, knowing that ordinal values are not meaningful in a scale, using logit values generated by a Rasch analysis can provide a sound picture of the tool's real scale.

Conversion tables can be generated, partially illustrated in Table 12-4, that show equivalent scores at different logit values. These conversion scores enable the clinician to estimate a patient's ability along the person-item map ability scale. This can inform intervention planning, targeting items at the right level of challenge for their patient and guiding progression of skill.

For example, the hierarchy shown on the person-item map for the FGA does not match the order of administration of the scale items (see Table 12-2). Considering the order of difficulty of items can allow for a more efficient process so that the test can start with easier or more difficult items to match a patient's ability, potentially making the test shorter.

The score conversion also helps the clinician interpret cutoff scores such as those related to fall risk. For example, Beninato and Ludlow[74] superimposed a score of 22,

which has been previously identified as a cutoff FGA score associated with fall risk in older adults, on the person-item map at logit +1.7 logits (see Fig. 12-4). This falls between items 8 and 7. Therefore, if a patient succeeds on item 8, there is a high probability that we could rule out fall risk. Such scores can identify which tasks will be most challenging for those near the fall risk criterion score (see Focus on Evidence 12-2).

Differential Item Functioning

Item functioning is intended to be *invariant* with respect to irrelevant characteristics of those who are measured. This means that an item's difficulty should be related to ability, regardless of other factors that are not related to the task. **Differential item functioning (DIF)** refers to potential item bias in the fit of data to the Rasch model. It occurs when there are differences across subgroups within a sample who respond differently to individual items despite their having similar levels of the latent trait being measured. Even though individuals may be expected to respond differently to an item because of their age, for example, the expectation is that this difference will only be due to an actual difference in ability, not because they differ in age.[4] DIF can reduce the validity of the scale. Typical factors that can contribute to DIF are age, gender, ethnicity, language, or cultural differences.

For example, researchers have evaluated scoring of the FIM in patients with strokes, finding significant DIF across six European countries.[86] Item difficulty varied across countries, in part because of different cultural norms. For instance, "transfer to tub/shower" was more difficult in some countries than others, seemingly due to preferential use of tubs versus showers in certain cultures.

Table 12-4	Abridged Conversion Table for FGA Scores[74]				
FGA SCORE	**LOGIT**	**SE**	**FGA SCORE**	**LOGIT**	**SE**
5	−2.66	0.57	20	1.15	0.51
10	−1.30	0.49	25	2.67	0.61
15	−0.10	0.49	30	6.70	1.93

SE = standard error

Focus on Evidence 12–2
Are We Measuring the Same Thing?

One of the advantages of Rasch analysis is the ability to translate scores across instruments by converting measurements to a common metric. For example, a score ≤22 points on the FGA has been used as a cutoff to indicate individuals at risk for falls.[20] Beninato and Ludlow[74] translated this score to a logit of +1.7 (see Figure 12-7). The BBS, another assessment of fall risk that uses a different scoring system, has identified ≤45 points on that scale as the cutoff.[8] In their Rasch analysis of the BBS, Kornetti et al[80] found that this matched a logit of +1.5. Because these logits represent a common construct, these close values support the validity of the scales for assessing balance and fall risk, as well as support their common construct.

It is important to realize, however, that the hierarchy of items may not be consistent across different patient groups, depending on their specific motor control impairments. For example, one might expect that someone with hemiparesis from a stroke would approach a balance task with different limitations than someone with bilateral peripheral neuropathy. This is illustrated in Rasch analyses of the BBS, which have shown different results in studies with patients with lower limb amputations versus older military veterans.[80,84] When items were compared across these two patient groups, 8 of 14 items changed location in the order of item difficulty. In another study of patients with PD, the BBS required substantial modification to meet the unidimensionality assumption and demonstrated a ceiling effect because it did not adequately represent postural control impairments typical of PD.[85] These findings demonstrate the important contribution of Rasch analysis to understanding a scale's application, especially if we want to assess patients with different conditions or in different settings, or if we monitor patients across the continuum of care, where different instruments are often used to assess function.[69]

The important lesson in this analysis is the caution in pooling data or comparing FIM scores across countries unless adjustments are made to account for DIF.

Identification of DIF may be addressed using factor analysis (see Chapter 31), regression analysis (see Chapter 30), or Rasch analysis. The individuals in different groups would be matched on their scores and their responses compared for each item so that variant patterns can be observed. Further discussion of DIF analysis methods is beyond the scope of this book, but many good references are available.[87-90]

Computer Adaptive Testing

Computer adaptive tests (CATs) are designed to adjust the level of difficulty of items or questions based on the responses provided to match the knowledge and ability of a test-taker. CATs were originally designed for educational evaluation using the IRT framework, and more recently have been used in the administration of health status questionnaires as a way of potentially reducing the number of items that need to be tested for any one individual.

You may be familiar with CAT through licensing exams or standardized achievement tests (like the GRE), when the test is taken on a computer.[91] Based on the algorithm used, some test-takers may be given different questions and different numbers of questions to complete the test. The goal of CATs is to match the level of item difficulty to the ability level of the examinee. Using a complex algorithm, each response, correct or incorrect, is used to adapt further questions to the appropriate level. This process can reduce the total number of questions needed, as easier items can be eliminated for someone who correctly passes the harder items.

Development of a CAT is based on an item bank of questions on a particular topic or related to a common construct, which are then ordered by level of difficulty. This ordering can be established through Rasch analysis. The items are then tailored to the individual by first administering an item of midrange difficulty. The response is used to derive an estimated score. The test algorithm then selects the next item from the bank to refine the estimated score. This process continues for each successive item until a specified measurement level is reached or the maximum number of questions has been administered. By tailoring content to the respondent, questions are omitted that are not relevant to the respondent's level of skill.

COMMENTARY

Measure what is measurable, and make measurable what is not so.

—Galileo Galilei (1564–1642)

Italian philosopher and astronomer

Creating scales to measure latent traits presents a formidable challenge, with considerable implications for evidence-based practice. The descriptions of reliability and validity testing in Chapters 9 and 10 are important in the design of a health status measure. As examples in those chapters illustrate, the process of developing a new tool is not simple or quick. The steps in development of a measuring instrument include several stages of planning, test construction, reliability testing, and validation. Those who are inexperienced in this process should consult experts who can provide guidance, including statistical support.

Part of the validation process for a new scale will involve establishing criterion-related validity against another similar measurement. It will be relevant to ask, therefore, why a new instrument is needed. For example, the new scale may be more efficient or easier to administer, or it may relate to the construct in a different way, such as focusing on a different target population. Clinicians often develop "home-grown" scales that meet their local need, but these are not typically subjected to the rigorous validation procedures that are needed to assure measures are meaningful. It is advisable to look for existing instruments that have gone through this process whenever possible.

The Rasch approach is often applied during scale development as a means of informing construction of a scale to determine which items should be included or excluded.[73,92] However, it can also be applied after a scale is developed to investigate the psychometric properties of its items.[72] Many widely used health measures have been subjected to validity testing, but recent attention to IRT has led to their reappraisal. The Rasch model has provided a way to examine the internal construct validity of a measure, including ordering of categories, unidimensionality, and whether items are biased across subgroups. Clinical use of these scales can be greatly enhanced by understanding how these measurement properties influence interpretation of scores.

REFERENCES

1. Gordon DB. Acute pain assessment tools: let us move beyond simple pain ratings. *Curr Opin Anaesthesiol* 2015;28(5):565–569.
2. Melzack R. The McGill Pain Questionnaire: major properties and scoring methods. *Pain* 1975;1(3):277–299.
3. Roland M, Fairbank J. The Roland-Morris Disability Questionnaire and the Oswestry Disability Questionnaire. *Spine* 2000; 25(24):3115–3124.
4. McDowell I. *Measuring Health: A Guide to Rating Scales and Questionnaires.* 3 ed. New York: Oxford University Press, 2006.
5. Beck AT, Steer RA, Carbin MG. Psychometric properties of the Beck Depression Inventory: twenty-five years of evaluation. *Clin Psychol Rev* 1988;8(1):77–100.
6. Mahoney FI, Barthel DW. Functional evaluation: the BARTHEL Index. *Md State Med J* 1965;14:61–65.
7. Oczkowski WJ, Barreca S. The Functional Independence Measure: its use to identify rehabilitation needs in stroke survivors. *Arch Phys Med Rehabil* 1993;74:1291–1294.
8. Berg KO, Wood-Dauphinee SL, Williams JI, Maki B. Measuring balance in the elderly: validation of an instrument. *Can J Public Health* 1992;83 Suppl 2:S7–S11.
9. Ware JE, Sherbourne CD. The MOS 36-item Short Form Health Survey (SF-36). I. Conceptual framework and item selection. *Med Care* 1992;30:473–483.
10. Jenkinson C, Layte R, Jenkinson D, Lawrence K, Petersen S, Paice C, et al. A shorter form health survey: can the SF-12 replicate results from the SF-36 in longitudinal studies? *J Public Health Med* 1997;19(2):179–186.
11. Ware JE. *How to Score and Interpret Single-Item Health Status Measures: A Manual for Users of the SF-8 Health Survey (with a Supplement on the SF-6 Health Survey).* Boston, MA: Quality-Metric, Inc; Health Assessment Lab, 2001.
12. Ware JE. Conceptualizing and measuring generic health outcomes. *Cancer* 1991;67(Suppl):774–779.
13. Meenan RF, Mason JH, Anderson JJ, Guccione AA, Kazis LE. AIMS2. The content and properties of a revised and expanded Arthritis Impact Measurement Scales Health Status Questionnaire. *Arthritis Rheum* 1992;35(1):1–10.
14. Schipper H, Clinch J, McMurray A, Levitt M. Measuring the quality of life of cancer patients: the Functional Living Index-Cancer: development and validation. *J Clin Oncol* 1984;2(5): 472–483.
15. Tulsky DS, Kisala PA, Victorson D, Tate DG, Heinemann AW, Charlifue S, et al. Overview of the Spinal Cord Injury–Quality of Life (SCI-QOL) measurement system. *J Spinal Cord Med* 2015;38(3):257–269.
16. Desai AD, Zhou C, Stanford S, Haaland W, Varni JW, Mangione-Smith RM. Validity and responsiveness of the pediatric quality of life inventory (PedsQL) 4.0 generic core scales in the pediatric inpatient setting. *JAMA Pediatr* 2014; 168(12):1114–1121.
17. Bowling A, Stenner P. Which measure of quality of life performs best in older age? A comparison of the OPQOL, CASP-19 and WHOQOL-OLD. *J Epidemiol Community Health* 2011;65(3):273–280.
18. Nelson, Wasson J, Kirk J, Keller A, Clark D, Dietrich A, et al. Assessment of function in routine clinical practice: Description of the COOP chart method and preliminary findings. *J Chronic Dis* 1987;40(Suppl 1):55S–63S.
19. Szabo S. The World Health Organization quality of life (WHOQOL) assessment instrument. In: Spilker B, ed. *Quality of Life and Pharmacoeconomics in Clinical Trials.* Philadelphia: Lippincott-Raven, 1996:355–362.
20. Wrisley DM, Kumar NA. Functional gait assessment: concurrent, discriminative, and predictive validity in community-dwelling older adults. *Phys Ther* 2010;90(5):761–773.
21. Kuzon WM, Jr., Urbanchek MG, McCabe S. The seven deadly sins of statistical analysis. *Ann Plast Surg* 1996;37(3): 265–272.
22. Likert R. A technique for the measurement of attitudes. *Arch Psychol* 1932;22(140):5–55.
23. Vagias WM. *Likert-type scale response anchors.* Clemson University: Clemson International Institute for Tourism & Research Development, Department of Parks, Recreation and Tourism Management, 2006. Available at https://www.uc.edu/content/dam/uc/sas/docs/Assessment/likert-type%20response%20anchors.pdf. Accessed May 20, 2018.
24. Zhu W, Updyke WF, Lewandowski C. Post-hoc Rasch analysis of optimal categorization of an ordered-response scale. *J Outcome Meas* 1997;1(4):286–304.
25. Stone MH, Wright BD. Maximizing rating scale information. *Rasch Meas Transactions* 1994;8(3):386. Available at https://www.rasch.org/rmt/rmt83r.htm. Accessed September 20, 2018.
26. Wallston KA. The validity of the multidimensional health locus of control scales. *J Health Psychol* 2005;10(5):623–631.
27. Wallston KA. Multidimensional Health Locus of Control (MHLC) scales. Available at https://nursing.vanderbilt.edu/projects/wallstonk/. Accessed September 16, 2018.
28. Wallston KA, Stein MJ, Smith CA. Form C of the MHLC scales: a condition-specific measure of locus of control. *J Pers Assess* 1994;63(3):534–553.
29. Wallston KA, Wallston BS, DeVellis R. Development of the Multidimensional Health Locus of Control (MHLC) scales. *Health Educ Monogr* 1978;6(2):160–170.
30. Wewers ME, Lowe NK. A critical review of visual analogue scales in the measurement of clinical phenomena. *Res Nurs Health* 1990;13(4):227–236.
31. Bijur PE, Silver W, Gallagher EJ. Reliability of the visual analog scale for measurement of acute pain. *Acad Emerg Med* 2001;8(12):1153–1157.
32. Jensen MP, Chen C, Brugger AM. Interpretation of visual analog scale ratings and change scores: a reanalysis of two clinical trials of postoperative pain. *J Pain* 2003;4(7): 407–414.
33. Hjermstad MJ, Fayers PM, Haugen DF, Caraceni A, Hanks GW, Loge JH, et al. Studies comparing numerical rating scales, verbal rating scales, and visual analogue scales for assessment of pain intensity in adults: a systematic literature review. *J Pain Symptom Manage* 2011;41(6):1073–1093.
34. Scheffer AC, Schuurmans MJ, vanDijk N, van der Hooft T, de Rooij SE. Reliability and validity of the visual analogue scale for fear of falling in older persons. *J Am Geriatr Soc* 2010;58(11):2228–2230.
35. Crossley KM, Bennell KL, Cowan SM, Green S. Analysis of outcome measures for persons with patellofemoral pain: which are reliable and valid? *Arch Phys Med Rehabil* 2004; 85(5):815–822.
36. Boonstra AM, Schiphorst Preuper HR, Reneman MF, Posthumus JB, Stewart RE. Reliability and validity of the visual analogue scale for disability in patients with chronic musculoskeletal pain. *Int J Rehabil Res* 2008;31(2):165–169.
37. Roland M, Morris R. A study of the natural history of back pain. Part I: development of a reliable and sensitive measure of disability in low-back pain. *Spine* 1983;8(2):141–144.
38. Kim E, Lovera J, Schaben L, Melara J, Bourdette D, Whitham R. Novel method for measurement of fatigue in multiple sclerosis: Real-Time Digital Fatigue Score. *J Rehabil Res Dev* 2010;47(5):477–484.
39. Tittle MB, McMillan SC, Hagan S. Validating the brief pain inventory for use with surgical patients with cancer. *Oncol Nurs Forum* 2003;30(2):325–330.
40. Webel AR, Longenecker CT, Gripshover B, Hanson JE, Schmotzer BJ, Salata RA. Age, stress, and isolation in older adults living with HIV. *AIDS Care* 2014;26(5):523–531.
41. Appukuttan D, Vinayagavel M, Tadepalli A. Utility and validity of a single-item visual analog scale for measuring dental anxiety in clinical practice. *J Oral Sci* 2014;56(2):151–156.
42. Levy O, Amit-Vazina M, Segal R, Tishler M. Visual analogue scales of pain, fatigue and function in patients with various

rheumatic disorders receiving standard care. *Isr Med Assoc J* 2015;17(11):691–696.

43. Wehby GL, Naderi H, Robbins JM, Ansley TN, Damiano PC. Comparing the Visual Analogue Scale and the Pediatric Quality of Life Inventory for measuring health-related quality of life in children with oral clefts. *Int J Environ Res Public Health* 2014; 11(4):4280–4291.

44. Pickard AS, Lin HW, Knight SJ, Sharifi R, Wu Z, Hung SY, et al. Proxy assessment of health-related quality of life in African American and white respondents with prostate cancer: perspective matters. *Med Care* 2009;47(2):176–183.

45. Pang PS, Collins SP, Sauser K, Andrei AC, Storrow AB, Hollander JE, et al. Assessment of dyspnea early in acute heart failure: patient characteristics and response differences between likert and visual analog scales. *Acad Emerg Med* 2014;21(6): 659–666.

46. Kleiner-Fisman G, Khoo E, Moncrieffe N, Forbell T, Gryfe P, Fisman D. A randomized, placebo controlled pilot trial of botulinum toxin for paratonic rigidity in people with advanced cognitive impairment. *PLoS One* 2014;9(12):e114733.

47. Bienkowski P, Zatorski P, Glebicka A, Scinska A, Kurkowska-Jastrzebska I, Restel M, et al. Readiness visual analog scale: A simple way to predict post-stroke smoking behavior. *Int J Environ Res Public Health* 2015;12(8):9536–9541.

48. Lansing RW, Moosavi SH, Banzett RB. Measurement of dyspnea: word labeled visual analog scale vs. verbal ordinal scale. *Respir Physiol Neurobiol* 2003;134(2):77–83.

49. Lucas C, Romatet S, Mekies C, Allaf B, Lanteri-Minet M. Stability, responsiveness, and reproducibility of a visual analog scale for treatment satisfaction in migraine. *Headache* 2012; 52(6):1005–1018.

50. Wong DL, Baker CM. Pain in children: comparison of assessment scales. *Pediatr Nurs* 1988;14(1):9–17.

51. Keck JF, Gerkensmeyer JE, Joyce BA, Schade JG. Reliability and validity of the Faces and Word Descriptor Scales to measure procedural pain. *J Pediatr Nurs* 1996;11(6):368–374.

52. Stuppy DJ. The Faces Pain Scale: reliability and validity with mature adults. *Appl Nurs Res* 1998;11(2):84–89.

53. Garra G, Singer A, Taira BR, Chohan C, Cardoz H, Chisena E, et al. Validation of the Wong-Baker FACES Pain Rating Scale in pediatric emergency department patients. *Acad Emerg Med* 2010;17(1):50–54.

54. Decruynaere C, Thonnard JL, Plaghki L. How many response levels do children distinguish on FACES scales for pain assessment? *Eur J Pain* 2009;13(6):641–648.

55. Gift AG. Validation of a vertical visual analogue scale as a measure of clinical dyspnea. *Rehabil Nurs* 1989;14(6):323–325.

56. Stroke Impact Scale, version 3.0. Available at https://www.strokengine.ca/pdf/sis.pdf. Accessed November 5, 2018.

57. Amico KR, Fisher WA, Cornman DH, Shuper PA, Redding CG, Konkle-Parker DJ, et al. Visual analog scale of ART adherence: association with 3-day self-report and adherence barriers. *J Acquir Immune Defic Syndr* 2006;42(4):455–459.

58. Ramachandran S, Lundy JJ, Coons SJ. Testing the measurement equivalence of paper and touch-screen versions of the EQ-5D visual analog scale (EQ VAS). *Qual Life Res* 2008; 17(8):1117–1120.

59. Altenburg J, Wortel K, de Graaff CS, van der Werf TS, Boersma WG. Validation of a visual analogue score (LRTI-VAS) in non-CF bronchiectasis. *Clin Respir J* 2016;10(2): 168–175.

60. Gothwal VK, Wright TA, Lamoureux EL, Pesudovs K. Guttman scale analysis of the distance vision scale. *Invest Ophthalmol Vis Sci* 2009;50(9):4496–4501.

61. Green BF. A method of scalogram analysis using summary statistics. *Psychometrika* 1956;21(1):79–88.

62. Tractenberg RE. Classical and modern measurement theories, patient reports, and clinical outcomes. *Contemp Clin Trials* 2010;31(1):1–3.

63. DeMars C. *Item Response Theory*. New York: Oxford University Press, 2010.

64. Boone WJ, Staver JR, Yale MS. *Rasch Analysis in the Human Sciences*. New York: Springer, 2014.

65. Boone WJ. Rasch analysis for instrument development: Why, when, and how? *CBE Life Sci Educ* 2016;15(4):pii: rm4.

66. Bond TG, Fox CM. *Applying the Rasch Model: Fundamental Measurement in the Human Sciences*. 3 ed. New York: Routledge, 2015.

67. Embretson SE, Reise SP. *Item Response Theory for Psychologists*. Mahwah, NJ: Lawrence Erlbaum Associates, 2000.

68. Tesio L. Measuring behaviours and perceptions: Rasch analysis as a tool for rehabilitation research. *J Rehabil Med* 2003;35(3): 105–115.

69. Velozo CA, Kielhofner G, Lai JS. The use of Rasch analysis to produce scale-free measurement of functional ability. *Am J Occup Ther* 1999;53(1):83–90.

70. Wright BD, Masters GN. *Rating Scale Analysis*. Chicago: MESA Press, 1982.

71. Cappelleri JC, Jason Lundy J, Hays RD. Overview of classical test theory and item response theory for the quantitative assessment of items in developing patient-reported outcomes measures. *Clin Ther* 2014;36(5):648–662.

72. Tennant A, Conaghan PG. The Rasch measurement model in rheumatology: what is it and why use it? When should it be applied, and what should one look for in a Rasch paper? *Arthritis Rheum* 2007;57(8):1358–1362.

73. Rasch G. *Probabilistic Models for Some Intelligence and Attainment Tests*. Copenhagen: Danish Institute of Educational Research, 1960.

74. Beninato M, Ludlow LH. The Functional Gait Assessment in older adults: validation through Rasch modeling. *Phys Ther* 2016;96(4):456–468.

75. Wrisley DM, Marchetti GF, Kuharsky DK, Whitney SL. Reliability, internal consistency, and validity of data obtained with the functional gait assessment. *Phys Ther* 2004;84(10): 906–918.

76. Sick S: Rasch Analysis Software Programs. *JALT Testing and Eval SIG Newsletter*;13(3):13–16. Available at http://hosted.jalt.org/test/PDF/Sick4.pdf. Accessed August 13, 2018.

77. WINSTEPS & Facets Rasch Software. Available at http://www.winsteps.com/index.htm. Accessed July 23, 2018.

78. Andrich D, Lyne A, Sheriden B, Luo G. RUMM 2020. Perth, Australia: RUMM Laboratory, 2003.

79. Linacre JM. Rasch analysis of rank-ordered data. *J Appl Meas* 2006;7(1):129–139.

80. Kornetti DL, Fritz SL, Chiu YP, Light KE, Velozo CA. Rating scale analysis of the Berg Balance Scale. *Arch Phys Med Rehabil* 2004;85(7):1128–1135.

81. Silverstein B, Fisher WP, Kilgore KM, Harley JP, Harvey RF. Applying psychometric criteria to functional assessment in medical rehabilitation: II. Defining interval measures. *Arch Phys Med Rehabil* 1992;73(6):507–518.

82. Chiu YP, Fritz SL, Light KE, Velozo CA. Use of item response analysis to investigate measurement properties and clinical validity of data for the dynamic gait index. *Phys Ther* 2006; 86(6):778–787.

83. White LJ, Velozo CA. The use of Rasch measurement to improve the Oswestry classification scheme. *Arch Phys Med Rehabil* 2002;83(6):822–831.

84. Wong CK, Chen CC, Welsh J. Preliminary assessment of balance with the Berg Balance Scale in adults who have a leg amputation and dwell in the community: Rasch rating scale analysis. *Physical Therapy* 2013;93(11):1520–1529.

85. La Porta F, Giordano A, Caselli S, Foti C, Franchignoni F. Is the Berg Balance Scale an effective tool for the measurement of early postural control impairments in patients with Parkinson's disease? Evidence from Rasch analysis. *Eur J Phys Rehabil Med* 2015;51(6):705–716.

86. Lundgren-Nilsson A, Grimby G, Ring H, Tesio L, Lawton G, Slade A, et al. Cross-cultural validity of functional independence measure items in stroke: a study using Rasch analysis. *J Rehabil Med* 2005;37(1):23–31.

87. Tennant A, Pallant JF. DIF matters: a practical approach to test if Differential Item Functioning makes a difference. *Rasch Meas Transactions* 2007;20(4):1082–1084. Available at https://www.rasch.org/rmt/rmt204d.htm. Accessed August 7, 2018.

88. Badia X, Prieto L, Linacre JM. Differential item and test functioning (DIF & DTF). *Rasch Meas Transactions* 2002;16(3):889. Available at https://www.rasch.org/rmt/rmt163g.htm. Accessed August 7, 2018.

89. Holland PW, Wainer H. *Differential Item Functioning*. New York: Routledge, 1993.

90. Krabbe PFM. *The Measurement of Health and Health Status: Concepts, Methods and Applications from a Multidisciplinarhy Perspective*. London: Academic Press, 2017.

91. Seo DG. Overview and current management of computerized adaptive testing in licensing/certification examinations. *J Educ Eval for Health Prof* 2017;14:17.

92. Ludlow LH, Matz-Costa C, Johnson C, Brown M, Besen E, James JB. Measuring engagement in later life activities: Rasch-based scenario scales for work, caregiving, informal helping, and volunteering. *Meas Eval Counsel Dev* 2014;47(2):127–149.

PART 3

Designing Clinical Research

CHAPTER 13 **Choosing a Sample** 180

CHAPTER 14 **Principles of Clinical Trials** 192

CHAPTER 15 **Design Validity** 210

CHAPTER 16 **Experimental Designs** 227

CHAPTER 17 **Quasi-Experimental Designs** 240

CHAPTER 18 **Single-Subject Designs** 249

CHAPTER 19 **Exploratory Research: Observational Designs** 271

CHAPTER 20 **Descriptive Research** 285

CHAPTER 21 **Qualitative Research** 297

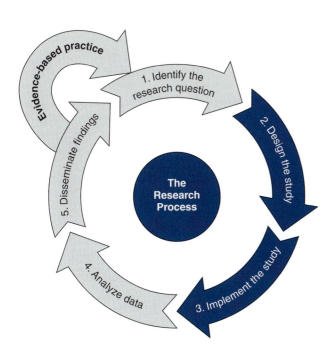

Choosing a Sample

Our daily lives are filled with generalizations. Cook a good steak and decide if it's done by tasting a small piece—you don't eat the whole steak. Try out a new therapy with one patient and decide if you will use it again based on its effectiveness—you don't test it on every patient. Researchers use this same principle in studying interventions, tests, and relationships. They obtain data on a group of subjects to make generalizations about what will happen to others with similar characteristics in a similar situation. To make this process work, we have to develop a plan to select appropriate individuals for a sample in a way that will allow us to extrapolate beyond that group's performance for the application of research evidence to others.

Whether developing a sampling plan for a research study or determining if published evidence is relevant for clinical practice, we need to understand how study samples are recruited and how these methods impact our ability to generalize findings. The purpose of this chapter is to describe various sampling techniques and how they influence generalizations from representative subjects to make predictions about the larger world.

■ Populations and Samples

If we wanted to be truly confident in the effectiveness of an intervention, we would have to test it on every patient in the world for whom that treatment is appropriate. This larger group to which research results will be applied is called the **population**. It is the aggregate of persons or objects that meet a specified set of criteria and to whom we wish to generalize results of a study. For instance, if we were interested in studying the effects of various treatments for osteoarthritis, the population of interest would be all people in the world who have osteoarthritis.

Of course, it is not practical to test every person who has osteoarthritis, nor could we access them. Working with smaller groups is generally more economical, more time efficient, and potentially more accurate because it affords better control of measurement. Therefore, through a process of *sampling*, a researcher chooses a subgroup of the population, called a **sample**. This sample serves as the reference group for estimating characteristics of and drawing conclusions about the population.

Populations are not necessarily restricted to human subjects. Researchers may be interested in studying characteristics of institutions or geographical areas, and these may be the units that define the population. In test–retest reliability studies, the "population" will consist of all possible trials and the "sample" would be the actual measurements taken. Industrial quality control studies use samples of items from the entire inventory of a particular manufacturing lot. Surveys often sample households from a population of housing units. A population can include people, places, organizations, objects, or any other unit of interest.

Target and Accessible Populations

The first step in planning a study is to identify the overall group of people to which the researcher intends to generalize findings. This universe of interest is the **target population**.

> ➤ **CASE IN POINT #1**
> Researchers were interested in studying the association between depression and risk factors for dementia in patients with type 2 diabetes.[1] They accessed data from medical records for patients with diabetes between 30 and 75 years of age who were enrolled in a large integrated healthcare system.

Because it is not possible to gain access to every person with diabetes in this age range, some portion of the target population that has a chance to be selected must be identified. This is the **accessible population**. It represents the people you have access to and from which the actual sample will be drawn (see Fig. 13-1).

> ➤ For the study of depression and dementia, the accessible population was all patients enrolled in one healthcare system who were included in the diabetes registry. The units within this population were the individual patients.

Strictly speaking, a sample can only be representative of the accessible population. For example, there may be differences in healthcare practices in different systems, and not all people with diabetes would be receiving the same type of care. Such differences can complicate generalizations to the target population. Geographic differences, such as climate, socioeconomic characteristics, or cultural patterns are often a source of variation in samples.

When the differences between the target and accessible populations are potentially too great, it may be necessary to identify a more restricted target population. For example, we could specify that our target population is people with type 2 diabetes who are enrolled in large managed-care systems. The results of the study would then be applicable only to people meeting this criterion. Because the validity of the accessible population is not readily testable, researchers must exercise judgment in assessing the degree of similarity with the target population.

Selection Criteria

In defining the target population, an investigator must specify selection criteria that will govern who will and will not be eligible to participate. Samples should be selected in a way that will maximize the likelihood that the sample represents the population as closely as possible. Inclusion and exclusion criteria should be fully described in the methods section of a research report.

Inclusion Criteria

Inclusion criteria describe the primary traits of the target and accessible populations that will make someone eligible to be a participant. The researcher must consider the variety of characteristics present in the population in terms of clinical findings, demographics, and geographic factors, as well as whether these factors are important to the question being studied.

> ➤ Subjects in the diabetes study were included if they were part of the diabetes registry. The investigators identified 20,188 eligible participants with type 2 diabetes between the age of 30 to 75 years.

Exclusion Criteria

Exclusion criteria are those factors that would preclude someone from being a subject. These factors will generally be considered potentially confounding to the results and are likely to interfere with interpretation of the findings.

> ➤ In the diabetes study, subjects were excluded if they had a prior diagnosis of dementia, or if they had type 1 diabetes.

Exclusion criteria for randomized controlled trials are often extensive, eliminating patients with comorbidities and other various health or demographic traits that could confound examination of relationships among the study variables. Patients may also be excluded if they have a medical condition that would put them at risk with the experimental treatment. If the study requires understanding instructions or completing

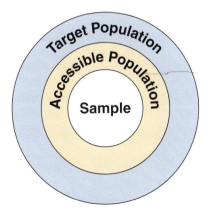

Figure 13–1 Levels of the sampling process.

a survey in English, for example, subjects may be excluded if they are not fluent in that language. As research progresses, however, these limitations may be quite artificial in terms of the patients who are typically seen in the clinic, thereby decreasing the ability to generalize results.

One of the challenges to evidence-based practice is the difficulty in generalizing from research studies to patients, especially when exclusion criteria rule out a good portion of the people for whom the study question would be relevant. Pragmatic clinical trials (PCTs) generally have fewer exclusion criteria, allowing "real" patients to be part of a study. PCTs must be interpreted with recognition of the analysis and interpretation issues that arise with more heterogeneous samples (see Chapter 2).

Recruitment

Once an accessible population is identified, the researcher must devise a plan for subject recruitment, inviting individuals to participate. This process may involve written invitations mailed to potential subjects' homes, telephone calls, posting announcements in public places or by emails, or personal contacts in the clinical setting. All members of the accessible population may be approached, or a smaller subgroup may be targeted.

The Final Sample

It is not unusual for fewer subjects to agree to enter the study than originally projected. Not all invited individuals will be eligible based on stipulated inclusion/exclusion criteria, and some may not be interested or willing to participate (see Focus on Evidence 13-1). With survey questionnaires, many subjects will not respond.

Focus on Evidence 13–1
The Framingham Heart Study

The Framingham Heart Study is one of the most prominent longitudinal cohort studies, begun in 1948 and still going on today into its third generation.[2,3] Its initial focus was on arteriosclerotic and hypertensive cardiovascular disease (CVD), but has expanded greatly over the decades to include neurological,[4] musculoskeletal,[5,6] and functional disorders,[7] as well as other conditions such as diabetes.[8]

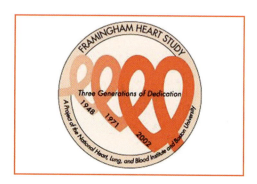

The site chosen for the study was a suburban area outside of Boston, the town of Framingham, Massachusetts, a primarily middle-class white community in 1948.[9] Although the investigators recognized that it would have been ideal to study several different areas, the logistics were sufficiently challenging to start with one town. Framingham was deemed to be of adequate size, with a variety of socioeconomic and ethnic subgroups, a relatively stable population, and a strong medical infrastructure.[10] The town had also been the site of a tuberculosis study nearly 30 years before that had had successful participation by the townspeople.

Given the intent to describe population risk factors, the sampling plan was to select a random group of participants from the community within the age range that CVD was likely to develop, with the original intent of following them for 20 years.[11] The researchers determined that they could complete 6,000 examinations every 2 years, and therefore this was their target sample size out of a town population of 10,000.

The official sampling process focused on the population aged 30 to 59 years according to the town census, divided into eight precincts. Within each precinct, lists were arranged by family size and then by address. Using a systematic sampling procedure, two of every three families were selected, and all family members within the eligible age range were invited to participate. This generated a sample of 6,507 subjects—but only 69%, or 4,469, actually came in for an examination. It turned out that respondents tended to be healthier than nonrespondents. This was considered a biased sample with a low response rate. Therefore, researchers had to use volunteers to obtain their desired sample size, which violated their random strategy.

Although the town's population has become more diverse, and later cohorts have been included to increase ethnic diversity, the Framingham investigators were well aware that the community may not have been fully representative of the U.S. population.[2,9] To address concerns about potential sampling biases, there has been a concerted effort, over several decades and generations of participants, to draw comparisons with other studies that have included subjects from many areas with varied ethnic, geographic, and socioeconomic profiles.[12-15] These have continued to show substantial agreement with the Framingham findings, which has supported the study's generalizability.

Courtesy of the Framingham Heart Study, National Heart, Lung, and Blood Institute.

In the study of type 2 diabetes, researchers invited 29,639 patients to participate, with 20,188 consenting. Of these, 801 were excluded based on not meeting eligibility criteria, and 148 were eventually excluded because of lack of any follow-up, leaving a final study cohort of 19,239 patients.

It is important to understand why subjects choose not to participate, as these reasons can influence interpretation of results. An investigator should have a contingency plan in mind, such as recruiting subjects from different sites or expanding inclusion criteria, when the sample size falls substantially short of expectations.

> In the end, the sample used for data analysis may be further reduced because of errors in data collection or dropouts for various reasons. The relevant concern is whether those who do not complete the study are different in any substantive way from those who remain, changing the profile of the final sample. Participants may differ from nonparticipants in ways that could affect the variables being studied, such as education, employment, insurance, age, gender, or health beliefs.[16-18] It is especially important to know if subjects drop out because of something they experienced as part of the study and if those reasons are not randomly distributed across groups. Strategies to address these issues will be discussed in Chapter 15.
>
> Researchers will often compare baseline and demographic characteristics of those who do and do not participate to determine if there is a difference between them as a way of estimating the effect on sample bias.

Reporting Subject Participation

A flowchart that details how participants pass through various stages of a study should be included in a research report. Figure 13-2 shows a generic chart for this purpose, with expected information about how many subjects were included or excluded at the start of the study, how many left the study (and their reasons), and finally how many completed the study. Guidelines for reporting such data have been developed by the Consolidated Standards of Reporting Trials (CONSORT) workgroup.[19]

See Figure 15-3 in Chapter 15 for a similar flowchart with actual study data. The CONSORT guidelines for reporting research are discussed further in Chapter 38.

Sample Size

A question about the number of subjects needed is often the first to be raised as a researcher recruits a sample. The issue of sample size is an essential one, as it directly affects the statistical power of the study. **Power** is the ability to find significant effects when they exist. It is

influenced by several factors, including the variability within the sample, the anticipated magnitude of the effect, and the number of subjects. With a small sample, power tends to be low and a study may not succeed in demonstrating the desired effects.

Issues related to sample size and power will be addressed in Chapter 23 and subsequent chapters.

■ Sampling

Sampling designs can be categorized as probability or nonprobability methods. **Probability samples** are created through a process of **random sampling** or **selection**. Random is not the same as haphazard. It means that every unit in the population has an equal chance, or "probability," of being chosen. Therefore, the sample should be free of any bias and is considered representative of the population from which it was drawn. Because this process involves the operation of chance, however, there is always the possibility that a sample will not reflect the spread of characteristics in its parent population. The selection of **nonprobability samples** is made by nonrandom methods. Nonprobability techniques are probably used more often in clinical research out of necessity, but we recognize that their outcomes require some caution for generalization.

> **HISTORICAL NOTE**
> Much of our knowledge of prehistoric times comes from artifacts such as paintings or burial sites created in caves nearly 40,000 years ago. Any paintings or relics made outdoors would have washed away, and so we have no record of them. Therefore, our understanding of prehistoric people is associated with caves because that is where the data still exist, not necessarily because that's where they lived most of their lives. Using cave data as representative of all prehistoric behavior is likely an example of sampling bias, what has been termed the "caveman effect."[20]

Sampling Error

If we summarize sample responses using averaged data, this average will most likely be somewhat different from the total population's average responses, just by chance. The difference between sample values, called **statistics**, and population values, called **parameters**, is **sampling error**, or sampling variation.

In most situations, of course, we don't actually know the population parameters. We use statistical procedures to estimate them from our sample statistics, always understanding there will likely be some error. The essence

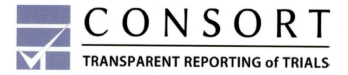

CONSORT 2010 Flow Diagram

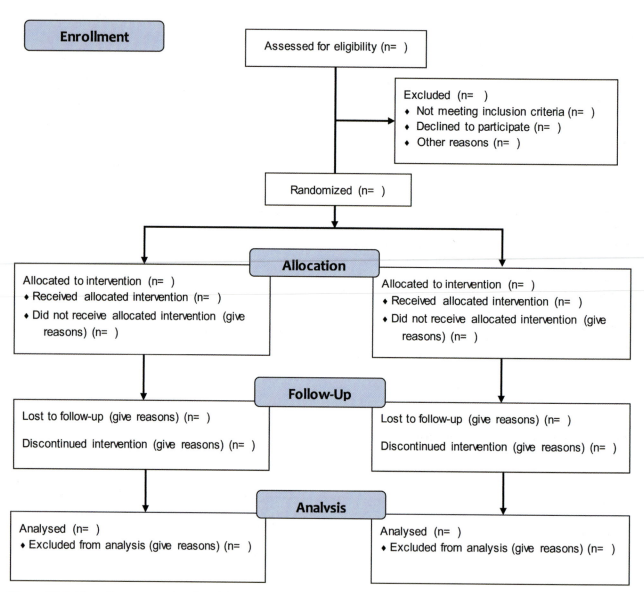

Figure 13–2 Flow diagram template for subject progression in a randomized trial, including data on those who withdrew or were lost to follow-up. From the CONSORT 2010 guidelines.[19]

of random sampling is that these sampling differences are due to chance and are not a function of any human bias, conscious or unconscious.

Although it is not perfect, random selection affords the greatest possible confidence in the sample's validity because, in the long run, it will produce samples that most accurately reflect the population's characteristics. In non-probability samples, the probability of selection may be zero for some members of the population and unknown for other members. Consequently, the degree of sampling error cannot be estimated. This limits the ability to generalize outcomes beyond the specific sample studied.

> Sampling *error* is a measure of chance variability between a sample and population. The term "error" in statistics does not mean a mistake but is another word for unexplained variance (see Chapter 23). This must be distinguished from *bias*, which is not considered a matter of chance.

Sampling Bias

To make generalizations, the researcher must be able to assume that the responses of sample members will be representative of how the population members would respond in similar circumstances. Human populations are, by nature, heterogeneous, and the variations that exist in behavioral, psychological, or physical attributes should also be present in a sample. Theoretically, a good sample reflects the relevant characteristics and variations of the population in the same proportions as they exist in the population. Although there is no way to guarantee that a sample will be representative of a population, sampling procedures can minimize the degree of bias or error in choosing a sample.

Sampling bias occurs when the individuals selected for a sample overrepresent or underrepresent certain population attributes that are related to the phenomenon under study. Such biases can be conscious or unconscious. Conscious biases occur when a sample is selected purposefully. For example, a clinician might choose only patients with minimal dysfunction to demonstrate a treatment's effectiveness, eliminating those subjects who were not likely to improve.

Unconscious biases might occur if an interviewer interested in studying attitudes of the public toward the disabled stands on a busy street corner in a downtown area and interviews people "at random," or haphazardly. The interviewer may unconsciously choose to approach only those who look cooperative on the basis of appearance, sex, or some other characteristics. Persons who do not work or shop in that area will not be represented.

The conclusions drawn from such a sample cannot be useful for describing attitudes of the "general public."

The validity of generalizations made from a sample to the population depend on the method of selecting subjects. Just getting a larger sample won't necessarily control for bias. A small representative sample of 50 may be preferable to an unrepresentative sample of 1,000. Therefore, some impartial mechanism is needed to make unbiased selections.

HISTORICAL NOTE

Large samples do not necessarily mean better representation. In the 1936 presidential election, the *Literary Digest* predicted that Alf Landon would beat Franklin Roosevelt with 57% of the vote. The prediction was based on responses from over 2 million voters (only 23% of those actually contacted), culled from lists of magazine readers, automobile owners, and telephone directories. Roosevelt ended up winning by a 3:2 margin, but his support came from lower-income voters, most of whom did not own cars or phones!

In contrast, in the 1968 presidential election, with better sampling methods, Gallup and Harris polls predicted that Richard Nixon would receive 41% to 43% of the popular vote, based on a random sample of only 2,000 voters. Nixon actually received 42.9%.[21]

■ Probability Sampling

In probability sampling, every member of a population has an equal opportunity, or probability, of being selected. A truly random sample is *unbiased* in that each selection is independent and no one member of the population has any more chance of being chosen than any other member. Several approaches are used, each with a different strategy, but all aimed at securing a representative sample (see Table 13-1).

> Often used for large surveys, polls, and epidemiologic studies, probability sampling is essential for accurately describing variables and relationships in a population. It is less practical in clinical research, except when using large databases. For clinical experiments, where samples are smaller and the focus is more on comparisons or explaining relationships, researchers often do not have access to true random samples.

Simple Random Sampling

In a simple random sample, subjects are drawn from the accessible population, often taken from a listing of persons, such as membership directories or census lists. For example, in the study of type 2 diabetes, researchers had

Table 13-1   Summary of Probability and Non-Probability Sampling Methods

PROBABILITY METHODS

Simple Random Sampling	Each member of the defined accessible population has an equal chance of being selected.
Systematic Sampling	Persons are randomly chosen from unordered lists using a fixed sampling interval, such as every 10th person. The interval is determined by the desired sample size and the number of persons on the list. As long as lists have no biased order, this is considered a random process.
Stratified Random Sampling	A particular sample characteristic is used to partition members of a population into non-overlapping subsets or strata, and random samples are drawn from each stratum based on the proportion of the population within each stratum.
Cluster Sampling	With especially large populations, samples are randomly chosen at multiple stages, such as counties, city blocks, households, and individuals.
Disproportional Sampling	A form of stratified sampling, disproportional sampling is used when certain strata are underrepresented in the population, which leads to their having small representation within the total sample. These strata are *oversampled* to provide stronger representation, and weights are used to adjust data to correct for this bias.

NON-PROBABILITY METHODS

Convenience Sampling	Also called accidental sampling, subjects are chosen on the basis of their availability. For example, they may be recruited as they enter a clinic or they may volunteer through advertising.
Quota Sampling	A form of stratified sampling that is not random, where subjects are recruited to represent various strata in proportion to their number in the population.
Purposive Sampling	Subjects are hand-picked and invited to participate because of known characteristics.
Snowball Sampling	Small numbers of subjects are purposively recruited and they help to identify other potential participants through networking. This approach is used when subjects are difficult to identify, especially when dealing with sensitive topics.

access to the full membership list of the healthcare system. Once a listing is available, a random sampling procedure can be implemented.

Suppose we wanted to choose a sample of 100 patients to study the association between depression and dementia with diabetes, taken from patient lists from 10 area hospitals. Conceptually, the simplest approach would be to place each patient's name on a slip of paper, place these slips into a container, and blindly draw 100 slips—not a very efficient process! A more realistic method involves the use of a *table of random numbers*, which can be found in most statistics texts or generated by computers (see Appendix A-6). They are comprised of thousands of digits (0 to 9) with no systematic order or relationship. The selections made using a table of random numbers are considered unbiased, as the order of digits is completely due to chance. More conveniently today, computer programs can be used to generate random choices from a list of participants.

This procedure involves *sampling without replacement*, which means that, once a subject is chosen, he is no longer eligible to be chosen again when the next random selection is made.

See the *Chapter 13 Supplement* for a description of the process for using a random numbers table and for generating a random sample using SPSS.

The terms *random sampling (selection)* and *random assignment* are often confused. Sampling or selection is the process of choosing participants for a study. Assignment is the allocation of participants to groups as part of a study design once they have been recruited.

Systematic Sampling

Random sampling can be a laborious technique, especially with large samples. When lists are arranged with no inherent order that would bias the sample (such as alphabetical order), an alternative approach can be used that simplifies this procedure, called **systematic sampling**. To use this sampling technique, the researcher divides the total number of elements in the accessible population by the number of elements to be selected.

Therefore, to select a sample of 100 from a list of 1,000 patients, every 10th person on the list is selected, with a random starting point. This approach was used in the Framingham Heart Study described earlier.

The interval between selected elements is called the *sampling interval* (in this case, 10). This approach is usually the least time-consuming and most convenient way to obtain a sample from an available listing of potential subjects. Systematic sampling is generally considered equivalent to random sampling, as long as no recurring pattern or particular order exists in the listing.

Stratified Random Sampling

In random and systematic sampling, the resulting distribution of characteristics of the sample can differ from that of the population from which it was drawn just by chance because each selection is made independently of all others. You could end up with an older sample, or more men than women. It is possible, however, to modify these methods to improve a sample's representativeness (and decrease sampling error) through a process called stratification.

Stratified random sampling involves identifying relevant population characteristics and partitioning members of a population into homogeneous, nonoverlapping subsets, or *strata*, based on these characteristics. Random samples are then drawn from each stratum to control for bias. Therefore, although subjects are differentiated on the basis of the stratified variable, all other factors should be randomly distributed across groups.

> ▶ In the study of depression and risk of dementia in patients with type 2 diabetes, researchers were concerned about racial/ethnic diversity and wanted their sample to reflect the distribution in their community. The researchers wanted a sample of 20,000 patients. They stratified their sample into four groups based on their accessible population, which was 23% African American, 15% Caucasian, 24% Latino, and 38% identified as Other/Unknown.

Rather than leave the distributions in the final sample to chance, they used a *proportional stratified sample* by first separating the population into the four categories and then drawing random samples from each one based on the proportion in the population (see Fig. 13-3). Therefore, to obtain a sample of 20,000, they chose 4,600 African Americans, 3,000 Caucasians, and so on. The resulting sample would intuitively provide a better estimate of the population than simple random sampling.

Cluster Sampling

In many research situations, especially those involving large dispersed populations, it is impractical or impossible to obtain a complete listing of a population or to

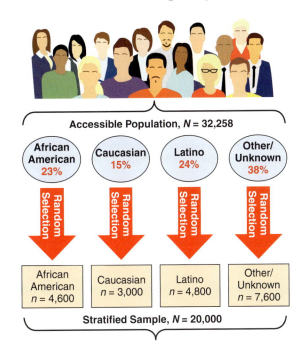

Figure 13–3 Schematic representation of proportional stratified sampling for a study of depression as a risk factor for dementia.[1]

consider recruiting a random sample from the entire population.

> ▶ **CASE IN POINT #2**
>
> The *National Health and Nutrition Examination Survey (NHANES)* is a program of interviews and physical examination studies designed to assess the health and nutritional status of adults and children in the United States.[22] Begun in the early 1960s, the survey examines a nationally representative sample of about 5,000 persons each year in counties across the country.
>
> The NHANES gathers demographic, socioeconomic, dietary, and health-related information and collects data on medical, dental, and physiological measurements. Findings are used to determine the prevalence of major diseases and risk factors associated with health promotion and disease prevention in the U.S. population.

For a study like the NHANES and other national surveys, which seek to represent the U.S. population, a strategy is needed that will link members of the population to some already established grouping that can be sampled. One approach is called **cluster sampling**, which involves grouping or clustering individuals according to some common characteristic and then randomly choosing specific clusters to study. For instance, we could divide the U.S. into eight different geographic areas, each composed of several states, and then randomly choose four of these clusters. From there, we can either sample all residents in those states or randomly choose subjects from each cluster. This approach is often used with surveys to condense the total population into a workable subset.

Multi-Stage Cluster Sampling

With large datasets, like the NHANES, a more common approach is called **multistage sampling**. This involves several successive phases of sampling to arrive at a representative sample (see Fig. 13-4).

> ➤ The NHANES uses a four-stage model. The first stage is identification of the *primary sampling units*, in this case counties across the country. The randomly chosen counties are divided into segments, typically city blocks, and, in stage 2, segments are randomly selected. The third stage is a random selection of households within each chosen segment, and finally individuals are randomly selected within households.

Sampling Techniques

Survey researchers often use multistage sampling to generate random samples of households. One technique, called *area probability sampling*, allows a population to be sampled geographically. The total target land area is divided into mutually exclusive sections. A list is then made of housing units in each section and a sample is drawn from these lists.

Another technique, called *random-digit dialing*, involves the generation of random numbers and may be based on lists of landlines or cell phones using multistage sampling of area codes and telephone exchanges.[23] Most of us have had experience with this type of survey (usually around dinner time!). Many studies in marketing research use this approach. This method presents many problems in terms of whose phones are listed and who

answers the phones. For certain survey research questions, however, random-digit dialing is most useful for generating a sizable sample over a large area.

Disproportional Sampling

The benefits of stratified and cluster sampling can be nullified when the researcher knows in advance that subgroups within the population are of greatly unequal size, creating a situation where one or more groups may provide insufficient samples for making comparisons. In such situations, certain groups may be *oversampled*, creating what is called a **disproportional sample**.

> ➤ Over the years, the NHANES has oversampled different groups as part of its selection procedures, such as African Americans, Mexican Americans, low-income white Americans, adolescents, and persons over 60 years old.[22]

This disproportional representation presents an analysis challenge because the sample no longer reflects the true proportions of population diversity. To correct for this, a *sample weight* is assigned to each person, based on the number of people in the population represented by that subject. These weights correct for the bias in the sampled groups.

> See the *Chapter 13 Supplement* for a description of the process for determining weights for disproportional samples.

■ Nonprobability Sampling

In practice, it is often difficult, if not impossible, to obtain a true random sample. Clinical researchers are often forced to use **nonprobability samples**, created when samples are chosen on some basis other than random selection. Because all the elements of the population do not have an equal chance of being selected under these circumstances, we cannot readily assume that the sample represents the target population. In fact, there may be characteristics of the population that are not known that could influence the likelihood of being selected. The probability exists that some segment of the population will be disproportionately represented.

> Researchers and clinicians make many generalizations based on nonprobability samples, out of pragmatic necessity. It is left to the judgment of those who interpret the evidence to decide if the obtained sample is sufficiently similar to the target population. For example, geographic, ethnic, or socioeconomic differences may limit generalizations.

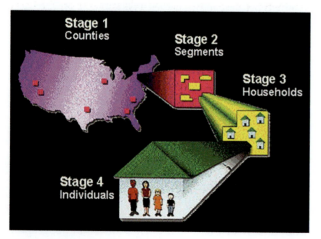

Figure 13–4 Four-stage multistage sampling process for the NHANES. Courtesy of cdc.gov/nchs.

Convenience Sampling

The most common form of nonprobability sample is a **convenience sample**, or *accidental sample*. With this method, subjects are chosen on the basis of availability.

> Investigators performed a trial to study the effectiveness of an exercise intervention for decreasing fatigue severity and increasing physical activity in individuals with pulmonary arterial hypertension.[24] A convenience sample was recruited from local outpatient pulmonary clinics between 2009 and 2012. Inclusion criteria included being between 21 and 82 years of age, not pregnant, and tobacco free. Several physiological and functional criteria were specified for exclusion.

Consecutive Sampling

A practical approach to convenience sampling is **consecutive sampling**, which involves recruiting all patients who meet the inclusion and exclusion criteria as they become available, often as they enter a clinic for care. The sample is usually defined by a time period within which patients become enrolled.

> Researchers looked at the effectiveness of screening spirometry for early identification of patients with chronic obstructive pulmonary disease (COPD) among a cohort of asymptomatic smokers.[25] Data were obtained by recruiting subjects consecutively as they participated in a routine screening examination. Participants had to be ≥30 years old with a smoking history of ≥5 pack-years. Exclusions included a prior diagnosis of asthma, COPD, or another chronic respiratory condition.

Use of Volunteers

The use of volunteers is also a commonly used convenience sampling method because of its expedience. Researchers who put up signs in schools or hospitals to recruit subjects with specific characteristics are sampling by this method.

> A study was done to determine whether a 6-week educational program on memory training, physical activity, stress reduction, and healthy diet could improve memory performance in older adults.[26] Researchers recruited a volunteer sample by posting advertisements and flyers in two continuing care retirement communities. To be eligible, participants had to be at least 62 years of age, living independently, and expressing complaints about memory loss. They were excluded if they had a history of dementia or were unable to exercise.

The major limitation of this method is the potential bias of *self-selection*. It is not possible to know which attributes are present in those who offer themselves as subjects, as compared with those who do not, and it is unclear how these attributes may affect the ability to generalize experimental outcomes. Those who volunteered for the memory study may be atypical of the target population in terms of motivation, prior activity level, family history, and other correlates of health. It is also not possible to know if those interested in participating were those who did or did not already experience memory problems.

Although all samples, even random samples, are eventually composed of those who participate voluntarily, those who agree to be part of a random sample were not self-selected. Therefore, characteristics of subjects in a random sample can be assumed to represent the target population. This is not necessarily a safe assumption with volunteer samples.

Quota Sampling

Nonprobability sampling can also incorporate elements of stratification. Using a technique called **quota sampling**, a researcher can control for the potential confounding effect of known characteristics of a population by guiding the sampling process so that an adequate number of subjects are obtained for each stratum. This approach requires that each stratum is represented in the same proportion as in the population. The difference between this method and stratification is the lack of random selection. There is an assumption that the quota sample is representative on the factors that are used as strata, but not on other factors that cannot be accounted for. Although this method still faces the potential for nonprobability biases, it does improve on the process by proportionally representing each segment of the population in the sample.

Purposive Sampling

A third nonprobability approach is **purposive sampling**, in which the researcher hand-picks subjects on the basis of specific criteria. The researcher may locate subjects by chart review or interview patients to determine if they fit the study. A researcher must exercise fair judgment to make this process meaningful.

> Because of the health consequences of excessive alcohol use in older adults, researchers were interested in gaining an in-depth understanding of experiences of and attitudes toward support for alcohol-related health issues in people aged 50 and over.[27] They designed a qualitative study that included in-depth interviews of 24 participants. Staff from several local alcohol service clinics identified clients of various ages, varied self-reported drinking habits, and both genders, and invited them to participate.

Purposive sampling is similar to convenience sampling but differs in that specific choices are made, rather than simple availability. This approach has the same limitations to generalization as a convenience sample in that it can result in a biased sample. However, in many instances, purposive sampling can yield a sample that will be representative of the population if the investigator wisely chooses individuals who represent the spectrum of population characteristics.[28]

> 📌 Purposive samples are commonly used in qualitative research to assure that subjects have the appropriate knowledge and will be good informants for the study (see Chapter 21).[29]

Snowball Sampling

Snowball sampling is a method that is often used to study sensitive topics, rare traits, personal networks, and social relationships. This approach is carried out in stages. In the first stage, a few subjects who meet selection criteria are identified and tested or interviewed. In the second stage, these subjects are asked to identify others they know who have the requisite characteristics. This process of "chain referral" or "snowballing" is continued until an adequate sample is obtained. The researcher must be able to verify the eligibility of each respondent to ensure a representative group.[30,31]

Snowball sampling is used extensively, for example, in studies involving individuals who are difficult to identify, such as homeless persons, substance abusers, or individuals with mental health issues.[32–35] This approach also lends itself well to qualitative studies, especially when dealing with sensitive topics.[36]

> Researchers were interested in understanding the causes and effects of postpartum depression.[37] They recruited 13 mothers through a hospital network who complained of feeling depressed after giving birth. These 13 mothers assisted by referring 17 other mothers to the study. Inclusion criteria included self-identification as postpartum depressed and giving birth within the past year. Mothers were excluded if they had a former history of depression.

As this example illustrates, snowball sampling is most useful when the population of interest is rare, unevenly distributed, hidden, or hard to reach.

COMMENTARY

All generalizations are false, including this one.

—Mark Twain (1835–1910)

American writer and humorist

With all apologies to Mark Twain, without the ability to generalize, research would be a futile activity. However, generalization is an "ideal," a goal that requires a leap from a derived sample to a defined population. Even though random selection is the best way to assure a representative sample, it does require a large enough sample to truly characterize a population. The reality is that final samples are seldom truly random and our assumptions are, therefore, always flawed to some extent.

For clinical studies, particularly those focused on comparing interventions, the main purpose is not application to the population, but more so on whether the treatment works. The primary concern is avoiding bias in comparing groups to each other, rather than comparing the sample to the population. For example, research has shown that criteria for choosing participants for an randomized controlled trial (RCT) are highly selective and, therefore, samples tend to exclude patients with comorbidities.[38] This effectively eliminates many of the patients who are typically seen in a healthcare practice. From an evidence-based practice perspective, this limits the understanding of how treatments may be relevant to a particular patient. PCTs, introduced in Chapter 2, have broad inclusion and fewer exclusion criteria, with a goal of recruiting subjects who represent the full spectrum of the population for which treatment will be used.[39,40] Samples can still be chosen at random, but they may have broader criteria, allowing for better generalization. The implications of RCTs and PCTs will be addressed in future chapters.

REFERENCES

1. Katon W, Lyles CR, Parker MM, Karter AJ, Huang ES, Whitmer RA. Association of depression with increased risk of dementia in patients with type 2 diabetes: the Diabetes and Aging Study. *Arch Gen Psychiatry* 2012;69(4):410–417.
2. Mahmood SS, Levy D, Vasan RS, Wang TJ. The Framingham Heart Study and the epidemiology of cardiovascular disease: a historical perspective. *Lancet* 2014;383(9921):999–1008.
3. Dawber TR, Meadors GF, Moore FE, Jr. Epidemiological approaches to heart disease: the Framingham Study. *Am J Public Health Nations Health* 1951;41(3):279–281.
4. Dufouil C, Beiser AS, McClure LA, Wolf PA, Tzourio C, Howard VJ, et al. A revised Framingham stroke risk profile to reflect temporal trends. *Circulation* 2017;135(12):1145–1159.
5. Menz HB, Dufour AB, Riskowski JL, Hillstrom HJ, Hannan MT. Foot posture, foot function and low back pain: the Framingham Foot Study. *Rheumatology* 2013;52(12):2275–2282.
6. Kalichman L, Li L, Kim DH, Guermazi A, Berkin V, O'Donnell CJ, et al. Facet joint osteoarthritis and low back pain in the community-based population. *Spine (Phila Pa 1976)* 2008;33(23):2560–2565.
7. Guccione AA, Felson DT, Anderson JJ, Anthony JM, Zhang Y, Wilson PW, et al. The effects of specific medical conditions on the functional limitations of elders in the Framingham Study. *Am J Public Health* 1994;84(3):351–358.
8. Wilson PW, Meigs JB, Sullivan L, Fox CS, Nathan DM, D'Agostino RB, Sr. Prediction of incident diabetes mellitus in middle-aged adults: the Framingham Offspring Study. *Arch Intern Med* 2007;167(10):1068–1074.
9. D'Agostino RB, Kannel WB: Epidemiological background and design: The Framingham Study. Proceedings of the American Statistical Association Sesquicentennial Invited Paper Sessions, 1988–1989. Available at https://biolincc.nhlbi.nih.gov/static/studies/framcohort/Epidemiological_Background_and_Design.pdf. Accessed March 17, 2017.
10. Feinleib M. The Framingham Study: Sample selection, follow-up and methods of analysis. National Cancer Institute Monograph No. 67, 1985. National Center for Health Statistics, Hyattsville, MD.
11. Wong ND, Levy D. Legacy of the Framingham heart study: rationale, design, initial findings, and implications. *Glob Heart* 2013;8(1):3–9.
12. ARIC Investigators. The Atherosclerosis Risk in Communities (ARIC) study: design and objective. *Am J Epidemiol* 1989;129(5):687–702.
13. Fried LP, Borhani NO, Enright P, Furberg CD, Gardin JM, Kronmal RA, et al. The Cardiovascular Health study: design and rationale. *Ann Epidemiol* 1991;1(3):263–276.
14. Friedman GD, Cutter GR, Donahue RP, Hughes GH, Hulley SB, Jacobs DR, Jr., et al. CARDIA: study design, recruitment, and some characteristics of the examined subjects. *J Clin Epidemiol* 1988;41(11):1105–1116.
15. Knuiman MW, Vu HT. Prediction of coronary heart disease mortality in Busselton, Western Australia: an evaluation of the Framingham, national health epidemiologic follow up study, and WHO ERICA risk scores. *J Epidemiol Comm Health* 1997;51(5):515–519.
16. Friedman LM, Furberg CD, DeMets DL. *Fundamentals of Clinical Trials*. 4 ed. New York: Springer, 2010.
17. Velicer WF, Keller S, Friedman RH, Fava JL, Gulliver SB, Ward RM, et al. Comparing participants and nonparticipants recruited for an effectiveness study of nicotine replacement therapy. *Ann Behav Med* 2005;29(3):181–191.
18. Moura LM, Schwamm E, Moura Junior V, Seitz MP, Hsu J, Cole AJ, et al. Feasibility of the collection of patient-reported outcomes in an ambulatory neurology clinic. *Neurology* 2016;87(23):2435–2442.
19. CONSORT (CONsolidated Standards of Reporting Trials) 2010 guidelines. Available at http://www.consort-statement.org/consort-2010. Accessed March 14, 2017.
20. Sampling bias. Wikipedia. Available at https://en.wikipedia.org/wiki/Sampling_bias. Accessed March 14, 2017.
21. Babbie ER. *Survey Research Methods*. Belmont, CA: Wadsworth, 1973.
22. National Center for Health Statistics, Centers for Disease Control and Prevention: *National Health and Nutrition Examination Survey*. Available at https://www.cdc.gov/nchs/nhanes/. Accessed March 15, 2017.
23. Pew Research Center: Sampling. Random digit dialing. Available at http://www.pewresearch.org/methodology/u-s-survey-research/sampling/. Accessed May 27, 2018.
24. Weinstein AA, Chin LM, Keyser RE, Kennedy M, Nathan SD, Woolstenhulme JG, et al. Effect of aerobic exercise training on fatigue and physical activity in patients with pulmonary arterial hypertension. *Respir Med* 2013;107(5):778–784.
25. Wisnivesky J, Skloot G, Rundle A, Revenson TA, Neugut A. Spirometry screening for airway obstruction in asymptomatic smokers. *Aust Fam Physician* 2014;43(7):463–467.
26. Miller KJ, Siddarth P, Gaines JM, Parrish JM, Ercoli LM, Marx K, et al. The memory fitness program: cognitive effects of a healthy aging intervention. *Am J Geriatr Psychiatry* 2012;20(6):514–523.
27. Haighton C, Wilson G, Ling J, McCabe K, Crosland A, Kaner E. A qualitative study of service provision for alcohol related health issues in mid to later life. *PLoS One* 2016;11(2):e0148601.
28. Hahn GJ, Meeker WQ. Assumptions for statistical inference. *Am Statistician* 1993;47:1–11.
29. Palinkas LA, Horwitz SM, Green CA, Wisdom JP, Duan N, Hoagwood K. Purposeful sampling for qualitative data collection and analysis in mixed method implementation research. *Adm Policy Ment Health* 2015;42(5):533–544.
30. Biernacki P, Waldorf D. Snowball sampling: problems and techniques of chain referral sampling. *Sociol Methods Res* 1981;10:141.
31. Lopes CS, Rodriguez LC, Sichieri R. The lack of selection bias in a snowball sampled case-control study on drug abuse. *Int J Epidemiol* 1996;25:1267–1270.
32. Barati M, Ahmadpanah M, Soltanian AR. Prevalence and factors associated with methamphetamine use among adult substance abusers. *J Res Health Sci* 2014;14(3):221–226.
33. Orza L, Bewley S, Logie CH, Crone ET, Moroz S, Strachan S, et al. How does living with HIV impact on women's mental health? Voices from a global survey. *J Int AIDS Soc* 2015;18(Suppl 5):20289.
34. Boys A, Marsden J, Strang J. Understanding reasons for drug use amongst young people: a functional perspective. *Health Educ Res* 2001;16(4):457–469.
35. Heimer R, Clair S, Grau LE, Bluthenthal RN, Marshall PA, Singer M. Hepatitis-associated knowledge is low and risks are high among HIV-aware injection drug users in three US cities. *Addiction* 2002;97(10):1277–1287.
36. Goncalves JR, Nappo SA. Factors that lead to the use of crack cocaine in combination with marijuana in Brazil: a qualitative study. *BMC Public Health* 2015;15:706.
37. Ugarriza DN. Postpartum depressed women's explanation of depression. *J Nurs Scholarsh* 2002;34(3):227–233.
38. Kennedy-Martin T, Curtis S, Faries D, Robinson S, Johnston J. A literature review on the representativeness of randomized controlled trial samples and implications for the external validity of trial results. *Trials* 2015;16:495.
39. Godwin M, Ruhland L, Casson I, MacDonald S, Delva D, Birtwhistle R, et al. Pragmatic controlled clinical trials in primary care: the struggle between external and internal validity. *BMC Med Res Methodol* 2003;3:28.
40. Tunis SR, Stryer DB, Clancy CM. Practical clinical trials: increasing the value of clinical research for decision making in clinical and health policy. *JAMA* 2003;290(12):1624–1632.

CHAPTER

14

Principles of Clinical Trials

A clinical trial is a study designed to test hypotheses about comparative effects. Trials are based on experimental designs, within which the investigator systematically introduces changes into natural phenomena and then observes the consequences of those changes. The randomized controlled trial (RCT) is the standard explanatory design, intended to support a cause-and-effect relationship between an intervention (the independent variable) and an observed response or outcome (the dependent variable).

The purpose of this chapter is to describe the basic structure of clinical trials using the RCT as a model and to discuss the important elements that provide structure and control for both explanatory and pragmatic studies.

■ Types of Clinical Trials

One of the most important influences in the advancement of scientific research over the past 60 years has been the development of the clinical trial as a prospective experiment on human subjects (see Box 14-1). Clinical trials have been classified as *explanatory*, focusing on efficacy, and *pragmatic* designs, focusing on effectiveness, differing in their degree of internal control and external generalizability (see Chapter 2). The National Institutes of Health (NIH) define a clinical trial as:

A research study in which one or more human subjects are prospectively assigned to one or more interventions

(which may include placebo or other control) to evaluate the effects of those interventions on health-related biomedical or behavioral outcomes.[1]

Trials are primarily conducted to evaluate therapies, diagnostic or screening procedures, or preventive strategies.

- *Therapeutic trials* examine the effect of a treatment or intervention on a particular disease or condition.

Begun in the 1970s, 25 years of clinical trials have shown that radical mastectomy is not necessary for reducing the risk of recurrence or spread of breast cancer, and that limited resection can be equally effective in terms of recurrence and mortality.[2]

- *Diagnostic trials* help to establish the accuracy of tests to identify disease states. Although these tests are often assessed using observational studies based on comparison with a reference standard, clinical trials can establish a test's clinical importance and its relative efficacy and efficiency against similar tests.[3]

Randomized trials have compared selective tests for suspected deep venous thrombosis (DVT), showing that different strategies can be used with equal accuracy.[4]

- A *preventive trial* evaluates whether a procedure or agent reduces the risk of developing a disease.

One of the most famous preventive trials was the field study of poliomyelitis vaccine in 1954, which covered 11 states.[5] The incidence of poliomyelitis in the vaccinated group was reduced by more than 50% compared to those receiving the placebo, establishing strong evidence of the vaccine's effectiveness.

Box 14-1   Clinical Trials Registries

Clinical trials registries are Web-based resources that catalog information on publicly and privately supported clinical studies. In the United States, *ClinicalTrials.gov* includes more than 300,000 trials.[6] Registries are also available in more than 20 countries.[7] The database was developed by NIH through the National Library of Medicine (NLM) in collaboration with the Food and Drug Administration (FDA), allowing broad availability of information to those with medical conditions, members of the public, healthcare providers, and researchers.

The intent of a clinical registry is to help patients find trials for which they may be eligible, to enhance the design of clinical trials, and to prevent duplication of unsuccessful or unsafe trials. It is also intended to improve the evidence base that informs clinical care, increase efficiency of drug and device development, improve clinical research practices, and build public trust in clinical research.[8]

Researchers can voluntarily register their studies when they begin using a Web-based entry system called the *Protocol Registration and Results System (PRS)*.[9] Not all studies must be registered, but those involving drug or device interventions are required to do so, and must also submit their results.[10] Researchers are responsible for updating and maintaining accuracy of information, such as when the study is recruiting subjects, when results are obtained, and when the study is complete. Protocols for trials are also published, giving details about study methods. Trials are assigned a number which can be used to search for specific studies and will be identified in PubMed citations.

⊚ FUN FACT

I actually participated in the original polio trial when I was in the first grade. I can remember standing outside the gym waiting in line for my shot with the other kids, feeling really nervous. Mostly I remember the lollipop I got and a little blue card stating that I was a "Polio Pioneer." Of course, I was bummed to find out later that I got the placebo and had to come back for another shot! But at least I got another lollipop!

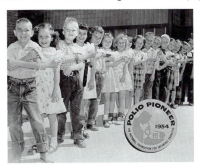

Source unknown.

The Randomized Controlled Trial

The **randomized controlled trial (RCT)** is considered the gold standard for experimental research because its structure provides a rigorous balance to establish cause-and-effect relationships. From an evidence-based practice perspective, the RCT is generally considered the highest form of evidence to support an intervention.

The basic structure of an RCT includes two groups, each getting a different treatment condition, with measurements taken before and after intervention to compare outcomes (see Fig. 14-1). The different groups within an RCT may be designated as experimental and control groups. They are also referred to as the **treatment arms** of the study. When two independent groups are compared in this way, the design is also considered a **parallel group** study. An RCT qualifies as a true experiment because of three requisite design characteristics: manipulation of independent variables, random assignment, and the use of a control group.

Several variations of the RCT are possible, and these will be described in Chapter 16.

■ Manipulation of Variables

Manipulation of variables refers to a deliberate operation performed by the investigator, imposing a set of predetermined experimental conditions, the independent variable, on at least two groups of subjects. The

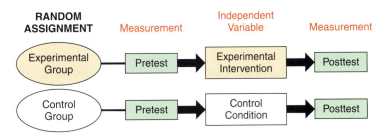

Figure 14–1 Basic structure of an RCT.

experimenter manipulates the levels of the independent variable by assigning subjects to varied conditions, usually administering the intervention to one group and withholding it from another.

> ➤ **CASE IN POINT #1**
>
> The *CopenHeart_VR Trial* was done to explore the effect of cardiac rehabilitation on physical capacity and mental health of patients following heart valve replacement (VR) surgery.[11] A 12-week rehabilitation program consisting of physical exercise and educational consultations was compared to usual care without structured physical exercise or education. The primary outcome was physical capacity measured by VO_2 peak, and a secondary outcome was self-reported mental health as measured by the mental component scale (MCS) of the Short Form-36 (SF-36) health status questionnaire. Patients were followed for 24 months, measured at six time points.

In this cardiac rehabilitation example, investigators incorporated two levels of the independent variable—exercise/education and usual care—and were able to assign the treatment conditions to two groups of patients.

📌 The acronym **PICO**, introduced in Chapter 3, is applied to clinical trials to designate the population being studied (**P**), intervention (**I**) and comparison (**C**) (levels of the independent variable), and the dependent variable or outcome (**O**). For the CopenHeart_VR Trial,

P = patients with valve replacement surgery
I = exercise/education
C = usual care
O = physical capacity and mental health

Active and Attribute Variables

Independent variables can be distinguished as either active or attribute factors. An **active variable** is one that is manipulated by the experimenter so that subjects are assigned to levels of the independent variable.

> ➤ In the cardiac study, patients were assigned to receive the exercise/education program or usual care. Therefore, treatment was an active variable.

An **attribute variable** is a factor that cannot be assigned because it is an inherent characteristic of the participants, such as age, gender, or diagnosis. Attribute variables cannot be manipulated by the experimenter. Therefore, when only the effect of one or more attribute variables is studied, the research cannot be considered a true experiment. If active and attribute variables are combined in one study, it would qualify as an

experiment because the researcher is able to manipulate the assignment of treatment levels for at least one independent variable.

■ Random Assignment

In Chapter 13, we discussed the importance of random *selection* for choosing subjects for a sample to ensure representation of the target population. Once a sample is selected, it is important to continue the process of randomization in *assigning* subjects to groups. **Random assignment**, also called **random allocation**, means that each subject has an equal chance of being assigned to any group.

Random assignment is an essential feature of an RCT (as its name clearly implies), providing the greatest confidence that no systematic bias exists with respect to a group's collective attributes that might differentially affect the dependent variable. If we can assume that groups are equivalent at the start of an experiment, then we can have confidence that differences observed at the end of the study are due to the experimental intervention and not other confounding factors.

Balancing Out Variability

The concept of random assignment means that groups are as much alike as possible at the start, making the independent variable the only substantive difference between them. This does not mean that every subject in one group is exactly equal to another subject in the other group. It does mean that any differences between the groups have been distributed as a function of chance alone. We can think of subjects as composites of personal characteristics such as motivation, intellectual ability, attitude, medical history, and so on. With random assignment, subjects with high or low values of these variables are just as likely to be assigned to one group or the other.

Random assignment is also expected to control for random events that might affect subjects during the course of the study. For instance, subjects in both groups should be equally likely to experience illness, scheduling problems, or any other nonsystematic event that might affect the dependent variable. Thus, *overall*, intersubject differences should balance out.

Baseline Characteristics

Although random assignment should balance study groups, it does not guarantee that groups will be similar at baseline. The concept of randomization is theoretical in that it applies to the probability of outcomes in the proverbial "long run." In other words, if we use random assignment to divide an infinitely large sample, the groups' average scores should not be different. However, because clinical samples tend to be limited in size, random assignment could result in groups that are quite disparate on certain important properties.

Researchers often use statistical means to compare groups on initial values that are considered relevant to the dependent variable to determine if the allocation plan did balance out extraneous factors.

▶ In the cardiac study, investigators gathered data on the two treatment groups upon enrollment, looking at age, gender, type of surgery, classification of heart disease at baseline, and a variety of comorbid conditions and physiological measures. They were then able to establish that the baseline values were balanced across the two groups.

When random assignment does not successfully balance the distribution of intersubject differences, there are several design and statistical strategies that can be used (see Chapter 15). This issue is only relevant, however, if characteristics influence treatment outcomes. In that case, a stratified randomization strategy, to be described shortly, can be used.

Assigning Subjects to Groups

Once a sample has been chosen, and subjects have agreed to participate following informed consent, a randomization scheme must be implemented to assure that assignment to groups is unbiased. The process of assigning subjects to groups can be carried out in several ways (see Table 14-1).

Simple Random Assignment

In **simple random assignment**, every member of the population has an equal chance of being chosen for either group. Many computer programs can generate random sequences to simplify this process.

▶ Researchers for the CopenHeart_{VR} Trial recruited subjects by approaching eligible patients 2 days following surgery to invite them to participate.[12] For those who consented, baseline measures were taken within 5 days post-surgery, and patients were randomly allocated to groups using a computer-generated sequence carried out by a centralized trials registry.

With smaller samples, a table of random numbers can also be used. To illustrate this process, we will use a portion of a table, shown in Table 14-2. Suppose we have a sample of 18 subjects and we want to assign them to two treatment groups, 1 (experimental) and 2 (control). The simplest approach is to create a stack of 18 sequentially numbered envelopes, each with a blank slip of paper.

We enter the table anywhere by placing our finger randomly at one spot—for this example, we will start at the second digit in row two (in red). Because we only have two groups, and digits run from 0 to 9, we will arbitrarily designate group 1 as odd and group 2 as even (ignoring zeros). Therefore, since our first number is 2,

Table 14-1	Summary of Random Assignment Strategies
Simple Random Assignment	Each member of the population has an equal chance of being chosen. Subjects are assigned to groups using a form of randomization.
Block Random Assignment	Subjects are randomly divided into even-numbered subgroups, called blocks. Within each block, subjects are randomly assigned to treatment arms. This assures an equal number of subjects within each treatment group.
Stratified Random Assignment	Members of the population are grouped by a relevant characteristic into different strata. Members within each stratum are then randomly assigned to groups, assuring that each group has a similar number of subjects from each stratum.
Cluster Random Assignment	Clusters of subjects are identified, typically by site. Each site is randomly assigned to a treatment group and all individuals at that site get the same treatment.
Random Consent Design	Potential subjects are assigned randomly to groups before seeking consent to participate. Only those assigned to the experimental group are approached for consent. Those assigned to standard care do not supply consent. Outcomes for both groups are compared.[15]
Assignment by Patient Preference	Subjects are given a choice of experimental interventions. Those who express no preference are randomly assigned to either group and their results examined. Those who express a preference are assigned to that treatment and their results are analyzed separately.
Run-In Period	As a way of assuring compliance, all subjects are given a placebo during a run-in period. They are monitored to determine adherence to the protocol. Only those who comply are then randomized to be part of the study.

Table 14-2	Random Numbers Table		
61415	00948	80901	36314
62758	49516	23459	23896
50235	20973	19272	66903
78049	46489	29853	30228
75380	06409	99961	21275

A complete version of a random numbers table can be found in Appendix Table A-6.

we will write "control" on a slip of paper and put it in the envelope numbered 1. The next digit is 7, so we write "experimental" on a slip of paper and put it in the second envelope. This process continues until all 18 envelopes are filled. The list of subjects is numbered and, as each one enters the trial, their envelope is opened to reveal their group assignment.

📌 If we had more than two groups, we could use the random numbers table a little differently. Suppose we have four groups. We locate all digits of 1, 2, 3, and 4 in the table (ignoring other digits). We would then assign subjects to groups as the digits occur. For instance, using Table 14-2, the first six subjects would be assigned to groups 2, 4, 1, 2, 3, 4, and so on.

 Random assignment must be distinguished from *random selection* (see Chapter 13). Random assignment can occur with or without random selection.

Block Randomization

The problem with simple random assignment is that it is possible to arrive at an uneven group allocation. In fact, if we continued with the method above, we would actually end up with 10 subjects in group 1 and 8 in group 2. If we want to assure that groups will be equal in number, we can use a process called **block randomization**, which distributes subjects evenly among treatment groups within small, even-numbered subgroups or "blocks."[14,15]

For example, with two groups, we can designate blocks of two, and the 18 envelopes are divided into two piles of 9. After the first envelope in pile 1 is filled, the first envelope in pile 2 is automatically assigned to the opposite group. This continues for each pair of envelopes, thereby assuring that the groups will be evenly distributed. Larger blocks can be designated for larger samples or with more than two groups. The cardiac rehabilitation study used this method with varying block sizes of eight, six, and four subjects.[11]

Specific sequences of assignments can also be designated in advance for each block. For instance, with blocks of four, subject assignments can cycle through each unique sequence: ABAB, AABB, ABBA, BAAB, and so on.[15]

Stratified Random Assignment

When a particular characteristic is considered a potential confounder in the comparison of treatments, one effective strategy is to stratify the sample on that variable. For example, if an intervention affects men and women differently, gender becomes a confounding variable. Therefore, rather than hope that random assignment will evenly distribute subjects by gender, we can stratify the sample to assure an equal distribution. This technique was described for the *selection* of subjects for the sample (see Chapter 13) and can also be applied to the *assignment* of subjects to groups. **Stratified random assignment** is accomplished by first dividing subjects into strata, and then within each stratum randomly assigning them to groups.

▶ In the CopenHeart$_{VR}$ Trial, the sample was stratified by left ventricular ejection fraction (<45% vs ≤45%) and type of valve surgery prior to randomization into the two treatment arms.

This technique is especially useful with smaller samples, when simple random assignment may not assure a reasonable distribution of subjects on a relevant variable.

Cluster Random Assignment

A different randomization strategy can be employed when multisite studies are designed. Randomizing participants across settings can be logistically difficult and can present contamination problems if subjects assigned to different groups intermingle within a setting. To correct for this possibility, a **cluster random assignment** process can be used, whereby the site, representing a "cluster" of subjects, is randomly assigned to an intervention and all individuals at that site receive that treatment.

Occupational therapists in the U.K. wanted to evaluate the benefit of therapy in maintaining functional capacity in care home residents living with stroke-related disabilities.[16] They randomly assigned 228 care homes to receive either a 3-month targeted program of occupational therapy or usual care, resulting in a total sample of 1,042 participants. The primary outcome was the score on the Barthel Index of Activities of Daily Living, with data collected by blinded assessors.

This method is distinguished from simple random allocation because the clusters represent natural groupings. Although the clusters were randomized to treatment, the residents were the unit of analysis and outcomes were collected for each individual. At the point of random assignment, all residents within one home had an equal opportunity of being allocated to the intervention or control conditions. Clusters may be other types of naturally occurring groups, such as communities or clinical practice settings, that can be chosen at random to represent a large population.

Assignment by Patient Preference

Another common concern arises when participants consent to take part in a study but then withdraw after randomization when they get assigned to a treatment they do not want, or they may comply poorly. Those who get the treatment they wanted may comply better than average, biasing the treatment effect.

An alternative method is the use of a *partially randomized patient preference* approach, in which all participants are asked if they have a preference for one treatment condition and only patients who have no preference are randomized. The others are assigned to their preferred treatment arm.[17]

> Researchers studied the difference between oral and topical ibuprofen for chronic knee pain in people aged 50 years and older.[18] The primary outcome was the score on the Western Ontario and McMaster Universities (WOMAC) Osteoarthritis Index. Eligible patients in 26 general practices were approached and provided consent. They were then asked if they preferred one treatment or the other. Those who did not care were assigned in a randomized study and those who joined the preference arm selected their treatment. The data from the two studies were analyzed separately and compared.

Not surprisingly, the researchers found that, in the randomized study, groups looked similar at baseline, but this was not the case for the preference groups. By essentially carrying out two studies, they were able to look at a controlled situation and to examine results under more pragmatic conditions that might be considered more like a true clinical experience where patients do get to choose treatments.[19] Obviously, the potential for bias must be considered with preference groups and separate analyses should be carried out.[17]

Randomized Consent Design

The process of random assignment in clinical trials is often seen as problematic for participants who are reluctant to give informed consent without knowing if they will be assigned to a treatment or control group. To address this issue, Marvin Zelen, a statistician, proposed an alternative approach called a **randomized consent design** (also called a *Zelen design*), which involves randomizing participants to experimental treatment or standard care prior to seeking consent and then only approaching those who will be assigned to the experimental intervention.[13] Those who will receive standard care do not supply consent.

> Researchers were interested in the effect of a personalized program of physical and occupational therapy on disability for patients with systemic sclerosis.[20] The experimental intervention was a 1-month individualized program of standardized exercises and splinting, followed by home visits. This was compared with usual care based on physician management. The primary outcome was performance on the Heath Assessment Questionnaire Disability Index (HAQ-DI) at 12 months. Patients from four clinical centers were assigned to the experimental or usual care group by an independent statistician. Only those assigned to the experimental group were informed about the study and asked to provide consent. All others received their standard care.

The researchers used a Zelen design to avoid the possibility that those assigned to usual care would feel they were getting less than optimal care and seek more rigorous exercise opportunities.

A main reason for using this approach is to limit bias in recruitment, as those who prefer one treatment may withdraw once they learn of their assignment.[21] It has not been used extensively, however, and remains controversial, primarily because of ethical concerns.[22,23] Zelen[13] addresses this concern by suggesting that every patient expects to get the best standard of care and therefore usual care patients are receiving the therapy they would otherwise have gotten.

Run-In Period

Investigators are often concerned about participants being cooperative, motivated. and adherent to study protocols. One way to ensure an efficient trial is to establish a **run-in period**, during which all subjects receive a placebo. Only those who demonstrate that they can adhere to the regimen are then randomized to be part of the study.[24] This approach has been useful to reduce dropout, identifying issues that can improve compliance.[25] It may reduce sample size and can dilute or enhance the clinical applicability of the results of a clinical trial, depending on the patient group to whom the results will be applied.[26]

Allocation Concealment

An important component of a randomization scheme is **allocation concealment**, ensuring that group assignment is done without the knowledge of those involved in the experimental process, thereby providing another assurance that bias is not involved in group formation.

Evidence suggests that a breakdown in concealment can create a substantial bias in estimates of treatment effect.[27]

Concealment can be accomplished in several ways. A common method is the use of sealed envelopes that contain a participants' group assignment, described earlier, so that investigators are not involved in the assignment process. An alternative technique is the use of personnel from an external service that is separate from the research institution. They generate the sequence of assignments and call the participants so that researchers have no involvement.

> In the cardiac rehabilitation study, the allocation sequence was generated by the Copenhagen Trial Unit, a centralized agency that collaborates with researchers to foster clinical trials.[28] They maintained the patient assignment lists, which remained concealed from the investigators for the duration of the study.

■ Control Groups

An essential design strategy for ruling out extraneous effects is the use of a control group against which the experimental group is compared. Subjects in a control group may receive a placebo or sham treatment, a standard treatment that will act as a basis of comparison for a new intervention, or no intervention at all. To be effective, the difference between the groups should only be the essential element that is the independent variable.

Inactive Controls

A placebo control is similar in every way to the experimental treatment except that it does not contain the active component that comprises the intervention's action (see Box 14-2).[29] For a drug study, for example, a pill can look exactly like the actual medication but not contain the active ingredient.

A sham treatment is analogous to a placebo but is used when treatments require physical or mechanical intervention. A sham is similar to the active treatment but has a benign effect. With a mechanical device, for instance, it could be "going through the motions" of treatment application without actually turning the machine on.

For a physical activity, like an exercise program, researchers often incorporate an *attention control* group, which provides some type of social or educational activity for the control group, to rule out the possible impact of the exercise group's interaction or the attention that a treatment group would receive.

Wait List Controls

Another strategy is the use of a wait list control group in which the experimental treatment is delayed for the control subjects. The control subjects may be asked to refrain from any activities that would mimic the treatment and are measured as control subjects during the first part of the study. They are then scheduled to receive the treatment following completion of the study. This approach has appeal when it is considered unethical to deny treatment, as long as the delay is not of unreasonable length.[33]

Active Controls

The use of a placebo or sham may be unfeasible in clinical situations, for practical or ethical reasons. Therefore, clinical researchers often evaluate a new experimental treatment against active controls, which are conventional methods of care or established standards of practice. Active controls can be used to show the efficacy of a treatment that may have large placebo effects, or to demonstrate the equivalence or superiority of the new treatment compared to established methods.

 Comparative effectiveness research (CER), using pragmatic trials, is based on the head-to-head comparison of two treatments, not including a placebo. CER addresses the need to establish which treatments will work better for various types of patients. Usual care is typically the "control" condition.

Box 14-2   Uncertainty and Placebos

Placebo effects can occur with the use of placebos or sham treatments when the patient believes their assigned intervention is working. These effects may be psychological, but nonetheless may produce real changes that benefit the patient. The changes cannot, however, be attributed to the experimental intervention.[30]

There is an ethical concept in the design of clinical trials called equipoise, which means that we should only conduct trials under conditions of uncertainty when we do not already have sufficient evidence of the benefit of a treatment.[24] This concept also means that placebos must be used judiciously. The *Declaration* of Helsinki specifically states that placebos are permissible "when no proven intervention exists" or when a compelling scientific rationale for a placebo can be provided, with the assurance that control subjects will not be at risk.[31]

Trials should always include a comparison with standard care or other recognized interventions as one of the treatment arms, as long as such treatment is available.[32] It is also considered unethical to include an alternative therapy that is known to be inferior to any other treatment.[24]

Using an active control does not diminish the validity or usefulness of the study, but it does change the question to be asked of the data. Instead of assessing whether the new treatment *works*, this approach assesses whether the new treatment is more or less effective than standard methods. Typically, the standard treatment has previously been tested against a control, which is how it got to be the standard! These standards are usually incorporated into guidelines for a given condition.

> In the cardiac rehabilitation study, it would not be reasonable for patients postsurgery to receive no follow-up care. Therefore, the control group received standard care according to accepted guidelines for management of patients following heart valve surgery.[34]

■ Blinding

The potential for observation bias is an important concern in experimental studies. The participants' knowledge of their treatment status or the investigator's expectations can, consciously or unconsciously, influence performance or the recording and reporting of outcomes.

Protection against this form of bias is best achieved by **blinding**, also called *masking*, assuring that those involved in the study are unaware of a subject's group assignment. The strongest approach is a **double-blind study**, where neither the subjects nor the investigators know the identity of treatment groups until after data are collected.

The necessity for and feasibility of blinding depends on the nature of the experimental treatment and the response variables. To blind subjects, the control condition must be able to be offered as a placebo or sham, or it must not be distinguishable from an active control. To blind investigators, the treatment must be offered in an unobtrusive way. For many active rehabilitation and surgical procedures, for instance, this is not possible. In that case, a **single-blind study** can be carried out, where only the subject is blinded.

In its most complete form, a blind design can be triple or quadruple blinded by hiding the identity of group assignments from subjects, from those who provide treatment, from those who measure outcome variables, and from those who will reduce and analyze the data.[35] It is also advisable to blind those responsible for treatment and assessment from the research hypothesis so that they do not approach their tasks with any preconceived expectations and so that such knowledge cannot influence their interactions with the subjects. To whatever extent is possible within an experiment, blinding will substantially strengthen the validity of conclusions.

📌 Because the terminology used to describe blinding is not consistent, the design can be misunderstood. Rather than using "single" or "double" blind as a descriptor, guidelines suggest being specific as to whether participants, care givers, those who measure outcomes, or others involved in the research are blind to group assignment.[36]

Preserving Blinding

The technique of blinding requires that treatments be coded so that, when data collection is complete, the code can be broken and group assignments revealed. The codes should be kept secure, either locked away or offsite, so that there is no access to those on the research team. Because the potential for biases in data collection is so strong, blindness should be rigorously and carefully preserved during the course of the study.

There are circumstances when researchers are obligated to *break the blind* code for a single patient when an adverse event has occurred that is considered relevant to the intervention being studied. When adverse events are not related to the study, the event should be handled without having to expose group assignment. The criteria for determining when "unmasking" is needed should be specified as part of the study protocol.[35]

Open-Label Trials

Sometimes it is not logistically or ethically reasonable to blind subjects or researchers to group assignments. In an **open-label trial** or *open trial*, both the researchers and participants know which treatment is being administered. Open label trials obviously create opportunities for bias.[37] **Detection bias**, also called *ascertainment bias*, can create a systematic difference in how outcomes are measured when assessors know group assignment. **Performance bias** occurs when there is a difference in the care that is provided or exposure to other factors outside the actual intervention, which can influence participants' behavior.

> In the CopenHeart$_{VR}$ Trial, clinicians and participants were not blinded. Because the intervention required physical activity, it was impossible to blind them to the rehabilitation program. The researchers did, however, blind the personnel who performed outcome assessments, data management, and all statistical analyses.

Open-label trials do have value in a pragmatic sense. Although they do not provide the same level of control as a blinded study, they do more accurately reflect usual care in clinical practice where both patients and providers are aware of treatment protocols. This can contribute to greater external validity, but with a tradeoff for decreased internal validity (see Chapter 15).[38]

■ Ideal Versus Pragmatic

The RCT Ideal

In the effort to control for confounding factors, and therefore have strong confidence in comparative data, RCTs incorporate two important restrictions in their design. The first is the strict and often broad specification of exclusion criteria for subjects, and the second is the specification of a standardized protocol so that the intervention and control conditions are administered in the same way to all participants within each group.

> ► Patients in the CopenHeart$_{VR}$ Trial were excluded if they had known ischemic heart disease prior to surgery, current participation in other rehabilitation programs, diseases of the musculoskeletal system, comorbidities affecting physical activity, pregnancy or breast feeding, or participation in competitive sports.
>   The intervention group received a standardized physical exercise program, which was comprised of 3 weekly sessions for 12 weeks. Adherence was monitored using programmed watches. All participants were engaged in the same protocol, which was identical across sites. The educational component was based on a prepared consultation guide, with five monthly sessions conducted by trained nurses.

These stipulations are essential control features to logically interpret outcomes in an RCT. But they present a challenge to clinicians who want to generalize the results of the study to their patients—people who have had valve replacement surgery, but who may also have various comorbidities that were excluded from this study, or who may not be fully adherent to a set protocol, both of which are real-life scenarios.

The Pragmatic Reality

Pragmatic clinical trials (PCTs), also called *practical clinical trials*, have several defining characteristics that counter RCT constraints.[39-41]

- The PCT incorporates a diverse patient population, with minimal exclusion criteria.
- Participants are recruited directly from various practice settings.
- Controls are active, often based on usual care or other commonly used interventions.
- Treatment proceeds as it would in typical clinical situations.
- Data collection focuses on important clinical outcomes such as patient satisfaction, quality of life, mobility and function.

This approach is based on the understanding that, when we apply treatments in practice, we do so without being able to control the environment, all treatment circumstances, or the characteristics of our patients. Therefore, our results may not be the same as those obtained with a randomized trial. PCTs allow for more direct application to clinical practice with stronger generalizability.

Importantly, however, PCTs still adhere to the basic principles of a controlled trial. They incorporate manipulation of the independent variables, using a randomization scheme to assign subjects, including allocation concealment strategies. They use a control condition, typically an active variable or usual care, and include blinding to the extent possible.

PCTs often incorporate analysis processes to correct for lack of adherence or other confounding that can take place because of naturally occurring practices. Their interpretation is more challenging because of heterogeneous samples and practice settings, but their data will have greater applicability to clinical practice (see Table 14-3).

Refer to a full discussion about PCTs and effectiveness research in Chapter 2.

 Pragmatic trials can also be designed using observational research approaches, rather than a randomized trial (see Chapter 19). These designs have been shown to have similar outcomes to randomized trials in many situations.[42]

The Pragmatic–Explanatory Continuum

Trials are rarely purely pragmatic or explanatory. There may be different levels of control incorporated into a design based on feasibility, such as the extent to which an intervention can be delivered in the exact same way for every subject, or the degree to which the researcher or participant adheres to the experimental protocol. Technically, an RCT violates its own design as soon as its first eligible patient refuses to be randomized. Therefore, rather than viewing these two approaches as a dichotomy, it is more reasonable to think about them along a continuum.

Thorpe et al[43] developed a tool called the *pragmatic–explanatory continuum indicator summary (PRECIS)* to provide a framework for estimating the degree to which a trial meets criteria for an explanatory or pragmatic trial. The tool is intended to provide guidance during planning stages for researchers to determine if the design meets their intended purpose, but may also be used to analyze a completed study to determine how well it met anticipated goals.

The tool is composed of a wheel with nine spokes, each representing one of the criteria for distinguishing

Table 14-3	Criteria for Distinguishing Explanatory and Pragmatic Trials	
CRITERION	**EXPLANATORY**	**PRAGMATIC**
Eligibility Criteria	Highly selective, stringent eligibility criteria, often restricted to those who are likely to respond to intervention, and excluding those at high risk with comorbidities.	Includes all participants who have the condition for which the intervention is intended, regardless of risk, responsiveness, comorbidities, or past compliance.
Flexibility of Experimental Intervention	Inflexible with strict instructions and protocols; monitored for consistency.	Highly flexible, with leeway for practitioners to determine how to best apply intervention to an individual patient.
Practitioner Expertise - Experimental Intervention	Intervention applied by researchers with training and documented expertise.	Intervention applied by full range of practitioners in typical clinical settings.
Flexibility of Comparison Intervention	Restricted flexibility; may use placebo instead of alternative or standard intervention.	Usual practice or alternative intervention.
Practitioner Expertise - Comparison Intervention	Practitioner has expertise in applying comparison for maximal benefit.	Applied by the full range of practitioners in typical clinical settings.
Follow-Up Intensity	Subjects followed with frequent updates.	May not include formal follow-up visits.
Outcomes	Primary outcome known to be a direct consequence of intervention; may be clinically meaningful, or may be a surrogate marker of a later anticipated outcome.	Primary outcome objectively measured and clinically meaningful to study participants, often including function, quality of life, and other relevant health outcomes.
Participant Compliance	Participant compliance with protocol monitored closely, and may be required to participate.	Unobtrusive or no measurement of compliance, and no special strategies to maintain compliance.
Practitioner Adherence to Protocol	Close monitoring of how well practitioners adhere to detailed protocol and procedures.	Unobtrusive or no measurement of practitioner adherence.
Primary Analysis	An intention-to-treat analysis is usually performed; may use per-protocol analysis, completer analysis, or other subgroup analyses.	Analysis uses intention-to-treat, including all patients regardless of compliance. All data included under usual conditions.

Adapted from Thorpe et al[43] and Gartlehner et al.[47]

between efficacy and effectiveness trials (see Table 14-3). Although varied scales have been used, each component is typically graded on a 4- or 5-point scale, scored 0 for explanatory characteristics at the center. The wider the web on the wheel, the more pragmatic the trial; the closer the web is to the hub of the wheel, the more the study has explanatory qualities (see Focus on Evidence 14-1). Scoring is based on judgments of researchers and has been evaluated for reliability.[44,45] Variations of the model have also been proposed.[46]

■ Phases of Clinical Trials

In the investigation of new therapies, including drugs, surgical procedures, and electromechanical devices, clinical trials are classified by phases. The sequential phases of trials are intended to provide different types of information about the treatment in relation to dosage, safety, and efficacy, with increasingly greater rigor in demonstrating the intervention's effectiveness and safety (see Fig. 14-2).[49] In early phases, the focus is on minimizing

Focus on Evidence 14–1
Explanatory or Pragmatic—or Somewhere in Between

The *pragmatic-explanatory continuum indicator summary (PRECIS)* provides a useful planning tool to help researchers assess the degree to which a study fits its intended purpose.[43] The figure shows results of a PRECIS analysis performed by an interprofessional team designing a study of intervention for pain-coping skills in patients undergoing total knee arthroplasty (TKA).[48] The team included investigators from biostatistics, internal medicine, orthopedic surgery,

physical therapy, psychology, and rheumatology, all with varying degrees of experience in RCTs and pragmatic trials.

The study was planned as a three-arm multicenter randomized trial. Patients were to be randomized to pain-coping skills training, an educational control condition, or usual care.

The team went through three rounds of analysis. The "initial" rating by individual investigators followed the development of a tentative study design. The "ideal" rating captured each investigator's own opinion about the best design, which showed a preference for a more pragmatic design. The "final" rating (in blue) reflected consensus among the team on the final design.

The results showed that the final design was closer to an explanatory study than pragmatic, with several items close to the hub of the wheel. For example, the rating for practitioner expertise in providing the experimental treatment ended up closer to explanatory than originally intended. Similarly, the researchers proposed eligibility criteria to be more flexible, but in the final design they agreed that, because this intervention had not been studied in this population before, they needed to be more restrictive in their sampling criteria.

These researchers found this visual approach to be particularly helpful in raising awareness of specific issues to consider in finalizing the design, several of which resulted in revisions from the original plan. Importantly, the graph shows that studies are not purely explanatory or pragmatic, and consideration must be given to all aspects of a study in terms of feasibility as well as desired outcomes.

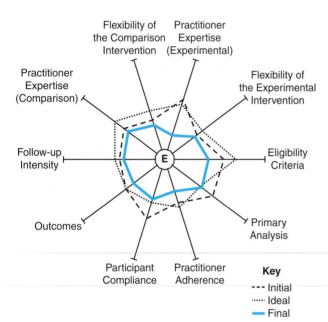

Key
- - - Initial
····· Ideal
—— Final

Adapted from Riddle DL, Johnson RE, Jensen MP, et al. The Pragmatic-Explanatory Continuum Indicator Summary (PRECIS) instrument was useful for refining a randomized trial design: experiences from an investigative team. *J Clin Epidemiol* 2010;63(11):271–275. Figure 2, p. 1274. Used with permission.

---

risk to subjects and insuring that resources are used responsibly. Studies progress to establish efficacy and then to demonstrate effectiveness under real-world conditions—with the ultimate goal of establishing the intervention as a new standard.

The definitions of trial phases are not clearly distinct and there can be significant overlap, depending on the type of treatment being studied. Some trials will not fit neatly into one category and many will not specify a phase in their reports. The important element is the progression of evidence that either supports adoption or merits discontinuing a treatment based on sound comparisons and analyses.

At any point in this sequence, a trial may be stopped if adverse events become too common or if the treatment's

benefit is so clear that it warrants immediate implementation (see Focus on Evidence 14-2).

Trial phases were introduced as part of the description of translational research (see Fig. 2-1 in Chapter 2). It will be useful to review that information as a context for this discussion.

• Preclinical Phase

Before a new therapy is used on humans, it is tested under laboratory conditions, often using animal models, as part of **preclinical** or **basic research**. The purpose of this type of research is to explore if and how the new treatment works, and to establish its physiological properties or mechanism of action. When a new drug or device

A 10-Year Journey to Approval

Preclinical Research
In 2001, researchers investigated the effects of roflumilast on airway inflammation in guinea pigs and rats.[53] They found that the drug demonstrated a combination of bronchodilatory, antiallergic, and anti-inflammatory properties that supported its potential efficacy in humans.

Phase I Trials
Multiple phase I studies were conducted in healthy volunteers to establish the safety and dosage constraints of the drug.[54] Men and women between 18-45 years of age were tested in small cohorts of less than 20 subjects. Findings revealed no food interactions and no effect on blood pressure or lab values. Up to 2.5 mg was safe, but above 1.0 mg there were many side effects, including headache, dizziness, nausea, and diarrhea. The limit of tolerability appeared to be 1.0 mg dose.

Phase II Trials
A phase II trial was conducted with 516 patients with COPD. Using a randomized placebo-controlled study, results showed that roflumilast at 500 µg/day significantly improved FEV1 at 24 weeks compared with placebo.[55] Data continued to demonstrate safety and adverse effects of nausea.

Phase III Trials
In randomized, double-blind, placebo-controlled studies, roflumilast was able to stabilize or improve lung function in patients with COPD.[56] Once a day dose of 500 µg was most effective, and quality-of-life measures have also shown improvement.

Phase IV Trials
Phase IV studies have examined the effectiveness of roflumilast in patients with different levels of exacerbations. They found that the drug was most effective in improving lung function and reducing exacerbations in participants with frequent exacerbations and/or hospitalization episodes.[57] These trials have continued to document safety in the overall population.

Figure 14–2 Progression of the development of a new drug from preclinical to phase IV trials. Roflumilast (marketed as Daliresp® in the U.S.) was approved by the FDA in 2011 for treatment of moderate to severe chronic obstructive pulmonary disease (COPD).[56,58]

shows promise at this phase, researchers will then request permission to begin human trials from the FDA.

- **Phase I Trials**

Is the Treatment Safe?
In a **phase I trial**, researchers work to show that a new therapy is safe. The treatment is tested on small groups of people, usually around 20 healthy volunteers, to understand its mechanisms of action, determine a safe dosage range, and identify side effects.

- **Phase II Trials**

Does the Treatment Work?
Once a therapy has been shown to be safe in humans, it is studied in a **phase II trial** to explore its efficacy by measuring relevant outcomes. These trials continue to monitor adverse effects and optimal dosage. Also done on relatively small samples of 100 to 300 patients, these trials may take several years. Subjects in these

studies are patients with the condition the therapy is intended to treat.

These trials may be further classified as *phase IIa* to study dosage and *phase IIb* to focus on efficacy. These may be randomized, double-blind studies that include a placebo control, or they may focus on cohorts of patients who all receive varied dosages of a drug. Phase II trials tend to have a relatively low success rate, with only 31% moving on to a phase III trial in 2015.[50,51]

- **Phase III Trials**

How Does this Treatment Compare with Standard Care?
Phase III trials build on prior research to establish efficacy through randomized controlled studies, which may include thousands of patients in multiple sites over many years. These studies will compare the new treatment to standard care to confirm its effectiveness, monitor side effects, and continue to study varied dosages. Successful

Focus on Evidence 14–2
When Things Don't Go as Planned—for Better or Worse

When studies are scheduled to run for many years, independent *data monitoring boards* are tasked with reviewing data along the way to monitor for adverse effects. When evidence is accumulated that demonstrates an important health finding, these boards can make recommendations for early termination. Two prominent examples that have had significant influence on healthcare practice demonstrate the importance of this process for public health—for positive and negative reasons.

The Women's Health Initiative: Between 1993 and 1998, 16,608 postmenopausal women between 50 and 79 years of age were enrolled in the Women's Health Initiative (WHI) study of the risks and benefits associated with estrogen plus progestin therapy.[59] Women were randomly assigned to a daily dose of estrogen plus progestin or to a placebo, with a primary outcome of coronary heart disease (CHD). Hip fracture was designated as a secondary outcome and invasive breast cancer was considered a primary adverse outcome. The study was scheduled to run until 2005.

An interim review in 2002 revealed that, although there was a one-third reduction in hip fracture rates, there were between 20% to 40% increases in strokes, heart attacks, blood clots, and cardiovascular disease (CVD), as well as a 26% increase in the number of cases of invasive breast cancer in the group receiving hormone therapy.[60]

Therefore, after an average follow-up of 5.2 years, the National Heart, Lung and Blood Institute stopped the trial, stating that the evidence of overall health risks exceeded any benefits, and that this regimen should not be initiated or continued for primary prevention of CHD. The health risks for breast cancer were still observed 3 years following cessation of the study.[61]

The Physicians' Health Study: In 1982, 22,071 male physicians were recruited for a randomized study of the effect of aspirin and beta carotene on primary prevention of CVD and cancer.[62] Subjects were assigned to one of four groups: aspirin and beta carotene taken every other day, aspirin placebo and beta carotene, aspirin and beta carotene placebo, or aspirin placebo and beta carotene placebo. The trial was planned to run until 1995.

At the end of 1987, interim review of data showed an extreme beneficial effect on nonfatal and fatal myocardial infarction, with a 44% reduction in risk, specifically among those who were 50 years of age or older.[63] The effect was present at all levels of cholesterol, but greatest at lower levels. Therefore, a recommendation was made to terminate the aspirin component of the trial and participants were informed of their aspirin group assignment. Data for strokes and mortality were inconclusive because too few subjects demonstrated these endpoints. The trial continued for the beta carotene arm until the scheduled end in 1995, at which time it was established that the supplement provided neither benefit nor harm in terms of the incidence of malignant neoplasms, CVD, or death from all causes.[64]

---

outcomes will lead to seeking approval from the FDA or another agency as appropriate.

Although typically designed as RCTs, phase III trials may be developed as PCTs to better reflect the "real-world" effectiveness of the new treatment.[52]

- **Phase IV Trials**

What Else Do We Need to Know?

Sometimes called postmarketing trials, **phase IV trials** are done after an intervention has been approved. Their purpose is to gather information on the treatment's effect in various populations or subgroups, under different clinical conditions, to explore side effects associated with long-term use, and to learn about risk factors, benefits, and optimal use patterns. These studies may be randomized trials or observational studies.

> 🔑 Early trial phases are typically geared toward studies of drug therapies or devices that require approval by the FDA. Studies of many therapeutic treatments will not require documentation of safety or licensing, but will be more appropriate for phase III and IV studies to demonstrate effectiveness.

■ Comparing Treatments: Better or No Worse?

Clinical trials are driven by research hypotheses put forth at the start of the trial. These hypotheses will stipulate the expected outcome in a comparison between the experimental treatment and control condition. When an intervention is new and untested, this comparison may be made against a placebo to demonstrate that the treatment has an effect and is safe. Once that initial hurdle is passed, however, active comparisons are more common, typically against previously established therapies.

> 📌 There are three possible forms of hypotheses to be addressed when comparing new and established treatments:
> 1. New therapy is *better than* standard care.
> 2. New therapy is *no worse than* (at least as good as) standard care.
> 3. New therapy is *equivalent to* standard care (no better and no worse).

Superiority Trials

When the purpose of a clinical study is to show that one treatment is better than another, it is called a **superiority trial**. This is probably the most familiar goal of a clinical trial. Finding a significant difference between the treatment groups provides evidence that the experimental intervention is superior to the control condition.

> 📌 It is important to note that finding no significant difference does not mean the new treatment does not work—just that the evidence from the trial is not sufficient to show a difference. See Box 5-2 in Chapter 5 for a discussion of the distinction between *absence of evidence* and *evidence of absence*.

> ➤ The CopenHeart$_{VR}$ Trial is an example of a superiority trial. The researchers hypothesized that cardiac rehabilitation would improve physical capacity and mental health better than usual care in patients following heart valve surgery.

Non-Inferiority Trials

Over time, research has supported many advances in the provision of healthcare, making it harder to improve on already-established care standards.[65] Therefore, when a new treatment is proposed for a condition, it is not always with the intention that the outcome will be superior to established therapy. It may be with the purpose of showing that the new treatment is just as effective as the standard.

Typically, the reason for proposing a new treatment, then, is because of ancillary benefits—it is safer, costs less, is more efficient or convenient, has fewer side effects, and so on. Therefore, even if outcomes remain the same, the new therapy would be preferable. When the goal of a trial is to show that a new treatment is as good as standard care, it is classified as a **non-inferiority trial**.[66]

> ➤ **CASE IN POINT #2**
> Physical therapy (PT), comprised of stretching and strengthening exercises, is a common evidence-based nonpharmacologic intervention for chronic low back pain (cLBP).[67] Yoga has also been shown to be an effective intervention for this condition.[68] Saper et al[69] designed a randomized, single-blind, non-inferiority trial to study the effects of yoga, PT, and self-care education for adults with cLBP, hypothesizing that yoga would be non-inferior to PT and both would be superior to education alone.

Establishing Non-Inferiority

A well-designed non-inferiority trial that successfully shows no difference between treatments cannot be distinguished, on the basis of data alone, from a superiority trial that fails to find a true difference.[70] Therefore, non-inferiority trials must reduce the possibility of confounding through strong controls such as assuring compliance, reliability of measurements, and unbiased outcomes.

> Although blinding is a cornerstone of control for superiority trials, it is actually problematic for non-inferiority studies. In a superiority trial, blinded investigators cannot influence results by assuming that the experimental treatment is better. However, in a non-inferiority trial, blinding does not offer this same protection if investigators believe both treatments are comparable, as they could assign similar ratings to both groups.[70]

The Non-Inferiority Margin

Where superiority trials are based on statistically significant differences, showing that one treatment has a larger effect than the other, the non-inferiority trial has the opposite function—wanting to show no important difference—or more precisely, that the new treatment is *no worse* than standard care.

Because of the nature of clinical research and the variability among participants, statistical testing is always subject to some element of chance. Therefore, it is fundamentally impossible to prove that two treatments will have the same exact effect. The best we can do is to demonstrate that a new treatment will differ by no more than a specified amount from standard care. Therefore, the concept of "no worse" requires a definition in terms of a **non-inferiority margin**, or what would be the biggest negative difference that would be acceptable to consider the new treatment a reasonable substitute for the standard therapy (see Fig. 14-3). Any bigger negative difference would mean that the new treatment was not as good. Non-inferiority margins are determined by a researcher's judgment regarding the maximum difference that would represent no practical difference between effects.

There are two approaches to establishing the non-inferiority margin. One common method is based on the smallest amount of change in a variable that is considered meaningful, called the **minimal clinically important difference (MCID)** (see Chapters 10 and 32). To be conservative, researchers have used half or two-thirds of the MCID to designate a non-inferiority margin.[32,71,72] A second method of determining the non-inferiority margin involves the use of historical data from placebo-controlled trials of the standard treatment. This is often based on a fraction of the effect size difference, such as 50%, or the lower bound of a confidence interval.[71]

Difference in treatment effect

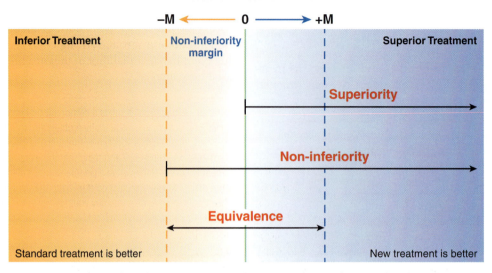

Figure 14–3 Relationship of superiority, non-inferiority, and equivalence trials. The negative and positive margins (-M and +M) represent the confidence intervals to establish the effect of the intervention.

 The primary outcomes in the cLBP study were changes in function measured on the modified Roland Morris Disability Questionnaire (RMDQ) and pain intensity on a 0 to 10 numerical scale. To demonstrate that yoga was *at least as good* as PT, researchers set a non-inferiority margin of 1.5 points on the RMDQ and 1 point on the pain scale, both derived by halving the MCIDs for these measures.

If you can get past the double negatives, this means that as long as the patients getting yoga had RMDQ scores that were no more than 1.5 points less than observed with PT, and pain scores no more than 1 point less than with PT, yoga would be considered non-inferior. The data showed that both yoga and PT were comparable, and both were better than self-care education.

Researchers try to be conservative about the specified margin to avoid the possibility of concluding that a new treatment is non-inferior when it is actually worse than standard care. This is why the preferred margin will be smaller than the MCID or documented effect sizes. Because the non-inferiority trial is only concerned about whether the new treatment performs *no worse* than the standard, the analysis will focus on one direction only.

 A conclusion of non-inferiority does not exclude a possible superiority of the tested treatment.[73]

For further discussion of statistical considerations in non-inferiority trials, see Chapter 23. MCID is discussed further in Chapter 32. For those interested in exploring analysis issues for non-inferiority trials, several good references are available.[66,72,74–76]

Equivalence Trials

A third type of trial is called an **equivalence trial**, which is focused on showing that the new treatment is no better and no worse than the standard therapy. This approach is used less often, primarily in what is called a *bioequivalence trial*, in which a generic drug is compared to the original commercial drug to show that they have the same pharmacokinetic properties.[76] These trials are not considered appropriate for therapeutic studies.[74]

Non-inferiority and equivalence trials are sometimes lumped under one classification as "equivalence trials" because they both focus on no difference between treatments. However, they are actually distinct and will use different analysis strategies.

COMMENTARY

An experiment is a question which science poses to Nature, and a measurement is the recording of Nature's answer.

—*Max Planck (1858-1947)*

German physicist, 1918 Nobel Prize in Physics

The rules of the "research road" for studies of interventions make clear the need to control for the effect of extraneous factors that can bias results. Clinicians understand, however, that such controls will often limit the ability to generalize findings to real patients and real treatment situations. This is especially true in rehabilitation contexts, for several reasons. The need for controls is problematic, as it would be unethical to deny adaptive activity to patients who require rehabilitation.[77] Another challenge is the inherent patient–clinician interaction that influences intervention and outcome, as well as the use of combinations of approaches that are used to develop treatment regimens.[78] In addition, treatments are not always protocol driven, requiring flexibility to meet unique patient needs. These issues have led to concerns about the feasibility of clinical trials in rehabilitation fields. Defining the active element of these interventions is much more difficult than characterizing a pharmacologic or surgical intervention. This presents a dilemma because clinical trials should allow replication of effectiveness by others.

Clinical trials are, however, necessary to build an evidence base for interventions and the use of this design is becoming more prevalent in rehabilitation.[79] Clinicians must consider the need to build treatments according to theory so that protocols can be designed according to standardized guidelines that would make it reproducible.[80–82] Although the specifics of the intervention may be personalized, the decision-making process can be made clear by delineating the rationale upon which treatments are based.[83] Using the *International Classification of Functioning, Disability and Health (ICF)* provides a consistent framework for delineating variables and choosing interventions and outcome measures.[84] Clinical trials will not be appropriate to answer every clinical question, but the PCT provides an important alternative to account for the real-time differences that will be encountered in clinical practice.

REFERENCES

1. National Institutes of Health. NIH's Definition of a Clinical Trial. Available at https://grants.nih.gov/policy/clinical-trials/definition.hrm. Accessed March 7, 2019.
2. Fisher B, Jeong JH, Anderson S, Bryant J, Fisher ER, Wolmark N. Twenty-five-year follow-up of a randomized trial comparing radical mastectomy, total mastectomy, and total mastectomy followed by irradiation. *N Engl J Med* 2002;347(8):567–575.
3. Rodger M, Ramsay T, Fergusson D. Diagnostic randomized controlled trials: the final frontier. *Trials* 2012;13:137.
4. Linkins L, Bates SM, Lang E, Kahn SR, Douketis JD, Julian Jet al. Selective D-dimer testing for diagnosis of a first suspected episode of deep venous thrombosis: A randomized trial. *Annals of Internal Medicine* 2013;158(2):93–100.
5. Francis T, Korns RF, Voight RB, Boisen M, Hemphill FM, Napier JA, et al. An evaluation of the 1954 poliomyelitis vaccine trials: summary report. *Am J Public Health* 1955;45(5, Part 2):1–63.
6. ClinicalTrials.gov. Available at https://clinicaltrials.gov/. Accessed April 31, 2018.
7. Office of Human Research Protections. Listing of clinical trial registries. Available at https://www.hhs.gov/ohrp/international/clinical-trial-registries/index/html. Accessed April 6, 2019.
8. Clinical trials and results information submission. Final Rule. *Fed Regist* 2016;81(183):64981-65157.
9. ClinicalTrials.gov. Protocol Registration and Results System. *PRS User's Guide.* Available at https://prsinfo.clinicaltrials.gov/prs-users-guide.html. Accessed April 6, 2019.
10. ClinicalTrial.gov. Checklist for evaluating whether a clinical trial or study is an application clinical trial (ACT). Available at https://prsinfo.clinicaltrials.gov/ACT_Checklist.pdf. Accessed April 6, 2019.
11. Sibilitz KL, Berg SK, Rasmussen TB, Risom SS, Thygesen LC, Tang L, et al. Cardiac rehabilitation increases physical capacity but not mental health after heart valve surgery: a randomised clinical trial. *Heart* 2016;102(24):1995–2003.
12. Sibilitz KL, Berg SK, Hansen TB, Risom SS, Rasmussen TB, Hassager C, et al. Effect of comprehensive cardiac rehabilitation after heart valve surgery (CopenHeartVR): study protocol for a randomised clinical trial. *Trials* 2013;14:104.
13. Zelen M. A new design for randomized clinical trials. *N Engl J Med* 1979;300(22):1242–1245.
14. Kim J, Shin W. How to do random allocation (randomization). *Clinics in Orthopedic Surgery* 2014;6(1):103–109.
15. Kepler CK. Randomization strategies. *Clin Spine Surg* 2017;30(3):120–121.
16. Sackley CM, Walker MF, Burton CR, Watkins CL, Mant J, Roalfe AK, et al. An occupational therapy intervention for residents with stroke-related disabilities in UK Care Homes (OTCH): cluster randomised controlled trial with economic evaluation. *Health Technol Assess* 2016;20(15):1–138.

17. Torgerson D, Sibbald B. Understanding controlled trials: what is a patient preference trial? *BMJ* 1998;316(7128):360.

18. Underwood M, Ashby D, Cross P, Hennessy E, Letley L, Martin J, et al. Advice to use topical or oral ibuprofen for chronic knee pain in older people: randomised controlled trial and patient preference study. *BMJ* 2008;336(7636):138–142.

19. Sedgwick P. What is a patient preference trial? *BMJ* 2013;347.

20. Rannou F, Boutron I, Mouthon L, Sanchez K, Tiffreau V, Hachulla E, et al. Personalized physical therapy versus usual care for patients with systemic sclerosis: a randomized controlled trial. *Arthritis Care Res* 2017;69(7):1050–1059.

21. Adamson J, Cockayne S, Puffer S, Torgerson DJ. Review of randomised trials using the post-randomised consent (Zelen's) design. *Contemp Clin Trials* 2006;27(4):305–319.

22. Homer CS. Using the Zelen design in randomized controlled trials: debates and controversies. *J Adv Nurs* 2002;38(2):200–207.

23. Torgerson DJ, Roland M. What is Zelen's design? *BMJ* 1998;316(7131):606.

24. Stanley K. Design of randomized controlled trials. *Circulation* 2007;115(9):1164–1169.

25. Fukuoka Y, Gay C, Haskell W, Arai S, Vittinghoff E. Identifying factors associated with dropout during prerandomization run-in period from an mHealth Physical Activity Education study: the mPED trial. *JMIR Mhealth Uhealth* 2015;3(2):e34.

26. Pablos-Mendez A, Barr RG, Shea S. Run-in periods in randomized trials: implications for the application of results in clinical practice. *JAMA* 1998;279(3):222–225.

27. Schulz KF, Grimes DA. Allocation concealment in randomised trials: defending against deciphering. *Lancet* 2002;359 (9306):614–618.

28. Centre for Clinical Intervention Research: Copenhagen Trial Unit. Available at http://www.ctu.dk/. Accessed March 24, 1017.

29. Sedgwick P, Hooper C. Placebos and sham treatments. *BMJ* 2015;351:h3755.

30. Kaptchuk TJ, Miller FG. Placebo effects in medicine. *New England Journal of Medicine* 2015;373(1):8–9.

31. WMA Declaration of Helsinki: Ethical Principles for Medical Research Involving Human Subjects. Amended October, 2013. Available at http://www.wma.net/en/30publications/10policies/b3/. Accessed March 27, 2017.

32. D'Agostino RB, Sr., Massaro JM, Sullivan LM. Non-inferiority trials: design concepts and issues – the encounters of academic consultants in statistics. *Stat Med* 2003;22(2):169–186.

33. Elliott SA, Brown JS. What are we doing to waiting list controls? *Behav Res Ther* 2002;40(9):1047–1052.

34. Butchart EG, Gohlke-Barwolf C, Antunes MJ, Tornos P, De Caterina R, Cormier B, et al. Recommendations for the management of patients after heart valve surgery. *Eur Heart J* 2005;26(22):2463–2471.

35. Food and Drug Administration: *Guidance for Industry. E9: Statistical Principles for Clinical Trials.* September, 1998. Available at https://www.fda.gov/downloads/drugs/guidancecompliance regulatoryinformation/guidances/ucm073137.pdf. Accessed March 23, 2017.

36. Moher D, Hopewell S, Schulz KF, Monton V, Gotzsche PC, Devereaux PJ, et al. CONSORT 2010 explanation and elaboration: updated guidelines for reporting parallel group randomised trials. *BMJ* 2010;340:c869.

37. Cochran Bias Methods Groups: Assessing risk of bias in included studies. Available at http://methods.cochrane.org/bias/assessing-risk-bias-included-studies. Accessed March 24, 2017.

38. Beyer-Westendorf J, Buller H. External and internal validity of open label or double-blind trials in oral anticoagulation: better, worse or just different? *J Thromb Haemost* 2011;9(11):2153–2158.

39. Horn SD, Gassaway J. Practice-based evidence study design for comparative effectiveness research. *Med Care* 2007;45(10 Supl 2):S50–S57.

40. Glasgow RE, Magid DJ, Beck A, Ritzwoller D, Estabrooks PA. Practical clinical trials for translating research to practice: design and measurement recommendations. *Med Care* 2005;43(6):551–557.

41. Tunis SR, Stryer DB, Clancy CM. Practical clinical trials: increasing the value of clinical research for decision making in clinical and health policy. *JAMA* 2003;290(12):1624–1632.

42. Bolland MJ, Grey A, Gamble GD, Reid IR. Concordance of results from randomized and observational analyses within the same study: a re-analysis of the Women's Health Initiative Limited-Access Dataset. *PLoS One* 2015;10(10):e0139975.

43. Thorpe KE, Zwarenstein M, Oxman AD, Treweek S, Furberg CD, Altman DG, et al. A pragmatic-explanatory continuum indicator summary (PRECIS): a tool to help trial designers. *CMAJ* 2009;180(10):E47–E57.

44. Glasgow RE, Gaglio B, Bennett G, Jerome GJ, Yeh HC, Sarwer DB, et al. Applying the PRECIS criteria to describe three effectiveness trials of weight loss in obese patients with comorbid conditions. *Health Serv Res* 2012;47(3 Pt 1):1051–1067.

45. Selby P, Brosky G, Oh PI, Raymond V, Ranger S. How pragmatic or explanatory is the randomized, controlled trial? The application and enhancement of the PRECIS tool to the evaluation of a smoking cessation trial. *BMC Med Res Methodol* 2012;12:101.

46. Loudon K, Treweek S, Sullivan F, Donnan P, Thorpe KE, Zwarenstein M. The PRECIS-2 tool: designing trials that are fit for purpose. *BMJ* 2015;350:h2147.

47. Gartlehner G, Hansen RA, Nissman D, Lohr KN, Carey TS. Criteria for distinguishing effectiveness from efficacy trials in systematic reviews. Technical Review 12. AHRQ Publication No. 06-0046. Rockville, MD: Agency for Healthcare Research and Quality. April, 2006. Available at https://www.ncbi.nlm.nih.gov/books/NBK44029/pdf/Bookshelf_NBK44029.pdf. Accessed March 27, 2017.

48. Riddle DL, Johnson RE, Jensen MP, Keefe FJ, Kroenke K, Bair MJ, et al. The Pragmatic-Explanatory Continuum Indicator Summary (PRECIS) instrument was useful for refining a randomized trial design: experiences from an investigative team. *J Clin Epidemiol* 2010;63(11):1271–1275.

49. US National Library of Medicine: FAQ: Clinical Trials.gov - Clinical Trial Phases. Available at https://www.nlm.nih.gov/services/ctphases.html. Accessed March 23, 2017.

50. Wechsler J: Low success rates persist for clinical trials. May 27, 2016. *Applied Clinical Trials*. Available at http://www.applied clinicaltrialsonline.com/low-success-rates-persist-clinical-trials. Accessed March 24, 2017.

51. Harrison RK. Phase II and phase III failures: 2013–2015. *Nat Rev Drug Discov* 2016;15(12):817–818.

52. Sonnad SS, Mullins CD, Whicher D, Goldsack JC, Mohr PE, Tunis SR. Recommendations for the design of Phase 3 pharmaceutical trials that are more informative for patients, clinicians, and payers. *Contemp Clin Trials* 2013;36(2):356–361.

53. Bundschuh DS, Eltze M, Barsig J, Wollin L, Hatzelmann A, Beume R. In vivo efficacy in airway disease models of roflumilast, a novel orally active PDE4 inhibitor. *J Pharmacol Exp Ther* 2001;297(1):280–290.

54. Center for Drug Evaluation and Research: Application Number 022522Orig1s000, 2011. Clinical Pharmacology and Biopharmaceutics Reviews. Available at https://www.accessdata.fda.gov/drugsatfda_docs/nda/2011/022522Orig1s000ClinPharmR.pdf. Accessed March 26, 2017.

55. Roflumilast: APTA 2217, B9302-107, BY 217, BYK 20869. *Drugs R D* 2004;5(3):176–181.

56. Wagner LT, Kenreigh CA. Roflumilast: the evidence for its clinical potential in the treatment of chronic obstructive pulmonary disease. *Core Evidence* 2005;1(1):23–33.

57. Martinez FJ, Rabe KF, Sethi S, Pizzichini E, McIvor A, Anzueto A, et al. Effect of Roflumilast and Inhaled Corticosteroid/Long-Acting beta2-Agonist on Chronic Obstructive Pulmonary Disease Exacerbations (RE(2)SPOND). A randomized clinical trial. *Am J Respir Crit Care Med* 2016;194(5):559–567.

58. Food and Drug Administration: Highlights of Prescribing Information: DALIRESP® (roflumilast) tablets. Available at https://www.accessdata.fda.gov/drugsatfda_docs/label/2015/022522s006lbl.pdf. Accessed March 26, 2017.

59. Writing Group for the Women's Health Initiative Investigators. Risks and benefits of estrogen plus progestin in healthy post-menopausal women: principal results from the Women's Health Initiative randomized controlled trial. *JAMA* 2002;288(3):321–333.

60. NIH News Release. July 9, 2002. NHLBI stops trial of estrogen plus progestin due to increase breast cancer risk, lack of overall benefit. Available at https://www.nhlbi.nih.gov/whi/pr_02-7-9.pdf. Accessed March 24, 2017.

61. Heiss G, Wallace R, Anderson GL, Aragaki A, Beresford SA, Brzyski R, et al. Health risks and benefits 3 years after stopping randomized treatment with estrogen and progestin. *JAMA* 2008;299(9):1036–1045.

62. Hennekens CH, Eberlein K. A randomized trial of aspirin and beta-carotene among U.S. physicians. *Prev Med* 1985;14(2):165–168.

63. Steering Committee of the Physicians' Health Study Research Group. Final report on the aspirin component of the ongoing Physicians' Health Study. *N Engl J Med* 1989;321(3):129–135.

64. Hennekens CH, Buring JE, Manson JE, Stampfer M, Rosner B, Cook NR, et al. Lack of effect of long-term supplementation with beta carotene on the incidence of malignant neoplasms and cardiovascular disease. *N Engl J Med* 1996;334(18):1145–1149.

65. Hills RK. Non-inferiority trials: No better? No worse? No change? No pain? *Br J Haematol* 2017;176(6):883–887.

66. Kaul S, Diamond GA. Good enough: a primer on the analysis and interpretation of noninferiority trials. *Ann Intern Med* 2006;145(1):62–69.

67. Hayden JA, van Tulder MW, Malmivaara AV, Koes BW. Meta-analysis: exercise therapy for nonspecific low back pain. *Ann Intern Med* 2005;142(9):765–775.

68. Wieland LS, Skoetz N, Pilkington K, Vempati R, D'Adamo CR, Berman BM. Yoga treatment for chronic non-specific low back pain. *Cochrane Database Syst Rev* 2017;1:Cd010671.

69. Saper RB, Lemaster C, Delitto A, Sherman KJ, Herman PM, Sadikova E, et al. Yoga, physical therapy, or education for chronic low back pain: a randomized noninferiority trial. *Ann Intern Med* 2017;167(2):85–94.

70. Snapinn SM. Noninferiority trials. *Curr Control Trials Cardiovasc Med* 2000;1(1):19–21.

71. Wiens BL. Choosing an equivalence limit for noninferiority or equivalence studies. *Control Clin Trials* 2002;23(1):2–14.

72. Jones B, Jarvis P, Lewis JA, Ebbutt AF. Trials to assess equivalence: the importance of rigorous methods. *BMJ* 1996;313(7048):36–39.

73. Pinto VF. Non-inferiority versus equivalence clinical trials in assessing biological products. *Sao Paulo Med J* 2011;129(3):183–184.

74. Lesaffre E. Superiority, equivalence, and non-inferiority trials. *Bull NYU Hosp Jt Dis* 2008;66(2):150–154.

75. Head SJ, Kaul S, Bogers AJJC, Kappetein AP. Non-inferiority study design: lessons to be learned from cardiovascular trials. *Europ Heart J* 2012;33(11):1318–1324.

76. Hahn S. Understanding noninferiority trials. *Korean J Pediatr* 2012;55(11):403–407.

77. Fuhrer MJ. Overview of clinical trials in medical rehabilitation: impetuses, challenges, and needed future directions. *Am J Phys Med Rehabil* 2003;82(10 Suppl):S8–S15.

78. Whyte J. Clinical trials in rehabilitation: what are the obstacles? *Am J Phys Med Rehabil* 2003;82(10 Suppl):S16–S21.

79. Frontera WR. Clinical trials in physical medicine and rehabilitation. *Am J Phys Med Rehabil* 2015;94(10 Suppl 1):829.

80. Hart T, Tsaousides T, Zanca JM, Whyte J, Packel A, Ferraro M, et al. Toward a theory-driven classification of rehabilitation treatments. *Arch Phys Med Rehabil* 2014;95(1 Suppl):S33–S44.e2.

81. Silverman WA. *Human Experimentation: A Guided Step into the Unknown*. New York: Oxford University Press, 1985.

82. Whyte J. Contributions of treatment theory and enablement theory to rehabilitation research and practice. *Arch Phys Med Rehabil* 2014;95(1 Suppl):S17–S23.e2.

83. Johnston MV. Desiderata for clinical trials in medical rehabilitation. *Am J Phys Med Rehabil* 2003;82(10 Suppl):S3–S7.

84. VanHiel LR. Treatment and enablement in rehabilitation research. *Arch Phys Med Rehabil* 2014;95(1 Suppl):S88–S90.

CHAPTER 15

Design Validity

Research designs are intended to provide structure that allows for logical conclusions about the relationship between independent and dependent variables. The investigator must have confidence that extraneous factors have not influenced the outcome. Even with a design that fulfills the requirements of an experiment, such as a randomized controlled trial (RCT), researchers must be vigilant regarding many potential sources of confounding that can obscure the effects of an intervention. Confounders may be extrinsic factors that emerge from the environment and the research situation, or they may be intrinsic factors that represent personal characteristics of the subjects of the study.

In Chapter 10, we addressed the importance of validity for measurements to have confidence in the meaning of a measured outcome. Here, we are concerned about validity in relation to the design of a research study and interpretation of results. The purpose of this chapter is to examine issues of control that must be addressed in the design and analysis of research. Although these concerns will be presented in the context of explanatory studies, they are also relevant to quasi-experimental and observational designs.

■ Validity Questions

Regardless of the care we take in the design of research, we know that clinical studies seldom have the ability to completely eliminate confounding effects. Although causality can never be demonstrated with complete certainty, the experimental method provides the most convincing evidence of the effect of one variable on another.

The goals of explanatory research correspond to four types of design validity (see Fig.15-1). These form a framework for evaluating experiments: statistical conclusion validity, internal validity, construct validity, and external validity (see Table 15-1).[1]

■ Statistical Conclusion Validity

Is there a relationship between the independent and dependent variables?

Statistical conclusion validity concerns the appropriate use of statistical procedures for analyzing data, leading to conclusions about the relationship between independent and dependent variables. Some specific threats to statistical conclusion validity are listed here. Because these threats involve concepts of statistical inference that will be covered later in the text (see Chapter 23 and beyond); only brief definitions are provided here.

- *Statistical Power.* The power of a statistical test concerns its ability to document a real relationship between independent and dependent variables. A study with low power may not be able to identify a statistical relationship even when one exists. Sample size is often the primary limiting

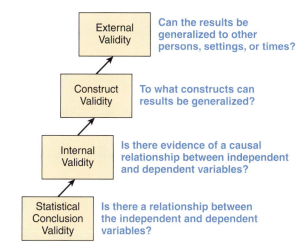

Figure 15–1 Four types of design validity. Each form is cumulatively dependent on the components below it.

factor when studies show no differences. The converse can also be true, when very large samples are used. In that case statistical differences may be found, even though they may not be meaningful.
- *Violated Assumptions of Statistical Tests.* Most statistical procedures are based on a variety of assumptions about levels of measurement and variance in the data or sample from which they are collected. If these assumptions are not met, statistical outcomes may lead to erroneous inferences.
- *Reliability and Variance.* Statistical conclusions are threatened by any extraneous factors that increase variability within the data, such as unreliable measurement, failure to standardize the protocol, environmental interferences, or heterogeneity of subjects.
- *Failure to Use Intention to Treat (ITT) Analysis.* When data are missing or subjects do not adhere to random group assignments, analysis procedures are designed to maintain the important element of randomization. This concept will be discussed later in this chapter.

Validity threats that impact design are often given the most press when we evaluate studies, focusing on concerns such as randomization, control groups, and operational definitions. The appropriate use of statistics is often assumed, perhaps because of a lack of understanding of statistical concepts. However, statistical outcomes may be erroneous or misleading if not based on valid procedures, potentially with serious implications for how conclusions are drawn. Evidence must be understood from a variety of perspectives, and statistical conclusion validity cannot be ignored.

Table 15-1 Threats to Design Validity

1. **Statistical Conclusion Validity:** Appropriate use of statistical procedures
   - Low statistical power
   - Violated assumptions of statistical tests
   - Reliability and variance
   - Failure to use intention to treat

2. **Internal Validity:** Potential for confounding factors to interfere with the relationship between independent and dependent variables

Internal Threats		Social Threats
• History	• Instrumentation	• Diffusion or imitation
• Maturation	• Regression	• Compensatory equalization
• Attrition	• Selection	• Compensatory rivalry
• Testing		• Demoralization

3. **Construct Validity:** Conceptualization of variables
   - Operational definitions
   - Time frame
   - Multiple treatment interactions
   - Experimental bias

4. **External Validity:** Extent to which results can be generalized
   - Influence of selection
   - Influence of settings
   - Influence of history

■ Internal Validity

Given a statistical relationship between the independent and dependent variables, is there evidence that one causes the other?

> ➤ **CASE IN POINT #1**
>
> Researchers designed *A Very Early Rehabilitation Trial (AVERT)* to study the efficacy and safety of early mobilization within 24 hours of stroke onset.[2] Patients were recruited from 56 stroke units in five countries. In a single-blind, pragmatic randomized trial, they assigned 2,104 patients to receive either usual care or early out-of-bed mobilization focusing on sitting, standing, and walking. The primary outcome, measured 3 months after stroke, was the patient's score on the modified Rankin Scale (mRS), an assessment based on the level of independence or assistance needed for functional activities.[3] The researchers hypothesized that more intensive, early out-of-bed activity would improve functional outcome at 3 months, reduce immobility-related complications, and accelerate walking recovery.

Internal validity focuses on cause-and-effect relationships. This is the paramount issue when testing for the success of interventions. The assumption of causality requires three components:

- *Temporal Precedence.* First, we must be able to document that the cause precedes the effect; that is, any change in outcome must be observed only after a treatment is applied. This is not a problem with randomized trials, where the independent variable is controlled by the investigator. It can be an issue in observational studies when independent and dependent variables are observed at the same time, and it may not be possible to know if the exposure preceded the outcome (see Chapter 19).
- *Covariation of Cause and Effect.* Second, we must be able to document that the outcome only occurs in the presence of the intervention, or that the degree of outcome is related to the magnitude of the intervention. This type of relationship is clear with an observed change in a treatment group and no change in a control group.
- *No Plausible Alternative Explanations.* Finally, we must be able to demonstrate that alternative explanations for observed change are not plausible. **Confounding variables** present threats to internal validity because they offer competing explanations for the observed relationship between the independent and dependent variables; that is, they interfere with cause-and-effect inferences. Several types of alternative explanations present potential threats to internal validity.

Internal Threats

Internal validity can be threatened by events or changes that occur during a study that may affect the relationship between the independent and dependent variables. Many of these threats can be mitigated when two or more groups are compared following random assignment, which allows the assumption that these threats will be equally distributed across groups. Studies that do not have control groups or that do not use random assignment are most vulnerable (see Chapter 19).

History

Did unanticipated events occur during the study that could affect the dependent variable?

History refers to the confounding effect of specific events, other than the experimental treatment, that occur after the introduction of the independent variable or between a pretest and posttest.

> ➤ In the AVERT trial, we would be concerned if the clinical staff changed during the course of the trial, or if patients were involved in other activities during the trial that could affect their outcomes. We would also be concerned if patients were receiving other treatments, such as occupational therapy, which could influence their functional recovery.

Maturation

Were changes in the dependent variable due to normal development or the simple passage of time?

A second threat concerns processes that occur simply as a function of the passage of time and that are independent of external events. **Maturation** may cause subjects to respond differently on a second measurement because they have grown older or more experienced, or if healing has occurred.

> ➤ For example, depending on the severity and type of stroke, patients in the AVERT trial could have improved within days of onset by virtue of neurological recovery.

Maturation is a relevant concern in many areas of clinical research, especially in studies where intervals between measurements are long. Those who study children often encounter physical and mental developmental changes, unrelated to therapeutic intervention, that may influence performance. Wound healing, remission of arthritic symptoms, and postoperative recovery are all examples of potential maturation effects.

Attrition

Is there a differential loss of subjects across groups?

Clinical researchers are often faced with the fact that subjects drop out of a study before it is completed.

Attrition, also called *experimental mortality*, is of concern when it results in a differential loss of subjects; that is, dropouts occur for specific reasons related to the experimental situation.

Studies with long follow-up periods are especially prone to attrition. Researchers may be able to compare pretest scores for those who remain and those who drop out to determine if there is a biasing effect. When subjects drop out for nonrandom reasons, the balance of individual characteristics that was present with random assignment may be compromised.

> ➤ Over the 3-month follow-up period in the AVERT trial, 21 patients dropped out, 6 for unknown reasons and 15 who refused to continue participation. There was no indication that their decisions were related to their group assignment.

Attrition is one of the few internal validity threats that cannot be controlled by having a comparison group because it can occur differentially across groups. This threat must be addressed through ITT analysis.

Testing

Did the pretest affect scores on the posttest?

Testing effects concern the potential effect of pretesting or repeated testing on the dependent variable. In other words, the mere act of collecting data changes the response that is being measured. Testing effects can refer to improved performance or increased skill that occurs because of familiarity with measurements.

For example, in educational tests, subjects may actually learn information by taking a pretest, thereby changing their responses on a posttest, independent of any instructional intervention. If a coordination test is given before and after therapy, patients may get higher scores on the posttest because they were able to practice the activity during the pretest. Testing effects also refer to situations where the measurement itself changes the dependent variable. For instance, if we take repeated measurements of range of motion, the act of moving the joint through range to evaluate it may actually stretch it enough to increase its range.

Reactive effects can occur when a testing process influences the response, rather than acting as a pure record of behavior. This can occur, for instance, when taping a session if the subject's responses are affected by knowing they are being recorded.

Instrumentation

Did the dependent variable change because of how it was measured?

Instrumentation effects are concerned with the reliability of measurement. Observers can become more experienced and skilled at measurement between a pretest and posttest. For example, if assessors in the AVERT trial were not equally trained in applying the mRS, the scores could be unreliable.

Changes that occur in calibration of hardware or shifts in criteria used by human observers can affect the magnitude of the dependent variable, independent of any treatment effect. Mechanical and bioelectronic instruments can threaten validity if linearity and sensitivity are not constant across the full range of responses and over time. This threat to internal validity can also bias results if the measurements are not the same for all groups, also called **detection bias**. These threats can be addressed by calibration and documenting test–retest and rater reliability to assure that measurement issues affect both groups equally.

Regression to the Mean

Is there evidence of regression from pretest to posttest scores?

Regression to the mean is also associated with reliability of a test (see Chapter 9). When there is substantial measurement error, there is a tendency for extreme scores on the pretest to regress toward the mean on the posttest; that is, extreme scores tend to become less extreme over time. This effect may occur even in the absence of an intervention effect. Statistical regression is of greatest concern when individuals are selected on the basis of extreme scores.

The amount of statistical regression is directly related to the degree of measurement error in the dependent variable. This can occur when the baseline and final scores are not correlated, when high baselines scores match to lower final scores, and vice versa. This effect is best controlled by including a control group in a study.

🖋 HISTORICAL NOTE

The term *regression* isn't intuitive. It was introduced by the English scientist Sir Frances Galton (1822–1911), who was an explorer, geographer, meteorologist, psychologist, inventor of fingerprint identification—and a statistician. With an interest in heredity, he used a linear equation to describe the relationship between heights of parents and children. He noticed that very tall fathers tended to have sons who were shorter than they were and very short fathers tended to have sons who were taller than they were.[4] He called this phenomenon "regression towards mediocrity," which has become known as regression to the mean.

Selection

Is there bias in the way subjects have been assigned to experimental groups?

The ability to assign subjects to groups at random is an essential strategy to have confidence that the primary difference between the intervention and control groups is the treatment. The threat of **selection** refers to factors other than the experimental intervention that can influence outcomes when groups are not comparable at baseline. This leaves open the potential for threats to internal validity that may affect the groups differentially.

Selection can interact with all the other threats to internal validity. For example, *selection–history effects* may occur when experimental groups have different experiences between the pretest and posttest. *Selection–maturation effects* occur when the experimental groups experience maturational change at different rates. Similar interactions can occur with attrition, testing, instrumentation, and regression.

Selection threats become an issue when intact groups are used, when subjects self-select groups, or when the independent variable is an attribute variable. Designs that do not allow random assignment are considered **quasi-experimental**, in that differences between groups cannot be balanced out (see Chapter 17). There may be several reasons that subjects belong to one group over another, and these factors can contribute to differences in their performance. Researchers can exert some degree of control for this effect when specific extraneous variables can be identified that vary between the groups. The

strategy of matched pairs or the **analysis of covariance (ANCOVA)**, to be discussed shortly, may be able to address these initial group differences.

Social Threats

Research results are often affected by the interaction of subjects and investigators. **Social threats** to internal validity refer to the pressures that can occur in research situations that may lead to differences between groups. These threats have also been called **performance bias**, occurring because those involved are aware of the other groups' circumstances or are in contact with one another.

Diffusion or Imitation of Treatments

Are subjects receiving interventions as intended?

Sometimes an intervention involves information or activities that are not intended to be equally available to all groups. Because the nature of many interventions makes blinding impractical, control subjects are often aware of the interventions intended for another group, and may attempt to change their behaviors accordingly.[5] This would diffuse the treatment effect and make it impossible to distinguish the behaviors of the two groups (see Focus on Evidence 15-1).

Focus on Evidence 15–1
The Lesson of MRFIT

Understanding validity in experimental design requires that we consider results within the social context of the intervention. Perhaps one of the most classic examples of this is the *Multiple Risk Factor Intervention Trial*, popularly known as MRFIT, which was conducted from 1973 to 1982. The trial was designed to test whether lowering elevated serum cholesterol and diastolic blood pressure, as well as ceasing cigarette smoking, would reduce mortality from coronary heart disease (CHD).[8] Over 360,000 men from 20 cities were screened, and more than 12,000 at highest risk for death from CHD were selected to be randomly assigned to either a special intervention (SI) program consisting of medication for hypertension, counseling for cigarette smoking, and dietary advice for lowering cholesterol levels, or to their source of usual care in the community.

Over an average follow-up period of 7 years, the mortality from CHD for the SI group was 17.9 deaths/1,000 men, and for the usual-care group was 19.3 deaths/1,000 men, a difference that was not significant. The difference in mortality for all causes was only 2%, also not significant. Although reductions in cholesterol and smoking were similar in both groups, after 6 years, 65% of the participants were still smoking, only 50% had blood pressure under control, and dietary changes were too small to summarize.[9]

In retrospect, researchers attributed the lack of significant differences between the two groups to the fact that men in both groups were originally selected in part because they were willing

to participate in a risk-factor modification program, knowing they could be assigned to either an intervention or control group. They all received information on their own health risks, but the usual-care group did not get further support. It is likely, however, that the subjects and their care providers were aware of widespread public health efforts in the 1970s to educate people about the benefits of risk-factor modification, which would have made usual care as good as the experimental intervention.[10] The death rates were also much smaller than expected and therefore markedly reduced the power of the study, even with such a large sample. At a cost of well over $180 million, this was an expensive experimental lesson.

There is another important lesson in this story, however, for evidence-based practice. These negative results unfortunately stymied efforts for many years to take advantage of preventive measures that were considered ineffective because of these findings.[11] For instance, the tobacco industry used these findings to erroneously support no connection between smoking and CHD.[12] Over the years, however, researchers have continued to examine these variables, many using observational designs, to demonstrate that behavioral changes can be preventive. Studies have looked at the more than 350,000 men who were originally screened for MRFIT and analyzed outcomes to show the relationship between cholesterol and CHD mortality.[13] Analyses of subgroups within the original cohort have also shown important relationships.[14,15] Despite the initial perceived "failure" of MRFIT, it has much to offer still.

➤ As a pragmatic trial, investigators in the AVERT trial were not prescriptive about usual care mobilization practices, which changed during the trial. They found that 60% of patients in the usual care group had actually started out-of-bed therapy within 24 hours after stroke onset. It was not clear if this was a consequence of contamination from the trial protocol, or a response to changes in attitudes about early mobilization. Regardless, this clearly diffused the effect of the early intervention.

Compensatory Equalization

Are researchers adhering to the protocol for all groups?

When an experimental treatment is considered a desirable service or condition, those who work with and care for the participants may try to even out experiences by providing compensatory services to the control group. For instance, clinicians in the AVERT trial may have given patients in the control group some additional activities within the first 24 hours to compensate for not getting them out of bed earlier. The effect of such compensatory attention will be to make the groups look more alike, and obscure the experimental effects of treatment.

Compensatory Rivalry or Resentful Demoralization

Are subjects' responses influenced by their knowledge of other group treatments?

These two effects represent opposite reactions to the same situation. Compensatory rivalry occurs when one group's assigned treatment is perceived as more desirable than the other's and subjects receiving the less desirable treatment try to compensate by working extra hard to achieve similar results. This is similar to compensatory equalization, described earlier, except that here the subject is responsible for equalizing effects.

In an alternative reaction to this type of situation, demoralization occurs when subjects receiving less desirable treatments become disheartened or resentful. Their reaction may be to respond at lower levels of performance. The effect of such responses will be to artificially inflate group differences, which may then be incorrectly attributed to a significantly greater treatment effect.

One way to control these effects is to be sure that there is no interaction among subjects. Sometimes this is difficult, depending on the experimental environment. Cluster random assignment is one strategy to account for this potential effect (see Chapter 14).

HISTORICAL NOTE

John Henry was an African-American folk hero, known as a "steel drivin' man" who worked on the railroads around 1870, hammering steel into mountainsides to set up explosions for building tunnels.[14] According to legend, he went head to head with a steam drill, which was introduced to improve productivity. He outperformed the steam drill, but worked so hard that he died of overexertion. The "John Henry effect" has been described as seeing above average performance by members of a control group who want to do as well as those in the experimental group, a form of compensatory rivalry.[15]

Ruling Out Threats to Internal Validity

Threats to internal validity are likely to be present in every study to some degree. The task of ruling out alternative explanations for observed changes and documenting the effect of the independent variable is not a small one. Many threats, such as history, maturation, selection, regression, testing, instrumentation, and selection interactions, can be ruled out by the use of random assignment and control groups. These issues are canceled out when both groups are equivalent at the start and are equally likely to be affected by events occurring during the course of the study.

Random assignment cannot rule out the effects of attrition, imitating treatments, or compensatory reactions. Blinding subjects and investigators, however, will control many of these effects.

The researcher must examine all possible threats and eliminate them or recognize their influence when they are inevitable. This can be done through stratification or statistical manipulation, but the investigator must specifically identify these variables at the start and collect data on them.

 As consumers of research evidence, we are responsible for making judgments about the degree of internal validity of a study, and the extent to which we consider findings relevant and useful. When internal validity is severely threatened, conclusions can be considered suspect. We might assume that peer review would prevent publication of such studies, but that is not necessarily the case—*caveat emptor*!

■ Construct Validity

Given that a cause-and-effect relationship is probable, to which constructs can the results be generalized?

Threats to design validity can also be characterized in terms of the construct validity of the independent and dependent variables (see Chapter 10). Construct validity related to design concerns how variables are conceptualized, and how well experimental results can be generalized within the desired clinical context.[1] Studies that are internally sound may have no practical application beyond the experimental situation if the researcher has not taken the time to explore conceptual questions and the theoretical basis for asking them.

Threats to construct validity are related to how variables are operationally defined within a study and to potential biases introduced into a study by subjects or experimenters.

Operational Definitions

Most of the treatments and responses that are used in clinical research are based on constructs that must be operationally defined by the researcher. The levels of the independent variable and measurement methods for the dependent variable will delimit their relationship.

> ➤ The independent variable of early mobilization in the AVERT trial was based on three elements: 1) beginning within 24 hours after stroke onset; 2) focusing on sitting, standing, and walking as out-of-bed activities; and 3) at least three additional out-of-bed sessions beyond usual care, with continued functional interventions based on protocol guidelines. Intervention lasted 14 days or until discharge.
> The primary dependent variable was score on the mRS, which is an ordinal scale ranging from 0 (no disability) to 5 (severe disability). A score of 6 was used to indicate death. The researchers defined a favorable outcome as a score of 0 to 2 (no or minimum disability) and a poor outcome as scores of 3 to 6 (moderate or severe disability or death).

Results of a study can only be interpreted within the contexts of these operational definitions.

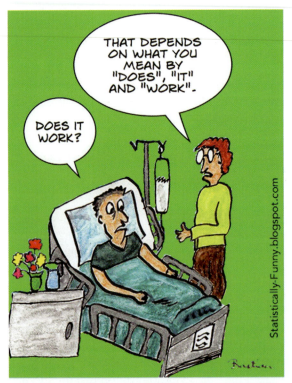

THINGS GOT REALLY INTERESTING WHEN THE STATISTICIAN STARTED DOING WARD ROUNDS.

Cartoon courtesy of Hilda Bastian.

Comprehensive Measurements

Cook and Campbell[1] suggest that full explication of most constructs requires use of multiple forms of measurement. When studies incorporate only one type of measurement, the results will apply only to a limited aspect of the construct.

> ➤ In addition to measuring function on the mRS, investigators in the AVERT trial measured secondary outcomes of time taken to achieve unassisted walking over 50 meters, the proportion of patients achieving functional unassisted walking by 3 months, and the number of fatal and non-fatal adverse events within 3 months, including cardiovascular events, falls, infections, and depression. These outcomes helped to further clarify the effect of early mobilization.

These additional data are important for clinical application, as they relate to many considerations in treatment, prevention, and outcome measurement.

Subgroup Differences

Threats to construct validity can also occur when some levels of the independent variable interact differently with various types of dependent variables. Many investigators will look at subgroup analyses to determine if the responses should be interpreted differently.

> ➤ Analysis in the AVERT trial included looking at the primary outcome for subgroups based on age, severity of stroke, type of stroke, time to first mobilization (in hours), and geographic region (Australia and New Zealand versus Asia versus the United Kingdom).

Understanding these variations is essential for clinicians to generalize findings and apply evidence to clinical decisions for different types of patients.

Time Frame

The timing of a study is important in determining the effect of intervention. How long a treatment lasts, when the treatment is begun relative to a patient's diagnosis, and how long patients are followed are examples of elements that must be defined for a study. For example, in the AVERT trial, patients were treated within the first 2 weeks and then followed for 3 months.

Basing decisions on short-term data can be misleading if the observed effects are not durable or if they are slow to develop. For instance, if in the AVERT trial follow-up was only carried out for 1 month, there would have been no way to determine if the outcome would have been different if carried out over a longer period. The construct validity of the independent variable must include reference to the time frame used for data collection.

Multiple Treatment Interactions

Construct validity is also affected when a study involves the administration of multiple treatments. Generalization is limited by the possibility of *multiple-treatment interaction*, creating carryover or combined effects. When treatment components are combined, the researcher cannot generalize findings to a situation where only a single treatment technique is used.

Multiple treatment interactions may be of particular concern when complex combinations of techniques are used, as is often the case in rehabilitation. Interpretations of findings must take these potential interactions into account, taking care to base conclusions on the full operational definitions of the variables being studied. This can be an issue when one component of a treatment is examined in isolation, especially if the potential influence of other components on the outcome is ignored.

Experimental Bias

A fourth aspect of construct validity concerns biases that are introduced into a study by expectations of either the subjects or the investigators. Subjects often try their best to fulfill the researcher's expectations or to present themselves in the best way possible; therefore, responses are no longer representative of natural behavior (see Box 15-1).

Those who provide intervention or measure outcomes may also have certain expectations that can influence how subjects respond. Researchers may react more positively to subjects in the experimental group or give less attention to those in the control group because of an emotional or intellectual investment in their hypothesis. Rosenthal[16] described several types of **experimenter effects** in terms of the experimenter's a*ctive behavior* and interaction with the subject, such as verbal cues and smiling, and *passive behaviors*, such as those related to appearance. This threat to construct validity can be avoided by employing testers and treatment providers who are blinded to subject assignment and the research hypothesis.

■ External Validity

Can the results be generalized to persons, settings, and times that are different from those employed in the experimental situation?

External validity refers to the extent to which the results of a study can be generalized beyond the internal specifications of the study sample. Whereas internal validity is concerned specifically with the relationship

---

Box 15-1   A Myth Too Good to Be Untrue

From 1924 to 1927, a series of experiments were run at the Hawthorne plant of the Western Electric Company, located outside of Chicago.[21,22] Managers were interested in studying how various levels of illumination affected workers' output. The primary test group consisted of five women who worked in the relay assembly test room. Their task was to complete relay switches and drop them down a chute that recorded their productivity—every 40 to 50 seconds, 8 hours a day.[23]

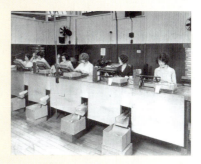

From Special Collections, Baker Library, Harvard Business School

What they found was that whether they lowered or raised lights, the workers increased production. Further studies involved introducing changes in work schedules, coffee breaks, shorter work week, temperature, even wages, all resulting in better output, even when conditions were made worse or later returned to original schedules! No matter what they did, productivity in regular and test groups increased.[24] This phenomenon became widely known as the *Hawthorne effect*, which is defined as the tendency of persons who are singled out for special attention to perform better merely because they know they are being observed.

---

between the independent and dependent variables within a specific set of circumstances, external validity is concerned with the usefulness of that information outside of the experimental situation. The generalizability of a study is primarily related to the specific patient context and conditions under investigation.[29] Threats to external validity involve the interaction of treatment with the type of subjects tested, the setting in which the experiment is carried out, or the time in history when the study is done.

Influence of Selection

One of the major goals of clinical research is to apply results to a target population, the individuals who are not experimental subjects but who are represented by them (see Chapter 13). If subjects are sampled according to specific characteristics, those characteristics define the target population. For instance, subjects may be restricted to a limited age range, one gender, a specific diagnosis, or a defined level of function. Because patient characteristics and eligibility requirements can vary, generalizability will depend on how closely the study sample represents the clinical situation.

External validity is threatened when documented cause-and-effect relationships do not apply across subdivisions of the target population; that is, when specific interventions result in differential treatment effects, depending on the subject's characteristics. Studies are especially vulnerable to this threat when volunteers are used as subjects. Those who choose to volunteer may do so because of certain personal characteristics that ultimately bias the sample. When studies demonstrate conflicting results, it is often because of the differences within the accessible populations.

Adherence

A related effect can occur if subjects do not comply with the experimental protocol. A study that is internally valid may still be compromised in relation to external validity under these circumstances. Researchers should examine adherence as they interpret findings to determine if results are realistic and have clinical applicability.[30]

From a sampling perspective, some investigators screen potential subjects prior to randomizing them to groups to eliminate those who are not adherent (see Chapter 14). For example, the Physicians' Health Study, which investigated the effect of aspirin and beta carotene in the prevention of ischemic heart disease, used an 18-week "run-in period" and eliminated 33% of the subjects from the final study based on non-compliance.[31] This practice may help to build a compliant study sample, but it may also dilute external validity of the findings. It is the researcher's responsibility to evaluate its potential effect in demonstrating the applicability of the findings.[32]

Influence of Setting

If a study demonstrates a causal relationship between treatment and outcome, can we generalize those findings to settings other than where the study was performed? Are there societal or administrative differences that could influence how treatments work? Studies that are done in laboratories, for instance, may not be easily translated to practice settings. Differences across types of treatment settings and geographic variations in practice are also examples of this threat.

> ➤ The AVERT study was carried out in 56 stroke units in five countries, including Australia, New Zealand, Malaysia, Singapore, and the United Kingdom (England, Scotland, Northern Ireland, and Wales).

This type of multi-site study has strong external validity relative to settings. As a pragmatic study, it represents sites that will have varied practice cultures, healthcare systems, and educational structures.

Ecological Validity

In an extension of external validity, **ecological validity** refers to the generalizability of study findings to real-world conditions, societal and cultural norms, and the health of populations. Pragmatic clinical trials, which are intended to be carried out in natural clinical settings, will have stronger ecological validity than studies that are done under controlled clinical conditions.

Influence of History

This threat to external validity concerns the ability to generalize results to different periods of time. It is actually an important consideration in evidence-based practice (EBP) because older studies may have limited application based on contemporary practices, such as reimbursement policies, available drugs, newer surgical procedures, updated guidelines, or changes in theoretical foundations for practice.

> ➤ Researchers in the AVERT study faced a dilemma regarding shifts in early mobilization practices that had changed over time in practice guidelines. Therefore, clinicians in the control group had gotten many patients moving earlier, mimicking the experimental intervention.

This does not mean that older studies have no value. Their findings may indeed stand up to the test of time, or they may provide important background to how treatments or theories have changed. Clinical judgment and expertise are important for interpreting the applicability of such studies.

■ Strategies to Control for Subject Variability

Clinical research is often influenced by confounding factors that may be personal traits of those being studied. Several design strategies can be incorporated into a study that will control for these intrinsic variables.

> ➤ **CASE IN POINT #2**
> Let's use a hypothetical study to illustrate strategies for controlling intersubject differences. Suppose we are interested in the effect of two types of lower extremity orthoses on step length. We randomly assign 40 subjects to two treatment groups. When we compare the subjects' step lengths, we find that the average step for those wearing orthosis A is longer than the average step for those wearing orthosis B.

We would like to attribute this difference to the type of orthosis being worn. However, step length is also related to characteristics such as height and leg length. Therefore, if the subjects in group A happen to be taller than those in group B, the observed difference in step length may be a function of height, not orthosis.

Random Assignment

Of course, the most fundamental strategy to eliminate bias across groups is to employ random assignment. We could randomly assign subjects to either orthosis, and assume a balance of factors, including height. However, as we have discussed before, random assignment is not perfect, especially with smaller samples, and may result in groups that are not balanced on important variables. When one or two extraneous factors are of special concern, the researcher may not want to depend on randomization.

Several methods can be used to address specific concerns about confounding factors in the design of a study. For these techniques to be effective, however, the researcher must be able to identify which variables are relevant in advance and collect data on those variables. For some strategies, this determination is made prior to recruiting a sample. For others, adjustments are made within the study design.

Homogeneous Samples

When a researcher suspects that specific subject traits may interfere with the dependent variable, the simplest way to control for them is to eliminate them by choosing subjects who are homogeneous on those characteristics, thereby eliminating them as confounders.

If we think males and females will respond differently to the wearing of the orthoses, we can choose only male subjects for our sample. We could also control for height by choosing only subjects who fit within a certain height range.

Once a homogeneous group of subjects is selected, those subjects can be randomly assigned to treatment conditions. Because there is no variability on that variable, the effects of the potential confounder are essentially eliminated. The major disadvantage of this approach is that the research findings can be generalized only to the type of subjects who participate in the study, in this case to men of a certain height. This will limit external validity and application of results.

Blocking Variables

Another means of controlling for extraneous effects is to systematically manipulate attribute variables by building them into the experimental design as an independent variable. If we are concerned with the effect of height, we could build that variable into the design so we could compare individuals within specified height ranges (short, medium, tall) as a second independent variable. Each category of height is called a *block*, and the attribute variable of height is called a **blocking variable**. This procedure lets us analyze the differential effect of height on treatment.

Creating a blocking variable is not the same as stratification, which was described in Chapter 13. With stratification, subjects are randomly assigned to groups within strata so that the variable of concern is distributed evenly across groups. In that way, the variable is effectively eliminated as a source of bias. A blocking variable is actually built into the design as an independent variable so that the differences between the blocks can be compared (see Chapter 16).

Matching

Another strategy for dealing with extraneous variables involves **matching** subjects on the basis of specific characteristics. If we were concerned with the effect of height on our dependent variable, we could use a matching procedure to guarantee an equivalent group of taller and shorter subjects in the experimental and control groups.

Studies that use identical twins to compare outcomes are using the ultimate matching process.

Matching also limits interpretation of research findings because the differential effect of the matching variables cannot be analyzed. For example, if we match subjects on height, then we cannot determine if the effect of treatment is different across height ranges. For most clinical studies, matching is not recommended when other methods of controlling extraneous variables are appropriate and practical.

When a researcher wants to control for several variables in a design, matching is more complicated. A technique of matching using **propensity scores** is often used in exploratory studies to match subjects on a set of potential confounders. This process uses multivariate regression modeling to develop a single combined score that can then be used as the measure of confounding to match subjects. This technique will be discussed further in Chapter 19.

Repeated Measures

Research designs can be structured to facilitate comparisons between independent groups of subjects, or they may involve comparisons of responses across treatment conditions within a subject. When the levels of the independent variable are assigned to different groups, with an active or attribute variable, the independent variable is considered an **independent factor**. When all levels of the independent variable are experienced by all subjects, the independent variable is considered a **repeated factor** or a **repeated measure**. The use of a repeated measure is often described as *using subjects as their own control*.

> ➤ We could ask each subject to wear both orthoses, and then compare their step lengths. The independent variable of "orthosis" would then be a repeated factor because both levels are experienced by all subjects.

A repeated measures design is one of the most efficient methods for controlling intersubject differences. It ensures the highest possible degree of equivalence across treatment conditions. Because subjects are essentially matched with themselves, any observed differences should be attributable solely to the intervention.

Issues related to the design of repeated measures studies are explored further in Chapter 16.

> The term *independent factor* should not be confused with *independent variable*. An independent variable can be either an "independent factor" or a "repeated factor" depending on how its levels are defined within the study design.

Analysis of Covariance

The last method of controlling for confounding effects does not involve a design strategy, but instead uses a statistical technique to equate groups on extraneous variables. The ANCOVA is based on concepts of analysis of variance and regression (see Chapter 30). Without going into details of statistical procedure at this time, let us consider the conceptual premise for ANCOVA using the hypothetical study of step length in patients wearing two types of lower extremity orthoses.

The purpose of the ANCOVA is to statistically eliminate the influence of extraneous factors so that the effect of the independent variable can be seen more clearly. These identified extraneous variables are called **covariates**. Conceptually, the ANCOVA removes the confounding effect of covariates by making them statistically equivalent across groups and then estimating what the dependent variable *would have been* under these equivalent conditions.

> ➤ If the patients wearing orthosis A happen to be taller than those in the other group, the ANCOVA can be used to predict what the step lengths *would have been* had the heights been equally distributed. The analysis of differences between the two groups will then be based on these *adjusted scores*.

The ANCOVA can also be used when baseline scores on the outcome variables are different between groups. In that case, researchers will specify the baseline score as a covariate and compare the outcome scores using the ANCOVA. This effectively makes the groups equivalent on their baseline values so that differences can be more clearly seen between groups on the outcome measure.[33,34]

■ Non-compliance and Missing Data

In addition to controlling for confounding variables in a design, it is important to maximize adherence to the research protocol. Investigators in randomized trials often face two complications that affect analysis: non-compliance and missing data. These situations can occur for several reasons.

> ➤ **CASE IN POINT #3**
> Researchers evaluated the efficacy of an exercise intervention (EI) to reduce work-related fatigue.[35] Subjects were recruited from various industries and work settings. They were randomly allocated to either a 6-week EI or a wait-list control (WLC) group. The primary outcome measure was work-related fatigue, defined as three concepts, each measured by a validated questionnaire: emotional exhaustion, overall fatigue, and short-term recovery. They were measured at baseline (T0) and post-intervention (T1). Subjects in the exercise group were also measured at 6-week (T2) and 12-week (T3) follow-up.

As shown in Figure 15-2, 362 subjects were screened for eligibility, with 265 excluded because of not meeting eligibility requirements or declining participation. The remaining 96 subjects were randomly assigned to the two treatment groups. Not all these subjects, however, completed the study as planned.

Compliance refers to getting the assigned treatment, being evaluated according to the protocol, and adherence to protocol requirements.[36] Subjects may also drop out,

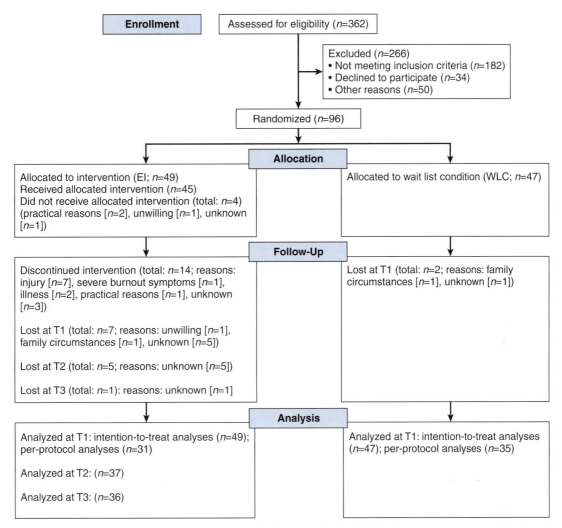

Figure 15–2 Flowchart of patient recruitment and allocation for the RCT of exercise to reduce work-related fatigue. From de Vries JD, van Hooff ML, Guerts SA, Kompier MA. Exercise to reduce work-related fatigue among employees: a randomized controlled trial. *Scand J Work Environ Health* 2017;43(4):337–349. Figure 1, p. 2.

miss a test session, or leave survey questions unanswered, creating missing data.

➤ The flow diagram shows that four subjects in the EI did not comply following allocation. We can also see that 14 additional exercise subjects discontinued their intervention during the follow-up period for various reasons.

- **Subjects may refuse the assigned treatment after allocation.** A patient may initially consent to join a study, knowing that she may be assigned to either group, but after assignment is complete, the patient decides she wants the other treatment. Ethically, these patients must be allowed to receive the treatment they want.

- **Subjects may cross over to another treatment during the course of the study.** This situation may be due to patient preference or a change in a patient's condition.
- **Subjects may not be compliant with assigned treatments.** Although they may remain in a study, subjects may not fulfill requirements of their group assignment, negating the treatment effect.

➤ A condition of eligibility for the fatigue study was that subjects did not exercise more than 1 hour/day. The control subjects were asked to maintain that level, but 10 control subjects increased their exercise activity during the wait period of the study.

- **Subjects may drop out of the study or terminate treatment before the study is complete.** Those who remain in a study often differ in an important way from those who drop out.[37] Subjects in the experimental group may find the commitment onerous, for example. Loss to follow-up is a concern when data collection extends over several measurement periods, potentially creating bias in the remaining sample.

> In the fatigue study, a total of 14 subjects in the exercise group discontinued their intervention over the course of the study, with 7 lost at the first post-intervention measure (T1). Two subjects were lost in the control group. Researchers in the fatigue study compared baseline scores for those who completed and did not complete the intervention. Their analysis showed no differences between them in either of the test groups.

Some research protocols call for random assignment prior to the point where eligibility can be determined. If subjects are later excluded from the study because of ineligibility, the balance of random assignment will be distorted. The issue of *post-randomization exclusion* is distinguished from patients dropping out because of non-compliance, withdrawal, or loss to follow-up.[38]

Per-Protocol Analysis

Each of the situations just described causes a problem for analysis, as the composition of the groups at the end of the study is biased from the initial random assignment, especially if the number of subjects involved is large. There is no clean way to account for this difficulty.

At first glance, it might seem prudent to just eliminate any subjects who did not get or complete their assigned treatment, and include only those subjects who sufficiently complied with the trial's protocol. This is called **per-protocol analysis**.

> Based on the subjects who did not comply with their assigned interventions, researchers in the fatigue study did a per-protocol analysis with 31 subjects in the intervention group and 35 in the control group. Using this approach, they found that the exercise group scored significantly lower at T1 on emotional exhaustion and overall fatigue compared to the WLC group, suggesting a positive effect of the exercise program.

Generally, the per-protocol approach will bias results in favor of a treatment effect, as those who succeed at treatment are able to tolerate it well and are most likely to stick with it.[39,40] For example, in the fatigue study, it

is possible that those who complied with the exercise regimen were those who tended to see positive results, and those who stopped exercising were not seeing any benefits or found the activity inconvenient. Therefore, when analyzing the data using only those subjects who complied, the exercise program would look more successful compared to the control group.

Intention to Treat Analysis

A more conservative approach uses a principle called **intention to treat (ITT)**, which means that data are analyzed according to original random assignments, regardless of the treatment subjects actually received, if they dropped out or were non-compliant; that is, we analyze data according to the way we *intended* to treat the subjects. This analysis ideally includes all subjects.

Purposes of Intention to Treat Analysis

The ITT approach is important because the effectiveness of a therapy is based on a combination of many factors beyond its biological effect, including how it is administered, variations in compliance and adherence to the study protocol, adverse events, and other patient characteristics that are related to the outcome.[41] All of these factors are assumed to be balanced across groups through random assignment, which needs to be maintained to obtain an unbiased estimate of the treatment effect.

The ITT approach, therefore, serves two main purposes:

- It guards against the potential for bias if dropouts are related to outcomes or group assignment, and preserves the original balance of random assignment.
- It reflects routine clinical situations, in which some patients will be non-compliant. This is most relevant to pragmatic trials, where the design is intended to incorporate real-world practice.

Reporting Intention to Treat Results

The ITT principle is considered an essential process for the interpretation of randomized controlled trials. Current guidelines for reporting randomized trials have been endorsed by an international community of medical journals, recommending use of ITT analysis whenever possible, with a flow diagram that documents how subjects were included or excluded through different phases of the study, as shown in Figure 15-2 (see Chapter 38).[42] This approach should be used with explanatory and pragmatic trials.

Interpreting ITT Analysis

As might be expected, an ITT analysis can result in an underestimate of the treatment effect, especially if the number of subjects not getting their assigned treatment is large. This will make it harder to find significant differences but is still considered a better representation of what would happen in practice. To be safe then, many researchers will analyze data using both ITT and per-protocol analyses.

> ▶ Using an ITT analysis, results of the fatigue study did not show a significant difference between groups on the primary outcome of fatigue. The authors attributed these findings to the fact that many of the exercise subjects had stopped exercising prior to the end of the trial, and some of the control subjects increased their level of exercise. Therefore, the treatment effect was diffused.
>
> In contrast, a per-protocol analysis, run on the "pure" groups of completers and true controls, did show the effect of exercise on reducing work fatigue. The authors interpreted this discrepancy in findings to suggest that exercise was effective for reducing fatigue, but that compliance was necessary to observe the beneficial effects.

When outcomes are the same using both analysis approaches, the researcher will have strong confidence in the results.[43] If the two methods yield different results, however, the researcher is obliged to consider which factors may be operating to bias the outcome and to offer potential explanations.

Because the chance of systematic bias is reduced with ITT, the per-protocol results may be less valid. Therefore, the researcher must be cautious in this interpretation, considering the role of confounding, in this example the role of compliance. Data should be collected to determine how this variable contributes to the outcome.

■ Handling Missing Data

Studies often end up with some missing data for various reasons. This can present a challenge for analysis in RCTs and observational studies because they can create bias that reduces validity of conclusions. The consequences of bias with missing data can depend on the reasons they are missing. Three types of "missingness" have been described.[44-46]

- ***Missing Completely at Random (MCAR).*** Data are assumed to be missing because of completely unpredictable circumstances that have no connection to the variables of interest or the study design, such as records getting lost or equipment failure. In this case, it is reasonable to assume that the subjects with missing data will be similar to those for whom full data are available.

- ***Missing at Random (MAR).*** Missing data may be related to the methodology of the study, but not to the treatment variable. For example, in the fatigue study, clinicians from different sites may have missed certain data points. In this case, missing data should also have no inherent bias.

- ***Missing Not at Random (MNAR).*** Sometimes the missing data will be related to group membership, such as patients dropping out because a treatment is not working, or not showing up because of inconvenience. This type of missing data is most problematic because it creates a bias in the data.

Strategies for handling missing data should be specified as part of the research plan. The approach may vary depending on the type of missing data. Sometimes, carrying out more than one strategy is helpful to see if conclusions will differ.

Completer Analysis

The most direct approach to handling missing data is to exclude subjects, using only the data from those who completed the study, called **completer analysis**, or *complete case analysis*. This analysis will represent efficacy of an intervention for those who persist with it but may be open to serious bias.

Using only complete cases can be justified if the number of incomplete cases is small and if data are MAR; that is, missing data are independent of group assignment or outcome. However, if those with missing data differ systematically from the complete cases, marked bias can exist. If a large number of cases are missing, this approach will reduce sample size, decreasing the power of the study.

Data Imputation

To maintain the integrity of a sample and to fulfill assumptions for ITT, missing data points can be replaced with estimated values that are based on observed data using a process called **imputation**. Analyses can then be run on the full dataset with the missing values "filled in" and conclusions drawn about outcomes based on those estimates. Of course, there is always some level of uncertainty in how well the imputed scores accurately represent the unknown true scores. This brief introduction will include several of the more commonly used techniques to determine what this replacement value should be. Validity of results will vary depending on how imputed values are generated.

Non-Completer Equals Failure

When the outcome of a study is dichotomous, subjects can be classified as "successes" or "failures." For an ITT analysis, then, those who drop out can be considered a "failure." This is the most conservative approach; thus, if the treatment group is better, we can be confident that the results are not biased by dropouts.[47] If the results show no difference, however, we would not know if the treatment was truly ineffective or if the dropouts confounded the outcome because they were classified as failures.

Last Observation Carried Forward

When data are measured at several points in time, a technique called **last observation carried forward (LOCF)** is often used. With this method, the subject's last data point before dropping out is used as the outcome score. With multiple test points, the assumption is that patients improve gradually from the start of the study until the end; therefore, carrying forward an intermediate value is a conservative estimate of how well the person would have done had he remained in the study. It essentially assumes that the subject would have remained stable from the point of dropout, rather than improving.[48] If the subject drops out right after the pretest, however, this last score could be the baseline score.

Although it is still often used, the LOCF approach has fallen into disfavor because it can grossly inflate or deflate the true treatment effect.[49,50] This is especially true when the number of dropouts is greater in the treatment group.[48] It does not take into account that some dropouts may have shown no change up to their last assessment, but might have improved had they continued.

Mean Value Imputation

Another approach involves the use of the distribution average, or mean, for the missing variable as the best estimate. For example, in the fatigue study, missing data for a control subject for the emotional exhaustion outcome could be replaced by the mean of that variable for those in the control group with complete data. This method assumes that the group mean is a "typical" response that can represent an individual subject's score. However, this approach can result in a large number of subjects with identical scores, thereby reducing variability, artificially increasing precision, and ultimately biasing results.[51]

Multiple Data Imputation

The LOCF and mean imputation techniques use a single value as the imputed score, leaving a great deal of uncertainty in how well the score represents the individual subject's true score. An approach called **multiple imputation** is considered a more valid method to estimate missing data.[52]

This procedure involves creating a random dataset using the available data, predicting plausible values derived from observed data. This procedure involves *sampling with replacement*, which means that the selected values are returned to the data and are available for selection with further sampling. This sampling procedure is repeated several times, each time using a different random dataset, and therefore resulting in different imputed values. The data from each dataset are then subjected to the planned statistical analysis to see what the differences are in the results. One value is then derived, usually by taking a mean of the several outcomes to get a pooled estimate for the missing values.

Multiple imputation techniques require sophisticated methodology that is beyond the scope of this book, and a statistician should be consulted. Several excellent references provide comprehensive reviews of these issues.[44,46,53-55] Most statistical programs include options for this process.

Pairwise and Listwise Deletion

Statistical programs provide several options for handling missing data in analysis. *Listwise deletion* means that a case is dropped if it has a missing value for one or more data points, and analysis will be run only on cases with complete data. *Pairwise deletion* can be used when a particular analysis does not include every score and cases are omitted only if they are missing any of the variables involved in the specific procedure (see Appendix C).

Trying to Limit Missing Data

Because missing data can create potentially biased outcomes in results of a clinical trial, researchers should take purposeful steps to limit this problem in the design and conduct of a study.[36] Efforts should be made to reduce non-compliance, drop outs, crossover of subjects, or loss to follow-up. Eligibility criteria should be as specific as possible to avoid exclusions. This process is important because those who are lost may differ systematically from those who remain on treatment.

A thorough consent process, including adequate warning of potential side effects and expectations, may help to inform subjects sufficiently to avoid non-compliance. Ongoing support for subjects during a trial, such as periodic check-ins, may also foster continuous participation. Researchers must also consider how they can follow up with subjects even if they withdrew early. It is often possible to obtain a final measurement at the end of the study period, even if subjects have been delinquent in their participation.[47]

COMMENTARY

The real purpose of the scientific method is to make sure that nature hasn't misled you into thinking you know something you actually don't know.

—Robert Pirsig (1928–2017)

Author, Zen and the Art of Motorcycle Maintenance

Because there are so many potential threats to validity, researchers must make judgments about priorities. Not all threats to validity are of equal concern in every study. When steps are taken to increase one type of validity, it is likely that another type will be affected. Because clinical trials focus on control to improve interpretation of outcomes, internal validity often receives the most press. However, the application of evidence to clinical practice requires an appreciation for all validity issues and the ability to judge when findings will have applicability.

For instance, if we attempt to control for extraneous factors by using a homogeneous sample, we will improve internal validity, but at the expense of external validity. Pragmatic studies face unique challenges because their purpose specifically negates controlling for many variables for the purpose of improving external validity and construct validity, often at the expense of internal validity. If we increase statistical conclusion validity by limiting variability in our data, we will probably reduce external and construct validity. Similarly, if we work toward increasing construct validity by operationalizing variables to match clinical utilization, we run the risk of decreasing reliability of measurements.

After describing all the above threats, we might wonder—is it ever possible to design a completely valid study? In fact, there is probably no such thing. Every study contains some shortcomings. Clinical researchers operate in an environment of uncertainty and it is virtually impossible to conduct experiments so that every facet of behavior, environment, and personal interaction is exactly the same for every subject.

Because clinical studies cannot be perfectly controlled, authors should provide sufficient details on the design and analysis of the study that will allow clinicians to judge how and to whom results can be reasonably applied. Limitations of a study should be included in the discussion section of a research report so that readers have a complete understanding of the circumstances under which results were obtained. Researchers must be able to justify the study conditions and analysis procedures as fair tests of the experimental treatment within the context of the research question. When important extraneous factors cannot be controlled, to the point that they will have a serious impact on the interpretation and validity of outcomes, it is advisable to consider alternatives to experimental research, such as observational approaches. Guidelines have been developed to assure consistency in reporting of clinical trials. These will be discussed in Chapter 38.

REFERENCES

1. Cook TD, Campbell DT. *Quasi-experimentation: Design and Analysis Issues for Field Settings*. Boston: Houghton Mifflin, 1979.
2. AVERT Trial Collaboration Group. Efficacy and safety of very early mobilisation within 24 h of stroke onset (AVERT): a randomised controlled trial. *Lancet* 2015;386(9988):46–55.
3. Banks JL, Marotta CA. Outcomes validity and reliability of the modified Rankin scale: implications for stroke clinical trials: a literature review and synthesis. *Stroke* 2007;38(3):1091–1096.
4. Galton F. Regression towards mediocrity in hereditary stature. *J Anthropological Institute of Great Britain and Ireland* 1886;15:246–263.
5. Kramer MS, Shapiro SH. Scientific challenges in the application of randomized trials. *JAMA* 1984;252(19):2739–2745.
6. Multiple Risk Factor Intervention Trial Research Group. Multiple risk factor intervention trial. Risk factor changes and mortality results. *JAMA* 1982;248(12):1465–1477.
7. Syme SL. Community participation, empowerment, and health: Development of a wellness guide for California. In: Jamner MS, Stokols D, eds. *Promoting Human Wellness: New Frontiers for Research, Practice, and Policy*. Berkeley, CA: University of California Press, 2000:78–98.
8. Lundberg GD. MRFIT and the goals of The Journal. *JAMA* 1982;248(12):1501.
9. University of Minnesota: Heart Attack Prevention. Multiple Risk Factor Intervention Trial (MRFIT). Available at http://www.epi.umn.edu/cvdepi/study-synopsis/multiple-risk-factor-intervention-trial-mrfit/. Accessed March 20, 2015.
10. Myers M. RJ Reynolds vs. the government; business can speak out in other ways. *The New York Times*, Business Day, July 6, 1986. Available at http://www.nytimes.com/1986/07/06/business/rj-reynolds-vs-the-government-business-can-speak-out-in-other-ways.html. Accessed April 1, 2017.
11. Stamler J, Neaton JD. The Multiple Risk Factor Intervention Trial (MRFIT)—importance then and now. *JAMA* 2008;300(11):1343–1345.
12. Stamler J, Neaton JD, Cohen JD, Cutler J, Eberly L, Grandits G, et al. Multiple risk factor intervention trial revisited: a new perspective based on nonfatal and fatal composite

endpoints, coronary and cardiovascular, during the trial. *J Am Heart Assoc* 2012;1(5):e003640.

13. Grundy SM. Cholesterol and coronary heart disease. A new era. *JAMA* 1986;256(20):2849–2858.

14. Nelson SR. *Steel Drivin' Man: John Henry, the Untold Story of an American Legend*. Oxford: Oxford University Press, 2006.

15. Saretsky G. The OEO P.C. experiment and the John Henry effect. *Phi Delta Kappa* 1972;53:579.

16. Rosenthal R. *Experimenter Effects in Behavioral Research*. New York: Appleton-Century-Crofts, 1966.

17. Roethlisberger J, Dickson WJ. *Management and the Worker*. Cambridge, MA: Harvard University Press, 1966.

18. Gillespie R. *Manufacturing Knowledge: A History of the Hawthorne Experiments*. New York: Cambridge University Press, 1991.

19. Gale EA. The Hawthorne studies-a fable for our times? *Qjm* 2004;97(7):439–449.

20. Kompier MA. The "Hawthorne effect" is a myth, but what keeps the story going? *Scand J Work Environ Health* 2006;32(5):402–412.

21. Questioning the Hawthorne effect. *The Economist*, June 4, 2009. Available at http://www.economist.com/node/13788427. Accessed April 1, 2017.

22. Kolata G. Scientific myths that are too good to die. *The New York Times*. December 6, 1998. Available at http://www.nytimes.com/1998/12/06/weekinreview/scientific-myths-that-are-too-good-to-die.html. Accessed March 31, 2017.

23. McCambridge J, Witton J, Elbourne DR. Systematic review of the Hawthorne effect: new concepts are needed to study research participation effects. *J Clin Epidemiol* 2014;67(3):267–277.

24. Cizza G, Piaggi P, Rother KI, Csako G. Hawthorne effect with transient behavioral and biochemical changes in a randomized controlled sleep extension trial of chronically short-sleeping obese adults: implications for the design and interpretation of clinical studies. *PLoS One* 2014;9(8):e104176.

25. Gould DJ, Creedon S, Jeanes A, Drey NS, Chudleigh J, Moralejo D. Impact of observing hand hygiene in practice and research: a methodological reconsideration. *J Hosp Infect* 2017;95(2):169–174.

26. On the magnitude and persistence of the Hawthorne effect–evidence from four field studies. Proceedings of the 4th European Conference on Behaviour and Energy Efficiency (Behave 2016); 2016.

27. De Amici D, Klersy C, Ramajoli F, Brustia L, Politi P. Impact of the Hawthorne effect in a longitudinal clinical study: the case of anesthesia. *Control Clin Trials* 2000;21(2):103–114.

28. Zinman R, Bethune P, Camfield C, Fitzpatrick E, Gordon K. An observational asthma study alters emergency department use: the Hawthorne effect. *Pediatr Emerg Care* 1996;12(2):78–80.

29. Gartlehner G, Hansen RA, Nissman D, Lohr KN, Carey TS: Criteria for distinguishing effectiveness from efficacy trials in systematic reviews. Technical Review 12. AHRQ Publication No. 06-0046. Rockville, MD: Agency for Healthcare Research and Quality. April, 2006. Available at https://www.ncbi.nlm.nih.gov/books/NBK44029/pdf/Bookshelf_NBK44029.pdf. Accessed March 27, 2017.

30. Guyatt GH, Sackett DL, Cook DJ. Users' guides to the medical literature. II. How to use an article about therapy or prevention. B. What were the results and will they help me in caring for my patients? Evidence-Based Medicine Working Group. *JAMA* 1994;271(1):59–63.

31. Hennekens CH, Buring JE, Manson JE, Stampfer M, Rosner B, Cook NR, et al. Lack of effect of long-term supplementation with beta carotene on the incidence of malignant neoplasms and cardiovascular disease. *N Engl J Med* 1996;334(18):1145–1149.

32. Pablos-Mendez A, Barr RG, Shea S. Run-in periods in randomized trials: implications for the application of results in clinical practice. *JAMA* 1998;279(3):222–225.

33. Rausch JR, Maxwell SE, Kelley K. Analytic methods for questions pertaining to a randomized pretest, posttest, follow-up design. *J Clin Child Adolesc Psychol* 2003;32(3):467–486.

34. Vickers AJ, Altman DG. Statistics notes: Analysing controlled trials with baseline and follow up measurements. *BMJ* 2001;323(7321):1123–1124.

35. de Vries JD, van Hooff ML, Geurts SA, Kompier MA. Exercise to reduce work-related fatigue among employees: a randomized controlled trial. *Scand J Work Environ Health* 2017;43(4):337–349.

36. Heritier SR, Gebski VJ, Keech AC. Inclusion of patients in clinical trial analysis: the intention-to-treat principle. *Med J Aust* 2003;179(8):438–440.

37. Mahaniah KJ, Rao G. Intention-to-treat analysis: protecting the integrity of randomization. *J Fam Pract* 2004;53(8):644.

38. Fergusson D, Aaron SD, Guyatt G, Hebert P. Post-randomisation exclusions: the intention to treat principle and excluding patients from analysis. *BMJ* 2002;325(7365):652–654.

39. Hollis S, Campbell F. What is meant by intention to treat analysis? Survey of published randomised controlled trials. *BMJ* 1999;319:670–674.

40. Stanley K. Evaluation of randomized controlled trials. *Circulation* 2007;115(13):1819–1822.

41. Detry MA, Lewis RJ. The intention-to-treat principle: how to assess the true effect of choosing a medical treatment. *JAMA* 2014;312(1):85–86.

42. CONSORT Website. Available at http://www.consort-statement.org/. Accessed April 5, 2017.

43. Motulsky H. *Intuitive Biostatistics*. New York: Oxford University Press, 1995.

44. Sterne JAC, White IR, Carlin JB, Spratt M, Royston P, Kenward MG, et al. Multiple imputation for missing data in epidemiological and clinical research: potential and pitfalls. *BMJ* 2009;338:b2393.

45. Little RJA, Rubin DM. *Statistical Analysis with Missing Data*. New York: John Wiley and Sons, 1987.

46. Li P, Stuart EA, Allison DB. Multiple imputation: a flexible tool for handling missing data. *JAMA* 2015;314(18):1966–1967.

47. Streiner D, Geddes J. Intention to treat analysis in clinical trials when there are missing data. *Evid Based Ment Health* 2001;4(3):70-71.

48. Molnar FJ, Hutton B, Fergusson D. Does analysis using "last observation carried forward" introduce bias in dementia research? *CMAJ* 2008;179(8):751–753.

49. Lachin JM. Fallacies of last observation carried forward analyses. *Clin Trials* 2016;13(2):161–168.

50. Shoop SJW. Should we ban the use of 'last observation carried forward' analysis in epidemiological studies? *SM J Public Health Epidemiol* 2015;1(1):1004.

51. Newgard CD, Lewis RJ. Missing data: how to best account for what is not known. *JAMA* 2015;314(9):940–941.

52. Schafer JL. Multiple imputation: a primer. *Stat Methods Med Res* 1999;8(1):3–15.

53. National Research Council. *The Prevention and Treatment of Missing Data in Clinical Trials*. Panel on Handling Missing Data in Clinical Trials. Committee on National Statistics, Division of Behavioral and Social Sciences and Education. Washington, DC: The National Academies Press, 2010.

54. Donders AR, van der Heijden GJ, Stijnen T, Moons KG. Review: a gentle introduction to imputation of missing values. *J Clin Epidemiol* 2006;59(10):1087–1091.

55. Gelman A, Hill J. *Data Analysis Using Regression and Multilevel/Hierarchical Models. Chapter 25: Missing-data imputation*. Cambridge: Cambridge University Press, 2007.

Experimental Designs

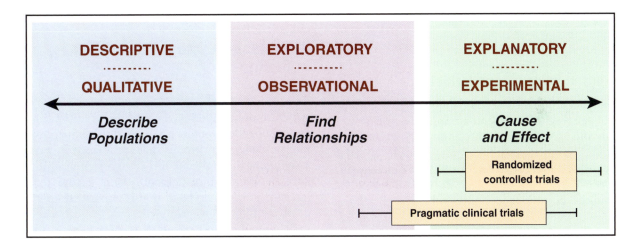

In the study of interventions, experimental designs provide a structure for evaluating the cause-and-effect relationship between a set of independent and dependent variables. In explanatory and pragmatic trials, the researcher manipulates the levels of the independent variable within the design to incorporate elements of control so that the evidence supporting a causal relationship can be interpreted with confidence.

The purpose of this chapter is to present basic configurations for experimental designs and to illustrate the types of research situations for which they are most appropriate. For each design, the discussion includes strengths and weaknesses in terms of internal and external validity, and the most commonly used statistical procedures are identified, all of which are covered in succeeding chapters. This information demonstrates the intrinsic relationship between analysis and design.

■ Design Classifications

Although experimental designs can take on a wide variety of configurations, the important principles can be illustrated using a few basic structures. A basic distinction among them is the degree to which a design offers experimental control.[1,2] In a *true experiment*, participants are randomly assigned to at least two comparison groups. An experimental design is theoretically able to exert control over most threats to internal validity, providing the strongest evidence for causal relationships.

Randomization Schemes

Experimental designs may be differentiated according to how subjects are assigned to groups. In **completely randomized designs**, also referred to as **between-subjects** designs, subjects are assigned to independent groups using a randomization procedure. A design in which subjects act as their own control is called a **within-subjects design** or a **repeated measures design** because treatment effects are associated with differences observed within a subject across treatment conditions, rather than between subjects across randomized groups.

> 📌 Designs are not considered true experiments if they do not include random assignment or control groups. When either of these conditions is not met, quasi-experimental designs can be used. These will be described in Chapter 17.

Number of Independent Variables

Experimental designs can also be described according to the number of independent variables, or *factors*, within the design. A **single-factor design** has one independent variable with any number of levels. Also called a **one-way design**, such a study may include one or more dependent variables. **Multi-factor designs** contain two or more independent variables.

■ Selecting a Design

Once a research question is formulated, the researcher must decide on the most effective design for answering it. Although experimental designs represent the highest standard in scientific inquiry for establishing a causal relationship between independent and dependent variables, they are not necessarily the best choice in every situation. When the independent variable cannot be manipulated by the experimenter, or when important extraneous factors cannot be controlled, an observational design may be more feasible (see Chapter 19).

When an experimental design is deemed appropriate, the choice of a specific design will depend on the answers to six critical questions about how the study is conceptualized:

1. How many independent variables are being tested?
2. How many levels does each independent variable have, and are these levels experimental or control conditions?
3. How many groups of subjects are being tested?
4. How will subjects be assigned to groups?
5. How often will observations of responses be made?
6. What is the temporal sequence of interventions and measurements?

When each of these issues is considered, the range of potential designs will usually be narrowed to one or two appropriate choices. As specific designs are presented, these questions will be addressed within the context of research questions from the literature.

> 🔑 Experimental designs can be applied to explanatory or pragmatic trials. The degree of control for internal and external validity may vary, which can require variations in analysis procedures. The essential design structures, however, can be used for both types of studies.

■ Pretest–Posttest Control Group Designs

The **pretest–posttest control group design** is the basic structure of a randomized controlled trial (RCT) with one independent variable. It is used to compare two or more independent groups that are formed by random assignment to determine if there is a significant difference between group outcomes from before to after intervention. This type of trial is also called a **parallel groups study**. One group receives the experimental variable and the other acts as a control, receiving no treatment, a placebo or sham, usual care, or another treatment (see Fig. 16-1).

Because groups are assigned at random, theoretically they differ only on the basis of what occurs between measurements. Therefore, within limits of internal validity, changes from pretest to posttest that appear in the experimental group but not the control group can be reasonably attributed to the intervention. This design is considered the scientific standard in clinical research for establishing a cause-and-effect relationship.

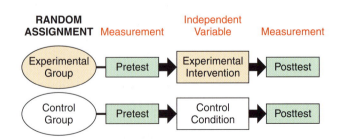

Figure 16–1 Pretest–posttest control group design, the basic structure of an RCT. The control condition may be no treatment, placebo or sham, usual care, or other intervention.

Experimental designs are classified according to the number of independent variables. Several dependent variables can be incorporated into one design, all measured at pretest and posttest.

Control Groups

Placebo Control

The basic pretest–posttest design incorporates a control group that receives no treatment, placebo, or sham.

Researchers conducted an RCT to study the effect of a supervised exercise program for improving venous hemodynamics in patients with chronic venous insufficiency.[3] They randomly assigned 31 patients to two groups. The experimental group practiced specific exercises for calf strengthening and joint mobility. The control group received no exercise intervention. Both groups received compression hosiery. Dynamic strength, calf pump function, and quality of life were assessed at baseline and after 6 months.

Measurements for the control group are taken within intervals that match those of the experimental group. The independent variable has two levels; in this case, exercise intervention and control. The absence of an experimental intervention in the control group is considered a level of the independent variable.

Treatment Control

The pretest–posttest design can also be used when the comparison group receives a second form of intervention, which may be usual care. Researchers use this approach when a control condition is not feasible or ethical, often comparing a "new" treatment with an "old" standard or alternative treatment. The standard treatment is considered a control. This design still provides a high level of experimental control because of the initial equivalence between groups formed by random assignment.

Researchers conducted an RCT to study the effect of semantic treatment on verbal communication in patients who experienced aphasia following a stroke.[4] They randomly assigned 58 patients to two groups. Speech-language pathologists provided semantic treatment to the experimental group. The control group received speech therapy focused on word sounds. Verbal communication was assessed using the Amsterdam Nijmegen Everyday Language Test. Both groups were assessed at the start of the study and following 7 months of treatment.

In this example, the word sound group acted as a control for the semantic treatment group and vice versa. If one group improves more than the other, we can attribute that difference to the fact that one treatment must have been more effective than the other. This design is appropriate when the research question specifically addresses interest in a difference between two treatments, but it does not allow the researcher to show that treatment works better than no intervention or sham intervention. However, usual care has typically been established as effective through previous study against a placebo.

Multigroup Design

The *multigroup pretest–posttest control group design* allows researchers to compare several treatment and control conditions.

Researchers wanted to determine the effectiveness of aquatic and on-land exercise programs on functional fitness and activities of daily living (ADLs) in older adults with arthritis.[5] Participants were 30 volunteers, randomly assigned to either aquatic exercise, on-land exercise, or a control group. The control group was asked to refrain from any new physical activity for the duration of the study. Outcomes included fitness and strength measures, and functional assessments before and after an 8-week exercise program.

As these examples illustrate, the pretest–posttest control group design can be expanded to accommodate any number of levels of one independent variable, with or without a traditional control group.

 It is important to distinguish the *levels* of an independent variable from the *number of independent variables*. For instance, in the study of aquatic and on-land exercise, there were three levels (aquatic, on-land, control), but only one independent variable.

Cluster Randomized Studies

The pretest–posttest design can be applied to cluster randomized studies, where multiple sites or communities are used to recruit subjects. Rather than randomizing individuals to experimental groups, sites are randomly assigned to interventions, and all individuals at that site receive the same treatment. This design is often used in pragmatic studies, especially when implementation questions are of interest (see Focus on Evidence 16-1). The unit of analysis may be the individual response or it can refer to cohorts, depending on the nature of the research question.[6]

Design Validity

The pretest–posttest design is strong in internal validity. Pretest scores provide a basis for establishing initial

The concept of knowledge translation is important in the consideration of experimental designs, as we strive to implement evidence-based strategies and guidelines into practice. Pragmatic trials are typically used to assess the effectiveness of interventions, often at the community level, to answer practical questions about interventions that have already been shown to be efficacious in RCTs.

For example, studies have established that decreases of 10 mm Hg in systolic blood pressure or 5 mm Hg in diastolic blood pressure can significantly reduce cardiovascular disease (CVD).[7] However, strategies to implement preventive programs to reduce hypertension are often largely ineffective.[8] In 2011, Kaczorowski et al[9] described the Cardiovascular Health Awareness Program (CHAP), which evaluated the effectiveness of community-based intervention to reduce cardiovascular admissions.

Using a cluster randomized design, the researchers identified 39 communities in Ontario with populations of at least 10,000 and stratified the communities by size and geographic area, randomly assigning them to receive the CHAP intervention (n = 20) or usual care (n = 19). The study was based on the following PICO question:

(P) Among midsized Ontario communities, for those >65 years old, (I) does a community-based program of blood pressure and CVD risk assessments with education and referral of all new or uncontrolled hypertensives to a source of continuing care, (C) compared with usual care, (O) reduce community rates of hospitalization for acute myocardial infarction, stroke, or congestive heart failure over 12 months?

The researchers acknowledged that this trial was highly pragmatic.[8] For instance, all municipalities of sufficient size were included, and all members of the communities over 65 years old were eligible to participate, regardless of comorbidities. Interventions were provided within community clinics and primary care settings by regular practitioners. Patient compliance was recorded but not controlled.

The results showed a modest but significant effect of the intervention, with a 9% relative reduction in hospitalizations compared to the prior 2 years, which translated to 3.02 fewer admissions/ 1,000 people. Although this seems small, the authors note that it could mean hundreds of thousands of fewer admissions across the general population.

The relevance of this trial to our discussion of design is based on the need to consider the research question and how validity would be viewed. Because the study did not include blinding, and provision of services was maintained within the natural health-care environment, internal validity could be suspect. However, the study was not about the efficacy of taking blood pressure measurements or educational programs to reduce CVD risk—that was established in earlier studies. Rather, its focus was on the effectiveness of organizing services in a community setting to influence outcomes, strengthening external validity.

---

equivalence of groups, strengthening the evidence that the causal effects of treatment must have brought about any measured group differences in posttest scores. Selection bias is controlled because subjects are randomly assigned to groups. History, maturation, testing, and instrumentation effects should affect all groups equally in both the pretest and posttest. Threats that are not controlled by this design are attrition and differential social threats.

The primary threat to external validity in the pretest–posttest design is the potential interaction of treatment and testing. Because subjects are given a pretest, there may be reactive effects, which would not be present in situations where a pretest is not given.

Analysis of Pretest–Posttest Designs. Pretest–posttest designs are often analyzed based on the change from pretest to posttest using *difference scores.*

With interval–ratio data, difference scores are usually compared using an unpaired *t*-test (with two groups) or a one-way analysis of variance (with three or more groups). The pretest–posttest design can also be analyzed as a two-factor design, using a two-way analysis of variance with one repeated factor, with treatment as one independent variable and time (pretest and posttest) as the second (repeated) factor.

With ordinal data, the Mann–Whitney *U*-test can be used to compare two groups, and the Kruskal–Wallis analysis of variance by ranks is used to compare three or more groups.

The analysis of covariance can be used to compare posttest scores, using the pretest score as the covariate. Discriminant analysis can also be used to distinguish between groups with multiple outcome measures.

■ Posttest-Only Control Group Design

The **posttest-only control group design** (see Fig. 16-2) is identical to the pretest–posttest design, with the obvious exception that a pretest is not administered to either group.

A study was designed to test the effectiveness of a computer-based counseling tool on reproductive choices in community family planning clinics in North Carolina.[10] A total of 340 women were randomly assigned to receive the Smart Choices packet or usual counseling over a 3-month period. Outcomes included

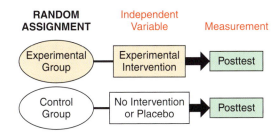

Figure 16–2 Posttest-only control group design.

the patients' confidence in choosing a contraceptive method that was right for them, ability to engage in shared decision-making with their provider, and their perception of the quality of the counseling experience.

In this study, researchers used the posttest-only design because the outcomes could only be assessed following the intervention condition. This design is a true experimental design that, like the pretest–posttest design, can be expanded to include multiple levels of the independent variable, with a control, placebo, or alternative treatment group.

The posttest-only design can also be used when a pretest is either impractical or potentially reactive. For instance, in surveys of attitudes, we might ask questions on a pretest that could sensitize subjects in a way that would influence their scores on a subsequent posttest. The posttest-only design avoids this form of bias, increasing the external validity of the study.

Design Validity

Because the posttest-only control group design involves randomization and comparison groups, its internal validity is strong, even without a pretest; that is, we can assume groups are equivalent prior to treatment because they have been randomly assigned. Because there is no pretest score to document the results of randomization, this design is most successful when the number of subjects is large so that the probability of truly balancing interpersonal characteristics is increased.

> **Analysis of Posttest-Only Designs**. With two groups, an unpaired t-test is used with interval–ratio data, and a Mann–Whitney U-test test with ordinal data.
>
> With more than two groups, a one-way analysis of variance or the Kruskal–Wallis analysis of variance by ranks should be used to compare posttest scores.
>
> An analysis of covariance can be used when covariate data on relevant extraneous variables are available. Regression or discriminant analysis procedures can also be applied.

■ Factorial Designs for Independent Groups

The designs presented thus far have involved the testing of one independent variable with two or more levels. Although easy to develop, these single-factor designs may impose an artificial simplicity on many clinical and behavioral phenomena; that is, they do not account for simultaneous and often complex interactions of several variables within clinical situations.

Interactions are generally important for developing a theoretical understanding of behavior and for establishing the construct validity of clinical variables. Interactions may reflect the combined influence of several treatments or the effect of several attribute variables on the success of a particular treatment.

A **factorial design** incorporates two or more independent variables, with independent groups of subjects randomly assigned to various combinations of levels of the variables. Although such designs can theoretically be expanded to include any number of independent variables, clinical studies usually involve two or three at most. As the number of variables increases, so does the number of experimental groups, creating the need for larger and larger samples, which are typically impractical in clinical situations.

Dimensions

Factorial designs are described according to their dimensions or number of factors so that a *two-way* or two-factor design has two independent variables, a *three-way* or three-factor design has three independent variables, and so on.

These designs can also be described by the number of levels within each factor so that a 3×3 design includes two independent variables, each with three levels, and a $2 \times 3 \times 4$ design includes three independent variables, with two, three, and four levels, respectively.

Factorial Diagrams

A factorial design is most easily diagrammed using a matrix that indicates how groups are formed relative to levels of each independent variable. Uppercase letters, typically A, B, and C, are used to label the independent variables and their levels. The number of groups is the product of the digits that define the design. For example, $3 \times 3 = 9$ groups; $2 \times 3 \times 4 = 24$ groups. Each cell of the matrix represents a unique combination of levels. In this type of diagram, there is no indication if measurements within a cell include pretest–posttest scores or posttest scores only. This detail is generally described in words.

Many clinical questions have the potential for involving several independent variables because response variables can be influenced by a multitude of factors. In this respect, the compelling advantage of multidimensional factorial designs is their more comprehensive construct validity.

Two-Way Factorial Design

A *two-way factorial design* (see Fig. 16-3A) incorporates two independent variables, *A* and *B*.

> ### ▶ CASE IN POINT #1
> Researchers were interested in studying the effect of joint protection and exercise on hand function in patients with osteoarthritis (OA).[11] All patients received leaflets with information on self-management of hand OA. Joint protection included occupational therapy sessions on management of joint stresses and pain. Exercises included stretching and strengthening. Patients ($N = 257$) were randomly assigned to one of four groups. The primary outcome was pain and function measured on the Australian/Canadian Hand Osteoarthritis Index.

In this example, the two independent variables are joint protection (*A*) and hand exercise (*B*), each with two levels (2 × 2). One group (A_1B_1) received both joint protection and exercise sessions. A second group (A_2B_1) received exercise only. The third group (A_1B_2) received joint protection only. And the fourth group (A_2B_2) received only the leaflet.

In this study, the two independent variables are *completely crossed*, which means that every level of one factor is represented at every level of the other factor. Each of the four groups represents a unique combination of the levels of these variables, as shown in the individual cells of the diagram in Figure 16-3A.

> ➤ This design allows us to ask three questions of the data:
> 1. Is there a differential effect of joint protection training versus information leaflet?
> 2. Is there a differential effect of hand exercises versus information leaflet?
> 3. What is the interaction between joint protection training and exercise?

Main Effects

The answers to the first two questions are obtained by examining the **main effect** of each independent variable, with scores collapsed across the second independent variable, as shown in Figure 16-3B. This means that we can look at the overall effect of the joint protection program without taking into account any differential effect of exercise. The main effect of exercise can also be analyzed without differentiating joint protection. Each main effect is essentially a single-factor experiment.

Interaction Effects

The third question addresses the **interaction effect** between the two independent variables. This question represents the essential difference between single-factor and multifactor experiments. Interaction occurs when the effect of one variable varies at different levels of the second variable. For example, we might find that the best response occurs with the combination of joint protection

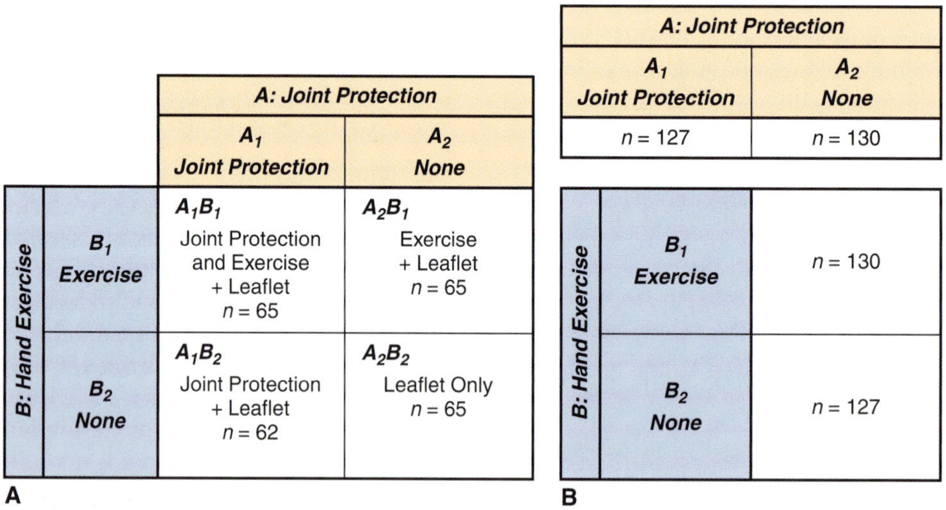

Figure 16–3 **A.** A two-way factorial design for a study of joint protection and hand exercise for patients with OA. All patients received the information leaflet as a control condition. **B.** Main effects for the two-way factorial design.

and exercise. Or we could find that exercise is most effective regardless of participation in the joint protection program.

This example illustrates the major advantage of the factorial approach, which is that it gives the researcher important information that could not be obtained with any one single-factor experiment. The ability to examine interactions greatly enhances the generalizability of results.

📌 Factorial designs can be extended to include more than two independent variables. In a *three-way factorial design*, a two-way design is essentially crossed on a third factor. For example, we could use a $2 \times 2 \times 2$ design, where subjects would be assigned to one of eight independent groups. We could examine the main effects of each independent variable, as well as their two-way and three-way interactions.

📊 ***Analysis of Factorial Designs.*** A two-way or three-way analysis of variance is most commonly used to examine the main effects and interaction effects of a factorial design.

Randomized Block Design

When a researcher is concerned that an extraneous factor might influence differences between groups, one way to control for this effect is to build the variable into the design as an independent variable. The **randomized block design** is used when an attribute variable, called a **blocking variable**, is crossed with an active independent variable. Groups of subjects from each of these "blocks" are randomly assigned to each of the treatment arms. The randomized block design helps ensure that participants who are similar with respect to the blocking variable are present in equal proportions across the groups. This serves to increase confidence that any measured group differences following treatment have resulted from the effects of the assigned treatments and not from other participant differences. In the following example, the study is based on a 2×3 randomized block design, with a total of six groups.

Researchers were interested in the effect of positioning on control of orofacial musculature for functional speech and coordinated swallowing.[12] They measured tongue pressure in upright and supine positions. They also questioned whether there were gender differences in the level of control. They tested 20 adults in a randomized block design, using gender as the blocking variable, randomly assigning men and women to the two positions. Subjects performed various oromotor tasks and outcomes included tongue pressures during difference speech tasks.

In studying the effect of position, the researchers were concerned that men and women would respond differently. They accounted for this potential effect by using gender as an independent variable and thereby eliminating it as a confounder.

We can think of the randomized block design as two single-factor randomized experiments, with each block representing a different subpopulation. Subjects are grouped by blocks and then random assignment is made within each block to the treatment conditions.

When the design is analyzed, we will be able to examine possible interaction effects between the treatment conditions and the blocking variable. When this interaction is significant, we will know that the effects of treatment do not generalize across the block classifications; in this case, across genders. If the interaction is not significant, we have achieved a certain degree of generalizability of the results.

📊 ***Analysis of Randomized Block Designs.*** Data from a randomized block design can be analyzed using a two-way analysis of variance, multiple regression, or discriminant analysis.

■ Repeated Measures Designs

All the experimental designs we have considered so far have involved at least two independent groups, created by random assignment or blocking. There are many research questions, however, for which control can be substantially increased by using a **repeated measures design**, where one group of subjects is tested under all conditions and each subject acts as his own control.

Advantages of Repeated Measures Designs

The major advantage of the repeated measures design is the ability to control for the potential influence of individual differences. It is a fairly safe assumption that important subject characteristics, such as age, sex, motivation, and intelligence, will remain constant throughout the course of an experiment. Therefore, differences observed among treatment conditions are more likely to reflect treatment effects, and not variability between subjects. Using subjects as their own control provides the most equivalent "comparison group" possible.

One-Way Repeated Measures Design

The simplest form of repeated measures design involves a single-factor experiment, where one group of subjects is exposed to all levels of one independent variable (see Fig. 16-4).

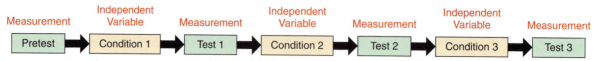

Figure 16–4 One-way repeated measures design. The order of test conditions may be randomized.

Researchers were interested in the effect of using a cane on the same side or contralateral side in patients with knee OA.[13] They studied women walking across a force platform unaided and using a cane on the same and opposite side to their arthritic knee. They measured knee and hip forces, speed, and cadence. A 5-minute rest period was permitted between each walking condition. The order of testing of the three walking conditions was randomized.

In this study, the researchers wanted to examine force and gait activity with all subjects exposed to all three walking conditions. It would be possible to use a randomized design to investigate this question by assigning different groups to each condition, but it does not make logical sense. By using a repeated measures format, we can be assured that differences across conditions are a function of cane use and not individual gait differences. This design is referred to as a *one-way repeated measures design*.

Because one-way repeated measures designs do not incorporate randomized comparison groups, they technically do not qualify as true experiments. However, they may be considered experiments when they incorporate randomization in the order of application of repeated conditions and the comparison of one condition or intervention to another within one subject.

> 📌 Repeated measures designs can also be used to look at time as a repeated factor when subjects are measured across several time periods. When time is the only independent variable, however, the design is considered quasi-experimental, as it is not possible to randomize order (see Chapter 17). Examples using time as an independent variable within an experimental design will be described under the section on multi-factor repeated measures models.

📉 ***Analysis of One-Way Repeated Measures Designs.*** The one-way repeated measures analysis of variance is used to test for differences across levels of one repeated factor.

Effects of Repeated Measurements

Because each participant experiences repeated measurements in this type of design, it should only be used when the outcome measure will revert back to baseline between interventions. In the OA study of cane use, for example, we assume that rest periods are sufficient to allow the gait parameters to be consistent across trials.

There are many treatments, however, for which carryover cannot be eliminated. With variables that produce permanent or long-term physiological or psychological effects, repeated measures designs are not appropriate. An exception to this caveat is the use of time as a repeated factor. In that case, when the purpose of the study is to observe trends in changes over several time periods, there is an expectation that the outcome measure will continue to change (see Chapter 26).

Practice Effects

One disadvantage of the repeated measures approach is the potential for **practice effects**, or the learning effect that can take place when one individual repeats a task over and over. For instance, in the OA study, it would be possible for subjects to become more accustomed to using the canes and walking on the force platform. The researchers controlled for this effect by randomizing the order of trials.

Carry Over Effects

Another disadvantage is the potential for **carryover effects** when one subject is exposed to multiple-treatment conditions. Carryover can be reduced by allotting sufficient time between successive treatment conditions to allow for complete dissipation of previous effects. In the cane study, the three walking conditions do not present a problem of carryover that would preclude one subject participating at all three levels. However, if we were to study the effect of these three walking conditions on fatigue, we may need to repeat testing on different days to be sure that tissues have returned to resting levels.

Order Effects

Because subjects are exposed to multiple-treatment conditions in a repeated measures design, there must be some concern about the potentially biasing effect of test sequence; that is, the researcher must determine if responses might be dependent on which condition preceded which other condition. Effects such as fatigue, learning, or carryover may influence responses if subjects are all tested in the same order.

One solution to the problem of order effects is to randomize the order of presentation for each subject, as was done in the OA study. This can be done by the flip of a coin or other randomization scheme so that there is no bias involved in choosing the order of testing. This approach does theoretically control for order effects. However, there is still a chance that some sequences will be repeated more often than others, especially if the sample size is small.

One solution for order effects involves use of a Latin square, which is a matrix composed of equal numbers of rows and columns, designating random permutations of sequence combinations. For example, in the cane study, if we had 30 subjects, we could assign 10 subjects to each of three sequences, as shown in Figure 16-5. Using randomization, we would determine which group would get each sequence, and then assign each testing condition to A, B, or C. This design is sometimes considered a randomized block design, with the blocks being the specific sequences.

Crossover Design

When only two levels of an independent variable are repeated, a preferred method to control for order

effects is to *counterbalance* the treatment conditions so that their order is systematically varied. This creates a crossover design in which half the subjects receive treatment A followed by B, and half receive B followed by A (see Fig. 16-6). Two subgroups are created, one for each sequence, and subjects are randomly assigned to one of the sequences.

> Researchers were interested in comparing the effects of prone and supine positions on stress responses in mechanically ventilated preterm infants.[14] They randomly assigned 28 infants to a supine/prone or prone/supine position sequence. Infants were placed in each position for 2 hours. Stress signs were measured following each 2-hour period, including startle, tremor, and twitch responses.

A crossover design should only be used in trials where the patient's condition or disease will not change appreciably over time. It is not a reasonable approach in situations where treatment effects are slow, as the treatment periods must be limited. It is similarly impractical where treatment effects are long term and a reversal is not likely.

Washout Period

The crossover design is especially useful when treatment conditions are immediately reversible, as in the positioning of infants in the previous example. When the treatment has cumulative effects, however, a washout period is essential, allowing a common baseline for each treatment condition (Fig. 16-6). The washout period must be long enough to eliminate any prolonged effects of the treatment.

> Researchers were interested in the effectiveness of a cranberry supplement for preventing urinary tract infections in persons with neurogenic bladders secondary to spinal cord injury.[15] They treated 21 individuals, evaluating responses based on urinary bacterial counts and white blood cell counts. Subjects were randomly

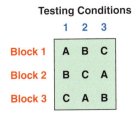

Testing Conditions

	1	2	3
Block 1	A	B	C
Block 2	B	C	A
Block 3	C	A	B

Figure 16–5 A 3 x 3 Latin Square.

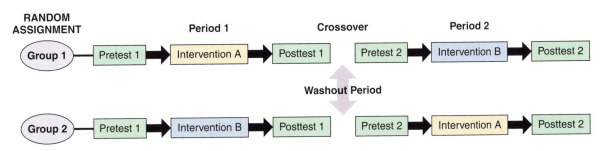

Figure 16–6 Crossover design. At the point of crossover, the study may incorporate a washout period.

assigned to standardized 400-mg cranberry tablets or placebo three times a day for 4 weeks. After 4 weeks, they imposed a 1-week "washout period," after which participants were crossed over to the other treatment condition.

In this example, 1 week was considered sufficient for removal of effects from the patient's system.

Analysis of Crossover Designs. In the analysis of a crossover design, researchers will usually group scores by treatment condition, regardless of which order they were given. A paired *t*-test can then be used to compare change scores, or a two-way analysis of variance with two repeated measures can be used to compare pretest and posttest measures across both treatment conditions. The Wilcoxon signed-ranks test should be used to look at change scores when ordinal data are used.

In some situations, the researcher may want to see if order did have an effect on responses and subjects can be separated into independent groups based on sequence of testing. This analysis may include a two-way analysis of variance with one repeated measure, with sequence as an independent factor and treatment condition as a repeated measure.

Two-Way Design with Two Repeated Measures

Repeated measures can also be applied to studies involving more than one independent variable.

Researchers were interested in studying the validity of wearable tracking devices to monitor heart rate and physical activity.[16] They asked 62 participants to wear three different types of wrist devices during a 16-minute ramped-up treadmill exercise. Measurements of heart rate were taken at four time periods during the exercise. Results for the three devices were compared following the exercise protocol.

This study was based on a 3 × 4 design, called a *two-way design with two repeated measures*: type of wrist device (3 levels) and measures over time (4 levels). Each subject was exposed to all test conditions and all time measures. When subject responses are compared over successive time periods, time becomes an independent variable.

Analysis of Two-Way Repeated Measures Designs. The two-way analysis of variance with two repeated measures is used to analyze differences across main effects and interaction effects.

Mixed Design

A **mixed design** is created when a study incorporates two independent variables, one repeated across all subjects, and the other randomized to independent groups.

A study was designed to evaluate the effectiveness of a program of stabilizing exercises for patients with pelvic girdle pain after pregnancy.[17] Eighty women with pelvic girdle pain were assigned randomly to two treatment groups for 20 weeks. One group received physical therapy with a focus on specific stabilizing exercises. The other group received individualized physical therapy without specific stabilizing exercises. Assessments were administered by a blinded assessor at baseline, after intervention, and at 1-year postpartum. Main outcome measures were pain, functional status, and quality of life.

In the comparison of the two exercise programs, subjects were randomly assigned to treatment groups. Each subject was tested three times (pretest and two posttests). The variable of exercise program is considered an *independent factor* because its levels have been randomized, creating independent groups. The variable of time is a *repeated factor* because all subjects are tested at each of the three levels.

Therefore, this design is called a *two-way design with one repeated measure*, or a 2 × 3 *mixed design*. This example illustrates a commonly used approach, where researchers want to establish if the effects of intervention are long-lasting and not just present immediately following completion of the program.

The description of a research design must specify if a variable is a repeated measure. Generally, independent variables are assumed to be independent factors unless otherwise indicated. In a two-way design, the number of repeated measures should be stated. When a study is termed a mixed design, indicating a combination of repeated and independent factors, the number of repeated measures should be specified if there are more than two factors.

Analysis of Mixed Designs. A two-way analysis of variance with one repeated measure is used to analyze main effects and interaction effects with a two-way mixed design.

■ Sequential Clinical Trials

The RCT presents practical challenges for clinical research because a large sample needs to be gathered at the start and results can only be analyzed at the end, regardless of whether the experimental treatment has been successful. The **sequential clinical trial** is an alternative approach to the RCT, which allows for continuous analysis of data as they become available, instead of waiting until the end of the experiment to compare groups. Results are accumulated as each subject is tested so that the experiment can be stopped at any point as soon as the evidence is strong enough to determine a significant difference between treatments. Consequently, it is possible that a decision about treatment effectiveness can be made earlier than in a fixed sample study, leading to a substantial reduction in the total number of subjects needed to obtain valid statistical outcomes and avoiding unnecessary administration of inferior treatments.

Allard et al[18] used a sequential design to study the effect of opioids to relieve dyspnea in patients with cancer. They compared 25% and 50% supplementary dosage regimens and measured intensity and frequency of respiratory problems following administration of the drug. Pairs of patients were alternately assigned to one dose and preference was based on the subjective assessment of a better outcome.

Sequential trials incorporate specially constructed charts that provide visual confirmation of statistical outcomes, without the use of formal statistical calculations (see Fig. 16-7). Upper, lower, and middle boundaries are constructed and successive pair preferences are charted in a continuous line, moving toward one of the boundaries, indicating if results are in favor of one treatment or the other, or show no preference. For instance, in the study of dyspnea and opioids, the first four pairs showed a preference for the 50% dose, the next three preferred the 25% dose, and further pairs alternated between the two outcomes. After 15 pairs were evaluated, the results showed no difference between the dose regimens, as the line that charted the preferences moved progressively toward the middle boundary.

Because of the ongoing sequential analysis, a major advantage of this approach is the potential ability to make a decision about treatment effectiveness earlier than in a fixed sample study, leading to a substantial reduction in the total number of subjects needed to obtain valid statistical outcomes and avoiding unnecessary administration of inferior treatments. For example, in a retrospective sequential analysis of data that

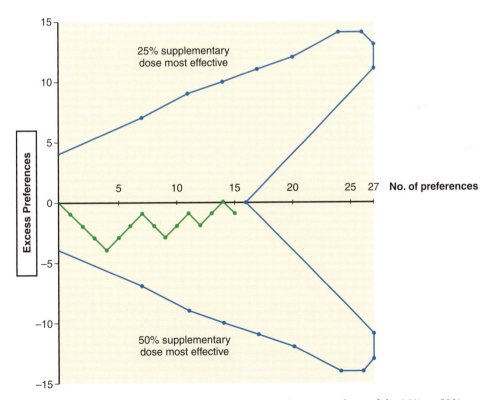

Figure 16–7 Sequential analysis diagram of paired preferences in favor of the 25% or 50% supplementary dose of opioids to reduce dyspnea in patients with cancer. From Allard P, Lamontagne C, Bernard P, et al. How effective are supplementary doses of opioids for dyspnea in terminally ill cancer patients? A randomized continuous sequential clinical trial. *J Pain Symptoms Manage* 1999;17(4):256–265. Figure 2, p. 260. Used with permission.

were collected in a clinical trial, researchers found that the sequential design would have reduced the trial sample by 234 patients and shortened its duration by 3 to 4 months.[19]

Although the sequential trial design has great appeal, it has been used primarily in drug trials. However, it has

potential for creating an efficient design in other types of clinical trials.

 See the *Chapter 16 Supplement* for a full description of sequential trials.

COMMENTARY

To consult a statistician after an experiment is finished is often merely to ask him to conduct a post mortem examination. He can perhaps say what the experiment died of.

—*Sir Ronald Fisher (1890-1962)*

British statistician

The importance of understanding concepts of design cannot be overemphasized in the planning stages of an experimental research project. There is a logic in these designs that must be fitted to the research question and the scope of the project so that meaningful conclusions can be drawn once data are analyzed. The choice of a design should ultimately be based on the intent of the research question:

> . . . *the question being asked determines the appropriate research architecture, strategy, and tactics to be used—not tradition, authority, experts, paradigms, or schools of thought.*[20]

The underlying importance of choosing an appropriate research design relates to consequent analysis issues that arise once data are collected. Many beginning researchers have had the unhappy experience of presenting their data to a statistician, only to find out that they did not collect the data appropriately to answer their research question. Fisher[21] expressed this idea in his classical work, *The Design of Experiments*:

> *Statistical procedure and experimental design are only two different aspects of the same whole, and that whole*

comprises all the logical requirements of the complete process of adding to natural knowledge by experimentation.

Although the clinical trial is considered a "gold standard" for establishing cause and effect, it is by no means the best or most appropriate approach for many of the questions that are most important for improving practice. The real world does not operate with controls and schedules the way an experiment demands. Quasi-experimental and observational studies, using intact groups or nonrandom samples, play an important role in demonstrating effectiveness of interventions.[22] These differences can be appreciated as the divergence between "evidence-based practice" and "practice-based evidence" (see Chapter 2). As we continue to examine outcomes as a primary focus of clinical research, we must consider many alternatives to the traditional clinical trial in order to discover the most "effective" courses of treatment.[23]

REFERENCES

1. Campbell DT, Stanley JC. *Experimental and Quasi-experimental Designs for Research*. Chicago: Rand McNally, 1963.
2. Cook TD, Campbell DT. *Quasi-experimentation: Design and Analysis Issues for Field Settings*. Boston: Houghton Mifflin, 1979.
3. Padberg FT Jr, Johnston MV, Sisto SA. Structured exercise improves calf muscle pump function in chronic venous insufficiency: a randomized trial. *J Vasc Surg* 2004;39(1):79–87.
4. Doesborgh SJ, van de Sandt-Koenderman MW, Dippel DW, van Harskamp F, Koudstaal PJ, Visch-Brink EG. Effects of semantic treatment on verbal communication and linguistic processing in aphasia after stroke: a randomized controlled trial. *Stroke* 2004;35(1):141–146.
5. Suomi R, Collier D. Effects of arthritis exercise programs on functional fitness and perceived activities of daily living measures in older adults with arthritis. *Arch Phys Med Rehabil* 2003;84(11): 1589–1594.

6. Donner A, Klar N. Pitfalls of and controversies in cluster randomization trials. *Am J Public Health* 2004;94(3):416–422.

7. Murray CJ, Lauer JA, Hutubessy RC, Niessen L, Tomijima N, Rodgers A, et al. Effectiveness and costs of interventions to lower systolic blood pressure and cholesterol: a global and regional analysis on reduction of cardiovascular-disease risk. *Lancet* 2003;361(9359):717–725.

8. Thabane L, Kaczorowski J, Dolovich L, Chambers LW, Mbuagbaw L. Reducing the confusion and controversies around pragmatic trials: using the Cardiovascular Health Awareness Program (CHAP) trial as an illustrative example. *Trials* 2015; 16:387.

9. Kaczorowski J, Chambers LW, Dolovich L, Paterson JM, Karwalajtys T, Gierman T, et al. Improving cardiovascular health at population level: 39 community cluster randomised trial of Cardiovascular Health Awareness Program (CHAP). *BMJ* 2011;342:d442.

10. Koo HP, Wilson EK, Minnis AM. A computerized family planning counseling aid: a pilot study evaluation of smart choices. *Perspect Sex Reprod Health* 2017;49(1):45–53.

11. Dziedzic K, Nicholls E, Hill S, Hammond A, Handy J, Thomas E, et al. Self-management approaches for osteoarthritis in the hand: a 2x2 factorial randomised trial. *Ann Rheum Dis* 2015; 74(1):108–118.

12. Dietsch AM, Cirstea CM, Auer ET Jr, Searl JP. Effects of body position and sex group on tongue pressure generation. *Int J Orofacial Myology* 2013;39:12–22.

13. Chan GN, Smith AW, Kirtley C, Tsang WW. Changes in knee moments with contralateral versus ipsilateral cane usage in females with knee osteoarthritis. *Clin Biomech* 2005; 20(4):396–404.

14. Chang YJ, Anderson GC, Lin CH. Effects of prone and supine positions on sleep state and stress responses in mechanically ventilated preterm infants during the first postnatal week. *J Adv Nurs* 2002;40:161–169.

15. Linsenmeyer TA, Harrison B, Oakley A, Kirshblum S, Stock JA, Millis SR. Evaluation of cranberry supplement for reduction of urinary tract infections in individuals with neurogenic bladders secondary to spinal cord injury. A prospective, double-blinded, placebo-controlled, crossover study. *J Spinal Cord Med* 2004; 27(1):29–34.

16. Dooley EE, Golaszewski NM, Bartholomew JB. Estimating accuracy at exercise intensities: a comparative study of self-monitoring heart rate and physical activity wearable devices. *JMIR Mhealth Uhealth* 2017;5(3):e34.

17. Stuge B, Laerum E, Kirkesola G, Vollestad N. The efficacy of a treatment program focusing on specific stabilizing exercises for pelvic girdle pain after pregnancy: a randomized controlled trial. *Spine* 2004;29(4):351–359.

18. Allard P, Lamontagne C, Bernard P, Tremblay C. How effective are supplementary doses of opioids for dyspnea in terminally ill cancer patients? A randomized continuous sequential clinical trial. *J Pain Symptom Manage* 1999;17(4):256–265.

19. Bolland K, Weeks A, Whitehead J, Lees KR. How a sequential design would have affected the GAIN International Study of gavestinel in stroke. *Cerebrovasc Dis* 2004;17(2-3):111–117.

20. Sackett DL, Wennberg JE. Choosing the best research design for each question. *BMJ* 1997;315:1636.

21. Fisher RA. *The Design of Experiments*. 9 ed. New York: Macmillan, 1971.

22. Gartlehner G, Hansen RA, Nissman D, Lohr KN, Carey TS: Criteria for distinguishing effectiveness from efficacy trials in systematic reviews. Technical Review 12. AHRQ Publication No. 06-0046. Rockville, MD: Agency for Healthcare Research and Quality. April, 2006. Available at https://www.ncbi.nlm. nih.gov/books/NBK44029/pdf/Bookshelf_NBK44029.pdf. Accessed March 27, 2017.

23. Concato J, Shah N, Horwitz RI. Randomized, controlled trials, observational studies, and the hierarchy of research designs. *N Engl J Med* 2000;342(25):1887–1892.

Quasi-Experimental Designs

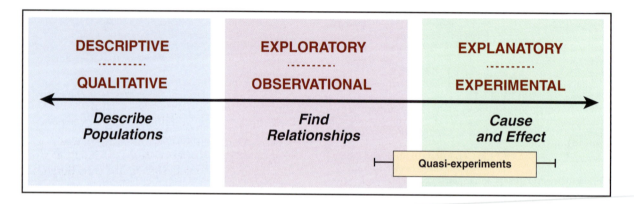

Although the randomized trial is considered the optimal design for testing cause-and-effect hypotheses, the necessary restrictions of a randomized trial are not always possible within the clinical environment. Depending on the nature of the treatment under study and the population of interest, use of randomization and control groups may not be possible.

Quasi-experimental designs utilize similar structures to experimental designs, but lack either random assignment, comparison groups, or both. Even with these limitations, these designs represent an important contribution to clinical research because they accommodate for the limitations of natural settings, where scheduling treatment conditions and random assignment are often difficult, impractical, or unethical. They are often used in pragmatic studies because of the logistic limitations that occur in practice. The purpose of this chapter is to describe time series designs and nonequivalent group designs, the two basic structures of quasi-experimental research.

■ Validity Concerns

Because quasi-experimental designs lack at least one of the requirements for controlled trials, they cannot rule out threats to internal validity with the same confidence as experimental studies. Nonequivalent groups may differ from each other in many ways in addition to differences between treatment conditions. Therefore, the degree of control is reduced.

Quasi-experimental designs present reasonable alternatives to the randomized trial as long as the researcher carefully documents subject characteristics, controls the research protocol, and uses blinding as much as possible. The conclusions drawn from these studies must take into account the potential biases of the sample, but may provide important information, nonetheless.

■ Time Series Designs

Many research questions focus on the variation of responses over time. In such a design, time becomes an independent variable with several levels and researchers will look for differences across time intervals. Such designs can be configured in several ways, with varying degrees of control.

One-Group Pretest–Posttest Design

The **one-group pretest–posttest design** is a quasi-experimental design that involves one set of repeated measurements taken before and after treatment on one group of subjects (see Fig. 17-1). The effect of treatment is determined by measuring the difference between pretest and posttest scores.

In this design, the independent variable is time, with two levels (pretest and posttest). Treatment is not an independent variable because all subjects receive the intervention.

> A study was designed to examine the effect of four-direction shoulder stretching exercises for patients with idiopathic adhesive capsulitis.[1] All subjects received the same exercise protocol. Researchers studied the effects of treatment on pain, range of motion (ROM), function, and quality of life measures. Comparisons were made between pretest scores and final scores at follow-up, with a mean duration of 22 months.

In this study, the researchers saw significant improvements in outcome variables and concluded that the treatment was successful.

Design Validity

We must be cautious in drawing conclusions from this design, however. The design is weak because it has no comparison group, making it especially vulnerable to threats to internal validity. Although the researcher can demonstrate change in the dependent variable by comparing pretest and posttest scores, there is always the possibility that some events other than the experimental treatment occurred within the time frame of the study that caused the observed change. External validity is also limited by potential interactions with selection because there is no comparison group.

The one-group pretest–posttest design may be defended, however, in cases where previous research has documented the behavior of a control group in similar circumstances. For instance, other studies may have shown that shoulder pain does not improve in this population over a 4-week period without intervention. On that basis, we could justify using a single experimental group to investigate just how much change can be expected with treatment. This documentation might also allow us to defend the lack of a control group on ethical grounds.

The design is also reasonable when the experimental situation is sufficiently isolated so that extraneous environmental variables are effectively controlled, or where the time interval between measurements is short so that temporal effects are minimized.[2] In studies where data collection is completed within a single testing session, temporal threats to internal validity will be minimal, but testing effects remain uncontrolled. Under all circumstances, however, this design is not considered a true experiment and should be expanded whenever possible to compare two groups. It is often possible to use an alternative treatment as a control.

📊 **Analysis of One-Group Pretest–Posttest Designs.** A paired *t*-test is usually used to compare pretest and posttest mean scores. With ordinal data or small samples, the sign test or the Wilcoxon signed-ranks test can be used.

Repeated Measures Design

Many research questions that deal with the effects of treatment on physiological or psychological variables are concerned with how those effects are manifested over time. As an extension of the pretest–posttest design, the repeated measures design is naturally suited to assessing such trends. Multiple measurements of the dependent variable are taken within prescribed time intervals. The intervention may be applied once or it may be repeated in between measurements (see Fig. 17-2).

> Researchers studied the effects of constraint-induced movement therapy (CIMT) on spasticity and upper extremity function in patients with chronic hemiplegia.[3] They studied 20 patients, taking measurements before

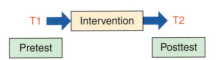

Figure 17–1 A one-group pretest–posttest design. The independent variable is time, with two levels (T1 and T2).

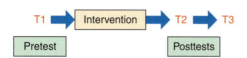

Figure 17–2 One-way pretest–posttest repeated measures design over time. Because there is only one group, the independent variable in this design is time, depicted here with three levels. The intervention may be applied in between the two posttests.

and after a 2-week CIMT program, with a follow-up at 6 months. Outcome measures reflected impairment and activity domains of the International Classification of Functioning, Disability and Health (ICF), including the Modified Ashworth Scale, ROM, grip strength, and several hand function tests. Improvements were noted following treatment, which persisted at 6 months.

Because there is only one treatment condition, treatment cannot be an independent variable. Therefore, time is the independent variable. Every subject is evaluated at each time interval, making it a repeated measure. The design is quasi-experimental because there is no comparison group.

Design Validity

Like the pretest–posttest design, internal validity is threatened without a control group. Therefore, it is not possible to discern if changes would have occurred over time without the intervention. However, this design can be extended to include multiple pretests or posttests, which may allow trends to be observed.

> **Analysis of Repeated Measures Designs Over Time.** When time is the independent variable, a one-way repeated-measures analysis of variance can be performed. Analysis may also include polynomial contrasts to describe trends over time (see Chapter 26).

Interrupted Time Series Design

Time series designs can incorporate multiple measurements, before and after intervention, to document patterns or trends of behavior. These designs are often used to study community interventions and the effects of organizational policy changes.

The **interrupted time series (ITS) design** is so named because it involves a series of measurements over time that are "interrupted" by one or more treatment occasions (see Fig. 17-3). It is considered a quasi-experimental design because only one group is studied. The independent variable is time. The research question concerns trends across these time intervals (see Focus on Evidence 17-1).

The number of observations in an ITS design can vary, depending on the stability of the dependent variable. In some studies, researchers may extend pretest or posttest periods if the data are very variable, in an effort to stabilize responses before initiating treatment or ending the observations.

Data Patterns

The ITS design is most effective when serial data can be collected at evenly distributed intervals, avoiding confounding by extraneous temporal factors.[5] To illustrate, consider several possible outcomes for an ITS design, where a series of observations are taken at times 1 through 8 (T_1–T_8), with the introduction of intervention at point X (see Fig. 17-4).

Consider the data from T_4 to T_5 for all three patterns, which show a similar increase in the dependent variable. In pattern A, we would be justified in assuming that intervention has an effect, as no change occurred prior to intervention and the level of response increased following intervention.

In pattern B, however, it would be misleading to make this interpretation, as the responses are already increasing within the baseline measures, before any intervention is implemented, and the same trend continues into the intervention period. Although pattern C also shows an increase in the dependent variable from T_4 to T_5, which would look like a treatment effect if these were the only two measurements taken, we can see from the erratic pattern changes before and after treatment that this conclusion is unwarranted.

These types of patterns would not be apparent in a pretest–posttest design. The primary benefit of an ITS is its ability to show such trends over extended periods of time.

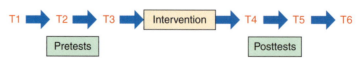

Figure 17–3 Interrupted time series design, with multiple pretests and posttests. The intervention can also be applied during the posttest period between measurements.

Focus on Evidence 17–1
Documenting Trends

Taking blood cultures is an important diagnostic tool in emergency departments. However, false positives from contamination can lead to unnecessary morbidity, invasive procedures, antibiotic therapy, and healthcare costs. Laboratory standards recommend that hospitals maintain a contamination rate of less than 3%.

One hospital found that its contamination rate was consistently above 4%, and developed an interdisciplinary task force to design a QI effort to achieve a sustainable rate below the 3% benchmark.[4] They used an ITS analysis to compare contamination rates prior to and after implementation of an intervention, shown in the figure. From March through December 2009, they documented their process of blood culture collection as a baseline. They found many factors that contributed to a high contamination rate, including significant variation in practice. This led to development of a standardized collection protocol and training sessions that were implemented across the hospital over a 2-month period (blue area).

Following the training period, the intervention was fully implemented. The data were analyzed using a *segmented linear regression model*, which looked at trends by dividing the study periods into 2-week intervals (segments), so that they had 24 time points each across baseline and intervention periods.

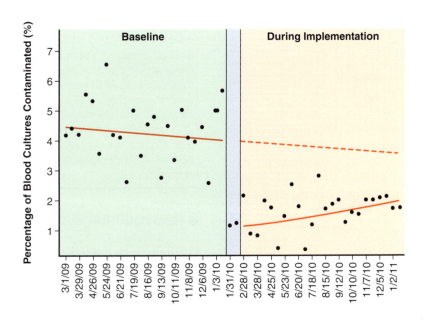

Using a forecasting model, the baseline trend was projected into the intervention period (dashed line) to estimate what the contamination rate would have been had the intervention not been implemented. During the baseline period, an average of 4.3% of cultures were contaminated, compared to 1.7% during the intervention period. The intervention was associated with an immediate 2.9% (95% CI = 2.2% to 3.2%) absolute reduction in contamination, which was significant. The contamination rate was maintained below 3% throughout the year of the monitored intervention period.

The ITS design is often used for this kind of QI project because it allows investigators to observe trends throughout the testing periods.

As shown in this example, the variability in data can be further explored to determine factors that impacted outcomes. Simple pretest–posttest designs cannot provide this level of information that can be extremely useful for decision-making and policy implementation.

From Self WH, Speroff T, Grijalva CG, et al. Reducing blood culture contamination in the emergency department: an interrupted time series quality improvement study. *Acad Emerg Med* 2013;20(1):89–97. Adapted from Figure 4, p. 94. Used with permission.

🖈 A time series design does involve repeated measures, but it is distinguished from standard repeated measures designs by the large number of measurements that are taken continuously across baseline and intervention phases.

Design Validity

The ITS design is an extension of the one-group pretest–posttest design. It offers more control, however, because the multiple pretests and posttests act as a pseudocontrol condition, demonstrating maturational trends that naturally occur in the data or the confounding effects of

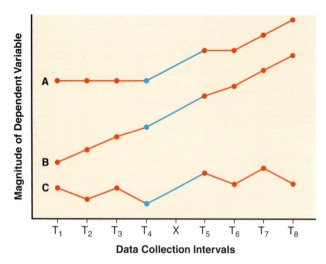

Figure 17–4 Illustration of three possible outcome patterns in the interrupted time series design. The change from T4 to T5 is the same in all three, although they show very different patterns that would warrant different conclusions.

extraneous variables. Therefore, trends that are present during the baseline phase can be accounted for.

The greatest threat to internal validity in the time series design is history. There is no control over the possible coincidental occurrence of some extraneous event at the same time that treatment is initiated. The level and trend of the preintervention data, however, do present a form of control for the postintervention segment.[6]

Most other threats to internal validity are fairly well controlled by the presence of multiple measurements; that is, their effects are not eliminated, but we can account for them. For instance, if instrumentation or testing effects are present, we should see changes across the pretest scores. External validity of a time series design is limited to situations where repeated testing takes place.

Design Variations

Several variations can be applied to the time series design. Comparisons may include two or more groups. Intervention may be administered one time only with follow-up measurements, or intervention may be continued throughout the posttest period, as it did in the blood-contamination study.

In a third variation, treatment may be started after a series of pretest measurements, and then withdrawn after a specified time period, with measurements continuing into the withdrawal period. The *withdrawal design* does help to account for history effects. If the behavior improves with treatment, and reverts back to baseline levels when treatment is withdrawn, a strong case can be made that extraneous factors were not operating.

📌 The structure of the interrupted time series design, which is geared toward the study of large groups or organizations, can also be applied to individuals using single-subject designs (SSDs), which will be described in Chapter 18.

📈 **Analysis of Time Series Designs.** Many researchers use graphic visual analysis as the primary means of interpreting time series data, although there is considerable disagreement as to the validity of this approach. One approach, related to quality improvement (QI), is the use of **statistical process control** techniques (see Chapter 18).

Statistical techniques for time series analysis involve multivariate methods. A model called the *autoregressive integrated moving average (ARIMA)* is often used to accommodate for serial scores and weighs heavily on the observations that fall closer to the point at which intervention is introduced. To be effective, the ARIMA procedure requires at least 25 data points in each phase.[7] Descriptions of this method can be found in several references.[2,8]

A technique called *segmented regression analysis* has also been used to look at patterns of change over time in the level and slope of regression lines for different segments of the data.[9]

■ Nonequivalent Group Designs

There are many research situations in the social, clinical, and behavioral sciences where groups are found intact or where participants are self-selected. The former case is common in a clinic or school where patients or students belong to fixed groups or classes. The latter case will apply when attribute variables are studied or when volunteers are recruited.

Nonequivalent Pretest–Posttest Control Group Design

The *nonequivalent pretest–posttest control group design* (see Fig. 17-5) is similar to the pretest–posttest experimental

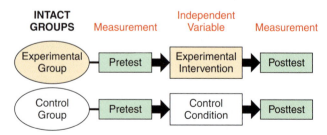

Figure 17–5 The nonequivalent pretest–posttest control group design. Subjects may be members of intact groups, or they may express preferences for a particular group.

design, except that subjects are not assigned to groups randomly. This design can be structured with one treatment group and one control group or with multiple treatment and control groups.

Intact Groups

A study was done to determine the effectiveness of an individualized physical therapy intervention in treating neck pain.[10] One treatment group of 30 patients with neck pain completed physical therapy treatment. The control group of convenience was formed by a cohort group of 27 subjects who also had neck pain but did not receive treatment for various reasons, such as delay in insurance approval, time constraints, or exacerbations.

There were no significant differences between groups in demographic data or the initial test scores of the outcome measures. A physical therapist rendered an intervention to the treatment group based on a clinical decision-making algorithm. Treatment effectiveness was examined by assessing changes in ROM, pain, endurance, and function. Both the treatment and control groups completed the initial and follow-up examinations, with an average duration of 4 weeks between tests.

In this study of therapy for neck pain, the patients are members of intact groups by virtue of their personal circumstances.

Subject Preferences

A study was designed to examine the influence of regular participation in chair exercises on postoperative deconditioning following hip fracture.[11] Patients were distinguished by their willingness to participate and were not randomly assigned to groups. A control group received usual care following discharge. Physiological, psychological, and anthropometric variables were measured before and after intervention.

In the chair exercise study, subjects self-selected their group membership. Because groups are not randomly assigned, bias is a concern in these designs.

Design Validity

Although the nonequivalent pretest–posttest control group design is limited by the lack of randomization, it still has several strengths. Because it includes a pretest and a control group, there is some control over history, testing, and instrumentation effects. The pretest scores can be used to test the assumption of initial equivalence on the dependent variable, based on average scores and measures of variability.

The major threat to internal validity is the interaction of selection with history and maturation. For instance, if those who chose to participate in chair exercises were stronger or more motivated patients, changes in outcomes

may have been related to physiological or psychological characteristics of subjects. These characteristics could affect general activity level or rate of healing. Such interactions might be mistaken for the effect of the exercise program. These types of interactions can occur even when the groups are identical on pretest scores.

Design Strategies for Nonequivalent Groups

When subjects cannot be assigned to groups, researchers are often concerned about whether confounding variables are balanced across groups at baseline. Several design and analysis strategies can be incorporated into a nonequivalent group design that help to balance groups.

Designs can incorporate stratification or a blocking variable, whereby a confounder is built into the design as an independent variable. For example, subjects can be divided into groups by age or gender. This allows the confounding variable to be controlled in comparisons within and across strata (see Chapter 14). This technique can only be effectively used with one or two variables at most.

A statistical strategy is the use of matching to equate groups on baseline scores that may present substantial confounding effects. For instance, subjects may be matched on age or gender to assure a balance of these factors. This is a challenge, however, when many variables may have a confounding effect, making one-on-one matching unfeasible. Researchers often use a technique of deriving **propensity scores** for this purpose. Through the use of regression analyses, a single variable is created that statistically represents a set of several confounders. This propensity score can then be used to match subjects so that observed covariates are balanced across groups (see Chapter 31).[12]

Analysis of Nonequivalent Pretest–Posttest Designs. Several statistical methods are suggested for use with nonequivalent groups, including the unpaired *t*-test (with two groups), analysis of variance, and analysis of covariance. Analyses can also include matched scores.

Ordinal data can be analyzed using the Mann–Whitney *U*-test. Nonparametric tests may be more appropriate with nonequivalent groups, as variances are likely to be unequal. Preference for one approach will depend in large part on how groups were formed and what steps the researcher can take to ensure or document initial equivalence.

Tests such as the *t*-test, analysis of variance, and chi square are often used to test for differences in baseline measures. Regression analysis or discriminant analysis may be the most applicable approach to determine how the dependent variable differentiates the treatment groups, while adjusting for other variables. Statistical strategies must include mechanisms for controlling for group differences on potentially confounding variables.

Historical Controls

Another strategy for comparing treatments involves the use of **historical controls** who received a different treatment during an earlier time period.

> Concern exists that prednisone-free maintenance immunosuppression in kidney transplant recipients will increase acute and/or chronic rejection. Over a 5-year period from 1999 to 2004, researchers worked with 477 kidney transplant recipients who discontinued prednisone on postoperative day 6, followed by a regimen of immunosuppressive therapy.[12] The outcomes were compared with that of 388 historical controls from the same institution (1996 to 2000) who did not discontinue prednisone. Outcomes included changes in serum creatinine levels, weight, and cholesterol, as well as patient and graft survival rates.

As this example illustrates, a nonconcurrent control group may best serve the purpose of comparison when ethical concerns may preclude a true control group. When the researcher truly believes that the experimental intervention is more effective than standard care, the use of historical controls provides a reasonable alternative.[13]

This approach has often been used in cancer trials, when protocols in one trial act as a control for subsequent studies.[14] The major advantage of this approach is its efficiency. Because all subjects are can be assigned to the experimental condition in the subsequent study, the total sample will be smaller and the results can be obtained in a shorter period of time.

Design Validity

The disadvantages of using historical controls must be considered carefully, however. Studies that have compared outcomes based on historical controls versus randomly allocated controls have found positive treatment effects with historical controls that randomized trials have not been able to replicate.[15,16] The most obvious problem, therefore, is the potential for confounding because of imbalances in characteristics of the experimental and historical control groups.

For this approach to work, then, the researcher must be diligent in establishing a logical basis for group comparisons. This means that the historical controls should not simply be any patients described in the literature, or those treated at another time or another clinic.[14,17] It is reasonable, however, as in the kidney transplant example, to consider using groups that were treated within the same environment, under similar conditions, where records of protocols were kept and demographics of subjects can be obtained. This approach may prove useful as large clinical data bases are accumulated within a given treatment setting.

Analysis of Designs With Historical Controls.
Researchers often use the independent samples *t*-test to compare current subjects with historical subjects, although there is an inherent flaw in this approach because there is no assumption of equivalence between the groups.

The Mann–Whitney *U*-test may be used with ordinal data. Chi square will allow the researcher to determine if there is an association among categorical variables.

Multiple regression, logistic regression, or discriminant analysis can be done, using group membership as a variable, to analyze differences between the groups while accounting for other variables.

Nonequivalent Posttest-Only Control Group Design

Nonequivalent designs are less interpretable when only posttest measures are available. The *nonequivalent posttest-only control group design* (see Fig. 17-6) is a quasi-experimental design that can be expanded to include any number of treatment levels, with or without a control group. This design uses existing groups that have and have not received treatment.

> Researchers were interested in studying the effects of a cardiac rehabilitation program on self-esteem and mobility skill in 152 patients who received cardiac surgery.[18] They studied 37 subjects who participated in a 2-month exercise program, and another 115 subjects who chose not to attend the program, forming the control group. Measurements were taken at the end of the 2-month study period. Outcomes were based on the Adult Source of Self-Esteem Inventory and the New York Heart Association classification.

Design Validity

To draw conclusions from this comparison, we would have to determine if variables other than the exercise program could be responsible for outcomes. Confounding factors should be identified and analyzed in relation to the dependent variable. For instance, in the cardiac

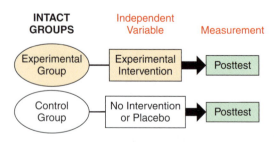

Figure 17–6 The nonequivalent posttest-only control group design.

rehabilitation example, researchers considered the subjects' age, years of education, and occupational skill.[18]

Although this comparison does have a control group, internal validity is severely threatened by selection biases and attrition. This design is inherently weak because it provides no evidence of equivalence of groups before treatment. Therefore, it should be used only in an exploratory capacity, where it may serve to generate hypotheses for future testing. It is essentially useless in the search for causal relationships.

> **Analysis of Nonequivalent Posttest-Only Designs.** Because this design does not allow interpretation of cause-and-effect, the most appropriate analysis is a regression approach, such as discriminant analysis. Essentially, this design allows the researcher to determine if there is a relationship between the presence of the group attribute and the measured response. An analysis of covariance may be used to account for the effect of confounding variables.

COMMENTARY

The only relevant test of the validity of a hypothesis is comparison of its prediction with experience.

—Milton Friedman (1912-2006)

American Economist, 1976 Nobel Memorial Prize in Economic Sciences

In the pursuit of evidence-based practice, clinicians must be able to read research literature with a critical eye, assessing not only the validity of the study's design, but also the generalizability of its findings. Published research must be applicable to clinical situations and individual patients to be useful. The extent to which any study can be applied to a given patient is always a matter of judgment.

Purists will claim that generalization of intervention studies requires random selection and random assignment—in other words, an RCT. In this view, quasi-experimental studies are less generalizable because they do not provide sufficient control of extraneous variables. In fact, such designs may be especially vulnerable to all the factors that affect internal validity.

One might reasonably argue, however, that the results of the RCT may not apply to a particular patient who does not meet all the inclusion or exclusion criteria, or who cannot be randomly assigned to a treatment protocol. Many of the quasi-experimental models will provide an opportunity to look at comparisons in a more natural context.

In the hierarchy of evidence that is often used to qualify the rigor and weight of a study's findings, the RCT is considered the highest level (see Chapter 5). But the quasi-experimental study should not be dismissed as a valuable source of information. As with any study, however, it is the clinician's responsibility to make the judgments about the applicability of the findings to the individual patient.

REFERENCES

1. Griggs SM, Ahn A, Green A. Idiopathic adhesive capsulitis. A prospective functional outcome study of nonoperative treatment. *J Bone Joint Surg Am* 2000;82-A(10):1398–1407.
2. Cook TD, Campbell DT. *Quasi-experimentation: Design and Analysis Issues for Field Settings*. Boston: Houghton Mifflin, 1979.
3. Siebers A, Oberg U, Skargren E. The effect of modified constraint-induced movement therapy on spasticity and motor function of the affected arm in patients with chronic stroke. *Physiother Can* 2010;62(4):388–396.
4. Self WH, Speroff T, Grijalva CG, McNaughton CD, Ashburn J, Liu D, et al. Reducing blood culture contamination in the emergency department: an interrupted time series quality improvement study. *Acad Emerg Med* 2013;20(1):89–97.
5. Matowe LK, Leister CA, Crivera C, Korth-Bradley JM. Interrupted time series analysis in clinical research. *Ann Pharmacother* 2003;37(7–8):1110–1116.
6. Ansari F, Gray K, Nathwani D, Phillips G, Ogston S, Ramsay C, et al. Outcomes of an intervention to improve hospital antibiotic prescribing: interrupted time series with segmented regression analysis. *J Antimicrob Chemother* 2003;52(5):842–8.
7. Ottenbacher KJ. Analysis of data in idiographic research: Issues and methods. *Am J Phys Med Rehabil* 1992;71:202–208.
8. Harrop JW, Velicer WF. A comparison of alternative approaches to the analysis of interrupted time-series. *Multivariate Behav Res* 1985;20(1):27–44.
9. Wagner AK, Soumerai SB, Zhang F, Ross-Degnan D. Segmented regression analysis of interrupted time series studies in medication use research. *J Clin Pharm Ther* 2002;27(4):299–309.
10. Wang WT, Olson SL, Campbell AH, Hanten WP, Gleeson PB. Effectiveness of physical therapy for patients with neck pain: an individualized approach using a clinical decision-making algorithm. *Am J Phys Med Rehabil* 2003;82(3):203–218; quiz 19–21.

11. Nicholson CM, Czernwicz S, Mandilas G, Rudolph I, Greyling MJ. The role of chair exercises for older adults following hip fracture. *S Afr Med J* 1997;87(9):1131–1138.

12. Matas AJ, Kandaswamy R, Humar A, Payne WD, Dunn DL, Najarian JS, et al. Long-term immunosuppression, without maintenance prednisone, after kidney transplantation. *Ann Surg* 2004;240(3):510–516; discussion 16–17.

13. Moser M. Randomized clinical trials: alternatives to conventional randomization. *Am J Emerg Med* 1986;4(3):276–285.

14. Viele K, Berry S, Neuenschwander B, Amzal B, Chen F, Enas N, et al. Use of historical control data for assessing treatment effects in clinical trials. *Pharm Stat* 2014;13(1):41–54.

15. Sacks HS, Chalmers TC, Smith H, Jr. Sensitivity and specificity of clinical trials. Randomized v historical controls. *Arch Intern Med* 1983;143(4):753–755.

16. Micciolo R, Valagussa P, Marubini E. The use of historical controls in breast cancer. An assessment in three consecutive trials. *Control Clin Trials* 1985;6(4):259–270.

17. Bridgman S, Engebretsen L, Dainty K, Kirkley A, Maffulli N. Practical aspects of randomization and blinding in randomized clinical trials. *Arthroscopy* 2003;19(9):1000–1006.

18. Ng JY, Tam SF. Effect of exercise-based cardiac rehabilitation on mobility and self-esteem of persons after cardiac surgery. *Percept Mot Skills* 2000;91(1):107–114.

Single-Subject Designs

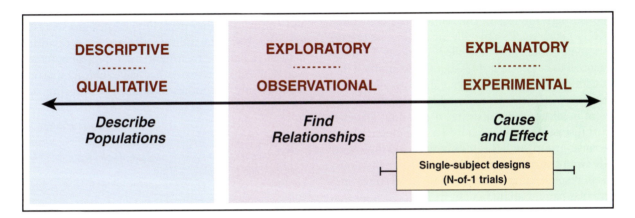

DESCRIPTIVE	EXPLORATORY	EXPLANATORY
··········	··········	··········
QUALITATIVE	OBSERVATIONAL	EXPERIMENTAL
Describe Populations	*Find Relationships*	*Cause and Effect*

Single-subject designs
(N-of-1 trials)

The demands of traditional experimental methods are often seen as barriers to clinical inquiry because of their rigorous structure, requiring control groups and large numbers of homogenous subjects, typically unavailable in clinical settings. The experimental model also deals with averages and generalizations across groups of individuals, which may not allow the researcher to differentiate characteristics of those patients who responded favorably to treatment from those who did not improve. Therefore, although group generalizations are important for explaining behavioral phenomena, clinicians understand that group performance is relevant only if it can contribute to making decisions about individual patients.

Single-subject designs (SSDs) involve serial observations of individuals before, during, and after interventions, providing feedback that reflects clinical outcomes. As a patient-level investigation, this pragmatic approach can facilitate evidence-based practice (EBP) by providing clinicians with practical information to improve decision-making within a clinical environment and to assess the impact of programs of care.[1–4] The purpose of this chapter is to describe a variety of SSDs and to explore issues related to their structure, application, analysis, and interpretation of treatment effectiveness.

■ Focus on the Individual

Consider the following clinical research scenario:

Several years ago, a study was done to determine if the occurrence of stuttering would be different if adults read aloud at "usual" or "fast-as-possible" rates.[5] A group of 20 adults was tested in a repeated measures design and no significant difference was seen between the two conditions based on a comparison of means.

Okay, so reading rate had no effect on stuttering—or did it? It turns out that a closer look at individual results showed that 8 subjects actually decreased their frequency of stuttering, 1 did not change, and 11 demonstrated an increase during the faster speaking condition. By drawing conclusions from average treatment effects, an important differentiation among individual performances was obscured, potentially affecting clinical outcomes.

Limitations of Randomized Trials

Because the application of research findings is often viewed through the lens of the randomized controlled trial (RCT), such studies generally incorporate large samples, randomization, and controlled protocols. Findings are assumed to be generalizable—but the assumption that one treatment's effect can be generalized to all patients is rarely true.[2] (If it were, we would not need so many different medications for arthritis, depression, diabetes, or heart disease—as evidenced by TV commercials!)

Because group studies typically take measurements at only two or three points in time, they may miss variations in response that occur over time. And sometimes a particular patient might benefit from a treatment that is shown to be inferior in a randomized trial. Therefore, randomized group studies can be ambiguous for purposes of clinical decision-making for an individual patient.

Individualized Care

In the spirit of EBP, there is an increasing recognition among providers that healthcare is not a "one-size-fits-all" process. The concept of "personalized" or "individualized" care is gaining acceptance, especially with the availability of relevant genetic information.[6] The personalized approach seeks to identify subgroups within populations to better understand how an individual's characteristics may affect treatment effectiveness and risks.[7]

Another aspect of this concept is a shift in the relationship between patient and provider. In addition to patients being "subjects" in research studies that will produce data to inform future care, there is a growing focus on patient involvement in studying issues that are most relevant to their lives, the idea of **patient-centered outcomes research** (see Chapter 2). Giving patients an opportunity to engage in the decision-making about their individual care allows all involved to take the unique circumstances of each patient into account. Therefore, there is a need to bring the search for evidence to the individual patient.

Single-subject studies provide an alternative approach that allows us to draw conclusions about the effects of treatment based on the responses of individuals under controlled conditions, with the flexibility to observe change before, during, and after treatment. By focusing on the individual patient, this approach provides information about which treatment works, for whom, and under which conditions.

The Research Question

Single-subject research can be used to study comparisons among several treatments, between components of treatments, or between treatment and no-treatment conditions. These designs are considered experimental because they require the same attention to logical design and control as other experimental designs. A research hypothesis should indicate the expected relationship between a defined treatment and a clinical outcome, as well as the characteristics that make subjects appropriate for the study. Hypotheses can be directional or nondirectional (see Chapter 3).

📌 Single-subject designs have also been called *single-case designs*, *single-system strategies*, *N-of-1 trials*, *small-N designs*, and *time series designs*.

■ Structure of Single-Subject Designs

SSDs are structured around two core elements: repeated measurement and design phases.

Repeated Measurement

An SSD involves the systematic collection of repeated measurements of a behavioral response for one individual and is therefore considered a **within-subjects design**. The outcome response, or **target behavior**, is measured at frequent and regular intervals, such as at each treatment session or over days. These repeated assessments are required to observe response patterns, evaluate variability of the behavioral response, and modify the intervention as necessary while the study progresses.

Design Phases

The second core element is the delineation of at least two testing periods, or phases: a *baseline phase*, prior to treatment, and an *intervention phase*. The target behavior is measured repeatedly across both phases.

The baseline phase provides information about responses during a period of "no treatment," or a control condition. The assumption is that baseline data reflect the natural state of the target behavior over time along with ongoing effects of background variables, such as daily activities, other treatments, and personal characteristics. When treatment is initiated, changes from baseline to the intervention phase should be attributable to intervention. Therefore, baseline data provide a standard of comparison for evaluating the potential cause-and-effect relationship between the intervention and target behavior.

 It is important to differentiate an SSD from a case report (see Chapter 20), which is an after-the-fact intensive description of a patient's episode of care. A case report is intended to identify patterns and generate hypotheses, but does not include systematic manipulation of variables or serial measurements under controlled treatment conditions.[1,8]

Graphing Responses

Data are plotted on a chart showing baseline and intervention phases, as shown in Figure 18-1, with magnitude of the target behavior along the *Y*-axis and time (sessions, trials, days, weeks) along the *X*-axis. Besides serving as research documentation, this process provides a clinically useful method for visualizing patterns of change and progress over time. This hypothetical data will be used for various illustrations throughout this chapter.

Using conventional notation, the baseline period is represented by the letter *A* and the intervention period by the letter *B*. To facilitate description, this design, with

one baseline phase and one intervention phase, is called an *A–B design*.

Collecting Baseline Data

The collection of baseline data is the single feature of an SSD that particularly distinguishes it from clinical practice, case reports, and traditional experimental designs, where treatment is initiated immediately following assessment, making it impossible to determine which components of treatment actually caused observed changes. More importantly, it is not possible to determine if observed changes would have occurred without intervention. Just as we need a control group to validate group comparisons, we must have a control period to make these determinations for a single-subject experiment (see Box 18-1).

Two characteristics of baseline data are important for interpretation of clinical outcomes: *stability*, which reflects the consistency of response over time, and *trend* or *slope*, which shows the direction and rate of change in the behavior (see Fig. 18-2).

The most desirable baseline pattern demonstrates a *stable baseline*, with constant level of behavior with minimal variability, indicating that the target behavior is not changing. Therefore, changes that are observed after the intervention is introduced can be confidently attributed to a treatment effect. If treatment has no effect, we would expect to see this baseline pattern continue into the intervention phase.

A *variable baseline* can present a problem for interpretation. When this type of pattern emerges, it is generally advisable to continue to collect baseline data until some

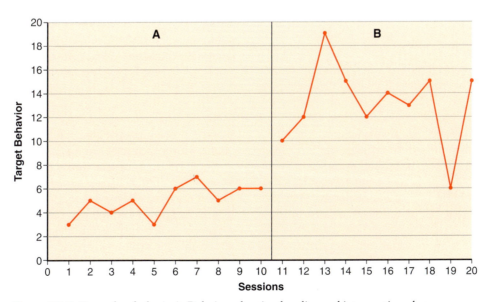

Figure 18–1 Example of a basic A–B design, showing baseline and intervention phases.

Box 18-1   Being All Right With Baseline Data

Ethical objections often arise when the baseline concept is introduced, just as they do when a control group is proposed for a group comparison study. Two points must be made in this regard. First, we can argue that it is not unethical to withhold treatment for a relatively short period when we are unsure about the effectiveness of the intervention in the first place. Indeed, it may actually be unethical to continue to provide an inferior or ineffective treatment without testing it experimentally. Second, collecting baseline data does not mean that the clinician is denying all treatment to the patient. It only means that one portion of the patient's total treatment is being isolated for study while all other treatments and activities are continued as background.

Measuring baseline data, however, may not be an appropriate approach for studying every type of intervention, such as treatments for critical or life-threatening situations, where treatment effects are not questioned and withholding treatment would be harmful.

Although single-subject studies are designed to incorporate intervention within the framework of clinical treatment, informed consent is required from all patients participating in single-subject trials.

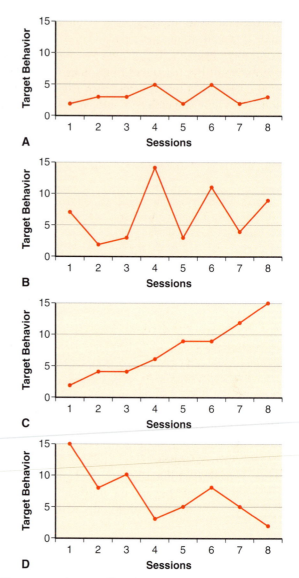

Figure 18–2 Types of baselines that may be encountered in single-subject designs: A) Stable, level baseline; B) Variable baseline; C) Stable accelerating trend; D) Variable decelerating trend.

stability is achieved. With extreme variability, the researcher is obliged to consider which factors might be influencing the target behavior to create such an erratic response.

Trending baselines, either accelerating or decelerating, indicate that the target behavior is changing without intervention. Either type of trend may represent improvement or deterioration, depending on the target behavior. Trends can also be characterized as stable or unstable; that is, the rate of change may be constant or variable.

Length of Phases

One of the first considerations when planning single-subject experiments concerns how long phases should be. There is some flexibility in these choices, allowing for consideration of the type of patient, the type of treatment, and the expected rate of change in the target behavior. This flexibility differentiates the SSD from traditional designs where onset and duration of treatment are established and fixed prior to experimentation, regardless of how the patient responds. There are some guidelines that can be followed to assist in these decisions.

Because trend is an important characteristic of repeated measurements, a minimum of five data points is recommended in each phase.[9] The application of some

analysis procedures is enhanced by having 12 or more points within each phase to establish stability.[10]

Phase length must take into account the time needed to see a meaningful change in the target behavior. If possible, it is generally desirable to use relatively equal phase lengths to control for potential time-related factors such as maturation or the motivational influence of continued attention over prolonged treatment periods. Many researchers set shorter baseline phases because of clinical considerations in treating the patient.

Despite these plans, however, it is usually advisable to extend baseline or intervention phases until stability is achieved, or at least until one is sure that responses are representative of the true condition under study. The decision on length, then, can rest with the researcher as a function of the subject's response, and may change during the course of the study.[11]

■ Defining the Research Question

Just like any other experiment, SSDs require rigor in the design protocol to assure confidence in observed effects of treatment. The intervention, or independent variable, should be operationally defined so that others could replicate it.

Some interventions, like drugs, can be controlled with placebos and can be easily blinded. That is not the case with many types of clinical interventions that require direct interaction between clinician and patient. Therefore, the strategies for treatment must be carefully delineated so that they are well understood by all those involved, including patients and families.

An important feature of SSDs is the ability to make adjustments in the intervention as the study progresses based on the subject's performance.[4] For instance, if the subject is not responding to treatment, it would be fruitless to continue to collect data without trying to vary aspects of intervention that might be successful.[12] This flexibility provides a valuable practical approach to understanding treatment effectiveness.

■ Measuring the Target Behavior

Because single-subject studies provide an individualized approach, target behaviors can be specified that reflect impairments as well as activity and participation restrictions in ways that are clinically relevant to the patient and practitioner. Like all studies, these measures must be operationally defined, reliable, observable, quantifiable, and a valid indicator of treatment effectiveness. Ideally, the behaviors will be stable and the degree of expected change will be meaningful.

Although patients usually present with several clinical problems, target behaviors should focus on a primary response. Is it how often a patient can perform a particular task, or how long a behavior can be maintained? Is it a score on a functional scale? Is the number of correct responses of interest? Or is it simply whether or not the behavior occurred? The answers to these questions should be based on the outcomes that are most meaningful to the patient, particularly activity and participation measures.

The most common techniques for measuring behaviors within SSDs are frequency, duration, and magnitude measures.

Frequency

A *frequency* count indicates the number of occurrences of a behavior within a fixed time interval or number of trials. Frequency can be expressed as a *percentage*, by dividing the number of occurrences of the target behavior by the total number of opportunities for the behavior to occur. This method is often used in studies in which accuracy of performance (percentage correct) is of primary interest.

Interval Recording

A useful procedure for measuring repetitive behavior is called *interval recording*, which involves breaking down the full measurement period into preset time intervals and determining if the behavior occurs or does not occur during each interval.

Xin et al[13] used an SSD to study the effects of using a customized iPad app on self-monitoring behaviors in four students who were classified with autism spectrum disorder (ASD). Students were observed during 20-minute periods to determine if they were able to remain seated, pay attention to the teacher, and focus their work on a given assignment. Behaviors were observed in 2-minute intervals across the 20-minute sessions, with measures recorded as "+" for an occurrence of the target behavior or "−" for a nonoccurrence in each interval.

The frequency of occurrences was summed over the 20-minute period and this sum was considered the child's score for that session. This study illustrates the importance of operational definitions for frequency counts, specifying exactly what constitutes an occurrence and nonoccurrence of the behavior.

Duration

Target behaviors can also be evaluated according to how long they last. *Duration* can be measured either as the cumulative total duration of a behavior during a treatment session or as the duration of each individual occurrence of the behavior. For example, this could include how long it takes to complete a task, how long one can maintain a certain posture, or how long pain lasts after an activity. Operational definitions for duration measures must specify criteria for determining when the behavior starts and ends.

Quantitative Scores

Many clinical variables are measured using some form of instrumentation that provides a quantitative score, which may be a summary score, a subscale score, or a single test value. When treatments are geared toward function or participation measures, scale scores can be used as the target behavior.

■ Limitations of the A–B Design

The element that most clearly characterizes an experimental research design is its ability to control for threats to internal validity. Unfortunately, the basic A–B design is limited in this respect because it provides no control comparison. Consider a scenario in the iPad study where we could look at only one student and, following intervention, we observe a meaningful change in behavior. Would we be confident in ascribing this change to the intervention? Could other events or changes within the subject have occurred coincidentally at the same time treatment was initiated that would have accounted for the observed change? For example, changes may be related to other treatments the child is receiving, or to maturation as the child develops across the year. Testing effects could be present with repeated assessment. In other words, is this conclusion internally valid? With an A–B design, it is impossible to conclude that the treatment is the causative factor for change.

> Another important element of internal validity is blinding. However, as is often the case in clinical studies like the iPad study, it is not possible to blind the patient, clinician, or assessor. Depending on the nature of the treatment and outcome variables, blinding should be attempted as much as possible.

Replication of Effects

To strengthen internal validity of the SSD without a control condition, we must include another form of evidence that the treatment was indeed responsible for observed changes, evidence that will discredit alternative hypotheses for explaining treatment outcomes. Within a single-subject strategy, this additional control is provided by *replication of effects*, which can be accomplished in three ways.

- Phases can be repeated by withdrawing and reinstating baseline and treatment conditions.
- Effects can be replicated across more than one subject or within one subject across multiple conditions, behaviors, or settings.
- Two or more interventions can be compared.

The more often an effect can be replicated within a design, the stronger the design controls against potential threats to internal validity. These strategies form the basis for structuring single subject experiments.

■ Withdrawal Designs

One way to achieve experimental control within an SSD is through withdrawal of intervention to demonstrate that the target behavior occurs only in the presence of treatment. The **withdrawal design** includes a second baseline period but may also include a second intervention period.

A–B–A Design

The *A–B–A design* replicates one baseline phase following intervention. The premise of this design lies in its ability to show that changes in the target behavior are not maintained during the second baseline period, allowing the conclusion that treatment was the factor causing the changes observed during the intervention phase.

Internal validity is controlled in the A–B–A design based on the assumption that it is unlikely that confounding factors would inadvertently occur at both the onset and cessation of treatment, what Barlow and Hersen[14] have called "the principle of unlikely successive coincidences." If other variables were responsible for changes seen in the target behavior during the first two phases, the behavior would not be expected to revert back to baseline levels during the withdrawal phase.

> Researchers studied the effects of an aquatic aerobic exercise program on function and endurance in a 5-year-old girl with cerebral palsy.[15] Following a 6-week baseline period, the intervention was carried out three times/week over 12 weeks. A 13-week follow-up period was also assessed. The 6-minute walk test (6MWT) was used to assess endurance.

The results of this study are shown in Figure 18-3. Clear improvement was seen during the intervention phase with minimal variability. A decrement in performance back to the original baseline level was seen when the intervention was removed.

Limitations of the A–B–A Design

There are two apparent concerns with the A–B–A design. One is that it seems clinically untenable to take away a treatment that is working. It also requires that the behavior is reversible, which is often not the case. Any response that is learned or that creates permanent change will not show a decrement when treatment is withdrawn.

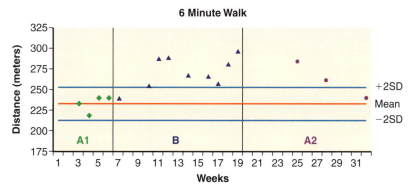

Figure 18–3 Example of an A–B–A design, showing endurance using the 6MWT in a child with cerebral palsy. The intervention was an aquatic-based aerobic exercise program. The horizontal bands represent 2 standard deviations (SD) above and below the mean of the first baseline scores. From Retarekar R, Fragala-Pinkham MA, Townsend EL. Effects of aquatic aerobic exercise for a child with cerebral palsy: single-subject design. *Pediatr Phys Ther* 2009;21(4): 336–344. Figure 4, p. 341. Used with permission of the Section on Pediatrics of the American Physical Therapy Association.

📌 The basic withdrawal design can be reversed to begin with a treatment phase, using a B–A–B configuration. This may be useful when it is not possible or ethical to start with a baseline period. Treatment can then be withdrawn to see if its effects are maintained.

A–B–A–B Design

Experimental control and clinical relevance can be further strengthened through additional replication using an *A–B–A–B design*, which includes a second intervention phase. The major advantage of this design is that it provides two opportunities to evaluate the effects of the intervention. If effects can be replicated during two separate intervention phases, controlling for internal validity, the evidence is quite strong that behavioral change was directly related to the treatment.

Researchers examined the effect of an activity-based therapy regimen on symmetric weight bearing in three adult subjects with hemiplegia.[16] The intervention program was introduced for 30 minutes each day during the intervention phase. Quantitative measurements of weight distribution over the affected leg were taken with a balance system. Each phase lasted 7 days with measures taken each day.

Figure 18-4 shows results for one subject in this study. Weight distribution was plotted as a ratio of the percent weight on the affected limb over total body weight. Therefore, the goal was to achieve higher ratios. Although the performance shows some variability, there is clearly a declining ratio during both baseline phases and an increasing ratio during both intervention phases.

The A–B–A–B design faces the same limitations as the A–B–A design, in that behaviors must be reversible to see treatment effects. If, however, the target behavior does not revert to original baseline values, but stays level during the second baseline, the A–B–A–B strategy can still document further improvement during the second intervention phase.

■ Multiple Baseline Designs

The use of withdrawal is limited in situations where ethical considerations prevail or where behaviors are either nonreversible or prone to carryover effect. When withdrawal is not practical, a **multiple baseline design** can be used.

The most common application of this approach is replication of effects across subjects, but the design can also look at one subject across behaviors or in multiple settings. At least three comparisons should be used within a study.[17] The multiple baseline approach allows for use of the basic A–B format as well as withdrawal variations.

Multiple Baseline Across Subjects

The multiple baseline design demonstrates experimental control by comparing three or more subjects, each of whom is assigned a baseline of a different length. One intervention is applied to the same target behavior across

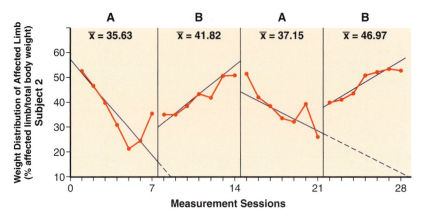

Figure 18–4 Example of an A–B–A–B design, showing the effect of an activity-based therapy on weight distribution over the affected limb in a patient with hemiplegia. These data are from one of three patients in the study. The superimposed lines in each phase are split-middle lines, showing data trends. From Wu S, Huang H, Lin C, Chen M. Effects of a program on symmetrical posture in patients with hemiplegia: a single-subject design. *Am J Occup Ther* 1996;50(1):17–23. Figure 1, p. 20. Reprinted with permission of the American Occupational Therapy Association.

three or more individuals who share common relevant characteristics.

All subjects begin with a concurrent collection of baseline data, which is then followed by a staggered introduction of the intervention. By allowing each baseline to run for a different number of data points, systematic changes in the target behavior that are correlated with the onset of intervention can be reliably attributed to a treatment effect.

Educators studied the effect of a student-centered precision teaching model on the development of basic reading skills and word building in three children with reading disorders.[18] They used a multiple baseline design with staggered introduction of the teaching strategy to study reading comprehension and fluency.

Results are shown in Figure 18-5. Each of the baselines shows minimal variability, but changes were obvious for each child following onset of the intervention. The authors concluded that training improved student performance. Each student showed initial decrement during a follow-up period, but performance rebounded back to intervention levels within a few weeks. When multiple baseline designs use the A–B format, internal validity is controlled because the results are replicated across three conditions at staggered times, making it unlikely that external factors could coincidentally occur at the time each treatment was initiated to cause the response change. One of the major advantages of the multiple-baseline approach is that replication and

experimental control can be achieved without withdrawal of treatment.

Other Multiple Baseline Designs

Multiple baseline designs can also be used to test the influence of environment. In the *multiple baseline design across settings*, one individual is monitored in multiple settings, with the same treatment applied sequentially across two or more environmental conditions testing the same intervention and behavior.

Sometimes, it is of interest to study the effect of one intervention on several related clinical behaviors. In the *multiple baseline design across behaviors*, the researcher monitors a minimum of three similar yet functionally independent behaviors in the same subject. Behaviors are addressed using the same intervention, which is introduced sequentially. This design requires that the targeted behaviors are similar enough that they will all respond to one treatment approach and that they are functionally independent of one another so that baselines will remain stable until treatment is introduced.

A basic premise of the multiple baseline design is that baseline data are available for all subjects simultaneously so that temporal effects cannot contaminate results. A variation, called a *nonconcurrent multiple baseline design*, can be used in the common clinical situation when similar subjects are not available for concurrent monitoring.[19] This approach requires that the researcher arbitrarily determines the length of several baselines and assigns them to subjects at random as they become available

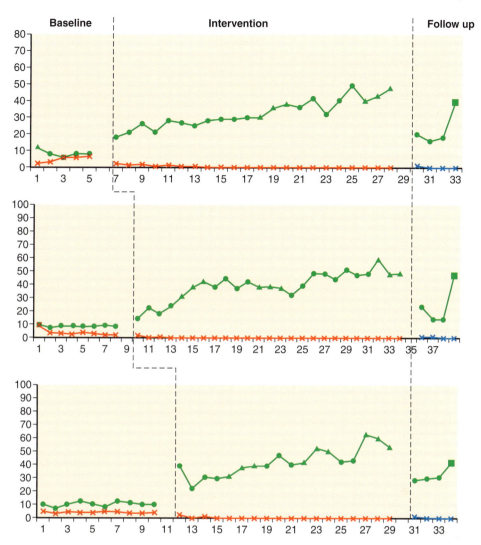

Figure 18–5 Example of a multiple baseline design across three subjects, showing the number of correct responses in building words during reading tests before, during, and after a student-centered precision teaching program. The A–B design incorporated staggered baselines. Green points represent correct responses; red points represent incorrect responses. From Bonab BG, Arjmandnia AA, Bahari F, Khoei BA. The impact of precision teaching on reading comprehension in students with reading disabilities. *J Educ Soc Sci* 2016;4:366–376. Figure 2, p. 375. Reprinted with permission.

for the study. This is a practical but weaker design because external factors related to the passage of time may be different for each subject.

 See the *Chapter 18 Supplement* for description of multiple baseline studies across settings and behaviors, and the noncurrent multiple baseline design.

■ Designs With Multiple Treatments

Single-subject strategies can also be used to compare the effects of two or more treatments.

Alternating Treatment Design

One strategy for studying multiple treatments involves the **alternating treatment design**. The essential feature of this design is the rapid alternation of two or more interventions or treatment conditions, each associated with a distinct stimulus. Treatment can be alternated within a treatment session, session by session, or day by day.

This design can be used to compare treatment with a control or placebo, but is more commonly used to compare two different interventions to determine which one will be more effective. Data for each treatment condition are plotted on the same graph, allowing for comparison of data points and trends between conditions.

A study was done to show the effect of service dog partnerships on energy conservation in individuals with mobility challenges.[20] Researchers compared duration and perceived effort to complete functional tasks in 12 sessions over 6 weeks. Subjects worked with dogs to train them in the tasks in different settings, with a randomized order of testing with and without the service dog.

Figure 18-6 illustrates the outcome for one subject with a spinal cord injury, showing the time and effort needed to pick up a fanny pack from the floor while seated in her wheelchair. The upper line represents effort without the service dog.

The alternating treatment design has a primary focus on comparison of data points between treatment conditions at each session. For instance, we see that the effort with the service dog at each session was consistently lower than without, even though the performance showed some variability.

It is actually unnecessary to include a baseline phase in an alternating treatment design, as seen here, just as a control group may not be included in group designs in which two treatments are compared. Baseline data can, however, be useful in situations where both treatments turn out to be equally effective to show that they are better than no treatment at all.

Because target behaviors are measured in rapid succession, the alternating treatment design is appropriate where treatment effects are immediate and where behavior is a clear consequence of one specific condition. The target behavior must be capable of reflecting differences with each intervention and the interventions must be able to trigger those changes as they are applied and switched. The major advantage of the alternating treatment design is that it will usually provide answers to questions of treatment comparison in a shorter time frame than designs that require introduction and withdrawal of multiple treatment phases over time.

Scheduling of alternating treatments will depend on the potential for carryover from trial to trial. Because treatment conditions are continuously alternated, sequence effects are of primary concern. This must be addressed either by random ordering of the treatment applications on each occasion or by systematic counterbalancing. In addition, other conditions that might affect the target behavior, such as the clinician, time of day, or setting, should be counterbalanced.

Multiple Treatment Designs

Using a variation of the withdrawal design, a *multiple treatment design* typically involves the application of one treatment (B) following baseline, the withdrawal of that treatment, and introduction of one or more additional treatments (C), using various configurations of an *A–B–A–C design*.

As a reflection of everyday practice, single-subject studies can also be used to examine the interactive or joint effect of two or more treatments as they are applied individually or as a treatment package. This can be done by starting with a combined treatment and then systematically dropping one component, or by adding successive components to treatment.[21] Designs can be arranged,

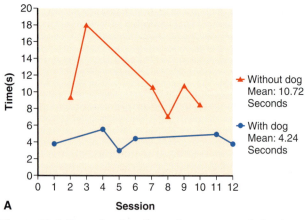

A   Session

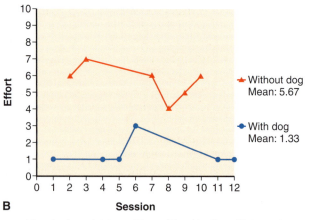

B   Session

Figure 18–6 Example of an alternating treatment design in a patient with spinal cord injury. Time (A) and effort (B) in picking up a fanny pack from the floor were measured with and without the assistance of a service dog. From Crowe TK, Perea-Burns S, Sedillo JS, et al. Effects of partnerships between people with mobility challenges and service dogs. *Am J Occup Ther* 2014; 68(2):194–202. Figure 1, p. 198. Reprinted with permission of the American Occupational Therapy Association.

for instance, as A–B–A–(B+C), or A–(B+C)–A–B, where B+C represents the combined application of interventions B and C. The intent is to determine the extent to which the effects of individual components are independent or if their combination has an additive effect.

Changing Criterion Design

Another approach is needed when treatments require adjustment over time to change as the patient improves. A design variation called a *changing criterion design* provides the opportunity for incrementally increasing goals as the patient progresses.[1,22] In this design, the treatment phase is broken down into multiple stages, each representing a new predetermined criterion, such as expected time to complete a task. Each criterion serves as a bar from which the researcher determines whether behavior gradually changes over time. As performance stabilizes and meets each consecutive criterion, the "bar" is raised and behavioral responses to criterion changes are measured repeatedly over time.[23]

> See the *Chapter 18 Supplement* for description of multiple treatment and changing criterion designs.

■ N-of-1 Trials

Single-subject methodology, with origins in the behavioral sciences, has been used in behavioral and rehabilitation research for decades to investigate systematic variations in treatment and their effect on patient responses. A somewhat different approach has been adopted in clinical medicine using a design commonly called an **N-of-1 trial**. Considered a form of single-subject investigation, this approach takes its origins from principles of RCTs, applying a randomized crossover design to an individual patient.

Clinicians and patients are often faced with the need to choose among several available interventions when existing evidence does not provide clear directive for one over others, whether because of conflicting studies or lack of objective data. The N-of-1 trial provides a structure for identifying the best treatment for an individual patient, thereby serving as a clinical decision tool.[24] Although the N-of-1 trial has largely been used to study the effectiveness of drugs, it can be applied to any discrete intervention that does not have carryover effects.[8] It can be used to compare two treatments or a treatment and placebo.

 Although they have the same basic premise and the terms are often used interchangeably, single-subject and N-of-1 designs are distinguished by their purpose. Single-subject studies are designed to explore treatment effects over time to answer the question, "Does this treatment work?" In contrast, the N-of-1 trial is used as an active decision-making tool to answer the question, "Which of these treatments should I use for this patient?" Although it can be used to inform further research, an N-of-1 trial typically ends with a decision to use one treatment or the other for the patient's continued care.

The Crossover Design

N-of-1 trials are based on a crossover design (see Chapter 16) in which the treatment and a placebo are systematically and randomly alternated until the patient and clinician reach a decision on preference for one, or satisfaction that both are equally effective or ineffective. More and longer measurement periods are recommended in situations where confounding effects are likely.

A washout period is an essential control for potential carryover effects. Some investigators use a run-in period prior to randomizing the order of treatment to assess the patient's commitment to the protocol (see Chapter 14).

An important element is using a double-blind design whenever possible. For drug trials, the assistance of a pharmacist is needed to create identical placebos.

> Because randomizing the order of treatment could result in certain sequences being more common, trials will often use block randomization or a counterbalanced Latin Square procedure (see Chapter 16).

Patient Engagement

The primary purpose of N-of-1 trials is to assist with individual treatment decisions about the optimum approach for a single patient. The study typically involves self-report data collected by the patient during the trial. The decision as to which treatment works best, then, is based directly on that patient's information.

An important part of the planning involves cooperation from the patient as well as a shared commitment from both patient and clinician in the design of the study and choice of relevant outcome measures. Because the success of the trial depends on adherence to a schedule and consistent assessment of outcomes, patients often have to be trained regarding expectations. This includes providing support for interpreting results to understand meaningful improvement or ambiguous effects.[25] Informed consent is required from all patients participating in N-of-1 trials.

When searching for evidence to guide decision-making, a relevant high-quality N-of-1 trial, along with systematic reviews of RCTs, is considered a high level of evidence for documenting effects of intervention (see Chapter 5).[26]

Appropriate Use of N-of-1 Trials

Like other types of single-subject experiments, N-of-1 trials are not suitable for all research questions. Several criteria have been proposed to decide if an N-of-1 trial is appropriate:[7,27]

- There is uncertainty of the effectiveness of a treatment for an individual patient.
- The condition is chronic or slowly progressing, with frequently occurring symptoms.
- A washout period is safe and feasible.
- The treatment effect has a rapid onset with no carryover.
- The patient and clinician can be blinded to the intervention.
- A clinically relevant outcome can be identified and measured, including symptoms or functional activities.
- The patient is motivated to participate and is expected to be compliant.
- Resources are available to cover costs of intervention and time commitments.
- The study is ethical.

Choosing a Primary Outcome

A primary outcome should be identified that will be used to make a determination about success of treatment. Although multiple outcomes can be assessed, especially as they reflect measures of importance to the patient, to avoid arbitrary decisions, one measure should be designated as the primary outcome as an indicator of success. The number and length of crossover periods is dictated by the nature of the outcome and intervention, the natural history of the disorder, the anticipated differential effect, and logistic constraints of healthcare costs and patient burden.[28,29]

Charting and Analyzing Results

Plotting results on a chart provides a visual medium for patients and practitioners to see results and understand patterns of response. Patients typically keep a daily or weekly log to chart repeated assessments, or clinical tests can be taken at appropriate intervals. To maintain blinding, cumulative results are not provided to patients or clinicians until the trial is completed. At that time, the clinician and patient will analyze the results and make a decision about which intervention is most effective.

Combining N-of-1 Trials

N-of-1 trials are essentially individualized crossover RCTs, in effect a personalized version of comparative effectiveness research. Analysis procedures for individual N-of-1 trials are similar to those used in other forms of SSDs. However, by adhering to a basic design paradigm, these trials provide an opportunity for synthesis of findings using meta-analytic techniques to estimate average treatment effects over a large number of patients.[30]

Combined results can be compared to findings from previous RCTs to determine if population estimates hold up with individual patients. Pooled results from several individual trials allow conclusions beyond the particular patient and help to characterize a subset of responders to a specific treatment or clarify the heterogeneity of the condition (see Focus on Evidence 18-1).[31]

Analysis of combined trials often incorporates statistical tests that are typical in RCTs, such as paired *t*-tests or tests of proportions, although many other procedures have also been proposed. Several useful references are available to provide detailed guidance on these methods.[24,28,32–34]

■ Visual Data Analysis

Analysis in single-subject data is often based on visual evaluation of measurements within and across design phases to determine if behaviors are changing and if observed changes during intervention are associated with the onset of treatment. Visual analysis is intuitively meaningful and can identify patterns or trends in responses within or between phases. These comparisons are based on changes in two characteristics of the data: level and trend. Figure 18-7 shows several common data patterns that reflect different combinations of these characteristics. Importantly, *phase comparisons can be made only across adjacent phases.*

Level

The **level** of data refers to the value of the dependent variable, or magnitude of performance, at the start or end of a phase. Changes in level are assessed by comparing the value of the target behavior at the last data point of one phase with its value at the first data point of the next adjacent phase. For example, Figures 18-7A and B show a change in level from the end of baseline to the start of the intervention phase.

Level can also be described in terms of the *mean* or average value of the target behavior within a phase, shown by dotted lines in graphs A and C. This value is computed by taking the sum of all data points within a phase and dividing by the number of points. Mean levels

Focus on Evidence 18–1
Gathering Evidence—One Patient at a Time

Fatigue is a common problem for patients with cancer, related to both treatment and the disease itself. One approach to treating this effect is the use of psychostimulants. In a systematic review of five RCTs, however, evidence on the effectiveness of these drugs was inconclusive—some studies showing benefits (large and small) and some showing none.[35]

In light of this uncertainty, Mitchell et al[36] developed a series of N-of-1 trials to study the effect of methylphenidate hydrochloride (MPH), a central nervous system stimulant, for alleviating fatigue in patients with advanced cancer. They recruited 43 patients from

six palliative care services to participate in 18-day trials, with three 6-day cycles: 3 days taking MPH alternating with 3 days on a placebo. The first day of each period was considered a washout period, and only 2 days were used for data collection. The order of treatment was determined by computer randomization.

The primary outcome was the score on the Functional Assessment of Chronic Illness Therapy-Fatigue (FACIT-F) subscale, a 13-item scale (0 to 52) with higher scores indicating less fatigue. A change of 8 points was considered to be meaningful based on previous research, and therefore was considered the threshold to determine a favorable response. Patients also kept a daily diary to record their symptoms.

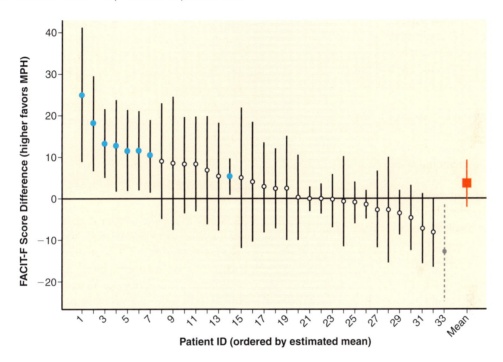

Patient ID (ordered by estimated mean)

Data analysis included looking at each individual's response, as well as combining all trials. The figure shows the mean change for each patient and the aggregated mean (shown in red). The circles represent the difference between MPH and placebo for each patient. The solid dots (in blue) represent those patients who had a positive response to MPH for all three cycles; the open circles represent those who did not have a response; and the grey circle indicates a negative response. The lines drawn on either side of the circle are the 95% *credible intervals*, which shows the degree of variability around the difference score.* If an interval crosses the center line (at zero difference), there is no significant difference between the two treatments for that patient. The data show that there was no significant difference for most patients as well as the aggregated mean.

The aggregated results of this study can be viewed in the same way as a full RCT, given the consistent protocol used by all patients. Therefore, the researchers concluded that MPH had no effect on fatigue in this population.

However, the N-of-1 methodology made it possible for them to identify eight patients who did respond favorably to MPH. Their credible intervals do not cross the center line, with seven of those above the 8-point threshold. These data allowed clinicians to make meaningful decisions for those individuals immediately after the trial—an opportunity that would have been missed using traditional evidence with aggregated data in a group trial.

---

* A credible interval is analogous to a confidence interval, but based on a different probability concept. It is a range of values within which an observed parameter value falls with a particular subjective probability.[37]

From Mitchell GK, Hardy JR, Nikles CJ, et al. The effect of methylphenidate on fatigue in advanced cancer: an aggregated N-of-1 trial. *J Pain Symptom Manage* 2015;50(3):289–296. Adapted from Figure 3, p. 294. Used with permission.

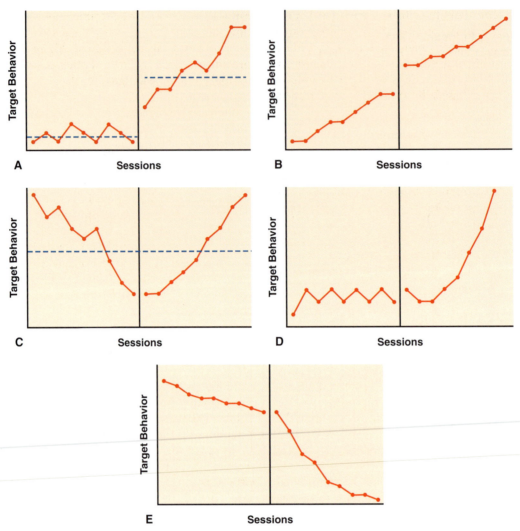

Figure 18–7 Examples of data patterns across baseline and intervention phases, showing changes in level and trend: A) Change in level and trend (dotted lines represent means for each phase); B) Change in level, no change in trend; C) Change in trend; D) Change in trend, with a curvilinear pattern during phase B; E) No change in level or trend, but a change in slope.

can be compared across adjacent phases as a method of summarizing change.

Means are useful for describing stable data that have no slope, such as graph A, as stable values will tend to cluster around the mean. However, when data are very variable or when they exhibit a sharp slope, means can be misleading. For instance, based on means in graph C, one might assume that performance did not change once intervention was introduced. Obviously, this is not the case. Mean values should always be shown on a graph of the raw data to reduce the chance of misinterpretation.

Trend

Trend refers to the direction of change within a phase. Trends can be described as accelerating or decelerating and may be characterized as stable (constant rate of change) or variable. Trends can be linear, shown in all graphs in Figure 18-7 except for graph D, which shows a curvilinear pattern.

A trend in baseline data does not present a serious problem when it reflects changes in a direction opposite to that expected during intervention. One would then anticipate a distinct change in direction once treatment is initiated, as seen in graph C. It is a problem, however, when the baseline trend follows the direction of change expected during treatment. If the improving trend is continued into the intervention phase, it would be difficult to assess treatment effects, as the target behavior is already improving without treatment (graphs B and E). It is important to consider what other factors may be contributing to this baseline change. Perhaps changes reflect maturation, a placebo effect, or the effect of other treatments. Instituting treatment under these conditions would make it difficult to draw definitive conclusions. When such a trend occurs, it is usually advisable to extend the baseline phase in hopes of achieving a plateau or reversal.

Slope

The **slope** of a trend refers to its angle, or rate of change within the data. Slope can only be determined for linear trends. In graph B, trends in both phases have approximately the same slope (although their level has changed). In graph E, both phases exhibit a decelerating trend, but the slope within the intervention phase is much steeper than that in the baseline phase. This suggests that the rate of change in the target behavior increased once treatment was initiated.

■ Statistical Analysis

There is controversy among researchers as to the validity and reliability of visual analysis in single-subject research.[2,38,39] Understanding the implications of various analysis strategies is important to critically examine the validity of conclusions. In most situations, a combination of visual and statistical analyses will provide the clearest interpretation.[40–43]

Several methods of statistical analysis can be applied to single-subject data. Because these varied approaches can lead to different results, it is important to consider how they approach the data.[44] A few of the most common methods will be presented. Many excellent texts provide thorough coverage of other techniques that can be applied to these designs.[17,40,45]

The Split-Middle Line

The reliability of assessing trend is greatly enhanced by drawing a straight line that characterizes rate of change.[46–49] A popular method involves drawing a line that represents the linear trend and slope for a data series. This procedure results in a **celeration line**, which describes trends as accelerating or decelerating. A celeration line is considered a **split-middle line** when it divides the data within a phase equally above and below the line, with an equal number of data points on or above and on or below the line (a median line). This method was used, for example, in the study of weight distribution shown in Figure 18-5.

 See the *Chapter 18 Supplement* for a full description of the method for drawing a split-middle line.

In Figure 18-8, a split-middle line has been drawn for baseline data. We can see that four points fall above and below the line, with two points directly on the line. By extending the line from the baseline phase into the intervention phase, the line can be used to test the null hypothesis that there is no difference in behavior between two adjacent phases. If there is no difference between the phases, then the split-middle line for baseline

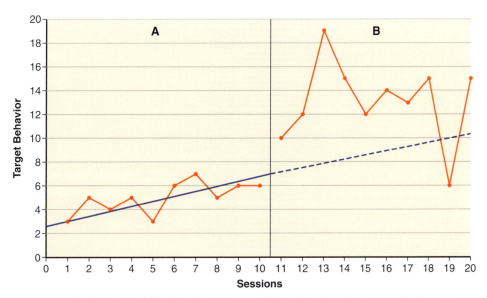

Figure 18–8 The split-middle line is drawn for baseline data. The line is extended into the intervention phase to test the null hypothesis. One point in the intervention phase falls below the extended line.

data should also be the split-middle line for the intervention phase. Therefore, 50% of the data in the intervention phase should fall on or above that line, and 50% should fall on or below it. If treatment has caused a real change in observed behavior, then the extended baseline trend should not fit this pattern.

Statistically, we propose a null hypothesis (H_0), which states that there is no difference across phases; that is, any changes observed from baseline to the intervention phase are due to chance, not treatment. Our intent, of course, is to discredit the null hypothesis, and so we also propose an alternative (H_1), which can be phrased as a nondirectional or directional hypothesis. For example, we can propose that there will be an increase in response to intervention for the study shown in Figure 18-8.

The Binomial Test

To test H_0, we apply a procedure called the **binomial test**, which is used when outcomes of a test are dichotomous; in this case, data points are either above or below the split-middle line. To do the test, we count the number of points in the intervention phase that fall above and below the extended line (ignoring points that fall directly on the line).

In our example, one point falls below and nine points fall above the extended line. Clearly, this is not a 50–50 split. On the basis of these data, we would like to conclude that the treatment did effect a change in response. However, we must first pose a statistical question: Could this pattern, with one point below and nine points above the line, have occurred by chance? Or can we be confident that this pattern shows a true treatment effect?

We answer this question by referring to Table 18-1, which lists probabilities associated with the binomial test. Two values are needed to use this table. First, we find the appropriate value of n (down the left side), which is the total number of points in the intervention phase that fall *above and below* the line (not including points *on the line*). In this case, there are a total of 10 points. We then determine if there are *fewer* points above or below the extended line. In our example, there are fewer points (one) below the line. The number of fewer points is given the value x. Therefore, $x = 1$. The probability associated with $n = 10$ and $x = 1$ is .011; that is, $p = .011$.

The probabilities listed in the table are *one-tailed probabilities*, which means they are used to evaluate directional alternative hypotheses, as we have proposed in this example. If a nondirectional hypothesis is proposed, a *two-tailed test* is performed, which requires *doubling* the probabilities listed in the table. If we had proposed a nondirectional hypothesis for this example, we would use $p = .022$.

Table 18-1	Abridged Table of Probabilities Associated With the Binomial Test					
				x		
n	0	1	2	3	4	5
5	.031	.188	.500	.812	.969	–
6	.016	.109	.344	.656	.891	.984
7	.008	.062	.227	.500	.773	.938
8	.004	.035	.145	.363	.637	.855
9	.002	.020	.090	.254	.500	.746
10	.001	.011	.055	.172	.377	.623
15	–	–	.004	.018	.059	.151
20	–	–	–	.001	.006	.021

This table is an abridged version for purposes of illustration. Probabilities are one-tailed values, and must be doubled for a two-tailed test.

The probability value obtained from the table is interpreted in terms of a conventional upper limit of $p = .05$. Probabilities that exceed this value are considered *not significant*; that is, the observed pattern could have occurred by chance. In this example, our probability is less than .05 ($p = .011$) and, therefore, is considered significant. The pattern of response in the intervention phase is significantly different from baseline (see Chapter 23).

 See the *Chapter 18 Supplement* for the full table of probabilities associated with the binomial test. See Chapter 27 for further discussion of the use of the binomial test.

Serial Dependency

It is possible to use conventional statistical tests, such as the *t*-test and analysis of variance (see Chapters 24 and 25) to test for significant changes across phases. With time series data, however, these applications are limited when large numbers of measurements are taken over time. Under these conditions, data points can be interdependent, as is often the case in single-subject research.[50,51] This interdependence is called **serial dependency**, which means that successive observations in a series of data points are correlated; that is, the level of performance at one point is related to the value of subsequent points in the series. Serial dependency can violate assumptions of several statistical procedures and may also be a problem for making inferences based on visual analysis.[52,53]

The degree of serial dependency is reflected by the *autocorrelation* in the data, or the correlation between successive data points. The higher the value of autocorrelation, the greater the serial dependency in the data. Ottenbacher[45] presents a method for computing autocorrelation by hand, but the process is easily performed by computer, especially with large numbers of data points.

The *C statistic* can be used to establish a difference in trends between baseline and intervention phases with as few as eight points in each phase. It is not affected by autocorrelation. This statistic first looks at baseline data to establish that there is no trend and, if so, it combines baseline and intervention scores to determine if there is a difference between them.[45,54]

 See the *Chapter 18 Supplement* for calculation of the *C* statistic.

Two Standard Deviation Band Method

Another useful method of analysis is the **two standard deviation band method**. This process involves calculating the mean and standard deviation (SD) of data points within the baseline phase (see Chapter 22 for calculation methods for these statistics). This procedure is illustrated in Figure 18-9. The solid line represents the mean level of performance for the baseline phase and the broken lines above and below this line represent ±2 SD from the mean.

As shown in the figure, these lines are extended into the intervention phase. If *at least two consecutive data points in the intervention phase fall outside the two standard deviation band*, changes from baseline to intervention are considered significant.

In this example, the mean response for baseline data is 5.0 with SD = ±1.33. The shaded areas show 2 SD above and below the mean (±2.66). Eight consecutive points in the intervention phase fall above this band. Therefore, we conclude that there is a significant change from the baseline to the intervention phase.

The two standard deviation band method is also illustrated in Figure 18-3.

Depending on the variability in the data, the two standard deviation band method might not be useful, especially if the width of the band takes scores below zero. Alternative analysis methods, like the binomial test, should be considered.

Statistical Process Control

Pfadt et al[55] introduced a unique statistical model to evaluate variability in single-subject data. This model, called **statistical process control (SPC)**, was actually developed in the 1920s as a means of quality control in manufacturing.[56] The basis of this process lies in the desire to reduce variation; that is, in manufacturing, product consistency is desirable.

One can always expect some variation in quality. Cars come off the assembly line with some defects; clothing will have irregularities. A certain amount of variation is

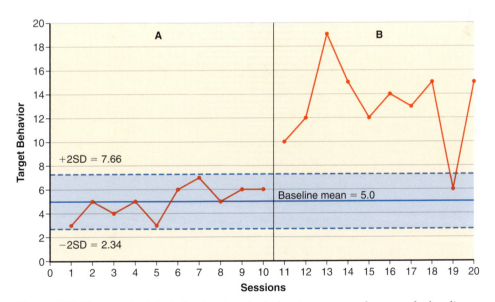

Figure 18–9 Two standard deviation band method, showing mean performance for baseline (solid line) and 2 SDs above and below the mean (broken lines). Because more than two consecutive points in the intervention phase fall outside of this band, the difference between phases is considered significant.

to be expected. This variation is considered background "noise," or what has been termed *common cause variation*.[57] Statistically, such variation is considered to be "in control," random, predictable, and tolerable.

There will be a point, however, at which the variation will exceed acceptable limits and the product will no longer be considered satisfactory. Such deviation is considered "out of control" or nonrandom, and is called *special cause variation*. This is variation that is not part of the normal process and has some cause that needs to be addressed. We can think of this variation in the context of reliability. How much variation is random error, and how much is meaningful, due to true changes in response?

> Think about variations in your own signature. If you sign your name 10 times there will be a certain degree of expected (common cause) variation, due to random effects such as fatigue, distraction, or shift in position. If, however, someone comes by and hits your elbow while you are writing, your signature will look markedly different—a special cause variation.

Applying SPC to Single-Subject Data

We can apply this model to single-subject data in two ways. First, by looking at baseline data, we can determine if responses are within the limits of expected random variability (common cause variation).[55] This would allow us to assess the degree to which the data represent a reasonable baseline.

Using the SPC model, intervention is a form of "special cause." We expect a change in the subject's response

because of the intervention, not simply due to random variation. SPC offers a mechanism to determine if variations in response are sufficiently different from baseline to warrant interpretation as special cause.[57]

Control Charts

SPC is based on analysis of graphs called *control charts*. These are the same as the graphs we have been using to show the results of single-subject data, although some differences exist depending on the type of data being measured.

In SPC, the interpretation of data is based on variability around a mean baseline value. A central line is plotted, representing the mean baseline response. An *upper control limit (UCL)* and *lower control limit (LCL)* are then plotted at 3 SDs above and below the mean. Regardless of the underlying distribution, if the process is in "statistical control," almost all data will fall within this range around the mean (see Chapter 22).[58] Therefore, these boundaries define the threshold for special cause.

This process is illustrated in Figure 18-10. The baseline data fall within the upper and lower control limits, demonstrating common cause. Even though there is some variability in the baseline data, it can be considered random.

We then extend the control limits into the intervention phase. If only common cause variation is operating (the treatment has no real effect), the intervention data should also fall within these limits. We can see, however, that 9 points fall outside the UCL and all 10 points are above the baseline mean, indicating that there is a significant difference in the response during the intervention phase.

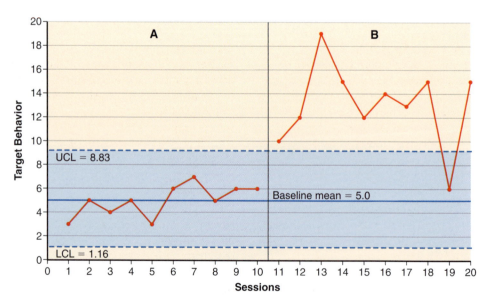

Figure 18–10 Statistical control chart showing upper (UCL) and lower (LCL) control limits. The mean of 10 baseline scores is 5.0, which is extended into the intervention phase.

As a process for total quality control, SPC can be used within healthcare settings to monitor variation in service delivery and health outcomes. The reader is encouraged to consult several excellent references that discuss this application.[58–64]

 See the *Chapter 18 Supplement* for calculation and interpretation of upper and lower control limits using the SPC method.

Effect Size

In the analysis of quantitative studies, a standardized **effect size index** is often used to characterize the strength of changes seen with intervention. These indices are based on differences between group means and variance within and across groups (see Chapter 32). Important benefits of this approach include the ability to judge the importance of results, compare or combine studies, and develop an evidence-based summary of findings that can be applied to clinical judgment (see Chapter 37).[65]

Using the approaches to visual analysis and the statistical methods described thus far, SSDs do not allow such judgments. Even when results show a significant change from baseline to intervention, the assessment of change is primarily descriptive and, in many cases, may be difficult to interpret because of variability. These types of results also preclude comparisons across studies. The advantage of using a standardized effect size is that it can be applied to comparisons of data in different units and with different sample sizes.

Nonoverlapping Scores

One approach for establishing effect size for single-subject research is based on the concept of *nonoverlap*.[66] If we look at the number of points in the intervention phase that *do not overlap* with values in the baseline phase, we get an idea of how different the two sets of scores are. The *percent of nonoverlapping data (PND)* is a reflection of the treatment effect.[67] When all the intervention points overlap with baseline scores, there is 0% nonoverlap. In that case, the distributions of scores in both phases are conceptually superimposed, indicating no treatment effect.

As an example, consider the hypothetical data in Figure 18-10. If we were to draw a horizontal line at the highest point in the baseline phase (try it), we can count how many points fall above that line in the intervention phase. (If the intent of the treatment was to decrease performance, the line would be drawn at the lowest point.) Then we can determine the proportion of data points above this line in the B phase. In this case, 9/10 points would be above it. Therefore, PND is 90%.

Scruggs et al[66] suggest the following interpretation of treatment effectiveness for nonoverlap:

Above 90%	Very effective
70-90%	Effective
50-70%	Questionable
Below 50%	Not effective

These are guidelines, not absolute thresholds, that should be used to make judgments about how important a treatment effect is. However, this approach provides a standardized common metric that can be used to compare studies of different sample size, different phase lengths, and different treatment presentations.

If we look back at the study of endurance measured using the 6MWT in Figure 18-3, we can see that eight of nine or 89% of data points in phase B are nonoverlapping with the baseline phase (one point is overlapped)—a strong effect. However, consider the data in Figure 18-4 for the study of weight distribution. With replicated phases, the total proportion of nonoverlapped intervention scores can be used.[11] In this example, all intervention points overlap with baseline points—there is 0% nonoverlap. This suggests that the effect size is small, even though there is an obvious change in direction based on the split-middle lines.

Several useful references provide detailed descriptions of other effect size measures for SSDs, including nonparametric statistical methods for determining confidence intervals.[42,43,66,68–73]

■ Generalization

The special appeal of single-subject research is that it focuses on clinical outcomes and can provide real-time data for clinical decision-making. The strongest criticism of this method, however, suggests that results cannot be generalized beyond the individual patient, limiting its value as a research approach.[74,75]

Although it certainly would be unreasonable to generalize findings from one individual to a population, one might argue that the reverse can be equally precarious, to generalize from a group to an individual patient. In fact, one might contend that a single-subject case can provide superior evidence compared to group studies for certain types of conditions and interventions.[8,14] The concept of pragmatic trials is based on a need to make research more reflective of actual practice, a good fit for single-subject research under the appropriate circumstances.

But, of course, all research has the ultimate goal of informing clinical decisions beyond those being studied.

With this intent, then, it is not sufficient just to demonstrate outcomes on a few patients during an experimental period. It is also necessary to show that improvements or changes in behavior will occur with other individuals and that improvement will be sustained after the intervention has ended.

Phases of Replication

Through a process of replication across subjects, settings, and clinicians, the single-subject study can establish generalizability. Three successive phases have been described to strengthen external validity.[14]

- **Direct replication** involves repeating single-subject experiments across several subjects. The setting, treatment conditions, and patient characteristics should be kept as constant as possible. Three successful replications are considered sufficient to demonstrate that findings are not a result of chance.[14,76] Multiple baseline designs provide direct replication.
- **Systematic replication** is intended to demonstrate that findings can be observed under conditions different from those encountered in the initial study. It is, in essence, a search for exceptions.[14] It involves the variation of one or two variables from the original study to allow generalization to other similar, but not identical, situations. It may include involvement of various clinicians, application in different settings, or patients with varied characteristics.
- **Clinical replication** is perhaps most important for generalization to complex clinical environments. It involves the replication of effects in typical clinical situations where treatment plans may be based on various combinations of techniques or approaches. In the long run, the true applicability of research data will depend on our ability to demonstrate that treatment packages can be successfully applied to patients with multiple behaviors that tend to cluster together.

Beyond the question of external validity, which concerns generalization of findings to different subjects and settings, researchers are also interested in the importance of treatment effects within a practical context. The term *social validity* has been used to indicate the application of single-subject study findings, including the applicability of procedures in real-world settings.[77]

The single-subject approach can readily demonstrate the meaningfulness of the goals of interventions, the acceptability of procedures by target groups, and the importance of a treatment's impact. This methodology is also ideally suited to demonstrate implementation of clinical procedures that have been studied using RCTs, as a form of pragmatic trial.

COMMENTARY

One example is worth a thousand arguments.

—*William E. Gladstone (1809–1898)*

British politician

EBP is about trying to find the right approach for the individual patient. Although clinical research has an important role in generalizing findings, single-subject studies provide a unique opportunity to discover which factors are necessary to expect certain outcomes.[11,78] Understanding a treatment's effectiveness is important even if it applies only to a narrow range of conditions, as long as we know what those condition are.[79]

The maturation of single-subject research and N-of-1 methodology has been an important step in the development of clinical research. It provides an opportunity for the practitioner to evaluate treatment procedures within the context of clinical care, as well as to share insights about patient behavior and response that are typically ignored or indiscernible using traditional group research approaches. The process of single-subject research should eventually diminish the role of trial and error in clinical practice and provide useful guidelines for making clinical choices.

Of course, SSDs are not a panacea for all clinical research woes. Many research questions cannot be answered adequately using these designs. Single-subject studies can be limited in that they require time to document outcomes. They are not readily applicable to acute situations in which baseline periods are less reasonable and treatment does not continue for long periods. In addition, researchers often find that patient responses are too unstable, making attempts at analysis frustrating. Nonetheless, SSDs serve a distinct purpose in the ongoing search for scientific documentation of therapeutic effectiveness. This process will force us to challenge clinical theories and to document the benefits of our interventions in a convincing scientific way, for ourselves and for others. Generalization does not always mean that the results of one study have to apply to everyone in a target population. Single-subject strategies provide an important perspective with the ultimate purpose of finding what works for the individual patient.

REFERENCES

1. Graham JE, Karmarkar AM, Ottenbacher KJ. Small sample research designs for evidence-based rehabilitation: issues and methods. *Arch Phys Med Rehabil* 2012;93(8 Suppl):S111–S116.
2. Ottenbacher KJ, Hinderer SR. Evidence-based practice: methods to evaluate individual patient improvement. *Am J Phys Med Rehabil* 2001;80(10):786–796.
3. Bloom M, Fisher J, Orme JG. *Evaluating Practice: Guidelines for the Accountable Professional.* 2 ed. Boston: Allyn and Bacon, 1995.
4. Zhan S, Ottenbacher KJ. Single subject research designs for disability research. *Disabil Rehabil* 2001;23(1):1–8.
5. Kalinowski J, Armson J, Stuart A. Effect of normal and fast articulatory rates on stuttering frequency. *Fluency Disord* 1995; 20:293–302.
6. Schork NJ. Personalized medicine: Time for one-person trials. *Nature* 2015;520(7549):609–611.
7. Davidson KW, Peacock J, Kronish IM, Edmondson D. Personalizing behavioral interventions through single-patient (N-of-1) trials. *Soc Personal Psychol Compass* 2014;8(8):408–421.
8. Backman CL, Harris SR. Case studies, single-subject research, and N of 1 randomized trials: comparisons and contrasts. *Am J Phys Med Rehabil* 1999;78(2):170–176.
9. Horner RH, Carr EG, Halle J, McGee G, Odom S, Wolery M. The use of single-subject research to identify evidence-based practice in special education. *Exceptional Children* 2005;71(2): 165–179.
10. Wheeler DJ. *Understanding Variation: The Key to Managing Chaos.* 2 ed. Knoxville, TN: SPC Press, 2000.
11. Dallery J, Cassidy RN, Raiff BR. Single-case experimental designs to evaluate novel technology-based health interventions. *J Med Internet Res* 2013;15(2):e22.
12. Lane JD, Gast DL. Visual analysis in single case experimental design studies: brief review and guidelines. *Neuropsychol Rehabil* 2014;24(3–4):445–463.
13. Xin JF, Sheppard ME, Brown MS. Brief report: using iPads for self-monitoring of students with autism. *J Autism Dev Disord* 2017;47(5):1559–1567.
14. Barlow DH, Hersen M. *Single Case Experimental Designs: Strategies for Studying Behavior Change.* 2 ed. New York: Pergamon Press, 1984.
15. Retarekar R, Fragala-Pinkham MA, Townsend EL. Effects of aquatic aerobic exercise for a child with cerebral palsy: single-subject design. *Pediatr Phys Ther* 2009;21(4):336–344.
16. Wu S, Huang H, LIn C, Chen M. Effects of a program on symmetrical posture in patients with hemiplegia: a single-subject design. *Am J Occup Ther* 1996;50(1):17–23.
17. Kazdin AE. *Single-Case Research Designs: Methods for Clinical and Applied Settings.* 2 ed. New York: Oxford University Press, 2010.
18. Bonab BG, Arjmandnia AA, Bahari F, Khoei BA. The impact of precision teaching on reading comprehension in students with reading disabilities. *J Educ Soc Sci* 2016;4:366–376.
19. Watson PJ, Workman EA. The nonconcurrent multiple baseline across individuals design: an extension of the traditional multiple baseline design. *J Behav Ther Exp Psychiatry* 1981; 12:257.
20. Crowe TK, Perea-Burns S, Sedillo JS, Hendrix IC, Winkle M, Deitz J. Effects of partnerships between people with mobility challenges and service dogs. *Am J Occup Ther* 2014;68(2): 194–202.
21. Ward-Horner J, Sturmey P. Component analyses using single-subject experimental designs: a review. *J Appl Behav Anal* 2010; 43(4):685–704.
22. Kazdin AE. *Single-Case Research Designs: Methods for Clinical and Applied Settings.* New York: Oxford University Press, 1982.
23. Cowan RJ, Hennessey ML, Vierstra CV, Rumrill PD, Jr. Small-N designs in rehabilitation research. *J Vocat Rehabil* 2004;20(3):203–211.
24. Duan N, Kravitz RL, Schmid CH. Single-patient (n-of-1) trials: a pragmatic clinical decision methodology for patient-centered comparative effectiveness research. *J Clin Epidemiol* 2013;66(8 Suppl):S21–S28.
25. Kaplan HC, Gabler NB, and the DEcIDE Methods Center N-of-1 Guidance Panel. User engagement, training, and support for conducting N-of-1 trials. In: Kravitz RL, Duan N, and the DEcIDE Method Center N-of-1 Guidance Panel, eds. *Design and Implementation of N-of-1 Trials: A User's Guide.* AHRQ Publication No 13(14)-EHC122-EF. Rockville, MD: Agency for Healthcare Research and Quality 2014:71–81. Available at www.effectivehealthcare.ahrq.gov/N-1-Trials.cfm. Accessed April 25, 2017.
26. Centre for Evidence-Based Medicine: OCEBM Levels of Evidence. Available at http://www.cebm.net/ocebm-levels-of-evidence/. Accessed April 28, 2017.
27. Sackett DL, Haynes RB, Guyatt GH, Tugwell P. *Clinical Epidemiology: A Basic Science for Clinical Medicine.* 2 ed. Boston: Little, Brown & Co., 1991.
28. Lillie EO, Patay B, Diamant J, Issell B, Topol EJ, Schork NJ. The n-of-1 clinical trial: the ultimate strategy for individualizing medicine? *Per Med* 2011;8(2):161–173.
29. Johannessen T, Petersen H, Kristensen P, Fosstvedt D. The controlled single subject trial. *Scand J Prim Health Care* 1991; 9(1):17–21.
30. Zucker DR, Schmid CH, McIntosh MW, D'Agostino RB, Selker HP, Lau J. Combining single patient (N-of-1) trials to estimate population treatment effects and to evaluate individual patient responses to treatment. *J Clin Epidemiol* 1997;50(4): 401–410.
31. Madsen LG, Bytzer P. Review article: Single subject trials as a research instrument in gastrointestinal pharmacology. *Aliment Pharmacol Ther* 2002;16(2):189–196.
32. Kravitz RL, Duan N, and the DEcIDE Method Center N-of-1 Guidance Panel, eds. *Design and Implementation of N-of-1 Trials: A User's Guide.* AHRQ Publication No 13(14)-EHC122-EF. Rockville, MD: Agency for Healthcare Research and Quality 2014:71–81. Available at www.effectivehealthcare.ahrq.gov/ N-1-Trials.cfm. Accessed April 25, 2017.
33. McAlister FA, Straus SE, Guyatt GH, Haynes RB. Users' guides to the medical literature: XX. Integrating research evidence with the care of the individual patient. Evidence-Based Medicine Working Group. *JAMA* 2000;283(21):2829–2836.
34. Scuffham PA, Nikles J, Mitchell GK, Yelland MJ, Vine N, Poulos CJ, et al. Using N-of-1 trials to improve patient management and save costs. *J Gen Intern Med* 2010;25(9):906–913.
35. Minton O, Richardson A, Sharpe M, Hotopf M, Stone PC. Psychostimulants for the management of cancer-related fatigue: a systematic review and meta-analysis. *J Pain Symptom Manage* 2011;41(4):761–767.
36. Mitchell GK, Hardy JR, Nikles CJ, Carmont SA, Senior HE, Schluter PJ, et al. The effect of methylphenidate on fatigue in

advanced cancer: an aggregated N-of-1 trial. *J Pain Symptom Manage* 2015;50(3):289–296.

37. Haskins R, Osmotherly PG, Tuyl F, Rivett DA. Uncertainty in clinical prediction rules: the value of credible intervals. *J Orthop Sports Phys Ther* 2014;44(2):85–91.

38. Harbst KB, Ottenbacher KJ, Harris SR. Interrater reliability of therapists' judgements of graphed data. *Phys Ther* 1991;71(2): 107–115.

39. Brossart DF, Parker RI, Olson EA, Mahadevan L. The relationship between visual analysis and five statistical analyses in a simple AB single-case research design. *Behav Modif* 2006; 30(5):531–563.

40. Kratochwill RT, Levin JR. *Single-Case Intervention Research: Methodological and Statistical Advances.* Washington, DC: American Psychological Association, 2014.

41. Orme JG, Cox ME. Note on research methodology. Analyzing single-subject design data using statistical process control charts. *Social Work Res* 2001;25(2):115–127.

42. Parker RI, Vannest KJ, Brown L. The improvement rate difference for single-case research. *Exceptional Children* 2009; 75(2):135–150.

43. Brossart DF, Vannest KJ, Davis JL, Patience MA. Incorporating nonoverlap indices with visual analysis for quantifying intervention effectiveness in single-case experimental designs. *Neuropsychol Rehabil* 2014;24(3–4):464–491.

44. Nourbakhsh MR, Ottenbacher KJ. The statistical analysis of single-subject data: a comparative examination. *Phys Ther* 1994; 74(8):768–776.

45. Ottenbacher KJ. *Evaluating Clinical Change: Strategies for Occupational and Physical Therapists.* Baltimore: Williams & Wilkins, 1986.

46. Bobrovitz CD, Ottenbacher KJ. Comparison of visual inspection and statistical analysis of single-subject data in rehabilitation research. *Am J Phys Med Rehabil* 1998;77:94–102.

47. Hojem MA, Ottenbacher KJ. Empirical investigation of visual-inspection versus trend-line analysis of single-subject data. *Phys Ther* 1988;68(6):983–988.

48. Johnson MB, Ottenbacher KJ. Trend line influence on visual analysis of single-subject data in rehabilitation research. *Int Disabil Stud* 1991;13(2):55–59.

49. Ottenbacher KJ. Interrater agreement of visual analysis in single-subject decisions: quantitative review and analysis. *Am J Ment Retard* 1993;98(1):135–142.

50. Ottenbacher KJ. Analysis of data in idiographic research: issues and methods. *Am J Phys Med Rehabil* 1992;71:202–208.

51. Jones RR, Baught RS, Weinrott MR. Time-series analysis in operant research. *J Appl Behav Anal* 1977;10:151.

52. Jones RR, Weinrott MR, Vaught RS. Effects of serial dependency on the agreement between visual and statistical inference. *J Appl Behav Anal* 1978;11:277.

53. Bengali MK, Ottenbacher KJ. The effect of autocorrelation on the results of visually analyzing data from single-subject designs. *Am J Occup Ther* 1998;52(8):650–655.

54. Janosky JE, Leininger SL, Hoerger M, P., Libkuman TM. *Single Subject Designs in Biomedicine.* New York: Springer, 2009.

55. Pfadt A, Cohen IL, Sudhalter V, Romanczyk RG, Wheeler DJ. Applying statistical process control to clinical data: an illustration. *J Appl Behav Anal* 1992;25(3):551–560.

56. Berwick DM. Controlling variation in health care: a consultation from Walter Shewhart. *Med Care* 1991;29(12):1212–1225.

57. Callahan CD, Barisa MT. Statistical process control and rehabilitation outcome: The single-subject design reconsidered. *Rehabil Psychol* 2005;50(1):24–33.

58. Benneyan JC, Lloyd RC, Plsek PE. Statistical process control as a tool for research and healthcare improvement. *Qual Saf Health Care* 2003;12(6):458–464.

59. Hantula DA. Disciplined decision making in an interdisciplinary environment: some implications for clinical applications of statistical process control. *J Appl Behav Anal* 1995;28(3): 371–377.

60. Solodky C, Chen H, Jones PK, Katcher W, Neuhauser D. Patients as partners in clinical research: a proposal for applying quality improvement methods to patient care. *Med Care* 1998; 36(8 Suppl):As13–20.

61. Diaz M, Neuhauser D. Pasteur and parachutes: when statistical process control is better than a randomized controlled trial. *Qual Saf Health Care* 2005;14(2):140–143.

62. Mohammed MA. Using statistical process control to improve the quality of health care. *Qual Saf Health Care* 2004;13(4): 243–245.

63. Karimi H, O'Brian S, Onslow M, Jones M, Menzies R, Packman A. Using statistical process control charts to study stuttering frequency variability during a single day. *J Speech Lang Hear Res* 2013;56(6):1789–1799.

64. Eslami S, Abu-Hanna A, de Keizer NF, Bosman RJ, Spronk PE, de Jonge E, et al. Implementing glucose control in intensive care: a multicenter trial using statistical process control. *Intensive Care Med* 2010;36(9):1556–1565.

65. Shire SY, Kasari C. Train the trainer effectiveness trials of behavioral intervention for individuals with autism: a systematic review. *Am J Intellect Dev Disabil* 2014;119(5):436–451.

66. Scruggs TE, Mastropieri MA. Summarizing single-subject research. Issues and applications. *Behav Modif* 1998;22(3): 221–242.

67. Cohen J. *Statistical Power Analysis for the Behavioral Sciences.* 2 ed. Hillsdale, NJ: Lawrence Erlbaum 1988.

68. Van den Noortgate W, Onghena P. The aggregation of single-case results using hierarchical linear models. *Behav Anal Today* 2007;8(2):196–209.

69. Lanovaz MJ, Rapp JT. Using single-case experiments to support evidence-based decisions: how much is enough? *Behav Modif* 2016;40(3)377–395.

70. Campbell JM. Statistical comparison of four effect sizes for single-subject designs. *Behav Modif* 2004;28(2):234–246.

71. Cushing CC, Walters RW, Hoffman L. Aggregated N-of-1 randomized controlled trials: modern data analytics applied to a clinically valid method of intervention effectiveness. *J Pediatr Psychol* 2014;39(2):138–150.

72. Nikles CJ, McKinlay L, Mitchell GK, Carmont SA, Senior HE, Waugh MC, et al. Aggregated n-of-1 trials of central nervous system stimulants versus placebo for paediatric traumatic brain injury—a pilot study. *Trials* 2014;15:54.

73. Zucker DR, Ruthazer R, Schmid CH. Individual (N-of-1) trials can be combined to give population comparative treatment effect estimates: methodologic considerations. *J Clin Epidemiol* 2010;63(12):1312–1323.

74. Francis NA. Single subject trials in primary care. *Postgrad Med J* 2005;81(959):547–548.

75. Newcombe RG. Should the single subject design be regarded as a valid alternative to the randomised controlled trial? *Postgrad Med J* 2005;81(959):546–547.

76. Chambless DL, Hollon SD. Defining empirically supported therapies. *J Consult Clin Psychol* 1998;66(1):7–18.

77. Wolf MM. Social validity: The case for subjective measurement or how applied behavior analysis is finding its heart. *J Appl Behav Anal* 1978;11:203.

78. Branch MN, Pennypacker HS. Generality and generalization of research findings. In: Madden GJ, Dube W, Hackenberg TD, Hanley GP, Lattal KA, eds. *APA Handbook of Behavior Analysis.* Washington, DC: American Psychological Association, 2011.

79. Johnston JM, Pennypacker HS. *Strategies and Tactics of Behavioral Research.* 3 ed. New York: Routledge, 2008.

Exploratory Research: Observational Designs

—with K. Douglas Gross

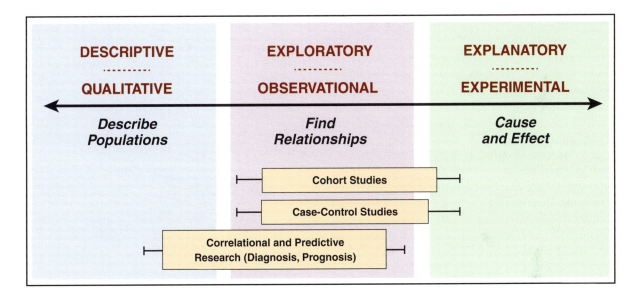

In contrast to experimental trials that test the effectiveness of interventions using variable manipulation and controlled comparisons, **observational studies** characterize unmodified relationships, analyzing how existing factors or individual characteristics are associated with health outcomes. Observational studies explore the causes, consequences, and predictors of disease or disability. They also characterize the impact of exposure to risk factors on individual or community health. This research approach may be regarded as **exploratory** since it often probes data about personal, environmental, behavioral, or genetic influences that may explain health outcomes.

The purpose of this chapter is to describe basic approaches to observational research with a focus on cohort and case-control study designs, and to discuss considerations that are relevant to using these designs for evidence-based practice. Analysis procedures for these designs will be covered in Chapter 34.

■ Exploring Relationships

Observational research may be classified as descriptive or analytic. The purpose of *descriptive research* is to characterize populations by examining the distribution of health-related variables within them, often with the intention of generating hypotheses about factors that may give rise to observed differences across population groups (see Chapter 20). *Analytic research* focuses on examining those group differences in order to demonstrate how personal, environmental, behavioral, or genetic **exposures** help explain why one group's outcomes differ from another's. Analytic studies are typically motivated by hypotheses that specify the particular exposures and outcomes to be studied and clarify the interpretations that will be offered for any found associations.

In experimental research, participants are assigned to an intervention or control group for the purpose of demonstrating what outcomes are expected when the trial treatment is provided or withheld. Similarly, observational investigators are interested in comparing the outcomes of subjects who are exposed or unexposed to hypothesized causal agents. However, an observational researcher plays no part in the assignment of subjects to exposed or unexposed conditions. Instead, existing groups of subjects are identified by their shared history or current health status. Although experimental designs offer the best option for demonstrating treatment effectiveness, observational studies are frequently undertaken to derive models that predict the likelihood that a particular treatment will succeed in the presence of one or more prognostic indicators.

📌 Observational studies are also used to derive clinical prediction rules for prognosis and to identify diagnostic indicators that accurately signal the presence or absence of a target condition. The accuracy of a set of diagnostic indicators may be modeled as a clinical diagnostic rule (see Chapter 33).

Estimating Risk

Perhaps the most common use of an observational design is to draw causal inferences about the effects of a hypothesized **risk factor**. This is done by comparing outcomes of a group of subjects who have been exposed to a risk factor to the outcomes of those who remain unexposed (see Chapter 34). Risks can refer to factors related to the occurrence or prevention of a disorder. Risk factors may include personal characteristics, behaviors, or environmental exposures, as the following examples illustrate.

In an investigation into the effects of asthma, Shen et al[1] found that adults with asthma had 2.5 times greater risk of developing chronic obstructive sleep apnea than adults who did not have asthma.

Investigators in this non-experimental study obviously played no part in determining which subjects were exposed to the effects of asthma. Yet, their observational findings suggested that asthma may play a causal role and should be regarded as a risk factor for sleep apnea.

Diet has been shown to be related to many diseases or disorders. In a study of older adults during a 5-year period, researchers documented that those with healthier diets had a 24% lower rate of cognitive decline than those with less healthy diets, thus establishing diet as a possible risk factor.[2]

No effort was undertaken to alter existing dietary habits in this observational study. Investigators merely compared rates of cognitive decline across extant groups of subjects whose reported dietary habits were judged to be either healthy or unhealthy.

Resnick et al[3] studied the association between exposure to ambient smoke during wildfires and emergency department (ED) visits. They found that 20- to 60-year-olds who were exposed to high levels of particulate matter from wildfire smoke had between a 1.5 and 2.6 times greater chance of visiting the ED for pulmonary or cardiovascular disorders.

As these examples illustrate, some risk factors, such as asthma or poor air quality, are suspected of contributing to increased disease occurrence, while others, like a healthy diet, may be protective. Although none of these observational studies assessed the effects of a treatment, their findings could suggest possible avenues for preventative intervention.

What's the Cause?

The goal of many observational studies is to implicate factors that contribute to health outcomes. In the examples above, asthma is a potential cause of sleep apnea, poor diet is a potential cause of cognitive decline, and poor air quality is a potential cause of cardiopulmonary problems. Individually, observational studies rarely provide conclusive evidence of a direct causal link. By comparison, explanatory trials have greater potential to provide compelling evidence of causation and are the preferred means of confirming the effectiveness of investigator-applied interventions.

Because observational designs investigate existing relationships and do not provide opportunities for variable manipulation or controlled comparisons, we can never fully exclude the possibility that the observed groups differ in other ways that could explain their unequal health outcomes. Despite the comparative advantages of experimental trial designs for etiologic research, there are many situations in which investigator-mandated group assignment is infeasible. Consider the practical and ethical difficulties of assigning subjects to a group that will be exposed to wildfire smoke or to an unhealthy diet. In such situations, observational designs offer the only plausible method of investigating the causal impact of a potentially deleterious exposure.

Especially where there is a preponderance of evidence, observational studies can strengthen support for hypothesized causal relationships (see Focus on Evidence 19-1). For example, the repeated finding of an association between tobacco smoking and lung cancer was eventually sufficiently compelling that the surgeon general changed the required warning label on cigarette cartons from "smoking may cause cancer" to "smoking causes cancer." A more recent example is the emerging relationship between concussions and chronic traumatic encephalopathy (CTE). A variety of design and analytic strategies can be applied to observational studies to strengthen causal inference in the absence of random group assignment.

Interpreting Causation

To support a causal hypothesis, the observational researcher must first strive to minimize concerns about bias, confounding, and chance variation. Several principles have been proposed to support a purported cause-and-effect association.[4-6]

- **Temporal Sequence.** An essential criterion for causation is the establishment of a time sequence confirming that the causative exposure clearly preceded its supposed outcome or effect. Without this pattern, a relationship cannot be causal.
- **Strength of Association**. Observational researchers often evaluate the magnitude of the association between an exposure and an outcome using a statistical measure of relative risk. The greater the measured association, the more likely it is that a true causal relationship exists which cannot be explained away entirely by hidden biases.
- **Biological Credibility**. The researcher should be able to postulate a plausible mechanism by which the exposure might reasonably alter the risk of developing an outcome. This explanation may be theoretical, depending on the current state of knowledge, but conclusions are more credible if they are grounded in a realistic model and research evidence.
- **Consistency.** Findings are more credible when they are consistent with other studies. The more times a similar relationship is documented by different researchers using different samples, conditions, and study methods, the more likely it is true.
- **Dose-Response.** Lastly, the presence of a **dose-response relationship** can lend support to a

---

Focus on Evidence 19–1
"The Woman Who Knew Too Much" [7]

The history of x-rays, from their discovery in 1895, is one of rapid advancement and varied applications, which eventually led them to become commonplace in doctor's offices by the 1930's. Older readers may remember x-rays being used in shoe stores to assure a good fit,[8] or when pregnant women were routinely subjected to pelvic x-rays, purportedly to establish baseline measures in case there were complications later in the pregnancy. The medical community believed that there was a threshold of safety, with a dosage that was small enough to avoid harm.[9]

Following WWII, an English physician, Alice Stewart (1935-2002), one of the youngest women to be elected to the Royal College of Physicians in Oxford, became aware of an increasing incidence of leukemia in children and began looking for an environmental cause. She interviewed mothers of children with and without the disease, not knowing what to look for, and asked questions about everything she could think of, like exposure to infection, inoculations, pets, fried foods, highly colored drinks, sweets—and whether they had had an x-ray.[7]

Starting in 1956, and over several years,[10] Stewart submitted a series of letters and manuscripts to the *Lancet* and the *British Medical Journal*, sharing data that showed that twice as many cancer deaths occurred before the age of 10 among children whose mothers had received a series of pelvic x-rays while pregnant.[11-16] This claim sparked a barrage of criticism, with some detractors rejecting her data on the grounds that it was acquired from observational and retrospective study and so could not provide evidence of causation.[17-21] Stewart continued to argue that even low doses of radiation might be harmful, a view that put her at odds with physicians and the emerging nuclear industry. It was not until late into the 1970's that her admonitions were finally heeded.[22] Today, the health effects of radiation exposure are better understood, but with a lack of appreciation for the strength of observational data, it took decades for clinical practice to catch up with the research evidence.

For those interested in this remarkable history, two wonderful videos provide great background, one with her coworkers and one with Alice Stewart telling her own story.[23,24]

hypothesized causal association. Dose-response means that the risk of the outcome changes, not only with the presence or complete absence of an exposure, but also with varying levels of graded exposure. If the risk of developing an outcome does not vary in response to increasing or decreasing intensities of exposure, it raises doubts about whether the exposure is a true cause.

There are circumstances under which verifiable causal associations do not adhere to one or more of these principles. For example, a dose-response relationship may not be evident for all causal associations. If a linear dose-response pattern were evident in the association of diet with cognitive decline, cognitive decline would be most common in those with the poorest diets, moderately common in those with moderately healthy diets, and least common in those with the healthiest diets. It is plausible, however, that a person's diet needs only to achieve a minimum requirement for essential vitamin and mineral content without exceeding safe levels of saturated fats and sugars. Once these simple thresholds are satisfied, it may be that no additional protection is afforded by further dietary alterations. In this scenario, the relationship between diet and cognitive decline, although still causal, would not follow the typical dose-response pattern.

Similarly, although biological plausibility and consistency with previous research findings certainly increase confidence in the veracity of a reported causal association, firm grounding in current scientific knowledge is sometimes lacking for newly discovered causes. Of the five criteria cited, temporal sequence may be the only criterion that is universally required for causation. Interpretation of all other criteria should be made within context using logic and relevant information from prior research (see Box 19-1).[6]

■ Longitudinal Studies

Observational studies are characterized by the timing of data collection relative to the occurrence of exposures and outcomes (see Fig. 19-1). In a **longitudinal study**, researchers follow subjects through time, acquiring measurements at prescribed intervals. An advantage of the longitudinal method is its ability to document change and establish the correct time sequence of events, including confirmation that a suspected risk factor preceded its supposed outcome or effect. Longitudinal studies can be carried out prospectively, looking forward in time, or retrospectively, looking backward.

Box 19-1   Necessary or Sufficient?

What does it mean when we say that an exposure causes a condition? When we consider cause, we are often thinking of something that is "the" cause, but it is not that simple. We also need to know if the exposure will *always* cause the outcome, *sometimes* cause it, or does it require that other factors also need to be in place? Causation needs to be considered in terms of the nature of the association between an exposure and outcome. Therefore, we must understand if causes are necessary, sufficient or both.

A *necessary* exposure *must* be in place for an outcome to occur. The condition will never develop without the exposure. A *sufficient* exposure is one that *can* cause the outcome but other factors may also be involved. These two concepts create four categories of causation:

- **Necessary and sufficient.** Without the exposure, the condition never develops. With the exposure the condition always develops. The Tay-Sachs gene mutation is an example. The disease only occurs in the presence of the mutation, and if it is present, the individual will always develop the disease.
- **Necessary but not sufficient.** The exposure is necessary for the condition to develop, but the condition may not develop if other factors are not present. An example is exposure to tuberculosis. Specific bacteria are necessary for infection, but not everyone who is exposed will get the disease. Other health or environmental factors can influence whether the disease will occur.
- **Sufficient but not necessary.** The exposure alone can cause the condition, but other factors can also cause it in the absence of the exposure. For example, lack of exercise can result in weight gain, but other factors can also cause weight gain, such as an unhealthy diet.
- **Neither necessary nor sufficient.** Sometimes the condition will develop with the exposure, but other times the condition will fail to develop despite exposure. The condition can also develop from other causes. For example, lung cancer can be caused by smoking, but those who smoke do not all get lung cancer, and lung cancer can be caused by other factors.

These concepts are based on logic, and are relevant as we examine various exposures, and how we draw conclusions from observational studies regarding how we might intervene to prevent or improve a condition.

Prospective Studies

In a **prospective study**, information about one or more exposure variables (potential risk factors) is acquired through direct recording at the start of the study. Exposed and unexposed subjects are identified, and both groups are followed forward in time to monitor subsequent outcomes. With investigators involved from the

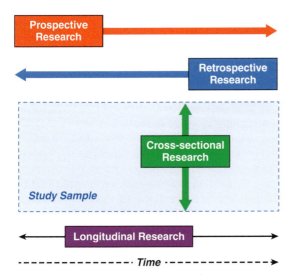

Figure 19–1 Graphic representation of the direction of inquiry for prospective and retrospective designs and the relationship between longitudinal and cross-sectional designs.

outset, data collection and measurement procedures can be tailored to ensure that the constructs of greatest relevance to the current study question are accurately captured.

In prospective studies, exposure status is determined at the start of the study, without foreknowledge of any participant's eventual outcome. This is a strength of the prospective design since the lack of investigator or participant knowledge of the outcome minimizes the threat of biased data collection or reporting.

On the other hand, the investigator's inability to precisely anticipate how many participants will eventually develop the target outcome or how long it may take for the outcome to become apparent can render the prospective design impractical for investigations into rare or slowly developing health conditions. The prospective approach is most useful when the target outcome can be expected to occur fairly frequently and without an excessively long period of monitoring before detection is possible.

Longitudinal studies may use a *closed design*, wherein a set period of follow-up time is established for all participants. Generalization of findings, then, are relevant only to that particular time period. Therefore, the failure to confirm increased risk of an outcome during a 1-year closed study period does not exclude the possibility that an increased risk would be evident during a 10-year follow-up. In an *open design*, each participant contributes a variable length of time under observation (see Chapter 34). From open design data, it may be possible to calculate the instantaneous rate at which an outcome occurs during various lengths of follow-up.

> **► CASE IN POINT #1**
> De Ryck et al[25] conducted a closed design prospective cohort study to determine incidence and risk factors for poststroke depression (PSD). They performed a baseline examination of 135 patients during the first week after stroke and then followed the cohort over a year and a half, testing for PSD at 1, 3, 6, 12, and 18 months. Results indicated an increased risk of developing PSD in patients with greater baseline impairments in mobility, cognition, or speech.

Challenges in Prospective Studies

Researchers using a longitudinal approach face many practical difficulties, most notably the long-term commitment of time, funds, and resources. Some health outcomes require a long period of incubation after exposure before they become evident, making prospective study of these outcomes a lengthy and sometimes unrealistic commitment.

Challenges to the internal validity of prospective studies include those related to measurement and confounding (see Chapter 15). Measurement validity can be threatened by testing effects since subjects undergoing repeated assessments may develop familiarity with testing procedures that could distort their performance. Attrition is also a potential threat in prospective studies involving a long period of monitoring. In the depression study, 32 patients were lost during the 18-month follow-up period as a result of death, unavailability, or unwillingness to continue. To minimize attrition, it is advisable to maintain regular contact with all prospective study participants.

Confounding is a ubiquitous threat in observational research. In prospective designs, investigators must consider the possibility that other risk factors for the same health outcome may be unequally distributed across exposed and unexposed groups.

> ► Because a history of depression pre-stroke is a likely risk factor for developing PSD, investigators were careful to assess all baseline participants for a history of pre-stroke depression so that they could adjust for this confounding factor as needed during analysis.

If pre-stroke depression was found to be more common or less common among participants with baseline exposure to mobility, cognition, or speech impairments, then the study's findings would be confounded. Efforts to control for confounding can be undertaken during the design or analysis phases of a prospective study, but potential confounding variables must always be enumerated prior to data collection so that appropriate procedures can be implemented to ascertain their presence (see Chapter 15).

Retrospective Studies

Retrospective studies involve the examination of data that were previously collected. Investigators may obtain previously recorded data from medical records, databases, completed surveys, or prior public health censuses (see Box 19-2). Available data must be sufficient to clearly establish each subject's exposure history and outcome status. When the target outcome is a transient condition, confirmation of prior outcome status can be challenging.

> ### ➤ CASE IN POINT #2
> Unhealthy weight gain during pregnancy creates many problems for both mother and child. Lindberg et al[26] designed a retrospective cohort study to evaluate insufficient and excess weight change among pregnant women who received prenatal care in a statewide health system. From the electronic medical records of 7,385 women, they determined whether maternal age, race/ethnicity, pre-pregnancy BMI, smoking status, insurance payor, and socioeconomic status were risk factors for unhealthy weight change.

Challenges in Retrospective Studies

Retrospective studies tend to be cheaper and faster than prospective studies, offering a more efficient way to investigate diseases with long latency or incubation periods. However, retrospective designs present several challenges. Medical records and historical records may be incomplete, and a retrospective researcher is unable to exert direct control over the procedures that were used previously to measure target variables. Consequently, measurements may not align perfectly with the current study question or with current expectations for accuracy.

> ➤ Researchers defined weight change as the difference between pre-pregnancy weight and weight within 8 weeks of delivery. Unfortunately, immediate pre-pregnancy weight measurements were missing for many women and had to be estimated using weight data from prior ambulatory visits.

Because the outcome status of participants is often known at the start of a retrospective study, investigators need to take action to protect against biased reporting or assessment. By assessing pre-pregnancy smoking status using medical records inscribed prior to the pregnancy, investigators hoped to avoid potentially biased reporting from mothers or doctors already aware of

> ### Box 19-2   Secondary Analysis
>
> Retrospective research often involves **secondary analysis**, when a researcher uses existing data sets to re-examine variables and answer questions other than those for which the data were originally collected. Investigators may analyze subsets of variables or subjects, or they may be interested in exploring new relationships among the variables. Secondary analysis has become increasingly common in recent years because of the accessibility of large data sets.
>
> Advantages of secondary analyses include their minimal expense, the ability to study large samples, and the elimination of the most time-consuming part of the research process—data collection. After formulating hypotheses, researchers can proceed without delay to test them. Retrospective researchers often develop their study questions after reviewing the existing data to determine what variables can be defined using available information. Alternatively, researchers may search for a database that can provide necessary information to answer their preformulated study question.
>
> A variety of large databases are supported by data libraries such as the Archive of the Inter-University Consortium for Political and Social Research at the University of Michigan.[27] The US government also sponsors continued collection of health-related data through the National Center for Health Statistics (NCHS),[28] which includes data from questionnaires such as the National Health Interview Survey[29] and the National Nursing Home Survey.[30] These studies include longitudinal data that are used by researchers in public health, rehabilitation, medicine, and social science to document changes in healthcare utilization, the health status of various age groups, and the association of personal and lifestyle characteristics with health outcomes. With increasing availability of data through electronic access, secondary analyses are an increasingly important research option.

pregnancy weight changes that they might incorrectly attribute to prior health or smoking habits.

■ Cross-Sectional Studies

In a **cross-sectional study**, the researcher takes a "snapshot" of a population, studying a group of subjects at one point in time (see Fig. 19-1). Variables are measured concurrently, meaning that their time sequence cannot be confirmed. In cross-sectional studies investigating potential causal factors, the designation of predictor (exposure) and outcome variables depends solely on the hypothesis that is proposed.

Cross-sectional data can provide useful insight into the current health status of a population, informing decisions about how best to allocate public resources. For example, in 2016 the prevalence of deaths from liver disease was found to be higher in New Mexico than other states., alerting public officials to a greater need for dialysis services there.[31]

A cross-sectional approach is often used because of its efficiency. Data about the exposure and outcome variables are collected concurrently, eliminating the need to follow subjects over long periods.

> ➤ In the television viewing study, parents were asked to estimate their child's weekly TV watching time and indicate their child's current height and weight. In some centers, height and weight estimates were confirmed using a stadiometer and scale.

Challenges in Cross-Sectional Studies

In establishing cause and effect, the time sequence of predictor and outcome variables is vitally important, a situation that can be clarified in longitudinal studies. In cross-sectional studies, however, it may not be possible to know whether the presumed cause (exposure) truly preceded the outcome.

> ➤ In the television viewing study, researchers found that the prevalence of obesity/overweight among children who watched

3 to 5 hours of TV per day was 37% greater than the prevalence among children who watched less than 1 hour. However, it was not possible to know if the hours of sedentary television watching were responsible for children becoming obese or if already obese children were simply inclined to forego more social activities in favor of watching television.

This is an example of potential **reverse causation**, wherein the variable designated as the "outcome" may actually cause the "exposure." For instance, the finding that liver disease was highly prevalent in New Mexico left unanswered the question of whether the New Mexican lifestyle was an antecedent cause of liver disease in that state, or whether, as some have suggested, persons already at risk of liver disease were simply immigrating or retiring to this sunny border state. When examining cross-sectional relationships, researchers must exercise caution in drawing conclusions about cause and effect relationships (see Focus on Evidence 19-2).

Cross-Sectional Validity Studies

Cross-sectional designs are commonly employed in the investigation of diagnostic test accuracy (see Chapter 33) and other studies of concurrent validity (see Chapter 10). When determining the accuracy of a diagnostic test to detect the presence or absence of a target health condition, the investigational test should be administered in close temporal proximity to the criterion test used to confirm the diagnosis. Diagnostic studies may be retrospective in so far as results from the index and reference tests are collected in the past (such as using medical records). Other diagnostic studies are prospective when data are not yet available

Focus on Evidence 19–2
When Genius Errs[33]

Sir Ronald Fisher (1890-1962) is generally considered the father of modern statistics—he invented a little thing called the analysis of variance and a few other important statistical concepts. In addition to his reputation for statistical discovery, however, he was also known for his strong voice disputing the relationship between smoking and lung cancer, despite clear evidence to the contrary. As early as 1950, this relationship had been well documented.[34]

As a smoker, Fisher's argument was that we could not know if smoking caused cancer or cancer caused smoking.[35] Their undeniable mutual occurrence, he proposed, could reflect a precancerous state that caused a chemical irritation in the lungs that was relieved by smoking, leading to an increased use of cigarettes. He later suggested that the association was most likely due to a third factor, a genetic predisposition, which made people more susceptible to lung cancer,

and at the same time created personality types that would lead to smoking. Fisher became a consultant for the tobacco companies in 1960 and was apparently instrumental in blocking many law suits at that time.

Fisher's arguments flew in the face of numerous studies that documented higher rates of lung cancer and mortality among smokers.[36,37] Bolstered by Fisher's learned opinions and statistical arguments, however, tobacco companies argued that there was no proof of causation, as this could only legitimately be achieved through experimental studies—and of course, there were none.[38]

This regrettable story illustrates the need to keep focused on logic and science, and to continue to question and examine relationships to truthfully understand clinical phenomena. Observational studies provide an invaluable source of data to explore hypothesized relationships for many health-related questions. It remains our job to identify the theoretical premise that justifies our conclusions.

from the index test, and must be newly collected by the investigators. In either instance, a diagnostic study is typically cross-sectional because current index test results are compared to current outcomes from the reference standard test.

While it is not always feasible to administer both tests during the same clinic visit, it is important to keep the interval between test administrations brief so that a participant's health status does not fluctuate. Likewise, when estimating the concurrent validity of a measurement tool, recorded values are compared to values obtained using a reference standard instrument that is administered at approximately the same time. The cross-sectional design of these studies reflects an expectation that the health status of participants will remain unaltered during the brief interval between test administrations.

■ Cohort Studies

In clinical research, a cohort is a group of individuals who are followed over time. A **cohort study**, also called a *follow-up study*, is a longitudinal investigation in which the researcher identifies a group of subjects who do not yet have the outcome of interest. Subjects are interviewed, examined, or observed to determine their exposure to factors hypothesized to alter the risk of developing the target outcome. Exposed and unexposed cohort members are then monitored for a period of time to ascertain whether they do, in fact, develop the outcome. Comparisons are made of the frequency of newly developed outcomes across exposed and unexposed groups, indicating whether the hypothesized association is supported by the data.

Types of Cohort Studies

Cohort studies can be either prospective or retrospective. If the investigation is initiated after some individuals have already developed the target outcome, the study is considered retrospective. More commonly, the investigator contacts participants before any of them have developed the target condition, in which case, the cohort study it is considered prospective (see Fig. 19-2).

An **inception cohort** is a group that is assembled early in the development of a disorder, for example, at the time of diagnosis. Although the disorder is already present in all members of an inception cohort, examination findings and subject characteristics present at the time of diagnosis can be studied for their longitudinal association with incident outcomes, including incidence of disease progression or remission.

Cohorts can be identified in different ways. *Geographic cohorts* are based on area of residence, such as a particular

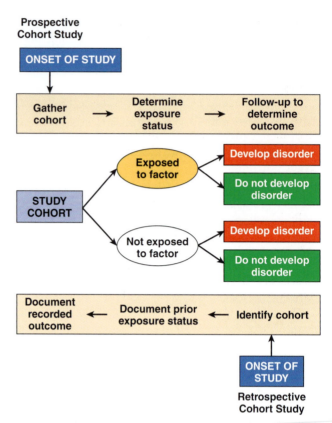

Figure 19–2 The design of prospective and retrospective cohort studies. Participants are chosen based on their membership in a defined cohort. In a prospective study, the investigator enters the study to determine exposure status and follows subjects to determine who develops the disorder of interest. In a retrospective study, the investigator enters after exposure status has been determined, and tracks data from the past to determine outcomes.

city, town, or neighborhood. *Birth cohorts* represent generational groups, such as baby boomers or millennials. An *historical cohort* includes individuals who experience common events, such as veterans of the Vietnam war. Victims who are survivors of natural disasters would be considered members of *environmental cohorts*. *Developmental cohorts* are based on life changes, such as getting married or moving into a nursing home.

> ➤ **CASE IN POINT #4**
>
> Dale and colleagues[39] undertook a prospective cohort study to determine the relation of self-reported physical work exposures to risk of carpal tunnel syndrome (CTS) among clerical, service, and construction workers during 3 years of follow-up. CTS was confirmed using nerve conduction velocity (NCV) tests.

Cohort studies may be purely descriptive, with the intent of chronicling the natural history of a disease (see Chapter 20). More often, however, they are analytic, endeavoring to estimate the magnitude of the risk associated with an exposure. This estimate is derived by comparing the incidence of new outcomes across groups of exposed and unexposed subjects. This is the strategy used in the study of CTS.

One advantage of a cohort study is the certainty that it affords in establishing the correct temporal sequence of events. Cohort studies involve only participants who, at the time exposure is ascertained, are free of the target outcome. Given this, we can be certain that a subject's baseline exposure status will have preceded any new occurrence of the outcome during the follow-up period.

> ➤ In the study of CTS, only workers who tested negative for existing nerve conduction impairment at the screening visit were eligible to participate. Investigators prospectively evaluated risk factors for developing incident CTS. Over 3 years of follow-up among 710 cohort members, 31 new cases of CTS were confirmed by NCV tests. Workers exposed to at least 4 hours per day of activities involving forceful gripping, use of vibrating tools, or lifting objects had two to three times the odds of developing symptomatic CTS.

A disadvantage of the cohort design is that it offers little assurance at the start of the study that the targeted outcome will occur with sufficient frequency to permit robust statistical comparisons of exposed and unexposed groups.

> ➤ Only eight subjects developed bilateral CTS, making it difficult to estimate the relation of physical work exposures to risk of bilateral CTS.

For this reason, the prospective cohort design may be inappropriate for studying rare outcomes. Large numbers of subjects would have to be followed over a long period to document new cases for analysis. To investigate risk factors for rare or slowly developing disorders, the case–control design is more appropriate, to be described shortly.

Cohort Subject Selection

The first step in subject selection for a prospective cohort study is identification of the target population. Eligible subjects are typically recruited from communities, health-care practices, or professional groups. The subjects must be free of the target outcome at baseline but susceptible to developing it during the follow-up period.

> ➤ CTS occurs most frequently in occupations involving upper extremity physical work. To generalize findings to this target population, participants in the CTS study were recruited from eight employers and three trade unions where workers spent time in activities requiring forceful use of arms, hands, and fingers. Workers who had a history of carpal tunnel release were excluded because they were no longer at risk for developing new CTS.

Once a cohort is assembled, subjects are classified by their level of exposure to the hypothesized risk factor. In the CTS study, subjects were classified as exposed to a physical stressor if they were engaged in that activity for an average of at least 4 hours per day.

For common outcomes, cohorts may be recruited from the general population. For outcomes that are less common in the general population, special cohorts may be assembled from professions that have high rates of occupational exposure, as was done in the CTS study, from residents living near sources of environmental contamination, or from patients that share an alternative risk factor for the same outcome.

To facilitate a valid comparison, the unexposed group should be as similar as possible to the exposed group in all factors related to the outcome except for the specific exposure under study. No subject in either group should be immune to the outcome.

Challenges for Cohort Studies

Misclassification of Exposure

The first task of any cohort study is to accurately classify subjects by their exposure status. If an exposed person is mistakenly classified as unexposed or vice versa, the error is referred to as *exposure misclassification*. When this occurs randomly, as when exposed and unexposed subjects are misclassified with equal frequency, it is considered *nondifferential*. Unreliable measurement tools are susceptible to random errors that can cause nondifferential misclassification. Clinical cohort studies, especially those that rely on unreliable clinical assessments to ascertain exposure status, are particularly susceptible to this type of misclassification. When exposure misclassification is both nondifferential and independent of the outcome for participants, the true relationship between exposure and outcome may be diluted, resulting in findings that are biased "towards the null."

Conversely, when errors are not randomly distributed across groups, the resulting misclassification may be *differential* or *dependent* on outcome status. These types of errors can result in an exaggeration of the true relationship between exposure and outcome. Such bias "away from the null" can occur, for example, when classification of exposure status is based on the inaccurate self-report of study participants.

➤ In the study of CTS, physical work exposures were ascertained by self-report. Investigators acknowledged a potential for workers to overreport or underreport their true exposure status, potentially resulting in misclassification error and biased findings.

In the CTS study, differential misclassification would have occurred if those who did not actually engage in heavy work consistently overreported their exposure to physical stressors. Since it seems unlikely that workers who truly are engaged in heavy work would underreport their own high levels of activity with equal frequency, differential misclassification errors may have biased the findings away from the null.

Bias and Attrition

The longitudinal nature of prospective cohort studies makes them prone to attrition. Bias will result if the loss of subjects is related to either their exposure status, their outcome status, or both. Unfortunately, it can be difficult to know if a subject who departed the study went on to develop the outcome or not.

➤ Of the 1,107 subjects recruited for the study of CTS, only 751 (67.8%) completed the follow-up physical examination. It was not known whether any of the subjects lost to attrition developed CTS during what remained of the follow-up period.

Researchers generally take great pains to avoid attrition by maintaining good rapport and regular communication with all cohort participants. When possible, researchers look at the baseline measures among those who dropped out to see if they are different from those who were retained. In the CTS study, for instance, the researchers found no significant difference in the baseline age, gender, body mass index (BMI), medical history, or job category between those who were lost to attrition and those who completed follow-up.

■ Case-Control Studies

A **case–control study** is a method of observational investigation in which groups of individuals are purposely selected on the basis of whether or not they have the health condition under study. *Cases* are those who have the target condition, while *controls* do not. The investigator then looks to see if these two groups differ with respect to their exposure history or the presence of a risk factor. The comparison of cases to controls can be made cross-sectionally by looking at current characteristics, or by looking backward in time via interview, questionnaire, or chart review (see Fig. 19-3).

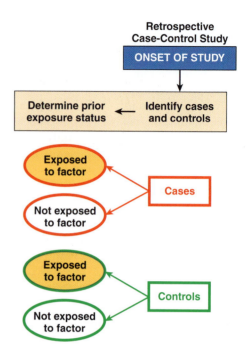

Figure 19–3 Design of a retrospective case-control study. Participants are chosen based on their status as a case or control, and then prior exposure status is ascertained.

➤ **CASE IN POINT #5**

Exercise is recognized as an important component of a healthy lifestyle but can also lead to physical injury. Using a case-control design, Sutton et al[40] tested the hypothesis that development of knee osteoarthritis (OA) was related to past participation in sports and exercise. Data were obtained from a large national fitness survey in England. They identified 216 eligible cases of knee OA, including 66 men and 150 women.

The case–control design is especially useful for studying rare disorders or conditions with long latency or incubation periods. For instance, knee OA develops slowly and may remain undetected for years, so a longitudinal study would require following subjects for many years before they could detect a sufficient number of knee OA cases. Greater efficiency is achieved using a retrospective case-control design that compares the past sporting histories of seniors who currently have knee OA (cases) to seniors who do not (controls).

➤ The only strong risk factor identified for knee OA was prior knee injury. Knee OA cases were 8 times as likely to report a previous sports-related knee injury than controls. The authors concluded that evidence did not support the popular belief that, absent a knee injury, participation in sports or exercise increased risk of knee OA later in life.

Selection of Cases

The internal validity of a case–control study is dependent on several design issues. Perhaps most obvious are the effects of case definition and case selection. **Case definition** refers to the diagnostic and clinical criteria that identify someone as a case (see Box 19-3). As with any diagnostic processes, false positives and false negatives can lead to misclassification errors and biased results.

> ➤ Cases of knee OA were identified by self-report on a questionnaire. To be identified as a case, subjects had to indicate that they currently had symptomatic arthritis with recurrent or continuous knee symptoms that did not also affect hands or wrists, and that they were at least 40 years old at the onset of these arthritis symptoms.

Unfortunately, the questionnaire did not include a specific item about knee OA. Instead, investigators derived logical criteria from the limited set of questions that were asked about symptoms and self-reported arthritis. The accuracy of these criteria cannot be known since it was not feasible to confirm or refute the self-report of the survey participants.

Recruiting Cases

Cases can be recruited from several sources. A **population-based study** uses cases obtained from the general population. This method can be used to study disorders that are prevalent in the population or where access to data on large numbers of people can be affordably obtained. The knee OA study included a large sample from the adult population of England that participated in the national fitness survey.

Box 19-3   Redefining Cases

Case definitions for many diseases have been developed by the Centers for Disease Control and Prevention (CDC) and the World Health Organization (WHO). At times, these definitions are revised to reflect recent medical findings. For example, in 1998 the criterion for type 2 diabetes was lowered from a threshold fasting plasma glucose level of >140mg/dl to 126mg/dl, a change that greatly increased the number of people who were considered to have the disease.[41,42] Similar changes have been made in the case definition of HIV infection over many years, responding to advances in diagnostic techniques.[43,44] Clinical diagnoses are sometimes more difficult to define or standardize. For instance, disorders such as birth defects, hemiplegia, cerebral palsy, and low back pain can be manifested in many different forms. Therefore, the specific characteristics that qualify an individual as having the disorder for research purposes must be spelled out in detail.

In a **hospital-based study**, cases are enlisted from patients in a medical institution. Compared to a population-based sample, hospital-based subjects tend to be relatively easy to contact and recruit, and information on a participant's health history is readily obtained. While the population-based approach may support broader generalizability of the study's findings, it can be expensive and logistically challenging to verify a case diagnosis or confirm an exposure history.

Selection of Controls

A critical and often underappreciated aspect of designing a valid case–control study is the selection of an appropriate control group. The purpose of the control group is to demonstrate how common the exposure is among people in the population from which the cases emerged. To serve this purpose, a useful question to ask is "Would the control subjects in this study have been eligible to serve as case subjects if they had developed the same target disorder?" Any restrictions or criteria used to select the cases should, therefore, also be used to select controls.

Recruiting Controls

Controls can be obtained from general population resources, such as using random-digit dialing, voter registration logs, membership directories, or Medicare beneficiary lists.[45] Sometimes special groups can provide viable controls, such as family members, friends, or neighbors of the case subjects. Controls selected in this manner typically resemble the cases with respect to ethnic and lifestyle characteristics, thereby reducing the threat that these factors might confound a comparison of cases to controls during the analysis.

Controls can also be recruited from the same hospital or clinic as cases. Hospital-based controls are chosen from among patients who have been admitted for health conditions other than the one under investigation. An advantage of using hospital-based controls is that patients are readily available and similarly motivated. A possible disadvantage is that, like the cases, they too are ill.

It is important to consider that a single exposure may be implicated in the etiology of more than one disease. Therefore, investigators in a hospital-based case-control study must ensure that a comparison of the exposure histories of ill cases to ill controls is not distorted by the dual role that exposure plays in both illnesses. Selecting hospital controls from among patients whose illnesses have a distinct etiology from that of the case subjects may be challenging, but it is essential to ensure a valid comparison.

Challenges in Case-Control Studies

Selection Bias

The analysis of case–control studies requires attention to bias in the selection and classification of subjects and in the ascertainment of exposure status. Because subjects are purposefully selected based on whether a target disorder is present or not, **selection bias** is a special concern.

Cases and controls must be chosen regardless of their exposure histories. If they are differentially selected on some variable that is related to the exposure of interest, it will not be possible to determine if the exposure is truly related to the disorder. When samples are composed of subjects who have volunteered to participate, self-selection biases can also occur.

> ▶ Out of 4,316 adults who completed the fitness survey, 216 cases of knee OA were identified, leaving 4,100 adults who were potentially eligible to serve as controls. Even after narrowing the list of potential control subjects to include only those who matched to a case on age and gender, the list of potential controls still exceeded what was required. To minimize the threat of bias, matching controls were selected randomly from among those who were eligible.

Observation Bias

In a case-control study, the outcome of each participant is known. Foreknowledge of the outcome renders the design particularly susceptible to biased measurement by the assessor or biased reporting by the participant. **Observation bias** occurs when there is a systematic difference in the way information about the exposure is obtained from the study groups.

Interviewer bias can occur when the individual collecting data elicits, records, or interprets information differently for controls than for cases. For example, an interviewer may be aware of the research hypothesis and might ascertain information to support this hypothesis. Because so many epidemiologic studies involve an interview or observation, this type of bias must be explicitly addressed by blinding interviewers to group and hypothesis, and by making data collection as objective as possible.

Recall Bias

Recall bias occurs when case subjects who have experienced a particular disorder remember their exposure history differently than control subjects who have not experienced the disorder. It is not unusual for individuals who have a disease to analyze their habits or past experiences with greater depth or accuracy than those who are healthy. This bias may result in an underestimate or an overestimate of the risk associated with a particular exposure.

> ▶ Individuals with painful knee OA might be more inclined to remember a past knee injury, whereas healthy control subjects could easily forget.

When cases are selected from hospitalized patients and controls are drawn from the general population, the problem of recall bias may be especially potent.

Confounding

Another factor that may interfere with analytic interpretations of case–control data is the confounding effect of extraneous variables that are related to the exposure of interest and that independently affect the risk of developing the disorder. For example, previous data have shown that women have an increased likelihood of developing knee OA. Female seniors are also less likely to have participated in sports than their male peers. Since gender is related to both the outcome (knee OA) and the exposure, sporting history or gender could confound the results. To examine the potential contribution of confounders, investigators must collect data on them and analyze their association with both the exposure and the disease.

Matching

When sufficient numbers are available, researchers often attempt to match control subjects to a case on one or more characteristics, such as age, gender, neighborhood, or other characteristics with potential to alter the risk of the outcome. Greater similarity between controls and cases facilitates more valid comparison of their exposure histories. This is an effective method of reducing or eliminating the possibility that the matched factors will confound the results. Matching on a small number of factors does not, however, eliminate the possibility that other differences between case and control groups may persist.

> ▶ In the knee OA study, each case was matched to four control subjects according to gender and age. It was possible to pick multiple controls for each case owing to the large number of people completing the health survey who did not have knee OA.

Matching the control group to the cases on gender and age eliminates the possibility that these differences could confound a comparison of their past sporting histories.

> 🔑 When feasible, researchers will try to recruit more than one control subject for each case to minimize bias and increase statistical precision during analysis. Matching may be difficult when many variables are relevant, such as gender, age, weight, or other health conditions. An alternative strategy for this purpose is the use of **propensity score** matching. These values are composite scores that represent a combination of several confounding variables. Scores are derived through a statistical process of logistic regression and can help to equate groups on baseline variables (see Chapter 30).

COMMENTARY

Smoking is one of the leading causes of statistics.

—Fletcher Knebel (1911-1993)

American author

In a classic tongue in cheek 2003 article by Smith and Pell,[46] they described their attempt at a systematic review to determine whether parachutes are effective for preventing major trauma related to gravitational challenge. They based their research question on the observation that parachutes appear to reduce the risk of injury when jumping from an airplane, with data showing increased morbidity and mortality with parachute failure or free fall.[47,48] The authors satirically noted, however, that as an intervention, parachute effectiveness had never been "proven" in any controlled trial. Using death or trauma as the primary outcome, the authors attempted a comprehensive literature search but found no randomized controlled trials of the parachute. They asserted that, despite this lack of formal evidence, the parachute industry continues to profit from the belief that their product is effective, a belief that is likely to remain unchallenged given the difficulty of finding volunteers willing to serve as control subjects in a randomized trial!

Even though observational studies are not able to establish direct cause-and-effect relationships with the same degree of control as in an RCT, they play an important role in clinical research, especially considering the lack of documented evidence that exists concerning most clinical phenomena. Before one can begin to investigate causal factors for behaviors and responses using experimental methods, one must first discover which variables are related and how they occur in nature. As several examples have shown, our understanding of the causes of an outcome can only move ahead if we recognize how those phenomena manifest themselves with regard to concurrent variables.

This chapter provides an introduction to issues that are relevant to observational designs. Analysis procedures will be discussed in more detail in succeeding chapters. Readers can refer to many excellent epidemiology texts to find more comprehensive discussions of observational designs that go beyond the scope of this chapter.[49-51]

REFERENCES

1. Shen TC, Lin CL, Wei CC, Chen CH, Tu CY, Hsia TC, Shih CM, Hsu WH, Sung FC, Kao CH. Risk of obstructive sleep apnea in adult patients with asthma: A population-based cohort study in Taiwan. *PLoS One* 2015;10(6):e0128461.
2. Smyth A, Dehghan M, O'Donnell M, Anderson C, Teo K, Gao P, Sleight P, Dagenais G, Probstfield JL, Mente A, et al. Healthy eating and reduced risk of cognitive decline: A cohort from 40 countries. *Neurology* 2015;84(22):2258-2265.
3. Resnick A, Woods B, Krapfl H, Toth B. Health outcomes associated with smoke exposure in Albuquerque, New Mexico, during the 2011 Wallow fire. *J Public Health Manag Pract* 2015;21 Suppl 2:S55-61.
4. Hill AB. The environment and disease: association or causation? *Proc Royal Soc Med* 1965;58(5):295-300.
5. Susser M. *Causal Thinking in the Health Sciences: Concepts and Strategies in Epidemiology*. New York: Oxford University Press; 1973.
6. Kundi M. Causality and the interpretation of epidemiologic evidence. *Environ Health Perspect* 2006;114(7):969-974.
7. Greene G. *The Woman Who Knew Too Much: Alice Stewart and the Secrets of Radiation*. Ann Arbor, MI: University of Michigan Press 2001.
8. Lapp DR. The x-ray shoe fitter — an early application of Roentgen's 'new kind of ray'. *The Physics Teacher* 2004;42(6): 354-358.
9. Wasserman H, Solomon N. The use and misuse of medical X rays. In Wasserman H, Solomon N. *Killing Our Own: The Disaster of America's Experience with Atomic Radiation*. New York: Dell Publishing Company; 2012: Chapter 6.
10. Stewart AM. Risk of childhood cancer from fetal irradiation: 1. *Br J Radiol* 1997;70(835):769-770.
11. Stewart A, Webb J, Hewitt D. A survey of childhood malignancies. *Br Med J* 1958;1(5086):1495-1508.
12. Stewart A, Webb J, Giles D, Hewitt D. Malignant disease in childhood and diagnostic irradiation in utero. *Lancet* 1956;268(6940):447.
13. Stewart A, Webb JW, Giles D, Hewitt D. X-rays and leukemia. Letter to the Editor. *Lancet* 1957;269(6967):528.
14. Stewart A, Kneale GW. Changes in the cancer risk associated with obstetric radiography. *Lancet* 1968;1(7534):104-107.
15. Stewart A. Prenatal x-ray exposure and childhood neoplasms. *Br J Radiol* 1972;45(538):794.
16. Kneale GW, Stewart AM. Mantel-Haenszel analysis of Oxford data. II. Independent effects of fetal irradiation subfactors. *J Natl Cancer Inst* 1976;57(5):1009-1014.
17. Court Brown WM, Doll R, Hill RB. Incidence of leukaemia after exposure to diagnostic radiation in utero. *BMJ* 1960; 2(5212):1539-1545.
18. Rabinowitch J. X-rays and leukemia. *Lancet* 1956;268(6955): 1261-1262.
19. Rabinowitch J. X-rays and leukemia. *Lancet* 1957;269(6961): 219-220.

20. Reid F. X-rays and leukemia. *Lancet* 1957;269(6965):428.
21. Lindsay DW. Effects of diagnostic irradiation. *Lancet* 1963; 281(7281):602-603.
22. Greene G. Richard Doll and Alice Stewart: reputation and the shaping of scientific "truth". *Perspect Biol Med* 2011;54(4): 504-531.
23. Medical Sleuth: Detecting Links Between Radiation and Cancer. City Club of Portland. Available at https://www.youtube.com/watch?v=H4l6frw8Uk8. Accessed May 20, 2017.
24. Alice Stewart: The woman who knew too much. Available at https://www.youtube.com/watch?v=proyrn2AAMA. Accessed August 23, 2016.
25. De Ryck A, Brouns R, Fransen E, Geurden M, Van Gestel G, Wilssens I, De Ceulaer L, Marien P, De Deyn PP, Engelborghs S. A prospective study on the prevalence and risk factors of poststroke depression. *Cerebrovasc Dis Extra* 2013;3(1):1-13.
26. Lindberg S, Anderson C, Pillai P, Tandias A, Arndt B, Hanrahan L. Prevalence and predictors of unhealthy weight gain in pregnancy. *WMJ* 2016;115(5):233-237.
27. ICPSR. Available at https://www.icpsr.umich.edu/icpsrweb/. Accessed December 5, 2017.
28. National Center for Health Statistics. Centers for Disease Control and Prevention. Available at https://www.cdc.gov/nchs/index.htm. Accessed December 5, 2017.
29. Centers for Disease Control and Prevention (CDC). National Health Interview Survey. National Center for Health Statistics. Available at https://www.cdc.gov/nchs/nhis/data-questionnaires-documentation.htm. Accessed June 30, 2017.
30. National Nursing Home Survey. National Center for Health Statistics. Centers for Disease Control and Prevention. Available at https://www.cdc.gov/nchs/nnhs/index.htm. Accessed December 5, 2017.
31. Centers for Disease Control and Prevention. National Center for Health Statistics. Stats of the State of New Mexico. Available at https://www.cdc.gov/nchs/pressroom/states/newmexico/newmexico.htm. Accessed March 7, 2019.
32. Braithwaite I, Stewart AW, Hancox RJ, Beasley R, Murphy R, Mitchell EA. The worldwide association between television viewing and obesity in children and adolescents: cross sectional study. *PLoS One* 2013;8(9):e74263.
33. Stolley PD. When genius errs: R.A. Fisher and the lung cancer controversy. *Am J Epidemiol* 1991;133:416-425.
34. Doll R, Hill AB. Smoking and carcinoma of the lung; preliminary report. *Br Med J* 1950;2(4682):739-748.
35. Gould SJ. The smoking gun of eugenics. *Nat Hist* 1991(12): 8-17.
36. United States Public Health Service. Smoking and Health. Report of the Advisory Committee to the Surgeon General of the Public Health Service. Public Health Service Publication No. 1103. Available at https://profiles.nlm.nih.gov/ps/retrieve/ResourceMetadata/NNBBMQ. Accessed October 16, 2017. Washington, DC: Office of the Surgeon General, 1964.
37. Proctor RN. The history of the discovery of the cigarette–lung cancer link: evidentiary traditions, corporate denial, global toll. *Tobacco Control* 2012;21(2):87-91.
38. Brandt AM. Inventing conflicts of interest: a history of tobacco industry tactics. *Am J Public Health* 2012;102(1):63-71.
39. Dale AM, Gardner BT, Zeringue A, Strickland J, Descatha A, Franzblau A, Evanoff BA. Self-reported physical work exposures and incident carpal tunnel syndrome. *Am J Ind Med* 2014; 57(11):1246-1254.
40. Sutton AJ, Muir KR, Mockett S, Fentem P. A case-control study to investigate the relation between low and moderate levels of physical activity and osteoarthritis of the knee using data collected as part of the Allied Dunbar National Fitness Survey. *Ann Rheum Dis* 2001;60(8):756-764.
41. Report of the expert committee on the diagnosis and classification of diabetes mellitus. *Diabetes Care* 2003;26 Suppl 1:S5-20.
42. Woolf SH, Rothemich SF. New diabetes guidelines: a closer look at the evidence. *Am Fam Physician* 1998;58(6):1287-1288, 1290.
43. Center for Disease Control and Prevention. Revised surveillance case definition for HIV infection—United States, 2014. Morbidity and Mortality Weekly Report, April 11, 2014. Available at https://www.cdc.gov/mmwr/preview/mmwrhtml/rr6303a1.htm. Accessed December 10, 2017.
44. World Health Organization. AIDS and HIV Case Definitions. Available at http://www.who.int/hiv/strategic/surveillance/definitions/en/. Accessed December 9, 2017.
45. Bertone ER, Newcomb PA, Willett WC, Stampfer MJ, Egan KM. Recreational physical activity and ovarian cancer in a population-based case-control study. *Int J Cancer* 2002; 99:431-436.
46. Smith GC, Pell JP. Parachute use to prevent death and major trauma related to gravitational challenge: systematic review of randomised controlled trials. *BMJ* 2003;327(7429):1459-1461.
47. Highest fall survived without a parachute. *Guinness Book of World Records*, 2002. Available at http://www.guinnessworldrecords.com/world-records/highest-fall-survived-without-parachute/. Accessed May 19, 2017.
48. Belmont PJ, Jr., Taylor KF, Mason KT, Shawen SB, Polly DW, Jr., Klemme WR. Incidence, epidemiology, and occupational outcomes of thoracolumbar fractures among U.S. Army aviators. *J Trauma* 2001;50(5):855-861.
49. Rothman KJ. *Epidemiology: An Introduction*. 2nd ed. Oxford: Oxford University Press; 2012.
50. Merrill RM. *Introduction to Epidemiology*. 7th ed. Burlington, MA: Jones and Bartlett; 2017.
51. Rothman KJ, Greenland S, Lash TL. *Modern Epidemiology*. Philadelphia: Lippincott Williams & Wilkins; 2008.

Descriptive Research

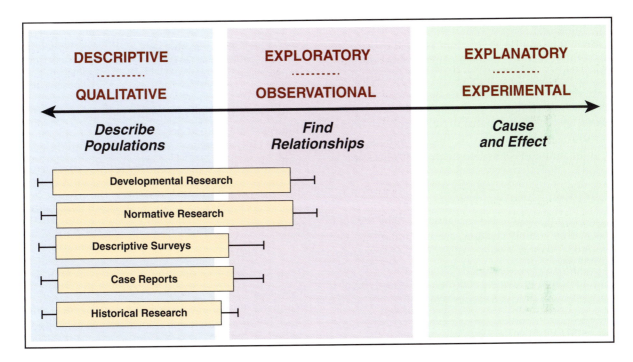

Descriptive research is an observational approach designed to document traits, behaviors, and conditions of individuals, groups, and populations. Descriptive and exploratory elements are often combined, depending on how the investigator conceptualizes the research question. These studies document the nature of existing phenomena using both quantitative and qualitative methods and describe how variables change over time. They will generally be structured around a set of guiding questions or research objectives, often to serve as a basis for research hypotheses or theoretical propositions that can be tested using exploratory or explanatory techniques.

Descriptive studies may involve prospective or retrospective data collection and may be designed using longitudinal or cross-sectional methods. Surveys and secondary analysis of clinical databases are often used as sources of data for descriptive analysis. Several types of research can be categorized as descriptive based on their primary purpose, including developmental research, normative research, case reports, and historical research.

■ Developmental Research

Concepts of human development, whether they are related to cognition, perceptual-motor control, communication, physiological change, or psychological processes, are important elements of a clinical knowledge base. Valid interpretation of clinical outcomes depends on our ability to develop a clear picture of those we treat, their characteristics, and performance expectations under different conditions. Developmental research involves the description of developmental change and the sequencing of behaviors in people over time.

Developmental studies have contributed to the theoretical foundations of clinical practice in many ways. For example, the classic descriptive studies of Gesell and Amatruda[1] and McGraw[2] provide the basis for much of the research on sequencing of motor development in infants and children. Erikson's studies of life span development have contributed to an understanding of psychological growth through old age.[3] Understanding how behavior naturally changes provides a basis for creation of measuring instruments to determine if an individual's development is progressing as expected.

Longitudinal Studies

Developmental studies can be characterized by the time period within which changes are documented. The longitudinal method involves collecting data over an extended period to document behaviors as they vary over time. The nature of the population must be specified to define the group to which results will apply.

> **HISTORICAL NOTE**
> One of the earliest developmental studies was actually a longitudinal case report of data collected between 1759 and 1777, chronicling the physical growth of a child at 6-month intervals from birth to 18 years.[4] These data still represent one of the most famous records of human growth.

Intellectual growth has been the subject of many longitudinal studies in children[5] and adults.[6] Changes that occur in psychological and physiological processes as people age are best described using longitudinal methods (see Focus on Evidence 20-1).

> Researchers have described longitudinal patterns of development in infant heart transplant recipients.[7] They studied 39 children, following them for up to 3 years. They identified mild motor delays between 18 to 35 months, speech-language delays at 18 months, and abstract reasoning deficits from 28 to 36 months.

This age-dependent variability provides important understanding of risk factors in this patient population, suggesting a concern for early intervention.

Natural History

An important type of longitudinal research is the documentation of the natural history of a disease or condition. This type of research documents the course of a condition, often from onset to its eventual resolution, which can range from cure to death. Understanding natural history is a fundamental precursor to prevention, intervention and establishing causality.

> In classic studies, Munsat and colleagues[8] followed 50 patients with amyotrophic lateral sclerosis (ALS) over 6 years to document the rate and pattern of motor deterioration. They described a linear and symmetric rate of motoneuron loss. The rate of deterioration was comparable across genders, ages at onset, and proximal and distal muscles.

By providing this important descriptive foundation, clinicians gained an understanding of the progressive nature of ALS, which was essential for study of its management. For instance, these data have been used to generate hypotheses about specific drug interventions to slow the progression.[9-12] Without the natural history data, it would not be possible to determine whether drug trials are effective.

Cross-Sectional Studies

With the cross-sectional method, the researcher studies various developmental levels within a particular group of subjects and describes differences among those levels as they exist at a single point in time. For this reason, this approach is often considered a "snapshot" of a population.

> Researchers from the Multi-Center Orthopaedic Outcome Network (MOON Group)[13] used a prospective cross-sectional design to describe symptom characteristics of rotator cuff tears. They studied 450 patients with full-thickness tears, dividing them into four groups according to duration of symptoms: ≤3 months, 4 to 6 months, 7 to 12 months, and >12 months. Their analysis showed that the longer duration of symptoms did not correlate with more severe tears, including weakness, limited range and other outcome measures.

The results of this study have to be considered within the limitations of a cross-sectional design, because the patients were not followed over time to determine the pattern or rate of symptom change. By looking at measurements only at one point in time, an

Focus on Evidence 20–1
Developmental Trajectories in Children with Autism

Autism spectrum disorders (ASD) are a group of neurodevelopmental disorders characterized by deficits in communication and social interaction. Researchers continue to look for etiology, as well as trying to understand the developmental trajectory.

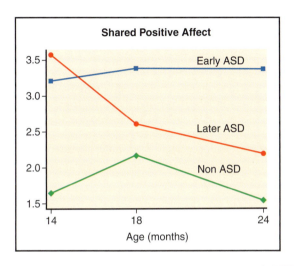

Landa et al[14] used a prospective longitudinal approach to study 204 infants who were siblings of children with autism and 31 infants with no family history, considered at low risk. Children were evaluated six times over 3 years. The results identified three groups: early ASD diagnosis (before 14 months), later ASD diagnosis (after 14 months), and no ASD. They found that despite the children exhibiting similar developmental levels at 6 months, the groups exhibited atypical trajectories thereafter in social, language, and motor skills. The figure illustrates one behavior, shared positive affect (smiling and eye contact), showing greater impairments from 14 to 24 months in the early diagnosed group (results are expressed as standardized scores, with higher values indicating greater impairment). Although similar at 14 months, the late diagnosed group improved over the 2 years, whereas the behavior of the early diagnosed group stayed steady. This type of descriptive study is essential for advancing theories about ASD, developing screening tools, and early detection to improve access to early intervention.

From Landa RJ, Stuart EA, Gross AL, Faherty A. Developmental trajectories in children with and without autism spectrum disorders: the first 3 years. *Child Dev* 2013;84(2):429-442. Figure 1, p. 436. Used with permission.

assumption is made that all patients with similar duration would have similar symptom development, which may not be true.

Pragmatically, the cross-sectional method makes it easier to sample large representative groups than a longitudinal study does. If, however, the primary interest is the study of patterns of change, the longitudinal method is preferred, as only that method can establish the validity of temporal sequencing of behaviors and characteristics.[15]

 Cross-sectional studies measure *prevalence* of a condition in a population, which is a measure of how many individuals are affected at any one point in time. This approach cannot measure *incidence*, which is a measure of the number of new cases within a period of time (see Chapter 34). Therefore, the cross-sectional design is not suited to studying the natural history of a disease or for drawing inferences about causes or prognosis.

Cohort Effects

Many of the extraneous variables that interfere in cross-sectional studies pertain to cohort effects, effects that are not age specific but are due to a subject's generation, or period effects, related to the particular time of observation. For instance, subjects can differ in their exposure to information about health or historical events that influence life choices and practices.

Reither et al[16] studied 1.7 million participants in the 1976-2002 National Health Interview Surveys to determine differences in the prevalence of obesity in different birth cohorts. They found that obesity at age 25 increased by 30% for cohorts born between 1955 and 1975. However, independent of birth cohort, the period of observation had a significant influence on the likelihood of obesity at age 25, with a predicted probability of 7% in 1976 to 20% in 2002.

The findings in this obesity study demonstrate both cohort and period effects, suggesting that changes such as societal norms, differences in food practices, and lifestyle choices have had an increasing influence on the rise in obesity.

The use of cross-sectional studies for analytic observational studies was described in Chapter 19.

■ Normative Studies

The utility of evaluative findings in the assessment of a patient's condition is based on the comparison of those findings with known standards. Clinicians need these standards as a basis for documenting the presence and severity of disease or functional limitations and as a guide for setting goals. The purpose of **normative research** is to describe typical or standard values for characteristics of a given population. Normative studies are often directed toward a specific age group, gender, occupation, culture, or disability. Norms are usually expressed as averages within a range of acceptable values.

Physiological Standards

Over time, studies have provided the basis for laboratory test standards that are used to assess normally or abnormally functioning systems. For example, hematocrit or serum blood glucose are used to determine the presence of anemia or diabetes. Physiological measures such as normal nerve conduction velocity (NCV) are used to diagnose or explain weakness or pain associated with neural transmission.

Norms can vary across studies, often based on the characteristics of the sample or the laboratory practices employed. For example, studies have resulted in different values for normal NCV based on how the measurements were taken and the quality of the study.[17-19] There are also correction factors which may need to be applied, such as corrections for limb temperature,[20] age, and height[21] in measures of NCV.

Normal values may be updated periodically, as indicators of disease are reevaluated. For instance, acceptable hemoglobin A1c levels, used to monitor type 2 diabetes, have been lowered and later raised, as new medical information has become available.[22-24] Such changes often result in a documented increase in the incidence of the disease in the population—not because the disease is occurring more often, but because more people are diagnosed.

Standardized Measures of Performance

Norms can also represent standardized scores that allow interpretation of responses with reference to "normed" value. For example, the Wechsler Intelligence Scales scores are normed against a mean of 100 and a standard deviation of 15.[25] Several tests of balance have set standards for fall risk, and norms have been established for developmental milestones. The influence of joint motion on functional impairment is based on values "within normal limits."

The importance of establishing the validity of normative values is obvious. The estimation of "normal" behavior or performance is often used as a basis for prescribing corrective intervention or for predicting future performance. Data collected on different samples or in different settings may result in variations of normal values.

If the interpretation of assessments and the consequent treatment plan are based on the extent of deviation from normal, the standard values must be valid reflections of this norm. Because no characteristics of a population can be adequately described by a single value, normal values are typically established in ranges with reference to concomitant factors.

As an example, several studies have established normative values for grip strength in children based on age and hand dominance.[26-28]

Häger-Ross and Rösblad[29] studied 530 boys and girls aged 4 through 16 and found that there was no difference in grip strength between the genders until age 10, after which the boys were significantly stronger than the girls. Another study established norms for 5- to 15-year-olds based on age, gender, and body composition.[30] Normative data for grip strength in adults[31] and older persons[32] is also distinguished by gender and level of fitness activity.

These data provide a reference for making clinical decisions about the management of hand problems and for setting goals after hand injury or surgery.

There is still a substantial need for normative research in health-related sciences. As new measurement tools are developed, research is needed to establish standards for interpretation of their scores. This is especially true in areas where a variety of instruments are used to measure the same clinical variables, such as balance, pain, function and quality of life assessments. It is also essential that these norms be established for a variety of diagnostic and age groups, so that appropriate standards can be applied in different clinical situations.

> Researchers should be aware of the great potential for sampling bias when striving to establish standard values. Samples for normative studies must be large, random, and representative of the population's heterogeneity. The specific population of interest should be delineated as accurately as possible. Replication is essential to this form of research to demonstrate consistency and thereby validate findings.

Chapter 10 includes further discussion of norm-referenced and criterion-referenced tests.

■ Descriptive Surveys

Descriptive studies attempt to provide an overall picture of a group's characteristics, attitudes, or behaviors, with the purpose of describing characteristics or risk factors for disease or dysfunction. Data for such studies are often collected through the use of surveys (see Chapter 11).

> Jensen and coworkers[33] used a survey to examine the nature and scope of pain in persons with neuromuscular disorders. Their data demonstrated that while pain is a common problem in this population, there are some important differences between diagnostic groups in the nature and scope of pain and its impact.

Descriptive studies are a good source of data for development of hypotheses that can be tested further with analytic research methods.

Large-scale surveys are often used to establish population characteristics that can be used for policy and resource decisions. For example, the Centers for Disease Control and Prevention (CDC) conduct many surveys, like the *National Health Interview Survey* or the *National Ambulatory Medical Care Survey*, to gather data on health habits, function, and healthcare utilization.[34] These types of surveys are also used to document the occurrence or determinants of health conditions and to describe patterns of health, disease, and disability in terms of person, place, and time.

Designs related to descriptive epidemiology will be described in Chapter 34.

■ Case Reports

Clinicians and researchers have long recognized the importance of in-depth descriptions of individual patients for developing a clinical knowledge base, influencing practice and policy. From biblical times to modern day, healthcare providers have described interesting cases, often presenting important scientific observations that may not be obvious in clinical trials.[35] A **case report** is a detailed description of an individual's condition or response to treatment but may also focus on a group, institution or other social unit, such as a school, healthcare setting, or community.

> 📌 The terms *case report* and *case study* have often been used interchangeably, but the terms actually reflect important differences in the nature of inquiry, how data are collected, and how conclusions are drawn.[36-39] Unfortunately, terminology is not used consistently across journals. A case study is considered a qualitative research methodology, investigating broad questions related to individuals or systems (see Chapter 21). Although their contribution to evidence-based practice is well recognized, case reports are generally not considered a true form of research because the methodology is not systematic. Case reports must also be distinguished from single-subject and N-of-1 designs, which involve experimental control in the application of interventions (see Chapter 18).

Purposes of Case Reports

The purpose of a case report is to reflect on practice, including diagnostic methods, patient management, ethical issues, innovative interventions, or the natural history of a condition.[40] A case report can present full coverage of a patient's management or focus on different aspects of the patient's care. For example, case reports have focused on the first procedure for a hand transplant,[41] how the surgery was planned,[42] and how anesthesia was managed.[43]

A case report can be prospective, when plans are made to follow a case as it progresses, or it can be retrospective, reporting on a case after patient care has ended. Prospective studies have the advantage of being able to purposefully design the intervention and data collection procedures, providing a better chance that consistent and complete data will be available.

A *case series* is an expansion of a case report involving observations in several similar cases. As more and more similar cases are reported, a form of "case law" gradually develops, whereby empirical findings are considered reasonable within the realm of accepted knowledge and professional experience. Eventually, with successive documented cases, a conceptual framework forms, providing a basis for categorizing patients and for generating hypotheses that can be tested using exploratory or experimental methods.

Clinical case reports can serve many purposes.

- Case reports often emphasize unusual patient problems and outcomes or diagnoses that present interesting clinical challenges.

> Prognosis following traumatic brain injury (TBI) is considered challenging. Nelson et al[44] presented a case report of a 28-year-old male who experienced severe TBI following a motorcycle accident without wearing a helmet. His initial examination revealed findings that were typically predictive of mortality and debilitating morbidity. Despite these factors, however, after 1 year the patient was living at home, performing simple activities of daily living at a higher level than anticipated. The improvement could not be attributed specifically to any given treatment, but the outcome was an important reminder of the variability among patients that can challenge prognostication for TBI.

- Case reports may focus on innovative approaches to treatment.

> MacLachan et al[45] described the first case of the successful use of "mirror treatment" in a person with a lower limb amputation to treat phantom limb pain. This intervention involves the patient feeling movement in their phantom limb while observing similar movement

in their intact limb. They demonstrated that this approach, which had been successful with upper extremity amputation, was equally effective for reducing lower extremity phantom pain.

- Case reports can present newer approaches to diagnosis, especially with rare conditions, which may provide more efficient, more accurate or safer testing methods.

Posterior epidural migration of lumbar disc fragments (PEMLDF) is extremely rare. It is often confused with other posterior lesions and is usually diagnosed intraoperatively. Takano et al[46] describe the case of a 78-year-old man with acute low back pain, gait disturbance, and paresthesia in both legs. The initial diagnosis suggested malignancy, hematoma, epidural abscess, or migration of lumbar disc fragments. Using preoperative lumbar discography, a provocation technique to identify disc pain, they were able to detect the migration of disc fragments, which was consistent with subsequent surgical findings. They concluded that discography is useful for the definitive diagnosis PEMLDF prior to surgery.

- Treatment and diagnostic decisions frequently require reference to theory in the absence of more direct evidence. Case reports are especially helpful for demonstrating how clinical theories can be applied.

Rosenbaum and coworkers[47] described the case of a man who experienced widespread brain damage in a motorcycle accident 20 years earlier and who was followed because of his unusual memory impairment. The researchers documented how this patient's experiences contributed to several aspects of memory theory, including understanding episodic and semantic memory, and the distinction between implicit and explicit memory.

- Although case reports focus on the details of individual patients, the results can often highlight issues that require further inquiry, providing a rich source of research questions. One major contribution of the case report is its ability to provide information that can be used to generate inductive hypotheses, often leading to the discovery of relationships that were not obvious before. These hypotheses can be tested in other patients or under different conditions.

Reinthal et al[48] examined the effectiveness of a postural control program in an adolescent who had problems walking and talking simultaneously following traumatic brain injury. They hypothesized that her difficulty was due to excessive coactivation of trunk, extremity, and oral musculature. Following 2 years of speech and physical therapy, the patient was able to significantly improve her ability to communicate intelligibly while walking. The results suggested that improved postural control could be tested as a treatment to facilitate less rigid compensation of oral musculature.

Format of a Case Report

📌 This section will provide a general description of the format for case reports. *Instructions for Authors* for specific journals should be consulted to understand terminology used and the required format (see Chapter 38). Several references provide useful tips for writing case reports and reporting guidelines.[35,40,49-53]

A clinical case report is an intensive investigation designed to analyze and understand those factors important to the etiology, care and outcome of the subject's problems. It is a comprehensive description of the subject's background, present status, and responses to intervention.

> ➤ **CASE IN POINT #1**
>
> Changes in technology provide an excellent opportunity to demonstrate resourceful approaches to patient care that can contribute to successful patient outcomes. Fluet et al[54] described the decision making process used to develop a robot-based intervention for upper extremity (UE) training for an 85-year-old man with left hemiparesis secondary to a stroke 5 years earlier. They used simulations to address motor impairments related to movement patterns, speed, range of motion and task-specific parameters to maximize his UE control. They were able to document improvements in several functional and movement measures.

- **Title.** The title of the case report should be concise but sufficiently clear to allow readers to understand the focus of the report.

➤ The title of the robotic-based intervention case report was "*Robots integrated with virtual reality simulations for customized motor training in a person with upper extremity hemiparesis: a case study.*"

This title explicitly describes the intervention and the type of patient who is the focus of the report. Note that the term "case study" was used here but should have more accurately been called a case report.

- **Abstract.** The abstract is a summary of the case, providing a quick way for readers to understand the scope of the paper. Abstracts are short and narrative and therefore will only highlight important information. Authors must follow journal guidelines regarding required subheadings for a case report.

> ➤ The *Journal of Neurologic Physical Therapy,* where the robot study was published, requires an abstract for a case report to include headings of *Background and Purpose, Case Description, Intervention, Outcomes,* and *Discussion.*[55] The abstract is limited to 250 words.

- **Introduction.** A case report begins with an introduction that describes background literature on the patient problem, including theoretical or epidemiologic information needed to understand the scope and context of the disorder. This section will provide a rationale for the study—why this case report provides important information regarding patient care. This may be due to gaps in literature, conflicting reports, or new approaches improve on current practice, or documentation of an unusual condition. The purpose of the report should be described in terms of how this case contributes to the relevant knowledge base. A review of literature is essential for establishing the rationale and interpreting outcomes.

> ➤ The authors described literature supporting the use of virtual environments and repetitive practice for improving motor skills. However, studies using robotic technology to date had used standardized protocols that did not allow specification to a patient's impairments and individual goals.

- **Case Description.** A full description of the case starts with assessments and background information. A patient history and exam findings will delineate problems, symptoms, and prior treatments, as well as demographic and social factors that are pertinent to the subject's care and prognosis. A clinical impression should be included to clarify the patient's chief complaint and goals, providing a rationale for the choice of intervention.

> ➤ The patient was an 85-year-old gentleman with left hemiparesis secondary to a stroke 5 years prior to this examination. The authors described his medical and rehabilitation history and examination findings related to his upper extremity function. The patient lived at home, needing close guarding and supervision for functional activities. They provided a clinical impression to describe why this patient was appropriate for this intervention.

- **Intervention.** This information should be followed by a full description of all elements of the intervention. This will include necessary operational definitions, characteristics of the setting, how data were collected, and how progress was determined Where relevant, literature should be cited to support the rationale for treatment and interpretation of outcomes. The author should reference theoretical considerations and the process of clinical decision making used to develop the treatment and assessment plan.

> ➤ The authors described the details of the procedures used, including timing and duration of sessions over 4 weeks, providing a rationale for their choices. They provided detailed descriptions of the equipment used, strategies incorporated into the intervention, and the patient's responses.

- **Outcomes.** This section includes a full description of measurements, which may include reference to literature on reliability and validity. Given that there are usually many ways to measure clinical variables, the reasons for choosing specific assessments should be given. If special assessments are used, they should be described in functional detail. Some case reports are actually geared to describing the applicability of new or unusual assessment instruments for diagnosing certain problems.

  The patient's progress and level of improvement or decline should be described, often with data presented in tables, charts, or graphs. Literature may provide a basis for determining the minimally important clinical difference (MCID) to allow interpretation of the outcome effect.

> ➤ The authors described a series of outcome measures used to evaluate changes in impairments, functional abilities and participation activities.[56] They included reliability and validity assessments from the literature to support each measure. They provided details on the patient's improvements and challenges in the application of the intervention.

- **Discussion.** The discussion section of the report provides interpretation of outcomes and conclusions, including reference to research, theory, and other clinical information that may support or challenge the current findings. This section should include discussion of unique or special considerations in the patient's condition or responses that may explain unexpected outcomes, or that may distinguish the patient from others with the same condition. Authors should also describe limitations to the study that impact conclusions.

▶ The discussion in the robot study focused on how the patient performed and how those outcomes are supported by previous research and theories on motor learning. They highlighted factors that facilitated the patient's success and those that presented challenges. They described limitations related to nonblinded assessments and lack of follow-up.

- **Summary and Conclusions.** The end of a case report should include a summary of the findings and conclusion about the effectiveness of the intervention that can be derived from the outcomes. It also should present questions for further study, suggesting where the case report's findings may lead.

▶ The authors of the robot study indicated that this case report demonstrated how this type of intervention could be applied successfully with this type of patient. They suggest further study to document how this intervention can be implemented to support rehabilitation within the ICF framework.

 See the *Chapter 20 Supplement* for annotations of the robot study and additional information on writing and appraising case reports, including reporting guidelines, checklists, and links to references.

Ethics of Case Reports

Clinicians must take precautions to protect patient privacy in case reports. This is especially important when unique conditions are described that may compromise the identity of the subject. Patients must always give consent for use of photographs or other identifiable information.

Many journals require substantiation of informed consent and approval by an IRB (see Chapter 7). A statement to this effect is often included at the end of the introduction section. The rules on the use of informed consent and IRB review for clinical reports vary across institutions and journals. Retrospective studies may undergo expedited review if it is clear that all patient information is de-identified and no potentially sensitive information is involved. It is advisable to check with your institution and the journal in which you intend to publish, to be sure you are fulfilling their requirements.

▶ The authors in the robot study stated that the protocol had been approved by their institutions' IRBs, and that they had obtained informed consent from the patient prior to participation.

Generalizability of Case Reports

The case report is probably the most practical approach to clinical inquiry because of its direct applicability to

patient care, but it is also the least rigorous approach because of its inherent lack of control and limited generalizability. The interaction of environmental and personal characteristics and the effect of multiple interventions make the case study weak in internal validity. Therefore, it is important that conclusions do not make cause and effect claims.

Generalization from one case to a larger population is limited because the responses of one individual or social unit may bear little resemblance to those of others in similar circumstances. In addition, case studies are often concerned with exceptional situations or rare disorders, and subjects are generally not representative of the "typical" patient seen in the clinic. Therefore, external validity is also limited.

The validity of inferences from a case study can be enhanced, however, by taking steps to objectify treatment effects and to demonstrate them under different conditions. For instance, interpretations can be made stronger by direct quantified observation and by taking repeated measurements over the course of treatment. Treatment effects can be further supported by using multiple dependent variables and by choosing outcome measures that show large and immediate changes. Single-subject designs may be preferable if this type of conclusion is desired.

Generalization can also be enhanced by documenting the subject's behavior in more than one setting and by including information from follow-up visits to establish the long-range success of treatment. Literature should be used to demonstrate how previous studies support a particular theoretical approach to treatment.

Case Reports in Epidemiology

An *epidemiologic case report* is a description of one or more individuals, documenting a unique or unusual health occurrence or medical condition (see Chapter 34). The purpose of the case report is to present as complete a picture as possible about the characteristics of, and exposures faced by, that individual, often resulting in the presentation of a hypothesis about the causal factors that might account for the observed outcome. Many notable examples of this approach exist, demonstrating the far reaching importance of these initial reports:

- The original report of a patient with unique dementia characteristics by Alzheimer in 1905.[57]
- The single case report in 1961 of a 40-year-old premenopausal woman who developed a pulmonary embolism 5 weeks after starting to use oral contraceptives.[58]
- A series of reports documenting the first cases of AIDS in five young previously healthy homosexual males in Los Angeles.[59]

These prominent cases led to significant public health initiatives and to the formulation of important analytic hypotheses that have since been widely tested and supported.

As is true with clinical case reports, epidemiologic case reports do not provide sufficient control to allow for generalizations or conclusions about causality. They are intended to act as a catalyst for further study. As the preceding examples illustrate, case reports can be vitally important for identifying new public health hazards, facilitating further analytic research, and implementing new health policies

■ Historical Research

The lessons of history are often essential for understanding today's practices and patterns. **Historical research** involves the critical review of events, documents, literature, and other sources of data to reconstruct the past in an effort to understand how and why past events occurred and how that understanding can influence current practice.

This approach has its foundations in the discipline of history, where past world events are examined and analyzed to determine how present conditions evolved and, ultimately, to anticipate or prevent future events. In similar fashion, historical research can build a foundation for interpreting current clinical theory and practice, providing a context within which we can evaluate professional trends. Lusk[60] has presented a primer on historical research methodology that, although written in the context of nursing, provides comprehensive guidelines for all health professionals.

Historical Questions

The process of historical research starts with the determination of a research question that addresses a topic of interest within a particular time period.[61]

> ### ▶ CASE IN POINT #2
>
> Researchers and practitioners have long argued the merits and pitfalls of siderail use as safeguards against patient falls from hospital beds. Brush and Capezuti[62] were interested in the evolution of this practice and how it became embedded in hospital culture despite evidence that it did not provide the intended level of safety.

These types of questions can only be answered retrospectively within the historical perspective of events that precipitated change. Realistically, historical studies begin with general questions, as the scope of the topic may not be realized until after most of the relevant materials are identified.

> ▶ The authors considered historic changes in the use of siderails in American hospitals through the 20th century. They examined social, economic and legal influences, and explored how values and attitudes regarding siderails have shifted over time.

Historical research is not merely a collection of facts or dates, and it should be distinguished from a critical review of literature. The historical inquiry is meant to incorporate judgments, analyses, and inferences in the search for relationships by organizing and synthesizing data from the past, not just summarizing them.[60]

Sources of Historical Data

Historians use a variety of sources to accumulate data. The researcher must be critical in the acceptance of all that is read, recognizing that those who wrote in the past may have been selective in their presentation of facts or creative in their representation of the truth. For this reason especially, the historical researcher should distinguish between firsthand and secondhand sources of information.

For the historian, *primary sources* include original documents, such as letters, videotapes, photographs, or minutes of a meeting, eyewitness accounts, and direct recordings of events. *Secondary sources* may include biographies, textbooks, encyclopedias, literature reviews, newspaper accounts, and any summary of primary materials. As with all research, the historian should use primary sources whenever possible.

> ▶ Primary sources used in the bedrail study included medical equipment catalogs, hospital procedure manuals, newsletters, photographs, journal articles, government documents, and published histories of hospital bed design. Secondary sources included nursing textbooks.

Reliability and Validity of Historical Data

Historical data must also be evaluated for reliability and validity. Because historical information is subject to contamination, researchers will find that not all sources are of equal value.[63] The historian must be able to establish the authenticity of data by subjecting the material to *external criticism*. This may involve determination that papers were indeed written by the ascribed author (not ghost-written) or that documents have not been altered.

The data must also be subjected to *internal criticism*, which questions the truth or worth of the material's content within the context of the research question. Although it is not a scientifically rigorous procedure, to some extent internal validity of information can be examined on the basis of corroboration from other sources or by finding no substantial contrary evidence.[63] It is also important to understand the relevant definitions and concepts used during the historical period and to recognize that standards and terminology change over time.

> ➤ Documents in the siderail study were obtained from archival collections in medicine and nursing, and government guidelines published by the Food and Drug Administration and the US Department of Health and Human Services.

Synthesis of Historical Data

After the validity of historical data is established, the data must be synthesized and analyzed within an objective frame of reference. The researcher must be careful not to make assumptions about the past merely because no information can be found. The historian attempts to incorporate a scientific logic into this process, so that interpretations are made as objectively as possible.

> ➤ Through their historic research, Brush and Capezuti[62] documented how siderails became prominently used, despite incidents of injury and death attributed to patients climbing over

them. The practice continued because of legal actions, linking it to hospital policy. Newer ideas regarding the importance of mobility and the federal redefinition of siderails as restraints began to change attitudes and practice.

Because sources, measurements, and organization of data are not controlled, cause-and-effect statements cannot be made in historical research. One can only synthesize what is already known into systematized accounts of the past and discuss potential relationships between variables based on sequencing of events and associated underlying characteristics of variables.

> ➤ The authors argued that the use of bedrails was based on a gradual consensus between law and medicine, rather than empirical evidence. They concluded that changes in this practice would have to be driven by data and that alternative strategies would only become accepted once administrators, regulators, attorneys, patients, and clinicians understood why bedrails became common practice in the first place. This historical perspective is an important consideration as policy on the use of bedrails continues to be revisited.[64]

COMMENTARY

To do successful research, you don't need to know everything, you just need to know of one thing that isn't known.

—*Arthur Schawlow (1921-1999)*

American physicist

Descriptive research is often a first step to understanding what *exists*, often the "first scientific toe in the water" in new areas of inquiry.[65] Without this fundamental knowledge, it would be impossible to ask questions about behaviors or treatment effects or to propose theories to explain them. This approach is clearly contrasted with explanatory or observational research studies that seek to determine what *will* happen in a given set of circumstances. Clinical scientists must first discover how the world around them naturally behaves before they can manipulate and control those behaviors to test methods of changing them.

Even though descriptive studies do not involve manipulation of variables, they still require rigor in defining and measuring variables of interest, whether they emerge as narrative descriptions or quantitative summaries. Descriptive findings can be meaningful as a basis for explanation when they are the result of a well-designed

study and when they are interpreted within the context of an appropriate research question. The results of descriptive studies may provide essential evidence for understanding the benefits of clinical trials and for describing or explaining why some subjects respond differently than others.

Descriptive studies such as case reports are often the first foray into publishing for clinicians, who are best suited to provide a comprehensive account of patient management. These studies have direct impact on practice as first line reports of clinical decision making—an important form of communication within the clinical community.

With many behavioral and clinical concepts not yet fully understood, descriptive research presents a critical opportunity for the clinical researcher and a vital source of evidence for clinicians who seek to understand patient circumstances and characteristics.

REFERENCES

1. Gesell A, Amatruda CS. *The Embryology of Behavior*. New York: Harper & Brothers 1945.

2. McGraw MB. *The Neuromuscular Maturation of the Human Infant*. New York: Hafner 1963.

3. Erikson EH. *Childhood and Society*. 2nd ed. New York: Norton; 1963.

4. Tanner JM. Physical growth. In: Mussen PH, ed. *Carmichael's Manual of Child Psychology*. 3rd ed. New York: Wiley; 1970.

5. Honzik MP, MacFarland JW, Allen L. The stability of mental test performance between two and eighteen years. *J Exp Educ* 1949;17:309.

6. Horn JL, Donaldson G. Cognitive development: II. Adulthood development of human abilities. In: Brim OG, Kagan J, eds. *Constancy and Change in Human Development*. Cambridge, MA: Harvard University Press; 1980.

7. Freier MC, Babikian T, Pivonka J, Burley Aaen T, Gardner JM, Baum M, Bailey LL, Chinnock RE. A longitudinal perspective on neurodevelopmental outcome after infant cardiac transplantation. *J Heart Lung Transplant* 2004;23(7):857-864.

8. Munsat TL, Andres PL, Finison L, Conlon T, Thibodeau L. The natural history of motoneuron loss in amyotrophic lateral sclerosis. *Neurology* 1988;38(3):409-413.

9. Munsat TL, Taft J, Jackson IM, Andres PL, Hollander D, Skerry L, Ordman M, Kasdon D, Finison L. Intrathecal thyrotropin-releasing hormone does not alter the progressive course of ALS: experience with an intrathecal drug delivery system. *Neurology* 1992;42(5):1049-1053.

10. Miller RG, Bouchard JP, Duquette P, Eisen A, Gelinas D, Harati Y, Munsat TL, Powe L, Rothstein J, Salzman P, et al. Clinical trials of riluzole in patients with ALS. ALS/Riluzole Study Group-II. *Neurology* 1996;47(4 Suppl 2):S86-90; discussion S90-82.

11. Riviere M, Meininger V, Zeisser P, Munsat T. An analysis of extended survival in patients with amyotrophic lateral sclerosis treated with riluzole. *Arch Neurol* 1998;55(4):526-528.

12. DeLoach A, Cozart M, Kiaei A, Kiaei M. A retrospective review of the progress in amyotrophic lateral sclerosis drug discovery over the last decade and a look at the latest strategies. *Expert Opin Drug Discov* 2015;10(10):1099-1118.

13. Unruh KP, Kuhn JE, Sanders R, An Q, Baumgarten KM, Bishop JY, Brophy RH, Carey JL, Holloway BG, Jones GL, et al. The duration of symptoms does not correlate with rotator cuff tear severity or other patient-related features: a cross-sectional study of patients with atraumatic, full-thickness rotator cuff tears. *J Shoulder Elbow Surg* 2014;23(7):1052-1058.

14. Landa RJ, Gross AL, Stuart EA, Faherty A. Developmental trajectories in children with and without autism spectrum disorders: the first 3 years. *Child Dev* 2013;84(2):429-442.

15. Kraemer HC, Yesavage JA, Taylor JL, Kupfer D. How can we learn about developmental processes from cross-sectional studies, or can we? *Am J Psychiatry* 2000;157(2):163-171.

16. Reither EN, Hauser RM, Yang Y. Do birth cohorts matter? Age-period-cohort analyses of the obesity epidemic in the United States. *Soc Sci Med* 2009;69(10):1439-1448.

17. Ehler E, Ridzoň P, Urban P, Mazanec R, Nakládalová M, Procházka B, Matulová H, Latta J, Otruba P. Ulnar nerve at the elbow – normative nerve conduction study. *J Brachial Plex Peripher Nerve Inj* 2013;8:2-2.

18. Haghighat S, Mahmoodian AE, Kianimehr L. Normative ulnar nerve conduction study: comparison of two measurement methods. *Adv Biomed Res* 2018;7:47.

19. Chen S, Andary M, Buschbacher R, Del Toro D, Smith B, So Y, Zimmermann K, Dillingham TR. Electrodiagnostic reference values for upper and lower limb nerve conduction studies in adult populations. *Muscle Nerve* 2016;54(3):371-377.

20. Nelson R, Agro J, Lugo J, Gasiewska E, Kaur H, Muniz E, Nelson A, Rothman J. The relationship between temperature and neuronal characteristics. *Electromyogr Clin Neurophysiol* 2004;44(4):209-216.

21. Rivner MH, Swift TR, Malik K. Influence of age and height on nerve conduction. *Muscle Nerve* 2001;24(9):1134-1141.

22. Mayfield J. Diagnosis and classification of diabetes mellitus: new criteria. *Am Fam Physician* 1998;58(6):1355-1362, 1369-1370.

23. Sandoiu A. Type 2 diabetes: new guidelines lower blood sugar control level. Medical News Today, March 6, 2018. Available at https://www.medicalnewstoday.com/articles/321123.php. Accessed November 9, 2018.

24. Qaseem A, Wilt TJ, Kansagara D, Horwitch C, Barry MJ, Forciea MA. Hemoglobin A1c targets for glycemic control with pharmacologic therapy for nonpregnant adults with type 2 diabetes mellitus: a guidance statement update from the American College of Physicians. *Ann Intern Med* 2018;168(8):569-576.

25. Maddox T. *Tests: A Comprehensive Reference for Assessment in Psychology, Education and Business*. 5th ed. Austin, TX: Pro-Ed; 2001.

26. Lee-Valkov PM, Aaron DH, Eladoumikdachi F, Thornby J, Netscher DT. Measuring normal hand dexterity values in normal 3-, 4-, and 5-year-old children and their relationship with grip and pinch strength. *J Hand Ther* 2003;16(1):22-28.

27. Beasley BW, Woolley DC. Evidence-based medicine knowledge, attitudes, and skills of community faculty. *J Gen Intern Med* 2002;17:632-639.

28. Surrey LR, Hodson J, Robinson E, Schmidt S, Schulhof J, Stoll L, Wilson-Diekhoff N. Pinch strength norms for 5-to 12-year-olds. *Phys Occup Ther Pediatr* 2001;21(1):37-49.

29. Häger-Ross C, Rosblad B. Norms for grip strength in children aged 4-16 years. *Acta Paediatr* 2002;91(6):617-625.

30. Sartorio A, Lafortuna CL, Pogliaghi S, Trecate L. The impact of gender, body dimension and body composition on hand-grip strength in healthy children. *J Endocrinol Invest* 2002;25(5):431-435.

31. Hanten WP, Chen WY, Austin AA, Brooks RE, Carter HC, Law CA, Morgan MK, Sanders DJ, Swan CA, Vanderslice AL. Maximum grip strength in normal subjects from 20 to 64 years of age. *J Hand Ther* 1999;12(3):193-200.

32. Horowitz BP, Tollin R, Cassidy G. Grip strength: collection of normative data with community dwelling elders. *Phys Occup Ther Geriatr* 1997;15(1):53-64.

33. Jensen MP, Abresch RT, Carter GT, McDonald CM. Chronic pain in persons with neuromuscular disease. *Arch Phys Med Rehabil* 2005;86(6):1155-1163.

34. Centers for Disease Control and Prevention (CDC). Data & Statistics. Available at https://www.cdc.gov/DataStatistics/. Accessed November 10, 2018.

35. Cohen H. How to write a patient case report. *Am J Health Syst Pharm* 2006;63(19):1888-1892.

36. Jansen CWS. Case reports and case studies: A discussion of theory and methodolgy in pocket format. *J Hand Ther* 1999; 12(3):230-232.

37. Porcino A. Not birds of a feather: case reports, case studies, and single-subject research. *Int J Ther Massage Bodywork* 2016;9(3):1-2.

38. Ridder H. The theory contribution of case study research designs. *Business Res* 2017;10(2):281-305.

39. Salminen AL, Harra T, Lautamo T. Conducting case study research in occupational therapy. *Austr Occup Ther J* 2006; 53(1):3-8.

40. McEwen I. *Writing Case Reports: A How-To Manual for Clinicians*. 3 ed. Alexandria, VA: American Physical Therapy Association; 2009.

41. Amaral S, Kessler SK, Levy TJ, Gaetz W, McAndrew C, Chang B, Lopez S, Braham E, Humpl D, Hsia M, et al. 18-month outcomes of heterologous bilateral hand transplantation in a child: a case report. *Lancet Child Adolesc Health* 2017;1(1):35-44.

42. Galvez JA, Gralewski K, McAndrew C, Rehman MA, Chang B, Levin LS. Assessment and planning for a pediatric bilateral hand transplant using 3-dimensional modeling: Case report. *J Hand Surg Am* 2016;41(3):341-343.

43. Gurnaney HG, Fiadjoe JE, Levin LS, Chang B, Delvalle H, Galvez J, Rehman MA. Anesthetic management of the first pediatric bilateral hand transplant. *Can J Anaesth* 2016;63(6): 731-736.

44. Nelson CG, Elta T, Bannister J, Dzandu J, Mangram A, Zach V. Severe traumatic brain injury: a case report. *Am J Case Rep* 2016;17:186-191.

45. MacLachlan M, McDonald D, Waloch J. Mirror treatment of lower limb phantom pain: a case study. *Disabil Rehabil* 2004;26(14-15):901-904.

46. Takano M, Hikata T, Nishimura S, Kamata M. Discography aids definitive diagnosis of posterior epidural migration of lumbar disc fragments: case report and literature review. *BMC Musculoskelet Disord* 2017;18(1):151.

47. Rosenbaum RS, Kohler S, Schacter DL, Moscovitch M, Westmacott R, Black SE, Gao F, Tulving E. The case of K.C.: contributions of a memory-impaired person to memory theory. *Neuropsychologia* 2005;43(7):989-1021.

48. Reinthal AK, Mansour LM, Greenwald G. Improved ambulation and speech production in an adolescent post-traumatic brain injury through a therapeutic intervention to increase postural control. *Pediatr Rehabil* 2004;7(1):37-49.

49. Riley DS, Barber MS, Kienle GS, Aronson JK, von Schoen-Angerer T, Tugwell P, Kiene H, Helfand M, Altman DG, Sox H, et al. CARE guidelines for case reports: explanation and elaboration document. *J Clin Epidemiol* 2017;89:218-235.

50. Rison RA. A guide to writing case reports for the Journal of Medical Case Reports and BioMed Central Research Notes. *J Med Case Rep* 2013;7:239-239.

51. Sun Z. Tips for writing a case report for the novice author. *J Med Radiat Sci* 2013;60(3):108-113.

52. Green BN, Johnson CD. How to write a case report for publication. *J Chiropr Med* 2006;5(2):72-82.

53. Gagnier JJ, Kienle G, Altman DF, Moher D, Sox H, Riley D. The CARE guidelines: consensus-based clinical case reporting guideline development. *J Med Case Rep* 2013;7:223.

54. Fluet GG, Merians AS, Qiu Q, Lafond I, Saleh S, Ruano V, Delmonico AR, Adamovich SV. Robots integrated with virtual reality simulations for customized motor training in a person with upper extremity hemiparesis: a case study. *J Neurol Phys Ther* 2012;36(2):79-86.

55. Journal of Neurologic Physical Therapy. Instructions for Authors. Available at https://journals.lww.com/jnpt/Pages/InstructionsforAuthors.aspx. Accessed November 24, 2018.

56. World Health Organization. *International Classification of Functioning, Disability and Health*. Geneva: World Health Organization; 2001.

57. Alzheimer A, Stelzmann RA, Schnitzlein HN, Murtagh FR. An English translation of Alzheimer's 1907 paper, "Über eine eigenartige Erkankung der Hirnrinde." *Clin Anat* 1995;8(6): 429-431.

58. Jordan WM. Pulmonary embolism. *Lancet* 1961;2:1146.

59. Centers for Disease Control. Pneumocystis pneumonia—Los Angeles. *MMWR* 1981;30:250.

60. Lusk B. Historical methodology for nursing research. *Image J Nurs Sch* 1997;29(4):355-359.

61. Rees C, Howells G. Historical research: process, problems and pitfalls. *Nurs Stand* 1999;13(27):33-35.

62. Brush BL, Capezuti E. Historical analysis of siderail use in American hospitals. *J Nurs Scholarsh* 2001;33(4):381-385.

63. Christy TE. The methodology of historical research: a brief introduction. *Nurs Res* 1975;24(3):189-192.

64. O'Keeffe ST. Bedrails rise again? *Age Ageing* 2013;42(4): 426-427.

65. Grimes DA, Schulz KF. Descriptive studies: what they can and cannot do. *Lancet* 2002;359(9301):145-149.

Qualitative Research

—with Heather Fritz and Cathy Lysack

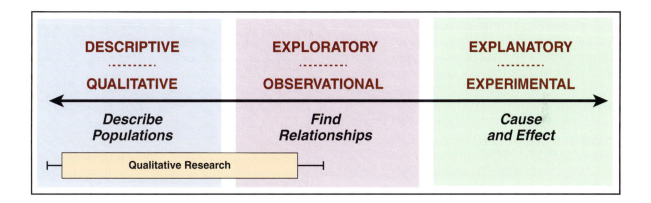

The types of research discussed thus far have included explanatory, exploratory and descriptive approaches, with one commonality—they have all been based on quantitative methods, using empirical data to answer questions about cause and effect or establishing linkages among variables based on statistical applications. An important limitation of the quantitative paradigm, however, is its inability to capture human experience in more nuanced contextual ways, including understanding the experience of patients, families, and healthcare providers who encounter illness and disability in clinical practice and daily life.

Qualitative research is based on the belief that all interactions are inherently social phenomena. It is used to provide evidence when the goal is to identify, describe, and ultimately understand human or organizational behaviors, attitudes, and experiences, and how they influence health. The purpose of this chapter is to provide an overview of qualitative research methods that will provide sufficient background to appreciate published qualitative studies.

Because the true complexity of qualitative research is beyond the scope of this text, readers who want to pursue qualitative study are encouraged to seek out expert consultants and to refer to many excellent references that provide more in-depth coverage of qualitative methods.[1-8]

■ Human Experience and Evidence

Concepts of research typically involve quantitative assumptions within which human experience is assumed to be limited to logical and predictable relationships. Linked to the philosophy of *logical positivism*, this approach to inquiry is deductive and hypothesis-based, requiring that the researcher operationally define the variables of interest in advance.

However, when we think about all the reasons that an intervention does or does not work, or why some patients adhere to therapeutic regimens while others do not, we realize that "counting" responses for groups is unlikely to bring us the full understanding that is needed to appreciate how personal differences impact outcomes. And while healthcare providers try to give patients the best care possible, they may be missing essential underlying elements that can influence outcomes.

In contrast, qualitative research favors a gestalt way of seeing the world that strives to represent social reality as it is found naturally. It goes beyond learning about individual beliefs and behaviors to more deeply discover and describe socioculturally constructed worldviews, values, and norms and how these are instilled, enacted, reinforced, or resisted and changed in everyday life. To obtain these insights, qualitative researchers must conduct inquiry in the natural settings where people interact and then find ways to systematically capture, mostly in narrative form, qualities that are often complex and difficult to measure. Where quantitative research is based on numbers and statistics, qualitative data are text-based, involving open-ended discussions and observation.

Whereas quantitative researchers try to control the influence of "extraneous variables" through standardized design and measurement, qualitative researchers work to capture as fully as possible the diverse experiences and events they study, so that the data gathered will be the truest possible representation of the real world, with all of its "messiness." The "insider view" of the individuals' world is particularly important for understanding the factors that are relevant to clinical assessment, care, and decision-making.

Qualitative research is generally considered an inductive process, with conclusions being drawn directly from the data. The value of qualitative methods lies in their ability to contribute insights and address questions that are not easily answerable by experimental methods.[9] In its broadest sense, qualitative research must be understood as the systematic study of social phenomena, serving three important purposes:[10]

- Describing groups of people or social phenomena
- Generating hypotheses that can be tested by further research
- Developing theory to explain observed phenomena

Complementary Traditions

As part of a broad understanding of research, it is useful to consider how quantitative and qualitative approaches are distinguished, as well as how they can serve complementary functions.[11] For example, qualitative research can be used as a preliminary phase in quantitative investigation, especially when there is a lack of prior research or theory. Understanding values and behaviors can help to identify relevant variables that can lead to generation of hypotheses, development and validation of instruments, setting a framework for evaluation, and developing research questions.[12]

Qualitative methods can also be used when a topic has been studied extensively with quantitative approaches, but the phenomenon is still not well understood and findings are contradictory. Qualitative research may be critical to "going deeper" to ask additional questions and may also help to explain unexpected findings of a randomized trial (see Focus on Evidence 21-1).

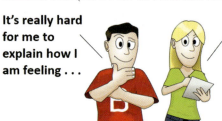

Courtesy of Publicdomainvectors.org.

Contributing to Evidence-Based Practice

Qualitative research addresses essential components of evidence-based practice. As described in Chapter 5, EBP requires attention to several sources of information, including patient preferences and providers' clinical judgments. These components require an understanding of how patients and care providers view their interactions with each other, family members, and colleagues within their social environments, and how those interactions influence care and health (see Fig. 21-1).

Qualitative designs are uniquely suited to clarify our understanding of patients' perspectives about treatment. There is increasing attention to the patient and family's perspectives today, as health systems recognize that outcomes are ultimately more positive if the patient's needs and preferences are considered throughout treatment planning and delivery.[19-20] A better understanding of patients' preferences can also give practitioners the opportunity to understand the concepts of health, illness, and disability from the direct perspective of the person who lives it.

Qualitative study can also contribute to understanding how providers' expertise, implicit behaviors, or professional cultures influence treatment encounters. For example, Jensen et al[21] developed a theoretical model related to what constitutes expert practice in physical therapy. They identified four dimensions of virtue, knowledge, movement, and clinical reasoning that become increasingly

Focus on Evidence 21–1
You Won't Find What You Aren't Looking For!

In 2015, Pakkarinen et al[13] reported on a randomized controlled trial of 201 patients comparing long-term weight loss with and without a maintenance program. The intervention consisted of a defined low-calorie diet for 17 weeks for both groups, and then the treatment group began a 1-year maintenance regimen, including behavioral modification and regular meetings of support groups. Follow up after 2 years showed no significant difference between the two groups, which the authors attributed to subject attrition, poor compliance with the weight-loss program, and a lack of sensitivity in their measuring tools.

Unfortunately, the authors neglected to consult evidence from qualitative research studies and thus did not consider several other factors known to influence weight-loss behavior, including self-efficacy. The authors also disregarded evidence from qualitative studies that showed how social and emotional factors enable or inhibit maintenance of weight loss. If they had considered these data, they may have reframed the intervention and gotten different results. For example, Cioffi[14] found that needing to come to classes and involvement with a group were inhibiting factors in weight-loss maintenance efforts. Other qualitative studies have shown that poor coping skills, inconsistent routines, unrealistic long-term goals, and social pressures all present challenges to weight-loss maintenance,[15-18] while social support, readiness to change, effective coping skills, and self-monitoring contribute to success.

After 2 years of involvement with 201 patients, as well as scores of personnel involved in delivering the long-term maintenance program, it is noteworthy that individual perceptions about weight loss went unnoticed. Qualitative studies that focus on personal rationales and intentions, as in this field, often hold the key to understanding complex health behavior, what factors may influence it, and how it can be studied.

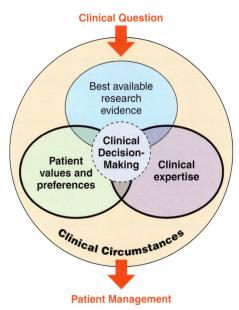

Figure 21–1 The model of evidence-based practice, emphasizing the role of patient preferences and clinical judgment, areas that are particularly relevant to qualitative study.

integrated as competence and expertise grow, moving from novice to expert through a well-developed philosophy of practice.

Informing Translational Research

Translational research has become important in the move to improve EBP, by considering the range of influences on clinical decision-making of healthcare professionals. A focus on knowledge translation and implementation research highlights the need for providers to apply evidence that is available (see Chapter 2). For example, clinicians may find it difficult to understand why a "proven" treatment program is not widely adopted by patients, even after RCTs have demonstrated positive outcomes. This challenge is heightened by the complexity of human behavior. New therapies may not be adopted because of treatment characteristics, the context where the intervention will be delivered, or even the attitudes and behaviors of providers themselves (see Focus on Evidence 21-2).[22]

■ The Research Question: Beyond "What" to "Why"

The first step in the research process is determining the study's aims and providing a rationale to justify the research question (see Chapter 3). Questions that lend themselves to qualitative inquiry often begin with curiosity about a particular topic, condition, or circumstance. A literature review is usually needed to understand the nature of knowledge on the topic, and to provide sufficient background to justify its importance through results of previous studies (see Box 21-1).

Qualitative research questions typically start out broad, seeking to understand how the dynamics of an experience or interaction influence subsequent behaviors or decisions, including why something happens, or does not.[23] This can be an iterative process, however, and additional questions can be added as data are collected. Irrespective of its particular disciplinary roots, qualitative studies focus on questions that are rarely specifiable as conventional hypotheses.

Focus on Evidence 21–2
Understanding the Provider-Patient Encounter

African Americans who have cancer tend to experience worse health and quality of life outcomes when compared to their Caucasian counterparts with similar disease burden.[24] Many factors can contribute to these disparities, including socioeconomic hardship, lack of health insurance, and environmental and behavioral risk factors. There are also disparities in how research supports care of different groups. For example, African Americans are often underrepresented in clinical trials that support state-of-the-art cancer treatment.[25]

Because oncologists play a central role in guiding patients with cancer through complex treatment decisions, it is important to consider the impact of provider behaviors in the clinical encounter. Qualitative studies using real-time video of provider-patient clinical interactions have provided important insights into how oncologists interact differently with Caucasians versus African Americans,

potentially contributing to differences in treatment, which then result in disparities in outcomes.

One such study showed that oncologists spent less time with and made fewer mentions of available clinical trials to their African American patients than to Caucasian patients.[25] Another study examined whether race or ethnicity was associated with the degree to which patients asked questions or raised treatment concerns when interacting with their oncologist.[26] That study found that African American patients asked fewer questions and stated fewer direct concerns. Consideration of these findings can contribute to providers becoming more aware of their own biases and the potential for race/ethnicity-based differences in patient communication styles. Through this understanding, providers can be more vigilant and work to improve knowledge-sharing during clinical encounters. It may also trigger development of educational programs to help patients understand the importance of their own participation in treatment decisions.

Box 21-1   Reviewing the Literature—or Not

One of the unique features of qualitative research is that the researcher will attempt to begin the study with as few preconceived hypotheses as possible. In some traditions, such as grounded theory, "purists" may prefer not to conduct a literature review at all, for fear that the existing literature could *a priori* shape their expectations about what the study will find.[27]

Most qualitative researchers will conduct a basic literature review, but it is rarely as exhaustive as in a quantitative study. If researchers prematurely limit themselves by paying too much attention to past research findings, they are not being true to

the intent of qualitative research which recognizes that data are generated and "meanings are made" as the phenomenon is happening in real time, and in the telling of that experience to others. Researchers must strike a balance between being aware of the problem and how it is discussed broadly in the scientific literature (and, of course, to make sure that someone else has not already conducted the study that they have in mind), and not prematurely narrowing the scope of their investigation. For those reasons, the best qualitative questions are often broad, to allow the researcher to query multiple dimensions of the phenomenon of interest.

Research questions for qualitative studies may be phrased as questions, or they may be stated as goals, aims, or the purpose of the study. They will often be embedded within a description of the rationale for the study related to previous research.

Depending on the nature of the question, different research methods will be applied. Qualitative research should be considered when the goals are to investigate complex phenomena that are not readily measured to generate data to understand a problem within a social context. This can involve individual relationships or organizational systems. Qualitative studies are also useful in the development of quantitative measurement scales and to provide insight into potential explanatory mechanisms.

Investigating Complex Phenomena

Sociocultural Influences

Qualitative approaches can add to the understanding of problems when quantitative data alone cannot provide the fine-grain detail needed to fully understand the situation. For example, Kayser-Jones and colleagues[28] studied dehydration and malnutrition in nursing homes:

> *There has been little research on the prevalence of borderline or overt dehydration. To our knowledge, there have been no qualitative studies that uncover, describe, and analyze the multiple but preventable factors that contribute to dehydration in nursing homes. The purpose of this 5-year anthropological study was to investigate the social, cultural, institutional, and clinical factors that influence eating behavior in nursing homes.*

These researchers observed what family caregivers and staff did to assist and support the older residents during meal times and took detailed notes about behaviors and gestures to encourage eating and drinking. In addition to the objective data of what residents ate and drank, data revealed widespread differences in patient health over that timeframe that could be directly linked to a systematic lack of time to provide support to eat. Detailed observations showed that many residents could eat and drink if someone were there to encourage and assist them.

Organizational Processes

Qualitative research is also well-suited to investigate complex activities and systems including organizational processes and cultures that are otherwise difficult to assess. In a study of operational failures in hospitals, Tucker and coworkers[29] stated this purpose:

> *Prior studies have found that explicit efforts to map the flow of materials in hospitals can identify opportunities for improvement. We build on these studies by explicitly examining underlying causes of operational failures in hospitals' internal supply chains. We looked at operational failures related to hospital room turnover, or the rate of getting a recently vacated hospital room ready for the next patient.*

Through observation and interviews on the hospital units, the authors were able to identify themes related to specific routines, knowledge, and collaboration mechanisms that could improve material flow and efficiencies across departments.

Exploring Special Populations

Qualitative studies can also provide insights into why individuals participate in research and why they do or do not adhere to protocols, contributing to more effective design of clinical trials.[30] Henshall et al[31] studied adults with recently diagnosed type 1 diabetes (T1D), to explore motivators and deterrents toward participating in clinical trials.

> *Barriers to participation in clinical trials are well documented, although no studies have looked at barriers to recruitment in people with T1D. We sought to determine the overall experiences of newly diagnosed adults with T1D in an exercise study, to understand issues that influence the retention of trial participants in such studies.*

They identified several themes that presented barriers, including too much study paperwork, long questionnaires, lack of feedback during a trial, and practical hurdles such as work pressures, travel time to appointments, and not liking blood tests. This information can be used to develop strategies to alleviate such barriers.

Developing Valid Measurements

Many measurement tools have been developed to quantify constructs such as quality of life, function, or pain (see Chapter 12). Qualitative information can provide essential insight into validity as such scales are developed (see Focus on Evidence 21-3).

Focus on Evidence 21–3
Fulfilling a PROMIS

No, it isn't misspelled. The *Patient Reported Outcomes Measurement Information System (PROMIS)* is the result of an NIH-funded 5-year cooperative group program of research designed to develop, validate, and standardize item banks to measure patient-reported outcomes (PROs) across common medical conditions (see Chapter 2). This was a completely new effort to standardize patient outcomes data so comparisons could be made more easily and the data could be exploited more cost-effectively.[33] The PROMIS Pediatric Working Group created self-report item banks for ages 8 to 17 years across five general health domains: emotional health, pain, fatigue, physical function, and social health, consistent with the larger PROMIS network.[33] Qualitative data were an important aspect of this initiative, to understand the issues that are faced by patients to inform what questions to ask and how they should be worded.[34]

As an example, one study specifically looked at items relevant to children with asthma.[35] Using focus groups with semi-structured interviews, the researchers spoke with 41 children aged 8 to 17 years old, 20 with asthma, to determine the unique difficulties and challenges of this population. They identified five themes relevant for the children with asthma: 1) They experienced more difficulty in physical activities; 2) They could experience anxiety about their asthma at any time; 3) They experienced sleep disturbances and fatigue; 4) Their asthma affected their emotional well-being; and 5) They often had insufficient energy to complete school activities.

These findings were then used to modify the questions being asked of this age group. For example, although questions did address sources of anxiety, there was no item on "fear of dying," which was a concern commonly expressed by the children with asthma. This item was added to capture the concerns that some children with asthma or other chronic diseases might have.

Based on these qualitative data, the item bank was expanded to include items that address broader issues faced by children with chronic disorders. Without this approach, it would not have been possible to create questions that truly reflect relevant outcomes.

Gaining Explanatory Insights

Qualitative research is also essential when the goal is to understand why a given intervention has a specific impact or why adverse outcomes occur.

The concept of causation is not directly applicable to qualitative research. However, qualitative findings can offer interpretations about possible explanatory factors since data are derived from social meanings using narrative data. Jackson and colleagues[32] studied factors that influenced the development of pressure ulcers in patients with spinal cord injury (SCI):

> *Previous research has documented numerous medical, demographic, and lifestyle variables that predict pressure ulcers within the population with SCI. However, a recent review suggests that additional evidence is needed to more adequately document the degree of ulcer-risk associated with psychological and behavioral factors that are relevant to primary and secondary intervention efforts. The aim of this article is to identify overarching principles that explain how daily lifestyle considerations affect pressure ulcer development as perceived by adults with SCI.*

The results of this study showed that far from forgetting what they had been taught, most patients worked diligently to adhere to their pressure relief protocols, despite obstacles. Data revealed, for example, instances where wheelchair equipment broke down or transportation services never arrived, challenging individuals' ability to take optimal care of their skin. The study reminded the therapists that "real life" poses major challenges to pressure ulcer prevention, and teaching patients to shift weight and use a properly inflated wheelchair cushion is not sufficient.

■ Perspectives in Qualitative Research

Once a research question or goal is identified, it is important to determine how it will be addressed. Qualitative researchers use several different methods to study health-related topics. The most common are ethnography, grounded theory, phenomenology, and case studies.[23,36] These approaches are often called *naturalistic inquiry* because they require substantial observation and interaction with research participants in their natural environments.

Although ethnography, grounded theory, phenomenology, and case studies are the most common qualitative research approaches, others include photovoice, participatory action research, and focus groups. Interested readers are encouraged to learn more about the kinds of research questions best suited to these approaches.[2,37,38]

Ethnography

Ethnography is a qualitative approach with a long history in anthropology. It is defined in large part by fieldwork where the investigators immerse themselves in the settings and activities studied. In classic anthropological research this means learning the local language and customs so that the activities, ways of life, and cultural beliefs of the group can be well described. In ethnographic research, study participants are often called "*informants*" (and not "subjects" as in the quantitative tradition) because they inform and teach the researcher about their lives and communities.

> ➤ **CASE IN POINT #1**
>
> Many adult day-care centers provide specialized services for older people with Alzheimer's disease. Hasselkus[39] studied the experience of being a staff person in such a setting, focusing on the structure of the day's activities, interactions between staff and clients, and the meanings of those activities. The day-care program's goal was to maximize the strengths of clients, to facilitate opportunities for their self-expression, and to affirm self-worth in a structured, safe, and caring environment.

This study illustrates how ethnography is distinguished from other forms of qualitative research in its exploration of naturally occurring viewpoints and cultural patterns of a particular group. These patterns may include habitual customs, systems of moral values, social structures, and symbolic meanings.

The Researcher and Participant

All forms of qualitative research must be attentive to the relationship between the researcher and the research participant, but in ethnographic research, strong ties of trust between the researcher and participants are essential. Without such bonds, study participants are unlikely to share details of the experiences of interest. This is especially true when the research topic is particularly sensitive or intimate, and putting the participant at ease is of utmost importance to obtain high quality data.

> ➤ **Case #1:** In the day-care study, the participants were the staff members, which included a nurse, a nurse's aide, a social worker, a certified occupational therapy (OT) assistant, and a program coordinator

Gaining access to the desired research setting and desired people may not be easy. Ethnographic researchers must learn how to identify and solidify relationships with gatekeepers and decision-makers with the authority to "open doors" and smooth the way.

Grounded Theory

A second common qualitative research approach is called **grounded theory**. As its name implies, theory derived from the study is "grounded" in the data. What distinguishes the grounded theory method from other qualitative approaches is the formalized process for simultaneous data collection and theory development. This method calls for a continuous interplay between data collection and interpretation leading to generalizations that are project-specific for that data.[40]

> ### ➤ CASE IN POINT #2
> Vascular leg amputations often occur in frail and vulnerable populations. Rehabilitation generally focuses on gait training, rather than the patient's experience. Madsen et al[41] designed a study to answer the question, "What is the main concern of patients shortly after having a leg amputated and how do they resolve it?" Understanding this experience can inform providers as to patient needs during hospitalization as well as planning for care post-discharge.

Constant Comparison

In the grounded theory tradition, the work of developing a theory or explanation from the data is built on a process of **constant comparison**. The process is one by which each new piece of information (a belief, explanation for an event, experience, symbol, or relationship) is compared to data already collected to determine where the data agree or conflict. As this iterative process continues, interrelationships between ideas begin to emerge. It continues until **saturation** occurs, a point where the researcher makes a judgment that additional data are yielding few new ideas or relationships.[42]

> ➤ **Case #2:** Researchers sought to build a theoretical model to explain patients' behavior shortly after having a leg amputated as a result of vascular disease. Through observation and interviews, researchers collected data using the constant comparative method, covering the period 4 weeks postsurgery in 11 patients. Data were examined for patterns until saturation occurred, yielding categories that focused on the patients' main concern: "How do I mange my life after having lost a leg?" These included being overwhelmed, facing dependency, managing consequences and building up hope.

Continuing to systematically compare categories, researchers put the pieces together to explain observed behavior, eventually leading to a theoretical premise.

> ➤ **Case #2:** The researchers identified that patients went through three phases as they realized they were experiencing

a life-changing event: losing control, digesting the shock, and regaining control. These categories supported a core theory they termed "Pendulating," describing how patients were swinging both cognitively and emotionally throughout the process.

This theory, illustrated in Figure 21-2, offers a tool for clinicians to recognize where patients are in their recovery process and how they can be best supported by recognizing their reactions.

Phenomenology

Phenomenology is built on the premise that lived experiences and meanings are fully knowable only to those who experience them. In daily life, we share these experiences using language and sometimes nonverbal behaviors. Thus, the skill of the qualitative researcher rests on the ability to identify an appropriate source of information, the ability to find the right words to use to elicit rich descriptions of their study participants' experiences, and the meanings they attribute to those experiences. Researcher must also have skills in a second step to find their own words to report those findings in written form.

> ### ➤ CASE IN POINT #3
> Hospitalized patients have significant medical and social issues that need to be considered in preparation for discharge, a process that is often time-consuming, inefficient, and complex. Pinelli and colleagues[43] conducted a phenomenological study to assess challenges in the discharge process in a teaching hospital from the perspectives of healthcare professionals and patients. They specifically explored communication practices between providers, awareness of colleagues' roles and responsibilities, factors inhibiting or promoting interprofessional collaboration, and potential improvements in the discharge process.

The task of data collection in the qualitative tradition is to engage in lengthy discussions with participants about their experiences, to listen carefully, and then to summarize common themes in their expressions of these experiences that convey a clear essential meaning.[44,45]

Finding the Participant's Voice

In phenomenology, observation and lengthy discussion style interviews are often used to "get inside" the experience of the study participant and describe it in a way that is as close as possible to how it is actually perceived. Qualitative researchers must interpret what the participants' actions and words mean.

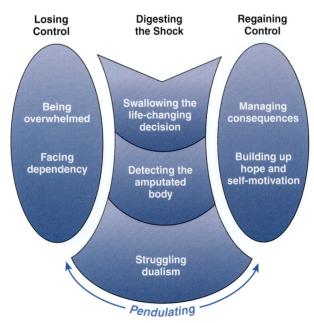

Losing Control	Digesting the Shock	Regaining Control
Being overwhelmed	Swallowing the life-changing decision	Managing consequences
Facing dependency	Detecting the amputated body	Building up hope and self-motivation
	Struggling dualism	

Pendulating

Figure 21–2 Illustration of the theory of "Pendulating," showing the three-phased process that patients go through shortly after having a leg amputated while realizing they are experiencing a life-changing event. Adapted from Madsen UR, Hommel A, Baath C, Berthelsen CB. Pendulating—a grounded theory explaining patients' behavior shortly after having a leg amputated due to vascular disease. *Int J Qual Stud Health Well-being* 2016; 11:32739, Figure 1. Used under Creative Commons Attribution 4.0 International License.

> **Case #3:** Researchers identified five barriers related to the discharge process and interprofessional collaboration, including system insufficiencies, lack of understanding of roles, information-communication breakdowns, patient issues such as difficulty following instructions and preferences, and a lack of perceived collaboration between members of the healthcare team. Patients' primary concerns related to worry that all members of the team were not communicating with each other and concern that the perceived fragmentation would impact their care following discharge.

Typically, a researcher using a phenomenological approach will be attentive to exploring and then writing up the results of the interviews addressing three dimensions.[46] *Spatiality* is the lived space, how people experience their day-to-day existence within a setting, such as home or hospital, which can elicit very different responses. For instance, in the discharge study, the hospital environment can present many stresses because of illness or lack of understanding what is happening. Going home can then present a different set of stressors and concerns.

Relationality refers to lived social relationships and how these interactions influence perceptions, fear, or other emotions. For example, this dimension can be affected by hospitalization that separates patients from family and the need to interact with many different professionals, particularly when care is seen as fragmented.

Temporality is a subjective sense of lived time, as opposed to clock time. Memories and perceptions can be influenced by how time is perceived under different circumstances. For instance, patient experiences during a hospital stay can affect how patients perceive the passage of time. It may feel like it takes forever for someone to help them. Providers may assess time differently in a busy and stressful environment, when it seems like there is never enough time. This can impact perception of the timeliness of discharge, for example.

Case Studies

Case study research is a mode of inquiry that investigates and describes a phenomenon in its real-life context.[5] With roots in the social sciences, case studies are used in many disciplines, including education, business, and psychology, often providing exemplars for program evaluation.

> 📌 Case studies must be distinguished from case reports, which provide comprehensive descriptions of a single patient or organization, based on a thorough account of history, management, and outcomes (see Chapter 20). Case reports are not considered true research because they lack the needed rigor. Case studies, however, are true research, structured as qualitative inquiry with specific design and analysis strategies.

Case studies can be useful for understanding individuals, institutional culture, and systems within their natural settings. It provides the framework to explore the subject's condition, beliefs, and past and present activities as they relate to the focus of the study.

> **▶ CASE IN POINT #4**
> Donnelly et al[47] used a multiple case study design to explore the role of occupational therapists (OTs) in an interprofessional model of primary care in Canada. They addressed the question: "What structures and processes support the integration of occupational therapy in Family Health Teams?"

The case study becomes a valuable source of information for evidence-based practice because it shares important aspects of experiences across a setting. Data for a case study may include qualitative and quantitative sources.

> **Case #4:** Based on in-depth interviews, document analyses, and questionnaires, the researchers described communication and

trust as key elements in the primary care environment, supported by strategies such as co-location, electronic medical records, and team meetings. They found that an understanding of OT was critical for integration into the team, and physicians were less likely to understand the OT's role than other health providers.

The authors also concluded that, with an increased emphasis on interprofessional primary care, integrating new professions into primary healthcare teams required an understanding of professional roles. This study illustrates the benefit of multiple sources of data, especially when looking at systems issues.

📌 These four cases will be used to illustrate varied concepts related to qualitative data collection and analysis throughout this chapter.

■ Methods of Qualitative Data Collection

In the qualitative tradition, the most common methods for gathering data are direct observation, interviews, and analysis of written documents or visual materials.

Observation

Field observation provides data about how social processes occur in real life situations, without the influence of the unnaturalness of a laboratory or controlled clinical setting. The observational record, frequently referred to as *field notes*, is composed of detailed, nonjudgmental, concrete descriptions of what is seen and heard. Field notes can be used as the sole source of data, or they can be used in combination with other forms of data.

When observing the environment, the researcher makes no special effort to have a particular role in the setting other than simply being an unobtrusive observer. The observer steps back and monitors behaviors with no interactions. Field notes are made either during or after the observation period or both. The notes record what was observed as well as potential questions for later follow-up. Ideas about the possible meanings of the observations can also be noted.

▶ **Case #2:** In the study of patients with leg amputations, Madsen et al[41] performed observations during the patients' hospital stay. Wanting to avoid interfering with any interactions, the researcher sat in the back of the hospital room when providers were evaluating the patient and when discussions focused on their care, such as fitting a prosthesis or discharge plans. Field notes were taken during these times with full notes being written immediately after.

Participant Observation

Qualitative researchers can also gather observational data while they are active participants in the group being studied. This technique is called **participant observation.** Often used in ethnographic research, the researcher becomes part of the community and setting being studied, with the idea that the data will be more informed because the researcher experiences are the same as those of the group being studied. The advantage is that the researcher is in a better position to recognize feelings and thoughts that emerge from the first-hand direct experience obtained.

▶ **Case #1:** In the study of day-care staff, a plan was developed for the author to participate as a member of the staff during different times of day across three weeks.[39] The staff were fully aware of her role. Handwritten field notes were recorded sporadically through the day.

Participant observation is inherently influenced and biased by the researcher's own preconceptions. While this is unavoidable, qualitative researchers take steps to mitigate undue influences on the data and to acknowledge this in reporting of study findings. There are situations when the only way to gain access to certain kinds of experiences is to be a part of them and then work to address the potential limitations that come with this "insider perspective." Participant observation increases the researcher's ability to describe results with conviction, using many examples of their personal experience with the social phenomenon.

Getting Close

Because closeness is inherent in participant observation, qualitative researchers must be especially attentive to the possibility of *reactive bias*, where participants may be influenced in some way that alters their behavior. Participants might want to "look good" in the eyes of the researcher or provide what they perceive to be as "the right answer."

For instance, by embedding herself in the day-care setting, Hasselkus[39] could not ignore her expertise as an occupational therapist, which could have intimidated some staff. With her functioning as a member of the staff, however, she was engaged in activities with them, making it easier for her to "fit in" and for staff to get used to her tracking their behaviors. Fortunately, research has shown that over time study participants become less concerned about the presence of the investigator and reveal their "true" thoughts and behaviors surprisingly quickly.[8]

Similarly, because of this same closeness, qualitative researchers must take care not to become "too close" to their participants and step out of the role of researcher and into the role of confidante or friend. This is not desirable as it renders the researcher unable to stand back and analyze the data in an objective way.

Sensitive Data

Participant observation, by its very nature, brings the researcher into closer proximity with the personal dimensions of participants' lives—closer to learning about sensitive and private topics, observing morally tenuous activities and, in rare situations, illegal activities.

Qualitative researchers must be well-prepared for these possibilities. They must understand the policies and laws applicable to the setting and have procedures to address them. For example, child abuse and elder abuse must be reported to authorities, and the researcher needs to be familiar with jurisdictional regulations. In fact, without such knowledge it would be unlikely that the researcher could design an appropriate informed consent form or gain ethical approval to conduct the research (see Chapter 7).

Leaving the Field of Study

A related challenge for those embedded in a setting is how best to "exit the field" at the conclusion of the study. Deep relationships of trust may have been established between the researcher and the participants in the course of the study, and participants often report that they find involvement in qualitative research helpful and therapeutic at some level because "someone was interested and listened to them." The end of the study means severing this bond. Care and time must be taken to debrief with research participants, thank them sincerely for their contributions of knowledge, and leave the research scene as it was before the researcher entered it.

Interviews

Interviews are most often conducted in face-to-face situations with one individual, although they can also be conducted by telephone, over the internet, or in a group situation. The goal of the qualitative interview is to delve deeply into a particular event, issue, or context. Interviews differ from participation and observation primarily in the nature of the interaction. In the *in-depth interview*, the purpose is to probe the ideas of the interviewees and obtain the most detailed information possible about the research topic of interest. Interviews vary with respect to their structure and in the latitude the interviewee has in responding to questions.

> The term *ethnographic interviewing* is often used to describe a method that combines immersive observation and interviews, with a focus on description of people, places, and events.

Unstructured Interviews

Unstructured interviews are generally "open-ended," proceeding more like a guided conversation. They typically include a short list of general questions, followed by more specific questions respecting how the interviewee frames and structures responses.

Answers may be brief or lengthy, and the interviewer accepts the words used and explanations as offered. The unstructured conversational style interview conveys the attitude that the participant's views are valuable and useful, and the task of the researcher is to capture these views as completely and accurately as possible. When appropriate, some probing follow-up questions may also be used. Optimally, probes are value neutral and function simply to elicit more information.

> ➤ **Case #2:** In Madsen's study of patients with leg amputations, open-ended interviews were conducted in the patients' homes 2 weeks postdischarge.[41] The session started with the question, *"Would you please start telling me what led to the amputation?"* This was followed by questions about experiences and concerns during the hospital stay. Incidents that were observed during the hospital stay were brought forward to explore feelings. Participants also talked about getting home and their present concerns.

A well-developed *interview guide* is key to collecting high-quality data. It is developed to suggest open-ended questions that can guide the interviewer's interaction with a participant. It can ensure that the same general areas of information are collected from each interviewee, still allowing flexibility in eliciting information.[48] Madsen used an interview guide to help the researchers cover the concepts of interest but customized it as data analysis developed to address concepts that arose in successive interviews.

Structured and Semi-Structured Interviews

Data collection methods should always match the goals of the research. In a *structured interview*, questions and response categories are predetermined, similar to a quantitative survey or questionnaire. These interviews elicit a standardized and narrow set of responses. This is useful when the goal of the study is to obtain data that needs to be compared or confirmed with other data.[49]

A *semi-structured interview* uses a combination of fixed-response and open-ended questions. Participants are asked the same questions, but they are worded so that responses are open ended, allowing participants to contribute detailed information as they desire.[50]

> ➤ **Case #4:** In the case study of integration of OT in primary care, Donnelly[47] used semi-structured interviews to cover five categories, including roles, physical space, community

collaborations, collaborative practice, and administrative processes. Additional questions were also included in the interview guide to fit the individual's position, such as the executive director who did not have clinical responsibilities.

Because researchers are seldom able to anticipate every aspect of an experience that would be important, semi-structured interviews allow respondents to introduce new ideas and opinions, still allowing for probing questions.

Designing Interview Questions

Designing good interview questions is more difficult than you might think. Clarity and brevity is essential, but questions should be asked in such a way that interviewees know what is meant and they can immediately begin to relate their personal experience.

Consider a question relevant to the amputation study:

Is it difficult to have experienced a leg amputation?

This is a poor question for several reasons. First, it sets up a "yes vs no" dichotomy in the mind of the respondent which immediately limits the richness of what the experience is really. It also provides no signal that the researcher is interested in all kinds of anecdotes and stories, which is the typical way that human beings naturally remember experiences and talk about them to others. Thus, a better question would be something like:

Tell me about how you think about your daily life now that you are home, and how it is different from before your surgery. Tell me about whatever comes to mind, big things or little. I am interested to learn about what you notice and how that is affecting you.

By asking this kind of "grand tour" question, the researcher is deliberately trying to "set the stage" to encourage the respondent to access relevant memories and feelings and know that the interviewer is genuinely interested to hear the response.

Focus Group Interviews

Focus group interviews bring together small groups of people to provide data about a specific topic. The topic may be patient experiences of receiving treatment or living with a particular health problem, but focus groups can also be used to study a wide variety of topics involving different people with unique perspectives to share.

> **Case #3:** In the discharge study, providers participated in several focus groups, exploring description of their roles in the discharge process, perceptions of others' roles, barriers to interprofessional communication, and strategies to improve collaboration.

The power of focus groups is facilitation of data that arise amid dynamic interactions between focus group members. This provides opportunity for new ideas to emerge as group members agree and disagree and provide additional examples of situations that add richness to the data. A pitfall is the potential for "groupthink," which can occur when members hesitate to voice conflicting opinions during the group discussion.

To conduct a rigorous focus group, the group facilitator must ensure that all members are heard, that those members who tend to dominate the conversation are kept in check, and that conflicting opinions are supported and encouraged. The text by Kreuger and Casey[51] is an excellent resource for those interested in conducting focus groups.

The Interviewer

Because qualitative data are often collected through conversations, how the interviewer engages during the interview is important. Becoming a good interviewer requires preparation, learning, and skill development. Interviewers can prepare by familiarizing themselves with the population and problem of interest, especially important when dealing with sensitive topics. They should also be familiar with the interview guide so that they understand the overall flow of the conversation that will take place during the interview. A skilled interviewer knows when to follow up on a lead, when the interviewee is becoming fatigued or disinterested, and how to manage conversations that go off topic.

Good interviews sometimes require moving off the predetermined question to follow-up on a particularly interesting or unexpected response. Interviewers must balance these opportunities for discovery with the need to cover all the intended interview topics.

Interviewers may engage in mock interviews amongst study team members to become comfortable with administering the interview guide. Mock interviews can also help determine the optimal wording and best way to ask questions or probe responses. There are a variety of Web-based resources, including video training and examples that novice investigators use to develop interview skills.

Establishing Rapport

All interviews involve personal interaction and cooperation, so trust and rapport between interviewer and interviewee are essential if the highest quality data are to be obtained.[52] Depending on the topic of study, interviewees may not be comfortable sharing all that the interviewer hopes to explore, at least at first. Techniques to enhance rapport include:

- Providing a clear explanation about the purpose of the research and the study participant's role as an expert contributor of data.

- Explaining why the topic is important to understand and how the data obtained will be used.
- Applying strong communication skills, empathy and personal sensitivity.
- Establishing safe and familiar surroundings to make participants as comfortable as possible.
- Demonstrating ease and familiarity with topic studied, and awareness of cultural norms and preferences.
- Expressing appreciation for participants' willingness to share their experiences, even when doing so is difficult.

Recording

Interviews and focus groups can be recorded using audio or video, providing a more comprehensive, accurate, and permanent record of the data. It also allows for other kinds of data analyses, including analysis of the structure and use of language, and with video a more detailed study of specific nonverbal body language and facial expressions. The ability to record data in a visual format is especially useful when the phenomenon being observed is fast-paced and difficult to detect without repeated review. Investigators should be aware that recording can detract from the naturalness of the observed behaviors. Participants must give their prior permission to be recorded as part of informed consent.

Written Documents

Important information can often be gathered through the use of existing documents or previously collected data, such as diaries, historical documents, and reports. These materials may be provided by individuals, or they may include program descriptions of organizations. The interpretation of data from these documents must be considered in context. Their information is clarified when supplemented with other data gathering methods.

> ▶ **Case #4:** In the case study of OT practice in primary care settings, data collection included document analyses, such as job descriptions, OT assessments, and statements of the team's mission and vision.[47] Web pages were consulted to provide demographic information about the practices. Each OT completed a profile that included information on education, background, and clinical experience.

Information from these documents was integrated with findings from interviews to provide a context for data analysis.

■ Sampling

Qualitative researchers use many different nonprobability sampling approaches, such as convenience, purposive, or snowball sampling (see Chapter 13).[53] The most common approach involves a purposive sample, as the investigator identifies individuals who will be most useful to study given the experiences that the researcher wishes to study, what Patton[8] has termed *information-rich cases*. When the researcher is interested in seeking a sample that represents a range of extremes related to the phenomenon under study, a technique called *maximum variation sampling* can be used. With this approach, the researcher selects a small number of cases that maximize the diversity relevant to the research question.

There are many ways to recruit a sample that reflects the study purpose and provides insights that can be strongly justified on the basis of previous research and theoretical understanding. Researchers may recruit participants through referrals from other health professionals, or they may identify participants through examination of medical records to find individuals with the appropriate characteristics.[52] Participants may also be enrolled by virtue of their being part of an organizational unit. For example, participants in the Alzheimer day-care study were current members of the staff.[39] Patients in the study of leg amputations and the discharge study were recruited from hospital units.[41,43]

In contrast to the goal of quantitative research, which seeks a sample size for probabilistic reasons related to prediction, the qualitative sample is guided by the goal of seeking richness and depth in the data, purposely finding participants who can provide insight into social phenomenon. The qualitative researcher asks, "Who, in what setting, will help me understand X?"

Sample Size

A common misconception is that all qualitative studies use small samples. However, samples that are too small will not support claims of having fully explored a phenomenon. On the other hand, samples that are too large will not permit the in-depth analysis that is the essence of qualitative inquiry. For example, five staff members participated in the day-care study,[39] 11 participants were identified in the study of patients with leg amputations,[41] and 87 patients and providers were interviewed in the study of discharge processes.[43]

Sandelowski[54] suggests that determining adequate sample size is a matter of judgment and experience in evaluating the quality of the information collected and the purpose of the research. A key consideration is the quality of the insights from previous research, whether a broader sample is needed to expand exploration of a well-studied topic or a smaller sample is needed to focus in an area that is not yet well understood.

Theoretical Sampling

In the development of theory, qualitative researchers try to collect data that fully capture the scope of the phenomenon being studied. When building a theory, however, researchers often apply a purposive strategy in a different way using a process called theoretical sampling. Once the research question is formulated, a small number of relevant participants are recruited and interviewed, and data are analyzed to identify initial concepts. As issues are brought up with early cases, new participants who are likely to expand or challenge those results are then interviewed, and further analysis is performed, leading to decisions about what additional questions should be added to the interview guide and queried in subsequent interviews.[55] Thus, as more cases are interviewed, additional questions are added to the interview guide. It is important to note that the research question does not change, only the questions in the guide that are used to collect data.

New participants continue to be interviewed and data analyzed, as components of the theory emerge and new perspectives are presented, continually reframing the theoretical premise. The process continues, moving back and forth between recruitment of new subjects, data collection and analysis, until the researcher determines that data have reached saturation.

> **Case #2:** In the study of patient behavior following leg amputation, researchers used principles of theoretical sampling.[41] Their interview guide was customized from interview to interview as analysis developed. They continued to recruit patients as they became accessible, until they found that the three components of the "pendulating" theory were explained.

■ Data Analysis and Interpretation

Qualitative data analysis is primarily an inductive process, with a constant interplay between data that represent the reality of the study participants and theoretical conceptualizations of that reality. Therefore, at least to some degree, analysis must be undertaken as data are collected. This is particularly true in observational studies and studies guided by grounded theory.

In studies using in-depth interviews, some analysis will be undertaken early on, but once the researchers are satisfied that they are getting high quality data and the

questions are yielding strong insights, it is not unusual to proceed with data collection and engage more heavily in analysis later in the process.

Data analysis involves systematic procedures to understand the meaning of the data.[45] Although the details of how to undertake qualitative data analysis are beyond the scope of this chapter, readers must be aware that there are an array of different analytic approaches. The techniques of data analysis can vary from purely narrative descriptions of observations to creating a detailed system of coding the data from which categories can be developed, and in a systematic way, patterns or themes develop from the mass of information.

Drawing Meaning from Narrative Data

Coding

Because qualitative data are textual, coding is an important process to make sense of the narratives. It provides the foundation for determining how themes or concepts emerge from the data by giving structure to the data. Codes are the smallest units of text that represents a common theme. Codes can be phrases or words. While some researchers will develop a coding scheme prior to data collection, it is more common to proceed in a deductive fashion by establishing codes as the data are reviewed.

Content analysis is a systematic technique used to draw inferences by interpreting and coding textual material. It involves counting the frequency of words in a text to analyze meanings and relationships of certain words, themes, or categories within the data.

> **Case #3:** In their analysis of discharge processes, Pinelli et al[43] used an inductive process to develop categories, integrating data from one-on-one and focus group interviews. After reading through transcripts to get a gestalt of the process, they reviewed words and phrases that recurred frequently to create an initial code book. The unit of analysis was phrases that contained one idea. The team met regularly to check progress of coding and made minor modifications as needed.

Five final categories were derived describing barriers related to the discharge process, a lack of understanding of roles, communication breakdowns, patient issues, and poor collaboration processes. Identified themes are typically illustrated in quotes from participant narratives. For example, one resident described the chaotic nature of the discharge process:

It's like trying to pack for a trip to Europe for two weeks. You have five minutes to do it and try to throw everything you can think of in the suitcase. But you're going to forget your toothbrush or something essential. Very often with discharges they evolve that way.

A consulting physician described the lack of delineation of responsibilities:

There's misunderstanding of who's going to do what. For example, when we say continue antibiotics for at least four weeks until your follow-up CT scan is done, who's scheduling that CT scan? We think the primary team is going to do it, the primary team thinks we're going to do it.

Content analysis benefits hugely from the power of computing to speed up the analysis and ensure a comprehensive enumeration of words. Bengtsson[56] provides a helpful review of the types of content analysis and the steps in conducting a rigorous content analysis study.

Volume of Data

Because observational and interview data are often recorded as narratives, qualitative data are typically voluminous. This is especially true with the common use of digital audio recordings along with written memos, which are then transcribed. It is not unusual for a 1-hour interview to yield 40 to 60 pages of single-spaced text.

Because of the volume of detailed data, analysis can be a time-consuming process. An experienced interviewer will need to distinguish between data that are relevant and data that are not central to the study aims. Because of time and cost, judgments may be made to set aside less relevant data and transcribe and analyze only the most important data. These are important decisions to make. No researcher wants to invest time and resources in collecting data that are not used. Similarly, no researcher wants to lose important insights by making poor judgments about what data matter and what do not.

Analysis of qualitative data by hand involves many hours of sifting through written texts. Data analysis software can help manage large amounts of narrative data, assisting in recording, storing, indexing, coding, and interconnecting text-based material.[57] Three of the more commonly used software packages for qualitative data analysis are NVIVO,[58] Atlas.ti[59], and QDA Miner.[60]

There is some debate about the use of computer programs for data analysis, but most acknowledge their value as a data organizing tool. The fundamental objections focus on the loss of intimacy with the data, and the criticism that an overreliance on software can result in mere quantification and counts of words in a text over more nuanced interpretations of the themes, and patterns. Computer software may be a valuable tool to assist in managing voluminous data, but it does not direct interpretive activity.[36] The researchers themselves are responsible for analyzing data, developing theory and drawing conclusions about the findings.

Evaluating Quality

Reliability and validity are issues of concern in qualitative research just as they are in all types of research. Because the data sources are words rather than numbers, different terms and techniques are used to describe rigor in terms of *trustworthiness* of the data. Though multiple frameworks have been proposed for assessing the quality of qualitative research,[61-63] the four criteria proposed by Lincoln and Guba[1] remain widely used: credibility, transferability, dependability, and confirmability (see Fig. 21-3).

🔖 Although the criteria of credibility, transferability, dependability, and confirmability reflect a substantially different paradigm from quantitative methods, they have been likened to internal validity, external validity, reliability, and objectivity, respectively.[1]

Credibility

Credibility refers to actions that are taken to ensure that the results of a qualitative study are believable—that there is confidence in "truth" of the findings. In planning the study, researchers use well-developed research methods, operationalize the phenomenon of interest, make

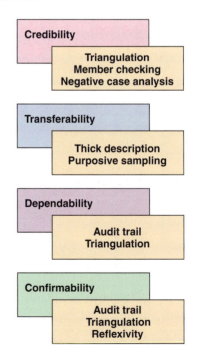

Figure 21-3 Techniques used to evaluate "trustworthiness" of qualitative studies. Based on the evaluative criteria developed by Lincoln and Guba.[1]

the sampling procedure clear, and ensure that they have the requisite training and expertise to conduct the study. Several techniques are used to establish credibility, but the most common include triangulation, member checking, and negative case analysis.

Triangulation involves comparing varying sources of data to validate findings. Most often this involves comparing results obtained through different methods, such as field notes from observations and interview transcripts. However, it may also include comparing interpretations of several data collectors or involving multiple persons in the data analysis. This technique is used to critically examine areas of convergence and divergence.

Negative case analysis involves discussing elements of data that do not support or appear to contradict explanations that are emerging from preliminary data. By identifying deviant cases, the researcher can refine the analysis until it can explain or account for a majority of cases.

Member checking involves opening up the analytical process to others, sharing preliminary findings and interpretations with research participants, allowing them to offer validation, feedback, critique, and alternative explanations that ultimately contribute to the credibility of findings.[64] Although controversial, Lincoln and Guba[1] suggest that this is the most crucial technique for establishing credibility to assess what the participant intended.

> **Case #1:** In the study of staff in adult day care, Hasselkus[39] checked her perceptions of meanings regularly against those of the staff.

> **Case #3:** In the discharge study, member checking included having participants read the coded data for accuracy.[43]

Transferability

No form of inquiry can yield insights that are "truths" for everyone in all situations. However, qualitative research should be *transferable*, meaning the results should be able to be applied in some way to other people in similar situations. This is an assessment of generalizability, similar to external validity in quantitative studies. This concept helps to direct choices of subjects through purposive sampling, to assure that participants will represent the type of individuals appropriate to the research question.

Researchers can increase the transferability of the work by *thick description*, reporting study details that make comparisons across studies possible, such as the participant characteristics, study setting, sources of data and collection techniques, and data collection period.[1]

> **Case #1:** In the day care study, Hasselkus[39] provides detailed description of the setting in terms of the staff makeup, client characteristics, the location, and the types of spaces available for daily activities. She also reports details about daily schedules and staff guidelines regarding monitoring clients.

The generalizability of results can also be strengthened by examining the same phenomenon under different conditions. Ideally, insights gained through qualitative investigations are reinforced when studies are replicated across multiple settings with different types of populations. Unfortunately, this type of replication work is seldom done in qualitative research.

Dependability

Dependability of data refers to how stable the data are over a span of time relevant to the study question at hand and the degree to which the study could be repeated with similar results. The experience of a health condition and its impact on daily life may change over time as individuals grow older, as the condition progresses, and as social roles change.

> **Case #2:** With their focus on patients' early reactions after leg amputation surgery, Madsen et al[41] recognized that patients gave insights during their hospital stay that were different from their perspectives weeks later when they had rationalized the experience after discharge and return home.

It is difficult, if not impossible, for a qualitative researcher to claim that their research findings at one moment in time are as "reliable" as a score on a standardized test that does not account for a range of personal and contextual factors that are not measured in the quantitative tradition.[36] Researchers can address dependability through triangulation, and by creating an audit trail.

Audit Trail

The **audit trail** concept stems from the idea of the fiscal audit, where independent auditors authenticate a firm's accounts and examine them for the possibility of error or fraud.[65] Lincoln and Guba[1] suggest that by implementing an audit trail, an auditor or second party who becomes familiar with the qualitative study, its methodology, findings and conclusions can audit the research decisions and the methodological and analytical processes of the researcher on completion of the study and thus confirm its findings.

In the simplest form, creating an audit trail involves documenting decisions and their rationale throughout all aspects of the study design and implementation so that other researchers can replicate the study and understand the rationale behind each of the methodological choices made. This includes articulation of rationales for sampling criteria, questions to ask participants, and analytical approach.

> Reporting checklists such as the Consolidated Criteria for Reporting Qualitative research (COREQ) have helped to standardize what is included in study audit trails and can aide in both transferability and dependability by making sure that the "nuts and bolts" of research studies are transparently reported (see Chapter 38).[62] Computer software can enhance dependability by creating a trail of decisions made throughout the data analysis, including a network of files and coding schemes.

Confirmability

Although qualitative research does not aim to be objective, researchers should strive to achieve *confirmability*, which refers to ensuring, as much as possible, that findings are due to the experiences and ideas of the participants rather than the characteristics and preferences of the researcher. Because it is impossible for researchers to enter into the research enterprise as blank slates, it is commonplace for qualitative researchers to document their own biases, assumptions, thoughts, and feelings throughout the research process. Doing so increases awareness of how investigator assumptions and bias may have influenced the study and findings. Strategies such as data triangulation, creating an audit trail, and addressing reflexivity can assist in confirmability.

Reflexivity

A researcher's experience can influence what is studied, methods used, and how findings are interpreted.[66] *Reflexivity* refers to systematic consideration of how researchers shape and are shaped by the qualitative research process.[67] Researchers can approach a question from different perspectives, with different understandings of meaning in the phenomenon they are studying.

Reflexivity can be fostered by involving multiple investigators who provide varied insights and by being transparent in reporting of preconceptions, assumptions, and values that are relevant to the research process.

> **Case #3:** In the study of the discharge process, the research team was composed of internal medicine physicians.[43] The team held regular sessions to achieve consensus on coding. They also addressed reflexivity by using an interdisciplinary team of physicians and behavioral scientists to review their analyses from multiple perspectives.

Levels of evidence for qualitative studies are described in Chapter 5. See Chapter 36 for discussion related to application of quality criteria for critical appraisal.

■ Mixed Methods

Because qualitative and quantitative approaches have complementary strengths, both methods can be used within a single study to increase the validity of the findings. By using a multiple methods approach, researchers can consider how measurable behaviors or attitudes relate to the nature of lived experience. This approach often involves working with multidisciplinary teams with diverse methodological expertise, incorporating diverse perspectives.

Two multiple methods approaches can be used to incorporate qualitative and quantitative data in one study, with a distinction based on how data are analyzed. In *multimethod* studies, different types of data are analyzed independently and results are reported separately. In contrast, in a **mixed methods** approach, a plan for combining data is set out in the proposal, with a rationale for how the different forms of data will inform each other.

> ➤ **CASE IN POINT #5**
>
> Despite the availability of effective interventions, individuals with type 2 diabetes (T2DM) often face barriers to self-management. Using a mixed-methods grounded theory approach, Fritz[68] examined the process by which low-income women develop the skills to integrate diabetes self-management (DSM) into daily life and the conditions that affect the process. Quantitative data were taken from the Diabetes Care Profile (DCP), a self-report assessment that includes questions on demographics, DSM practices, diabetes knowledge, and perception of support and barriers.[69] Qualitative methods included semi-structured interviews, photography, and a geographic diary.

A mixed methods approach is considered a formalized methodology that is distinct from both qualitative and quantitative research. Readers are urged to refer to texts that focus comprehensively on this design for more information.[23,53]

Mixed Methods Designs

The design and implementation of mixed methods research requires careful consideration, starting with the theoretical assumptions and research question. This approach requires attention to design principles for both qualitative and quantitative approaches, with careful consideration of the rationale for mixing, at what stage and in what way varying approaches are mixed, and how they improve our ability to draw inference from the results. Because it includes both components, the investigator formulates quantitative and qualitative questions or "hybrid" questions that combine elements of the two.[70]

> In the study of diabetes management, the overarching research question was, "To what extent do the qualitative findings confirm the quantitative results?" The authors hypothesized that those who scored lower on the Diabetes Care Profile would also be those who related more life context issues that interfered with their efforts to manage their diabetes.

Mixed Methods Typologies

Mixed methods researchers have developed design typologies helpful for organizing both research approaches within a single study. Though not an exhaustive list, the four basic mixed methods designs include convergent, sequential, embedded, and multiphase designs.[71,72]

- *Convergent designs* involve the collection, often simultaneously, of both qualitative and quantitative data, combining the data during the data analysis and interpretation phase.
- *Sequential designs* are useful when the intent is to have one dataset build on the other to enhance understanding of a phenomenon. For example, a researcher may collect and analyze survey data followed by in-depth interviews to better understand the quantitative findings.
- *Embedded designs* are especially useful in health sciences as researchers work to develop and refine interventions. Researchers may collect quantitative data to determine the efficacy of a trial while also using interviews or other qualitative approaches to better understand participants' experiences of being in the intervention.
- *Multiphase designs* are best suited for linked projects that are conducted over time and that require different types of knowledge generated at each stage for the project as a whole to advance.

Each of these study designs can further be classified as predominantly quantitative, predominantly qualitative, or equally balanced depending on the methods used.

> Data in the DSM study were gathered sequentially, starting with (1) the Diabetes Care Profile followed by an interview; (2) participant-generated photography followed by an interview; and then (3) a time geographic diary followed by an interview. Data were collected in this sequence for all participants.

Sampling

Mixed methods research also requires special consideration of sampling procedures that fit each qualitative and quantitative component. Quantitative studies generally involve larger samples to achieve sufficient power, while qualitative studies tend to require many fewer participants and may rely more on purposive sampling methods. For example, an investigator might purposively recruit a subsample from a large quantitative study to participate in a qualitative component of a study. Because sampling strategies can become quite elaborate depending on the study design, we recommend readers review the work by Teddlie and Yu,[72] which offers an excellent primer on mixed methods sampling with example typologies.

> Fritz[68] recruited a sample of 10 women for the DSM study from a list of participants who had previously participated in formal DSM classes. She intentionally recruited participants with a broad range of demographic characteristics including age, education, family size, and socioeconomic status.

Data Collection

Within mixed methods studies, researchers are free to use a wide and creative range of data collection methods, including the use of technology.

> Fritz[68] incorporated participant-generated photography, whereby participants were asked to "take photographs of the things you associate with diabetes self-management." These photos were then used as a source of discussion in a *photo-elicitation interview*.

She also asked participants to complete a time *geographic diary*, in which they were asked to record all of their daily activities, with the assumption that DSM would emerge as part of the daily routine. Follow-up interviews focused on why certain activities occurred in different locations and how the DSM activities competed with daily demands.

Coding and Analysis

Investigators must also consider how to treat the varied types of qualitative and quantitative data during analysis and interpretation. Mixing of research data may be one of the least clear aspects of mixed methods research, yet it is essential for assessing the quality of inferences made. The three most common approaches discussed in the literature are merging, connecting, and embedding.[71]

Merging, also referred to as integrating, involves combining qualitative and quantitative data in both the analysis and reporting of results. The goal of merging is to reveal where findings from each method converge, offer complementary information on the issue, or contradict each other.[73]

> Fritz[68] began analysis by coding text sources to develop themes. That process was followed by considering all data together through constant comparisons across cases and data types. For instance, the DCP data were compared with data obtained during interviews, allowing the researcher to explore convergence and divergence.

The grounded theory process resulted in the development of the Transactional Model of Diabetes Self-Management Integration, which depicts a process whereby participants accepted how aspects of diabetes education and management can become integrated within the context of their daily lives.

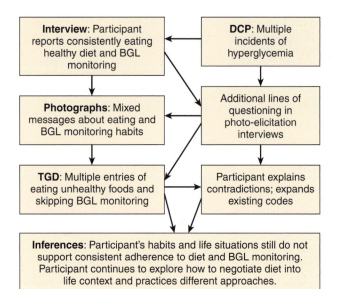

This process is summarized in Figure 21-4, showing how each method informed the other.

Connecting data consists of analyzing one dataset and then using the inferences generated from that analysis to inform subsequent data collection. This approach is especially useful in survey development because initial qualitative interviews about a phenomenon may generate data to suggest potential items for a quantitative instrument.

When *embedding* data, researchers integrate data of secondary priority into a larger principle dataset. For example, in a study of pain management, qualitative data were embedded within an intervention trial.[74] Even though the trial found a significant decrease in pain for the treatment group, qualitative data revealed that many patients still did not obtain satisfactory relief.

Figure 21–4 The process of integrating multiple data sources during data analysis. Note: BGL = blood glucose level, DCP = Diabetes Care Profile, and TGD = time geographic diary. From Fritz, H. Learning to do better: the Transactional Model of Diabetes Self-Management Integration. *Qual Health Res* 2015;25(7):875-886. Figure 1, p. 879. Used with permission.

COMMENTARY

You may have heard the world is made up of atoms and molecules, but it's really made up of stories.

—*William Turner (1508-1568)*

British scientist

The purpose of qualitative descriptive research is to characterize phenomena so that we know what exists. Without this fundamental knowledge, it would be impossible to ask questions about behaviors or treatment effects or to propose theories to explain them. This approach is essential for bridging the gap between scientific evidence and clinical practice. It can help us understand the limitations in applying research literature to clinical decisions. Most importantly, clinicians should recognize that different research methods are needed to address different questions.

Qualitative research is often viewed as lacking rigor, and generalizability is challenged because of the nature of data collection. This is a misguided characterization, however. The ever-increasing complexity of healthcare, including provider and organizational changes, requires new understandings of our environment and how patients and providers interact to develop optimal methods

of care.[11,75] Qualitative findings provide rigorous accounts of treatment regimens in everyday contexts.[9]

Without qualitative insights, we could not know what kinds of questions to ask in experimental situations, or what measurements would make sense of them.[76] The best answer to a research question will be achieved by using the appropriate design—and that will often call for a qualitative approach.

Just because it does not require statistical analysis, qualitative research is by no means easier than other approaches, and doing it well requires its own set of skills. Novice investigators are encouraged to work with an experienced qualitative researcher who can assist with planning, implementation, and analysis. Many decisions need to be made in the planning of a qualitative study, including the appropriate approach, availability of resources, data collection strategies, and understanding the potential influence of personal biases.[52]

This brief introduction to qualitative methods is by no means sufficient to demonstrate the scope of data collection and analysis techniques that are used. It should, however, provide a good foundation for understanding qualitative research studies and how their findings can be evaluated and applied. Many topics relevant to qualitative research are also addressed with other topics, including translational research (Chapter 2), developing research questions (Chapter 3), application of theory (Chapter 4), evidence-based practice (Chapter 5), informed consent (Chapter 7), writing proposals (Chapter 35), and critically appraising literature (Chapter 36).

REFERENCES

1. Lincoln YS, Guba EG. *Naturalistic Inquiry*. Newbury Park, CA: Sage; 1985.
2. Creswell JW, Poth CN. *Qualitative Inquiry and Research Design: Choosing Among Five Approaches*. 4th ed. Thousand Oaks, CA: Sage; 2018.
3. Creswell JW, Creswell JD. *Research Design: Qualitative, Quantitative, and Mixed Methods Approaches*. 5th ed. Thousand Oaks, CA: Sage; 2018.
4. Charmaz K. *Constructing Grounded Theory*. 2nd ed. Los Angeles: Sage; 2014.
5. Yin RK. *Case Study Research and Applications: Design and Methods*. 6th ed. Los Angeles: Sage; 2018.
6. Smith JA, Flowers P, Larkin M. *Interpretative Phenomenological Analysis: Theory, Method and Research*. Thousand Oaks, CA: Sage; 2009.
7. Pope C, Mays N. *Qualitative Research in Health Care*. Oxford: Blackwell; 2006.
8. Patton MQ. *Qualitative Research and Evaluation Methods: Integrating Theory and Practice*. 4th ed. Newbury Park, CA: Sage; 2015.
9. Green J, Britten N. Qualitative research and evidence based medicine. *BMJ (Clinical research ed)* 1998;316(7139):1230-1232.
10. Benoliel JQ. Advancing nursing science: qualitative approaches. *West J Nurs Res* 1984;6(3):1-8.
11. Meadows KA. So you want to do research? 3. An introduction to qualitative methods. *Br J Community Nurs* 2003;8(10):464-469.
12. Ailinger RL. Contributions of qualitative research to evidence-based practice in nursing. *Rev Lat Am Enfermagem* 2003;11(3):275-279.
13. Pekkarinen T, Kaukua J, Mustajoki P. Long-term weight maintenance after a 17-week weight loss intervention with or without a one-year maintenance program: a randomized controlled trial. *J Obes* 2015;2015:651460.
14. Cioffi J. Factors that enable and inhibit transition from a weight management program: a qualitative study. *Health Educ Res* 2002; 17(1):19-26.
15. Green AR, Larkin M, Sullivan V. Oh stuff it! The experience and explanation of diet failure: an exploration using interpretative phenomenological analysis. *J Health Psychol* 2009;14(7):997-1008.
16. McKee H, Ntoumanis N, Smith B. Weight maintenance: self-regulatory factors underpinning success and failure. *Psychol Health* 2013;28(10):1207-1223.
17. Rogerson D, Soltani H, Copeland R. The weight-loss experience: a qualitative exploration. *BMC Public Health* 2016;16:371.
18. Chambers JA, Swanson V. Stories of weight management: factors associated with successful and unsuccessful weight maintenance. *Br J Health Psychol* 2012;17(2):223-243.
19. Downing AM, Hunter DG. Validating clinical reasoning: a question of perspective, but whose perspective? *Man Ther* 2003;8(2):117-119.
20. Dougherty DA, Toth-Cohen SE, Tomlin GS. Beyond research literature: Occupational therapists' perspectives on and uses of "evidence" in everyday practice. *Can J Occup Ther* 2016;83(5):288-296.
21. Jensen GM, Gwyer J, Hack LM, Shepard KF. *Expertise in Physical Therapy Practice*, 2nd ed. St. Louis: Saunders; 2007.
22. Kane H, Lewis MA, Williams PA, Kahwati LC. Using qualitative comparative analysis to understand and quantify translation and implementation. *Transl Behav Med* 2014;4(2):201-208.
23. Creswell JC. *Qualitative Inquiry and Research Design: Choosing among Five Approaches*. 3rd ed. Thousand Oaks, CA: Sage; 2013.
24. National Cancer Institute. Cancer Disparities. Available at https://www.cancer.gov/about-cancer/understanding/disparities. Accessed February 28, 2019.
25. Eggly S, Barton E, Winckles A, Penner LA, Albrecht TL. A disparity of words: racial differences in oncologist-patient communication about clinical trials. *Health Expect* 2015;18(5):1316-1326.
26. Eggly S, Harper FW, Penner LA, Gleason MJ, Foster T, Albrecht TL. Variation in question asking during cancer clinical interactions: a potential source of disparities in access to information. *Patient Educ Couns* 2011;82(1):63-68.
27. Rubin HJ, Rubin IS. *Qualitative Interviewing: The Art of Hearing Data*. Thousand Oaks, CA: Sage 1995.
28. Kayser-Jones J, Schell ES, Porter C, Barbaccia JC, Shaw H. Factors contributing to dehydration in nursing homes: inadequate staffing and lack of professional supervision. *J Am Geriatr Soc* 1999;47(10):1187-1194.
29. Tucker AL, Heisler WS, Janisse LD. Designed for workarounds: a qualitative study of the causes of operational failures in hospitals. *Perm J* 2014;18(3):33-41.
30. Sanchez H, Levkoff S. Lessons learned about minority recruitment and retention from the centers on minority aging and health promotion. *Gerontologist* 2003;43(1):18-26.
31. Henshall C, Narendran P, Andrews RC, Daley A, Stokes KA, Kennedy A, Greenfield S. Qualitative study of barriers to clinical trial retention in adults with recently diagnosed type 1 diabetes. *BMJ Open* 2018;8(7):e022353.
32. Jackson J, Carlson M, Rubayi S, Scott MD, Atkins MS, Blanche EI, Saunders-Newton C, Mielke S, Wolfe MK, Clark FA. Qualitative study of principles pertaining to lifestyle and pressure ulcer risk in adults with spinal cord injury. *Disabil Rehabil* 2010;32(7):567-578.
33. Cella D, Yount S, Rothrock N, Gershon R, Cook K, Reeve B, Ader D, Fries JF, Bruce B, Rose M. The Patient-Reported Outcomes Measurement Information System (PROMIS): progress of an NIH Roadmap cooperative group during its first two years. *Med Care* 2007;45(5 Suppl 1):S3-S11.
34. Quinn H, Thissen D, Liu Y, Magnus B, Lai JS, Amtmann D, Varni JW, Gross HE, DeWalt DA. Using item response theory to enrich and expand the PROMIS(R) pediatric self report banks. *Health Qual Life Outcomes* 2014;12:160.
35. Walsh TR, Irwin DE, Meier A, Varni JW, DeWalt DA. The use of focus groups in the development of the PROMIS pediatrics item bank. *Qual Life Res* 2008;17(5):725-735.
36. Marshall C, Rossman GB. *Designing Qualitative Research*. 6th ed. Thousand Oaks, CA: Sage; 2016.
37. Harper D. *Visual Sociology*. New York: Routledge; 2012.
38. Wang C, Burris MA. Photovoice: concept, methodology, and use for participatory needs assessment. *Health Educ Behav* 1997;24(3):369-387.
39. Hasselkus BR. The meaning of activity: day care for persons with Alzheimer disease. *Am J Occup Ther* 1992; 46(3):199-206.

40. Corbin J, Strauss A. *Basics of Qualitative Research: Techniques and Procedures for Developing Grounded Theory*. 4th ed. Thousand Oaks, CA: Sage; 2015.

41. Madsen UR, Hommel A, Baath C, Berthelsen CB. Pendulating—A grounded theory explaining patients' behavior shortly after having a leg amputated due to vascular disease. *Int J Qual Stud Health Well-being* 2016;11:32739.

42. Saunders B, Sim J, Kingstone T, Baker SB, Waterfield J, Bartlam B, Burroughs H, Jinks C. Saturation in qualitative research: exploring its conceptualization and operationalization. *Qual Quant* 2018;52(4):1893-1907.

43. Pinelli V, Stuckey HL, Gonzalo JD. Exploring challenges in the patient's discharge process from the internal medicine service: A qualitative study of patients' and providers' perceptions. *J Interprof Care* 2017;31(5):566-574.

44. Schram TH. *Conceputalizing and Proposing Qualitatice Research*. 2nd ed. Upper Saddle River, NJ: Pearson; 2006.

45. Luborsky M. The identifications and analysis of themes and patterns. In: Gubrium J, Sankar A, eds. *Qualitative Methods in Aging Research*. New York: Sage; 1994.

46. Finlay L. Applying phenomenology in research: problems, principles and practice. *Br J Occup Ther* 1999;62(7):299-306.

47. Donnelly C, Brenchley C, Crawford C, Letts L. The integration of occupational therapy into primary care: a multiple case study design. *BMC Fam Pract* 2013;14:60.

48. Turner DW. Qualitative interview design: a practical guide for novice investigators. *Qual Report* 2010;15(3):754-760. Available at http://www.nova.edu/ssss/QR/QR715-753/qid.pdf. Accessed March, 2019.

49. Miller PR, Dasher R, Collins R, Griffiths P, Brown F. Inpatient diagnostic assessments: 1. Accuracy of structured vs. unstructured interviews. *Psychiatry Res* 2001;105(3):255-264.

50. Gall MD, Gall JP, Borg WR. *Educational Research: An Introduction*. 8th ed. New York: Pearson; 2006.

51. Krueger RA, Casey MA. *Focus Groups: A Practical Guide for Applied Research*. 5th ed. Thousand Oaks, CA: Sage; 2015.

52. Davies B, Larson J, Contro N, Reyes-Hailey C, Ablin AR, Chesla CA, Sourkes B, Cohen H. Conducting a qualitative culture study of pediatric palliative care. *Qual Health Res* 2009; 19(1):5-16.

53. Teddlie C, Tashakkori A. *Foundations of Mixed Methods Research: Integrating Quantitative and Qualitative Approaches in in the Social and Behavioral Sciences*. Thousand Oaks, CA: Sage; 2009.

54. Sandelowski M. Sample size in qualitative research. *Res Nurs Health* 1995;18(2):179-183.

55. Glaser BG, Strauss AI. *The Discovery of Grounded Theory: Strategies for Qualitative Research*. New York: Routledge; 1999.

56. Bengtsson M. How to plan and perform a qualitative study using content analysis. *Nursing Plus Open* 2016;2:8-14. Available at https://doi.org/10.1016/j.npls.2016.1001.1001, Accessed March 10, 2019.

57. Denzin NK, Lincoln YS. *Handbook of Qualitative Research*. 4th ed. Thousand Oaks, CA: Sage; 2011.

58. NVIVO. QSR International. Available at https://www.qsrinternational.com/nvivo/home. Accessed March 6, 2019.

59. ATLAS.ti. Available at https://atlasti.com/. Accessed March 6, 2019.

60. QDA Miner. Available at https://provalisresearch.com/products/qualitative-data-analysis-software/. Accessed March 6, 2019.

61. Spencer L, Ritchie J, Lewis J, Dillon L. Quality in qualitative evaluation: a framework for assessing research evidence. National Center for Social Research, 2003. Available at http://dera.ioe.ac.uk/21069/2/a-quality-framework-tcm6-38740.pdf. Accessed November 25, 2017.

62. Tong A, Sainsbury P, Craig J. Consolidated criteria for reporting qualitative research (COREQ): a 32-item checklist for interviews and focus groups. *Int J Qual Health Care* 2007;19(6):349-357.

63. Sandelowski M, Docherty S, Emden C. Focus on qualitative methods. Qualitative metasynthesis: issues and techniques. *Res Nurs Health* 1997;20(4):365-371.

64. Sandelowski M. Rigor or rigor mortis: the problem of rigor in qualitative research revisited. *Adv Nurs Sci* 1993;16(2):1-8.

65. Koch T. Establishing rigour in qualitative research: the decision trail. *J Adv Nurs* 1994;19(5):976-986.

66. Malterud K. Qualitative research: standards, challenges, and guidelines. *Lancet* 2001;358(9280):483-488.

67. Palaganas EC, Sanchez MC, Molintas MP, Caricativo RD. Reflexivity in qualitative research: a journey of learning. *Qual Report* 2017;22(2):426-438. Available at https://nsuworkss. nova.edu/tqr/vol422/iss422/425. Accessed March 410, 2019.

68. Fritz H. Learning to do better: the Transactional Model of Diabetes Self-Management Integration. *Qual Health Res* 2015; 25(7):875-886.

69. Fitzgerald JT, Davis WK, Connell CM, Hess GE, Funnell MM, Hiss RG. Development and validation of the Diabetes Care Profile. *Eval Health Prof* 1996;19(2):208-230.

70. Creswell JW, Tashakkori A. Developing publishable mixed methods manuscripts. *J Mixed Methods Res* 2007;1:107-111.

71. Creswell JC, Plano Clark VL. *Designing and Conducting Mixed Methods Research*. 3rd ed. Thousand Oaks, CA: Sage; 2018.

72. Teddlie C, Yu F. Mixed methods sampling: a typology with examples. *J Mixed Methods Res* 2007;1:77-100.

73. Farmer T, Robinson K, Elliott SJ, Eyles J. Developing and implementing a triangulation protocol for qualitative health research. *Qual Health Res* 2006;16(3):377-394.

74. Plano Clark VL, Schumacher K, West C, Edrington J, Dunn LB, Harzstark A, Melisko M, Rabow MW, Swift PS, Miaskowski C. Practices for embedding an interpretive qualitative approach within a randomized clinical trial. *J Mixed Methods Res* 2013;7(3):219-242.

75. Bachrach CA, Abeles RP. Social science and health research: growth at the National Institutes of Health. *Am J Public Health* 2004;94(1):22-28.

76. Sofaer S. Qualitative methods: what are they and why use them? *Health Serv Res* 1999;34(5 Pt 2):1101-1118.

PART 4

Analyzing Data

C H A P T E R 22 **Descriptive Statistics** 318

C H A P T E R 23 **Foundations of Statistical Inference** 333

C H A P T E R 24 **Comparing Two Means: The *t*-Test** 351

C H A P T E R 25 **Comparing More Than Two Means: Analysis of Variance** 365

C H A P T E R 26 **Multiple Comparison Tests** 383

C H A P T E R 27 **Nonparametric Tests for Group Comparisons** 400

C H A P T E R 28 **Measuring Association for Categorical Variables: Chi-Square** 415

C H A P T E R 29 **Correlation** 428

C H A P T E R 30 **Regression** 440

C H A P T E R 31 **Multivariate Analysis** 468

C H A P T E R 32 **Measurement Revisited: Reliability and Validity Statistics** 486

C H A P T E R 33 **Diagnostic Accuracy** 509

C H A P T E R 34 **Epidemiology: Measuring Risk** 529

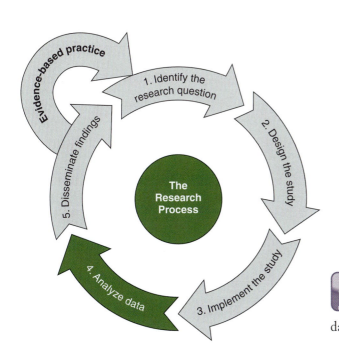

The Data Download icon in tables will indicate that the original data and full output for the data in that table are available in online supplements.

Descriptive Statistics

In the investigation of most clinical research questions, some form of quantitative data will be collected. Initially these data exist in *raw form*, which means that they are nothing more than a compilation of numbers representing empirical observations from a group of individuals. For these data to be useful as measures of group performance, they must be organized, summarized, and analyzed, so that their meaning can be communicated. These are the functions of the branch of mathematics called statistics.

Descriptive statistics are used to characterize the shape, central tendency, and variability within a set of data, often with the intent to describe a sample or population. Measures of population characteristics are called **parameters**. A descriptive index computed from sample data is called a **statistic**. When researchers generalize sample data to populations, they use statistics to estimate population parameters. In this chapter we introduce the basic elements of statistical analysis for describing quantitative data.

■ Frequency Distributions

Because the numerical data collected during a study exist in unanalyzed, unsorted form, a structure is needed that allows us to summarize trends or averages.

> ➤ **CASE IN POINT #1**
>
> Consider a set of hypothetical scores for the Coin Rotation Test (CRT), an assessment of motor dexterity.[1,2] Using a stop watch, a clinician determines the time it takes for the patient to rotate a nickel as rapidly as possible through consecutive 180° turns, using the thumb, index, and middle fingers for 20 rotations. A lower score (shorter time) indicates better dexterity.

Table 22-1A presents a set of hypothetical scores on the CRT for 32 patients with multiple sclerosis. The total set of scores for a particular variable is called a **distribution**. The total number of scores in the distribution is given the symbol N. In this sample, $N = 32$.

> 📌 An uppercase N is used to represent the total number of subjects in a sample. If the sample is divided into groups, a lowercase n is used to indicate the number of subjects in each group.

Although visual inspection of a distribution allows us to see all the scores, this list is long and unwieldy and inadequate for describing this group of patients or comparing them with any other group. We can begin to summarize the data by presenting them in a **frequency distribution**, a table of rank ordered scores that shows the number of times each value occurred, or its *frequency* (f).

The first two columns in Table 22-1B show the frequency distribution for the CRT scores. Now we can tell more readily how the scores are distributed. We can see the lowest and highest scores, where the scores tend to cluster, and which scores occurred most often. The sum of the numbers in the frequency column (f) equals N, the number of subjects or scores in the distribution.

Examining a frequency distribution is also useful as a screening process when first analyzing data. This type of

Table 22-1   Distribution of Scores for the Coin Rotation Test (in seconds) (N= 32)

A. Raw Data

	Score
1	9
2	21
3	23
4	26
5	10
6	16
7	15
8	22
9	30
10	24
11	18
12	32
13	13
14	20
15	21
16	29

	Score
17	19
18	28
19	24
20	15
21	17
22	23
23	20
24	25
25	21
26	26
27	18
28	20
29	19
30	27
31	21
32	22

B. Frequency Distribution

CRTScore

	Frequency	Percent	Cumulative Percent
9.00	1	3.1	3.1
11.00	1	3.1	6.3
13.00	1	3.1	9.4
15.00	2	6.3	15.6
16.00	1	3.1	18.8
17.00	1	3.1	21.9
18.00	2	6.3	28.1
19.00	2	6.3	34.4
20.00	3	9.4	43.8
21.00	4	12.5	56.3
22.00	2	6.3	62.5
23.00	2	6.3	68.8
24.00	2	6.3	75.0
25.00	1	3.1	78.1
26.00	2	6.3	84.4
27.00	1	3.1	87.5
28.00	1	3.1	90.6
29.00	1	3.1	93.8
30.00	1	3.1	96.9
32.00	1	3.1	100.0
Total	32	100.0	

Portions of the output have been omitted for clarity.

presentation can identify outliers (extreme scores) and values that are out of the appropriate range, which may indicate errors in data collection or recording. The number of scores can also be confirmed to match the numbers of subjects in the study.

Percentages

Sometimes frequencies are more meaningfully expressed as percentages of the total distribution. We can look at the percentage represented by each score in the distribution or at the *cumulative percent* obtained by adding the percentage value for each score to all percentages that fall below that score. For example, it may be useful to know that 4 patients, or 12.5% of the sample, had a score of 21, or that 56.3% of the sample had scores of 21 and below.

Percentages are useful for describing distributions because they are independent of sample size. For example, suppose we tested another sample of 200 patients and found that 25 individuals obtained a score of 21 seconds. Although there are more people in this second sample with this score than in the first sample, they both represent the same percentage of the total sample. Therefore, the samples may be more similar than frequencies would indicate.

Grouped Frequency Distributions

When continuous data are collected, researchers will often find that very few subjects, if any, obtain the exact same score, as seen with our CRT scores. Obviously, creating a frequency distribution can be an impractical process if almost every score has a low frequency. In this situation, a *grouped frequency distribution* can be constructed by grouping the scores into intervals, each representing a unique range of scores within the distribution. Frequencies are then assigned to each interval.

Table 22-2A shows a grouped frequency distribution for the CRT data. The intervals represent ranges of 5 seconds. They are *mutually exclusive* (no overlap) and *exhaustive* within the range of scores obtained. The choice of the number of intervals to be used and the range within each one is an arbitrary decision. It depends on the overall range of scores, the number of observations, and how much precision is relevant for analysis.

Although information is inherently lost in grouped data, this approach is often the only feasible way to present large amounts of continuous data. The groupings should be clustered to reveal the important features of the data. The researcher must recognize that the choice of the number of intervals and the range within each interval can influence the interpretation of how a variable is distributed.

Graphing Frequency Distributions

Graphic representation of data often communicates information about trends and general characteristics of distributions more clearly than a tabular frequency distribution. The most common methods of graphing frequency distributions are the histogram, line plot, and stem-and-leaf plot, illustrated in Table 22-2.

Histogram

A **histogram** is a type of bar graph, composed of a series of columns, each representing one score or group interval. A histogram is shown in panel B for the distribution of CRT scores. The frequency for each score is plotted on the Y-axis, and the measured variable, in this case CRT score, is on the X-axis. The bars are centered over the scores. This presentation provides a clear visual depiction of the frequencies.

The curve superimposed on the histogram shows how well the distribution fits a *normal curve*. This will be addressed later in this chapter.

Table 22-2 Various Methods to Display CRT Scores (from Table 22-1)

A. Grouped Frequency Distribution

	Frequency	Percent
5-9	1	3.1
10-14	2	6.3
15-19	8	25.0
20-24	13	40.6
25-29	6	18.7
30-34	2	6.3
Total	32	100.0

B. Histogram

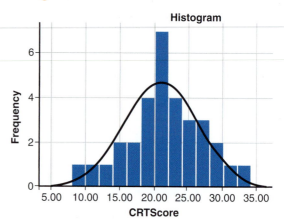

C. Line Plot (Grouped Data)

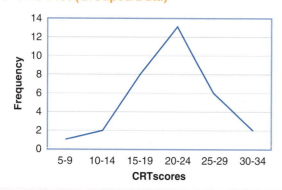

D. Stem-and-Leaf Plot

Frequency	Stem & Leaf
1.00	0 . 9
2.00	1 . 03
8.00	1 . 55678899
13.00	2 . 0001111223344
6.00	2 . 566789
2.00	3 . 02

Line Plot

A line plot, also called a *frequency polygon*, shows data points along a contiguous line. Panel C shows a line plot for the grouped CRT data. When grouped data are used, the points on the line represent the midpoint of each interval.

Stem-and-Leaf Plot

The stem-and-leaf plot is a grouped frequency distribution that is like a histogram turned on its side, but with individual values. It is most useful for presenting the pattern of distribution of a continuous variable, derived by separating each score into two parts. The *leaf* consists of the last or rightmost single digit of each score, and the *stem* consists of the remaining leftmost digits.

Panel D shows a stem-and-leaf plot for the CRT data. The scores have leftmost digits of 0 through 3. These values become the stem. The last digit in each score becomes the leaf. To read the stem-and-leaf plot, we look across each row, attaching each single leaf digit to the stem. Therefore, the first row represents the score 9; the second row, 10 and 13; the third row starts with 15, 15, 16, 17, and so on.

This display provides a concise summary of the data while maintaining the integrity of the original data. If we compare this plot with the grouped frequency distribution or the histogram, it is clear how much more information is provided by the stem-and-leaf plot in a small space and how it provides elements of both tabular and graphic displays.

> 📌 Graphic displays can be essential to a full understanding of data, and to generate hypotheses that may not be obvious from tabular data (see Focus on Evidence 22-1).

Focus on Evidence 22–1
A Picture is Worth a Thousand Words

Most researchers think of statistics as a way to test specific hypotheses, looking for statistical tests that will tell us whether a treatment was effective, or if we can predict certain outcomes. This approach is called *confirmatory data analysis,* which relies on pre-set assumptions about the relationship between independent and dependent variables. One caveat in this effort is the realization that summary values may not always provide meaningful information about individuals, and we must make generalizations and assumptions that allow us to apply such findings to clinical decision making.

In his classic work, Tukey[3] has urged researchers to consider a broader approach as a preliminary step in research, before hypotheses are generated. He has suggested a process called *exploratory data analysis (EDA)* to gain insight into patterns in data. EDA is often referred to as a philosophy as well as an approach to data analysis, requiring a "willingness to look for what can be seen, whether or not anticipated,"—along with flexibility and some graph paper![4]

EDA relies heavily on descriptive statistics and graphic representations of data, allowing researchers to examine variability in different subgroups and to see patterns that might not have otherwise been obvious.[5,6] To illustrate this, researchers were interested in studying the frequency of safety incidents reported in general practice in England and Wales from 2005 to 2013, to identify contributory factors.[7] They used the EDA approach to examine more than 13,000 reports, and found that that among 462 separate clinical locations that provided at least one incident report, over half of the reports originated from only 30 locations (52%), and 67 locations reported only one incident. Using a scatterplot, charting the number of incident reports (*X*-axis) against the degree of harm reported (*Y*-axis), they showed that some organizations did not report safety incidents at all, and that the top reporting locations tended to have incidents with lower harm.

These findings led them to look at thresholds for reporting. For instance, by looking at the dots high on harm but low on number of reports (upper left), the data suggested that some locations appear to file reports only if there is serious harm or deaths. It also shows that those sites with more frequent reporting tended to have less harmful incidents (bottom right). This approach illustrates how graphs can be more powerful than summary statistics to find gaps in scores within a certain range, to identify a particular score that is "somewhere in left field," or to show where there may be a "pile-up" of scores at one point in a distribution.[8] This type of analysis can be used to generate hypotheses, to suggest alternative questions of the data, or to guide further analysis. Other, more complex, statistical procedures can then be used to explore data structures, such as factor analysis and multiple regression (see Chapters 30 and 31).

From Carson-Stevens A, Hibbert P, Williams H. et al. Characterising the nature of primary care patient safety incident reports in the England and Wales National Reporting and Learning System: a mixed-methods agenda-setting study for general practice. *Health Serv Deliv Res* 2016;4(27). Figure 3, p. 15. Used with permission.

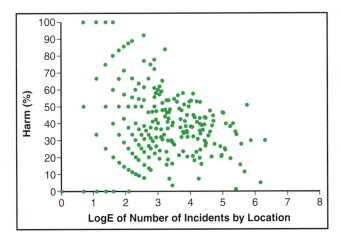

■ Shapes of Distributions

When graphs of frequency distributions are drawn, the distributions can be described by three characteristics: shape, central tendency, and variability. Let's first consider shape. Although real data seldom achieve smooth curves, minor discrepancies are often ignored in an effort to characterize a distribution.

The Normal Curve

Curve B in Figure 22-1 shows a symmetrical distribution called the **normal curve**. In statistical terminology, "normal" refers to a specific type of bell-shaped curve where most of the scores fall in the middle of the scale and progressively fewer fall at the extremes. The unique characteristics of this curve provide a foundation for statistical tests, and will be discussed in greater detail later in this chapter.

Skewed Distributions

A **skewed distribution** is asymmetrical, with fewer scores at one end forming a "tail." The degree to which the distribution deviates from symmetry is its *skewness*, which is described by the side of the longer tail.

Curve A in Figure 22-1 is *positively skewed*, or skewed to the right, because most of the scores cluster at the low end and only a few scores at the high end have caused the tail of the curve to point toward the right. If we were to plot a distribution of home values in the United States, for example, it would be positively skewed, because most homes have low to moderate value, with fewer at the high end.

When the curve "tails off" to the left, the distribution is *negatively skewed*, or skewed to the left, as in Curve C. We might see a negatively skewed distribution if we plotted scores for an easy exam on which most students achieved a high score.

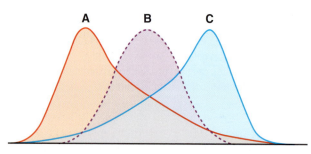

Figure 22–1 Shapes of frequency distributions. A) Skewed to the right, B) Symmetrical normal distribution, C) Skewed to the left.

■ Measures of Central Tendency

Although frequency distributions enable us to order data and identify group patterns, they do not provide a practical quantitative summary of a group's characteristics. Numerical indices are needed to describe the "typical" nature of the data and to reflect different concepts of the "center" of a distribution. These indices are called measures of **central tendency**, or *averages*. The term "average" can actually denote three different measures of central tendency: the mode, median, and mean.

The Mode

The **mode** is the score that occurs most frequently in a distribution. It is most easily determined by inspection of a frequency distribution. For instance, the frequency distribution in Table 22-1 shows that the mode for the CRT data is 21 because it occurs four times, more than any other score. We can also easily see this in the histogram and in the stem-and-leaf plot. When more than one score occurs with the highest frequency, a distribution is considered *bimodal* (with two modes) or *multimodal* (with more than two modes).

The mode has only limited application as a measure of central tendency for continuous data but is most useful in the assessment of categorical variables on nominal or ordinal scales. Many distributions of continuous variables do not have a mode.

The Median

The **median** of a series of observations is that value above which there are as many scores as below it, dividing a rank-ordered distribution into two equal halves.

For the following distribution

$$4, 5, 6, 7, 8$$

with an odd number of scores, the middle score, 6, is the median. With an even number of scores, the midpoint between the two middle scores is the median, so that for the series

$$4, 5, 6, 7, 8, 9$$

the median lies halfway between 6 and 7, or 6.5.

For the distribution of CRT scores given in Table 22-1, with $N = 32$, the median will lie midway between the 16th and 17th scores. As both of these are 21, the median is 21.

The advantage of the median as a measure of central tendency is that it is unaffected by the value of extreme scores. It is an index of average *position* in a distribution, not amount. It is therefore a useful measure in describing skewed distributions or distributions of ordinal scores.

The Mean

The **mean** is the sum of a set of scores divided by the number of scores, *n*. This is the value most people refer to as the "average." The symbol used to represent the mean of a population is the Greek letter mu, μ, and the mean of a sample is represented by $\bar{X}$. The formula for calculation of the sample mean from raw data is

$$\bar{X} = \frac{\sum X}{n}$$

where the Greek letter Σ (sigma) stands for "the sum of." This is read, "the mean equals the sum of *X* divided by *n*," where *X* represents each individual score in the distribution. For example, we can apply this formula to the CRT scores shown in Table 22-1. In this distribution of 32 scores, the sum of scores is 675. Therefore,

$$\bar{X} = \frac{675}{32} = 21.09$$

> 📌 The bar above the *X* indicates that the value is a mean score. Other statistics, with different letter designations, will also be expressed as means with a bar.

Comparing Measures of Central Tendency

Determining which measure of central tendency is most appropriate for describing a distribution depends on several factors. Foremost is the intended application of the data. The level of measurement of the variable is another important consideration. All three measures of central tendency can be applied to variables on the interval or ratio scales, although the mean is most useful. For data on the nominal scale, only the mode is meaningful. If data are ordinal, the median is most useful, but the mode can also be used. It is necessary to consider how the summary measure will be used statistically.

Of the three measures of central tendency, the mean is considered the most stable; that is, if we were to repeatedly draw random samples from a population, the means of those samples would fluctuate less than the mode or median.[9] Only the mean can be subjected to arithmetic manipulations, making it the most reasonable estimate of population characteristics. For this reason, the mean is used more often than the median or mode for statistical analysis of ratio or interval data.

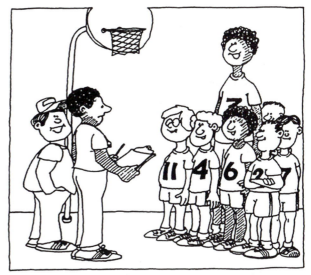

"Should we scare the opposition by announcing our mean height or lull them by announcing our median height?"

From Macmillan Publishing.

Central Tendency and Skewness

We can also consider the utility of the three measures of central tendency for describing distributions of different shapes. With normal distributions, the mean, median, and mode are the same value, and therefore any of the three averages can be applied with validity. With skewed distributions, however, the mean is limited as a descriptive measure because, unlike the median and mode, it is affected by the quantitative value of every score in a distribution and can be biased by extreme scores. For instance, in the example of CRT scores (Table 22-1), if subject #12 had obtained a score of 80 instead of 32, the mean would increase from 21.09 to 22.6. The median and mode would be unaffected by this change.

The curves in Figure 22-2 illustrate how measures of central tendency are typically affected by skewness. The median will usually fall between the mode and the mean in a skewed curve, and the mean will be pulled toward the tail. Because of these properties, the choice of which index to report with skewed distributions depends on what facet of information is appropriate to the analysis. It may be reasonable to report two or three of these values to present a complete picture of a distribution's characteristics.

> 🔑 The relationship between mean, median and mode in skewed distributions can vary from this typical pattern, especially when distributions are multimodal, where one tail is long but the other is heavy, or in discrete distributions where the areas to the left and right of the median are not equal.[10]

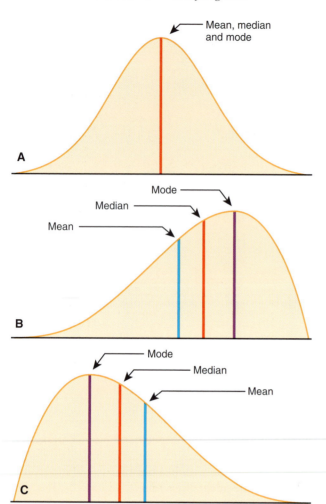

Figure 22–2 Typical relationship of the mean, median and mode in A) normal, B) negatively skewed, and C) positively skewed distributions. The mean is pulled toward the tail of skewed curves.

■ Measures of Variability

The shape and central tendency of a distribution are useful but incomplete descriptors of a sample. Consider the following dilemma:

You are responsible for planning the musical entertainment for a party of seven individuals, but you don't know what kind of music to choose — so you decide to use their average age as a guide.

The guests' ages are
3, 3, 13, 14, 59, 70, and 78 years

Mode = 3
Median = 14
Mean = 34.3

If you based your decision on the mode, you would bring in characters from Sesame Street. Using the median you might hire a heavy metal band. And according to the mean age of 34.3 years, you might decide to play soft rock, although nobody in the group is actually in that age range. And the Frank Sinatra fans are completely overlooked!

What we are ignoring is the spread of ages within the group. Consider now a more concrete example using the hypothetical CRT scores reported in Table 22-3 for two groups of patients. If we were to describe these two distributions using only measures of central tendency, they would appear identical. However, a careful glance reveals that the scores for Group B are more widely scattered than those for Group A. This difference in *variability*, or *dispersion* of scores, is an essential element in data analysis.

The description of a sample is not complete unless we can characterize the differences that exist *among* the scores as well as the central tendency of the data. This section will describe five commonly used statistical measures of variability: range, percentiles, variance, standard deviation, and coefficient of variation.

Range

The simplest measure of variability is the **range**, which is the difference between the highest and lowest values in a distribution. For the test scores reported in Table 22-3,

Group A range: 20–14 = 6
Group B range: 28–9 = 19

These values suggest that the Group A is more homogeneous.

Although the range is a relatively simple statistical measure, its applicability is limited because it is determined using only the two extreme scores in the distribution. It reflects nothing about the dispersion of scores between the two extremes. One aberrant extreme score can greatly increase the range, even though the variability within the rest of the data set is unchanged.

The range of scores also tends to increase with larger samples, making it an ineffective value for comparing distributions with different numbers of scores. Therefore, although it is easily computed, the range is usually employed only as a rough descriptive measure and is typically reported in conjunction with other indices of variability.

Rather than reporting range as the difference between scores, research reports will usually provide the actual minimum and maximum scores, which is more useful information to characterize a sample.

Table 22-3 Descriptive Statistics for CRT Scores (in seconds) for Two Groups

Group A

	Score
1	14
2	15
3	16
4	18
5	18
6	18
7	19
8	20

Descriptives

		Group A	Group B
N	Valid	8	8
Mean		17.250	17.250
Median		18.000	18.000
Mode		18.00	18.00
Std. Deviation		2.053	6.251
Variance		4.214	39.071
Range		6.00	19.00
Minimum		14.00	9.00
Maximum		20.00	28.00
Percentiles	25	15.250	11.000
	50	18.000	18.00
	75	18.750	21.250

Group B

	Score
1	9
2	10
3	14
4	18
5	18
6	19
7	22
8	28

Percentiles and Quartiles

Percentiles are used to describe a score's position within a distribution relative to all other scores. Percentiles divide data into 100 equal portions. A particular score is located in one of these portions. Percentiles are helpful for converting actual scores into comparative scores or for providing a reference point for interpreting a particular score. For instance, a child who fits in the 20th percentile (P_{20}) for weight in his age group can be evaluated relative to his peer group, rather than considering only the absolute value of his weight.

Most of us are familiar with the use of percentiles in standardized exams, like the SAT and GRE. If a student's score is in the 92nd percentile (P_{92}), that individual's score was higher than 92% of those who took the test.

Quartiles divide a distribution into four equal parts, or quarters. Quartiles Q1, Q2, and Q3 correspond to percentiles at 25%, 50%, and 75% of the distribution (P_{25}, P_{50}, P_{75}). The score at the 50th percentile or Q2, is the median. The distance between the first and third quartiles, Q3 – Q1, is called the **interquartile range**, which represents the spread of scores within the middle 50% of the data. As shown in the results in Table 22-3, the interquartile range, the difference from P_{25} to P_{75}, is 3.5 for Group A and 10.25 for Group B, again illustrating the difference in their variability.

Box Plots

A **box plot** graph is a useful way to visually demonstrate the spread of scores in a distribution, including the range, median and interquartile range. The plots in Figure 22-3 represent the scores for Groups A and B from Table 23-3. The "box" represents the interquartile range, and the horizontal line is the median or 50th percentile. Also called

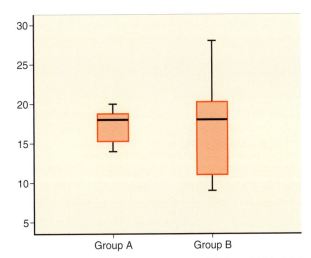

Figure 22–3 Box plots for Groups A and B from Table 22-3. Each box spans the interquartile range, and the horizontal line is the median score. The "whiskers" represent the minimum and maximum score in each group.

box-and-whisker plots, these graphs are usually drawn with "whiskers" representing the range of scores. Sometimes these will indicate the highest and lowest scores, or they can be drawn at the 90th and 10th percentiles (see Focus on Evidence 22-2). These plots clearly show that Group B is more variable than Group A, even though their medians are the same.

Variance

Measures of range have limited application as indices of variability because they are not influenced by every score in a distribution and are sensitive to extreme scores. To more completely describe a distribution, we need an index that reflects the variation within a full set of scores. This value should be small if scores are close together and large if they are spread out. It should also be objective so that we can compare samples of different sizes and determine if one is more variable than another. It is useful to consider how these values are derived to better understand their application.

Deviation Scores

We can begin to examine variability by looking at the deviation of each score from the mean. By subtracting the mean from each score in the distribution we obtain a *deviation score*, $X-\bar{X}$. Obviously, samples with larger deviation scores will be more variable around the mean. To illustrate this, let's just focus on the distribution of scores from Group B in Table 22-3. The deviation scores for this sample are shown in Table 22-4A. The mean of the distribution is 17.25. For the score $X = 9$, the deviation score will be $9 - 17.25 = -8.25$. Note that the first three deviation scores are negative values because these scores are smaller than the mean.

As a measure of variability, the deviation score has intuitive appeal, as these scores will obviously be larger as scores become more heterogeneous and farther from the mean. It might seem reasonable, then, to take the average of these values, or the *mean deviation*, as an index of dispersion within the sample. This is a useless exercise, however, because the sum of the deviation scores will always equal zero, as illustrated in the second column in Table 22-4A $[\Sigma(X - \bar{X}) = 0]$. If we think of the mean as a central balance point for a distribution, then it makes sense that the scores will be equally dispersed above and below that central point.

Focus on Evidence 22–2
The Plot Thickens

Box plots can provide useful visual clarification of how different groups compare in their variability and central tendency. For example, Morone et al[11] studied the use of the Wii video game system for balance exercise compared with standard balance therapy for patients who had experienced strokes. Functional outcome, based on the Barthel Index, was measured at three time intervals: baseline (T0), after 4 weeks of intervention (T1), and at follow-up (T2). The results showed that improvement was significantly greater for the group that used the Wii system.

Box plots were created for each group at each time period (T0 = white, T1 = green, T2 = blue). In this example, the whiskers indicate 10th and 90th percentiles, and circles beyond the whiskers indicate scores beyond these limits. These scores are considered outliers, which are scores that fall an abnormal distance from other values in a distribution.

The side-by-side box plots allow for easy comparisons, showing that the spread of scores was quite wide at baseline and decreased at T1 and T2 in both groups. This decreased variability was much more marked in the Wii group, however. Stars indicate significantly better improvement in the Wii group at T1 and T2.

Besides just determining that the groups are statistically different, researchers can use boxplots to provide important information for interpreting group differences. For instance, although the variability in the Wii group was certainly smaller than in the control group, there were also many more outliers in this group at T1, indicating that several patients did not respond with "average" scores. This variability did decrease, however, at T2, with only one outlier score.

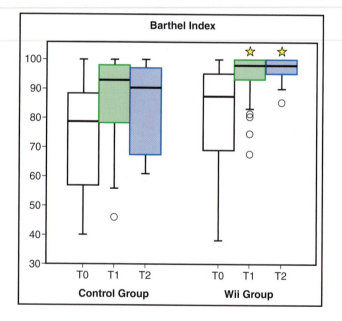

From Morone G, Tramontano M, Iosa M, et al. The efficacy of balance training with video game-based therapy in subacute stroke patients: a randomized controlled trial. *Biomed Res Int* 2014; Volume 2014, Article ID 580861, 6 pages, http://dx.doi.org/10.1155/2014/580861. Figure 2, p. 4. Used with permission.

| Table 22-4 | Calculation of Variance and Standard Deviation using Group B CRT Scores (from Table 22-3) | |

A. Data

X	$(X - \bar{X})$	$(X - \bar{X})^2$
9	−8.25	68.06
10	−7.25	52.56
14	−3.25	10.56
18	0.75	0.56
18	0.75	0.56
19	1.75	3.06
22	4.75	22.56
28	10.75	115.56
$\Sigma X = 138$	$\Sigma(X - \bar{X}) = 0.00$	$\Sigma(X - \bar{X})^2 = 273.48$
$\bar{X} = 17.25$		

B. Calculations

Variance:

$$s^2 = \frac{\Sigma(X - \bar{X})^2}{n - 1} = \frac{273.48}{7} = 39.07$$

Standard Deviation:

$$s = \sqrt{\frac{\Sigma(X - \bar{X})^2}{n - 1}} = \sqrt{39.07} = 6.25$$

Sum of Squares and Variance

Statisticians solve this dilemma by squaring each deviation score to get rid of the minus signs, as shown in the third column of Table 22-4A. The *sum of the squared deviation scores*, $\Sigma(X - \bar{X})^2$, shortened to **sum of squares (SS)**, will be larger as variability increases.

We now have a number we can use to describe the sample's variability. In this case,

$$\Sigma(X - \bar{X})^2 = 273.48$$

As an index of relative variability, however, the sum of squares is limited because it can be influenced by the sample size; that is, as *n* increases, the sum will also tend to increase simply because there are more scores. To eliminate this problem, the sum of squares is divided by *n*, to obtain the *mean of the squared deviation scores*, shortened to **mean square, (MS)**. This value is a true measure of variability and is also called the **variance**.

> Hold onto these concepts. The sum of squares (*SS*) and mean square (*MS*) will be used many times as we describe statistical tests in future chapters.

Population Parameters.
For population data, the variance is symbolized by σ^2 (lowercase Greek sigma squared). When the population mean is known, deviation scores are obtained by $X - \mu$. Therefore, the population variance is defined by

$$\sigma^2 = \frac{SS}{N} = \frac{\Sigma(X - \mu)^2}{N}$$

Sample Statistics.
With sample data, deviation scores are obtained using $\bar{X}$, not μ. Because sample data do not include all the observations in a population, the sample mean is only an estimate of the population mean. This substitution results in a sample variance slightly smaller than the true population variance. To compensate for this bias, the sum of squares is divided by $n-1$ to calculate the sample variance, given the symbol s^2:

$$s^2 = \frac{SS}{n - 1} = \frac{\Sigma(X - \bar{X})^2}{n - 1}$$

This corrected statistic is considered an *unbiased estimate* of the parameter σ^2. The descriptive statistics in Table 22-3 show that $s^2 = 4.21$ for Group A and $s^2 = 39.07$ for Group B. The variance for Group B is substantially larger than for Group A.

Standard Deviation

The limitation of variance as a descriptive measure of a sample's variability is that it was calculated using the squares of the deviation scores. It is generally not useful to describe sample variability in terms of squared units, such as seconds squared. Therefore, to bring the index back into the original units of measurement, we take the square root of the variance. This value is called the **standard deviation**, symbolized by *s*. As shown in Table 22-3, $s = 2.05$ for Group A, and $s = 6.25$ for Group B.

> Research reports may use *sd* or *SD* to indicate standard deviation.

The standard deviation of sample data is usually reported along with the mean so that the data are characterized according to both central tendency and variability. Therefore, a mean may be expressed as

$$\text{Group A: } \bar{X} = 17.25 \pm 2.05$$
$$\text{Group B: } \bar{X} = 17.25 \pm 6.25$$

The smaller standard deviation for Group A indicates that the scores are less spread out around the mean than the scores for Group B.

Variance and standard deviation are fundamental components in any analysis of data. We will explore the application of these concepts to many statistical procedures throughout the coming chapters.

> When means are not whole numbers, calculation of deviation scores can be biased by rounding. Computational formulae provide more accurate results. See the *Chapter 22 Supplement* for calculations using the computational formula for variance and standard deviations.

Coefficient of Variation

The **coefficient of variation (CV)** is another measure of variability that can be used to describe data measured on the interval or ratio scale. It is the ratio of the standard deviation to the mean, expressed as a percentage:

$$CV = \frac{s}{\bar{X}} \times 100$$

There are two major advantages to this index. First, it is independent of units of measurement because units will mathematically cancel out. Therefore, it is a practical statistic for comparing variability in distributions recorded in different units.

Second, the coefficient of variation expresses the standard deviation as a proportion of the mean, thereby accounting for differences in the magnitude of the mean. The coefficient of variation is, therefore, a measure of *relative variation*, most meaningful when comparing two distributions.

These advantages can be illustrated using data from a study of normal values of lumbar spine range of motion, in which data were recorded in both degrees and inches of excursion.[12] The mean ranges for 20- to 29-year-olds were

$$\text{Degrees: } \bar{X} = 41.2 \pm 9.6 \text{ degrees}$$
$$\text{Inches: } \bar{X} = 3.7 \pm 0.72 \text{ inches}$$

The absolute values of the standard deviations for these two measurements suggest that the measure of inches, using a tape measure, was much less variable—but because the means and units are substantially different, the standard deviations are not directly comparable.

By calculating the coefficient of variation, we get a better idea of the relative variation of these two measurements:

$$\text{Degrees: } \quad CV = \frac{9.6}{41.2} \times 100 = 23.3\%$$

$$\text{Inches: } \quad CV = \frac{0.72}{3.7} \times 100 = 19.5\%$$

Now we can see that the variability within these two distributions is actually fairly similar. As this example illustrates, the coefficient of variation is a useful measure for making comparisons among patient groups or different clinical assessments to determine if some are more stable than others.

■ The Normal Distribution

Earlier in this chapter, the symmetrical **normal curve** was described. This distribution represents an important statistical concept because many biological, psychological, and social phenomena manifest themselves in populations according to this shape.

Unfortunately, in the real world we can only estimate such data from samples and therefore cannot expect data to fit the normal curve exactly. For practical purposes, then, the normal curve represents a theoretical concept only, with well-defined properties that allow us to make statistical estimates about populations using sample data. For example, a normal curve was superimposed on the CRT data in Table 22-2.

> The normal distribution is called a *Gaussian distribution* after Carl Friedrich Gauss who identified its properties.

Proportions of the Normal Curve

The statistical appeal of the normal distribution is that its characteristics are constant and therefore predictable. As shown in Figure 22-4, the curve is smooth, symmetrical, and bell-shaped, with most of the scores clustered around the mean. The mean, median, and mode have the same value.

> The fact that the normal curve is important to statistical theory should not imply that data are not useful or valid if they are not normally distributed. Such data can be handled using statistics appropriate to non-normal distributions (see Chapter 27).

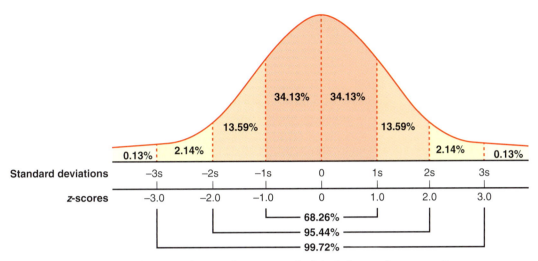

Figure 22–4 Areas under the normal curve, showing standard deviations and corresponding z-scores.

The vertical axis of the curve represents the frequency of data. The frequency of scores decreases steadily as scores move in a negative or positive direction away from the mean, with relatively rare observations at the extremes. Theoretically, there are no boundaries to the curve; that is, scores potentially exist with infinite magnitude above and below the mean. Therefore, the tails of the curve approach but never quite touch the baseline (called an *asymptotic curve*).

Because of these standard properties, we can also determine the proportional areas under the curve represented by the standard deviations in a normal distribution. Statisticians have shown that 34.13% of the area under the normal curve is bounded by the mean and the score one standard deviation above or below the mean. Therefore, 68.26% of the total distribution (the majority) will have scores within ±1 standard deviation (±1*s*) from the mean.

Similarly, ±2*s* from the mean will encompass 95.45%, and ±3*s* will cover 99.73% of the total area under the curve. At ±3*s* we have accounted for virtually the entire distribution. Because we can never discount extreme values at either end, we never account for the full 100%. This information can be used as a basis for interpreting standard deviations.

> ► **CASE IN POINT #2**
> For this next section, properties of the normal curve will be illustrated using hypothetical scores for pulse rates from a sample of 100 patients, with $\bar{X}$ = 68 and *s* = 10 beats per minute (bpm). Therefore, we can estimate that approximately 68% of the individuals in the sample have scores between 58 and 78 bpm.

Standardized Scores

Statistical data are meaningful only when they are applied in some quantitative context. For example, if a patient has a pulse rate of 58 bpm, the implication of that value is evident only if we know where that score falls in relation to a distribution of normal pulse rates. If we know that $\bar{X}$ = 68 and *s* = 10 for a given sample, then we also know that an individual score of 58 is one standard deviation below the mean. This gives us a clearer interpretation of the score.

When we express scores in terms of standard deviation units, we are using **standardized scores**, also called **z-scores**. For this example, a score of 58 can be expressed as a z-score of −1.0, the minus sign indicating that it is one standard deviation unit below the mean. A score of 88 is similarly transformed to a z-score of +2.0, or two standard deviations above the mean.

A z-score is computed by dividing the deviation of an individual score from the mean by the standard deviation:

$$z = \frac{X - \bar{X}}{s}$$

Using the example of pulse rates, for an individual score of 85 bpm, with $\bar{X}$ = 68 and *s* = 10,

$$z = \frac{85 - 68}{10} = \frac{17}{10} = 1.7$$

Thus, 85 bpm is 1.7 standard deviations above the mean.

The Standardized Normal Curve

The normal distribution can also be described in terms of standardized scores. The mean of a normal distribution of *z*-scores will always equal zero (no deviation from the mean), and the standard deviation will always be 1.0.

As shown in Figure 22-4, the area under the standardized normal curve between $z = 0$ and $z = +1.0$ is approximately 34%, the same as that defined by the area between the mean ($z = 0$) and one standard deviation. The total area within $z = \pm 1.00$ is 68.26%. Similarly, the total area within $z = \pm 2.00$ is 95.45%. Using this model, we can determine the proportional area under the curve bounded by any two points in a normal distribution.

Determining Areas under the Normal Curve

We can illustrate this process using our pulse rate example. Suppose we want to determine what percentage of our sample has a pulse rate above 80 bpm. First, we determine the *z*-score for 80 bpm:

$$z = \frac{80 - 68}{10} = \frac{12}{10} = 1.2$$

Therefore, 80 bpm is slightly more than one standard deviation above the mean. Now we want to determine the proportion of our total sample that is represented by all scores above 80, or above $z = 1.2$. This is the shaded area above 80 in Figure 22-5.

These values are given in Appendix Table A-1. This table is arranged in three columns, one containing *z*-scores and the other two representing areas either from 0 to *z* or above *z* (in one tail of the curve). For this example, we are interested in the area above *z*, or above 1.2. If we look to the right of $z = 1.20$ in Table A-1, we find that the area above *z* equals .1151. Therefore, scores above 80 bpm represent 11.51% of the total distribution.

For another example, let's determine the area above 50 bpm. First we determine the *z*-score for 50 bpm:

$$z = \frac{50 - 68}{10} = \frac{-18}{10} = -1.8$$

Therefore, 50 bpm is slightly less than two standard deviations below the mean.

Now we want to determine the proportion of our total sample that is represented by all scores above 50, or above $z = -1.8$. We already know that the scores above the mean (above $z = 0$) represent 50% of the curve, as shown by the dark green area in Figure 22-6. Therefore, we are now concerned with the light green area between 68 and 50, which is equal to the area from $z = 0$ to $z = -1.8$. Together these two shaded areas represent the total area above 50.

Table A-1 uses only absolute values of *z*. Because it includes standardized units for a symmetrical curve, the proportional area from 0 to $z = +1.8$ is the same as the area from 0 to $z = -1.8$. The area between $z = 0$ and $z = -1.8$ is .4641. Therefore, the total area under the curve for all scores above 50 bpm will be .50 + .4641 = .9641, or 96.41%.

Standardized scores are useful for interpreting an individual's standing relative to a normalized group. For example, many standardized tests, such as psychological, developmental, and intelligence tests, use *z*-scores to demonstrate that an individual's score is above or below the "norm" (the standardized mean) or to show what proportion of the subjects in a distribution fall within a certain range of scores.

The validity of estimates using the standard normal curve depends on the closeness with which a sample approximates the normal distribution. Many clinical samples are too small to provide an adequate approximation and are more accurately described as "non-normal."

With skewed distributions, values like means and standard deviations can be misleading and may contribute to statistical misinterpretations.[9] Areas under the curve are only relevant to the normal curve.

Goodness of fit tests can be applied to distributions to determine how well the data fit a normal curve (see Chapter 23).

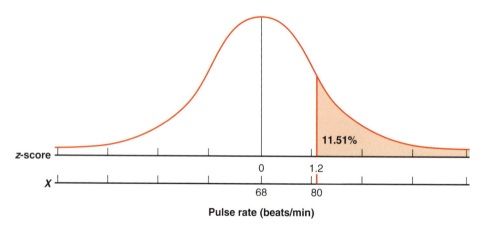

z-score

X

Pulse rate (beats/min)

11.51%

0   1.2

68   80

Figure 22–5 Distribution of pulse rates with $\bar{X} = 68$ and $s = 10$, showing the area under the normal curve above 80 bpm, or $z = 1.2$. The shaded area in the tail of the curve represents 11.51% of the curve (from Table A-1).

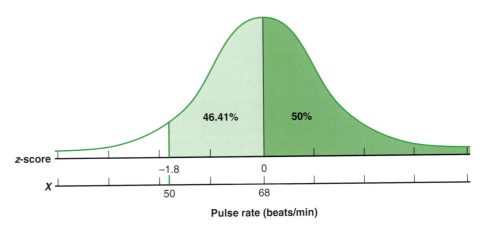

Figure 22–6 Distribution of pulse rates with $\bar{X} = 68$ and $s = 10$, showing the area under the normal curve above 50 bpm, or $z = -1.8$. The light green area represents $z = 0$ to $-1.8 = .4641$ (from Table A-1). The dark green area represents 50% of the distribution. Together, the shaded areas represent 96.41% of the total area under the curve.

COMMENTARY

A statistician is a person who lays with his head in an oven and his feet in a deep freeze, and says "on the average, I feel comfortable."

—*C. Bruce Grossman (1921-2001)*

Professor

Descriptive statistics are the building blocks for data analysis. They serve an obvious function in that they summarize important features of quantitative data. Every study will include a description of participants and responses using one or more measures of central tendency and variance as a way of profiling the study sample, understanding the variables being studied, and establishing the framework for further analysis.

Descriptive measures do not, however, provide a basis for inferring anything that goes beyond the data themselves. Such interpretations come from inferential statistics, which will be covered in following chapters. It is essential to understand, however, that these inferential tests are founded on certain assumptions about data such as central tendency, variance, and the degree to which the distribution approaches the normal curve. Examination of descriptive data through graphic representation can usually provide important insights into how the data are behaving and how they can best be analyzed.

The take-home message is the importance of descriptive statistics as the basis for sound statistical reasoning and the generation of further hypotheses.[9] Descriptive analyses are necessary to demonstrate that statistical tests are used appropriately and that their interpretations are valid.[13]

REFERENCES

1. Mendoza JE, Apostolos GT, Humphreys JD, Hanna-Pladdy B, O'Bryant SE. Coin rotation task (CRT): a new test of motor dexterity. *Arch Clin Neuropsychol* 2009;24(3):287-292.
2. Hill BD, Barkemeyer CA, Jones GN, Santa Maria MP, Browndyke JN. Validation of the coin rotation task: a simple, inexpensive, and convenient screening tool for impaired psychomotor processing speed. *The Neurologist* 2010;16(4): 249-253.
3. Tukey JW. *Exploratory Data Analysis*. Boston: Addison-Wesley; 1977.
4. Tukey JW. We need both exploratory and confirmatory. *Am Stat* 1980;34(1):23-25.
5. NIST/SEMATECH e-Handbook of Statistical Methods. Available at http://www.itl.nist.gov/div898/handbook/index.htm. Accessed May 19, 2017.
6. Hartwig F, Dearing BE. *Exploratory Data Analysis*. Thousand Oaks, CA: Sage Publications; 1979.
7. Cohen J. Things I have learned (so far). *Am Psychologist* 1990; 45(12):1304-1312.
8. Carson-Stevens A, Hibbert P, Williams H, Evans HP, Cooper A, Rees P, Deakin A, Shiels E, Gibson R, Butlin A, et al. Characterising the nature of primary care patient safety incident reports in the England and Wales National Reporting and Learning System: a mixed-methods agenda-setting study for general practice. *Health Serv Deliv Res*, 2016. Available at https://www.ncbi.nlm.nih.gov/books/NBK385186/. Accessed June 11, 2019.

9. Gonzales VA, Ottenbacher KJ. Measures of central tendency in rehabilitation research: what do they mean? *Am J Phys Med Rehabil* 2001;80(2):141-146.

10. von Hippel PT. Mean, median and skew: Correcting a textbook rule. *J Stat Educ* 2005;13(2):Available at http://ww2.amstat.org/publications/jse/v13n12/vonhippel.html. Accessed October 26, 2017.

11. Morone G, Tramontano M, Iosa M, Shofany J, Iemma A, Musicco M, Paolucci S, Caltagirone C. The efficacy of balance training with video game-based therapy in subacute stroke patients: a randomized controlled trial. *Biomed Res Int* 2014; 2014:580861.

12. Fitzgerald GK, Wynveen KJ, Rheault W, Rothschild B. Objective assessment with establishment of normal values for lumbar spinal range of motion. *Phys Ther* 1983;63(11): 1776-1781.

13. Findley TW. Research in physical medicine and rehabilitation. IX. Primary data analysis. *Am J Phys Med Rehabil* 1990;69(4): 209-218.

Foundations of Statistical Inference

In the previous chapter, statistics were presented that can be used to summarize and describe data. Descriptive procedures are not sufficient, however, for testing theories about the effects of experimental treatments, for exploring relationships among variables, or for generalizing the behavior of samples to a population. For these purposes, researchers use a process of *statistical inference.*

Inferential statistics involve a decision-making process that allows us to estimate unknown population characteristics from sample data. The success of this process requires that we make certain assumptions about how well a sample represents the larger population. These assumptions are based on two important concepts of statistical reasoning: probability and sampling error. The purpose of this chapter is to demonstrate the application of these concepts for drawing valid conclusions from research data. These principles will be applied across several statistical procedures in future chapters.

■ Probability

Probability is a complex but essential concept for understanding inferential statistics. We all have some notion of what probability means, as evidenced by the use of terms such as "likely," "probably," or "a good chance." We use probability as a means of prediction: "There is a 50% chance of rain tomorrow," or "This operation has a 75% chance of success."

Statistically, we can view probability as a system of rules for analyzing a complete set of possible outcomes. For instance, when flipping a coin, there are two possible outcomes. When tossing a die, there are six possible outcomes. An event is a single observable outcome, such as the appearance of tails or a 3 on the toss of a die.

Probability is the likelihood that any one event will occur, given all the possible outcomes.

We use a lowercase p to signify probability, expressed as a ratio or decimal. For example, the likelihood of getting tails on any single coin flip will be 1 out of 2, or 1/2, or .5. Therefore, we say that the probability of getting tails is 50%, or $p = .5$. The probability that we will roll a 3 on one roll of a die is 1/6, or $p = .167$. Conversely, the probability that we will not roll a 3 is 5/6, or $p = .833$. These probabilities are based on the assumption that the coin or die is unbiased. Therefore, the outcomes are a matter of chance, representing random events.

For an event that is certain to occur, $p = 1.00$. For instance, if we toss a die, the probability of rolling a 3 or not rolling a 3 is 1.00 ($p = .167 + .833$). These two events are *mutually exclusive* and *complementary* events because they cannot occur together and they represent all possible outcomes. Therefore, the sum of their probabilities will always equal 1.00. We can also show that the probability of an impossible event is zero. For instance, the probability of rolling a 7 with one die is 0 out of 6, or $p = 0.00$. In the real world, the probability for most events falls somewhere between 0 and 1. Scientists will generally admit that nothing is a "sure bet" and nothing is impossible!

Applying Probability to a Distribution

> ➤ **CASE IN POINT #1**
> Suppose we had access to records of birth weights for all live-born infants in the United States in the past year. This hypothetical distribution of millions of scores would likely approximate the normal curve. Assume we find that the population parameters for birth weight in the United States are $\mu = 7.5$ pounds with $\sigma = 1.25$. Let's see how these data can help us understand how samples and populations differ.

If we were to select one infant at random from this population, what is the probability that the infant's birth weight would be between 6.25 and 8.75 lbs, or within ±1 standard deviation of the mean? Based on the characteristics of the normal population, there is a 68% probability ($p = .68$) that any one infant we select will fall within this range (see Fig. 23-1).

Similarly, the probability of selecting an infant weighing more than 11.25 lbs (scores beyond +3 standard deviations) is .0013, as this area represents 0.13% of the total distribution, as shown by the orange area in the tail of the curve. Expectant mothers would be pleased to know that there is very little chance of this occurring!

Interpreting Probability

It is important to understand that probability implies uncertainty. It is predictive in that it reflects what *should* happen over the long run, not necessarily what will happen for any given trial or event. When a surgeon advises that an operation has a 75% probability of success, it means that in the long run, for all such cases, 75% can be expected to be successful. For any single patient the surgery will not be 75% successful—it will either be a success or not. Therefore, once an event occurs, it is no longer "probable." It either happened as

predicted or not. Probability applies to the proportion of time we can *expect* a given outcome to occur in the idealized "long run."

We use probability in research as a guideline for making decisions about how well sample data estimate the characteristics of a population. We also use probabilities to determine if observed effects are likely to have occurred *by chance*. We try to estimate what would happen to others in the population on the basis of our limited sample. To understand these applications of probability, we must first understand the statistical relationship between samples and populations.

■ Sampling Error

The estimation of population characteristics from sample data is based on the assumption that samples are random and valid representatives of the population (see Chapter 13). Even when truly random samples are used, however, we cannot be sure that one sample's characteristics will be identical to those of the population.

Suppose we measure the weights of 10 randomly selected infants and find that $\overline{X} = 6.8$ lbs and $s = 1.5$. Because selection was unbiased, this sample should be a good representative of the population. However, the sample mean and standard deviation are somewhat different from the population values and, therefore, do not provide accurate estimates. What would account for this difference?

If we were to choose a second sample of 10 infants, we would probably obtain yet a different mean and standard deviation. The tendency for sample values to differ from population values is called **sampling error**. *Sampling error of the mean* for any single sample is equal to the difference between the sample mean and the population mean ($\overline{X} - \mu$). In practice, sampling error is unpredictable

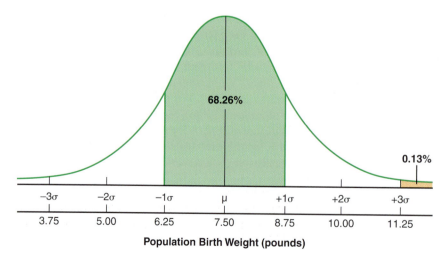

Figure 23–1 Hypothetical distribution of birth weights, with $\mu = 7.5$ and $\sigma = 1.25$. The green area represents ±1 σ, or 68.26% of the population. The orange area in the right tail represents ≥3 σ, or 0.13% of the population.

because it occurs strictly by chance, by virtue of who happens to get picked for any one sample.

Sampling Distributions

Theoretically, if we were to randomly draw an infinite number of samples from a population, each with $n = 10$, the means of these samples would exhibit varying degrees of sampling error. But because the majority of the population falls within ±1 standard deviation, we would expect, by chance, that most of the sample means would cluster around the population mean.

This set of sample means is called a *sampling distribution of means*. If we plotted all the sample means, we would find that the distribution would take the shape of a normal curve, and that the mean of the sample means would be equal to the population mean. Because no one goes through such a process in practice, sampling distributions are only theoretical. However, because of the predictable properties of the normal curve, we can use the concept of the sampling distribution to formulate a basis for drawing inferences from sample data.

Standard Error of the Mean

We can also establish the variance properties of a sampling distribution of means. The standard deviation is called the **standard error of the mean ($\sigma_{\bar{X}}$)**. This value is considered an estimate of the population standard deviation, σ. The histogram and curve in Figure 23-2A represent a hypothetical sampling distribution formed by repeated sampling of birth weights with samples of $n = 10$. The means of such small samples tend to vary, and in fact, we see a wide curve with great variability.

The sampling distribution in Figure 23-2B was constructed from the same population but with samples of $n = 50$. These sample means form a narrower distribution with less variability and therefore a smaller standard deviation. As sample size increases, samples become more representative of the population, and their means are more likely to be closer to the population mean; that is, their sampling error will be smaller. Therefore, the standard deviation of the sampling distribution is an indicator of the degree of sampling error, reflecting how accurately the various sample means estimate the population mean.

Because we do not actually construct a sampling distribution, we need a way to estimate the standard error of the mean from sample data. This estimate, $s_{\bar{X}}$, is based on the standard deviation and size of the sample:

$$s_{\bar{X}} = \frac{s}{\sqrt{n}}$$

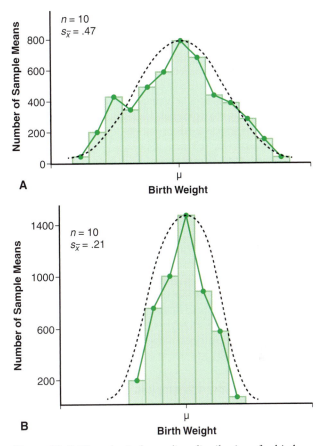

Figure 23–2 Hypothetical sampling distributions for birth weight. Curve A is drawn for samples with $n = 10$. Curve B is drawn for samples with $n = 50$, showing less variability among sample means.

Using our example of birth weights, for a single sample of 10 infants, with mean of 6.8 and a standard deviation of 1.5:

$$s_{\bar{X}} = \frac{1.5}{\sqrt{10}} = 0.47$$

With a sample of $n = 50$,

$$s_{\bar{X}} = \frac{1.5}{\sqrt{50}} = 0.21$$

As n increases, the standard error of the mean decreases. With larger samples the sampling distribution is expected to be less variable, and therefore a statistic based on a larger sample is considered a better estimate of a population parameter than one based on a smaller sample. A sample mean, together with its standard error, helps us imagine what the sampling distribution curve would look like.

🔑 Estimating population values from a sample requires that we make certain assumptions about the shape of the sampling distribution based on the sample. However, if we do not have a normal sample, it is not possible to know the shape of the sampling distribution unless our sample is quite large. You may see reference to two types of "resampling" methods in the literature, effectively using sample data for this purpose. A large number of smaller samples are drawn from the total sample using random selection (by a computer of course!). With a *bootstrap* procedure this is done *with replacement*, which means that each score is put back into a sample before another score is chosen (which means some scores could end up being in a sample more than once). A *jackknife* procedure is considered less cumbersome, using a *leave one out* method, sequentially deleting one observation from the data set for each sample drawn. With either method, the parameter of interest (such as a mean or any other statistic) is calculated for each smaller sample. Then the standard deviation of these scores can be used as the standard error of the parameter estimate or as an estimate of confidence limits. Essentially the total sample data are used to represent the population from which smaller samples are taken. These methods are considered useful for reducing bias in data to achieve more accurate population estimates.

■ Confidence Intervals

We can use our knowledge of sampling distributions to estimate population parameters in two ways. A *point estimate* is a single value obtained by direct calculation from sample data, such as using $\bar{X}$ to estimate μ. Using our sample of birth weights, the point estimate of μ is the sample mean, 6.8 lbs.

Because a single sample value will most likely contain some degree of error, it is more meaningful to use an *interval estimate*, by which we specify a range within which we believe the population parameter will lie. Such an estimate takes into consideration not only the value of a single sample statistic but the relative accuracy of that statistic as well.

For instance, we might guess that the population mean for birth weight is likely to be within 0.5 lbs of the sample mean, to fall within the interval 6.3 to 7.3 lbs. We must be more precise than guessing allows, however, in proposing such an interval, so that we can be "confident" that the interval is an accurate estimate.

A **confidence interval (CI)** is a range of scores with specific boundaries, or *confidence limits*, that should contain the population mean. The boundaries of the confidence interval are based on the sample mean and its standard error. The wider the interval we propose, the more confident we will be that the true population mean will fall within it. This degree of confidence is expressed as a probability percentage, typically 95% or 99% confidence.

Constructing Confidence Intervals

Let's illustrate the procedure for constructing a 95% confidence interval using the birth weight data, $\bar{X} = 6.8$, $s = 1.5$, $n = 50$, and $s_{\bar{X}} = 0.21$. The sampling distribution estimated from this sample is shown in Figure 23-3.

We know that 95.45% of the total distribution will fall within $\pm 2\, s_{\bar{X}}$ from the mean, which is equal to the boundaries of $z = \pm 2$. Therefore, to determine the proportion of the curve within 95%, we need to determine points just slightly less than $z = \pm 2$. By referring to Table A-1 in the Appendix, we can determine that .95 of the total curve (.475 on either side of the mean) is bounded by a z-score of ± 1.96, just less than 2 standard error units above and below the mean. Therefore, as shown in Figure 23-3, we are 95% sure that the population mean will fall within this interval. This is the *95% confidence interval*.

We obtain the boundaries of a confidence interval using the formula

$$CI = \bar{X} \pm (z)s_{\bar{X}}$$

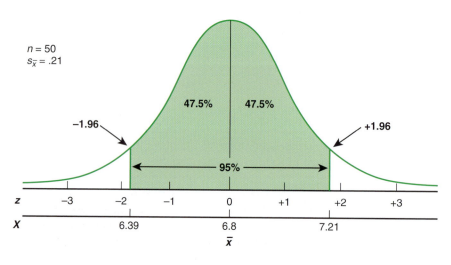

$n = 50$
$s_{\bar{x}} = .21$

Figure 23–3 95% confidence interval for a sampling distribution of birth weights.

For 95% confidence intervals, $z = \pm 1.96$.
For our data, therefore,

$$95\% \text{ CI} = 6.8 \pm (1.96)(0.21)$$
$$= 6.8 \pm 0.41$$
$$95\% \text{ CI} = 6.39 \text{ to } 7.21$$

Based on these sample data, we are 95% confident that the population mean of birth weights will fall between 6.39 and 7.21 lbs.

Interpreting Confidence Intervals

Because of sampling error, we know that different samples may have different means, even if they are all randomly chosen from the same population. The concept of 95% confidence limits indicates that if we were to draw 100 random samples, each with $n = 50$, we would expect 95% of them to contain the true population mean and 5% would not, as illustrated in Figure 23-4. In this example, 1 out of 20 (5%) does not contain the population mean.

Theoretically, this would occur just by chance, because the scores chosen for that one sample were too extreme and not good representatives of the population. In reality, however, we construct only one confidence interval based on the data from one sample. Therefore, we cannot know if our one sample would produce one of the correct intervals or one of the incorrect ones. Therefore, there is always a 5% chance that the population mean is not included in the obtained interval, that is, a 5% chance the interval is one of the incorrect ones.

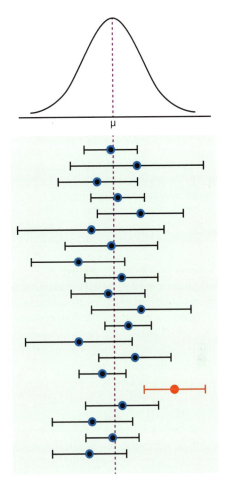

Figure 23–4 Hypothetical 95% confidence intervals for birth weights for 20 random samples of $n = 50$. The center line represents the population mean, μ, and the brackets represent the confidence limits. The center dot in each interval is the sample mean. Intervals vary in width, reflecting different sample variances. One interval does not contain the population mean (in red).

🔑 The correct interpretation of a confidence interval is that if we were to repeat sampling many times, 95% of the time our confidence interval would contain the true population mean. Therefore, we can say, given our sample data, we are 95% confident that the population mean for birth weight is between 6.4 and 7.2 lbs.

There are many ways to misinterpret these values. For instance, it is NOT correct to say:

- 95% of all infants will weigh between 6.4 and 7.2 lbs.
- We are 95% confident that a randomly selected infant will weigh between 6.4 and 7.2 lbs.
- 95% of the time the mean birth weight of a sample will be 6.8 lbs
- There is a 95% probability that the population mean falls between 6.4 and 7.2 lbs.

The population mean does not change. Each time we draw another sample, our data may or may not include the population mean—it is either in the confidence interval or not. The population mean remains constant (although unknown) and only the confidence interval varies around it.

Being More Confident

To be more confident in the accuracy of a confidence interval, we could use 99% as our reference, allowing only a 1% risk that the interval we propose will not contain the true population mean. Using Table A-1, we can determine that 99% of the area under the curve (0.495 on either side of the mean) is bounded by $z = \pm 2.576$. Therefore, for our data,

$$99\% \text{ CI} = 6.8 \pm (2.576)(0.21)$$
$$= 6.8 \pm 0.54$$
$$99\% \text{ CI} = 6.26 \text{ to } 7.34$$

We are 99% confident that the population mean falls between 6.26 and 7.34 lbs. Note that the 99% confidence limits are wider than 95%. We reduce the risk of being wrong by sacrificing precision. The choice of confidence interval depends on the nature of the variables being studied and the researcher's desired level of accuracy.

 By convention, the 90%, 95% and 99% confidence intervals are used most often. The corresponding z values are:

90%	$z = 1.645$
95%	$z = 1.96$
99%	$z = 2.576$

Confidence intervals can be obtained for most statistics, not just for means. The process will be defined in future chapters as different statistical procedures are introduced.

■ Statistical Hypothesis Testing

The estimation of population parameters is only one part of statistical inference. More often inference is used to answer questions concerning comparisons or relationships, such as, "Is one treatment more effective than another?" or "Is there a relationship between patient characteristics and the degree of improvement observed?" These types of questions usually involve the comparison of means, proportions, or correlations.

➤ CASE IN POINT #2

Researchers proposed a hypothesis that a single intervention session of soft-tissue mobilization would be effective for increasing external rotation in patients with limited shoulder mobility.[1] Experimental and control groups were formed through random assignment. Range of motion (ROM) measurements were taken and the improvement from pretest to posttest was calculated for each subject. The researchers found that the mean improvement in external rotation was 16.4 degrees for the treatment group and 1 degree for the control group.

On the basis of the difference between these means, should the researcher conclude that the research hypothesis has been supported? According to the concept of sampling error, we would expect to see some differences between groups even when a treatment is not at all effective. Therefore, we need some mechanism for deciding if an observed effect is or is not likely to be chance variation. We do this through a process of *hypothesis testing*.

The Null Hypothesis

Before we can interpret observed differences, we must consider two possible explanations for the outcome. The first explanation is that the observed difference between the groups occurred by chance. This is the **null hypothesis** (**H_0**), which states that the group means are not different—the groups come from the same population. No matter how the research hypothesis is stated, the researcher's goal will always be to statistically test the null hypothesis.

Statistical hypotheses are formally stated in terms of the population parameter, μ, even though the actual statistical tests will be based on sample data. Therefore, the null hypothesis can be stated formally as

$$H_0: \ \mu_A = \mu_B \quad (H_0: \ \mu_A - \mu_B = 0)$$

which predicts that the mean of Population A is not different from the mean of Population B, or that there will be no treatment effect. For the example of joint mobilization and shoulder ROM, under H_0 we would state:

➤ For patients with limited shoulder mobility, there will be no difference in the mean change in external rotation between those who do (μ_A) and do not (μ_B) receive mobilization.

The null hypothesis will either be true or false in any given comparison. However, because of sampling error groups will probably not have exactly equal means, even when there is no true treatment effect. Therefore, H_0 really indicates that observed differences are sufficiently small to be considered pragmatically equivalent to zero.[2] So rather than saying the means are "equal" (which they are not), it is more accurate to say they are *not significantly different*.

The Alternative Hypothesis

The second explanation for the observed findings is that the treatment is effective and that the effect is too large to be considered a result of chance alone. This is the **alternative hypothesis (H_1)**, stated as

$$H_1: \ \mu_A \neq \mu_B \quad (H_1: \ \mu_A - \mu_B \neq 0)$$

These statements predict that the observed difference between the two population means is not due to chance, or that the likelihood that the difference is due to chance is very small. The alternative hypothesis usually represents the research hypothesis (see Chapter 3). For the joint mobilization study, under H_1 we would state:

➤ For patients with limited shoulder mobility, the mean change in external rotation will be different for those who do and do not receive mobilization.

This is a *nondirectional* alternative hypothesis because it does not specify which group mean is expected to be larger. Alternative hypotheses can also be expressed in *directional* form, indicating the expected direction of difference between sample means. We could state

$$H_1: \ \mu_A > \mu_B \quad (H_1: \ \mu_A - \mu_B > 0)$$

or

$$H_1: \ \mu_A < \mu_B \quad (H_1: \ \mu_A - \mu_B < 0)$$

The mobilization study used a directional alternative hypothesis:

> ➤ For patients with limited shoulder mobility, the mean change in external rotation will be greater for those who receive mobilization than for those who do not receive mobilization.

📌 Note that a stated hypothesis should always include the four elements of PICO (see Chapter 3), including reference to the target population, the intervention and comparison conditions (levels of the independent variable), and the outcome (dependent variable). For the mobilization study: **P** = patients with limited shoulder disability, **I** = mobilization, **C** = no mobilization, **O** = change in external rotation range of motion.

"Disproving" the Null Hypothesis

We can never actually "prove" the null hypothesis based on sample data, so the purpose of a study is to give the data a chance of *disproving* it. In essence, we are using a decision-making process based on the concept of negative inference. No one experiment can establish that a null hypothesis is true—it would require testing the entire population with unsuccessful results to prove that a treatment has no effect. We can, however, discredit the null hypothesis by any one trial that shows that the treatment is effective. Therefore, the purpose of testing the statistical hypothesis is to decide whether or not H_0 is *false*.

There is often confusion about the appropriate way to express the outcome of a statistical decision. We can only legitimately say that we *reject* or *do not reject* the null hypothesis. We start, therefore, with the assumption that there is no treatment effect in a study (the null hypothesis). Then we ask if the data are consistent with this assumption (see Box 23-1). If the answer is yes, then we must acknowledge the possibility that no effect exists, and we *do not reject the null hypothesis*. If the answer is no, then

we have discredited that assumption. Therefore, there probably is an effect, and we *reject the null hypothesis*.

When we reject the null we can *accept* the alternative hypothesis—we say that the alternative hypothesis is consistent with our findings.

Superiority and Non-Inferiority

Chapter 14 introduced the concepts of superiority and non-inferiority trials. For most studies, the intent is to show that the experimental treatment is better than the control, hoping that H_0 will be rejected. There may be situations, however, where the researcher does not want to find a difference, such as trying to show that a new treatment is as effective as a standard treatment. In such a case, demonstrating "no difference" is a bit more complicated, and the roles of the null and alternative hypotheses are reversed. Box 23-2 addresses this seemingly "backwards" logic.

Box 23-1 What's the Verdict?

The decision to "reject" or "not reject" the null hypothesis is analogous to the use of "guilty" or "not guilty" in a court of law. We assume a defendant is innocent until proven guilty (the null hypothesis is true until evidence disproves it). A jury can reach a guilty verdict if evidence is sufficient (beyond a reasonable doubt) that the defendant committed the crime. Otherwise, the verdict is not guilty (H_0). The jury cannot find the defendant "innocent." Similarly, we cannot actually accept the null hypothesis. A "not guilty" verdict is expected if the evidence is not sufficient to establish guilt. But that doesn't necessarily mean the defendant is innocent!

Although not technically correct, researchers sometimes do say they "accept" the null hypothesis to indicate that it is probably true. The word "retained" has also been used to denote this outcome.[2]

Box 23-2 No Better, No Worse

Most of the time when researchers design a randomized trial, they are looking to show that a new intervention is more effective than a placebo or standard treatment. Such studies are considered **superiority trials** because their aim is to demonstrate that one treatment is "superior" to another. The process typically involves the statement of a null hypothesis and an alternative hypothesis asserting that there will be a difference. This may be directional or nondirectional, but in either case the intent is to reject the null and accept the alternative in favor of one treatment.

A **non-inferiority trial** focuses on demonstrating that the effect of a new intervention is the same as standard care, in an effort to show that it is an acceptable substitute. This approach is based on the intent to show no difference, or more precisely that the new treatment is "no worse" than standard care. It requires inverted thinking about how we look at significance. It is not as simple as just finding no difference based on a standard null hypothesis. Remember, it is not possible to "prove" no difference based on one study (see Chapter 5, Box 5-2).

The concept of "no worse" requires the specification of a **non-inferiority margin**, the largest difference between the two treatments that would still be considered functionally equivalent (see Chapter 14). If the difference between treatments is within that margin, then non-inferiority is established. The new treatment would be considered no worse than standard care, and therefore its preference for use would be based on its safety, convenience, cost or comfort.[3]

In the scheme of a non-inferiority trial, the roles of the alternative and null hypotheses are actually reversed. The null (the hypothesis we want to reject) says the standard treatment is better than the new approach, while the alternative (the hypothesis we want to accept) states that the new treatment is not inferior to the standard treatment. In this case, it is the non-inferiority margin that must be considered and the confidence interval around that margin. Further discussion is beyond the scope of this book, but several useful references provide more detailed explanation.[3-7]

■ Errors in Hypothesis Testing

Hypothesis testing will always result in one of two decisions: either reject or do not reject the null hypothesis. By rejecting the null hypothesis, the researcher concludes that it is *unlikely* that chance alone is operating to produce observed differences. This is called a *significant effect*, one that is probably not due to chance. When the null hypothesis is not rejected, the researcher concludes that the observed difference is probably due to chance and is *not significant*.

The decision to reject or not reject the null hypothesis is based on the results of objective statistical procedures, although this objectivity does not guarantee that a correct decision will be made. Because such decisions are based on sample data only, it is always possible that the true relationship between experimental variables is not accurately reflected in the statistical outcome.

Statistical Decisions

Any one decision can be either correct or incorrect. Therefore, we can classify four possible statistical decision outcomes, shown in Figure 23-5. If we *do not reject* H_0 when it is in fact true (observed differences are really due to chance), we have made a correct decision. If we *reject* H_0 when it is false (differences are real), we have also made a correct decision.

If, however, we decide to reject H_0 when it is true, we have made an error, called a **Type I error**. In this case, we have concluded that a difference exists, when in fact, it is due to chance. Having committed this type of statistical error, we might decide to use a treatment that is not really effective.

Conversely, if we do not reject H_0 when it is false, we have committed a **Type II error**. Here we would conclude that differences are due to chance when in fact they are real. In this situation, we might ignore an effective treatment or abandon a potentially fruitful line of research.

In any statistical analysis, we may draw a correct conclusion, or we may commit one of these two types of errors. We cannot make both types of errors in one comparison.

The seriousness of one type of error over the other is relative. Historically, statisticians and researchers have focused attention on Type I error as the primary basis of hypothesis testing. However, the consequences of failing to recognize an effective treatment may be equally important. Although we never know for sure if we are committing one or the other type of error, we can take steps to decrease the probability of committing one or both.

 Sometimes it may seem like there are double and triple negatives floating around! Long story short:

Type I error- Mistakenly finding a difference
Type II error- Mistakenly finding no difference

Using the court room analogy, Type I error is finding the defendant guilty when he is actually innocent, and Type II error is finding him not guilty when he is actually guilty.

We can also think of Type I error as a false-positive and Type II error as a false-negative finding.

■ Type I Error and Significance

Because we know that observed differences may be due to chance, we might ask how we can ever make a decision regarding the null hypothesis if we can never be certain if it is true or false. In fact, there will always be some uncertainty in this process. We must be willing to take some risk in making a mistake if we reject the null hypothesis when it is true. We must be able to set some criterion for this risk, a dividing line that allows us to say that a mistake in rejecting H_0 (a Type I error) is "unlikely."

Level of Significance

To determine the probability of committing a Type I error, we must set a standard for rejecting the null hypothesis. This standard is called the **level of significance**, denoted as **alpha (α)**. The level of significance represents a criterion for judging if an observed difference can be considered sampling error. The larger an observed difference, the less likely it occurred by chance. The probability that an observed difference did occur by chance is determined by statistical tests (which will be introduced later in this chapter and in the upcoming chapters).

For example, we might find that an analysis comparing two means yields $p = .18$. This means that there is an 18% probability that the difference between the means

REALITY

	H_0 is true	H_0 is false
Reject H_0	Type I Error α	✔ Correct
Do Not Reject H_0	✔ Correct	Type II Error β

DECISION

Figure 23–5 Potential errors in hypothesis testing.

occurred by chance alone. Therefore, if we decide to reject H_0 and conclude that the tested groups are different from each other, we have an 18% chance of being wrong, that is, an 18% chance of committing a Type I error.

Taking a Risk

The question facing the researcher is how to decide if this probability is acceptable. How much of a chance is small enough that we would be willing to accept the risk of being wrong? Is an 18% chance of being wrong acceptable?

For research purposes, the selected alpha level defines the *maximal acceptable risk* of making a Type I error if we reject H_0. Traditionally, researchers have set this standard at 5%, which is considered a small risk. This means that we would be willing to accept a 5% chance of *incorrectly rejecting H_0* or a 5% risk that we will reject H_0 when it is actually true. Therefore, for a given analysis, if p is *equal to or less than* .05, we would be willing to reject the null hypothesis. We then say that the difference is *significant*. If p is greater than .05, we would not reject the null hypothesis and we say that the difference is *not significant*.

For the earlier example, if we set $\alpha = .05$, we would not reject the null hypothesis at $p = .18$. The probability that the observed difference is due to chance is too great. If a statistical test demonstrates that two means are different at $p = .04$, we could reject H_0, with only a small acceptable risk (4%) of committing a Type I error.

What does it mean to take a risk? Let's personalize it: The weather report says that there is a 75% chance of rain today. Will you take your umbrella? If you decide NOT to take it, and it rains, you will be wrong and you will get wet! Now let's say that the report is for a 5% chance of rain. Are you more likely to leave your umbrella at home? What is the maximal risk you are willing to take that you will be wrong—that you will get wet—10% chance of rain, 25%, 50%? What is your limit? Of course, my bringing my umbrella is likely to make the probability 100% that it won't rain!

Choosing a Level of Significance

How does a researcher decide on a level of significance as the criterion for statistical testing? The conventional designation of .05 is really an arbitrary, albeit accepted, standard. A researcher may choose other criterion levels depending on how critical a Type I error would be.

For example, suppose we were involved in the study of a drug to reduce spasticity, comparing control and experimental groups. This drug could be very beneficial to patients with upper motor neuron involvement. However, the drug has potentially serious side effects and is very expensive to produce. In such a situation we would want to be very confident that observed results were not due to chance. If we reject the null hypothesis and recommend the drug, we would want the probability of our committing a Type I error to be very small. We do not want to encourage the use of the drug unless it is clearly and markedly beneficial.

We can minimize the risk of statistical error by lowering the level of significance to .025 or .01. If we use $\alpha = .01$ as our criterion for rejecting H_0, we would have only 1 out of 100 chances of making a Type I error. This would mean that we could have greater confidence in our decision to reject the null hypothesis.

Researchers should specify the minimal level of significance required for rejecting the null hypothesis prior to data collection. The decision to use .05, .01, or any other value, should be based on the concern for Type I error, not on what the data look like. If a researcher chooses $\alpha = .01$ as the criterion, and statistical testing shows significance at $p = .04$, the researcher would not reject H_0. If $\alpha = .05$ had been chosen as the criterion, the same data would have resulted in the opposite conclusion.

 If we want to be really confident in our findings, why not just set α really low, like .0001? That would certainly increase rigor in avoiding a Type I error—but practically it would also make finding significant differences very difficult, increasing risk of Type II error. For instance, a result at $p = .01$ would not be significant, although this represents a very low risk. Absent an otherwise compelling reason, using $\alpha = .05$ is usually reasonable to balance both Type I and Type II error.

Interpreting Probability Values

Researchers must be aware of the appropriate interpretation of p values:

> *The p value is the probability of finding an effect as big as the one observed when the null hypothesis is true.*

Therefore, with $p = .02$, even if there is no true difference, you would expect to observe this size effect 2% of the time. Said another way, if we performed 100 similar experiments, 2 of them would result in a difference this large, even if no true difference exists.

It is tempting to reverse this definition, to assume that there is a 98% probability that a real difference exists. This is not the case, however. The p value is based on the assumption that the null hypothesis is true, although it cannot be used to prove it. The p value will only tell us how *rarely* we would expect a difference this large in the population just by chance. It is not accurate to imply that a small p value means the observed result is "true."[8]

Confidence intervals are actually a more appropriate way to think about what the "true" value would be.

We must also be careful to avoid using the magnitude of *p* as an indication of the degree of validity of the research hypothesis. It is not advisable to use terms such as "highly significant" or "more significant" because they imply that the value of *p* is a measure of treatment effect, which it is not. We will revisit this important point again shortly when we discuss statistical power.

Significance as a Dichotomy

In conventional statistical practice, the level of significance is considered a point along a continuum that demarcates the line between "likely" and "unlikely." Once the level of significance is chosen, it represents a dichotomous decision rule: yes or no, significant or not significant. Once the decision is made, the magnitude of *p* reflects only the relative degree of confidence that can be placed in that decision.

That said, researchers will still caution that a nonsignificant *p* value is not necessarily the end of the story, especially if it is close to α.[9] We must, therefore, also consider the possibility of Type II error.

HISTORICAL NOTE

The history of statistics actually lies in agriculture, where significant differences were intended to show which plots of land, treated differently, yielded better crops. The ability to control the soil and common growing conditions made the use of probability practical in making decisions about best growing conditions. However, when dealing with the uncertainties of clinical practice and the variability in people and conditions, relying on a single fixed probability value does not carry the same logic. It is more reasonable to think of probability as a value that varies continuously between extremes, with no sharp line between "significant" and "nonsignificant."[9, 10]

■ Type II Error and Power

We have thus far established the logic behind classical statistical inference, based on the probability associated with rejecting a true null hypothesis, or Type I error. But what happens when we find no significant effect and we do not reject the null hypothesis? Does this necessarily mean that there is no real difference?

If we do not reject the null hypothesis when it is indeed false, we have committed a Type II error—we have found no significant difference when a difference really does exist. This type of error can have serious consequences for evidence-based practice.

The probability of making a Type II error is denoted by **beta (β)**, which is the *probability of failing to reject a false null hypothesis*. If β = .20, there is a 20% chance that we will make a Type II error, or that we will not reject H_0 when it is really false. The fact that a treatment really is effective does not guarantee that a statistically significant finding will result.

Statistical Power

The complement of β error, $1 - β$, is the statistical **power** of a test.

Power is the probability that a test will lead to rejection of the null hypothesis, or the probability of attaining statistical significance.

If β = .20, power = .80. Therefore, for a statistical test with 80% power, the probability is 80% that we would correctly demonstrate a statistical difference and reject H_0 if actual differences exist. The more powerful a test, the less likely one is to make a Type II error.

Power can be thought of as sensitivity. The more sensitive a test, the more likely it will detect important clinical differences that truly exist. Where α = .05 has become the conventional standard for Type I error, there is no standard for β, although β = .20, with corresponding power of 80%, represents a reasonable protection against Type II error.[11] If β is set at .20, it means that the researcher is willing to accept a 20% chance of missing a difference of the expected effect size if it really exists.

Just as we might lower α to reflect the relative importance of Type I error, there may be reasons to use a lower value of β to avoid Type II error. For instance, researchers may be interested in newer therapies that may only show small but important effects. In that case, β might be set at .10, allowing for 90% power.

The Determinants of Statistical Power

Power analysis involves four interdependent concepts (using the mnemonic PANE):

P = power $(1 - β)$
A = alpha level of significance
N = number of subjects or sample size
E = effect size

Knowing any three of these will allow determination of the fourth factor.

Power

Power can be measured following completion of a statistical analysis when there is no significant difference, to determine if there was sufficient power to detect a true difference. The researcher can also set the desired level of power during planning stages of the study.

Level of Significance

Although there is no direct mathematical relationship between α and β, there is trade-off between them.

Lowering the level of significance reduces the chance of Type I error by requiring stronger evidence to demonstrate significant differences. But this also means that the chance of missing a true effect is increased. By making the standard for rejecting H_0 more rigorous (lowering α), we make it harder for sample results to meet this standard.

Sample Size

The influence of sample size on power of a test is critical—the larger the sample, the greater the statistical power. Smaller samples are less likely to be good representations of population characteristics, and, therefore, true differences between groups are less likely to be recognized. This is the one factor that is typically under the researcher's control to affect power.

Effect Size

Power is also influenced by the size of the *effect* of the independent variable. When comparing groups, this effect will be the difference between sample means. In studies where relationships or measures of risk are of interest, this effect will be the degree of association between variables. This is the essence of most research questions: "How large an effect will my treatment have?" or "How strong is the relationship between two variables?" Studies that result in large differences or associations are more likely to produce significant outcomes than those with small or negligible effects. **Effect size (ES)** is a measure of the *degree to which the null hypothesis is false*.[11] The null hypothesis states that no difference exists between groups—that the effect is zero.

An **effect size index** is a unitless standardized value that allows comparisons across samples and studies. There are many types of effect size indices, depending on the specific test used. They can focus on differences between means, proportions, correlations, and other statistics. The index is a ratio of the effect size to the variance within the data. The power of a test is increased as the effect gets larger and variance within a set of data is reduced, showing distinct differences between groups. Different indices will be described in the context of statistical tests in upcoming chapters.

Power Analysis

We can analyze power for two purposes: To estimate sample size during planning stages of a study, and to determine the probability that a Type II error was committed when a study results in a nonsignificant finding.

A Priori Analysis: Determining Sample Size

One of the first questions researchers must ask when planning a study is, "How many participants are needed?" An easy answer may be as many as possible.

However, this is not helpful when one is trying to place realistic limits on time and resources for data collection. Many researchers have arbitrarily suggested that a sample size of 30 or 50 is "reasonable."[10] Unfortunately, these estimates may be wholly inadequate for many research designs or for studies with small effect sizes.

Sample size estimates should be incorporated in the planning stages of every experimental or observational study. The lack of such planning often results in a high probability of Type II error and needlessly wasted efforts. Institutional Review Boards will demand such estimates before approving a study (see Box 23-3).

> ### ▶ CASE IN POINT #3
> Nobles et al[17] studied the effect of a prenatal exercise intervention on gestational diabetes mellitus (GDM) among pregnant women at risk for GDM. They compared an individualized 12-week exercise program against a comparison wellness program. They hypothesized that participants in the exercise intervention would have a lower risk of GDM and lower screening glucose values as compared to a health and wellness control intervention.

By specifying a level of significance and desired power in the planning stages of a study, a researcher can estimate how many participants would be needed to detect a significant difference for an expected effect size. The smaller the expected effect size, the larger the required sample. This is considered *a priori* power analysis.

Box 23-3   Goldilocks and Power: Getting It "Just Right"
Because of established guidelines for reporting, most journals now require authors to substantiate their basis for estimating sample size and power as part of the planning process for recruitment.[12] Ethical issues related to power center on concern for participants and justification of resources.[13] Institutional Review Boards typically require this type of analysis before a study will be approved, to be sure that a study has a chance of success and is thereby worth the effort and potential risks.[14] However, some argue that small, underpowered trials are still defensible if they will be able to eventually contribute to estimates of effect size through meta-analyses (see Chapter 37).[15]
An equally serious concern has been expressed about samples that are too large, exposing more participants than necessary to potential risks.[16] By having a very large sample, thereby increasing the power of a test, even trivial differences can be deemed statistically significant. Using a power analysis to determine the ideal sample size prior to data collection can assure a reasonable number, not too small or too large—giving the researcher the most realistic and reasonable opportunity to see an effect. Information on how sample size was determined is typically reported in the methods section of a research paper.

> ▶ Based on previous literature and estimates of incidence of GDM, researchers in the exercise study determined that a sample size of 352 (176 per group) would have the ability to detect reductions in risk of 35% or larger with statistical significance based on $\alpha = .05$ for a two-sided test. For screening glucose, they set 80% power to detect a clinically significant mean difference as small as 5.99 ng/mL based on a standard deviation of 20 mg/dL.

Estimating Effect Size

To project the needed sample size, the researcher can readily specify α and β but must make an educated guess as to the expected effect size. This guess is often based on previous research or pilot data, as in the GDM study, or from meta-analyses. When relevant data are not available, the effect size estimate may be based on the researcher's opinion of a meaningful difference, or how large an effect would be considered clinically important. In the exercise study, for example, one might use clinical guidelines to determine the minimum difference in glucose levels that would have implications for patient management decisions.

When no clinical data are available to make a judgment about effect size, researchers can use *conventional effect sizes*, which have been defined for "small," "medium," and "large" effects.[11] These standardized values are different for varied effect size indices. They provide a default value that can be used in the absence of more specific estimates.

One way to conceptualize these definitions is to think of effect size in terms of variance. Using a simple framework involving two group means as an example, the difference between means would be considered small if it was 20% of one standard deviation (assuming both groups have the same standard deviation). A medium effect would be equivalent to half a standard deviation, and a large effect would be 80% of a standard deviation.

Cohen[11] stipulates that there is an inherent risk in setting these conventional values and that they should only be considered "relative," not just to each other, but to the specific field of study. The assessment of what is considered a large or small effect must be a judgment based on the types of variables used, an understanding of the measurement scale, clinically meaningful change, and research method being used. For instance, if the conventional effect size for a "large" effect is considered too small to be meaningful, Cohen recommends that different criteria be defined according to the nature of the data. Unfortunately, many researchers follow the proposed conventions without reference to what they are measuring.

When the sample size estimate is beyond realistic limits, a researcher may try to redesign the study by controlling variability in the sample or choosing a different dependent variable to increase effect size. Sometimes the researcher may decide not to conduct the study, given that significant results are so unlikely.

> 🔑 When studies involve more than one dependent variable, the proposed effect size for the primary outcome should be used to determine sample size. However, if several analyses are planned, the sample size should be large enough to support the smallest hypothesized effect.[18]

Post Hoc Analysis: Determining Power

What happens if we predict a large effect and choose the appropriate sample, but the actual scores reveal an effect smaller than expected, which turns out to be nonsignificant? Could we have committed a Type II error?

> ▶ Researchers in the GDM study found no significant difference between groups in any of the outcome variables. The exercise group had a lower mean glucose level by 1.95 mg/dL, but the difference was not significant ($p = .61$).

It is, of course, possible that the treatment was not effective. Just because we find no difference, doesn't automatically mean we committed a Type II error! However, we must also consider what level of power was actually achieved.

Even with good planning, results may not show the expected effect, or variance in scores could be greater than anticipated. The projected sample size may not be achieved because of subjects refusing to participate, ineligibility, or attrition. Therefore, by knowing the observed effect size, the level of significance used, and the actual sample size, the researcher can determine the degree of power that was achieved in the analysis.

> ▶ Researchers in the GDM study had planned for a sample of 352 but were able to recruit only 290 subjects, and only 251 were available for follow-up. Their results also showed a smaller effect than they had anticipated. This resulted in an actual power of about 13%.

Given the extremely low power that was achieved in this study, despite their planning, it was unlikely that a significant difference would be found. Many researchers will project potential attrition or recruitment problems and increase sample size estimates to account for possible dropouts. It is also possible that a study will result in an effect larger than expected, and a smaller sample would have sufficed!

Clinical Versus Statistical Significance

If power is low, the researcher must determine if the data support drawing tentative conclusions about the lack of significant treatment effect. When significance levels are close to α, investigators often talk about a "nonsignificant trend" toward a difference. This is a cautionary conclusion, however, and should probably only be supported when power is an issue, suggesting that a larger sample might have led to a significant outcome.[8] However, when effect sizes are considered small, as in the GDM study, there may be reason to consider that there is truly no difference (see Focus on Evidence 23-1).

It is also important to remember that power can be quite high with very large samples, even when effect sizes are small and meaningless. In our search for evidence, we must be able to distinguish clinical versus statistical significance. As clinicians, we should never lose sight of the role our clinical expertise and experience play in understanding mechanisms of interventions, theoretical underpinnings, relevant changes in patient performance, and the context of all available research on a topic.[19] Patient preferences can also help us to understand what outcomes are meaningful when evidence is not sufficient (see Focus on Evidence 23-2).[20]

Resources to determine power and sample size are available online and through statistical programs such as SPSS.[21,22]
G*Power is a widely-used free online program that will be illustrated in chapter supplements for various tests.[23]
See the *Chapter 23 Supplement* for an introduction to this process. References are also available for hand calculations.

Focus on Evidence 23–1
What does it mean when we DON'T find a significant difference...

Researchers and clinicians have long understood the difference between statistical significance and clinical relevance. This distinction has been part of the impetus for translational research, to make research findings more applicable to practice. In our eagerness to find evidence for practice decisions, however, sometimes this distinction can get lost.

The phrase *"Absence of evidence is not evidence of absence"* was introduced in Chapter 5, serving as a caveat to remind us that we don't know what we don't know! Just because we do not have evidence that something exists does not mean that we have evidence that it does not exist—an essential premise for evidence-based practice. Remember that, in fact, we can never actually prove no difference, which is why we cannot "accept" the null hypothesis.[24]

So when is it reasonable to claim that a study has "proved" there is no effect of an intervention? The correct answer is close to "never," because uncertainty will always exist,[25] although there needs to be some theoretical premise that warrants continued discovery. Missing the α threshold does not end the discussion. Unfortunately, when results are not significant, clinicians may assume that the experimental treatment was not effective and stop there. And compounding the dilemma, researchers and journal editors are often unable or unwilling to publish reports that end in nonsignificant outcomes, a problem called **publication bias** (see Chapter 37).[26-29]

The implications of this issue can be far-reaching. As practitioners and researchers, it is important for us to know about interventions that were and were not effective, and how to interpret such findings. Otherwise, we may be losing a great deal of valuable information, moving critically off course by ignoring potentially fruitful lines of research.

Focus on Evidence 23–2
... and what does it mean when we DO find a significant difference?

Several considerations are critical to understand results of significant statistical tests. The immediate interpretation will be to consider differences or relationships to be meaningful. This may certainly be true, but there is more to this interpretation than a simple "yes" or "no."

Even when significance is obtained, we must consider what the numbers mean. Looking at data plots is important to consider variability and confidence intervals to estimate the effect. Reliability and validity assessments may be relevant to determine if the measured change is clinically meaningful. Most importantly, it is the size of the effect that is going to indicate how important the results are, not statistical significance. There is no magic in $p = .05$!

We must also be careful not to confuse the significance level with size of the effect. Remember that probabilities only tell us the likelihood of appropriately rejecting a true null hypothesis. A lower probability does not indicate a larger effect size and a higher probability does not indicate a smaller effect—both are influenced by sample size. We can't compare *p* values across studies to say that one treatment is better than another, and a low *p* value doesn't mean the treatment effect was meaningful, especially if the sample is very large, which would increase power.

It is important to look at the size of the treatment effect, whether or not the null hypothesis is rejected. Effect size indices can help to assess the magnitude of the effect and will provide a basis for comparison across studies. Consider the effect size and confidence intervals in addition to statistical significance, to avoid discarding potentially important discoveries, especially with new treatment approaches.[30]

■ Concepts of Statistical Testing

Statistical procedures are used to test hypotheses through the calculation of a test statistic, or test ratio. Different statistics are used to test differences between means, correlations, and proportions. These statistics are used to determine if a significant effect is attained by establishing the probability that an effect would occur if H_0 were true. To illustrate these concepts, we will revisit the birth weight example for a one-sample test, comparing a sample mean against a population mean.

> ## ➤ CASE IN POINT #1- REVISITED
> Assume we are interested in comparing the average birth weight in a particular community with the national average. The community has limited access to healthcare, and we want to establish if this affects birth weights. From national studies, we know the population birth weight values: μ = 7.5 lbs with σ = 1.25. We draw a random sample of n = 100 infants from the community. Results show $\overline{X}$ = 7.2 lbs and s = 1.73.

The Null Hypothesis

If there is a difference between the sample mean and the known population mean, it may be the result of chance, or it may indicate that these children should not be considered part of the overall population. The null hypothesis proposes no difference between the sample and the general population. Therefore, we predict that the population from which the sample is drawn has a mean of 7.5.

$$H_0: \mu = 7.5$$

The alternative hypothesis states that the children come from another population with a mean birth weight different from 7.5, that is, different from the general population:

$$H_1: \mu \neq 7.5$$

This is a nondirectional hypothesis. We are not predicting if the sample mean will be larger or smaller than the population mean, only that it will be different. We begin by assuming that the null hypothesis is true, that the observed difference of 0.3 lbs is due to chance. We then ask, how likely is a difference of this size if H_0 is true? The answer to this question is based on the defined properties of the normal sampling distribution and our desired level of significance, α = .05. We must determine the probability that one would observe a difference as large as 0.3 lbs by chance if the population mean for infants in this community is truly 7.5.

The z-Ratio

Recall from Chapter 22 that we can determine the area beyond any point in a normal distribution using values of z, or standard deviation units. For an individual sample score, X, a z-score represents the distance between that score and the sample mean divided by the standard deviation of the distribution.

When z is applied to a sampling distribution of means, the ratio reflects the distance between an individual sample mean, $\overline{X}$, and the population mean, μ, divided by the standard error of the sample mean, $s_{\overline{X}}$:

$$Z = \frac{\overline{X} - \mu}{s_{\overline{X}}}$$

For our example, with $\overline{X}$ = 7.2, s = 1.73, n = 100, and μ = 7.5, we calculate

$$s_{\overline{X}} = \frac{1.73}{\sqrt{100}} = 0.173$$

Therefore,

$$z = \frac{7.2 - 7.5}{0.173} = \frac{-0.3}{0.173} = -1.73$$

This tells us that the sample mean is 1.73 standard error units below the population mean of 7.5. The question we must ask is: Does this difference represent a significant difference? Is the difference large enough that we would consider the mean birth weight in our community to be significantly different from 7.5?

 Importantly, the z-ratio can be understood in terms of a relationship between the difference *between* means (the numerator) and the variance *within* the sample (the denominator). The ratio will be larger as the difference between means increases and as variance decreases. This concept will be revisited in discussions of many statistical tests.

Applying Probability

Let us assume we could plot the sampling distribution of means of birth weight for the general population, which takes the form of the normal curve as shown in Figure 23-6. Using α = .05 as our criterion, we accept that any value that has only a 5% chance of occurring is considered "unlikely." So we look at the area under the curve that represents 95%, which we know is bounded by z = ±1.96. Therefore, there is a 95% chance that any one sample chosen from this population would have a mean within those boundaries.

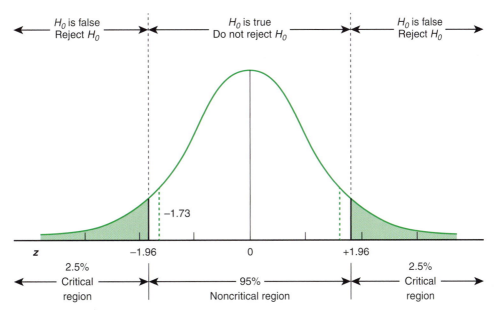

Figure 23–6 Standard normal distribution of z-scores showing critical values for a two-tailed (nondirectional) test at $\alpha_2 = .05$. The critical region falls in both tails, and 5% is divided between the two. The critical value is at ± 1.96. The calculated z-score for community birth weights ($z = -1.73$) does not fall within the critical region and is not significant.

Said another way, it is *highly likely* that any one sample chosen from this general population would have a mean birth weight within this range. Conversely, there is only a 5% chance that any sample mean would fall above or below those points. This means that it is *unlikely* that a sample mean from this general population would have a z-score beyond ± 1.96.

Therefore, if our sample yields a mean with a z-ratio beyond ± 1.96, it is unlikely that the sample is from the general population (H_1). If the sample mean of birth weights falls within $z = \pm 1.96$, then there is a 95% chance that the sample does come from the general population with $\mu = 7.5$ (H_0).

The Critical Region

The tails of the curve depicted in Figure 23-6, representing the area above and below $z = \pm 1.96$, encompass the **critical region**, or the *region of rejection* for H_0. This region, in both tails, equals a total of 5% of the curve, which is our criterion for significance. Therefore, this test is considered a **two-tailed test**, to indicate that our critical region is split between both tails. Because we proposed a nondirectional alternative hypothesis, we have to be prepared for the difference between means to be either positive or negative.

The value of z that defines the critical region is the **critical value**. When we calculate z for our study sample, it must be *equal to or greater than* the absolute critical value if H_0 is to be rejected. If a calculated z-ratio is less

than the critical value ($z < \pm 1.96$) it will fall within the *noncritical region*, representing a difference that may be due to chance. If a calculated z-ratio falls within the critical region ($z \geq \pm 1.96$), the ratio is *significant*.

 Remember that the values for z are symmetrical. The values in Table A-1 will apply to positive or negative z scores.

In our example, $z = -1.73$ for the sample mean of birth weights. This value is less than the absolute critical value of -1.96 and falls within the central noncritical region of the curve. Therefore, it is likely that this sample does come from the general population with $\mu = 7.5$. The observed difference between the means is not large enough to be considered significant at $\alpha = .05$ and we do not reject the null hypothesis.

 See the data files with supplemental materials for the data used in the birth weight example.

Directional Versus Nondirectional Tests

Two-Tailed Test

The process just described is considered *nondirectional* because we did not predict the direction of the difference between the sample means. Consequently, the critical region was established in both tails, so that a large enough positive or negative *z*-ratio would lead to rejection of the null hypothesis. For this two-tailed test, we can designate our level of significance as α_2 = .05, to indicate a two-tailed probability with $\alpha/2$ or .025 in each tail.

One-Tailed Test

In situations where a researcher has sufficient reason to propose an alternative hypothesis that specifies which mean will be larger, a *directional* test can be performed. For example, we could have hypothesized that the mean community birth weight is less than 7.5 lbs. This would be a directional hypothesis, and we would only be interested in outcomes that showed this direction of difference.

In that case, it is not necessary to locate the critical region in both tails, because we are only interested in a negative ratio. We anticipate either no difference or a negative difference. We are only interested in the left tail of the curve. Therefore, we would perform a **one-tailed test**. In this situation we can specify the level of significance as α_1 = .05 because the full 5% will be located in one tail of the curve. The critical value will now represent that point at which the area in the negative tail equals 5% of the total curve. Using Appendix Table A-1, we find that this area starts at *z* = −1.645, as shown in Figure 23-7. We are hypothesizing that there is only a 5% that any sample chosen from the general population would have a mean birth weight below *z* = −1.645. The absolute value of the calculated *z*-ratio must be less than or equal to −1.645 to be considered significant. Based on our example, *z* = −1.73 would now fall in the critical region and therefore be considered significant. With a one-tailed test, we would reject the null hypothesis.

📌 The critical value, against which the calculated *z*-ratio is compared, is determined according to the specified level of significance. According to Appendix Table A-1:

α_2 = .10 and α_1 =.05   Critical value = ±1.645
α_2 = .05 and α_1 =.025   Critical value = ±1.96
α_2 = .01 and α_1 =.005   Critical value = ±2.576

You have undoubtedly noticed that the *z*-ratio used in this example was significant with a one-tailed test but not with a two-tailed test. This happens because the critical value for the one-tailed test is smaller. Therefore, the one-tailed test is more powerful. The decision to use a one-tailed or two-tailed test, however, should be made based on the merits of the alternative hypothesis, not the statistical outcome. This will be discussed again in the next chapter.

🔑 Regardless of whether a directional or nondirectional alternative hypothesis has been proposed, once a significant difference is obtained, the results of the study are expressed in terms of the direction of the observed difference—which group had a significantly higher score than the other.

■ Parametric Versus Nonparametric Statistics

Statistics that are used to estimate population parameters are called **parametric statistics**. The validity of parametric tests is dependent on certain assumptions about the nature of data.

- *Samples are randomly drawn from a parent population with a normal distribution.*

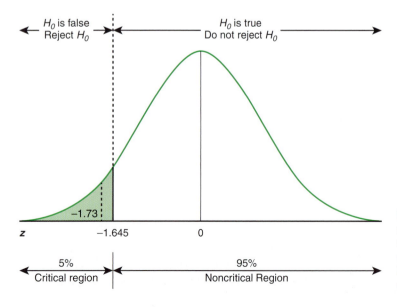

Figure 23–7 Standard normal curve of *z*-scores showing critical values for a one-tailed (directional) test at α_1 = .05. The critical value is at −1.645. The calculated *z*-score for community birth weights (*z* = −1.73) falls in the critical region and is significant.

Therefore, the sample should be a useful representation of population "parameters." With small samples, or with distributions that have not been previously described, it may be unreasonable to accept this assumption. Tests of "goodness of fit" can be performed to determine how well data match the normal distribution (see Box 23-4). Alternatively, data can be transformed to another scale of measurement, such as a logarithmic scale, to create distributions that more closely satisfy the necessary assumptions for parametric tests (see Appendix C).

- *Variances in the samples being compared are roughly equal, or homogeneous.*

A test for **homogeneity of variance** can substantiate this assumption (see Chapters 24 and 25).

- *Data should be measured on the interval or ratio scales.*

Therefore, scores can be subjected to arithmetic manipulations to calculate means and standard deviations.

When statistical conditions do not meet the assumptions for parametric statistics, **nonparametric tests** can be used. Nonparametric tests make fewer assumptions about population data and can be used when normality and homogeneity of variance criteria are not satisfied. They can be used effectively, therefore, with very small samples. In addition, they have been specifically developed to operate on data at the nominal and ordinal scales.

Several nonparametric tests have been designed as analogs of parametric procedures. The nonparametric tests tend to be less powerful than parametric procedures, but they can provide more valid analyses when the proper assumptions are not in place for parametric tests. Nonparametric procedures are described in Chapters 27, 28, and 29.

Box 23-4   What Is Normal?

Because many statistical procedures are based on assumptions related to the normal distribution, researchers should evaluate the shape of the data as part of their initial analysis. Alternative non-parametric statistical operations can be used with skewed data, or data may be transformed to better reflect the characteristics of a normal distribution.

Unfortunately, researchers often do not test for normality as part of their initial analysis, running the risk of invalid statistical conclusions.[31,32] "Goodness of fit" procedures can be applied to test for normality. The two most often applied tests are the *Kolmogorov-Smirnov (KS) Test* [33] and the *Shapiro-Wilk (SW) test*.[34] The SW test is considered more powerful, providing better estimates with smaller samples.[35]

Tests of Normality

	Kolmogorov-Smirnov			Shapiro-Wilk		
	Statistic	df	Sig.	Statistic	df	Sig.
Birthweight	.069	100	.200	.991	100	.741

The tests are based on the null hypothesis that the observed distribution does not differ from the pattern of a normal distribution. If the test is significant ($p \le .05$), then the null hypothesis is rejected, and the observed scores are not normally distributed. This may necessitate adjustments in the analysis strategy. If the test is not significant ($p > .05$), then the distribution is considered normal. To illustrate using the sample of birth weights, the results show that both the KS and SW tests were not significant (column labeled "Sig" is the probability). Therefore, the data are considered a good fit to the normal distribution.

COMMENTARY

Surely God loves the .06 nearly as much as the .05.

—*Ralph Rosnow (1936-) and Robert Rosenthal (1933-)*

American psychologists

The emphasis placed on significance testing in clinical research must be tempered with an understanding that statistical tests are tools for analyzing data and should never be used as a substitute for knowledgeable and critical interpretation of outcomes. A simple decision based on a *p* value is too simplistic for clinical application. A lack of statistical significance does not necessarily imply a lack of practical importance and vice versa.[9] The pragmatic difference in clinical effect with $p = .05$ or $p = .06$ may truly be negligible. What would be the difference in a clinical decision with an outcome at $p = .049$ versus $p = .051$?

Sir Ronald Fisher, who developed the concept of the null hypothesis and other statistical principles, cautioned against drawing a sharp line between "significant" and "nonsignificant" differences, warning that

> *…as convenient as it is to note that a hypothesis is contradicted at some familiar level of significance, … we do not ever need to lose sight of the exact strength which*

the evidence has in fact reached, or to ignore the fact that with further trial it might come to be stronger or weaker.[36]

To be evidence-based practitioners, we must all recognize the role of judgment as well as an understanding of statistical principles in using published data for clinical decision making. Understanding statistics and design concepts is important, but the statistics do not make decisions about what works—that is the judgment of the researcher and clinician who applies the information.

For example, being able to appreciate the information contained within a confidence interval will put a probability value within a context that can be more useful for clinical decision making.

Finally, we should always reflect on the collective impact of prior studies and critically assess the meaningfulness of the data in the aggregate. Interpreting results in the context of other studies requires that we recognize the need for replication and meta-analytic approaches (see Chapter 37).

REFERENCES

1. Godges JJ, Mattson-Bell M, Thorpe D, Shah D. The immediate effects of soft tissue mobilization with proprioceptive neuromuscular facilitation on glenohumeral external rotation and overhead reach. *J Orthop Sports Phys Ther* 2003;33(12):713-718.
2. Keppel G. *Design and Analysis: A Researcher's Handbook*. 4th ed. Englewood Cliffs, N.J.: Prentice Hall; 2004.
3. Hills RK. Non-inferiority trials: no better? No worse? No change? No pain? *Br J Haematol* 2017;176(6):883-887.
4. Lesaffre E. Superiority, equivalence, and non-inferiority trials. *Bull NYU Hosp Jt Dis* 2008;66(2):150-154.
5. Schumi J, Wittes JT. Through the looking glass: understanding non-inferiority. *Trials* 2011;12:106.
6. Head SJ, Kaul S, Bogers AJJC, Kappetein AP. Non-inferiority study design: lessons to be learned from cardiovascular trials. *Europ Heart J* 2012;33(11):1318-1324.
7. Kaul S, Diamond GA. Good enough: a primer on the analysis and interpretation of noninferiority trials. *Ann Intern Med* 2006;145(1):62-69.
8. Cohen HW. P values: use and misuse in medical literature. *Am J Hypertens* 2011;24(1):18-23.
9. Rosnow RJ, Rosenthal R. Statistical procedures and the justification of knowledge in pyschological science. *Am Psychol* 1989;44:1276-1284.
10. Cohen J. Things I have learned (so far). *Am Pyschologist* 1990;45(12):1304-1312.
11. Cohen J. *Statistical Power Analysis for the Behavioral Sciences*. 2nd ed. Hillsdale, NJ: Lawrence Erlbaum; 1988.
12. CONSORT Website. Available at http://www.consort-statement.org/. Accessed April 5, 2017.
13. Halpern SD, Karlawish JH, Berlin JA. The continuing unethical conduct of underpowered clinical trials. *JAMA* 2002;288(3):358-362.
14. Prentice R. Invited commentary: ethics and sample size—another view. *Am J Epidemiol* 2005;161(2):111-112.
15. Edwards SJ, Lilford RJ, Braunholtz D, Jackson J. Why "underpowered" trials are not necessarily unethical. *Lancet* 1997;350(9080):804-807.
16. Bacchetti P, Wolf LE, Segal MR, McCulloch CE. Ethics and sample size. *Am J Epidemiol* 2005;161(2):105-110.
17. Nobles C, Marcus BH, Stanek EJ, 3rd, Braun B, Whitcomb BW, Solomon CG, Manson JE, Markenson G, Chasan-Taber L. Effect of an exercise intervention on gestational diabetes mellitus: a randomized controlled trial. *Obstet Gynecol* 2015;125(5):1195-1204.
18. Knapp TR. The overemphasis on power analysis. *Nurs Res* 1996;45:379-380.
19. Clarke PJ, Notebaert L, MacLeod C. Absence of evidence or evidence of absence: reflecting on therapeutic implementations of attentional bias modification. *BMC Psychiatry* 2014;14:8.
20. Rozmovits L, Rose P, Ziebland S. In the absence of evidence, who chooses? A qualitative study of patients' needs after treatment for colorectal cancer. *J Health Serv Res Policy* 2004;9(3):159-164.
21. Inference for means: Comparing two independent samples. Available at https://www.stat.ubc.ca/~rollin/stats/ssize/n2.html. Accessed October 31, 2018.
22. ClinCalc. Sample size calculator. Available at http://clincalc.com/stats/samplesize.aspx. Accessed October 31, 2018.
23. G*Power: Statistical Power Analysis for Windows and Mac. Available at http://www.gpower.hhu.de/. Accessed October 31, 2018.
24. Lesaffre E. Use and misuse of the p-value. *Bull NYU Hosp Jt Dis* 2008;66(2):146-149.
25. Alderson P. Absence of evidence is not evidence of absence. *BMJ* 2004;328(7438):476-477.
26. Chan AW, Altman DG. Identifying outcome reporting bias in randomised trials on PubMed: review of publications and survey of authors. *BMJ* 2005;330(7494):753.
27. Ioannidis JP. Effect of the statistical significance of results on the time to completion and publication of randomized efficacy trials. *JAMA* 1998;279(4):281-286.
28. Chan AW, Krleza-Jeric K, Schmid I, Altman DG. Outcome reporting bias in randomized trials funded by the Canadian Institutes of Health Research. *CMAJ* 2004;171(7):735-740.
29. Krzyzanowska MK, Pintilie M, Tannock IF. Factors associated with failure to publish large randomized trials presented at an oncology meeting. *JAMA* 2003;290(4):495-501.
30. Altman DG, Bland JM. Absence of evidence is not evidence of absence. *BMJ* 1995;311:485.
31. Findley TW. Research in physical medicine and rehabilitation. IX. Primary data analysis. *Am J Phys Med Rehabil* 1990;69(4):209-218.
32. Gonzales VA, Ottenbacher KJ. Measures of central tendency in rehabilitation research: what do they mean? *Am J Phys Med Rehabil* 2001;80(2):141-146.
33. Siegel S, Castellan NJ. *Nonparametric Statistics for the Behavioral Sciences*. 2nd ed. New York: McGraw-Hill; 1988.
34. Shapiro SS, Wilk MB. An analysis of variance test for normality (complete samples). *Biometrika* 1965;52(3-4):591-611.
35. Razali N, Wah YB. Power comparisons of Shapiro-Wilk, Kolmogorov-Smirnov, Lilliefors and Anderson-Darling tests. *J Stat Modeling Anal* 2011;2(1):21-33.
36. Fisher RA. *The Design of Experiments*. 9th ed. New York: Macmillan; 1971.

Comparing Two Means: The *t*-Test

The simplest experimental comparison involves the use of two independent groups within a randomized controlled trial (RCT). This design allows the researcher to assume that all individual differences are evenly distributed between the groups at baseline, and therefore, observed differences after the application of an intervention to one group should reflect a significant difference, one that is unlikely to be the result of chance.

The statistical ratio used to compare two means is called the *t*-test, also known as *Student's t-test*. The purpose of this chapter is to introduce procedures that can be applied to differences between two independent samples or between scores obtained with repeated measures. These procedures are based on parametric operations and, therefore, are subject to assumptions underlying parametric statistics.

■ The Conceptual Basis for Comparing Means

The concept of testing for statistical significance was introduced in Chapter 23 in relation to a one-sample test. The process for comparing two sample means is similar, with some important variations. To illustrate this process, suppose we divide a sample of 100 subjects into two randomly assigned groups ($n=50$), one experimental and one control, to determine if an intervention makes a difference in their performance. Theoretically, if the treatment was ineffective (H_0), we would expect all subjects in both groups to have the same response, with no difference between groups.

But if the treatment is effective, all other factors being equal, we would expect a difference, with all subjects within the experimental group getting the same score, and all subjects within the control group getting the same score, but scores would be different between groups. This is illustrated in Figure 24-1A, showing that everyone in the treatment group performed better than everyone in the control group.

Now think about combining all 100 scores. If we were asked to *explain* why some scores in this sample were different, we would say that all differences were due to the effect of treatment. There is a difference *between the groups* but no variance *within the groups*.

Error Variance

Of course, that scenario is not plausible, so let's consider the more realistic situation where subjects within a group do not all respond the same way. As shown in Figure 24-1B, the scores within each group are variable, but we still tend to see higher scores among those in the experimental group.

Now if we look at the entire set of scores, and we were asked again to explain why scores were different, we would say that some of the differences can be *explained* by the treatment effect; that is, most of the higher scores were in the treatment group. However, the scores are also influenced by a host of other random factors that create variance within the groups, variance that is *unexplained* by the treatment. This unexplained portion is called error variance.

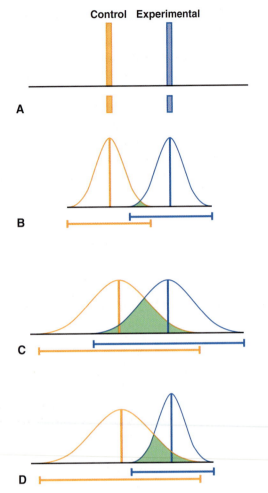

Control   Experimental

A

B

C

D

Figure 24–1 Four sets of hypothetical distributions with the same means but different variances. A) All subjects in each group have the same score, but the groups are different from each other. There is no variance within groups, only between groups. B) Subjects' scores are more spread out, but the control and experimental conditions are still clearly different. The variances of both groups are equal. C) Subjects are more variable in responses, with greater variance within groups, making the groups appear less different. D) The variances of the two groups are not equal.

> The concept of statistical "error" does not mean mistakes or miscalculation. It refers to all sources of variability within a set of data that cannot be explained by the independent variable.

The distributions in Figure 24-1B show two means that are far apart, with few overlapping scores at one extreme of each curve. The curves show that the individuals in the treatment and control groups behaved very differently, whereas subjects within each group performed within a narrow range (error variance is small). In such a comparison, the experimental treatment has

clearly differentiated the groups, and the difference between groups is unlikely to be the result of chance. Therefore, the null hypothesis would probably be rejected.

Contrast this with the distributions in Figure 24-1C, which shows the same means but greater variability within the groups, as evidenced by the wider spread of the curves. Factors other than the treatment variable are causing subjects to respond very differently from each other. Here we find more overlap, indicating that many subjects from both groups had the same score, regardless of whether or not they received the treatment. These curves reflect a greater degree of error variance; that is, the treatment does not help to fully explain the differences among scores. In this case, it is less likely that the treatment is differentiating the groups, and the null hypothesis would probably not be rejected. Any differences observed here are more likely to be due to chance variation.

The Statistical Ratio

These subjective guesses about the distributions in Figure 24-1 are not adequate, however, for making research decisions about the effectiveness of treatment. We must derive a more objective criterion to determine if observed differences between groups are large enough to reflect a treatment effect. In other words, how do we decide if we should reject the null hypothesis? This is what a test of statistical significance is designed to do.

The *t* Distribution

The properties of the normal curve provide the basis for determining if significant differences exist. Recall from Chapter 22 how the normal curve was used to determine the probability associated with choosing a single value out of a population. By knowing the variance and the proportions under the curve, we could know the probability of obtaining a certain value to determine if it was a "likely" or "unlikely" event. By converting a value to a z-score, we were able to determine the area of the curve above or below the value, and thereby interpret the probability associated with it.

We can use this same logic to determine if the *difference between two means* is a likely outcome. If we were to choose a random sample of individuals, divide them randomly into two groups and do nothing to them, theoretically we should find no difference between their means ($\bar{X}_1 - \bar{X}_2 = 0$). But because we might expect some difference just by chance, we have to ask if the observed difference is large enough to be considered significant.

The significance of the difference between two group means is judged by a ratio, the *t*-test, derived as follows:

$$t = \frac{\text{Difference } between \text{ means}}{\text{Variability } within \text{ groups}}$$

The numerator represents the separation *between* the groups, which is a function of all sources of variance, including treatment effects and error. The denominator reflects the variability *within* groups as a result of error alone.

> The *between* and *within* sources of variance are essential elements of significance testing that will be used repeatedly. It can be thought of as a signal to noise ratio, where the "signal" represents the difference between means, and the "noise" is all the other random variability. The larger the signal in proportion to the noise, the more likely the null hypothesis will be rejected. Most statistical tests are based on this relationship.

When H_0 is false (the treatment worked), the numerator will be larger and the denominator will be smaller—a greater variance between groups, less variance within groups. When H_0 is true (no treatment effect), the error variance gets larger and the t ratio will be smaller, approaching 1.0. If we want to demonstrate that two groups are significantly different, the value of t should be as large as possible. Thus, we would want the separation between the group means to be large and the variability within groups to be small—a lot of signal to little noise.

HISTORICAL NOTE

Following graduation from Oxford in 1899, with degrees in mathematics and chemistry, William S. Gosset (1876-1937) had the somewhat enviable job of working for the Guinness Brewery in Dublin, Ireland, with responsibility for assuring the quality of the beer. He began studying the results of his inspections on small samples and figured out that his accuracy improved when he estimated the standard error of his sample. With no computer to assist him, he worked for over a year, testing hundreds of random samples by hand—calculations we could do in seconds today—but he got it right!

It seems that another researcher at Guinness had previously published a paper that had revealed trade secrets, and Guinness prohibited its employees from publishing to prevent further disclosures. Gosset convinced his bosses that his information presented no threat to the company, and was allowed to publish, but only if he used a pseudonym. He chose "Student."[1] Gosset's landmark 1908 article, "The Probable Error of a Mean," became the foundation for the *t*-test, which is why it is also known as "Student's *t*."[2] Today a plaque hangs in the halls of the Guinness Brewery, honoring Gosset's historic contribution.

Statistical Hypotheses

The null hypothesis states that the two means are equal:

$$H_0: \mu_1 = \mu_2 \ (\mu_1 - \mu_2 = 0)$$

The alternative hypothesis can be stated in a nondirectional format,

$$H_1: \mu_1 \neq \mu_2 \ (\mu_1 - \mu_2 \neq 0)$$

or a directional format,

$$H_1: \mu_1 > \mu_2 \ (\mu_1 - \mu_2 > 0)$$

Depending on the direction of the difference between means, t can be a positive or negative value. Nondirectional hypotheses are tested using a two-tailed test, and directional hypotheses are tested using a one-tailed test (see Chapter 23).

> Even though we are comparing sample means, hypotheses are written in terms of population parameters.

Homogeneity of Variance

A major assumption for the *t*-test, and most other parametric statistics, is equality of variances among groups, or **homogeneity of variance**. While there is an expectation that some error variance will be present in each group, the assumption is that the degree of variance will be roughly equivalent—or *not significantly different*. This is illustrated by the curves in Figure 24-1B and C. However, in D we can see that the treatment group is much less variable than the control group, and the assumption of homogeneity of variance is less tenable.

Most statistical procedures include tests to determine if variance components are not significantly different; that is, if observed differences between the variances are due to chance. With random assignment, larger samples will have a better chance of showing equal variances than small samples. When variances are significantly different (they are not equal), adjustments can be made in the test to account for this difference.

■ The Independent Samples *t*-Test

To compare means from two independent groups, usually created through random assignment, we use an *independent* or **unpaired *t*-test**. Groups are considered independent because each is composed of different sets of subjects, with no inherent relationship derived from repeated measures or matching.

The test statistic for the unpaired *t*-test is calculated using the formula

$$t = \frac{\bar{X}_1 - \bar{X}_2}{s_{\bar{X}_1 - \bar{X}_2}}$$

The numerator of this ratio represents the difference *between* the independent group means. The term in the denominator is called the **standard error of the difference between the means**, representing the pooled variance *within* the groups.

🔑 To understand the concept of the *standard error of the difference between means*, think back to the description of sampling distributions in Chapter 23. The theoretical underpinning of this distribution is based on taking many samples from a population, dividing each into two random groups, and then taking the difference between the two means. Most of these samples will have mean differences at or close to zero, and some, just by chance, will have larger differences above and below zero. The standard error of the difference between means is the standard deviation of this sampling distribution.

This discussion will begin with procedures for comparisons with *equal variances*. The independent *t*-test involves adjustments if homogeneity of variance is not present, and the process for *unequal variances* will be described.

> ➤ **CASE IN POINT #1**
>
> Suppose we want to determine if a newly designed splint will improve hand function in patients with rheumatoid arthritis (RA) better than a standard splint, as measured by pinch strength in pounds (lbs). We design a two-group pretest-posttest design to compare the change in pinch strength over 2 weeks. We recruit a sample of 20 participants with RA with similar degrees of deformity in the hand and wrist. We hypothesize that there will be a difference between the two splints in the amount of improvement in pinch strength following the treatment period.
>
> Participants are randomly assigned to the new splint group (n_1 =10) or the standard splint group (n_2 =10). Pinch strength is measured at baseline and again after 2 weeks, and the change in strength is compared: For the new splint group $\overline{X}_1$ = 10.11 lbs, and for the standard group $\overline{X}_2$ = 5.45 lbs.

Equal Variances

Hypothetical results for the splint study are shown in Table 24-1A, including the means and standard deviations (*s*) for each group. The mean difference between groups is 4.66 lbs. We then ask:

What is the probability that we would find a difference this large if the treatment is not effective—if the null hypothesis is true?

The value of *t* is used to determine if this difference is significant (not likely due to chance). Calculations are shown in Table 24-1B to illustrate how these values result in the *t* ratio. Note how the denominator is calculated based on the *pooled variance* for the two groups. The *calculated t* = 2.718. Now we need to determine if this ratio is large enough to represent a significant difference.

📌 Most of you will be using computer programs to calculate statistics, so we won't spend a lot of time on the math. The focus will be on interpreting SPSS output for each test. However, calculations will be included in some tables to provide a conceptual foundation for basic tests, as understanding formulas can be helpful to clarify what statistical ratios mean. For more complicated procedures, however, we will focus on computer output only. Look for reference to online supplements in many chapters, where details on appropriate calculations are provided for those who want (or are required) to do the math. Data files are also available for all examples, and can be found with online resources at www.fadavis.com.

The Critical Value

We determine if a calculated *t* value is significant by comparing it with a **critical value** at a specified level of significance. Appendix Table A-2 shows critical values associated with *t* distributions for samples of various sizes. At the top of the table, levels of significance are identified for one-tailed (α_1) and two-tailed (α_2) tests. Because we proposed a nondirectional alternative hypothesis in this example, we will perform a two-tailed test.

The column along the left side of the table, labeled *df*, identifies the **degrees of freedom**, which is based on the size of the sample. Each group will have *n*-1 degrees of freedom. Therefore, the total degrees of freedom are:

$$df = (n_1 - 1) + (n_2 - 1) = (n_1 + n_2 - 2)$$

This can also be written $df = N - 2$, where *N* is the combined sample size. For the splint study, $df = 20 - 2 = 18$.

🔑 The concept of degrees of freedom is based on the number of components that are *free to vary* within a set of data. As an illustration, suppose we took five measurements with a sum of 30 and a mean of 6. Theoretically, any set of five numbers could be specified to equal a sum of 30. However, once four of the scores are known, the fifth is automatically determined. If we measured 8, 9, 10, and 11, the fifth score would have to be –8 to get a total of 30. Therefore, this set of data has four degrees of freedom. Four values are free to vary, given the restrictions imposed on the data, in this case a sum of 30 with a mean of 6. Therefore, the degrees of freedom will equal one less than the number of scores, or *n* – 1.

As other statistical tests are presented in the coming chapters, rules for determining degrees of freedom will be described.

For this study, using Table A-2, we look across the row for 18 *df* to the column labeled α_2 = .05 and find the critical value *t* (18) = 2.101. For notation purposes, the degrees of freedom are indicated in parentheses following the statistical symbol.

Table 24-1 **Results of the Unpaired *t*-Test (Equal Variances): Change in Pinch Strength (Pounds of Force) Following Hand Splinting**

A. Descriptive Data

Group Statistics

	group	N	Mean	Std. Deviation	Std. Error Mean
strength	New Splint	10	10.1100	3.71587	1.17506
	Standard Splint	10	5.4500	3.94722	1.24822

B. Calculation of *t*

Step 1: Calculate the pooled variance:
$$s_p^2 = \frac{s_1^2\,(n_1 - 1) + s_2^2\,(n_2 - 1)}{n_1 + n_2 - 2} = \frac{(3.7158)^2\,(10 - 1) + (5.45)^2\,(10 - 1)}{10 + 10 - 2} = 14.695$$

Step 2: Calculate the standard error of the difference between means:
$$s_{\bar{x}_1 - \bar{x}_2} = \sqrt{\frac{s_p^2}{n_1} + \frac{s_p^2}{n_2}} = \sqrt{\frac{14.695}{10} + \frac{14.695}{10}} = 1.714$$

Step 3: Calculate *t*:
$$t = \frac{\bar{x}_1 - \bar{x}_2}{s_{\bar{x}_1 - \bar{x}_2}} = \frac{10.11 - 5.45}{1.714} = 2.718$$

C. SPSS Output: Independent *t*-test (Equal Variances)

Independent Samples Test

Strength	Levene's Test for Equality of Variances		t-test for Equality of Means					95% Confidence Interval of the Difference ⑤	
	F	① Sig.	t	df	Sig. (2-tailed)	Mean Difference	Std. Error Difference	Lower	Upper
Equal variances assumed	.685	.419	2.718	18	② 0.14	③ 4.6600	④ 1.71430	1.05839	8.26161
Equal variances not assumed			2.718	17.935	0.14	4.6600	1.71430	1.05745	8.26255

① Levene's test compares the variances of the two groups. This difference is not significant (*p*=.419). Therefore, we will use the *t*-test for equal variances.

② The two-tailed probability for the the *t*-test is .014. This is a significant test, and we reject H_0. SPSS uses the term "Sig" to indicate *p* values, and only reports two-tailed values by default. If we had performed a one-tailed test, we would divide this value by 2, and it would be significant at *p* = .007.

③ The difference between the means of group 1 and 2 (the numerator of the *t*-test)

④ The standard error of the difference between the means (denominator of the *t*-test)

⑤ The 95% confidence interval does not contain the null value zero, confirming that the difference between the means is significant.

Notice in Table A-2 that as the degrees of freedom get larger, the critical value of *t* approaches *z*. For instance, with samples larger than 120, the critical value of *t* at α_2=.05 is 1.96, the same as *z*.

Figure 24-2 illustrates the critical value of *t* for 18 *df* at α_2 = .05. Because we are using a two-tailed test, each tail holds $\alpha/2$ or .025. The null hypothesis states that the difference between means will be zero, and therefore, the *t* ratio will also equal zero. The probability that a calculated *t* ratio will be as large or larger than (2.101 when means are only different by chance is 5% or less. Therefore, the critical value reflects the maximum difference under the null hypothesis. Anything larger would be

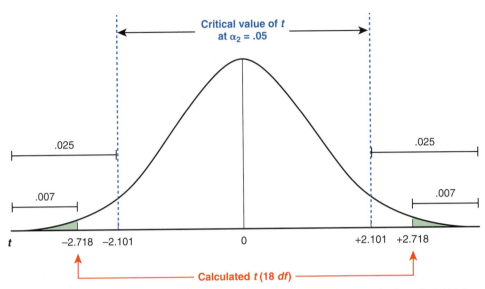

Figure 24–2 Curve representing a *t* distribution for 18 df, showing the critical value of ±2.101 for a two-tailed test at .05, with each tail representing .025 of the curve. The null hypothesis states that the *t* ratio will equal zero. The calculated value for the splint example is *t* = 2.718, which falls within the critical region beyond the critical value, and therefore is significant. This value demarcates an area in the two tails of the curve of 0.014, with .007 in each tail (from Table 24-1).

considered significant, and the null hypothesis would be rejected.

For a *t* ratio to represent a significant difference, the absolute value of the calculated ratio must be *greater than or equal to* the critical value. In this example, the calculated value *t* = 2.718 is greater than the critical value 2.101. Therefore, *p* < .05 for this calculated value, and the group means are considered significantly different. We reject H_0, accept H_1, and conclude that patients wearing the new splint improved more than those in the standard group.

The Sign of *t*

Critical values of *t* are absolute values, so that negative or positive ratios are tested against the same criteria. The sign of *t* can be ignored when a nondirectional hypothesis has been proposed. The critical region for a two-tailed test is located in both tails of the *t* distribution, and therefore either a positive or negative value can be considered significant (see Chapter 23). The sign will be an artifact of which group happened to be designated Group 1 or 2. If the group designations were arbitrarily reversed, the ratio would carry the opposite sign, with no change in outcome. For the current example, the ratio happens to be positive, because the experimental group was designated as Group 1 and $\bar{X}_1$ was larger than the mean improvement for the control group, $\bar{X}_2$.

The sign is of concern, however, when a directional alternative hypothesis is proposed. In a one-tailed test, the researcher is predicting that one specific mean will

be larger or smaller than the other, and the sign must be in the predicted direction for the alternative hypothesis to be accepted (see Box 24-1).

Computer Output

Table 24-1 shows the output for an unpaired *t*-test for the example of pinch strength and hand splints. Descriptive statistics are given for each group. This information is useful as a first pass, to confirm the number of subjects, and to see how far apart the means and variances are. We can see that the standard deviations are similar, although not exactly the same.

The test for homogeneity of variance will indicate if the difference between variances is large enough to be meaningful, and not the result of chance. When variances are significantly different (they are not equal), adjustments can be made in the *t* test that will account for these differences. **Levene's Test for equality of variances** compares the variances of the two groups. It uses the *F* statistic and reports a *p* value that indicates if the variances are significantly different. If Levene's test is significant ($p \leq .05$), the assumption of homogeneity of variance has been violated. If $p > .05$, we can assume the variances are not significantly different, that is, they are homogeneous.

Notice that there are actually two lines of output for the *t*-test reported in Table 24-1C, labeled according to whether the assumption of equal variances can be applied. Computer packages automatically run the *t*-test for both equal and unequal variances, and the researcher must choose which one to use for analysis.

Box 24-1   Two-Tailed or Not Two-Tailed? That is the Question

In Chapter 23, the difference between one- and two-tailed tests was demonstrated, showing that results with the same data can differ depending on which type of test is done. This situation has sparked many debates about the appropriate use of directional and nondirectional alternative hypotheses.

Some statisticians favor exclusive use of two-tailed (nondirectional) tests, based on a conservative and traditional approach to data analysis.[3] Because there is uncertainty in every study, they suggest there is always a possibility that differences will go in either direction. With this argument, one-tailed tests should only be used when it is impossible for the difference to go in the opposite direction.[4]

Others have argued that the rationale behind most research questions supports one-sided tests, especially in studies where a control or placebo group is involved.[5] These proponents argue that the ethics of research would demand that a study be based on a sound theoretical rationale that would identify an expected direction of difference.

The middle ground on this issue is probably most reasonable. Researchers are obliged to justify whether the alternative hypothesis is directional or nondirectional and use the appropriate statistical approach. Although you may assume that only one direction is possible, such assumptions may not always hold. For example, we may assume that strength training will increase strength, but there could be conditions when a reverse outcome might occur, such as over-training or the presence of muscle pathologies. It is important to realize that if a directional hypothesis is proposed, and results go in the opposite direction, H_0 cannot be rejected because it is not possible to accept the alternative. Therefore, one-tailed tests are more appropriately applied when the outcome of interest is solely in one direction, so if the difference turns out to be significant in the other direction, it will not be relevant.

Because statistical results can influence conclusions, and perhaps clinical judgments, the designation of a one-tailed test should be applied only when a sound rationale can be provided in advance. The choice of a one- or two-tailed test should be reported with published data.

As shown in Table 24-1C ❶, $p = .419$ for Levene's test. Because this value is greater than .05, we conclude that the variances are not significantly different. Therefore, we can use the first line of *t*-test data for "*Equal variances assumed*."

A test for homogeneity of variance can sometimes be confusing when it is performed in conjunction with a test for differences between means. Two different probability values are produced because two different tests are being done. First the test for homogeneity of variance determines if the variances are significantly different from each other. Then the *t*-test will determine if the means are significantly different. If the first test shows that variances are not equal ($p < .05$), an adjustment is made in the test for means, which is why different output is presented for unequal variances.

Tails

Using the data for our example, we performed a two-tailed test, which is the default (see Table 24-1C ❷). This represents the total area in both tails of the curve beyond $t = \pm 2.718$ (see Figure 24-2). Because *p* is less than .05, we reject the null hypothesis. There is only a .014 probability that we would see a ratio this large if H_0 were true—an unlikely event.

Note that if we had proposed a one-tailed test, we would have to divide the *p* value by 2. For a one-tailed test, this analysis would be significant at $p = .007$. Various statistical programs will handle this differently, so it is important to be aware of how *p* values are reported.

Confidence Intervals

Recall from Chapter 23 that a confidence interval specifies a range of scores within which the population mean is likely to fall. We can also use this approach to set a confidence interval to estimate the *difference between group means* that exists in the population as follows:

$$95\% \text{ CI} = (\bar{X}_1 - \bar{X}_2) \pm (t)s_{\bar{X}_1 - \bar{X}_2}$$

where $s_{\bar{X}_1 - \bar{X}_2}$ is the standard error of the difference between means (the denominator of the *t*-test), and *t* is the *critical value* for the appropriate degrees of freedom at $\alpha = .05$. We will be 95% confident that the true difference between population means will fall within this interval.

Consider again the data shown in Table 24-1 for changes in pinch strength, with a difference between means of 4.66 pounds. The independent *t*-test is significant at $p = .014$, and H_0 is rejected. Now let us examine how confidence intervals support this conclusion.

We create the 95% confidence interval using the critical value $t(18) = 2.101$ and the standard error of the difference between means, 1.714 (see Table 24-1 ❹). We substitute these values to determine the 95% confidence limits:

$$95\% \text{ CI} = (10.11 - 5.45) \pm 2.101 (1.714)$$
$$= 4.66 \pm 3.60$$
$$= 1.06 \text{ to } 8.26$$

We are 95% confident that the true mean difference, $\mu_1 - \mu_2$, lies between 1.06 and 8.26 (see Table 24-1C ❺). This interval provides important information regarding the clinical application of these data (see Focus on Evidence 24-1).

Focus on Evidence 24–1
Confidence by Intervals

Researchers in many disciplines have become disenchanted with the overemphasis placed on reporting *p* values in research literature.[3] The concern relates to the lack of useful interpretation of these values, which focus solely on statistical significance or the viability of the null hypothesis, rather than the magnitude of the treatment effect.[7] In an effort to make hypothesis testing more meaningful, investigators have begun to rely more on the confidence interval (CI) as a practical estimate of a population's characteristics. Many journals now require the reporting of confidence intervals, some to the exclusion of *p* values.

In hypothesis testing, we always wrestle with a degree of uncertainty. Confidence intervals provide an expression of that uncertainty, helping us understand a possible range of true differences, something the *p* value cannot do.[8] Although confidence intervals incidentally tell us whether an effect is "significant" (if the null value is not included), their more important function is to express the precision with which the effect size is estimated.[9,10] This information can then be used for evaluating the results of assessments and for framing practice decisions.

To illustrate this point, Obeid et al[11] were interested in studying sedentary behavior of children with cerebral palsy (CP), recognizing the metabolic and cardiovascular risks associated with lack of physical activity. They hypothesized that children with CP would spend more hours sedentary than their typically developing peers and would take fewer breaks to interrupt sedentary time. Using an independent *t*-test, they found that the difference between groups was significant as follows:

Each of these values was averaged over a measurement period of 6 days. The differences between groups are significant for both variables ($p < .05$), supported by CIs that do not contain zero. But how do the CIs help to interpret these outcomes? For sedentary time, a difference of 4 min/hr may seem small (with a small CI), but the authors suggest that this can add up over a day or week to a meaningful variation. However, looking at the number of breaks shows a different story, with a much wider CI. The degree to which these differences have a clinical impact must be interpreted in relation to the amount of sedentary time that would be considered detrimental to the child's health and how intervention might address activity levels. Clearly, there is substantial variability in the sample, which makes interpretation less certain.

Although confidence intervals and *p* values are linked, they are based on different views of the same problem. The *p* value is based on the likelihood of finding an observed outcome if the null hypothesis is true. Confidence intervals make no assumptions about the null hypothesis, and instead reflect the likelihood that the limits include the population parameter. Like *p* values, however, confidence intervals do not tell us about the importance of the observed effect. That will always remain a matter of clinical judgment.

From Obeid J, Balemans AC, Nooruyn SG, et al. Objectively measured sedentary time in youth with cerebral palsy compared with age-, sex-, and season-matched youth who are developing typically: an explorative study. *Phys Ther* 2014;94(8):1163-7. Adapted from Table, p. 1165. Used with permission of the American Physical Therapy Association.

Measure	CP Group (n = 17)	Non-CP Group (n = 17)	Difference	95% CI	t	p
Sedentary time (min/hr)	47.5 (4.9)	43.6 (4.2)	3.9	0.7 to 7.1	2.509	.02
Breaks (number/hr)	179 (70)	232 (61)	−53.0	−99.0 to −7.0	−2.356	.03

The null value for a difference between two means is zero. Because this confidence interval does not contain zero, we can reasonably reject H_0 with a 5% risk. This confirms the results of the *t*-test for these same data using the *p* value.

Unequal Variances

Studies have shown that the validity of the independent *t*-test is not seriously compromised by violation of the assumption of equality of variance when $n_1 = n_2$.[6] However, when sample sizes are unequal, differences in variance can affect the accuracy of the *t* ratio. If a test for equality of variance shows that variances are significantly different, the *t* ratio must be adjusted.

Computer Output

Consider the previous example in which we examined the effect of a hand splint on changes in pinch strength.

Table 24-2 shows alternative data for this comparison, with unequal sample sizes ($n_1 = 15$, $n_2 = 10$). Descriptive statistics are provided for the performance of each group.

We first look at the results of Levene's test, which shows that the variances in this analysis are significantly different ($p = .038$, Table 24-2 ❶). Therefore, for this analysis, we use the second line of data in the output, "*Equal variances not assumed.*"

Note that the degrees of freedom associated with the *t*-test for unequal variances are adjusted downward, so that the critical value for *t* is also modified. In this example, 20.6 degrees of freedom are used to determine the critical value of *t* (see Table 24-2 ❷). From Table A.2, we can find the critical value $t (21) = 2.080$.

Confidence Intervals

This test also includes a confidence interval for the mean difference (see Table 24-2 ❸). The standard error is

Table 24-2   Results of the Independent *t*-Test (Unequal Variances): Changes in Pinch Strength (Pounds of Force) Following Hand Splinting

A. Descriptive Data

Group Statistics

	group	N	Mean	Std. Deviation	Std. Error Mean
strength	Splint	15	10.8000	5.01711	1.29541
	Control	10	5.6500	2.21171	.69940

B. SPSS Output: Independent *t*-test (Unequal Variances)

Independent Samples Test

strength	Levene's Test for Equality of Variances		t-test for Equality of Means						95% Confidence Interval of the Difference	
	F	Sig. ①	t	df	Sig. (2-tailed)	Mean Difference	Std. Error Difference		Lower	Upper
Equal variances assumed	4.866	.038	3.039	23	.006	5.15000	1.69489		1.64386	8.65614
Equal variances not assumed			3.498	② 20.625	③ .002	④ 5.15000	⑤ 1.47216		2.08508	8.21492

---

① Levene's test is significant ($p=.038$). indicating that the variance of group 1 is significantly different from the variance of group 2. Therefore, we will use the *t*-test for unequal variances.

② With 25 subjects, the adjusted total degrees of freedom for the test of unequal variances is 20.625.

③ The two-tailed probability for the *t*-test is .002. This is significant, and we reject H_0.

④ The difference between the means of group 1 and 2 (numerator of the *t*-test)

⑤ Standard error of the difference (denominator of the *t*-test).

⑥ The 95% confidence interval does not contain zero, confirming that the difference between means is significant at $p < .05$.

---

different for the test of unequal variances, calculated as the denominator of the t-test (see Table 24-2 ⑤). For this analysis, we use the critical value $t(21) = 2.080$ for $\alpha_2=.05$.

$$95\% \text{ CI} = 10.8 - 5.65 \pm 2.080 (1.472)$$
$$= 5.15 \pm 3.062$$
$$= 2.088 \text{ to } 8.212$$

 See the *Chapter 24 Supplement* for calculations associated with the *t*-test for unequal variances.

■ Paired Samples *t*-Test

Researchers often use repeated measures to improve the degree of control over extraneous variables in a study. In these designs, subjects usually serve as their own controls, each being exposed to both experimental conditions and then responses are compared across these conditions. A repeated measures design may also be based on matched samples.

In these types of studies, data are considered *paired* or *correlated*, because each measurement has a matched value for each subject. To determine if these values are significantly different from each other, a **paired *t*-test** is performed. This test analyzes *difference scores* (*d*) within each pair, so that subjects are compared only with themselves. Statistically, this has the effect of reducing the total error variance in the data because most of the extraneous factors that influence data will be the same across both treatment conditions. Therefore, tests of significance involving paired comparisons tend to be more powerful than unpaired tests.

The paired *t*-test may also be called a test for *correlated, dependent,* or *matched* samples.

The test statistic for paired data is based on the ratio

$$t = \frac{\bar{d}}{s_{\bar{d}}}$$

where $\bar{d}$ is the mean of the difference scores, and $s_{\bar{d}}$ represents the **standard error of the difference scores**. Like the independent test, this t ratio reflects the proportional relationship of *between-* and *within-group* variance components. The numerator is a measure of the differences between scores in each pair, and the denominator is a measure of the variability within the difference scores.

In accordance with requirements for parametric statistics, the paired t-test is based on the assumption that samples are randomly drawn from normally distributed populations, and data are at the interval/ratio level. Because the number of scores must be the same for both levels of the repeated measure, it is unnecessary to test the assumption of homogeneity of variance.

> ➤ **CASE IN POINT #2**
>
> Suppose we set up a study to test the effect of using a lumbar support pillow on angular position of the pelvis in relaxed sitting. We hypothesize that pelvic tilt will be greater with a lumbar support pillow compared to sitting with no pillow, a directional hypothesis. We test eight subjects, each one sitting with and without the pillow, in random order. The angle of pelvic tilt is measured using a flexible ruler, with measurements transformed to degrees.
>
> The mean angle with the pillow was 102.375, and the mean without the pillow was 99.00, a difference of 3.375 degrees.

The Critical Value

With a directional hypothesis, this study applies a one-tailed test. We are predicting that the pelvic tilt will be greater with a pillow than without. Statistical hypotheses can be expressed as

$$H_0: \mu_1 = \mu_2 \text{ against } H_1: \mu_1 > \mu_2$$

where means represent repeated conditions. These hypotheses may also be expressed in terms of difference scores:

$$H_0: \bar{d} = 0 \text{ and } H_1: \bar{d} > 0$$

Hypothetical data are reported in Table 24-3A. A difference score is calculated for each pair of scores, and the mean ($\bar{d}$), and standard deviation (s_d) of the difference scores are calculated. By calculating the standard error, $s_{\bar{d}}$, and substituting values in the formula for the paired t-test, we obtain $t = -1.532$ (see Table 24-3B). The value of t is positive because we designated the Pillow condition as group 1.

Because a repeated measures design uses only one sample of subjects (not separate groups), the total *df*

associated with a paired t-test are $n - 1$, where n is the number of pairs of scores. The absolute value of the calculated ratio is compared with a critical value, in this case for a one-tailed test with $n - 1 = 7$ *df*: Using Appendix Table A-2, we find the critical value $t(7) = 1.895$ for $\alpha_1 = .05$. Because the calculated value is less than the critical value, these conditions are not considered significantly different.

The output in Table 24-3C ➅ shows that $p = .169$ for a two-tailed test. Because we proposed a directional hypothesis, however, we must divide this value by 2 to get a one-tailed value, so $p = .085$. Because this is greater than .05, H_0 is not rejected.

Confidence Intervals

For the paired t-test, a confidence interval is obtained using the formula:

$$95\% \text{ CI} = \bar{d} \pm t(s_{\bar{d}})$$

where t is the critical value for the appropriate degrees of freedom ($\alpha_2 = .05$), and $s_{\bar{d}}$ is the standard error of the difference scores. Even though we have proposed a one-tailed test, we use a two-sided test to determine high and low confidence limits. Table A-2 tells us that $t(7) = 2.365$. Therefore,

$$95\% \text{ CI} = 3.375 \pm 2.365 \, (2.203)$$
$$= 3.375 \pm 5.210$$
$$= -1.835 \text{ to } 8.585$$

We are 95% confidence that the true difference in pelvic angle between the pillow and non-pillow conditions is between −1.84 and 8.59 degrees (see Table 24-3C ➆). This means the population mean could be negative, positive, or even zero. When zero is contained within a confidence interval, means are not significantly different.

■ Power and Effect Size

Power analysis for the t-test is based on the effect size index, d, originally proposed by Cohen.[12] This index expresses the difference between the two sample means in standard deviation units (see Fig. 24-3), which is why it is sometimes called the **standardized mean difference (SMD)**. The calculation of d is specific to the type of t-test performed.

Conventional effect sizes for d are:

Small	$d = .20$
Medium	$d = .50$
Large	$d = .80$

These guidelines are intended to provide a way to interpret effect size along a continuum, not to serve as absolute cutoff values. They are open to interpretation

Table 24-3   Results of the Paired *t*-Test: Angle of Pelvis With and Without a Lumbar Support Pillow

A. Data

| | X_1 | X_2 | |
Subject	Pillow	No pillow	d
1	112	108	4
2	96	102	−6
3	105	98	7
4	110	112	−2
5	106	100	6
6	98	85	13
7	90	92	−2
8	102	95	7

$$\Sigma d = 27$$
$$\bar{d} = 3.375 \;\; ①$$
$$s_d = 6.232$$

B. Calculation of *t*

Step 1: Calculate the standard error of the different scores:

$$s_{\bar{d}} = \frac{s_d}{\sqrt{n}} = \frac{6.232}{\sqrt{8}} = 2.203 \;\; ②$$

Step 2: Calculate *t*:

$$t = \frac{\bar{d}}{s_{\bar{d}}} = \frac{3.375}{2.203} = 1.532 \;\; ③$$

C. SPSS Output: Paired *t*-test

Paired Samples Statistics

Pair 1	Mean ④	N	Std. Deviation	Std. Error Mean
Pillow	102.3750	8	7.40536	2.61819
NoPillow	99.0000	8	8.63548	3.05310

Paired Samples Correlations

Pair 1	N	Correlation	Sig.
Pillow & NoPillow	8	⑤ .708	.049

Paired Samples Test

| | Paired Differences | | | | | | | |
Pair 1	Mean ①	Std. Deviation	Std. Error Mean ②	95% Confidence Interval of the Difference ⑦ Lower	Upper	t ③	df	Sig. (2-tailed) ⑥
Pillow - NoPillow	3.37500	6.23212	2.20339	−1.83518	8.58518	1.532	7	.169

① The mean difference score, $\bar{d}$, is 3.375 (numerator of the *t*-test), with a standard deviation, s_d of 6.232.

② The standard error of the difference scores, $s_{\bar{d}}$, is 2.203 (denominator of the *t*-test)

③ The paired *t*-test results in $t = 1.532$.

④ Means are provided for each condition.

⑤ The paired *t*-test procedure includes the correlation of pillow and non-pillow scores and significance of the correlation.

⑥ Because a directional alternative hypothesis was proposed, a one-tailed test is used. Therefore, we must divide the 2-tailed significance value by 2, resulting in $p = .085$. This test is not significant.

⑦ 95% confidence interval of the difference scores contains zero, confirming no significant difference.

---

depending on the context of the variables being measured.

> Don't confuse the use of *d* to indicate both a difference score and the effect size index. Unfortunately, these are conventional designations, but they represent different values.

Effect Size for the Independent *t*-Test

For the independent *t*-test (with equal variances), the effect size index is

$$d = \frac{\bar{X}_1 - \bar{X}_2}{s}$$

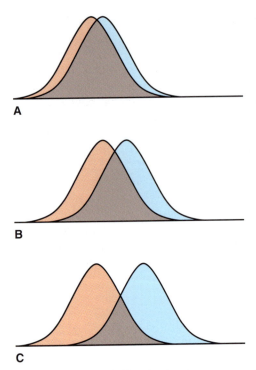

Figure 24–3 Illustration of effect size in relation to standard deviation units. A. Samples separated by .5 standard deviation, B. Samples separated by 1 standard deviation, C. Samples separated by 2 standard deviations.

where $\bar{X}_1$ and $\bar{X}_2$ are the group means, and s is their common standard deviation. Because the variances are not significantly different, we can use either group standard deviation or take the average of both group standard deviations. For the data in Table 24-1,

$$d = \frac{10.11 - 5.45}{3.83} = 1.22$$

Therefore, these samples differ by slightly more than one standard deviation unit. See Box 24-2 for an example of power analysis and sample size estimates for the pinch study data.

Including Effect Size in Results

Authors may present their results within tables or within the narrative *Results* section of an article. Whichever format is used, data should include group means and standard deviations, the difference between means, confidence intervals, the calculated test statistic, whether it was a one- or two-tailed test, degrees of freedom, and value of p. It has become common practice to also include the effect size index.

> ▶ **Results**
> The mean change in pinch strength was 10.11 pounds (±3.62) for the group using the new splint, and 5.45 pounds (±3.95) for the

---

Box 24-2　Power And Sample Size: Independent *t*-Test (Equal Variances)

Post Hoc Analysis: Determining Power

Because the results of the *t*-test in Table 24-1 were significant, we generally would not be interested in establishing power. For illustration, however, using G*Power, we must enter the effect size index *d*, the number of subjects in each group, and the alpha level used for a one- or two-tailed test. With $d = 1.22$, $\alpha_2 = .05$ and $n = 10$ per group, we have achieved 73% power (*see chapter supplement*). Although this is slightly less than the desired 80%, it is moot because the test was significant.

A Priori Analysis: Estimating Sample Size

Now suppose we were planning this study. Based on previous research, we propose that a difference of 5 pounds would be important with a standard deviation of 6.0. We might guess this based on a previous study with similar splints. Therefore, we estimate that $d = 5/6 = .833$. Using G*Power, we must enter the projected effect size index *d*, the desired alpha level for a one- or two-tailed test, and the desired level of power. For this study, we enter $d = .833$, $\alpha_2 = .05$ and 80% power, resulting in an estimated sample size of 24 *per group* (48 total) (*see chapter supplement*).

Knowing our outcome, this would have been an overestimate, because we had a higher effect size than was projected. Although we predicted the difference between means pretty accurately, we projected a larger standard deviation than observed, which resulted in a smaller effect size. Using G*Power with $d = 1.2$ (what the study actually achieved), we would have only needed 12 subjects per group for 80% power. Hindsight is 20/20!

Lehr[13] offers a practical alternative to estimate sample size for the independent *t*-test: $n = 16/d^2$, based on 80% power and $\alpha_2 = .05$ only. For our example, using $d = .833$, $n = 16/0.694 = 23$ subjects per group. Pretty close.

---

group using the standard splint. The mean difference between groups was 4.66 pounds (95% CI = 1.06 to 8.26). An independent, two-tailed *t*-test showed that the group using the new splint had a significantly larger change in strength than the group using the new splint ($t(18) = 2.718$, $p = .014$, $d = 1.2$).

This information allows the reader to understand the full context of the statistical outcome, including whether the effect was large or small, which is not evident from the p or t values alone.

Effect Size for the Paired *t*-Test

For the paired *t*-test, the effect size index requires a correction factor to account for correlated scores:

$$d = \frac{\bar{d}}{s_d}\sqrt{2}$$

where $\bar{d}$ is the mean and s_d is the standard deviation of the differences scores. For the data in Table 24-3,

$$d = \frac{3.375}{6.232}\sqrt{2} = .765$$

Box 24-3 illustrates the power analysis and sample size estimate for the lumbar pillow study.

> ### ▶ Results
> The mean difference in pelvic tilt angle between using and not using a lumbar pillow was 3.38 degrees ± 6.23 (95% CI = −1.84 to 8.58). A paired, one-tailed *t*-test showed that there was no significant difference between the two test conditions ($t(7) = 1.532$, $p = .169$, $d = .77$). A post hoc analysis showed that the test achieved 40% power.

 See the *Chapter 24 Supplement* for illustration of power analysis for unpaired and paired *t*-tests using G*Power.

■ Inappropriate Use of Multiple *t*-Tests

The *t*-test is one of the most commonly applied statistical tests. Unfortunately, it is also often misused. The sole purpose of the *t*-test is to compare two means. Therefore, when more than two means are analyzed within a single sample, the *t*-test is inappropriate. For instance, we could have designed the pinch strength study to compare three different splints. It would not be appropriate, then, to compare each pair of splints, which would result in three different comparisons (1-2, 2-3, 1-3).

The problem with using multiple *t*-tests within one set of data is that the more comparisons one makes, the more likely one is to commit a Type I error—to find a significant difference when none exists. Remember that α is the probability of committing a Type I error for any *single* comparison. For a significant test at α = .05, we are willing to take a 5% chance we will be in error when we say that group means are different. But if we do this for several comparisons, the potential *cumulative error* will actually be greater than .05.

Consider the interpretation that, for α = .05, if we were to repeat a study 100 times when *no difference really existed*, we could expect to find a significant difference five times, as a random event, just by chance. Five percent of our conclusions could be in error. For any one comparison, however, we cannot know if a significant finding represents one of the potentially correct or incorrect decisions. Theoretically, any one test could be in error.

Consider a relatively rare random event, such as a strike of lightning.[14] Suppose you had to cross a wide open field during a lightning storm. There may be only a small risk of getting struck (perhaps 5%?)—but would you prefer to cross the field just once, or several times? Would you consider the risk greater if you crossed the field 20 times? This same logic applies to repeated *t*-tests. The more we repeat comparisons within a sample, the greater are our chances that one or more of those comparisons will result in a random event, a false positive—even when a significant difference does not exist.

This problem can be avoided by using the more appropriate analysis of variance (ANOVA), which is a logical extension of the *t*-test specifically designed to compare more than two means. As an adjunct to the analysis of variance, multiple comparison procedures have been developed that control the Type I error rate, allowing valid interpretations of several comparisons at the desired α level. These procedures are discussed next in Chapters 25 and 26.

Box 24-3 Power and Sample Size: The Paired *t*-Test

Post Hoc Analysis: Determining Power
For the paired *t*-test, G*Power requires you to enter the value of d_z (not *d*) which is equal to $d/\sqrt{2}$, in this case $0.765/\sqrt{2} = 0.541$. With $d_z = 0.541$ for a one-tailed test for dependent samples at $\alpha_1 = .05$ and $n = 8$, power is 40% (*see chapter supplement*). Given that the effect size was large but power so low, it is not surprising that the test was not significant. We might think about running a larger study, although we would also have to consider whether a mean difference of 3.375 degrees is clinically meaningful. Finding no significant difference, even with low power, does not necessarily mean a Type II error has occurred.

A Priori Analysis: Estimating Sample Size
Let's see what we could have done differently in planning this study. Let's say that we did not have any prior data to help us estimate the effect size, and we therefore decided to use a medium effect size as our estimate, $d = .50$. Using G*Power, we have to convert *d* to d_z. Given our estimate $d = .50$, $d_z = 0.354$. For a one-tailed test for dependent samples at $\alpha_1 = .05$ and 80% power, the projected sample size will be $n = 51$ (*see chapter supplement*). Because this is a paired test, this is the number of subjects in the total sample. Clearly the sample size used was too small.

When the projected sample size is not feasible, we might look at different measurement methods that could result in larger effect sizes—or decide not to do the study, as it would be unlikely to have a meaningful result.

COMMENTARY

What the use of a p-value implies, is that a hypothesis that may be true may be rejected because it has not predicted observable results that have not occurred.

—*Harold Jeffreys (1891–1989)*

British mathematician and statistician

Author of *Theory of Probability, 1939*

The *t*-test has great appeal because of its simplicity—the basic comparison of two means, which is the foundation for the archetypical randomized clinical trial. Although the test is apparently straightforward, it still needs to be interpreted properly and reported clearly in a publication. Unfortunately, many authors do not provide adequate information to indicate what kind of test was run—whether it was independent or paired, one- or two-tailed, what values were used to estimate sample size (and how they were determined), and what level of significance was applied. Information on means, confidence intervals, exact *p* values, effect size and power should also be included with results. All of these descriptors are essential for a full understanding of an analysis, interpretation of results, and clinical application. If the literature is going to provide evidence for decision making, it must foster statistical conclusion validity so that we can be confident in the work and the meaning of the results.

REFERENCES

1. Zabell SL. On Student's 1908 article "The probable error of a mean." *J Am Stat Assoc* 2008;103(481):1-7.
2. Student. The probable error of a mean. *Biometrika* 1908;6:1-25.
3. Bailar JC, 3rd. Redefining the confidence interval. *Int J Occup Med Environ Health* 2004;17(1):123-129.
4. Ringwalt C, Paschall MJ, Gorman D, Derzon J, Kinlaw A. The use of one- versus two-tailed tests to evaluate prevention programs. *Eval Health Prof* 2011;34(2):135-150.
5. Peace KE. One-sided or two-sided p values: which most appropriately address the question of drug efficacy? *J Biopharm Stat* 1991;1(1):133-138.
6. Glass GV, Peckham PD, Sanders JR. Consequences of failure to meet assumptions underlying the fixed effects analysis of variance and covariance. *Rev Educ Res* 1972;42:237-288.
7. Borenstein M. A note on the use of confidence intervals in psychiatric research. *Psychopharmacol Bull* 1994;30(2):235-238.
8. Lesaffre E. Use and misuse of the p-value. *Bull NYU Hosp Jt Dis* 2008;66(2):146-149.
9. Streiner DL. Statistics Commentary Series: Commentary #14—Confidence Intervals. *J Clin Psychopharmacol* 2016;36(3):198-199.
10. Cohen J. Things I have learned (so far). *Am Pyschologist* 1990;45(12):1304-1312.
11. Obeid J, Balemans AC, Noorduyn SG, Gorter JW, Timmons BW. Objectively measured sedentary time in youth with cerebral palsy compared with age-, sex-, and season-matched youth who are developing typically: an explorative study. *Phys Ther* 2014;94(8):1163-1167.
12. Cohen J. *Statistical Power Analysis for the Behavioral Sciences.* 2nd ed. Hillsdale, NJ: Lawrence Erlbaum 1988.
13. Lehr R. Sixteen S-squared over D-squared: a relation for crude sample size estimates. *Stat Med* 1992;11(8):1099-1102.
14. Dallal GE. Multiple comparison procedures. *The Little Handbook of Statistical Practice.* Available at http://www.jerrydallal.com/LHSP/mc.htm. Accessed November 1, 2018.

Comparing More Than Two Means: Analysis of Variance

As knowledge and clinical theory have developed, clinical researchers have proposed more complex research questions, necessitating the use of elaborate multilevel and multifactor experimental designs. The **analysis of variance (ANOVA)** is a powerful analytic tool for analyzing such data when three or more groups or conditions are compared with independent groups or repeated measures. The ANOVA uses the *F* statistic, named for Sir Ronald Fisher, who developed the procedure.

The purpose of this chapter is to describe the application of the ANOVA for a variety of research designs. Although statistical programs can run the ANOVA easily, understanding the basic premise is important for using and interpreting results appropriately. An introduction to the basic concepts underlying analysis of variance is most easily addressed in the context of a single-factor experiment (one independent variable) with independent groups. Discussion will then follow with more complex models, including factorial designs, repeated measures and mixed designs.

■ ANOVA Basics

Recall from our discussion of the *t*-test (Chapter 24) that differences between means are examined in relation to the distance between group means as well as the error variance within each group—the signal to noise ratio. The analysis of variance is based on the same principle, except that it is a little more complicated because the ratio must now account for the relationships among more than two means.

Also like the *t*-test, the ANOVA is based on statistical assumptions for parametric tests, including homogeneity of variance, normal distributions, and interval/ratio data. When assumptions for parametric statistics are not met, there are nonparametric analogs that can be applied (see Chapter 27).

🖈 The ANOVA can be applied to two-group comparisons, but the *t*-test is generally considered more efficient for that purpose. The results of a *t*-test and ANOVA with two groups will be the same. The *t*-test is actually a special case of the analysis of variance, with the relationship $F = t^2$.

■ One-Way Analysis of Variance

The *one-way analysis of variance* is used to compare three or more independent group means. The descriptor "one-way" indicates that the design involves one independent variable, or *factor*, with three or more levels.

➤ CASE IN POINT #1

Consider a hypothetical study of the differential effect of four intervention strategies to increase pain-free range of motion (ROM) in patients with elbow tendinitis. Through random assignment, we create 4 independent groups treated with ice, a nonsteroidal anti-inflammatory drug (NSAID), a splint support, or rest. We measure ROM at baseline and after 10 days of intervention, using the change in pain-free ROM as our outcome. We recruit a sample of 44 patients with comparable histories of tendinitis and randomly assign 11 subjects to each of the four groups.

In this study, the independent variable modality has four levels, incorporated in a single-factor, multigroup pretest-posttest design (see Chapter 16). The dependent variable is change in pain-free elbow ROM, measured in degrees. Hypothetical data for this study are reported in Table 25-1A.

The one-way ANOVA provides an overall test of the null hypothesis that there is no significant difference among the group means:

$$H_0: \mu_1 = \mu_2 = \mu_3 = \dots = \mu_k$$

where k is the number of groups or levels of the independent variable. In our example, $k = 4$.

The alternative hypothesis (H_1) states that there will be a difference in the change in pain-free ROM between at least two of the four groups following the treatment period.

Partitioning the Variance

As we have discussed before, the total variance in a set of data can be attributed to two sources: a treatment

---

Table 25-1   One-Way ANOVA: Change in Pain-Free Elbow ROM Following Treatment for Tendinitis ($k = 4$, $N = 44$)

A. Data

Descriptive Statistics

ROM	N	Mean	Std. Deviation	95% CI for Mean Lower Bound	95% CI for Mean Upper Bound
Ice	11	44.18	10.870	36.88	51.48
NSAID	11	45.27	8.403	39.63	50.92
Splint	11	35.27	9.509	28.88	41.66
Rest	11	24.09	8.538	18.36	29.83
Total	44	❶ 37.20	12.487	33.41	41.00

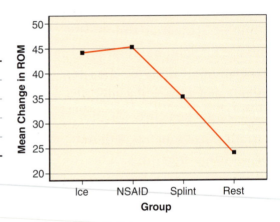

B. SPSS Output: One-Way ANOVA

Test of Homogeneity of Variances

		Levene Statistic	df1	df2	❷ Sig.
ROM	Based on Mean	.329	3	40	.804

ANOVA

ROM	Sum of Squares	❸ df	Mean Square	❹ F	❹ Sig.	Partial Eta Squared	Observed Power
Between Groups	3184.250	3	1061.417	12.058	.000	❻ .475	❻ .999
Within Groups ❺	3520.909	40	88.023				
Total	6705.159	43					

---

❶ The grand mean for all 44 subjects, $\bar{X}_G = 37.20$.

❷ The Levene statistic indicates that there is no significant difference among the variances of the four groups ($p = .804$). Therefore, the assumption of homogeneity of variance is supported.

❸ The between groups df are k-1 ($df_b = 3$), within groups $df = N$-k ($df_e = 43$), total df are N-1 ($df_t = 43$).

❹ The F statistic is significant. We reject H_0 and conclude that there is a significant difference among 4 groups. The actual probability is not zero, but SPSS only takes these values to three decimal places. Therefore, this is reported as $p < .001$.

❺ *Within Groups* is the term used for error variance in this analysis.

❻ The power analysis shows an effect size $\eta_p^2 = .475$. This is a large effect, resulting in more than 99% power. Although SPSS uses the term *partial eta squared*, for the one-way ANOVA this value is the same as *eta squared*.

This ANOVA was run using SPSS General Linear Model to obtain power and effect size. This analysis can also be run using Compare Means/One-Way ANOVA, but effect size and power are not options. Portions of the output have been omitted for clarity.

effect (*between* the groups), and unexplained or error variance among the subjects (*within* the groups). As its name implies, the analysis of variance partitions the total variance within a set of data into these two components (see Fig. 25-1).

To understand this concept with the ANOVA, we start by thinking of the entire combined sample as one group. This combined group has a mean, called the **grand mean,** $\bar{X}_G$ (see Fig. 25-2). We expect to see some variance between participants in all groups, but we want to determine if some groups are more alike than others. The *between-groups variance* reflects the spread of group means around the grand mean. The larger this effect, the greater the separation between the groups. For example, we can see that the means for groups 1 and 2 are close together, and both appear separated from groups 3 and 4. The mean for Group 4 demonstrates the largest deviation from the grand mean.

The within-groups variance reflects the spread of scores within each group around the group mean. We always expect some variability within a group but hope that it will be small so that treatment effects are clear. Based on the standard deviations in each group, the spread of scores for ice is highest.

Sum of Squares

The term **sum of square (*SS*)** is used to reflect variance. Recall that the *SS* is based on deviations of individual

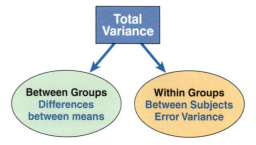

Figure 25–1 Partitioning the total variance in a one-way ANOVA.

scores from the group mean within a distribution (see Chapter 22). The larger the *SS*, the higher the variance. For an ANOVA, a total sum of squares (SS_t) is calculated for the combined sample around the grand mean, indicating the total variance within the entire sample. Now we want to know how much of this total variance can be explained by the treatment.

This total *SS* is partitioned into two parts: the between-groups variance (SS_b) indicating the spread of the four means, and the remaining unexplained error variance (SS_e). The larger the proportion of the total variance that is represented by the between group differences, the more likely a significant difference will be found.

See the *Chapter 25 Supplement* for calculations of sums of squares for a one-way ANOVA.

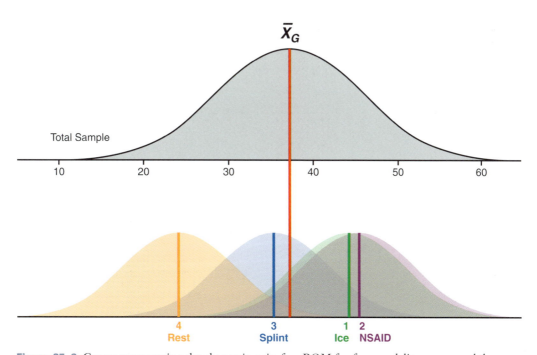

Figure 25–2 Curves representing the change in pain-free ROM for four modality groups and the combined sample. The center red line represents the grand mean, $\bar{X}_G$. The between-groups variance is the difference between group means and the grand mean.

Results of a One-Way ANOVA

Table 25-1B shows the output for comparison of the four modality groups.

Homogeneity of Variance

The first section of this output includes a test for homogeneity of variance to help us satisfy the parametric assumption that groups have equal variances. Levene's statistic is not significant ($p = .804$) (Table 23-1 ❷). Therefore, the assumption of homogeneity of variance is met.

With samples of equal size, the ANOVA is considered robust, in that reasonable departures from normality and homogeneity will not seriously affect validity.[1] With unequal sample sizes, however, gross violations of homogeneity of variance can increase the chance of Type I error. In such cases, when Levene's test is significant ($p < .05$), a nonparametric analysis of variance can be applied (see Chapter 27), or data can be transformed to a different scale that improves homogeneity of variance within the sample distribution (see Appendix C).

The ANOVA Summary Table

The general format for an ANOVA summary table is presented in Table 25-2, showing how each of the elements is derived.

Sum of Squares

The SS values are given for each source of variance with the *total sum of squares* (SS_t) partitioned into the between (SS_b) and error (SS_e) components. The total SS will be equal to the sum of the between and error components.

📌 Terminology used in the ANOVA table may vary among computer programs and research reports, but generally the sources of variance will represent *between*, *within*, and *total* variance components. Rather than listing "between groups" as a source of variance, some programs list the name of the independent variable. The error variance may be called the *within-groups variance, error, residual,* or *between-subjects variance.*

Degrees of Freedom

The total degrees of freedom (df_t) within a set of data will always be one less than the total number of observations, in this case $N - 1$. The df associated with the between-groups variability (df_b) is one less than the number of groups ($k - 1$). The df_e associated with the error term is $N - k$. The degrees of freedom for the separate variance components are additive, so that $(k - 1) + (N - k) = (N - 1)$. For the modality study, $N = 44$, $df_t = 43$, $k = 4$ and $df_b = 3$, and the error term, $df_e = N - k$, in this case $44 - 4 = 40$.

Mean Square

The sum of squares is converted to a variance estimate, or **mean square (MS)**, by dividing each SS by its respective degrees of freedom (see Chapter 22). A mean square can be calculated for the between (MS_b) and error (MS_e) variance components.

The F Statistic

The F ratio is the MS_b divided by MS_e. When H_0 is false and the treatment effect is significant, the between-groups variance is large, yielding an F ratio greater than 1.0. The larger the F ratio, the more likely it will be significant. In the modality study, $F = 12.06$, which is significant ($p < .001$) (Table 25-1 ❹). Therefore, we can conclude the there is a significant difference among the four group means, and we reject H_0.

🔑 Computer programs will often restrict p values to 3 decimal places. Therefore, if p is less than .001, the output will just say $p = .000$, as shown in Table 25-1 ❹. This does not mean the probability is zero, but only that the report does not generate values beyond that decimal place. Therefore, it should be reported as $p < .001$.

Critical Value

The calculated F ratio is compared to a critical value to determine its significance. Appendix Table A-3 contains critical values of F at $\alpha = .05$. The critical value is located in the table by df_b across the top and df_e along the side. For our example, $df_b = 3$ and $df_e = 40$ (always given in that order). The calculated value of F must be *greater than or equal to* the critical value to achieve statistical significance. The critical value for $F (3,40) = 2.84$. Because the calculated value ($F = 12.06$) is higher than the critical value, the test is significant.

Table 25-2   Components of a One-Way ANOVA Summary Table

SOURCE	SS	df	MS	F	Sig.
Between Groups	SS_b	$df_b = k-1$	$MS_b = SS_b/df_b$	MS_b/MS_e	p
Within Groups (Error)	SS_e	$df_e = N-k$	$MS_e = SS_e/df_e$		
Total	$SS_t = SS_b + SS_e$	$df_t = N-1$			

SS = sum of squares, k = number of groups, N = total sample, df = degrees of freedom, MS = mean square, p = probability. Subscripts b = between groups, e = error, t = total

You will note that we are not referring to one- or two-tailed tests with ANOVA. Because we are comparing more than two groups, we cannot predict differences in one direction.

Interpreting *F*

Finding a significant difference with an ANOVA is not the end of the story, however. It only tells us that there is a difference among the four means and does not indicate which groups are significantly different. The *F* test is called an *omnibus test* because it is based on the overall variance within the sample. A follow-up test must be done to determine exactly where the significant differences lie. Various **multiple comparison tests** are used for this purpose. When the *F* ratio is smaller than the critical value, H_0 is not rejected and no further analyses are appropriate.

These data will be used again in Chapter 26 to illustrate several multiple comparison tests. For now, we simply know that there is a difference somewhere among these four group means.

Power and Effect Size

Two forms of effect size indices are used with the one-way ANOVA, **eta squared, η^2**, and **Cohen's *f***. These indices represent the proportion of the total variance associated with the independent variable. These effect size indices can be calculated using the *SS* values in the ANOVA:

$$\eta^2 = \frac{SS_b}{SS_t} \qquad f = \sqrt{\frac{SS_b}{SS_e}}$$

They can be converted as follows:

$$f = \sqrt{\frac{\eta^2}{1-\eta^2}} \qquad \eta^2 = \frac{f^2}{1-f^2}$$

Different procedures for power analysis will use either of these values. SPSS uses η^2 as the effect size (see Table 25-1), and the online G*Power calculator uses *f*.

For the data in Table 25-1,

$$\eta^2 = \frac{3184.25}{6705.16} = 0.475 \qquad f = \sqrt{\frac{3184.25}{3520.91}} = 0.951$$

Conventional effect sizes have been proposed for these indices:[2]

Small	$\eta^2 = .01$	$f = .10$
Medium	$\eta^2 = .06$	$f = .25$
Large	$\eta^2 = .14$	$f = .40$

Using these criteria, both indices in this example show a substantially large effect.

As with other effect size indices, these conventions are intended to provide a way to interpret values along a continuum, not to serve as absolute values. They are open to interpretation depending on the context of the variables being measured. See Box 25-1 for an example of these analyses for the tendinitis data from Table 25-1.

Power and sample size calculations using G*Power are illustrated in the *Chapter 25 Supplement* for the ANOVA with independent and repeated measures.

You may see an alternative effect size measure for ANOVA, **omega squared, ω^2**. This value is calculated as:

$$\omega^2 = \frac{SS_b - (k-1)MS_e}{SS_t + MS_e}$$

It is considered to have less bias than η^2 and will typically result in lower power and higher required sample sizes.[4] It is not used as often in computer programs, however, which is why *f* and η^2 are more frequently reported in the literature.[5]

Box 25-1 Power and Sample Size for the One-Way ANOVA

Post Hoc Analysis: Determining Power

The ANOVA output presented in Table 25-1 includes effect size (partial eta squared) and power. This is an option that can be requested when running the ANOVA in SPSS, and therefore we do not need to do further analysis to determine power. In this case we have achieved 99.9% power (can't do much better than that!).

If we did not have this information, however, we could use G*Power, entering *f* = .951 (converting from η_p^2), α = .05, *N* = 44 with 4 groups, resulting in power = 99.9% (*see chapter supplement*).

A Priori Analysis: Estimating Sample Size

If we wanted to determine a reasonable sample size as part of planning this study, we would need to project an effect size, the number of groups in the design, α level, and the desired level of power. This requires some foundation based on prior research to estimate what can be expected. Assume we have found a systematic review that reports on several studies showing medium effect sizes after 8 weeks of treatment with various modalities.[3] Based on this information, we enter *f* = .25 (a medium effect), α = .05, four groups, and 80% power in G*Power, resulting in a total sample size of *N* = 180, or *n* = 45 per group (*see chapter supplement*).

In retrospect, we know we would not have needed that large a sample because our effect size was much larger than we projected. However, that is not something we would know beforehand—it's a best guess!

Reporting ANOVA Results

The ANOVA summary table may be included in the results section of an article, although many authors choose instead to report *F* ratios in the body of the text. When this is done, the calculated value of *F* is given, along with the associated degrees of freedom, probability, and effect size.

> ➤ **Results**
> A one-way ANOVA was run to compare the effect of ice, NSAIDs, splint, or rest on change in pain-free ROM. There was a significant difference among the four modality groups $(F(3,40) = 12.06, p < .001, f = .951)$.

Alternatively, the effect size may be reported as $\eta^2 = .475$. This statement would be followed by information about specific differences among the four means using a multiple comparison, which will be covered in Chapter 26.

■ Two-Way Analysis of Variance

Because of the complexity of human behavior and physiological function, many clinical investigations are designed to study the simultaneous effects of two or more independent variables. This approach is often more economical than testing each variable separately and provides a stronger basis for generalization of results to clinical practice.

> ➤ **CASE IN POINT #2**
> Let's take our elbow tendinitis example and extend its design. Assume we wanted to compare the effect of ice, splint, and rest but also consider whether NSAIDs would be helpful in combination with any of these modalities. For this study, we will assemble a sample of 60 participants.

This study includes two factors: modality (Factor A) with three levels (ice, splint, or rest), and medication (Factor B) with two levels (NSAID or no medication). Instead of looking at each of these factors separately, we can examine their combined influence using a **two-way factorial design** (see Chapter 16).

This is a 3 × 2 design with six treatment combinations, as shown in Figure 25-3. Each cell represents a unique combination of levels for A and B. With a total sample of 60 subjects, we can randomly allocate 10 subjects per cell. These two factors are considered *completely crossed*, because every level of factor A is paired with every level of factor B.

The appropriate statistical analysis for this design is a **two-way analysis of variance**. The descriptor "two-way" indicates that it involves two independent variables.

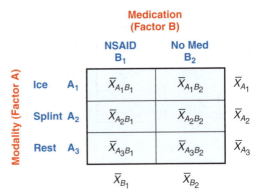

Figure 25–3 Two-way (3×2) factorial design testing the effect of (A) modality ($k =3$) and (B) medication ($k=2$) on change in pain free elbow ROM in patients with tendinitis. Sixty subjects are randomly assigned to each of six conditions ($n = 10$). The marginal means for each independent variable are obtained by pooling data across the second variable.

Partitioning the Variance

In a two-way ANOVA, the total variance is partitioned to account for the separate and combined effect of each independent variable. Therefore, we can ask three questions of these data:

(1) *What is the effect of modality, independent of medication?*
(2) *What is the effect of medication, independent of modality?*
(3) *What is the combined effect or interaction of modality and medication?*

Null hypotheses are generated for each of the three research questions. An alternative hypothesis can be proposed for each hypothesis, which states that there will be a difference among means.

The first two questions ask about the effect of each independent variable separately, essentially creating two single-factor experiments. These effects are called **main effects**, illustrated in Figure 25-4.

We can study the main effect of modality by pooling data for the two medication conditions. With 10 subjects in each of the original cells, we would now obtain a mean for 20 scores at each level of modality. The sum of squares associated with this main effect accounts for the separation among groups that received different forms of modality.

Similarly, we can collapse the three levels of modality to obtain two means for the main effect of medication with 30 scores per level. A second sum of squares will be calculated to account for the separation between these two groups.

The means for levels of the main effects are called **marginal means**. They represent the average separate

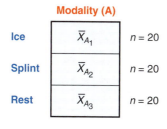

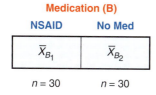

Figure 25–4 Main effects for modality and medication in a two-way factorial design with $N = 60$, showing marginal means for each group.

effect of each independent variable in the analysis. Comparison of the marginal means within each factor indicates how much of the variability in all 60 scores can be attributed to the overall effect of modality or medication alone.

In addition to main effects, the factorial design has the added advantage of being able to examine combinations of levels of each independent variable to determine if there are differential effects. These are referred to as **interaction effects**. Interaction is present when the effect of one variable is not constant across different levels of the second variable.

📌 The ANOVA can be expanded to include more than two independent variables, although it is rare to see analyses beyond three dimensions. A three-way ANOVA would generate three main effects, three double interactions, and one triple interaction across all three variables. Although this type of design does allow for more comprehensive comparisons, it can become overly complex, requiring a large sample to generate sufficient power.

No Interaction

To illustrate this concept, consider first the hypothetical means given for the six treatment groups in Table 25-3A. Each mean represents a unique combination of modality and medication condition. We can plot these means to more clearly illustrate these relationships (Table 25-3B). The plot on the left shows the three modality groups along the X-axis. The means for change in ROM for each medication condition are plotted at each level of modality, with lines representing each main effect.

Note that in this example, the lines are parallel, which means that the pattern of response at each medication condition is consistent across all levels of modality. We can reverse the plot, as shown on the right, with medication condition on the X-axis, demonstrating a similar constant pattern for each level of modality. These graphs demonstrate a situation where there is no interaction. Ice will generate the highest response under both medication conditions and the NSAID scores are higher across all levels of modality.

ANOVA Summary Table

The results of the two-way ANOVA are shown in Table 25-3C. Note that there are three between-groups sources of variance listed, two main effects and one interaction effect.

In a two-way ANOVA, these sources of variance are usually listed in the summary table according to the name of the independent variable. Thus, for our example, type of modality and medication condition are listed as main effects. The interaction between two variables may be signified by * or ×, such as modality * medication, read "modality by medication." The error term represents the unexplained variance among all subjects across all combinations of the two variables.

Degrees of Freedom

The degrees of freedom associated with each main effect is one less than the number of levels of that independent variable ($k - 1$). With two independent variables, we use ($A - 1$) degrees of freedom for Factor A, and ($B - 1$) for Factor B, where the letters A and B represent the number of levels of each factor. The number of degrees of freedom for the interaction is the product of the respective degrees of freedom for the two variables, ($A-1$)($B-1$).

The total degrees of freedom will always be one less than the total number of observations, $N - 1$. The error degrees of freedom can be determined by using (A)(B)($n-1$) with equal-size groups, or by subtracting the combined between-groups degrees of freedom from the total degrees of freedom.

For modality with three levels, $df = 2$. For medication with two levels, $df = 1$. Therefore, the interaction effect in the modality study has $2 \times 1 = 2$ degrees of freedom. With $N = 60$ ($n = 10$ per group), $df_t = 59$. For this example, $df_e = (3)(2)(9) = 59 - 5 = 54$.

The *F* Statistic

An *F* value is calculated for each main effect and interaction effect with an associated *p* value. The *F* ratio for each effect is calculated by dividing the MS_b for that effect by MS_e for the common error term.

Table 25-3   Two-Way ANOVA for the Effect of Medication and Modality on Pain-Free ROM: Showing No Interaction (*N* = 60)

A. Data

Medication Condition

Modality	NSAID	No Med	① Marginal Means
Ice	45.00	36.00	40.50
Splint	33.00	25.00	29.00
Rest	22.00	12.00	17.00
② Marginal Means	33.33	23.33	

B. SPSS Output: Mean Plots

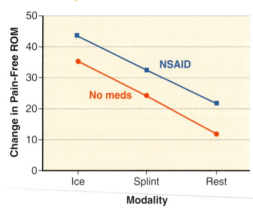

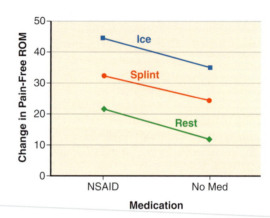

C. SPSS Output: Two-Way ANOVA

Tests of Between-Subjects Effects

Dependent Variable: ROMChange

Source	Sum of Squares	df	Mean Square	F	③ Sig.	Partial Eta Squared	Observed Power
Modality	5523.333	2	2761.667	231.568	.000	.896	1.000
Medication	1215.000	1	1215.000	101.879	.000	.654	1.000
Modality * Medication	10.000	2	5.000	.419	.660	④ .015	④ .115
Error	644.000	54	11.926				
Total	7392.333	59					

① The three marginal means for the main effect of Modality.

② The two marginal means for the main effect of Medication.

③ The two main effects of Modality and Med are significant (*p*<.001), but the interaction effect is not (*p*=.660)

④ The main effects have large effect sizes and high power, but partial eta squared for the interaction is quite small, showing that power was only 11.5%.

The ANOVA and plots were run using SPSS/General Linear Model. Portions of the output have been omitted for clarity.

Critical Value

By looking at the summary table, we can see that the probabilities associated with the two main effects are significant. The interaction effect is not significant ($p = .660$). This is not surprising given the pattern of means across the groups.

Each F ratio is compared to a critical value from Appendix Table A-3 based on the degrees of freedom for that effect (df_b) and the error term. For modality and modality*medication ($df = 2,54$), the critical value is approximately 3.15. For Medication ($df = 1,54$), the critical value is approximately 4.00. Because the table does not include all possible df values, these values are estimated using the closest value for $df_e = 60$.

The F ratios for the main effects of modality and medication are higher than the critical values. Therefore, this ANOVA demonstrates significant main effects. The F value for the interaction is smaller than the critical value, and is therefore, not significant. These conclusions are consistent with the p values listed in the table.

Interpreting *F*

We look at the outcome of a two-way ANOVA by considering the significance of each main and interaction effect. We focus on the interaction effect first, as the combination of variables is typically the primary reason for using the two-way design. If the interaction is not significant, as in this example, we then go to each main effect.

Further analysis requires a multiple comparison test to compare the three marginal means for the main effect of modality. There is no need for further tests for the medication condition since there are only two levels. The NSAID condition results in a significantly better improvement in ROM than no medication.

Interaction

Now consider a different set of results for the same study, given in Table 25-4. The plots for these data show lines that are not parallel—the pattern of one variable is not constant across all levels of the second variable. We can see in the plots that the combination of ice and NSAID has the greatest effect, whereas all the other conditions have means that are lower and fairly close.

 Researchers generally propose a factorial design when the research question focuses on the potential interaction between two variables. Therefore, when the interaction is significant, main effects are usually ignored.

When lines are not parallel or when they cross, as shown here, interaction is present ($p = .005$). In this example, it is not the use of one modality alone that makes the treatment more effective. It is the combination

of ice with an NSAID. Although the data clearly suggest that the ice/NSAID combination has a better outcome than all other combinations, we will have to use multiple comparison tests to determine which of these six means are significantly different from each other (see Chapter 26).

Power and Effect Size

For a two-way analysis, effect size and power estimates must be determined for each main and interaction effect. In a two-way design, the effect size indices f or η^2 have to be partitioned to represent the proportion of total variance that is accounted for by each effect. Therefore, we use **partial eta squared, η_p^2**, and f based on separate sums of squares:

$$\eta_p^2 = \frac{SS_b}{SS_b + SS_e} \qquad f = \sqrt{\frac{SS_b}{SS_e}}$$

where SS_b is the sum of squares for the particular effect being evaluated, and SS_e is the common error sum of squares.

The ANOVA summary tables show η_p^2 and power estimates for each of the three effects. Power analyses for data in Table 25-4 are illustrated in Box 25-2.

> **Results**
>
> A two-way ANOVA was used to analyze the effect of medication and modality on pain-free ROM. The ANOVA shows significant outcomes for the main effect of modality ($F(2,54) = 5.97$, $p = .005$, $\eta_p^2 = .181$), the main effect of medication ($F(1,54) = 5.77$, $p = .02$, $\eta_p^2 = .097$), and their interaction ($F(22,54) = 5.79$, $p = .005$, $\eta_p^2 = .177$).

Alternatively, a value for f can be reported instead of partial eta squared. This statement would be followed by results of a multiple comparison across the six interaction means (see Chapter 26).

■ Repeated Measures Analysis of Variance

Up to now we have discussed the ANOVA only as it is applied to completely randomized designs, also called *between-subjects designs* because all sources of variance represent differences between subjects. Clinical investigators, however, often use repeated factors to evaluate the performance of each subject under several experimental conditions. The repeated measures design is logically applied to study variables where practice or carryover effects are minimal and where differences in an individual's performance across levels are of interest.

Table 25-4	Two-Way ANOVA for the Effect of Medication and Modality on Pain-Free ROM Showing Interaction (N = 60)

A. Data

Medication

Modality	NSAID	No Med	Marginal Means
Ice	50.00	22.00	**36.00**
Splint	20.00	21.00	**20.50**
Rest	24.00	23.00	**23.50**
Marginal Means	**31.33**	**22.00**	

B. SPSS Output: Mean Plots

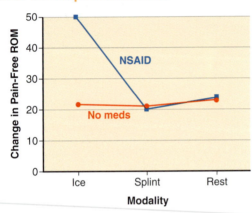

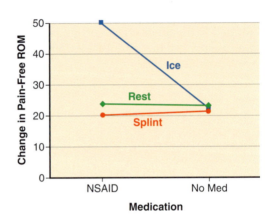

C. SPSS Output: Two-Way ANOVA

Tests of Between-Subjects Effects

Dependent Variable: ROMChange

Source	Sum of Squares	df	Mean Square	F	❶ Sig.	Partial Eta Squared	Observed Power
Modality	2703.333	2	1351.667	5.970	.005	❷ .181	❷ .867
Med	1306.667	1	1306.667	5.771	.020	.097	.655
Modality * Med	2623.333	2	1311.667	5.793	.005	.177	.851
Error	12226.000	54	226.407				
Total	18859.333	59					

❶ The two main effects and the interaction effect are significant. Interactions are illustrated in graphs.

❷ Using conventional effect sizes, values of η_p^2 for all three effects represent medium to large effects. The power for Modality and interaction is above 80%. Power for Medication is lower (65%), but this is irrelevant because the effect was significant

ANOVA and mean plots were run with General Linear Model/Univariate. Portions of the output have been omitted for clarity.

This type of study can involve one or more independent variables (see Chapter 16).

In a repeated measures design, all subjects are tested under *k* treatment conditions. The **repeated measures analysis of variance** is modified to account for the correlation among successive measurements on the same individual. For this reason, such designs are also called *within-subjects designs*. The statistical hypotheses proposed for repeated measures designs are the same as those for independent samples, except that the means represent treatment conditions rather than groups. The simplest repeated measures design involves one independent variable, where all levels of treatment are administered to all subjects.

Post Hoc Analysis: Determining Power

SPSS can generate η_p^2 and power estimates if requested as part of the ANOVA, in which case no further *post hoc* analysis is necessary. For the data in Table 25-3, showing no interaction, the two main effects have large effect sizes and power of 1.00. However, the interaction effect was small, with extremely low power of 11.5%.

For the data in Table 25-4, we found significant main and interaction effects. All three effect sizes were medium to large. The main effect of modality and the interaction effect both showed power above .80. The main effect of medication had lower power of 65.5%, but this is irrelevant because the effect was significant.

Data from Table 25-4 will be used to illustrate G*Power for *post hoc* analysis. We enter parameters including effect size *f*, total sample size (*N*) and the number of groups (*k*) for each main and interaction effect. Effect sizes are calculated using *SS* values from the ANOVA. G*Power will convert values of η_p^2 to *f* (*see chapter supplement for calculations*). For modality (*N*=60, *k*=3), *f* = .470,

power = .867; for medication (*N*=60, *k*=2), *f* = .327, power = .655; for the interaction (*N*=60, *k*=3), *f* = .463, power = .851.

A priori Analysis: Estimating Sample Size

In planning this study, we want to determine a total sample size to achieve sufficient power for the interaction means. Given that we are interested in comparing combinations of modality and medication, we focus this estimate on six groups. To use G*Power, we must specify parameters of effect size *f*, α = .05, power = .80, and the number of groups in the design, in this case for the interaction effect *k* = 6. If we propose a medium effect, *f* = .25, we generate a sample size estimate of *N* = 158, or 26 subjects per group (*see chapter supplement*). In retrospect, however we would not have needed that large a sample for the data in Table 25-4, as we saw a significant interaction, with *f* = .463 (η_p^2 = .177)—a much higher effect than we projected.

▶ CASE IN POINT #3

To illustrate the repeated measures approach, consider a single-factor experiment designed to look at differences in isometric elbow flexor strength with the forearm in three positions: pronation, neutral, and supination. The independent variable, forearm position, has three levels (*k* = 3).

Logically, this question warrants a repeated measures design, where each subject's strength is tested in each position. Hypothetical data for a sample of nine subjects are presented in Table 25-5. In a repeated measures design, we are interested in a comparison across treatment conditions *within each subject*. It is not of interest to look at averaged group performance at each condition. Therefore, statistically, each subject is considered a unique block in the design.

Partitioning the Variance

The repeated measures ANOVA will partition the total variance in the sample into variance *between-subjects* and variance *within-subjects*. The variance between-subjects is an error component, reflecting individual differences among subjects, which are expected and not of interest. The variance within-subjects consists of two components, the difference between the treatment conditions and error.

🖈 For the one-way ANOVA, the *between-subjects* effect was the difference between groups (treatment conditions), and the *within-subjects* effect was the error within groups. This is different for repeated measures because there are no independent groups. Therefore, the *within-subjects* effect is the variance of interest—how each subject's scores vary across the treatment conditions.

Like other forms of ANOVA, the *F* statistic for repeated measures is the ratio of the variance due to treatment conditions and the error variance, but in this case the variance due to subject differences has been removed from the total.

The statistical advantage of using repeated measures is that individual differences are controlled. When independent groups are compared, it is likely that groups will differ on extraneous variables and that these differences will be superimposed on treatment effects; that is, both treatment differences and error variance will account for observed differences between groups.

With repeated measures designs, however, we have only one group, and differences between treatment conditions should primarily reflect treatment effects. Because variance due to inter-subject differences is separated from the total, error variance in a repeated measures analysis will be smaller than in a randomized experiment. Statistically, this has the effect of reducing the size of the error term, which means that the *F* ratio will be larger. Therefore, the test is more powerful than when independent samples are used.

ANOVA Summary Table
Degrees of Freedom

The total degrees of freedom associated with a repeated measures design will equal one less than the total number of observations made, or $nk - 1$. The *df* associated with the main effects will be $k - 1$ for the independent variable, and $n - 1$ for subjects. The degrees of freedom for the error term are determined as they are for an interaction, so that $df_e = (k - 1)(n - 1)$.

For the elbow strength study, $df_t = (9)(3) - 1 = 26$. These are partitioned into three components: the main

Table 25-5   One-Way Repeated Measures ANOVA: Elbow Flexor Strength Tested in Three Forearm Positions ($N = 9$)

A. Data

Descriptive Statistics

	N	Mean	Std Deviation
Pronation	9	17.33	10.15
Neutral	9	27.56	10.42
Supination	9	29.11	11.34

B. SPSS Output: Repeated Measures ANOVA

Mauchly's Test of Sphericity

Within Subjects Effect	Mauchly's W	Approx Chi-Square	df	Sig. ❶	Epsilon ❷ Greenhouse-Geisser	Huynh-Feldt
POSITION	.664	2.861	2	.239	.749	.883

Tests of Within-Subjects Effects

Source	Sum of Squares	df	Mean Square	F	Sig. ❸	Partial Eta Squared	Observed Power
POSITION	736.889	2	368.444	50.338	.000	❹ .863	1.000
Error	117.111	16	7.319				

Tests of Between-Subjects Effects ❺

Measure: STRENGTH

Source	Sum of Squares	df	Mean Square	F	Sig.
Error	2604.000	8	325.500		

C. Combined Summary Table

This table is not part of SPSS output, but is created to show how the above data might be combined in a concise way in a research article.

Source		SS	df	MS	F	Sig. ❸	η_p^2	Power
Subjects	❺	2604.00	8	325.50				
Position		736.89	2	368.44	50.34	.000	.863	1.000
Error		117.11	16	7.32				

❶ Mauchly's Test of Sphericity is used to determine if adjustments are needed to degrees of freedom for the repeated measure. In this case, it is not significant ($p = .239$), and therefore, no further adjustment is necessary.

❷ If Mauchly's test is significant, two versions of epsilon are used for the adjustment of *df*. In this instance, they are not applied because the sphericity test is not significant. Separate output is provided showing *df* and *p* for the condition when sphericity is assumed, and with each of the correction factors, showing the change in the *df* and *p* values (see chapter supplement).

❸ The repeated measure of Forearm Position is significant.

❹ Power and effect size estimate for the repeated measures test.

❺ The effect of "subjects" as a source of variance is presented as "Between-Subjects Effects." The error term in this analysis is the Subjects effect. No *F* value is generated for this effect, but could be calculated by dividing *MS* for subjects by *MS* error. This effect is often omitted from ANOVA summary tables because it is not meaningful to the analysis.

This analysis was run in SPSS using the General Linear Model. Portions of output have been omitted for clarity.

effect of forearm position with three levels , $df_b = 2$, the within-subjects error, $df = (2)(8) = 16$, and the error component of between-subjects, $df = 9 - 1 = 8$.

The *F* Statistic

The sums of squares for the treatment effect and the error effect are divided by their associated degrees of freedom to obtain the mean squares. These *MS* values are then used to calculate the *F* ratio. For the data in Table 25-5, $F = 50.34$.

Critical Value

The critical value for the *F* ratio for treatment is located in Appendix Table A-3, using the degrees of freedom for treatment (df_b) and the degrees of freedom for the error term (df_e). Therefore, the critical value for this effect will be $F(2,16) = 3.63$. The calculated *F* ratio exceeds this critical value and, therefore, is significant.

The output for this analysis shows results for the between and within subjects sources of variance. The difference across the three positions is significant (p < .001, Table 25-5 ❸). We conclude that elbow flexor strength does differ across forearm positions. It will be appropriate at this point to perform a multiple comparison test on the three means to determine which forearm positions are significantly different from the others (see Chapter 26).

📌 We can calculate an *F* ratio for the between-subjects effect, but this is generally not a meaningful test. We expect subjects to differ from each other, and it is of no experimental interest to establish that they are different. The *F* ratio for between-subjects is often omitted from summary tables (Table 25-5 ❺), and this effect is typically ignored in the interpretation of data for a repeated measures test.

Although not important for experimental studies, the effect of subjects is of interest for some analyses, such as the intraclass correlation coefficient (see Chapter 32).

Variance Assumptions with Repeated Measures Designs

Past discussions have addressed the important assumption of homogeneity of variances among treatment groups. This assumption is also made with repeated measures designs, but we cannot examine variances of different groups because only one group is involved. Instead, the variances of interest reflect difference scores across treatment conditions within a subject. For example, with three repeated treatment conditions, a_1, a_2, a_3, we will have three difference scores:

$$a_1 - a_2 \qquad a_1 - a_3 \qquad a_2 - a_3$$

With this approach, the homogeneity of variance assumption is called the assumption of **sphericity**, which

states that the variances within each pair of difference scores will be relatively equal and correlated with each other.

Because independent tests with equal sample sizes are generally considered robust to violations of homogeneity of variance, one might think that violations of this assumption would be unimportant for repeated measures, where treatment conditions must have equal sample sizes.

This is not the case, however. Because the repeated measures test examines correlated scores across treatment conditions, it is especially sensitive to variance differences, biasing the test in the direction of Type I error. In other words, the repeated measures test is considered too liberal when variances are not correlated, increasing the chances of finding significant differences above the selected α level.

Tests of Sphericity

The sphericity assumption is evaluated using **Mauchly's Test of Sphericity** (Table 25-5B), which is tested using the chi-square statistic. This test is only relevant if the ANOVA results in a significant *F* ratio. If Mauchly's test is not significant, the sphericity assumption *is met*, and no further adjustment is necessary. This is the case in our example ($p = .239$, Table 25-5 ❶).

However, if Mauchly's test is significant ($p < .05$), the sphericity assumption is *not met*, and a correction is necessary. This is achieved by decreasing the degrees of freedom used to determine the critical value of *F*, thereby making the critical value larger. If the critical value is larger, then the calculated value of *F* must be larger to achieve significance. This compensates for bias toward Type I error by making it harder to demonstrate significant differences.

Sphericity Corrections

When Mauchly's test is significant, the degrees of freedom for the *F* ratio are adjusted by multiplying them by a correction factor given the symbol *epsilon*, ε (Table 25-5 ❷). Two different versions of epsilon are used: the **Greenhouse–Geisser correction**[6] and the **Huynh–Feldt correction**.[7]

Because the test for sphericity is not significant in our example, we are not concerned about this adjustment. If the test for sphericity had been significant, however, the df_b would be multiplied by ε, a different critical value would be applied, and a different *p* value would be used as the value for interpretation. Computer output for this analysis will generate results for each of these conditions, and the researcher can determine which results to use.

🔑 In studies that use a repeated measures ANOVA, authors should mention analysis of the sphericity assumption in their results section. Without such information, a significant finding cannot be properly interpreted.

▶ Results

A one-way repeated measures ANOVA was conducted to compare elbow flexor strength at three forearm positions. Results showed a significant difference among the three forearm positions ($F(2,16) = 50.34$, $p<.001$, $\eta_p^2 = .863$). Mauchley's test for sphericity was not significant ($\chi^2(2) = 2.86$, $p = .239$), and therefore, no adjustments were needed.

Two-Factor Repeated Measures Designs

The concepts of repeated measures analysis can also be applied to multifactor experiments. With two repeated factors, the within-subjects design is an extension of the single-factor repeated measures design.

▶ CASE IN POINT #4

Suppose we redesigned our previous example to study isometric elbow flexor strength with the forearm in three positions and with the elbow at two different angles. We would then be able to see if the position of the forearm had any influence on strength when combined with different elbow positions.

Because all subjects would be tested in all conditions, this is a two-way repeated measures design. In this 3×2 design with $n = 8$, each subject would be tested six times, for a total of 48 measurements. Results for hypothetical data are shown in Table 25-6.

With two repeated factors, variance is partitioned to include a main effect for each independent variable and their interaction. Each of these effects is listed as a source of variance in the ANOVA table (see Table 25-6 ❶). Like the one-way repeated measures ANOVA, the effect of between subject differences is first removed from the total variance. Each main and interaction effect is tested against its own error term, representing the random or chance variations among subjects for each treatment effect.

The assignment of degrees of freedom for each of these variance components follows the rules used for the regular two-way analysis of variance: for each main effect $df = k - 1$; for each interaction effect $df = (A - 1)(B - 1)$.

As shown in Table 25-6B, each repeated factor is essentially being tested as it would be in a single-factor experiment. By separating out an error component for each treatment effect, we have created a more powerful test than we would have with one common error term; that is, the error component is smaller for each separate treatment effect than it would be with a combined error term. Therefore, F ratios tend to be larger. In this example, the main effect of forearm and the interaction are significant (Table 25-6 ❷).

Power and Effect Size

Power and effect size estimates are calculated for repeated measures designs using the same process as for a two-way ANOVA.

$$\eta_p^2 = \frac{SS_b}{SS_b + SS_e} \qquad f = \sqrt{\frac{SS_b}{SS_e}}$$

where SS_b is the repeated factor and SS_e is the error term for that factor. For example, for the two-way repeated measures ANOVA (Table 25-6), for the effect of forearm position,

$$\eta_p^2 = \frac{1942.758}{1942.758 + 3236.576} = .375$$

$$f = \sqrt{\frac{1942.758}{3236.576}} = .775$$

These effect sizes would be considered large, and this effect was significant.

▶ Results

A two-way repeated measures ANOVA was used to look at the effect of forearm and elbow position on elbow flexor strength. The main effect of forearm position was significant ($F(2,20) = 6.003$, $p = .009$, $\eta_p^2 = .375$), there was no significant difference between the two elbow positions ($F(1,10) = 1.433$, $p = .259$, $\eta_p^2 = .125$). The interaction effect was significant ($F(2,20) = 3.559$, $p = .048$, $\eta_p^2 = .263$).

This analysis will be followed with a multiple comparison comparing the six means for combinations of forearm and elbow position. (see Chapter 26).

 Application of these values using G*Power for power and sample size estimates is illustrated in the *Chapter 25 Supplement*.

■ Mixed Designs

When a single experiment involves at least one independent factor and one repeated factor, the design is called a **mixed design**. A mixed ANOVA, also called a *split-plot ANOVA*, is therefore used. The overall format for the ANOVA is a combination of between-subjects (independent factors) and within-subjects (repeated factors) analyses. The independent factor is analyzed as it would be in a regular one-way ANOVA, pooling all data for the repeated factor. The repeated factor is analyzed using techniques for a repeated measures analysis.

Table 25-6	**Two-Factor Repeated Measures ANOVA: Elbow Flexor Strength in Three Forearm Positions and Two Elbow Positions ($N = 8$)**

A. Data

Forearm Position

Elbow Angle	Pronation	Neutral	Supination	Marginal Means
90°	25.00	33.00	34.38	**30.79**
45°	17.38	28.13	30.25	**25.25**
Marginal Means	**21.19**	**30.57**	**32.32**	

B. SPSS Output: Two-Way Repeated Measures ANOVA

Measure: Strength
Sphericity Assumed

Tests of Within-Subjects Effects

Source ❷	Sum of Squares	df	Mean Square	F	Sig.	Partial Eta Squared	Observed Power
Elbow	368.521	1	368.521	1.112	.327	.137	.150
Error	2319.979	7	331.426				
Forearm	1145.167	2	572.583	6.074	❶ .013	.465	.804
Error	1319.833	14	94.274				
Elbow x Forearm	27.167	2	13.583	.120	.888	.017	.065
Error	1587.833	14	113.417				

Measure: STRENGTH

Tests of Between-Subjects Effects ❸

Source	Sum of Squares	df	Mean Square	F	Sig.	Partial Eta Squared	Observed Power
Intercept	37688.021	1	37688.021	268.521	.000	.975	1.000
Error	982.479	7	140.354				

❶ Because the main effect of forearm position is the only significant effect, the marginal means for forearm position are the only means of interest.

❷ Each repeated measure is tested against its own error term, which is the interaction between that effect and the effect of subjects

❸ The between-subjects effect is often eliminated from the summary table in a research report. It does not provide important information to the interpretation of the main or interaction effects, but is used to determine the error term for each effect. This effect is expected to be significant, as it reflects that the subjects' scores were different from each other. In a repeated measures analysis, this is not of interest. The meaningful comparisons are across subjects within the repeated factors.

This analysis was run in SPSS using the General Linear Model. Some portions of the output have been omitted for clarity.

Repeated measures often reflect testing subjects at different levels of a treatment variable, as illustrated in previous examples (see Focus on Evidence 25-1). However, many research questions include follow-up measures to determine if outcomes change over time. A common approach utilizes a two-way mixed design to assess changes in the independent factor, with time being an independent variable that is a repeated measure, each interval representing a level of the independent variable.

> When reporting the analysis in a mixed design, the test should be clearly described as a mixed ANOVA or as a two-way ANOVA with one repeated measure.

▶ CASE IN POINT #5

Studies have shown that aerobic exercise training can benefit adolescents with mild traumatic brain injury (TBI).[8] Suppose we designed a study to look at the effect of a treatment program including aerobic exercise compared with a full-body stretching program and an educational control condition, on postinjury symptom improvement in this population. We randomly assign 24 subjects to one of the three conditions ($n = 8$ for each group), and the main outcome is a self-report symptom inventory, scored 0-50 (higher score is better). Measurements are taken at three intervals: baseline, after 6 months, and at a 12-week follow-up. We hypothesize that improvement in symptoms will be greater in those who participate in aerobic exercise as compared to the other two conditions, with improvement seen over time.

Hypothetical data are reported in Table 25-7. The first part of the analysis for this study is the *within-subjects* analysis of all factors that include the repeated factor (Table 25-7 **❶**). This section lists the main effect for time, the interaction between time and treatment, and a common error term to test these two effects. In this example, the main effect of time is significant ($p < .001$), but the interaction effect is not ($p = .073$).

The second part of the analysis addresses treatment as the independent factor. Each level of this factor is assigned to 8 different subjects. Comparison across these groups is a *between-subjects* analysis, shown in Table 25-7 **❷**. This is actually a one-way ANOVA for the effect of treatment. In this example, there is a no significant difference among the three levels of exercise ($p = .097$).

▶ Results

A two-way mixed ANOVA was used to examine the change in symptoms over time following TBI. The ANOVA showed a significant main effect of time ($F(2,42) = 40.32$, $p < .001$, $\eta_p^2 = .658$), with improvements increasing over the three time periods. There was no significant effect of treatment ($F(2,42 = 2.61$, $p = .097$, $\eta_p^2 = .199$) and no significant interaction ($F(4,42) = 2.32$, $p = .073$, $\eta_p^2 = .181$).

Given that time is the only significant effect, we will need to do a multiple comparison to assess differences across the three time periods (see Chapter 26).

Power and Effect Size

Power and effect size estimates for the two-way mixed design reflect the same components as repeated measures and independent designs.

Focus on Evidence 25–1
All Play and No Work...

The health benefits of physical activity in children are well documented, although studies suggest that children are not meeting the recommendation for 60 minutes of moderate to vigorous physical activity each day. Wood et al[9] were interested in the impact of school playing environment on the duration of vigorous physical activity during recesses. They developed a two-way mixed design to study the differential effect of gender and play environment—in school playgrounds versus natural field settings.

They studied 23 children between 8 and 9 years old in one elementary school in the United Kingdom. Using a crossover design, students were split into two groups, each participating in play in one of the two environments for 2 weeks and then switched to the other setting. Children wore accelerometers to monitor time of physical activity in minutes.

Results were presented by gender and play environment (mean and 95% CI):

	BOYS	GIRLS
Playground	15.4 (13.5-17.3)	9.6 (7.7-11.4)
Field	18.8(16.3-21.2)	16.1 (13.8-18.5)

Physical activity was higher in the field for both boys and girls, and boys were consistently more active than girls. The authors found significant main effects but no significant interaction:

- Environment ($p < .001$, $\eta_p^2 = .616$)
- Gender ($p = .002$, $\eta_p^2 = .371$)
- Gender × Environment ($p = .078$, $\eta_p^2 = .140$)

How meaningful are these findings? Is it worth considering changes in school-based activity? If we consider effect size, the environment had a significantly greater effect for boys and girls. However, we can also look at the actual values and confidence intervals, to determine if the observed differences are *important*. The actual difference in playtime between playground and field for boys, for example, is 3.4 minutes and for girls 6.5 minutes, with relatively small confidence intervals. With a goal of 60 minutes of physical activity each day, are these differences impactful? Do these differences warrant policy or financial considerations that would influence a school being able to offer alternative environments? These interpretations are not black and white. It is never just about significance—decisions must be put in context.

Data from Wood C, Gladwell V, Barton J. A repeated measures experiment of school playing environment to increase physical activity and enhance self-esteem in UK school children. *PLoS One* 2014;9(9):e108701.

Table 25-7 Two-Way (3 X 2) Mixed ANOVA: Symptom Improvement over Time With and Without Exercise (N = 24)

A. Data

Time

Intervention	Baseline	6 Weeks	Follow-up	Marginal Means
Exercise	23.63	30.88	45.38	33.09
Stretch	20.00	26.25	33.88	26.71
Control	17.38	28.13	30.25	25.25
Marginal Means	**20.34**	**28.42**	**36.50**	

B. SPSS Output: Two-Way Mixed ANOVA

Measure: STRENGTH
Sphericity Assumed

Tests of Within-Subjects Effects ❶

Source	Sum of Squares	df	Mean Square	F	Sig.	Partial Eta Squared	Observed Power
Time	3136.333	2	1568.167	40.320	.000	.658	1.000
Time* Treatment	360.833	4	90.208	2.319	.073	.181	.623
Error (Time)	1633.500	42	38.893				

Measure: STRENGTH
Sphericity Assumed

Tests of Between-Subjects Effects ❷

Source	Sum of Squares	df	Mean Square	F	Sig.	Partial Eta Squared	Observed Power
Treatment	881.083	2	440.542	2.612	.097	.199	.463
Error (Time)	3541.750	42	168.655				

C. Summary Table

This table is not part of SPSS output, but is created to show how the above data might be combined in a concise way in a research article.

Source	Sum of Squares	df	Mean Square	F	Sig.	Partial Eta Squared	Observed Power
Between subjects ❷							
Treatment	881.083	2	657.76	2.612	.097	.199	.463
Error	3541.750	42	168.655				
Within subjects ❶							
Time	3136.333	2	1568.167	40.320	.000	.658	1.000
Time × Treatment	360.833	4	90.208	2.319	.073	.181	.623
Error	1633.500	42	38.893				

❶ The within-subjects effect includes the repeated measure (Time) and the interaction of the repeated measure with the independent measure (Treatment). Only the main effect of time is significant ($p<.001$).

❷ The between-groups effect is computed for the main effect of Treatment, which is not significant ($p=.097$). This section is equivalent to a one-way analysis of variance.

This analysis was run in SPSS using the General Linear Model. Portions of the printout have been omitted for clarity

COMMENTARY

Sometimes the questions are complicated and the answers are simple!

—Theodor Geisel (Dr. Seuss) (1904-1991)

American author

To understand clinical phenomena, it is necessary to explore various approaches to treatment and how responses vary under different conditions or with different types of patients. Research questions can become more complicated when we try to incorporate several types of interventions or conditions at one time. We must be careful, however, not to make studies so complicated that we cannot make clear comparisons.

Understanding reports that include ANOVA can help to clarify the design of a study. For example, the number of subjects actually tested and the number of groups or measurements can be discerned from degrees of freedom. This is important because the data that are finally analyzed in a study are often different than originally intended in a design, especially when subjects drop out or data are lost. If effect sizes are not reported, they can often be calculated using data provided in a research report. These can be used for clinical interpretation of the results.

The analysis of variance provides researchers with a statistical tool that can adapt to a wide variety of design situations. This chapter has covered only the most common applications. Many other designs, such as nested designs, randomized blocks, and studies with unequal samples, require mathematical adjustments in the analysis that are too complex to cover here. As designs get more complicated, the nuances of analysis of variance can be substantial, and a statistician should be consulted to make sure that the right tests are being used.

When the analysis of variance results in a significant finding, researchers will want to pursue the analysis to determine which specific levels of the independent variables are different from each other. Multiple comparison tests, designed specifically for this purpose, are described in the next chapter.

REFERENCES

1. Ferguson GA. *Statistical Analysis in Psychology and Education.* 5th ed. New York: McGraw-Hill; 1981.
2. Cohen J. *Statistical Power Analysis for the Behavioral Sciences.* 2nd ed. Hillsdale, NJ: Lawrence Erlbaum; 1988.
3. Gaujoux-Viala C, Dougados M, Gossec L. Efficacy and safety of steroid injections for shoulder and elbow tendonitis: a meta-analysis of randomised controlled trials. *Ann Rheum Dis* 2009;68(12):1843-1849.
4. Lakens D. Calculating and reporting effect sizes to facilitate cumulative science: a practical primer for t-tests and ANOVAs. *Front Psychol* 2013;4:863.
5. Warner RM. *Applied Statistics.* Thousand Oaks, CA: Sage Publications; 2013.
6. Geisser S, Greenhouse SW. An extension of Box's results on the use of the F distribution in multivariate analysis. *Ann Math Statist* 1958;29:885.
7. Huynh H, Feldt LS. Estimation of the Box correction for degrees of freedom from sample data in the randomized block and split-plot designs. *J Educ Statist* 1976;1:69.
8. Kurowski BG, Hugentobler J, Quatman-Yates C, Taylor J, Gubanich PJ, Altaye M, Wade SL. Aerobic Exercise for Adolescents With Prolonged Symptoms after mild traumatic brain injury: An exploratory randomized clinical trial. *J Head Trauma Rehabil* 2017;32(2):79-89.
9. Wood C, Gladwell V, Barton J. A repeated measures experiment of school playing environment to increase physical activity and enhance self-esteem in UK school children. *PLoS One* 2014;9(9):e108701.

Multiple Comparison Tests

When an analysis of variance (ANOVA) results in a significant F ratio, the researcher is justified in rejecting the null hypothesis and concluding that not all means are equal. However, this outcome tells us nothing about which means are significantly different from which other means. The purpose of this chapter is to describe the most commonly used **multiple comparison tests** for a variety of designs. Several procedures are available, given names for the individuals who developed them. Each test involves contrasts of pairs of means which are tested against a critical value to determine if the difference is large enough to be significant. These tests can be run with one-way or multidimensional designs, with independent or repeated measures. The use of multiple comparisons will be illustrated using examples introduced in Chapter 25.

■ Corrections and Adjustments

At the end of Chapter 24 we discussed the inappropriate use of multiple *t*-tests when more than two comparisons are made within a single set of data. The ANOVA provides one solution to look at multiple means. However, if the ANOVA is significant, we are still faced with the need for multiple comparisons to determine which means are significantly different from each other.

This process is based on the desired protection against Type I error in an experiment, specified by α. At

α = .05, we limit ourselves to a 5% chance that we will experience the random event of finding a significant difference for a given comparison when none exists. We must differentiate this **per comparison error rate ($α_{PC}$)** from the situation where α is set at .05 for each of several comparisons in one experiment. If we test each one at α = .05, the potential cumulative error for the set of comparisons is actually greater than .05. This cumulative probability has been called the **familywise error rate ($α_{FW}$)** and represents the probability of making at least one Type I error in a set or "family" of statistical comparisons.

> ✎ Think of it this way—you are riding on a train. Quality testing has been performed on several components, all done by different inspectors. One found that there is only a 5% risk of failure for the engines. Ok, not bad. Knowing your statistics, you consider 5% a small risk. However, you didn't know that another inspector found a 5% possibility of a problem with the tracks, and still another found a 5% risk for failure of communication systems. How does it feel now? What is your *cumulative* risk that at least one problem would occur? It's a lot more than 5%.

Type I Error Rate

The Type I error rate for a family of comparisons, where each individual comparison is tested at α= .05, is equal to

$$α_{FW} = 1 - (1 - α)^c$$

where c represents the total number of comparisons. The maximum number of pairwise contrasts for any set of data will be $k(k - 1)/2$. For example, if we want to compare four means, testing each comparison at α = .05, we will perform $4(4 - 1)/2 = 6$ comparisons. Therefore,

$$α_{FW} = 1 - (1 - .05)^6 = .265$$

This means that in making these six comparisons, there is a greater than 26% chance that we will make a Type I error for at least one of these differences. As the number of comparisons increases, so does this probability. For example, with 5 means (10 comparisons), $\alpha_{FW}= .40$. These probabilities clearly exceed the generally accepted standard of 5% risk for Type I error.

Differences Among Tests

Following the ANOVA, a null hypothesis is proposed for individual comparisons, tested against a critical value that indicates if the difference between individual means is significant. Asking the right questions can help to identify which follow-up tests are most appropriate (see Box 26-1).

The purpose of multiple comparison tests is to examine several contrasts simultaneously, making adjustments to control Type I error. The major difference among various tests lies in the degree of that protection. More *liberal* procedures base their critical values on per comparison error rates, resulting in greater statistical power, but with the potential for more Type I errors. These tests will find significant differences with means closer together. More *conservative* tests base critical values on the entire family of comparisons, producing fewer Type I errors, but at the cost of power. Using a stricter standard, this requires that means be farther apart to find significant differences. There is no consensus about preferences for one approach over the other.

Researchers must determine if Type I or Type II error is of greater concern, which can influence the choice of a multiple comparison test. There are actually quite a number of tests, many with subtle statistical differences. It is useful to be familiar with their names and purposes so you can make judgments about results when reading research reports.

> Most computer packages include multiple comparison tests to follow up after the ANOVA, although some will require manipulation to get the appropriate results. This is one of those situations where it is useful to understand statistical procedures to appreciate differences among tests. Most multiple comparisons are simple enough to be carried out with a hand calculator once the analysis of variance data are obtained.

Bonferroni Correction

Because α_{FW} is dependent on the number of comparisons, one approach to correct for the inflation of α is to split it evenly among the set of contrasts, so that each contrast is tested at α_{FW}/c. This process of adjusting α to protect against Type I error is called the **Bonferroni correction** or *adjustment*. For example, if a researcher wants an overall probability of .05 for a set of six comparisons, each individual comparison would have to achieve significance at .05/6, or $p = .008$. This will allow the overall familywise probability across all comparisons to achieve .05.

The Bonferroni correction will decrease the risk of a Type I error but will also have the effect of increasing the possibility of Type II error, especially when the number of contrasts is large.

■ *Post Hoc* Multiple Comparisons

Most multiple comparison procedures are classified as *post hoc* because specific comparisons are decided *after* the ANOVA is completed. These are considered **unplanned comparisons** in that they are based on exploration of the outcome. Most tests involve comparison of all pairwise differences.

> Even though all pairwise comparisons can be made with *post hoc* tests, it is often relevant to limit the number to those that specifically support the purpose of the research. This helps to control for the inherent risk of Type I error with many comparisons.

Although several methods have been devised for testing the significance of *post hoc* comparisons, three of the most commonly used will be discussed here: Tukey's honestly significant difference, the Student-Newman-Keuls comparison, and the Scheffé comparison. Other *post hoc* tests, used less often, are shown in Table 26-1. Special tests have also been developed for use when equal variances cannot be assumed. All are available in SPSS.

 See the *Chapter 26 Supplement* for further examples and a description of multiple comparison tests for planned and unplanned contrasts.

Box 26-1   What Do You Want to Know?

There are two major approaches to multiple comparison testing that should be considered as part of the planning of a study.

Exploring the data for unexpected relationships. After data are collected, a researcher can examine all potential comparisons, looking for any interesting relationships among groups. These are *post hoc* tests based on *unplanned comparisons* that typically involve looking at many pairwise contrasts.

Testing specific questions. During the planning of a study, specific questions may be identified that involve a fixed number of comparisons. These are considered *a priori* or *planned comparisons*. Because they are planned in advance, these tests will have greater power.

Hypotheses may also be identified during planning that involve different combinations of variables. These are *complex contrasts* that use subsets of means, involving some or all groups.

Table 26-1   Commonly Used Multiple Comparison Tests

More Powerful / **Less Type I Error Protection**	**Fisher's Least Significant Difference (LSD)**	A *post hoc* test that is essentially application of multiple *t*-tests, making no adjustments for multiple comparisons. Generally considered too liberal.
	Duncan's New Multiple Range Test	Compares all pairwise differences using the *q* statistic. Considered a liberal *post hoc* test.
	Student-Newman-Keuls Test (SNK)	A step-down *post hoc* comparison of all pairwise means, using different critical values based on their distance apart. Considered liberal. Based on the studentized range, *q*.
	REGWF and REGWQ	A conservative modification of the SNK procedure, making less rapid adjustments at each step. Initials stand for developers Ryan-Einot-Gabriel-Welsh. REGWF uses the *F* statistic, and REGWQ uses the *q* statistic. Considered a good balance between Type I and II error.
	Dunnett's Correction	Comparisons that compare a control group mean to each other group mean. Uses the standard *t*-test, but with a more conservative critical value.
	Tukey's Honestly Significant Difference (HSD)	*Post hoc* comparison used to explore all pairwise differences. Uses one critical value for all differences. Considered a good protection against Type I error with reasonable balance of Type II error. Based on the studentized range, *q*.
	Sidak-Bonferroni Procedure	Uses a more restrictive calculation of α than the Bonferroni procedure, and is therefore slightly more powerful.
Less Powerful / **Greater Type I Error Protection**	**Bonferroni Correction**	A correction for Type I error by dividing alpha by the number of comparisons, thereby requiring a much smaller *p* value to attain significance. Used with the *t*-test for multiple comparisons but can be used with other tests as well.
	Scheffé's Method	*Post hoc* comparison considered most conservative, with highest protection against Type I error. Can be used with pairwise and complex contrasts. Recommended for use with unequal sample sizes. Based on the *F* statistic.

► CASE IN POINT #1

Recall the hypothetical study in Chapter 25 comparing the effects of ice, NSAID, splint, and rest for relieving pain in 44 patients with elbow tendinitis (see Table 25-1). Group means represent the change in pain-free range of motion (ROM) for the four treatment groups. Eleven subjects were tested in each group.

Results for this hypothetical study are shown in Table 26-2. The *F* ratio for these data is significant ($p < .001$), and it is now of interest to examine individual differences among the four means.

The Minimum Significant Difference

The process of testing differences among several means is fairly consistent for all multiple comparison procedures. In each test, differences between pairs of means are obtained, as shown in Table 26-2B. This triangular table shows the absolute differences between all pairs of means, with the means listed in ascending order. With *k* = 4, there will be a total of 6 comparisons.

Each pairwise comparison is tested against a **minimum significant difference (MSD)**. If the absolute difference between a pair of means is *equal to or greater than* the minimum significant difference, then the contrast is considered significant. If the absolute value of the pairwise difference is smaller than the MSD, the means are not significantly different from each other.

🔑 The minimum significant difference, MSD, should be distinguished from the minimal detectable change, MDC. Both of these values represent a threshold—the MSD for a significant difference, and the MDC for reliable change (see Chapter 32).

Table 26-2 One-Way ANOVA: Change in Pain-Free ROM with Treatment for Elbow Tendinitis ($N = 44$)

A. Group Means

ROM	N	Mean	Std. Deviation
Ice	11	44.18	10.870
NSAID	11	45.27	8.403
Splint	11	35.27	9.509
Rest	11	24.09	8.538
Total	44	37.20	12.487

B. Mean Differences

			4	3	2	1
			Rest	Splint	Ice	NSAID
		Means	24.09	35.27	44.18	45.27
4	Rest	24.09	—	11.18	20.09	21.18
3	Splint	35.27		—	8.91	10.00
1	Ice	44.18			—	1.09

C. SPSS Output: One-Way ANOVA

ANOVA

ROM	Sum of Squares	df	Mean Square	F	Sig.	Partial Eta Squared	Observed Power
Between Groups	3184.250	3	1061.417	12.058	.000	.475	.999
Within Groups ❺	3520.909	40	88.023				

These data are taken from Table 25-1 in Chapter 25.

Calculation of the MSD is based on the error mean square (MS_e) taken from the ANOVA, which reflects the degree of variance within groups (between subjects). For the example we are using, the error mean square (MS_e) is 88.023 (see Table 26-2C). The greater the variance within groups, the less likely we will see a significant difference between means.

Critical values for the MSD are used differently, depending on the number of means being compared and the type of error rate used (per comparison or family-wise).

Tukey's Honestly Significant Difference

Perhaps the most widely used multiple comparison test is Tukey's **honestly significant difference (HSD)** method.[1] This procedure sets a familywise error rate, so that α identifies the probability that one or more of the pairwise comparisons will be falsely declared significant. Therefore, this test offers generous protection against Type I error.

Tukey's HSD is calculated using the **studentized range** statistic, given the symbol q. Critical values of q are shown in Table 26-3. The q statistic is influenced by the overall number of means that are being compared. At the top of the table, the number or "range" of means being compared is given the symbol "r".

 In this case, r stands for *range*. This symbol should not be confused with the use of *r* as a correlation coefficient.

Logically, as the number of sample means increases, the size of the difference between the largest and smallest means will also increase, even when H_0 is true. The q statistic provides a mechanism for adjusting critical values to account for the effect of larger numbers of means. The relevant critical values are located according to the degrees of freedom associated with the error term in the ANOVA. For the current example, $df_e = 40$ (see Table 26-2C).

It is not uncommon to find that the exact value for the error degrees of freedom is not listed in these tables. In that case, it is usually sufficient to refer to the closest value for degrees of freedom for an approximate critical value. To be conservative, the next lowest value for degrees of freedom should be used

Minimum Significant Difference

The minimum significant difference for Tukey's HSD procedure is given by

$$MSD = q\sqrt{\frac{MS_e}{n}} = 3.79\sqrt{\frac{88.023}{11}} = 10.72$$

Table 26-3	Abridged Table of Critical Values of the Studentized Range Statistic, q (α = .05)			
			r	
df_e	2	3	4	5
10	3.15	3.88	4.33	4.65
20	2.95	3.58	3.96	4.23
30	2.89	3.49	3.85	4.10
40	2.86	3.44	3.79	4.04
60	2.83	3.40	3.74	3.98
120	2.80	3.36	3.68	3.92
∞	2.77	3.31	3.63	3.86

r = number of means (HSD) or comparison interval (SNK). This is an abridged version of this table for purposes of illustration. Refer to the Chapter 26 Supplement for the full table.

where n is the number of subjects *in each group* (assuming equal sample sizes), and q = 3.79 for r = 4 and df_e = 40 (see Table 26-3). The MSD is compared with each pairwise mean difference. Absolute differences that are equal to or greater than this value are significant.

 See the *Chapter 26 Supplement* for calculation of the harmonic mean, which is used to calculate the MSD when samples sizes are not equal.

Computer Output

SPSS uses two formats to display results of the Tukey HSD. In Table 26-4 ❷, multiple comparisons for each pairwise contrast include the mean difference and its significance, and a confidence interval (CI). If the mean difference is greater than 10.72, it is significant. For the Tukey procedure, the same MSD is applied for all comparisons.

The 95% confidence interval for each comparison is calculated using:

$$95\% \text{ CI} = \text{mean difference} \pm \text{MSD}$$

Confidence intervals for comparisons of the mean for rest with means for ice, splint, or NSAID do not contain zero and therefore represent significant differences. All others are not significant. For example, for the difference between ice and NSAID,

$$95\% \text{ CI} = -1.09 \pm 10.72$$
$$= -11.81 \text{ to } 9.63$$

This confidence interval contains zero, denoting no difference between means, which indicates that the difference between ice and NSAID means is not significant.

An alternative presentation shows *homogeneous subsets of means* (see Table 26-4 ❹). In this table, each subset listed in the same column represents means that are not significantly different. Means that are listed in separate columns are different from one another. Means are listed in ascending order. These results show that the mean for the rest group is significantly different from the three other means.

Results of multiple comparison tests are often reported in narrative form, although they may also be included in data tables in an article. Some authors include graphs showing which means are different from each other. Results should include the ANOVA outcome, followed by specific description of the multiple comparison test and significant differences among groups.

> ### ▶ Results
> The one-way ANOVA demonstrated a significant difference among the four group means ($F(3,40)$ =12.06, $p <$ .001, η^2 = .475). The *post hoc* Tukey multiple comparison procedure showed that the change in pain-free ROM was not significantly different across ice ($\bar{X}$ = 44.18 ± 10.87), NSAID ($\bar{X}$ = 45.27 ± 8.40) and splint ($\bar{X}$ = 35.27 ± 9.51) treatments. All three of these treatments produced significantly greater ROM change than the rest condition ($\bar{X}$ = 24.09 ± 8.54).

Student-Newman–Keuls Method

The **Student-Newman–Keuls (SNK) test** (also called *Newman–Keuls test*) is similar to the Tukey method, except that it uses an adjusted per comparison error rate. Therefore, α specifies the Type I error rate for each pairwise contrast rather than for the entire set of comparisons. The result is a more powerful test but with greater chances of Type I error, especially with a large number of comparisons.

Comparison Intervals

The SNK procedure is also based on the studentized range q. However, values of q are used differently for each contrast, depending on the number of *adjacent* means (r) within an ordered *comparison interval*.

This method is considered a *sequential* procedure because comparisons are made in a "step" fashion, starting with the two most extreme means and then examining successively smaller subsets. To illustrate how this is applied, consider the four sample means for the tendinitis study, ranked in ascending size order: (4) rest, (3) splint, (1) ice (2) NSAID (see Fig. 26-1).

If we compare the two smaller means, the comparison interval for rest → splint includes two adjacent means. Therefore, r = 2 for that comparison. If we compare the largest and smallest means, the interval for rest → NSAID contains four adjacent means (4-3-1-2), and so r = 4. Table 26-5B shows these intervals for each pair of means.

In contrast to Tukey's approach, which uses one critical difference for all comparisons, the SNK test will use

Table 26-4 **Significant Differences for Tukey's HSD (α=.05): Change in Pain-Free ROM with Elbow Tendinitis (N = 44)**

❶ MSD = 10.72

SPSS Output: Tukey's HSD

Multiple Comparisons

Dependent Variable: ROM

(I) Group	(J) Group	Mean Difference (I–J) ❷	Sig. ❷	95% Confidence Interval ❸ Lower Bound	Upper Bound
Ice	NSAID	−1.09	.993	−11.81	9.63
	Splint	8.91	.133	−1.81	19.63
	Rest	20.09*	.000	9.37	30.81
NSAID	Ice	1.09	.993	−9.63	11.81
	Splint	10.00	.075	−.72	20.72
	Rest	21.18*	.000	10.46	31.90
Splint	Ice	−8.91	.133	−19.63	1.81
	NSAID	−10.00	.075	−20.72	.72
	Rest	11.18*	.038	.46	21.90
Rest	Ice	−20.09*	.000	−30.81	−9.37
	NSAID	−21.18*	.000	−31.90	−10.46
	Splint	−11.18*	.038	−21.90	−.46

* The mean difference is significant at the 0.05 level

Homogeneous Subsets

Tukey HSD Group	N	Subset for alpha = .05 1	2
Rest	11	24.09	❹
Splint	11		35.27
Ice	11		44.18
NSAID	11		45.27
Sig		1.000	0.75

Means for groups in homogeneous subsets are displayed.

❶ All mean differences greater than the MSD 10.72 are significant.

❷ Each pairwise mean difference (labeled I − J) is listed with its corresponding *p* value. The table is redundant because each group is used as a reference. Minus signs are ignored. Significant effects are highlighted and tagged with an asterisk.

❸ 95% confidence intervals are presented for each mean difference. If the interval contains zero, it would indicate that the difference is not significant.

❹ Subsets in the same column are considered "homogeneous," indicating they are not different from each other. Means not in the same column are significantly different. Means for Splint, Ice, and NSAID are not different, but all three are different from Rest.

These data are taken from Table 26-2. Portions of the output have been omitted for clarity.

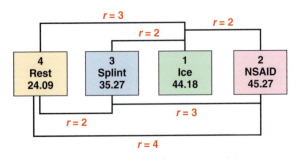

Figure 26-1 Comparison intervals for a set of four group means, arranged in size order. Based on data from Table 26-1.

a larger critical difference as the comparison interval increases. This adjusts for the fact that larger differences are expected with a greater range of means, even when H_0 is true.

Minimum Significant Difference

The minimum significant difference for the SNK comparison is

$$\text{MSD} = q_{(r)} \sqrt{\frac{MS_e}{n}}$$

where values of $q_{(r)}$ are obtained from Table 26-3 for each comparison interval. For the example we are using, we find q for $df_e = 40$ for comparison intervals of r = 2, 3, and 4. With MS_e = 88.023 and *n* = 11, we find the corresponding minimum significant differences, shown in Table 26-5A.

A table of mean differences helps us identify the difference for each pair of means (see Table 26-5B). The first "step" in the procedure is a comparison of the two extreme scores (r = 4), rest and NSAID. The difference between these means (21.18) is larger than the MSD, and therefore, these means are significantly different. We then go to the next two smaller subsets with r = 3. Each of these is significant, and so we continue with the three smallest subsets with r = 2. Two of these comparisons are significant. Only the difference between ice and NSAID is not significant.

Because means are in rank order, if at any step of the analysis we find no significant differences, we do not have to check smaller subsets. For instance, if none of the means with r = 3 were significant, we would not have to examine subsets for r = 2.

Computer Output

Results are shown in Table 26-5C for subsets of means. Because the mean for the rest group is listed in a column by itself, it is different from all other means. The same is true for the mean for the splint group. The means for ice and NSAID are listed in the same column, indicating that they are not different from each other. This pattern of differences shows a difference between splint and ice or NSAID, a difference that was not considered significant with the Tukey test.

▶ **Results**

The ANOVA showed a significant difference among the four group means ($F(3,40)$ = 12.06, $p < .001$, η^2 = .475). The *post hoc* Student-Newman-Keuls test showed that the change in pain-free ROM with rest was significantly less than the other three interventions. There was no significant difference between ice and NSAID. These two treatments also had significantly better results than using a splint.

Table 26-5 **Significant Differences for the Student-Newman-Keuls Test (α=.05): Change in Pain-Free ROM with Elbow Tendinitis (N = 44)**

A. Minimum Significant Differences ①

$$MSD = q_{(r)} \sqrt{\frac{MS_e}{n}} = q_{(r)} \sqrt{\frac{88.023}{11}}$$

MSD (r = 2) = 2.86 (2.83) = 8.09
MSD (r = 3) = 3.44 (2.83) = 9.73
MSD (r = 4) = 3.79 (2.83) = 10.72

B. Table of Mean Differences ②

			4	3	1	2
			Rest	Splint	Ice	NSAID
		Means	24.09	35.27	44.18	45.27
4	Rest	24.09	—	11.18* (r=2)	20.09* (r=3)	21.18* (r=4)
3	Splint	35.27		—	8.91* (r=2)	10.00* (r=3)
1	Ice	44.18			—	1.09 (r=2)

* indicates a significant difference.

C. SPSS Output: SNK Test

Homogeneous Subsets of Means ③

Student-Newman-Keuls		Subset for alpha = .05		
Group	N	1	2	3
Rest	11	24.09		
Splint	11		35.27	
Ice	11			44.18
NSAID	11			45.27
Sig		1.000	1.000	.786

SPSS provides only the homogeneous subsets of means as output for the SNK procedure.

These data are taken from Table 26-2.

① Minimum significant differences are calculated for each range of means. Values of *q* are obtained from Table 26-2 for values of r = 2, 3, and 4, for 40 degrees of freedom.

② The table of mean differences shows results for each pairwise comparison. The MSD used to determine significance for each comparison is based on the range of means, *r*. Significant differences are tagged with an asterisk.
This table is not generated by SPSS. It is created to illustrate how mean differences are used for comparison to MSD values. SPSS does not generate the table of mean differences for the SNK test.

③ The homogeneous subsets of means show that Ice and NSAID means are not significantly different, but they are both different from Rest and Splint. Rest and Splint means are also significantly different from each other.

You may have noted that the MSD for the SNK test with r = 4 is the same as the MSD used for Tukey's test (in this case 10.72). The Tukey procedure uses this one MSD for all comparisons, whereas the SNK test adjusts the MSD for smaller comparison intervals. Therefore, the MSD will be lower for some contrasts using the SNK method, resulting in more significant differences. Consequently, the SNK test is more powerful, and more likely to reveal significant differences between group means than the Tukey comparison. However, it will also produce a greater number of Type I errors than the Tukey method over the long run.

Scheffé Comparison

The **Scheffé comparison** is the most flexible and most rigorous of the *post hoc* multiple comparison tests.[2] It is also popular with many researchers because it is based on the familiar F distribution. It is a conservative test because it adopts a familywise error rate that applies to all contrasts. This provides strong protection against Type I error, but it also makes the procedure much less powerful than other tests. Scheffé has recommended using a less stringent level of significance, such as $\alpha = .10$, to avoid excess Type II error.[3]

Minimum Significant Difference

The minimum significant difference for the Scheffé comparison is given by

$$MSD = \sqrt{(k-1)F}\sqrt{\frac{2MS_e}{n}}$$

$$= \sqrt{(4-1)(2.84)}\sqrt{\frac{2(88.023)}{11}} = 11.68$$

where k is the total number of means involved in the set of comparisons, and F is the *critical value* for df_b and df_e obtained from Appendix Table A-3 (not the calculated value of F from the ANOVA). For the example we are using $k = 4$, and $F(3,40) = 2.84$ at $\alpha = .05$.

All differences between means must meet or exceed 11.68 to be significant. As shown in Table 26-6, this analysis results in two significant comparisons—fewer than with the Newman–Keuls or Tukey methods. This outcome demonstrates the lower power associated with the Scheffé comparison. According to this test, the rest and splint groups are not significantly different from each other, where they were considered significantly different with the other tests.

Using the Scheffé comparison, note that the rest group is significantly different from ice and NSAID groups but not from the splint group. However, the splint mean is not different from ice and NSAID. This

overlap may seem illogical, but there is a statistical explanation. It occurs because variance components from the different variables are not independent of each other (see Focus on Evidence 26-1). This result suggests that the Scheffé comparison is not the most useful approach to understand the relationships in these data.

■ *Post Hoc* Tests for Factorial Designs

Multiple comparison procedures are applicable to all analysis of variance designs. So far, we have described their use following an analysis with only one independent variable. When multifactor experiments are analyzed, the multiple comparison procedures can be used to compare means for main effects and interaction effects.

> ### ► CASE IN POINT #2
>
> To illustrate this application, refer back to Chapter 25 again, where we created a two-way design, looking at three treatments for elbow tendinitis combined with medication to increase pain-free ROM. Modality had three levels: ice, splint, and rest (see Table 25-4). Medication had two levels: NSAID and no medication. In this 3 x 2 design, 10 subjects were tested in each of the six treatment combinations.

Data for this hypothetical study are shown in Table 26-7.

Main Effects

The ANOVA shows a significant effect for main effects of modality and medication. These effects can be further analyzed using a multiple comparison test to look at differences among marginal means. For the main effect of modality, we would compare means for ice, splint, and rest, pooled on medication. It is not necessary to do a multiple comparison for medication because it has only two levels. Therefore, the marginal means can be used directly to describe differences.

Interaction Effects

In most cases, researchers develop factorial designs with the expectation of specific patterns of interaction between the independent variables. If this were not the case, the researcher could just as easily design separate one-way studies. When the interaction effect is significant, main effects are usually ignored.

It is reasonable to consider how multiple comparisons can help to understand the relationship among the various combinations of factors. In the modality study, with six groups, if we looked at all pairwise comparisons, we would perform 15 contrasts. However, not all of these

Table 26-6   Significant Differences for the Scheffé Comparison (α=.05): Change in Pain-Free ROM with Elbow Tendinitis (N = 44)

❶ MSD = 11.68

SPSS Output: Scheffé Test

Multiple Comparisons

Dependent Variable: ROM

(I) Group	(J) Group	Mean Difference (I–J)	❷ Sig.	95% Confidence Interval Lower Bound	95% Confidence Interval Upper Bound
Scheffe Ice	NSAID	−1.091	.995	−12.77	10.58
	Splint	8.909	.192	−2.77	20.58
	Rest	20.091*	.000	8.42	31.77
NSAID	NSAID	1.091	.995	−10.58	12.77
	Splint	10.000	.118	−1.67	21.67
	Rest	21.182*	.000	9.51	32.86
	Ice	−8.909	.192	−20.58	2.77
Splint	NSAID	−10.000	.118	−21.67	1.67
	Rest	11.182	.065	−.49	22.86
	Ice	−20.091*	.000	−31.77	−8.42
Rest	NSAID	−21.182*	.000	−32.86	−9.51
	Splint	−11.182	.065	−22.86	.49

* The mean difference is significant at the 0.05 level

Homogeneous Subsets of Means

Scheffé

Group	N	Subset for alpha = .05 1	Subset for alpha = .05 2
Rest	11	24.09	❸
Splint	11	35.27	35.27
Ice	11		44.18
NSAID	11		45.27
Sig		.065	.118

Means for groups in homogeneous subsets are displayed.

❶ The minimum significant difference is 11.68. Therefore, all mean differences greater than 11.68 are significant.

❷ Each pairwise mean difference (labeled I – J) and the significance of the difference is listed. Significant effects are highlighted and tagged with an asterisk.

❸ Means that are listed in the same column are not significantly different. In this case Rest and Splint are not different from each other, but both are different from Ice and NSAID. Splint, Ice, and NSAID are not significantly different from each other. This outcome is difficult to interpret because of the overlap of Splint in both subsets.

These data are taken from Table 26-2. Portions of the output have been omitted for clarity.

would be meaningful. For example, a comparison of ice/NSAID with splint/no med would not provide a clinically useful contrast. Because these comparisons involve completely different combinations, they cannot logically help us understand the differential effect of modality or medication.

Simple Effects

With a significant interaction, it is usually more meaningful to consider an analysis of combinations within rows or columns of the design. These separate analyses are called **simple effects**. Essentially, we convert the factorial design into several smaller "single-factor" experiments. The plots in Table 26-7 show the interaction between levels of modality and medication, with each

line representing a simple effect. Interaction is defined as a significant difference between simple effects.[5]

For example, we can look at the simple effect of modality for those who got the NSAID, represented by the blue line in plot A. Then we could look at the simple effect for those who got no medication, represented by the red line. Alternatively, we can look at the simple effect of medication for each level of modality, represented by the lines in plot B.

Simple effects are distinguished from main effects which are based on averaged values across a second variable. An analysis of simple effects will reveal differential patterns within each level of the independent variables.

Simple Comparisons

When there are three or more levels of an independent variable, as with modality, we can perform a separate ANOVA on the three means for each level of medication. These analyses for the NSAID and no med groups are shown in Table 26-7C. The modalities were significantly different for the NSAID group, but not for the no med group. A follow-up Tukey test for the NSAID group showed that the ice condition was significantly larger than the other two. This finding would have been expected according to the interaction plot.

▶ Results
The analysis of variance showed significant main effects for modality ($F(2,54) = 5.97$, $p = .005$, $\eta_p^2 = .181$) and medication ($F(1,54) = 5.77$, $p = .02$, $\eta_p^2 = .097$). The interaction was also significant ($F(2,54) = 5.79$, $p = .005$, $\eta_p^2 = .177$). A test of simple effects indicated that the ice treatment resulted in significantly more improvement for the group taking the NSAID ($p < .001$). All other combinations were not significantly different.

■ *Post Hoc* Tests for Repeated Measures

The standard *post hoc* multiple comparisons procedures just described are not generally applied for repeated measures analyses. Because repeated measures involve within-subject comparisons, the multiple comparison procedures do not logically fit, as they are based on overall group differences.

▶ CASE IN POINT #3
Let's reconsider the hypothetical repeated measures study described in Chapter 25 that examined elbow flexor strength in three forearm position for nine subjects (see Table 25-5). The mean for pronation was 17.33, for neutral 27.56, and for supination 29.11 pounds. Recall that the ANOVA showed a significant difference among the three means ($p < .001$).

The results of the repeated measures ANOVA are shown in Table 26-8A. A *post hoc* multiple comparison test is warranted to compare the three means.

The paired *t*-test can be used for these comparisons, with adjustments for the Type I error rate.[6,7] The pairwise comparisons can also be run using the General Linear Model to generate pairwise comparisons for all pairs. Table 26-8B presents the results of the three pairwise comparisons using a Bonferroni adjustment. The differences for pronation-neutral and pronation-supination are significant ($p < .001$), but the difference for neutral-supination is not ($p = .382$).

Table 26-7   Simple Effects for Interaction: Pain-Free ROM Across Levels of Modality and Medication

A. Means

Medication

Modality	NSAID	No Med
Ice	50	22
Splint	20	21
Rest	24	23

B. SPSS Output: Two-Way ANOVA

ANOVA

Source	Sum of Squares	df	Mean Square	F	❶ Sig.	Partial Eta Squared	Observed Power
Modality	2703.333	2	1351.667	5.970	.005	.181	.867
Med	1306.667	1	1306.667	5.771	.020	.097	.655
Modality* Med	2623.333	2	1311.667	5.793	.005	.177	.851
Error	12226.000	54	226.407				
Total	18859.333	59					

C. SPSS Output: Simple Effects

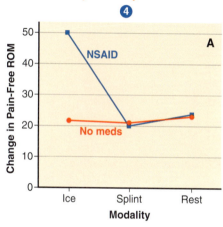

❹

Modality within Each Level of Medication

Pairwise Comparisons

Dependent Variable: ROMChange

❷ Med	(I) Modality	(J) Modality	Mean Difference (I–J)	Sig.	95% CI Lower Bound	95% CI Upper Bound
NSAID	Ice	Splint	30.000*	.000	16.509	43.491
	Ice	Rest	26.000*	.000	12.59	39.491
	Splint	Rest	−4.000	.555	−17.491	9.491
No Med	Ice	Splint	1.000	.882	−12.491	14.491
	Ice	Rest	−1.000	.882	−14.491	12.491
	Splint	Rest	−2.000	.767	−15.491	11.491

Medication within Each Level of Modality

Pairwise Comparisons

Dependent Variable: ROMChange

❸ Modality	(I) Med	(J) Med	Mean Difference (I–J)	Sig.	95% CI Lower Bound	95% CI Upper Bound
Ice	NSAID	No Med	28.000*	.000	14.509	41.491
Splint	NSAID	No Med	−1.000	.882	−14.491	12.491
Rest	NSAID	No Med	1.000	.882	−12.491	14.491

❶ The ANOVA shows a significant interaction effect ($p = .005$).

❷ To test simple effects for Modality, pairwise comparisons are made between the three modalities within each level of Medication. The Ice/NSAID combination resulted in a significantly greater change in ROM than any of the other combinations. Significant differences are tagged with an asterisk.

❸ To test simple effects for Medication, pairwise comparisons are made between the NSAID and No Med conditions within each level of Modality. The two medication groups are different only for the Ice treatment. Significant differences are tagged with an asterisk.

❹ The plots show how means differ for (**A**) the three modalities and (**B**) the two medication groups. The change in pain-free ROM was substantially higher in the Ice/NSAID combination than for any other combination. The pairwise comparisons confirm this.

These data are taken from Table 25-4 in Chapter 25. Analyses were run using GLM in SPSS. Portions of the output have been omitted for clarity.

Table 26-8	Pairwise Comparisons Following Repeated Measures ANOVA: Elbow Flexor Strength in Three Forearm Positions (*N*=9)

A. SPSS Output: One-Way Repeated Measures ANOVA

ANOVA

	Sum of Squares	df	Mean Square	F	Sig.	Partial Eta Squared	Observed Power
Subjects	2604.000	8	325.500				
Position	736.889	2	368.444	50.34	.000	.863	1.000
Error	117.111	16	7.319				

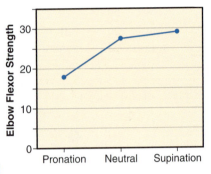

B. SPSS Output: Pairwise Comparisons

Pairwise Comparisons

(I) Position	(J) Position	Mean Difference (I–J)	Sig.b	95% Confidence Intervalb Lower Bound	Upper Bound
Pronation	Neutral	−10.222*	.000	−14.010	−6.435
	Supination	−11.778*	.000	−16.514	−7.042
Neutral	Pronation	10.222*	..000	6.435	14.010
	Supination	−1.556	.382	−4.314	1.203
Supination	Pronation	11.778*	.000	7.042	16.517
	Neutral	1.556	.382	−1.203	4.314

Based on estimated marginal means
*The mean difference is significant at the .05 level
b. Adjusted for multiple comparisons: Bonferroni

These data are taken from Table 25-5 in Chapter 25. Portions of the output have been omitted for clarity.

▶ **Results**

In the study of forearm position, there is a significant difference in strength among the three forearm positions ($F(2,16) = 50.34$, $p < .001, \eta_p^2 = .863$). Pairwise comparisons were run using a paired *t*-test with a Bonferroni adjustment. With 3 comparisons, all tests had to achieve significance at $\alpha = .017$. Results showed significant differences for means of pronation with neutral and supination ($p < .001$). The difference between neutral and supination was not significant ($p = .382$).

■ Planned Comparisons

As part of planning a study, researchers often identify a limited number of comparisons of interest. These contrasts usually relate to theoretical expectations of the data. When comparisons are planned in advance, *a priori* tests can be used. The rationale for valid application of planned comparisons must be established before data are

collected, so that the choice of specific hypotheses cannot be influenced by the results. The number of planned contrasts is usually small, given that they answer specific questions posed at the start of the study. This is in contrast to *post hoc* tests that focus on exploration of all possible contrasts.

Because the researcher is not interested in the overall null hypothesis with planned comparisons, it is actually unnecessary to run an ANOVA. Regardless of whether the ANOVA demonstrates a significant *F* ratio, planned comparisons can be made. Because these tests focus on specific questions, rather than all possible comparisons, they will generally have higher power. These contrasts are run using a *t*-test with no adjustments to the per comparison error rate.

 Planned comparisons are determined in advance, and there is usually an assumption that the contrasts are *orthogonal*, or independent of each other. This means that the variance in one measure cannot be predicted by the other.[8] Accordingly, the questions being answered can be considered in isolation, allowing them to be tested using the per comparison error rate with no further adjustments.[5,9] When contrasts are not orthogonal, adjustments are made to the comparisons.[10]

Complex Contrasts

The contrasts we have described so far in this chapter are considered *simple contrasts* because they involve the comparison of pairs of means. We can also specify contrasts in terms of differences between subsets of means. For example, in the study of treatment for elbow tendinitis, suppose we want to compare the group that receives ice with both groups that receive passive treatments of splint and rest. This is a *complex contrast* because it involves more than two means. The multiple comparison test will respond to the question, "Is the mean of Group 1 significantly different from the average mean for Groups 3 and 4?"

The null hypothesis for this comparison would be

$$H_0: \mu_1 = \frac{\mu_3 + \mu_4}{2}$$

This hypothesis indicates that the mean for ice (μ_1) will be equal to the average mean of splint and rest groups (μ_3 and μ_4). The mean for the NSAID group (μ_2) would not be included in the comparison.

Contrast Coefficients

To program complex comparisons, we must indicate which groups we want to compare using a set of weights called *contrast coefficients*. These coefficients define the two sides of the equation. One side of the equation is given positive weights and the other side negative weights, so that the total will be zero. It does not matter which side is positive or negative, but the means must be included in the order they are included in the data file. For example, in the elbow tendinitis study, with four means, we would use (2, 0, –1, –1).

Group 2 is given the coefficient 0 because it is not included in this comparison. Group 1 is given the weight of 2 so it will balance against the two means for groups 3 and 4—remembering that the total must be zero.

As the number of means in a study increases, the number of potential complex contrasts also increases. Complex contrasts are designed to answer specific questions in a research study that offer different theoretical explanations of the data. By looking at subsets of data, investigators can often clarify relationships that may not be evident with simple contrasts.

Trend Analysis

Multiple comparison tests are most often used in studies where the independent variable is qualitative or nominal and where the researcher's interest focuses on determining which categories are significantly different from the others. When an independent variable is quantitative, the treatment levels no longer represent categories but differing amounts of something, such as age, dosage, or time. When the levels of an independent variable are ordered along a continuum, the researcher is often interested in examining the shape of the response rather than differences between levels. This approach is called a **trend analysis**.

The purpose of a trend analysis is to find the most reasonable description of continuous data based on the number of turns or "ups and downs" seen across the levels of the independent variable. Because this approach is an integral part of the study design, it is considered a planned comparison.[5]

> ➤ **CASE IN POINT #4**
>
> Researchers have documented strength changes that occur with aging.[11,12] A study was designed to test maximum isometric strength of knee extension in women from the ages of 8 to 80. Data were obtained for 10 age groups, each with 10 subjects.

A hypothetical plot of such data is shown in Figure 26-2, and the ANOVA is shown in Table 26-9A. There is a significant difference among the age groups. A multiple comparison of means will not tell us about the directions of change across age, but a trend analysis will.

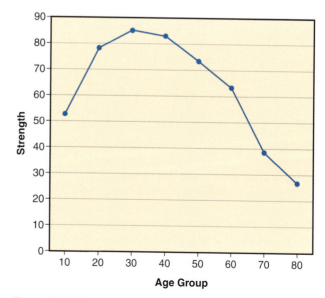

Figure 26-2 Plot of strength scores across 8 age groups.

Table 26-9   Example of an ANOVA with a Trend Analysis: Changes in Strength Across Eight Age Groups (N = 80)

A. SPSS Output: ANOVA

ANOVA

	Sum of Squares	df	Mean Square	F	➊ Sig.	Partial Eta Squared	Observed Power
Age	32426.550	7	4632.364	84.110	.000	.891	1.000
Error	3965.400	72	55.075				
Total	➍ 36391.950	79					

B. SPSS Output: Trend Analysis

ANOVA

			Sum of Squares	df	Mean Square	F	Sig.
Age			32426.550	7	4632.364	84.110	➊ .000
	Linear Term	Contrast	12355.438	1	12355.438	224.338	➋ .000
		Deviation	20071.112	6	3345.185	60.739	➌ .000
	Quadratic Term	Contrast	18229.260	1	18229.260	330.990	➋ .000
		Deviation	1841.852	5	368.370	3.389	.000
Error			3965.400	72	55.075		
Total			➍ 36391.950	79			

➊ The difference among age groups is significant ($p < .001$).

➋ The linear and quadratic trends are significant ($p < .001$).

➌ After the linear component is removed, there is still residual variance (Deviation) that is significant, indicating that there are other components that need to be accounted for.

➍ The total sample variance, reflected in the sum of squares for Age and the error term, are the same for the trend analysis as in the original ANOVA. The difference with the trend analysis is that the total variance in age is now partitioned into linear and quadratic components.

Shapes of Trends

Basically, trends are classified as either linear or nonlinear. In a *linear trend*, all data rise or fall at a constant rate as the value of the independent variable increases. This trend is characterized by a straight line, which can reflect positive or negative direction, as shown in Figure 26-3A. For example, researchers have documented a linear relationship between increases in HbA1c and peripheral neuropathies in patients with type 2 diabetes.[13]

A nonlinear trend demonstrates "bends" or changes in direction. This is most often characterized as a **quadratic trend**, shown in Figure 26-3B. Scores demonstrate a single turn upward or downward, creating a concave shape to the data. This means that following an initial increase or decrease in the dependent variable, scores vary in direction or rate of change. For instance, learning

curves are often characterized as quadratic, with strong improvement through early trials followed by deceleration or plateaus over time.[14,15]

Higher-order nonlinear trends are more complex and are often difficult to interpret. As shown in Figure 26-3C and D, a *cubic trend* involves a second change of direction and a *quartic trend* a third turn. As the number of levels of the independent variable increases, the number of potential trend components will also increase. There can be a maximum of $k-1$ turns, or trend components, within any data set.

The curves in Figure 26-3 are examples of pure trends. Real data seldom conform to these patterns exactly. Even with data that represent true trends, chance factors will produce dips and variations that may distort the observed relationship.

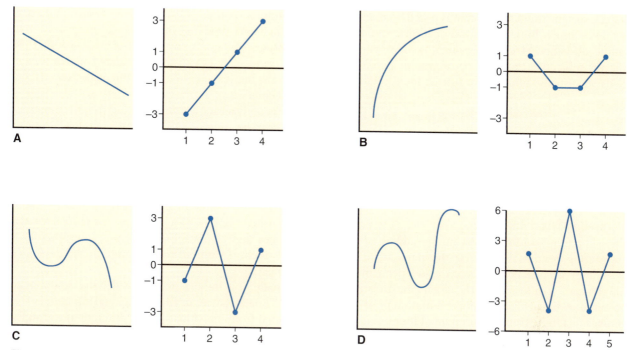

Figure 26-3 Examples of several types of trends: A) linear trend, B) quadratic trend, C) cubic trend, and D) quartic trend.

See Chapter 30 for further discussion of linear and quadratic trends associated with regression analysis.

Purpose of Trend Analysis

How one chooses to analyze data is directly related to how one frames the research question. When testing an ordered variable such as age or time, the research question would not be focused on whether one group or interval was different from another but rather would address how the dependent variable changes across the span.

> Trends can be run on an ordered variable with independent groups, as in the age/strength study, or it can also be run on a repeated measure, such as time.

The purpose of a trend analysis is to describe the overall tendency in the data using the least number of trend components possible. Some data can be characterized by a single trend, while others demonstrate more than one pattern within a single data set. The hypothetical data for strength and age illustrate this possibility. The portion of the data from 10 to 50 years shows a quadratic pattern, indicating that individuals tend to get stronger and then weaker as they grow within this age range. We can also see a linear component with a gradual but steady decline after age 40.

Significance of Trend Components

Trends are tested for significance as part of an analysis of variance. Table 26-9A shows the one-way ANOVA for the strength data, resulting in a significant difference across age groups ($p < .001$). However, this information does not help us clarify how the data vary across the age groups.

The ANOVA can be run to include a trend analysis, as shown in Table 26-9B. The variance, indicated by the sum of squares, for the variable of age is now broken into linear and quadratic trend components. Each of these components is tested for significance.

> **Results**
>
> An analysis of variance was used to assess the pattern of change in strength across age groups. This test resulted in a significant difference across age groups ($F(7,72) = 84.11$, $p < .001$). A trend analysis demonstrated significant linear and quadratic trends across the age groups ($p < .001$).

Because there are eight measurement intervals, we have the potential for seven trend components. However, testing beyond the quadratic component usually yields uninterpretable results. Therefore, variance attributable to all higher-order trends is included in the error term (called Deviation here). The researcher can define the number of trends to include in a test, which can be informed by looking at a plot of the data.

Each specific trend component is tested by an F ratio. In this example, both linear and quadratic trends are significant. When a trend component is statistically significant, subjective examination of graphic patterns of the data is usually sufficient for further interpretation.

📌 Just to make life interesting, some computer packages will refer to trend analyses as *orthogonal decomposition* or *orthogonal polynomial contrasts*. These terms derive from the types of equations that are used to characterize the trends, which you might remember from advanced algebra.

Interpreting Trend Analysis

Three important considerations must be addressed when interpreting trend analyses. First, the number and spacing of intervals between levels of the independent variable can make a difference to the visual interpretation of the curve. A linear trend requires a minimum of three points, a quadratic trend a minimum of four points, and so on. With larger spans in the quantitative variable, more intervals may be necessary.

Most investigators try to use equally spaced intervals to achieve consistency in the interpretation. Others will purposefully create unequal intervals to best represent the samples of interest. For instance, trends that are established over time may involve some intervals of hours and others of days. Most computer packages that perform trend analyses will accommodate equal or unequal intervals, but distances between unequal intervals must be specified.

A second caution for interpreting trend analysis is to avoid extrapolating beyond the upper and lower limits of the selected intervals. For example, based on Figure 26-3, if we had tested only individuals between 40 and 80, we would conclude that strength declines linearly with age, but we could not draw any conclusions about changes from ages 10 to 30. By limiting the range of intervals, we would have missed the quadratic function that more accurately describes the relationship. Therefore, interpretation of trends must be limited to the range of the dependent variable.

Finally, it is important to consider the design of the study. For instance, in the current example, data were collected from individuals in the different age groups at the same time. This is a *cross-sectional* design. This can be contrasted with a *longitudinal* study, in which we would have followed individuals across the lifespan to see if their strength actually did decrease over time (see Chapter 19).

COMMENTARY

Statistics: the only science that enables different experts using the same figures to draw different conclusions.

—*Evan Esar (1899 - 1995)*

American humorist

There are no widely accepted criteria for choosing one multiple comparison test over another, and the selection of a particular procedure is often made arbitrarily. Two basic issues should guide the choice of a multiple comparison procedure.

The first issue relates to the decision to conduct either planned or unplanned contrasts. This decision, made during planning phases of a study, will relate to theoretical expectations. With planned comparisons, the researcher asks, "Is *this* difference significant?" With *post hoc* tests the question shifts to, "*Which* differences are significant?" When the researcher is interested in exploring all possible combinations of variables, unplanned contrasts should be used.

The second issue concerns the importance of Type I or Type II error. Each multiple comparison test will control for these errors differently, depending on the use of per comparison or familywise error rates. Of the three *post hoc* comparisons described here, the Newman–Keuls test is the most powerful. Scheffé's comparison gives the greatest control over Type I error, but at the expense of power. Researchers often prefer Tukey's HSD because it offers a balanced option, both reasonable power and protection against Type I error. The power of the Newman–Keuls procedure is increased by using different comparison intervals but use of the per comparison error rate increases the risk of Type I error.

Other than these rather straightforward criteria, when there is no overriding concern for either Type I or Type II error, there may be no obvious choice for a specific test. This is probably why the Tukey procedure is so popular as a "middle of the road" test. A researcher is obliged to consider the rationale for comparing treatment conditions or groups and to justify the basis for making these comparisons. This rationale should be provided in an article for the reader but is rarely included.

Regardless of how the choice is made, consumers of research should make judgments about findings based on whether they think the author took too liberal or too conservative an approach. As we apply evidence to clinical decisions, this prerogative should be stressed, perhaps leading to only tentative use of findings. This emphasizes the importance of understanding the statistical procedures, so that an author's conclusions may be questioned based on their choice of analysis.

As the examples in this chapter illustrate, different outcomes can be achieved with different multiple comparison procedures with the same data—leading to different conclusions and perhaps different clinical decisions! This makes the choice of a test during planning stages of a study that much more meaningful. The choice should not be made after the results are available—and perhaps most importantly, should not be based on trying all of the possible alternatives to see what the results are! Pick your poison and interpret your data fairly!

REFERENCES

1. Tukey JW. *The Problem of Multiple Comparisons*. Ditto: Princeton University; 1953.
2. Scheffé HA. A method for judging all contrasts in the analysis of variance. *Biometrika* 1953;40:87.
3. Scheffé HA. *The Analysis of Variance*. New York: Wiley, 1959.
4. Dallal GE. Multiple comparison procedures. *The Little Handbook of Statistical Practice*. Available at http://www.jerrydallal.com/LHSP/mc.htm. Accessed November 1, 2018.
5. Keppel G. *Design and Analysis: A Researcher's Handbook*. 4th ed. Englewood Cliffs, N.J.: Prentice Hall; 2004.
6. Green SB, Salkind NJ. *Using SPSS for Windows and Macintosh: Analyzing and Understanding Data*. 8 ed. New York: Pearson; 2017.
7. Maxwell SE. Pairwise multiple comparisons in repeated measures designs. *J Educ Stat* 1980;5:269-287.
8. Hinkle DE, Wiersma W, Jurs SG. *Applied Statistics for the Behavioral Sciences*. 5th ed. Boston: Houghton Mifflin; 2003.
9. Hays WL. *Statistics*. 5th ed. Belmont, CA: Wadsworth; 1994.
10. Field A. *Discovering Statistics Using IBM SPSS Statistics*. 5th ed. Thousand Oaks, CA: Sage; 2018.
11. Keller K, Engelhardt M. Strength and muscle mass loss with aging process. Age and strength loss. *Muscles Ligaments Tendons J* 2014;3(4):346-350.
12. Borges O. Isometric and isokinetic knee extension and flexion torque in men and women aged 20-70. *Scand J Rehabil Med* 1989;21(1):45-53.
13. Yang CP, Lin CC, Li CI, Liu CS, Lin WY, Hwang KL, Yang SY, Chen HJ, Li TC. Cardiovascular risk factors increase the risks of diabetic peripheral neuropathy in patients with type 2 diabetes mellitus: The Taiwan Diabetes Study. *Medicine (Baltimore)* 2015;94(42):e1783.
14. Hayes H, Geers AE, Treiman R, Moog JS. Receptive vocabulary development in deaf children with cochlear implants: achievement in an intensive auditory-oral educational setting. *Ear Hear* 2009;30(1):128-135.
15. Mayer-Kress G, Newell KM, Liu YT. Nonlinear dynamics of motor learning. *Nonlinear Dynamics Psychol Life Sci* 2009; 13(1):3-26.

CHAPTER 27

Nonparametric Tests for Group Comparisons

In previous chapters several statistical tests have been presented that are based on certain assumptions about the parameters of the population from which the samples were drawn. These parametric tests are appropriate for use with ratio/interval data. In this chapter, we present a set of statistical procedures classified as **nonparametric**, which test hypotheses for group comparisons without normality or variance assumptions and are appropriate for analysis of nominal or ordinal data. For this reason, these methods are sometimes referred to as *distribution-free tests*. The data for these tests are reduced to ranks, and comparisons are based on distributions, not means.

The purpose of this chapter is to describe five commonly used nonparametric comparison procedures: the Mann-Whitney U test, the Kruskal-Wallis ANOVA, the sign test, the Wilcoxon signed-ranks test, and the Friedman ANOVA. Nonparametric tests for measures of association will be presented in Chapters 28 and 29.

■ Criteria for Choosing Nonparametric Tests

Nonparametric comparison tests are applied to designs that are analogous to their parametric counterparts using t and F tests (see Table 27-1). Two major criteria are generally adopted for choosing a nonparametric test over a parametric procedure. The first criterion is that data are measured on the nominal or ordinal scales. This makes nonparametric tests useful for analysis of data from many assessment tools that are based on ordinal ranks.

The second criterion is that assumptions of population normality and homogeneity of variance cannot be satisfied. Many clinical investigations involve variables

Table 27-1 Corresponding Parametric and Nonparametric Tests for Comparisons		
COMPARISON OF:	**PARAMETRIC TEST**	**NONPARAMETRIC TEST**
Two Independent Groups	Independent t-test	Mann-Whitney U test Wilcoxon Rank Sum Test
≥3 Independent Groups	One-way ANOVA (F)	Kruskal-Wallis ANOVA by ranks (H or χ^2)
Two Related Samples	Paired t-test	Sign test (x) Wilcoxon signed-ranks test (T)
≥3 Related Samples	One-way repeated measures ANOVA (F)	Friedman two-way ANOVA by ranks ((χ^2_r)

that are represented by skewed distributions rather than symmetrical ones. In addition, small clinical samples and samples of convenience cannot automatically be considered representative of larger normal distributions (see Focus on Evidence 27-1). The Kolmogorov-Smirnov and Shapiro-Wilk tests can be used to determine if data follow a normal distribution (see Chapter 23, Box 23-4).

In parametric tests like the *t*-test and analysis of variance, statistical hypotheses are based on a comparison of means. The expectation is that sample means will

Focus on Evidence 27–1
The Relevance of Being "Normal"

Measurement of pain has taken many forms, made difficult by the subjective nature of sensation.[1] As a way of incorporating objective quantitative data, the cold pressor test (CPT) has become a widely used assessment, performed by immersing the hand into an ice water container, usually for 1 minute, and measuring changes in blood pressure and heart rate as well as pain parameters. Outcomes include time to onset of pain, pain intensity, and tolerance.[2] Because this test results in continuous data, researchers have typically taken advantage of parametric statistical procedures to evaluate treatment effects.

In a review of 122 studies using the CPT as an outcome, Treister et al[3] found that although the vast majority of studies used parametric statistics, only 39% mentioned testing for normality, and among them, only 18% found cold-pain tolerance to be normally distributed. Forty-four percent transformed their data to try to improve normality (see Appendix C), but in most cases, it did not change the distribution sufficiently. In another set of studies, the authors found that 96% of CPT outcomes were non-normal, as illustrated in the figure.

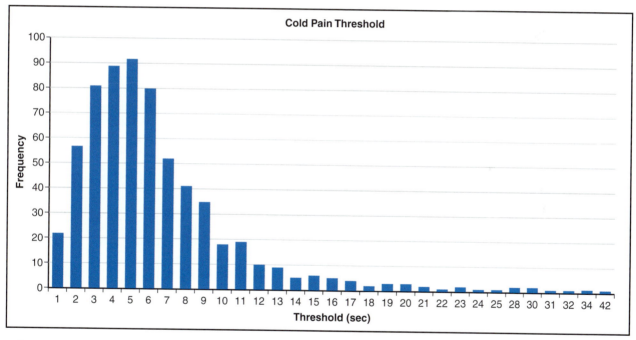

This situation suggests a strong need for researchers to consider normality in deciding which statistics to use. In comparing outcomes using *t*-tests versus the nonparametric Wilcoxon test, the nonparametric test is almost always more statistically powerful with non-normal data, meaning that applying *t*-tests to non-normal data sets might compromise study outcomes and lead to false negative conclusions, especially with smaller samples.[3] The Kolmorgorov-Smirnoff and Shapiro-Wilks tests for goodness of fit to a normal distribution were described in Chapter 23, Box 23-4.

Nonparametric tests are generally appropriate for use with ordinal data but may also be needed with continuous data with small samples or samples with non-normal distributions. Grant reviewers have become more aware of the need to consider appropriate analyses based on data characteristics. The importance of validating a normal distribution is often overlooked, or at least ignored, as part of a research report—but may be biasing important outcomes.

From Treister R, Nielsen CS, Stubhaug A, et al. Experimental comparison of parametric versus nonparametric analyses of data from the cold pressor test. *J Pain* 2015;16(6):537-48, From Figure 1A p. 542, Used with permission.

estimate population means because of assumptions of homogeneity and normality. In nonparametric tests, we are unable to make the same type of comparison because of the ranked nature of scores. The median score is often more meaningful but still may not reflect the full distribution. Therefore, the null and alternative hypotheses are stated more generally, based on a comparison of the distributions of scores. This will be illustrated for each of the examples that follow.

> Although nonparametric tests require fewer statistical assumptions than parametric procedures, this does not preclude the need for strong experimental design to avoid bias in the data. For example, whenever possible, random sample selection and random assignment to groups should be incorporated, and control groups and blinding should also be included.

The major disadvantage of nonparametric tests is that they generally cannot be adapted to complex clinical designs, such as factorial designs and tests of interactions. There are many newer tests, however, that have been developed to allow the application of regression procedures or tests of interaction effects. These are beyond the scope of this book but can be found in many recent texts.[4-6]

Power-Efficiency for Nonparametric Tests

Many researchers prefer to use parametric tests because they are considered more powerful. Nonparametric tests are less sensitive than parametric tests because most of them involve ranking scores rather than comparing precise metric changes. Nonparametric and parametric methods have been compared on the basis of their *power-efficiency*, which is a test's relative ability to identify significant differences for a given sample size.

Generally, an increase in sample size is needed to make a nonparametric test as powerful as an analogous parametric test. For instance, a nonparametric test may require a sample size of 50 to achieve the same degree of power as a parametric test with 30 subjects. This relationship can be expressed as a percentage that indicates the relative power-efficiency of the nonparametric test. With equal sample sizes, nonparametric tests will generally be less powerful than their parametric counterparts. However, with larger samples this discrepancy is minimized. Most of the nonparametric tests described here can achieve approximately 95% power-efficiency in comparison to their most powerful parametric analogs.[7-9] These figures apply to calculations based on comparisons of normal populations.

Estimating Sample Size

Researchers generally choose to use nonparametric tests when they are unable to make assumptions about the shape of or variance in underlying distributions. Unfortunately, however, without making explicit assumptions about a distribution, it is not possible to estimate sample size or power as we do with parametric tests.[10]

With very small samples, as with six subjects or less per group, many nonparametric tests will be as powerful as their parametric counterparts. With larger non-normal populations, the nonparametric statistics may actually be more powerful.[11] Lehman[10] suggests a rule of thumb: compute the sample that would be needed if you were doing a parametric test and add 15%. Of course, this requires an estimate of effect size, which will be described for different tests. Although most computer programs will not calculate effect sizes for nonparametric tests, they can be calculated quite easily by using information from the test result.

> Nonparametric statistics are generally easy to calculate by hand, and some calculations will be illustrated here to clarify the rationale behind the tests. Most statistical packages will provide analyses for nonparametric tests, however, and this chapter will focus on interpretation of those results.

> G*Power can be used to estimate sample size and power for the Mann-Whitney *U* test and the Wilcoxon signed-ranks test when data are continuous (not ranks). The process is the same as for the *t*-test (see the *Chapter 27 Supplement*).

■ Procedure for Ranking Scores

Most nonparametric tests are based on rank ordering of scores. The procedure for ranking will be illustrated using the two samples shown in Table 27-2. Scores are always ranked from smallest to largest, with the rank of 1 assigned to the smallest score. Algebraic values are taken into account, so that the lowest ranks are assigned to the largest negative values, if any. The highest rank

Table 27-2   Examples of Ranked Scores Without Ties (A) and with Ties (B) (*n*=8)

SAMPLE A		SAMPLE B	
Score	Rank	Score	Rank
6	4	8	3
2	3	11	5
8	5	3	1.5
9	6	17	8
−3	1	11	5
0	2	3	1.5
16	8	11	5
12	7	12	7

will equal *n*. As shown in Sample A, the rank of 1 is assigned to the smallest score (–3), the rank of 2 goes to the next smallest (0), and so on, until the rank of 8 is assigned to the highest score (16).

When two or more scores in a distribution are tied, they are each given the same rank, which is the average of the ranks they occupy. For instance, in Sample B, there are two scores with the smallest value (3). They occupy ranks 1 and 2. Therefore, they are each assigned the average of their ranks: $(1 + 2)/2 = 1.5$. The next highest value (8) receives the rank of 3, as the first two ranks are filled. The next highest value is 11, which appears three times. As we have already filled ranks 1, 2, and 3, we average the next three ranks: $(4 + 5 + 6)/3 = 5$. Each score of 11 is assigned the rank of 5. Having filled the first 6 rank positions, the last two values in the distribution are assigned ranks 7 and 8.

■ Tests for Independent Samples

Nonparametric procedures can be applied to studies using independent samples, with two or more groups. These groups may be randomly assigned, or they may represent intact groups.

The Mann-Whitney *U* Test

The **Mann–Whitney *U* test** is one of the more powerful nonparametric procedures, designed to test the null hypothesis that two independent samples come from the same population. The *U* test does not require that groups be of the same size. It is, therefore, an excellent alternative to the independent *t*-test when parametric assumptions are not met.

> ➤ **CASE IN POINT #1**
>
> A researcher is interested in the effect of vaginal versus cesarean section births on Apgar score, graded from 0-10, with higher scores indicating a healthier infant.[12] Scores are obtained at 5 minutes from newborns of 11 women. The researcher hypothesizes that the Apgar score will be different for the two types of delivery (a nondirectional hypothesis). A nonparametric test is chosen for analysis because the data are ordinal and the sample is small.

Procedure

Hypothetical data for this example are given in Table 27-3A. The first step is to combine scores from both groups and rank all 11 scores in order of increasing size. The ranks are then examined within each group, and the sum of the ranks is designated R_1 or R_2. The null hypothesis states that there will be no difference between the distributions of scores for vaginal or cesarean delivery. Under the null hypothesis, then,

we would expect the groups to be equally distributed with regard to high and low ranks, and the mean of the ranks would be the same for both groups. The test will determine if the difference between the rank sums is sufficiently large to be considered significant.

The sum of ranks for vaginal delivery is higher than for caesarean, but there are also more patients in the vaginal group. This difference in sample size is taken into account in the calculation of the test statistic.

The *U* Test Statistic

The test statistic, *U*, is calculated using each group as a reference, as shown in Table 27-3B, where n_1 is the smaller sample size, n_2 is the larger sample size, and R_1 and R_2 are the sums of the ranks for the groups. Designation of n_1 or n_2 is arbitrary if groups are of equal size.

These formulas will yield different values of *U*. For example, we obtain $U_1 = 8.5$ with Group 1 as the reference group and $U_2 = 21.5$ using Group 2 as the reference group. Either of these values will produce the same outcome. However, the smaller value of *U* is used with a table of critical values, so in this case we will use $U = 8.5$.

Test of Significance

Critical values of *U* are given in Table 27-4 for one- and two-tailed tests at $\alpha = .05$ based on n_1 and n_2. The calculated value of *U* must be *equal to or less than* the tabled value to be significant. Note that this is opposite to the way we analyzed critical values with parametric tests.

For the current example, we proposed a nondirectional alternative hypothesis. Using $\alpha_2 = .05$, with $n_1 = 5$, and $n_2 = 6$, the critical value of *U* is 3. Because the calculated value, $U = 8.5$, is larger than this critical value, we cannot reject H_0. Output for this analysis is shown in Table 27-3C.

Nonparametric tests may be subject to bias if there are many ties in the ranks. The analysis automatically generates an adjusted version. The *p* value can be affected if the number of ties is excessive.

Large Samples

With large samples (> 25), the value of *U* approaches a normal distribution and *U* is converted to *z*. Although the present example does not warrant it, we have used the data to illustrate this application in Table 27-3C. The calculated value of *z* must be *equal to or larger than the critical value* at the appropriate level of significance. Because we proposed a nondirectional hypothesis with $\alpha_2 = .05$, the critical value is 1.96.

Our calculated value is smaller than this critical value, and the null hypothesis is not rejected. We can also determine the exact *p* value associated with $z = 1.2$ using Appendix Table A-1. This score corresponds to .1151 in each tail, which corresponds to a two-tailed test at $p = .230$ (see Table 27-3 ❺).

Table 27-3   Mann–Whitney U Test: Difference in Apgar Score with Cesarean and Vaginal Delivery ($N = 11$)

A. Data

Cesarean Delivery ($n_1 = 5$)		Vaginal Delivery ($n_2 = 6$)	
Apgar	**Rank**	Apgar	**Rank**
7	**6**	6	**4**
4	**2**	5	**3**
3	**1**	9	**10**
8	**8.5**	10	**11**
7	**6**	8	**8.5**
		7	**6**

Ranks

	Delivery	N	Mean Rank	Sum of Ranks
Apgar	Cesarean	5	4.70	23.50
	Vaginal	6	7.08	42.50
	Total	11		

B. Calculations

$$U_1 = R_1 - \frac{n_1(n_1 + 1)}{2} = 23.5 - \frac{5(5 + 1)}{2} = 8.5$$

②

$$U_2 = R_2 - \frac{n_2(n_2 + 1)}{2} = 42.5 - \frac{6(6 + 1)}{2} = 21.5$$

C. Test for Large Samples

④
$$Z = \frac{U - \frac{n_1 n_2}{2}}{\sqrt{\frac{n_1 n_2 (n_1 + n_2 + 1)}{12}}} = \frac{8.5 - \frac{(5)(6)}{2}}{\sqrt{\frac{(5)(6)(5 + 6 + 1)}{12}}} = \frac{-6.5}{\sqrt{30}} = -1.19$$

D. SPSS Output: Mann-Whitney U Test

Test Statistics^a

		Apgar
Mann-Whitney U	**③**	8.500
Wilcoxon W	**③**	23.500
Z	**④**	−1.200
Asump. Sig. (2-tailed)	**⑤**	.230
Exact Sig. [2*(1-tailed Sig.)]	**⑤**	.247^b

a. Grouping Variable: Delivery
b. Not corrected for ties.

Portions of the output have been omitted for clarity.

① The rank sums and mean ranks are reported.

② Either value of U can be used with the same result in calculating the test statistic. For comparison to critical values, $U = 8.5$, the smaller of the values of U_1 or U_2.

③ Some statisticians prefer to use the *Wilcoxon Rank Sum Test* (W) to test the difference between two independent samples. This test is statistically equivalent to the Mann-Whitney U-test and will yield the same result. Both values are reported.

④ The negative sign can be ignored as it is a function of which value of U was used, not the direction of the difference. The result of the test will be the same using either value of U.

⑤ The test is not significant. Two p values are reported. The first value ($p = .230$) is corrected for ties, and will provide a more conservative test. The second value is the probability associated with z.

📌 Recall that for $\alpha_1 = .05$, the critical value of z is 1.645. For $\alpha_2 = .05$, the critical value is 1.96. At $\alpha_1 = .01$, the critical value of z is 2.326, and for $\alpha_2 = .01$ it is 2.576.

Effect Size for the Mann-Whitney U Test

The effect size for comparison of two groups is based on a correlation coefficient, r, that represents the strength of the association between the sample scores and group assignment (see Chapter 29).[13] For the Mann-Whitney U test, the correlation coefficient is based on the z score reported in the results:

$$r = \frac{z}{\sqrt{N}}$$

where N is the total number of observations on which the z score is based.[14] Cohen[15] suggests conventional effect sizes for r: small = .10, medium = .30, large = .50.

Table 27-4 Abridged Table of Critical Values for the *U* Statistic ($\alpha = .05$)

n_1		n_2 (larger sample)						
		4	**5**	**6**	**7**	**8**	**9**	**10**
4	α_1	1	2	3	4	5	6	7
	α_2	0	1	2	3	4	4	5
5	α_1	—	4	5	6	8	9	11
	α_2	—	2	3	5	6	7	8
6	α_1	—	—	7	8	10	12	11
	α_2	—	—	5	6	8	10	14
7	α_1	—	—	—	11	13	15	17
	α_2	—	—	—	8	10	12	14
8	α_1	—	—	—	—	15	18	20
	α_2	—	—	—	—	13	15	174

This table is an abridged version for purposes of illustration. See the Chapter 27 Supplement for the full table.

With $z = 1.20$ (see Table 27-3 ④),

$$r = \frac{1.19}{\sqrt{11}} = .36$$

which would be considered a medium effect. We can interpret this relative to the clinical significance of our findings. There was a difference between the mean ranks, but we can also see that there were both high and low scores in both groups (see Table 27-3A). Therefore, we may conclude that this is not an issue of power, as the effect is not substantial.

> **Results**
> The Mann-Whitney *U* test was used to compare Apgar scores for infants born through Cesarean ($n = 5$) or vaginal delivery ($n = 6$). This test was chosen because the sample was small and Apgar scores are considered ordinal measures. The test was not significant ($U = 8.5$, $p = .247$), and we conclude that there is no difference in Apgar scores for infants born by cesarean or vaginal delivery.

The Kruskal-Wallis Analysis of Variance

When three or more independent groups are compared ($k \geq 3$), a nonparametric analysis of variance is appropriate for the same reasons that an *F* test is used with parametric data. The **Kruskal–Wallis one-way analysis of variance by ranks** is a nonparametric analog of the one-way analysis of variance. It is a powerful alternative to the ANOVA when variance and normality assumptions for parametric tests are not met. When $k = 2$, this test is equivalent to the Mann–Whitney *U*-test. Multiple comparison procedures can also be applied.

> ➤ **CASE IN POINT #2**
> Researchers have been interested in the use of nonpharmacologic interventions to reduce chronic pain.[16] Consider a hypothetical study to assess the effect of three treatment strategies. We will randomly assign 17 subjects ($N = 17$) to receive yoga ($n = 6$), acupuncture ($n = 6$), or transcutaneous electrical nerve stimulation (TENS) ($n = 5$). Pain is measured on a VAS from 0 mm (pain-free) to 100 mm (worst pain imaginable). Scores are recorded as the change in level of pain (mm) from pretreatment to posttreatment levels over 1 month. We hypothesize that there will be a difference among the three strategies.

Procedure

Hypothetical data are reported in Table 27-5A. The procedure for the Kruskal–Wallis ANOVA is essentially an expansion of method used for the Mann–Whitney *U*-test. The first step is to combine data for all groups and rank scores from the smallest to the largest. The ranks are then summed for each group separately, as shown in Table 27-5A.

The null hypothesis states that the distributions from the three groups come from the same population. Our alternative hypothesis states that these distributions come from different populations. If the null hypothesis is true, we would expect an equal distribution of ranks under the three conditions.

The *H* Statistic

The test statistic for the Kruskal–Wallis test is *H*, calculated according to

$$H = \frac{12}{N(N+1)} \sum \frac{R^2}{n} - 3(N+1)$$

Table 27-5   Kruskal–Wallis One-Way Analysis of Variance By Ranks: Change in Pain (VAS in mm)
(N=14)

A. Data

Group 1 Yoga		Group 2 Acupuncture		Group 3 TENS	
Change Score	Rank	Change Score	Rank	Change Score	Rank
40	8	35	6	80	4
60	11	25	2.5	50	10
10	1	30	4.5	75	13
25	2.5	40	8	70	12
30	4.5	40	8		
❶ ΣR	27		29		49

Ranks ❶

	group	N	Mean Rank
Pain	Yoga	5	5.40
	Acupuncture	5	5.80
	TENS	4	12.25
	Total	14	

B. Calculations

$$H = \frac{12}{N(N+1)} \sum \frac{R^2}{n} - 3(N+1)$$

$$H = \frac{12}{14(14+1)} \left[\frac{(27)^2}{5} + \frac{(29)^2}{5} + \frac{(49)^2}{4} \right] - 3(14+1) = \frac{12}{210}[914.25] - 45 = 7.243 \quad ❷$$

C. SPSS Output: Kruskal-Wallis Test

❷ Test Statistics[a,b]

	Pain
Kruskal-Wallis H	7.340
df	2
Asymp. Sig.	.025

a. Kruskal Wallis Test
b. Grouping Variable: Group

❸ Homogeneous Subsets Based on Pain

		Subset	
		1	2
Sample[1]	Yoga	5.400	
	Acupuncture	5.800	
	TENS		12.250
Test Statistic		.102	
Sig. (2-sided test)		.750	
Adjusted Sig. (2-sided test)		.750	

Homogeneous subsets are based on asymptotic significances. The significance level is .05.

[1] Each cell shows the sample average rank of pain.

❶ The rank sums and mean ranks show a distinct spread between TENS and the other two interventions.

❷ The test statistic *H* is tested against χ^2 with 2 *df*. The overall test is significant (*p* = .025).

❸ The homogeneous subsets show a significant difference between TENS and both Yoga and Acupuncture.

Calculated values vary due to rounding differences. Portions of the output have been omitted for clarity.

where N is the number of cases in all samples combined, n is the number of cases in each individual sample, and R is the sum of ranks for each individual sample. This calculation is illustrated in Table 27-5B. For this example, $H = 7.243$.

Test of Significance

The H statistic is tested using the chi-square distribution with $k - 1$ degrees of freedom (see Chapter 28). With three groups we will have 2 *df*. Therefore, we test H against the critical value of $\chi^2(2) = 5.99$ (Appendix Table A-5). The calculated value must be *equal to or greater than* the critical value to be significant. Our calculated value of 7.243 is greater than the critical value, and therefore, H is significant, and we can reject H_0. The output for this analysis is shown in Table 27-5C, confirming this conclusion ($p = .025$).

Multiple Comparisons

Like the parametric ANOVA, this result does not indicate which groups are different. Some researchers will stop here, basing their interpretation of data on a subjective comparison of the mean ranks for each group. For example, we observe that ranks for the TENS group are higher than the other two groups (see Table 27-5 ❶). However, this subjective judgment can be misleading, and a multiple comparison procedure should be used to determine which groups are significantly different.

Dunn's multiple comparison is a nonparametric procedure used to perform pairwise comparisons for the Kruskal-Wallis test.[17] The Mann–Whitney U test can also be used as a multiple comparison procedure, but a Bonferroni correction should be applied to control for the increased risk of Type I error.

The results of this test are shown using homogeneous subsets based on mean ranks (see Table 27-5C ❸). Here we see that TENS is significantly better than both yoga and acupuncture, not unexpected given the difference among the ranks.

Effect Size for the Kruskal-Wallis ANOVA

The overall effect size index for the Kruskal-Wallis test is eta squared, η^2, based on the H statistic.[14] For the study of pain interventions:

$$\eta^2 = \frac{H - k + 1}{N - k} = \frac{7.340 - 3 + 1}{14 - 3} = .668$$

where k is the number of groups and N is the total sample. According to conventional effect sizes for η^2, this would be considered a large effect (see Chapter 25).

> **Results**

The Kruskal-Wallis test resulted in a significant difference in change in pain among the three interventions ($\chi^2(2) = 7.34$, $p = .025$, $\eta^2 = .67$). Dunn's test showed no significant difference between yoga and acupuncture groups. Improvement in pain was significantly better for the TENS groups compared to the other two interventions.

> See the *Chapter 27 Supplement* for further illustration of follow up tests for the Kruskal-Wallis test, including multiple comparison procedures.

■ Tests for Related Samples

Nonparametric procedures can be used with paired samples within a two-level repeated measures design, using either the sign test or the Wilcoxon signed-ranks test. These are analogous to the paired *t*-test. The Friedman Two-Way Analysis of Variance by Ranks can be used with three or more levels of the independent variable.

The Sign Test

The **sign test** is one of the simplest nonparametric tests because it requires no mathematical calculations. It is based on the binomial distribution and does not require that measurements be quantitative. As its name implies, the data are analyzed using plus and minus signs rather than numerical values. Therefore, this test provides a mechanism for testing relative differentiations such as more–less, higher–lower, or larger–smaller. It is particularly useful when quantification is impossible or unfeasible and when subjective ratings are necessary.

> ### CASE IN POINT #3

Researchers have been interested in the effect of psychostimulants on attention deficits in patients with traumatic brain injury (TBI).[18] A crossover study was designed to test the efficacy of a new drug versus a placebo. An attention task was administered to 10 patients under each test condition, in randomized order. A washout period was inserted between test conditions. The outcome was the number of correct responses out of 12 trials on an attention task. We hypothesize that there will be a difference in the attention task score between those who take the drug and those who take the placebo.

Procedure

Hypothetical data for this study are shown in Table 27-6A. The sign test is applied to the differences between each pair of scores, based on whether the direction of

Table 27-6   **Sign Test and Wilcoxon Signed-Ranks Test: Effect of Drug and Placebo on an Attention Deficit Task (*N* = 10)**

A. Data

Subject	Drug Condition Drug	Drug Condition Placebo	Sign	d	Rank of d
1	8	8	0	0	
2	10	11	−	−1	−1
3	7	7	0	0	
4	9	7	+	+2	+3
5	10	8	+	+2	+3
6	11	7	+	+4	+7
7	10	8	+	+2	+3
8	10	7	+	+3	+5.5
9	8	8	0	0	
10	10	7	+	+3	+5.5

❶ *x* = 1
Number of fewer signs

T = 1 ❶
Number of ranks with less frequent sign

B. SPSS Output: Sign Test

Frequencies

			N
Placebo − Drug	Negative Differences[a]		6
	Positive Differences[b]	❶	1
	Ties[c]		3
	Total		10

a. Placebo < Drug, b. Placebo > Drug, c. Placebo = Drug

Test Statistics[a]

	Placebo − Drug
Exact Sig. (2-tailed)	❷ .125[b]

a. Sign Test
b. Binomial distribution used.

C. SPSS Output: Wilcoxon Signed-Ranks Test

Ranks

		N	Mean Rank	Sum of Ranks
Placebo − Drug	Negative Ranks	6[a]	4.50	27.00
	Positive Ranks	1[b]	1.00	1.00
	Ties	3[c]		
	Total	10		

a. Placebo < Drug, b. Placebo > Drug, c. Placebo = Drug

Test Statistics[a]

	Placebo − Drug
Z	−2.217[b]
Asymp. Sig. (2-tailed)	❸ .027

a. Wilcoxon Signed Ranks Test
b. Based on positive ranks.

D. Calculation of *z*

• **Sign test** ❹

$$z = \frac{|D| - 1}{\sqrt{n}} = \frac{|5| - 1}{\sqrt{7}} = 1.51$$

• **Wilcoxon signed-ranks test** ❺

$$Z = \frac{T - \frac{n(n+1)}{4}}{\sqrt{\frac{n(n+1)(2n+1)}{24}}} = \frac{1 - \frac{7(7+1)}{4}}{\sqrt{\frac{7(7+1)(14+1)}{24}}} = -2.197$$

❶ The number of fewer signs (in this case negative signs) is 1. For the binomial sign test, *x* = 1. For the Wilcoxon test, *T* = 1.

❷ The two-tailed sign test is not significant (*p* = .125).

❸ The two-tailed Wilcoxon signed-ranks test is significant (*p* = .027).

❹ The standardized *z* score for the sign test is less than the critical value 1.96 (*p* = .05) and is not significant.

❺ The standardized *z* score for the Wilcoxon test is greater than the critical value 1.96 and is significant. The sign can be ignored with a two-tailed test.

Calculated values vary due to rounding differences. Portions of the output have been omitted for clarity.

difference is positive or negative. In this example, we will use the scores for the drug condition as the reference and record whether that score is greater (+), the same (0), or less (−) than the placebo score, always maintaining the same direction of comparison. This order is only relevant if we propose a directional hypothesis.

Under the null hypothesis, the distributions of scores under each condition are not different, and chance will be the determinant of which score is greater in each pair. Therefore, we would expect half the differences to be positive and half to be negative ($p = .50$). We will reject H_0 if one sign occurs sufficiently less often.

The alternative hypothesis states that the probability of one condition is greater than 50%. With a nondirectional hypothesis, it does not matter which value is used as the reference, as in our example. In the fourth column in Table 27-6A, the signs of the differences are listed. When no difference is obtained, a zero is recorded.

Test Statistic *x*

To proceed with the test, we count the number of plus signs and the number of minus signs. Ties, recorded as zeros, are discarded from the analysis, and *n* is reduced accordingly. In this example, 3 subjects showed no difference. Therefore, $n = 7$. There are six plus signs and one minus sign. We take the smaller of these two values, the *number of fewer signs*, and assign it the test statistic, *x*. In this case, $x = 1$, the number of minus signs.

Test of Significance

To determine the probability of obtaining *x* under H_0, we refer to Table 27-7. This table lists one-tailed probabilities associated with *x* for values up to $n = 20$, where *n* is the number of pairs whose differences showed direction. *Two-tailed tests require doubling the probabilities given in the table.*

| Table 27-7 | Abridged Table of One-Tailed Probabilities Associated with *x* in the Binomial Test | | | | | |

				x		
n	0	1	2	3	4	5
5	.031	.188	.500	.812	.969	—
6	.016	.109	.344	.656	.891	.984
7	.008	.062	.227	.500	.773	.938
8	.004	.035	.145	.363	.637	.855
9	.002	.020	.090	.254	.500	.746
10	.001	.011	.055	.172	.377	.623
15	—	—	.004	.018	.059	.151
20	—	—	—	.001	.006	.021

This is an abridged version for purposes of illustration. See the Chapter 27 Supplement for the full table.

For $x = 1$ and $n = 7$, the table shows $p = .062$. We double this value for a two-tailed test, $p = .124$. This is greater than the acceptable level of .05, and we do not reject H_0. The output for this test is shown in Table 27-6B, confirming these results.

> ### ➤ Results
> A sign test was run to compare the distributions of attention deficit under two drug conditions. There was no significant difference in performance on the attention task between drug and placebo conditions ($p = .125$).

📌 The determination of the probability associated with *x* is based on a theoretical distribution called the *binomial probability distribution*. A binomial outcome is one that can take only two forms, in this case either positive or negative. The binomial test determines the likelihood of getting the smaller number of plus or minus signs out of the total number of differences just by chance.

The binomial test was also described in Chapter 18 in relation to using the split middle line with single-subject designs.

Large Samples

With sample sizes greater than 30, *x* is converted to *z* and tested against the normal distribution according to the formula

$$z = \frac{|D| - 1}{\sqrt{n}}$$

where $|D|$ is the absolute difference between the number of plus and minus signs (excluding ties). This calculation is illustrated in Table 27-6 ❹ for data with six plus signs and one minus sign, resulting in $z = 1.51$. Using the critical value of $z = 1.96$ for $\alpha_2 = .05$, this outcome does not achieve significance, and we do not reject H_0. We can confirm that the exact two-tailed probability associated with $z = 1.51$ is .0655 from Table A-1.

The Wilcoxon Signed-Ranks Test

The sign test evaluates differences within paired scores based solely on whether one score is larger or smaller than the other. This is often the best approach with subjective clinical variables that offer no greater precision. However, if data provide information on the relative magnitude of differences, the more powerful **Wilcoxon signed-ranks test** can be used. This test examines both the direction of difference and the relative difference based on ranks.

Procedure

Consider the same example presented in the previous section. We obtain a difference score for each subject, labeled *d*. We proceed by ranking these difference scores, *without regard to sign*, discarding pairs with no difference. We then attach the sign of the difference to the obtained ranks. For instance, in our example, the rank of 1 is given to the smallest difference score (Subject 2), and then assigned – 1 because it reflects a negative difference. The direction of difference is only relevant if a directional hypothesis is proposed.

The null hypothesis states that there is no difference in the distributions of the two conditions. If the null hypothesis is true, we would expect to find an equal representation of positive and negative signs among the larger and smaller ranks. We reject H_0 if either of these sums is too small.

The *T* Statistic

We determine if there are fewer positive or negative ranks, and then sum the ranks for the *less frequent sign*. This sum is assigned the test statistic, *T*. In this example, there are fewer ranks with negative signs, with the sum of – 1. Therefore, *T* = 1. The absolute value of *T* is used to determine significance. The sign is not of concern because we proposed a nondirectional hypothesis, and we will perform a two-tailed test.

Test of Significance

Critical values of *T* are shown in Table 27-8 for one- and two-tailed tests, where *N* is the number of pairs with nonzero differences. The absolute calculated value of *T* must be *less than or equal to* the critical value to achieve significance. Note once again that this is opposite to the way most critical values are used.

For this analysis at $\alpha_2 = .05$ with *n* = 7, the critical value of *T* is 2. Therefore, our calculated value of *T* = 1 is significant. We can reject H_0.

This outcome is significant (*p* = .027), shown in Table 27-6 ❸. The value of *z* is usually reported, rather than *T*, as it is more easily interpreted.

📌 Note the difference in the outcomes of the Wilcoxon and sign test on the same data. The Wilcoxon procedure showed a significant difference because it is sensitive to relative differences, not just direction. Therefore, if data achieve adequate precision, the Wilcoxon test is more powerful and is recommended over the sign test.

Large Samples

With sample sizes ≥ 25, the absolute value of *T* can be converted to *z*, as shown in Table 27-6 ❺, where *n* is the number of paired observations. For this analysis, *z* = 2.20. The absolute value of *z* is greater than the standard critical value 1.96 at $\alpha_2 = .05$. According to Table A-1, the two-tailed significance associated with *z* = 2.20 is .0278. This is confirmed in the output for the *z* test (see Table 27-6 ❸).

Effect Size for the Wilcoxon Signed-Ranks Test

The effect size index for the Wilcoxon signed-ranks test is based on a correlation coefficient, using the same statistic as the *U* test. Based on data from Table 27-6 for the comparison of attention deficit with and without a drug:

$$r = \frac{z}{\sqrt{N}} = \frac{2.217}{\sqrt{20}} = .496$$

In this instance, *N* is the total number of observations, not people. Therefore with 10 subjects in a repeated measures design, we will have 20 observations. This would be considered a medium to strong effect.

➤ **Results**
The Wilcoxon signed-ranks test was used to compare performance on the attention task under drug and placebo conditions using a cross-over design. Results showed that there was a significant difference in attention scores (*z* = 2.217, *p* = .027, *r* = .473), with higher attention scores under the drug condition.

Friedman Two-Way Analysis of Variance

The **Friedman two-way analysis of variance by ranks** is a nonparametric test to analyze data from a single-factor repeated measures design with three or more experimental conditions. Although the test has the designation "two-way," it is equivalent to the one-way repeated measures ANOVA. The two-way designation refers to the interaction of subjects with the independent variable.

➤ **CASE IN POINT #4**
We are interested in measuring the effect of changing body position on blood pressure in six patients with chronic pulmonary

Table 27-8	Abridged Table of Critical Values of *T* for the Wilcoxon Signed-Ranks Test			
	α_2		α_1	
N	.05	.01	.05	.01
6	0	—	2	—
7	2	—	3	0
8	3	0	5	1
9	5	1	8	3
10	8	3	10	5

This is an abridged table for purposes of illustration. See the Chapter 27 Supplement for the full table.

disease. Each patient will be placed in three positions—level, head down, and head elevated—in random order. Blood pressure will be measured within 1 minute of assuming each position.

Even though blood pressure is considered a ratio level measure, we may choose to use a nonparametric form of analysis for this study because the sample is small, and because we do not have sufficient reason to assume that blood pressure for a population of patients with this disease will be normally distributed.

Procedure

Hypothetical data for this study are reported in Table 27-9A. Data are arranged so that rows represent subjects (n) and columns represent experimental conditions (k). In this example, $n = 6$ and $k = 3$. We begin by converting all scores to ranks. However, for this test, the ranks are assigned *across each row* (within a subject). Ties are assigned average ranks within a row. The highest rank within a row will equal k.

The next step is to sum the ranks within each column. If the null hypothesis is true, we would expect the distribution of ranks to be a matter of chance, and high and low ranks should be evenly distributed across all treatment conditions. Therefore, the rank sums within each column should be equal. If the alternative hypothesis is true, at least one pair of conditions will show a difference.

The χ_r^2 Statistic

The test statistic for the Friedman ANOVA is χ_r^2 (read "chi square r"). It is computed using the formula

$$\chi_r^2 = \frac{12}{nk(k+1)} \sum R^2 - 3n(k+1)$$

where n is the number of subjects (rows), k is the number of treatment conditions (columns), and ΣR^2 is the sum of the squared ranks for each column. Calculation is illustrated in Table 27-9B. For this analysis, $\chi_r^2 = 9.25$.

Test of Significance

The distribution of χ_r^2 follows the standard χ^2 distribution with $k - 1$ degrees of freedom (see Table A-5).

With 3 conditions, we have 2 *df*, and we compare our calculated value of 9.25 against the critical value $\chi^2(2) = 5.99$ at $\alpha = .05$. The calculated value must be *equal to or larger than* the critical value to be significant. Therefore, the test is significant.

Multiple Comparisons

The output shows that the overall analysis of variance is significant ($p = .008$) (see Table 27-9 ❷). At this point, we can use a multiple comparison procedure to determine which groups are significantly different. Although the Wilcoxon signed-ranks test is often used for this purpose with a Bonferroni adjustment, Dunn's test is appropriate for multiple comparisons with the Friedman ANOVA.[17] Results for homogeneous subsets are shown in Table 26-9.

> ### ▶ Results
>
> A Friedman ANOVA identified a significant difference in blood pressure among the three body positions ($\chi_r^2(2) = 9.65$, $p = .008$). Dunn's test showed no significant difference in blood pressure between elevated and head down positions. Blood pressure in the level position was significantly lower than in the other two positions.

Effect Size for Friedman ANOVA

The effect size index for the Friedman analysis of variance is the Kendall coefficient of concordance, W, a correlation of ranked data for more than two conditions.[14] Based on the χ_r^2 statistic from Table 27-9 for the comparison of blood pressure in three head positions:

$$W = \frac{\chi_r^2}{N(k-1)} = \frac{9.652}{6(3-1)} = .802$$

This represents the effect size for the overall test across three conditions and is interpreted using conventional effect sizes for correlation. Therefore, this would be considered a strong effect.

 See the *Chapter 27 Supplement* for further illustration of follow up tests for the Friedman ANOVA, including multiple comparison procedures and effect size measures for pairwise contrasts.

Table 27-9 Friedman Two-Way Analysis of Variance by Ranks: Blood Pressure in Three Positions (*N* = 6)

A. Data

Subject	(1) Level BP	Rank	(2) Elevated BP	Rank	Head Down BP	Rank
1	110	1	150	2	175	3
2	100	1.5	100	1.5	110	3
3	120	1	140	3	135	2
4	110	1	130	2	155	3
5	120	1	130	2	145	3
6	130	1	155	2	170	3
ΣR		6.5		12.5		17.0
❶ $\bar{R}$		1.08		2.08		2.83

Descriptive Statistics

	N	Mean	Std. Deviation
Level	6	115.0000	10.48809
Elevated	6	134.1667	19.60017
Down	6	148.3333	24.01388

Ranks

	Mean Rank
Level	1.08
Elevated	2.08
Down	2.83

B. Calculations

$$\chi_r^2 = \frac{12}{nk\,(k+1)} \sum (\Sigma R)^2 - 3n(k+1)$$

$$\chi_r^2 = \frac{12}{(6)(3)(3+1)} \;[42.25 + 156.25 + 289.00] - (3)(6)(3+1) = \frac{12}{72}\,[487.50] - 72 = 9.25$$

❷

C. SPSS Output: Friedman ANOVA

Test Statistics[a]

N	6
Chi-Square	9.652
df	2
Asymp. Sig. ❷	.008

a. Friedman Test

Homogeneous Subsets ❸

		Subset 1	Subset 2
Sample[1]	Level	1.083	
	Elevated		2.083
	HeadDown		2.833
Test Statistic			2.667
Sig. (2-sided test)			.102
Adjusted Sig. (2-sided test)			.102

Homogeneous subsets are based on asymptotic significances. The significance level is .05.

[1] Each cell shows the sample average rank.

❶ The rank sums and mean ranks show a distinct spread between Level and the other two positions.

❷ The test statistic is significant (*p* = 008).

❸ The table of homogeneous subsets shows mean ranks for each group. Blood pressure is significantly lower in the Level condition than either of the other two conditions.

Calculated values differ due to rounding differences. Portions of the output have been omitted for clarity.

COMMENTARY

There are three kinds of lies: lies, damned lies, and statistics.

—Attributed to Benjamin Disraeli (1804 - 1881)

British Prime Minister

There is a longstanding debate among researchers and statisticians regarding the use of nonparametric versus parametric statistical procedures. This discussion continues today, with no more consensus than 50 years ago.[19]

Many researchers prefer to use parametric tests because they believe they are more powerful than nonparametric counterparts. However, simulations have shown that this is not necessarily the case, especially when scores are not normally distributed or when samples are small.[8] In fact, nonparametric procedures like the Mann-Whitney and Wilcoxon signed rank tests have been shown to have greater power than the comparable *t*-test when normality is not established, even in larger samples.[3,11,20,21] This effect is most prominent with between-group studies, and less of an influence in repeated measures designs.[22]

Many misconceptions continue to influence choices between parametric and nonparametric statistical tests.[21] These include the classical view that nonparametric tests should only be used with ordinal measures or with small samples. As examples in this chapter have illustrated, these tests can be applied with continuous data when the conditions warrant their application. And we should remember the converse situations where parametric statistics are used with ordinal scores, when certain assumptions are appropriate regarding the nature of measurements and their intervals, such as use in cumulative scales (see Chapter 12).

The tests that have been described in this chapter are only a sampling of the most commonly applied nonparametric procedures that are available. Statisticians continue to develop and refine these tests and to expand the capabilities of nonparametric methods into areas such as regression and factorial designs. Many tests have been developed with very specific purposes, such as comparing several treatment groups with a single control or looking at differences in variable that have an inherent order. Nonparametric statistics can also be used for correlation procedures and for testing nominal scale data. These procedures are presented next.

REFERENCES

1. Dworkin RH, Turk DC, Katz NP, Rowbotham MC, Peirce-Sandner S, Cerny I, Clingman CS, Eloff BC, Farrar JT, Kamp C, et al. Evidence-based clinical trial design for chronic pain pharmacotherapy: a blueprint for ACTION. *Pain* 2011;152(3 Suppl): S107-115.
2. Modir JG, Wallace MS. Human experimental pain models 2: the cold pressor model. *Methods Mol Biol* 2010;617:165-168.
3. Treister R, Nielsen CS, Stubhaug A, Farrar JT, Pud D, Sawilowsky S, Oaklander AL. Experimental comparison of parametric versus nonparametric analyses of data from the cold pressor test. *J Pain* 2015;16(6):537-548.
4. Hollander M, Wolfe DA, Chicken E. *Nonparametric Statistical Methods*. 3rd ed. Hoboken, NJ: John Wiley & Sons; 2014.
5. Hettmansperger TP, McKean JW. *Robust Nonparametric Statistical Methods. Momographs on Statistics and Applied Probability 119*. 2nd ed. Boca Raton, FL: CRC Press; 2011.
6. O'Connell AA. *Logistic Regression Models for Ordinal Response Variables*. Thousand Oaks, CA: Sage Publications; 2005.
7. Winer BJ, Michels KM, Brown DR. *Statistical Principles in Experimental Design*. 3rd ed. New York: McGraw-Hill; 1991.
8. Siegel S, Castellan NJ. *Nonparametric Statistics for the Behavioral Sciences*. 2nd ed. New York: McGraw-Hill; 1988.
9. Daniel WW. *Applied Nonparametric Statistics*. 2nd ed. Independence, KY: Cengage Learning; 2000.
10. Lehmann EL. *Nonparametrics: Statistical Methods Based on Ranks*. New York: Springer Science; 2006.
11. Neave HR, Granger WJ. A Monte Carlo study comparing various two-sample tests for differences in means. *Technometrics* 1968; 10:509.
12. Jepson HA, Talashek ML, Tichy AM. The Apgar score: evolution, limitations, and scoring guidelines. *Birth* 1991; 18(2):83-92.
13. Field A. *Discovering Statistics Using IBM SPSS Statistics*. 5th ed. Thousand Oaks, CA: Sage; 2018.
14. Tomczak M, Tomczak E. The need to report effect size estimates revisited. An overview of some recommended measures of effect size. *Trends Sport Sci* 2014;1(21):19-25.
15. Cohen J. *Statistical Power Analysis for the Behavioral Sciences*. 2nd ed. Hillsdale, NJ: Lawrence Erlbaum; 1988.
16. Lin LA, Bohnert ASB, Jannausch M, Goesling J, Ilgen MA. Use of non-pharmacological strategies for pain relief in addiction treatment patients with chronic pain. *Am J Addict* 2017; 26(6):564-567.
17. Dinno A. Nonparametric pairwise multiple comparisons in independent groups using Dunn's test. *Stata J* 2015;15: 292-300.
18. Whyte J, Vaccaro M, Grieb-Neff P, Hart T, Polansky M, Coslett HB. The effects of bromocriptine on attention deficits after traumatic brain injury: a placebo-controlled pilot study. *Am J Phys Med Rehabil* 2008;87(2):85-99.

19. Altman DG, Bland JM. Parametric v non-parametric methods for data analysis. *BMJ* 2009;338:a3167.

20. Blair RC, Higgins JJ, Smitley WDS. On the relative power of the U and t tests. *Brit J Math Stat Psychol* 1980;33(1): 114-120.

21. Sawilowsky SS. Misconceptions leading to choosing the t-test over the Wilcoxon Mann-Whitney test for shift in location parameter. *J Mod Appl Stat Methods* 2005;4(2): 598-600.

22. Bridge PD, Sawilowsky SS. Increasing physicians' awareness of the impact of statistics on research outcomes: comparative power of the t-test and and Wilcoxon Rank-Sum test in small samples applied research. *J Clin Epidemiol* 1999;52(3): 229-235.

Measuring Association for Categorical Variables: Chi-Square

The statistical procedures that have been described thus far have focused on comparisons, generally applied to experimental and quasi-experimental designs. We will now begin to examine procedures for exploratory analysis, where the purpose of the research question is to evaluate the relationship between two or more measured variables. Where studies of group differences ask if group A is different from group B, measures of association ask, "What is the relationship between A and B?"

Many such research questions involve categorical variables that are measured on a nominal or ordinal scale. Rather than using means, these questions deal with analysis of proportions or frequencies within various categories. The purpose of this chapter is to describe the use of several nonparametric tests based on the chi-square distribution. These tests have many applications in clinical research, in both experimental and descriptive analysis, including tests of goodness of fit to determine if a set of observed frequencies differs from a theoretical distribution and tests

of independence to determine if two classification variables are related to each other.

■ Testing Proportions

Many research questions in clinical and behavioral science involve categorical variables that are measured on a nominal or ordinal scale. Such data are analyzed by determining if there is a difference between the proportions *observed* within a set of categories and the proportions that would be *expected* by chance.

For example, suppose we tossed a coin 100 times. The null hypothesis states that the coin is not biased, and therefore we would theoretically *expect* a 50:50 outcome—50 heads and 50 tails. But we actually *observe* 47 heads and 53 tails. Does this deviation from the null hypothesis occur because the coin is biased, or is it only a matter of chance? In other words, is the difference between the observed and expected frequencies sufficiently large to justify rejection of the null hypothesis?

Chi-Square

The **chi-square statistic, χ^2**, tests the difference between observed and expected frequencies:

$$\chi^2 = \sum \frac{(O - E)^2}{E}$$

where O represents the observed frequency and E represents the expected frequency. As the difference between observed and expected frequencies increases, the value of χ^2 will increase. If observed and expected frequencies are the same, χ^2 will equal zero.

Using the coin example, we calculate χ^2 by substituting values for each category.

For heads,

$$\frac{(O-E)^2}{E} = \frac{(47-50)^2}{50} = \frac{(-3)^2}{20} = .18$$

For tails,

$$\frac{(O-E)^2}{E} = \frac{(53-50)^2}{50} = \frac{(3)^2}{50} = .18$$

The sum of these terms for all categories is the value of χ^2. Therefore,

$$\chi^2 = \sum \frac{(O-E)^2}{E} = .18 + .18 = .36$$

Test of Significance

We analyze the significance of this value using critical values of χ^2 found in Appendix Table A-5. Along the top of the table we identify the desired α level, say .05. Along the side we locate the appropriate degrees of freedom. The rules for determining degrees of freedom for different statistical models will be described shortly. In this case, $df = k - 1$, where k is the number of categories. Therefore, with two categories (heads/tails), we have 1 degree of freedom. Chi-square tests do not distinguish between one- and two-tailed tests because no negative values are possible.

The calculated value of χ^2 must be *greater than or equal to* the critical value to be significant. In this example, the observed value $\chi^2 = .36$ is less than $\chi^2(1) = 3.84$. Therefore, H_0 is not rejected, and we would conclude that the coin toss was fair.

Assumptions

Analyses that involve frequency counts in categories are based on two general assumptions:

- **Frequencies represent individual counts.**

Frequencies are not based on ranks or percentages. Data in each category represent the actual number of persons, objects, or events in those categories, not a summary statistic.

- **Categories are exhaustive and mutually exclusive.**

Every subject can be assigned to an appropriate category, but only one. Any number of categories can be used, but repeated measurement or assignment is not appropriate. Therefore, no one individual should be represented in more than one category, and the characteristics being measured are independent.

■ Goodness of Fit

One use of χ^2 is to test for **goodness of fit**, where the researcher compares observed frequency counts with a theoretical or known distribution. The coin toss described earlier is essentially a test of goodness of fit to a theoretical 50:50 probability distribution. Chi-square will test the null hypothesis that the proportion of outcomes within each category will not differ significantly from the expected distribution; that is, the observed proportions will fall within random fluctuation of the expected proportions. This type of test is considered a *one-sample test* because there is only one variable being assessed.

HISTORICAL NOTE
The classical studies of heredity performed by Mendel illustrate the concept of goodness of fit. He observed the color and shape of several generations of peas and compared the frequencies of specific color and shape combinations with a theoretical distribution based on his predictions about the role of dominant and recessive genes. When the observed distributions matched the theoretical model, his genetic theory was supported.

Uniform Distributions

A uniform distribution is one in which we would expect an equal distribution across categories.

> ### ➤ CASE IN POINT #1
> Consider a study that was designed to determine if the incidence of ischemic stroke is greater in the right or the left hemispheres. Hedna et al[1] looked at the number of large-vessel strokes in a sample of 233 patients and found that these events were more common in the left hemisphere (57%) than in the right hemisphere (43%).

Procedure

Is this distribution significantly different from what we would expect by chance? If we assume that the causative factors of stroke are not biased to one side, then theoretically we would expect to see a uniform distribution in the population. By definition, the expected frequencies for a uniform distribution will be evenly divided among the categories. Therefore, with 2 categories, under the null hypothesis we would expect 50% of our sample, or 116.5 people, to have right hemisphere events, and 50%, or 116.5 people, to have left hemisphere events. If we had more than two categories, we would divide the total sample into equal portions to get the expected frequencies. Calculations are shown in Table 28-1A, resulting in $\chi^2 = 4.124$.

| Table 28-1 | Chi-Square Goodness of Fit to a Uniform Distribution: Frequency of Left-Sided and Right-Sided Stroke (N= 233)[1] |

A. Data and Computation

Side	O	E	O-E	(O-E)^2	$\frac{(O - E)^2}{E}$
Right	101	116.5	−15.5	240.25	2.062
Left	132	116.5	15.5	240.25	2.062
Total	233				

$$\chi^2 = \sum \frac{(O\_E)^2}{E} = 4.124 \ \text{①}$$

B. SPSS Output: Chi-Square One-Sample Case

Side

	Observed N	Expected N	Residual ④
Right	101	116.5	−15.5
Left	132	116.5	15.5
Total	233		

Test Statistics

	Side
Chi-Square	① 4.124^a
df	1
Asymp. Sig.	② .042

③ a. 0 cells (0.0%) have expected frequencies less than 5. The minimum expected cell frequency is 116.5.

① The calculated value of χ^2 is reported.

② The χ^2 test is significant ($p = .042$).

③ The χ^2 test requires adjustment if expected frequencies in any one category are less than 5. This is not an issue for this test.

④ The residuals reported here represent the simple difference between the observed and expected counts (O-E).

It may seem strange to be dealing with fractions of a count in expected frequencies, as we obviously cannot have a fraction of an individual in a category. However, these values represent theoretical values based on probabilities and are not interpreted as actual counts.

It is important to emphasize that a χ^2 test of significance establishes that the observed frequencies are different from expected values. It does NOT indicate that the number of counts within categories are different from each other.

Sample size for goodness of fit tests should be large enough that no expected frequencies are less than 5.0 (see Table 28-1 ③). When this criterion is not met, sample size should be increased or categories combined to create an appropriate distribution. Note that this criterion applies to the expected frequencies, not the observed counts.

Test of Significance

In the uniform distribution goodness of fit model, $df = k - 1$. With two categories (right and left), $df = 1$. Therefore, we compare the calculated value, $\chi^2 = 4.124$, with the critical value $\chi^2(1) = 3.84$, obtained from Table A-5. The calculated value is higher than the critical value, and we can reject the null hypothesis. The computer output for this test shows that the test is significant at $p = .042$ (see Table 28-1 ②).

The difference between the observed and expected frequencies is not likely to be a matter of chance, and the null hypothesis is rejected. By looking at the data, we can see that left-sided strokes occurred more often and right-sided strokes less often than expected. Therefore, researchers in this study concluded that left-hemispheric strokes were more common.[1]

▶ Results

The total number of patients with large vessel ischemic strokes was 233. The χ^2 test was used to examine the null hypothesis that there would be no difference in the proportion of left or right hemispheric strokes in this population. The results showed that left-hemispheric strokes (57%) were more common than right-hemispheric strokes (43%) ($\chi^2(1) = 4.68$, $p = .031$).

Known Distributions

A second goodness of fit model compares a sample distribution with a known distribution within an underlying population. This is one way to document how well a sample represents its parent population.

> ► **CASE IN POINT #2**
>
> Blood types are known to be unevenly distributed within the population. Investigators have suggested that venous thromboembolism (VTE) is more common in individuals with certain blood types.[2] If this is true, then we can expect to see those blood types represented among patients with VTE in higher percentages than in the overall population. Consider hypothetical data for a sample of 85 patients who have experienced a VTE. The null hypothesis states that VTE is not associated with blood type and that the distribution of blood types in the sample will be similar to that in the overall population.

Procedure

Data have shown the following distribution of blood types in the general population: A: 39%, B: 19%, AB: 5%, and O: 37%.[3] Therefore, we can use these proportions to determine how many of the patients should be expected to have each blood type under the null hypothesis. For example, 39% of the sample, or $(.39)(85) = 33.15$ patients, should have type A blood, and $(.05)(85) = 4.25$ patients should have type AB. Hypothetical data for all four categories are shown in Table 28-2A, resulting in $\chi^2 = 13.42$.

Test of Significance

With a known distribution, we test χ^2 with $k - 1$ degrees of freedom. In this case, with four categories, $df = 3$. The critical value is obtained from Table A-5, $\chi^2(3) = 7.82$.

Table 28-2 Chi-Square Goodness of Fit to a Known Distribution of Blood Types ($N = 85$)

A. Data and Computation

Blood Type	% in Population	O	E	❸ O-E	(O-E)²	(O − E)² / E	√E	❹ Std. Residual
A	**39%**	36	33.15	2.85	8.12	0.25	5.76	0.49
B	**19%**	22	16.15	5.85	34.22	2.12	4.02	1.46
AB	**5%**	9	4.25	4.75	22.56	5.31	2.06	2.30
O	**37%**	18	31.45	−13.45	180.90	5.75	5.61	−2.40
	Total	85				$\chi^2 = 13.42$ ❶		

B. SPSS Output: Chi-Square One-Sample Case

Bloodtype

	Observed N	Expected N	Residual ❸
A	36	33.1	2.9
B	22	16.2	5.8
AB	9	4.3	4.7
O	18	31.4	−13.4
Total	85		

Test Statistics

	Bloodtype
Chi-Square	13.266[a]
df	3
Asymp. Sig. ❶	.004

❷ a. 1 cells (25.0%) have expected frequencies less than 5. The minimum expected cell frequency is 4.3.

---

❶ The χ^2 test statistic is significant ($p = .004$), indicating that the observed frequencies do not fit the proportion of blood types in the population.

❷ Corrections can be applied to account for the small expected frequency for type AB (see discussion of Yates correction).

❸ The residuals reported here are not standardized. They are the simple difference between observed and expected frequencies (O-E). A negative residual tells us that the observed frequency was smaller than expected. These values are not comparable, however, because they do not account for the number of people in each category.

❹ Standardized residuals are obtained by $(O - E) / \sqrt{E}$. These values allow comparison across categories to indicate which contribute most to χ^2. These values are not generated by SPSS for the one-sample case. In this analysis, the categories of AB and O blood types have the largest standardized residuals. The proportion of type AB is more than expected, and type O is less than expected.

Calculated values vary due to rounding differences.

The calculated value of $\chi^2 = 13.42$ exceeds the critical value, and we can reject the null hypothesis. These hypothetical data do not follow the population distribution, and therefore there is reason to believe that this disorder has an association with blood type. So how do we interpret such a finding? We need some way to determine which category contributed substantially to this significant finding.

Standardized Residuals

With more than two categories, significant results of a chi-square test need to be further examined, to determine where important differences lie. We can examine the results subjectively, to determine which categories demonstrate the greatest discrepancy between observed and expected values. For this purpose we can look at a *residual* for each cell, which is the difference between the observed and expected frequencies, given in the column labeled O – E (see Table 28-2 ❸).

For the blood type study, for instance, the residual for type A is 2.85. This means that the observed proportion of type A blood in this sample was more than expected. For type O the residual is –13.45, indicating that this proportion was less than expected. These raw values may be difficult to interpret, however, as they are affected by the number of observed counts within each cell; that is, cells with larger counts are likely to have larger residuals. Therefore, **standardized residuals, R**, are often used to demonstrate the relative contribution of each cell to the overall value of chi-square:

$$R = \frac{O - E}{\sqrt{E}}$$

For example, using the data for type B, the standardized residual is

$$R = \frac{5.85}{\sqrt{16.15}} = 1.46$$

Standardized residuals for blood types are shown in Table 28-2 ❹. These residual values can be compared to determine which categories contributed most to the value of χ^2. Standardized residuals can be interpreted relative to a z score, with scores close to or greater than 1.96 being considered most important.[4,5] Therefore, the deviation of types AB and O from expected proportions are the most meaningful.

> ### ► Results
> The chi-square test showed a significant difference in proportions of blood types in a sample of patients with VTE compared to the known distribution of blood types in the population ($\chi^2(3) = 13.42$, $p = .004$). Standardized residuals showed that discrepancies for AB and O contribute significantly to this finding. For type O blood

the proportion of individuals with VTE is less than expected by chance, and type AB has a higher than expected frequency. This finding suggests that there is a relationship between O blood types and lower risk of VTE.[2]

■ Tests of Independence

The most common application of chi-square is in tests of independence. With this approach, researchers examine the association, or lack thereof, between two categorical variables. This association is based on the proportion of individuals who fall into each category. These data may be obtained from randomized experiments or from observational studies involving classification of subject characteristics (see Focus on Evidence 28-1).

> ### ► CASE IN POINT #3
> Many studies have shown a relationship between depression and dementia.[6] Suppose we designed a study to explore this relationship. We recruit a sample of 75 individuals from an elder residence community who have been evaluated for depression and dementia using two standardized tests. We hypothesize that there will be a greater proportion of depressed individuals among those with dementia than among those without dementia.

In this study we are looking at the relationship between two nominal variables. The null hypothesis states that the proportion of subjects observed in each category of dementia is independent of depression. If the null hypothesis is rejected following a significant χ^2 test, it indicates that an association between the variables is present.

Contingency Tables

To test the relationship between two categorical variables, data are arranged in a two-way matrix called a **contingency table**, or *crosstabulation*, with R rows × C columns. This study uses a 2 × 2 design (see Table 28-3). The data are recorded as frequency counts within each of the four cells. The cell designations of *a, b, c, d* are standard for calculation of many statistics using this format.

When data are arranged in a contingency table, the marginal frequencies can be generated in one of two ways. They may be *fixed effects*, in that the totals are determined by the experimenter. This happens, for instance, when researchers recruit or assign a certain number of individuals to groups. *Random effects* do not have predetermined marginal frequencies. Contingency tables may incorporate two fixed effects, two random effects, or a mixed model. The depression study is an example of a random model, in which the number of subjects with the two conditions was not specified in advance.

Focus on Evidence 28–1
Important Answers: Yes or No

Evidence-based respiratory therapy (RT) protocols, based on published guidelines, are used to standardize patient care in hospital settings, allowing timely assessment and management of patients, without waiting for a physician order. Studies have shown that this practice is cost-effective and safe, providing efficient utilization of resources.[7, 8] Werre et al[9] looked at the effectiveness of RT protocols on length of stay (LOS) and 30-day readmissions for patients with chronic obstructive pulmonary disease (COPD) who were admitted with a diagnosis of acute bacterial pneumonia in one hospital between 2007 and 2012.

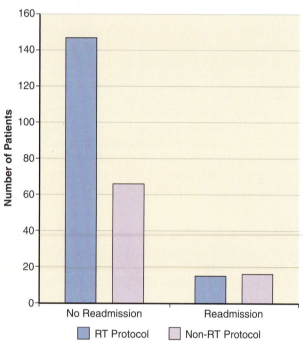

The researchers were interested in the effect of protocol type (RT or not), age (below or above 70), and severity index (based on presence of comorbidities, rated minor/moderate or major/severe) on LOS. Using a three-way ANOVA, they found that there was no difference in LOS regardless of age or use of RT protocol. Not surprisingly, they found that the only significant difference was the effect of severity.

They also used chi-square to determine whether readmission within 30 days of discharge was independent of RT protocol, and found that RT protocols were associated with fewer readmissions, as shown in the figure (p = .02). This type of graphic display is useful with a test of independence to visually demonstrate such differences in proportions. Based on these data, the researchers concluded that respiratory care delivered by RT protocols did not confer a disadvantage to patients in terms of hospital stay compared with physician-directed treatment, that treatment efficacy was not sacrificed regardless of disease severity, and 30-day post-discharge readmission rates were lower under RT protocols.

Creating dichotomous variables, as in this example, can be a useful way to look at differences, especially when outcomes can be converted to categories that are meaningful, like 30-day readmissions, a common marker in health service delivery studies. However, some information is lost when variables such as age and severity are reduced to two categories, and other statistical approaches may provide more precise estimates, such as regression analysis (see Chapter 31).

Data taken from Were ND, Boucher EL, Beachey WD. Comparison of therapist-directed and physician-directed respiratory care in COPD subjects with acute pneumonia. *Respir Care* 2015;60(2):151-4.

Table 28-3	Contingency Table Showing Relationship Between Presence of Dementia and Depression			
	No Dementia		**Dementia**	**Total**
Not Depressed	*a* 42		*b* 11	53
Depressed	*c* 7		*d* 15	22
Total	49		26	75

Procedure

The null hypothesis states that there is no association between depression and dementia. We begin our analysis by calculating the expected frequencies for each cell in the table. The expected frequencies essentially define the null hypothesis. This process of determining expected frequencies is somewhat more complicated than with one-sample tests because we cannot just evenly divide the total sample among the four cells. We must account for the observed *proportions* within each cell. Each cell expected frequency (E) is determined using the following formula:

$$E = (\text{row total} \times \text{column total})/N$$

Cell A   E = (53 × 49)/75 = 34.63

Cell B   E = (53 × 26)/75 = 18.37

Cell C   E = (22 × 49)/75 = 14.37

Cell D   E = (22 × 26)/75 = 7.62

Test of Significance

Table 28-4A shows the calculation of χ^2 using the depression data. These calculations proceed as in previous examples, with all observed and expected frequencies listed (order is unimportant). The test value, $\chi^2 = 15.43$, is compared with the critical value with $(R-1)(C-1)$ degrees of freedom. In this case, we have $(2-1)(2-1) = 1$ degree of freedom.

From Appendix Table A-5 we obtain the critical value $\chi^2(1) = 3.84$. Because the calculated value is higher than the critical value, χ^2 is significant and the null hypothesis is rejected. These variables are not independent of each other. There is a significant association between the presence of depression and dementia in this sample.

Interpreting Chi-Square

If χ^2 is not significant, our analysis ends, and we would conclude that there was no association between the variables. However, with a significant test, we can examine the frequencies within each cell to interpret these findings. The crosstabulation for this analysis is shown in Table 28-4B. Note that this table includes row and column percentages in addition to observed and expected frequencies. These values are helpful when trying to interpret proportions.

The frequency within each cell is given as a percentage of the column (% within Dementia) and the row (% within Depression). For instance, 15 patients who were depressed exhibited dementia. This represents 68.2% of all those who were depressed (the row %) and 57.7% of all those who had dementia (the column %). Those who had both dementia and depression represent 20.0% of the total sample.

If we examine the standardized residuals (R) for each cell (see Table 28-4 ❸), we can see that the two cells representing patients who were depressed contribute most to the significant outcome, with standardized residuals close to or greater than 1.96. For those who were depressed, the number of patients without dementia was *less* than expected by chance (R = –1.9), and the number of patients with dementia was *more* than expected by chance (R = 2.7). It is reasonable, then, to conclude that the presence of depression and dementia are related.

🔑 It is important to note that the presence of a relationship does *not* indicate that depression *causes* dementia or vice versa—only that there is a relationship, which may be due to other factors that were not examined. We do not know if one condition preceded the other (see Chapter 19).

Sample Size Considerations

Interpretation of chi-square is based on certain assumptions about the expected frequencies in each cell. Because of the continuous nature of the chi-square distribution,

there are limitations when samples are too small affecting the applicability of critical values and potentially increasing the risk of Type I error. No more than 20% of the cells should contain expected frequencies less than 5.[10] When this occurs, the researcher may choose to collapse the table (if it is larger than 2×2) to combine adjacent categories and increase expected cell frequencies, or consider increasing the sample size.

Yates' Continuity Correction

When samples are too small in a 2×2 contingency table, a correction can be applied. Yates proposed a **continuity correction** that involves subtracting .5 from the absolute value of (O-E) prior to squaring in the calculation of χ^2. This results in a more conservative test with a smaller value for χ^2. This test is automatically included with the output but would be ignored for the depression study because there are no cells with too small expected frequencies (see Table 28-4 ❹).

A number of statistical sources suggest that Yates' correction for continuity is too conservative and unduly increases the chance of committing a Type II error.[11-13] It has been suggested that χ^2 can provide a reasonable estimate of Type I error for 2×2 tables when random or mixed models are used with $N \geq 8$.[14]

Fisher's Exact Test

Because the chi-square distribution can be inaccurate with very small samples, another approach is use of **Fisher's exact test** for 2×2 tables. It is recommended when any expected frequency is less than 1, or 20% of expected frequencies are 5 or less. The test statistic is itself a probability value. The calculation of this test is quite cumbersome, but it is fortunately available in most statistical programs. This value can be requested as part of the results of the chi-square test, but would not be applied in the depression study because there are no cells with small expected frequencies.

🎯 **FUN FACT**

On a sunny afternoon in Cambridge, England, in the 1920s, a group of friends were sharing tea when Muriel Bristol claimed that she could tell whether milk was poured into tea or tea was poured into milk. The renowned statistician, Sir Ronald Fisher happened to be one of the guests, and of course he took on the challenge. He devised a now famous experiment, *The Lady Tasting Tea*, with 8 cups of tea, 4 each of the two conditions, and presented them to the lady in random order.[15,16] This exercise resulted in his development of Fisher's exact test to demonstrate the likelihood that she could identify the cups of tea correctly. It was a landmark advance in the principles of hypothesis testing and probability.

Although accounts disagree, according to legend the lady got them all correct!

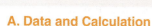

Table 28-4 Chi-Square Test of Independence: Association between Depression and Dementia ($N = 75$)

A. Data and Calculation

	❶ Category	O	E	O-E	(O-E)²	$\frac{(O-E)^2}{E}$	Std. Residual
Not Depressed	**No Dementia (A)**	42	34.63	7.37	54.32	1.57	1.25
	Dementia (B)	11	18.37	−7.37	54.32	2.96	−1.72
Depressed	**No Dementia (C)**	7	14.37	−7.37	54.32	3.78	−1.94
	Dementia (D)	15	7.63	7.37	54.32	7.12	2.67

$$\chi^2 = 15.43 \;❷$$

B. SPSS Output: Chi-Square Crosstabs

Depression * Dementia Crosstabulation

Depression		No Dementia	Dementia	Total
Not Depressed	Count	A 42	B 11	53
	Expected Count	34.6	18.4	53.0
❷	% within Depression	79.2%	20.8%	100.0%
	% within Dementia	85.7%	42.3%	70.7%
	% of Total	56.0%	14.7%	70.7%
	Standardized Residual	1.3	−1.7	
Depressed	Count	C 7	D 15	22
	Expected Count	14.4	7.6	22.0
❷	% within Depression	31.8%	68.2%	100.0%
	% within Dementia	14.3%	57.7%	29.3%
	% of Total	9.3%	20.0%	29.3%
	Standardized Residual	−1.9	2.7	
Total	Count	49	26	75
	Expected Count	49.0	26.0	75.0
	% within Depression	65.3%	34.7%	100.0%
	% within Dementia	100.0%	100.0%	100.0%
	% of Total	65.3%	34.7%	100.0%

❶ $\chi^2 = 15.43$

❷ Percentages can be confusing, so look at rows and columns. The row percentages are for depression, and column percentages are for dementia.

❸ Standardized residuals indicate that cells C and D provide the largest effects. Chi-square is significant ($p < .001$)

❹ The continuity correction is only applied when there are cells with expected frequencies less than 5. Therefore, it is not relevant here and we can ignore this value.

❺ Effect size indices can be requested, including phi, V, C, and the odds ratio.

Chi-Square Tests

	Chi	df	Asymptotic Sig. (2-sided)
Pearson Chi-Square	15.440ᵃ	1	❸ .000
Continuity Correctionᵇ	13.417	1	.000
N of Valid Cases	75		

❹ a. 0 cells (0.0%) have expected count less than 5. The minimum expected count is 7.63.
b. Computed only for a 2 × 2 table

Symmetric Measures ❺

		Value	Approx Sig.
Nominal by Nominal	Phi	.454	.000
	Cramer's V	.454	.000
	Contingency Coefficient	.413	.000
N of Valid Classes		75	

Risk Estimate ❺

		95% Confidence Interval	
	Value	Lower	Upper
Odds Ratio for Depression	8.182	2.680	24.977
N of Valid Cases	75		

Calculated values vary due to rounding differences. Portions of the output have been omitted for clarity.

■ Power and Effect Size

The chi-square statistic tests the hypothesis that observed proportions differ from chance. However, it does not provide a measure of effect size. Effect size indices for chi-square are interpreted as correlation coefficients, which reflect the strength of the association between two variables (see Chapter 29). There are several measures that can be used for nominal data, each with conventional effect sizes (see Table 28-5).[17] The choice of test depends on the design and type of categories.

Effect Size Indices

The effect size index, w, can be used with uniform and known distributions as well as contingency tables. This value is also called the **phi coefficient, ϕ,** which is used with 2 × 2 tables. For the data in Table 28-4,

$$w = \sqrt{\frac{\chi^2}{N}} = \frac{\sqrt{15.44}}{\sqrt{75}} = \mathbf{.454}$$

This is the effect size used in G*Power. These values will range from 0 to 1.0. See Box 28-1 for a description of the process for power analysis and sample size estimation using this index.

With symmetrical tables larger than 2 × 2, the *contingency coefficient, C,* is used. The range of possible values will differ depending on the size of the table. Therefore, values cannot be compared unless tables are of equal size. When tables are asymmetrical, *Cramer's V* is used, Conventional effect sizes vary depending on the smaller number of rows or columns (q).

These coefficients can be reported with chi-square output if requested (see Table 28-4). We can see that all of these indices are significant, approximating .45. Given the conventional effect sizes shown in Table 28-5, these would be considered close to large effects. It is the researcher's task to determine if this degree of relationship was meaningful in the context of the study of depression and dementia.

> 🔑 It is worth reinforcing Cohen's admonition that conventional effect sizes should not be used as absolutes, but must be put into the context of the variables being studied.[17,18]

Table 28-5 Effect Size Indices Used with Chi-Square

INDEX	FORMULA	APPLICATION
For all indices, N refers to the total sample size		
w	$w = \sqrt{\dfrac{\chi^2}{N}}$	Used with one-sample tests or contingency tables.
Phi ϕ	$\phi = \sqrt{\dfrac{\chi^2}{N}}$	For 2 × 2 tables
Contingency Coefficient C	$C = \sqrt{\dfrac{\chi^2}{N + \chi^2}}$	For symmetrical tables larger than 2 × 2
Cramer's V V	$V = \sqrt{\dfrac{\chi^2}{N(q-1)}}$	For asymmetrical tables (q = *smaller number of rows or columns*)

Conventional Effect Sizes			
	SMALL	**MEDIUM**	**LARGE**
w	.10	.30	.50
ϕ	.10	.30	.50
C	.10	.287	.447
V q = 3	.071	.212	.354
V q = 4	.058	.173	.150
V q = 5	.354	.289	.250

> ➤ **Results**
> The chi-square test identified a significant association between depression and dementia ($\chi^2(1)$ = 15.44, $p < .001$, phi = .45). Of those who were not depressed, 20.8% had dementia. Of those who were depressed, 68.2% had dementia. Of those who exhibited dementia, 57.7% were depressed. Standardized residuals indicate that the strongest relationship supported the mutual occurrence of dementia and depression.

Odds Ratio

Another useful measure of effect for categorical data is the **odds ratio, OR,** which is calculated from 2 × 2 tables.[5] This risk measure serves a useful purpose in describing how proportions differ among groups. The OR represents the odds that an outcome will occur given a particular exposure, compared to the odds of the outcome occurring in the absence of that exposure. For our current example, it would predict the odds of dementia occurring with and without depression.

Using the cell designations shown in Table 28-3, the odds ratio can be calculated as:

$$OR = \frac{ad}{bc}$$

The null value for an OR is 1.0, indicating no difference in proportions. A value higher or lower than 1.0 indicates increased or decreased likelihood. For instance, for the depression example, the OR = 8.18 (see Table 28-4 **5**). This means that the odds of having dementia with depression are 8 times higher than if they did not have depression.

> Other measures of association can be used with contingency tables when categorical variables are on the ordinal scale, including *Kendall's tau*, the *lambda coefficient*, and *gamma*.

> See the *Chapter 28 Supplement* for further description and calculation of these effect size indices, and how they are applied in the use of G*Power for power and sample size estimates for the examples in this chapter.

■ McNemar Test for Correlated Samples

One of the basic assumptions required for use of χ^2 is that variables are independent so that no one subject is represented in more than one cell. There are many research questions, however, for which this assumption will not hold. For instance, we could examine the effects of a particular treatment program by looking at the presence or absence of an outcome variable before and after treatment. These studies use categorical variables

but in a repeated measures design. The χ^2 test is not valid under these conditions.

The **McNemar test** is a form of the χ^2 statistic used with 2×2 tables that involve correlated samples, where subjects act as their own controls or where they are matched. This test is especially useful with pretest–posttest designs when the dependent variable is measured as a dichotomy on an ordinal or nominal scale.

> ➤ **CASE IN POINT #4**
>
> Researchers have studied the effect of percutaneous vertebroplasty on pain and function in patients with vertebral fractures.[19] Suppose we designed a study to assess whether patients were taking pain medications before and after the procedure in a sample of 70 patients. We hypothesize that the proportion of patients who stopped taking medication after the procedure will be greater than the proportion of patients who began taking medications afterwards.

Table 28-6A shows hypothetical data in a crosstabulation for the use of pain medications before and after vertebroplasty. In this situation, the cells are not independent, and each subject is represented twice.

Procedure

The cells in the correlated design follow the standard notation for a 2×2 table as shown. The number of patients who demonstrate a change in the use of pain medications following the vertebroplasty are reflected in shaded cells B and C. Patients in cell B did not use pain medications prior to the procedure but did use them afterwards. Those in cell C used pain medications prior to the procedure, but no longer used them post-surgery. Patients in cells A and D did not change their use (or nonuse) of medications.

As B and C represent the total number of patients who showed a change in their behavior, these are the only cells relevant to this analysis. Under the null hypothesis, the proportion of patients who changed in either direction will be the same. We test this hypothesis using the formula

$$\chi^2 = \frac{(B-C)^2}{B+C}$$

The McNemar test can be adjusted for small cell frequencies using a continuity correction, which involves subtracting 1 from the absolute value of B – C before squaring.[20] This is illustrated in Table 28-6 **2**, resulting in a corrected statistic of $\chi^2 = 2.857$.

Test of Significance

The McNemar statistic is tested against critical values of χ^2 with one degree of freedom (Appendix Table A-5).

Table 28-6   McNemar Test: Use of Pain Medications Before and After Vertebroplasty (*N*=53)

A. SPSS Output: McNemar Test

Before * After Crosstabulation ❶

			After		Total
			No Meds	Meds	
Before	No meds	Count	**A** 25	**B** 12	37
		% of Total	35.7%	17.1%	52.9%
	Meds	Count	**C** 23	**D** 10	33
		% of Total	32.9%	14.3%	47.1%
Total		Count	48	22	70
		% of Total	68.6%	31.4%	100.0%

Test Statistics[a]

		Before & After
N		70
Chi-Square[b]	❷	2.857
Asymp. Sig.	❸	.091

a. McNemar Test
b. Continuity Corrected

- Using the standard calculation

$$\chi^2 = \frac{(B - C)^2}{(B + C)} = \frac{(12 - 23)^2}{(12 + 23)} = 3.457$$

- Using the continuity correction ❷

$$\chi^2 = \frac{(|B - C| - 1)^2}{(B + C)} = \frac{(|12 - 23| - 1)^2}{(12 + 23)} = 2.857$$

❶ The four cells in a 2 × 2 design are labelled A, B, C, D. The only cells of interest are B and C, representing subjects who changed their status from before to after. Percentages indicate the proportion of the total sample in each cell. The effect size odds ratio is the ratio of the proportions for cells B and C (.171/.329 = .519).

❷ In SPSS, the McNemar chi-square test statistic is adjusted using the continuity correction. Other statistical programs may use the standard calculation.

❸ The test statistic is less than the critical value $\chi^2(1) = 3.84$.and is not significant (*p* = .091). Note that this result would still be nonsignificant if the uncorrected value was used.

This calculated value is less than the critical value $\chi^2(1) = 3.84$ and is not significant (see Table 28-6 ❸).

Power and Effect Size

The effect size for the McNemar test is based on the **odds ratio (OR)**. However, for this analysis we must account for the fact that the data are paired, not independent. With correlated samples OR = P_B/P_C, which is the ratio of the proportion (P) of cases in cells B and C, the cells that represent change. These cells denote *discordant pairs*. Cells A and D are considered *concordant pairs*, showing no change. For this analysis, P_B is 12/70 = .171, and P_C is 23/70 = .329. Therefore, OR = .171/.329 = .519. This value is used as an effect size index for the test.

This value is interpreted similarly to the standard OR. The null value is 1.0 (both B and C proportions are the same). With a value less than 1.0, as we see here, cell B has a smaller proportion than C, and with an OR above 1.0, cell B would have the larger proportion. In this example, a larger proportion of those who changed went from Med to No Meds than the reverse. See Box 28-2 for further discussion of power analysis for the McNemar test.

> **Results**
>
> The McNemar test was used to examine the proportion of patients who changed their medication status from before to after vertebroplasty. Of the total sample (*N* = 70), 47.1% were taking medications before surgery, which was reduced to 31.4% post-surgery. Of those using medications before (*n* = 33), 70% (*n* = 23) were no longer using medications after surgery. Of those not using medication before (*n* = 37), 32.4% (*n* = 12) started using medications post-surgery. Using a continuity correction, these associations were not significant ($\chi^2(1) = 2.857$, *p* = .091, OR = .52). Based on these results, the proportion of patients who changed their medication status was not different from what would be expected by chance.

Box 28-2   Power Analysis for the McNemar Test

Post Hoc Analysis: Determining Power

Using G*Power for *post hoc* power analysis, we enter the achieved OR, level of significance, actual sample size and the observed proportion of discordant pairs. For this analysis, OR = .519, α = .05, N = 70, and B and C (n = 35) represent .50 of the total sample *(see chapter supplement)*. This results in 58% power, so it is not surprising that we did not find a significant effect *(see chapter supplement)*.

A Priori Analysis: Estimating Sample Size

For estimation of sample size, we enter an estimated OR, level of significance, desired power and an estimate of the proportion of discordant pairs. In other words, we have to estimate what proportion of the total sample will change from before to after (in either direction). Let's assume we project an OR of .60, α = .05, 80% power, and

an estimate that 80% of the sample will change. This results in a required total sample of 128 *(see chapter supplement)*.

As we know in retrospect, this proposed OR is larger than what we actually found. This suggests that if there is an effect in this study, we probably need a larger sample to show it.

One- and Two-Tailed Tests

Power analysis for the McNemar test can be run with a one-tailed or two-tailed test. Typically, two-tailed tests are used, as we did here. But if we truly believed that the changes would be in one direction, such as mostly going from Meds to No Meds, we could propose a directional alternative hypothesis and use a one-tailed test. As we have discussed before, however, this can be a risky decision if it should not come out in the predicted direction (see Chapter 24).

COMMENTARY

Statistics are no substitute for judgment.

—*Henry Clay (1777-1852)*

American statesman

Clinical researchers can find many uses for the chi-square statistic when proportions are of interest for data analysis and for descriptive purposes. It is often useful as a way of establishing group equivalence following random assignment. For instance, once two groups have been assigned, it may be of interest to compare the numbers of males and females in each group to see if they were assigned in equal proportions. Or it may be important to determine if certain age groups are balanced across the groups. Chi-square can be used to make these determinations and confirm the validity of the randomization process.

Although chi-square seems like an uncomplicated test to run, its interpretation is not so simple. Analysis of proportions is not as straightforward as comparisons between groups. That is why effect sizes are relevant, so that there is some guide for judging the strength of an association. However, even then, it is a matter of translating the story that frequencies provide into clinically meaningful judgments.

REFERENCES

1. Hedna VS, Bodhit AN, Ansari S, et al. Hemispheric differences in ischemic stroke: Is left-hemisphere stroke more common? *J Clin Neurol* 2013;9(2):97-102.
2. Wu O, Bayoumi N, Vickers MA, et al. ABO(H) blood groups and vascular disease: a systematic review and meta-analysis. *J Thromb Haemost* 2008;6(1):62-9.
3. Blood types and facts. MemorialCare. Available at https://www.memorialcare.org/services/blood-donation/blood-types-and-facts. Accessed October 15, 2017.
4. Haberman SJ. The analysis of residulas in cross-classified tables. *Biometrics* 1973;29(1):205-20.
5. Field A. *Discovering Statistics Using IBM SPSS Statistics*. 5th ed. Thousand Oaks, CA: Sage; 2018.
6. Byers AL, Yaffe K. Depression and risk of developing dementia. *Nat Rev Neurol* 2011;7(6):323-31.
7. Kollef MH, Shapiro SD, Clinkscale D, et al. The effect of respiratory therapist-initiated treatment protocols on patient outcomes and resource utilization. *Chest* 2000;117(2):467-75.
8. Kallam A, Meyerink K, Modrykamien AM. Physician-ordered aerosol therapy versus respiratory therapist-driven aerosol protocol: the effect on resource utilization. *Respir Care* 2013; 58(3):431-7.
9. Werre ND, Boucher EL, Beachey WD. Comparison of therapist-directed and physician-directed respiratory care in COPD subjects with acute pneumonia. *Respir Care* 2015;60(2):151-4.
10. Cochran WG. Some methods for strengthening the common χ^2 tests. *Biometrics* 1954;10:417-51.
11. Sahai H, Khurshid A. On analysis of epidemiological data involving a 2 x 2 contingency table: an overview of Fisher's exact test and Yates' correction for continuity. *J Biopharm Stat* 1995;5(1):43-70.

12. Haviland MG. Yates's correction for continuity and the analysis of 2 × 2 contingency tables. *Stat Med* 1990;9(4):363-7; discussion 69-83.

13. Campbell I. Chi-squared and Fisher-Irwin tests of two-by-two tables with small sample recommendations. *Stat Med* 2007; 26(19):3661-75.

14. Mantel N, Benjamin E. The odds ratios of a 2 × 2 contingency table. *Am Stat* 1975;29(4):143-45.

15. Fisher RA. *The Design of Experiments*. 9th ed. New York: Macmillan; 1971.

16. Salsburg D. *The Lady Tasting Tea: How Statistics Revolutionized Science in the Twentieth Century*. New York: Henry Holt and Company; 2001.

17. Cohen J. *Statistical Power Analysis for the Behavioral Sciences*. 2nd ed. Hillsdale, NJ: Lawrence Erlbaum; 1988.

18. Cohen J. Things I have learned (so far). *Am Pyschologist* 1990;45(12):1304-12.

19. Evans AJ, Jensen ME, Kip KE, et al. Vertebral compression fractures: pain reduction and improvement in functional mobility after percutaneous polymethylmethacrylate vertebroplasty—retrospective report of 245 cases. *Radiology* 2003;226(2):366-72.

20. Siegel S, Castellan NJ. *Nonparametric Statistics for the Behavioral Sciences*. 2nd ed. New York: McGraw-Hill; 1988.

Correlation

Correlation is, by and large, a familiar concept. Pairs of observations, *X* and *Y*, are examined to see if they "go together." For instance, we generally accept that heart rate increases with physical exertion, that weight loss will be related to caloric intake, or that weight loss will increase as the frequency of exercise increases. These variables are correlated in that the value of one variable is systematically related to values of the second variable, although not perfectly and to differing degrees. With a strong correlation, we can infer something about the second value by knowing the first. In Chapter 28, chi-square was used to look at the association between nominal variables. The purpose of this chapter is to introduce several correlation statistics for use with ordinal and ratio/interval data that can be applied to a variety of exploratory research designs.

■ Concepts of Correlation

The basic purpose of correlation is to describe the association between two variables. These *bivariate* relationships are defined by the shared pattern within the two sets of data. For example, if we measure heart rate and physical exertion in several individuals, we would expect to see higher scores in heart rate with higher scores in exertion, and the same for low scores. This is a *positive* relationship. If we look at the association between weight and exercise duration, we might expect to see lower scores in weight with higher exercise time in a *negative* relationship.

Scatter Plots

Visualizing these data can help to clarify patterns using a scatter plot, as shown in Figure 29-1. Each dot represents the intersection of a pair of related observations. The points in Plot A show a pattern in which the values of *Y* increase in exact proportion to the values of *X*, in a perfect positive relationship with data points falling on a straight line. In Plot B the data demonstrate a perfect negative relationship, with lower values of *Y* associated with higher values of *X*.

More realistic results are shown in the other plots. The closer the points approximate a straight line, the stronger the association. Plots C and D show a positive relationship, but the correlation in Plot D is not as strong. Plot E shows a negative relationship with greater variance from a straight line. In Plot F the points have a seemingly random pattern, reflecting no relationship.

> Positive correlations are sometimes called *direct* relationships. Negative correlations may also be described as *indirect* or *inverse* relationships.

The Correlation Coefficient

Inspection of a scatter plot provides some idea about the nature of a relationship but is not adequate for summarizing it. Correlation coefficients are used to quantitatively describe the strength and direction of a relationship between two variables. Represented by a lowercase *r*, correlation can take values ranging from –1.00 for a perfect negative relationship, to 0.00 for no correlation, to +1.00 for a perfect positive relationship. Perfect relationships are truly rare, however, and values of *X* and *Y* will typically manifest variation, yielding coefficients that fall between 0.00 and ±1.00. These values are expressed as decimals, usually to two places, such as $r = .14$ or $r = -.70$.

The plots in Figure 29-1 represent a variety of potential outcomes. The magnitude of the coefficient indicates the *strength* of the association between X and Y. The closer the value is to ±1.00, the stronger the relationship (see Box 29-1). The sign of the correlation coefficient indicates the *direction* of the relationship.

 There is often misunderstanding of negative correlations as being weaker or less meaningful, but that is not the case. The sign only indicates direction.

Hypothesis Testing

Correlation coefficients can be tested against a population value to determine if they are significant. A significant correlation is unlikely to have occurred by chance. Typically, the null hypothesis will state that the population correlation will be zero.

An alternative hypothesis can be specified as nondirectional or directional. Nondirectional hypotheses are more common, analyzed using two-tailed tests, recognizing the potential for positive or negative outcomes.

There may be instances, however, when a one-tailed test is justified when only one direction is of interest.

Assumptions for Correlation

Meaningful interpretation of correlation coefficients can only be made when certain assumptions are met.

- Subjects' scores represent the underlying population, which is normally distributed.
- Each subject contributes a score for X and Y.
- X and Y are independent measures so that one score is not a component of the other. For instance, it would make no statistical sense to correlate a measure of gait velocity with distance walked, as distance is a component of velocity (distance/time). Similarly, it is fruitless to correlate a subscale score on a functional assessment with the total score, as the first variable is included in the second. In each case, correlations will be artificially high because part of the variance in each quantity is being correlated with itself.
- X values are observed, not controlled. It is not appropriate, for instance, to assign subjects to a particular intervention dosage to correlate with a response. If it is of interest to see the effect of a

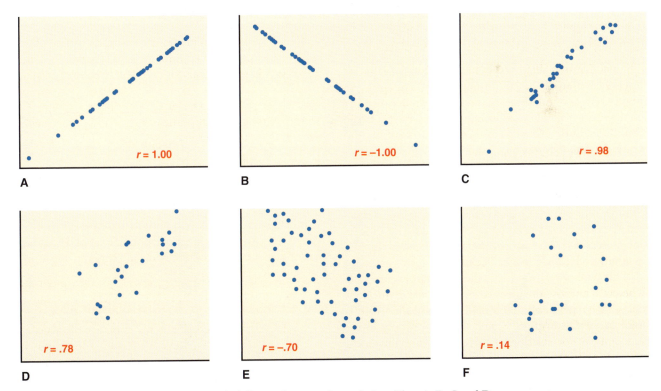

Figure 29–1 Examples of scatterplots with different degrees of correlation. Plots A, B, C and D represent strong positive correlations. Plot E shows a moderately strong negative correlation. Plot F shows a scatterplot with a random pattern and a correlation close to zero.

particular dosage of medication on an outcome, a regression procedure should be used (see Chapter 30).

- The relationship between X and Y must be linear. Most correlation coefficients cannot be meaningfully interpreted if there is a nonlinear pattern, although there are procedures to account for such relationships.

■ Linear and Curvilinear Relationships

The pattern of a relationship between two variables is often classified as linear or nonlinear. The plots in Figures 29-1A and B are perfectly linear because the points fall on a single straight line. Plots C-E can also be considered linear, although as they begin to deviate from a straight line their correlation decreases.

The coefficient r is a measure of *linear relationship* only. When a *curvilinear relationship* is present, the linear correlation coefficient will not be able to describe it accurately. For instance, a curvilinear shape typically characterizes the relationship between strength and age. As age increases so does strength, until a plateau is reached in adulthood, followed by a decline in elderly years.

This type of relationship is illustrated in Figure 29-2 where a strong systematic relationship is clearly evident between X and Y, although r = .58, suggesting only a moderate relationship. Because r measures only linear functions, the correlation coefficient for a curvilinear relationship can be small, even when X and Y are indeed related.

This should caution readers to be critical about the interpretation of correlation coefficients. It may not be reasonable to conclude that two variables are unrelated solely on the basis of a low correlation. By plotting a

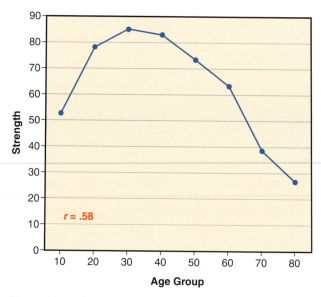

Figure 29-2 Illustration of a curvilinear relationship between age and strength. These data were also used in the explanation of quadratic trends in Chapter 26.

scatter diagram for all correlation analyses, researchers can observe whether the association in a set of data is linear or curvilinear and thereby decide if r is an appropriate statistic for analysis.

> The *eta coefficient* (η), also called the *correlation ratio*, is an index that does not assume a linear relationship between two variables. It can be interpreted in the same way as r, although η can only range from 0.00-1.00. This statistic requires that one variable is nominal.

> See the *Chapter 29 Supplement* for further description of the eta coefficient.

Pearson Product–Moment Correlation Coefficient

The most commonly reported measure of correlation is the **Pearson product–moment coefficient of correlation**, developed by the English statistician Karl Pearson. The statistic is given the symbol r for sample data and ρ (rho) for a population parameter. This is a parametric statistic and is appropriate for use when X and Y are continuous variables with underlying normal distributions on the interval or ratio scales.

> ➤ **CASE IN POINT #1**
>
> Researchers have studied several prognostic factors in children with traumatic brain injury (TBI).[3] Let's consider a study to examine the relationship between ambulatory function and cognitive status for 93 children who experienced a TBI. We hypothesize that there will be a relationship between these factors.

Hypothetical results for this study are shown in Table 29-1A. The null hypothesis states that there is no relationship between these two behaviors, making the correlation coefficient equal to zero in the population. The alternative hypothesis states that there will be a relationship, and the coefficient will not equal zero.

$$H_0: \rho = 0 \quad H_1: \rho \neq 0$$

Remember that even though we are using sample data, null hypotheses are written using population parameter designations, in this case ρ and not r. The alternative hypothesis can also be expressed as a directional hypothesis, indicating that the correlation coefficient will be greater or less than zero.

The *r* Statistic

Calculation of r is unwieldy, so we will focus on the output here, yielding $r = .348$ (see Table 29-1 ❷). This would be considered a relatively weak correlation, suggesting that there is a weak association between ambulation and cognitive status.

📌 For those with a need to know, the computational formula for the Pearson r is:

$$r = \frac{n\Sigma XY - (\Sigma X)(\Sigma Y)}{\sqrt{[n\Sigma X^2 - (\Sigma X)^2][n\Sigma Y^2 - (\Sigma Y)^2]}}$$

Although these calculations are cumbersome, they are straightforward.

🌐 See the *Chapter 29 Supplement* for calculation of the Pearson correlation coefficient.

DATA DOWNLOAD

Table 29-1	**Pearson Correlation Coefficient: Ambulation and Cognitive Status in Children with Traumatic Brain Injury (*N* = 93)**

A. Data: Scatterplot

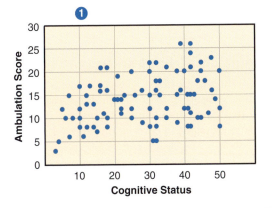

B. SPSS Output: Bivariate Correlation

Correlations

			Cognition		Ambulation
Cognition	Pearson Correlation	❸	1	❷	.348**
	Sig. (2-tailed)			❹	.001
	N		93		93
Ambulation	Pearson Correlation	❷	.348**	❸	1
	Sig. (2-tailed)		.001		
	N		93		93

**Correlation is significant at the 0.01 level (2-tailed).

❶ The scatterplot reveals a variable pattern with a positive linear trend, but does not approach a straight line.

❷ The Pearson correlation is .348. This matrix is redundant, showing the correlation of each variable with the other.

❸ The correlation of each variable with itself is 1.0.

❹ The correlation coefficient is significant at $p = .001$.

Test of Significance

The product–moment correlation coefficient can be subjected to a test of significance to determine if the observed value is significantly different from zero. Critical values of r are provided in Appendix Table A-4 for one- and two-tailed tests with $n - 2$ degrees of freedom. For this analysis, $df = 91$. The observed value of r must be *greater than or equal to* the tabled value to be significant.

In this case we will use a two-tailed test, since we proposed a nondirectional alternative hypothesis. Referring to the nearest value for df in the table, we will use the critical value $r(90) = .205$ for $\alpha_2 = .05$. The observed value, $r = .348$, is greater than this critical value, and H_0 is rejected. Computer output shows that $p = .001$ (see Table 29-1). These results indicate that the observed correlation is not likely to be the result of chance (see Box 29-2).

Clinical vs. Statistical Significance

The significance of a correlation coefficient does not mean that it represents a strong relationship or that it is clinically meaningful. Significance only indicates that an observed value is unlikely to be the result of chance. Correlation coefficients can be statistically powerful even with smaller samples.

As we can see in our example, the correlation of .348 is significant, even though it is not a strong value. The scatterplot shows a widely variable pattern. In fact, based on the critical value, even a correlation as small as .205 would be significant with this sample size. Looking at values in Table A-4, we can see that a sufficient increase in sample size can generate a significant correlation even if it is so small as to be a meaningless indicator of association.

Some authors are enamored with p values, often ignoring the strength of a relationship in their interpretation. But reporting significance is not useful to interpretation of correlations. Some authors *only* report p values, which gives no information about the strength of a relationship. Low correlations should not be discussed as clinically important just because they have achieved statistical significance. Such interpretations should be made on the basis of the magnitude of the correlation coefficient and its practical significance in the context of the variables being measured (See Focus on Evidence 29-1).

> **Results**
>
> In this sample of children who experienced a TBI, the Pearson correlation coefficient showed a significant relationship ($r(91) = .348$, $p = .001$) for a two-tailed test. Although the correlation was significant, the pattern of responses showed a weak relationship between ambulation and cognitive status.

Power Analysis and Effect Size

The correlation coefficient, r, is its own effect size index. The strength of the effect is indicated by the magnitude of the coefficient. Cohen[2] suggests that conventional effect sizes are:

Small $r = .10$
Medium $r = .30$
Large $r = .50$

As discussed in previous chapters, these values are not intended to serve as absolute cutoffs, and their use requires consideration of the context of the variables being studied. See Box 29-3 for illustration of power and sample size determinations using G*Power.

■ Correlation of Ranked Data

When ordinal data are used or when it is not reasonable to assume that data come from a normal distribution, nonparametric versions of correlation can be used.

Box 29-2   Correlation and Confidence

Most statistical packages do not calculate confidence intervals for the correlation coefficient, and the process is complex by hand.[4] Because values of r are restricted between 0 and 1, a transformation is needed to determine the confidence intervals. This process is called *Fisher's r to z transformation*, and tables can be found in most statistics texts and online. Fortunately, online calculators are available that facilitate this process without having to do the math.[5,6] For the data in Table 29-1, with $r = .348$ and $n = 93$,

$$95\% \ CI = .156 \ to \ .515$$

This interval does not cross zero, supporting the conclusion that this is a significant correlation. We are 95% confident that the true population correlation falls within this range. Given the wide interval within the low range of correlation, it will be a matter of judgment as to how clinically useful this measure would be.

> ### CASE IN POINT #2
>
> Researchers have established that reading comprehension difficulties appear to be critically dependent on a range of verbal language comprehension skills.[8] Suppose we designed a study to examine this relationship for a sample of 16 children with a learning disability. Scores are based on standardized tests using an ordinal scale (1–100). We hypothesize that there will be a positive correlation between these measures.

Focus on Evidence 29–1
Correlation and Validity: Defining "Useful"

There is growing interest in the study of sedentary behavior and its correlates, in an effort to develop interventions that will encourage more physical activity. Studies have used specially designed questionnaires to derive data on self-report sedentary time.

Two recent studies have established criterion validity of questionnaires by correlating self-report sedentary time with minutes of activity recorded by a movement monitoring device.[9,10] These studies examined activity in adolescents and adults, men and women. Both studies found their distributions were skewed and therefore used the nonparametric Spearman rank correlation (r_s) for analysis.

The studies found that participants overestimated their sedentary time compared to the minutes of activity logged by the device. They also found various differences between adolescents and adults and between men and women. Most relevant, however, is that they both documented significant correlations ranging from .02 to .52, predominantly around .30 and with narrow confidence intervals.

In summarizing findings, one study defined correlations as low, moderate or high using Cohen's conventional criteria.[10] Interestingly, they considered r_s = .52 as high, but both r_s = .49 and r_s = .38 as moderate. The other study compared findings to previous research, citing a systematic review that showed an average correlation of .30 in similar studies, suggesting that their findings of r_s = .30 in women and .25 in men indicated "above average" criterion validity.[9] One study involved 159 subjects[10] and the other tested 2,175 people,[9] assuring good power for their analyses. In their conclusions, both sets of authors said that the questionnaires would be "useful" and valid instruments for gathering information on sedentary behavior.

What does criterion validity mean, and how do correlation coefficients help to establish it? If the monitoring device is considered the "standard," is a correlation below .50 helpful in establishing the utility of the questionnaire? And how does one make judgments about high versus moderate correlations, when they vary by .03? You can draw your own judgments about how well validity has been established, but these findings illustrate why conventional criteria do not always make sense for clinical application. Authors should find the clinical relevance in their data, not take statistical "rules" too literally. And those who look to evidence for guidance must draw their own conclusions about how to use data in a meaningful way.

Box 29-3 Power and Sample Size: Pearson Correlation Coefficient

Post Hoc Analysis: Determining Power

The effect size index for the Pearson correlation coefficient is r. Therefore, no further calculations are needed to determine the index. To use G*Power, we must enter the effect size (the obtained value of r), the level of significance for a one- or two-tailed test, sample size, and the null value. For this analysis, r = .348, α_2 = .05, N = 93, and ρ = 0 under H_0. This results in 93% power (*see chapter supplement*). The power is quite high because we had a large sample, even though the actual correlation would not be considered strong.

Although conventional effect sizes suggest that this is a medium effect, it is possible that an important correlation between ambulation and cognitive status would be much higher. We might consider a medium effect to be .50, and large effect to be .70 or higher for our purposes. This is an important caveat with all power analysis, to identify the values that will provide meaningful interpretation and clinical application, regardless of power.

A Priori Analysis: Estimating Sample Size

If we were planning this study, we would first need to project an expected r based on prior studies or an estimate of what we would consider clinically meaningful. Let's assume in this case we determined that a correlation of at least .50 would be important. Using G*Power, we must enter the projected effect size r, level of significance for a one- or two-tailed test, desired power, and the null value. For r = .50, α_2 = .05, power = 80%, and ρ = 0 under H_0, the needed sample size is 29 subjects (*see chapter supplement*). A relatively small sample is needed to obtain a significant correlation at .50. A medium effect (r = .30) would generate a needed sample of 84 subjects. However, both of these effect size values may be too small to be clinically meaningful for this study. If we felt that a correlation of at least .80 would be meaningful, we would only need a sample of 9 subjects! If the effect size was that large, we would need few subjects to demonstrate it. However, if we don't attain that correlation, we would probably have too small a sample to show a significant effect.

Spearman Rank Correlation Coefficient

The **Spearman rank correlation coefficient**, given the symbol r_s (also called Spearman's rho), is a nonparametric analog of the Pearson r. The null hypothesis for the study of verbal and reading comprehension states that there is no association between these measures. The alternative hypothesis states that a positive correlation is expected:

$$H_0: r_s = 0 \quad H_1: r_s > 0.$$

Note that the hypothesis for the Spearman test uses r_s because this test does not approximate a population parameter.

The Spearman correlation is based on ranking X and Y scores. If there is a strong positive relationship between X and Y, we would expect these rankings to be consistent; that is, low ranks in X will correspond to low ranks in Y, and vice versa.

Test of Significance

Hypothetical data for this study are shown in Table 29-2. The Spearman correlation for these variables is high, $r_s = .92$. We can test the significance of r_s using critical values shown in Table 29-3. This table uses n rather than degrees of freedom to locate critical values. The observed value of r_s must be *greater than or equal to* the tabled value to achieve significance. For this example, we find the critical value $r_s(16) = .429$ at $\alpha_1 = .05$. Therefore, our calculated value of r_s is significant. The output in Table 29-2B indicates the actual $p < .001$.

> ▶ **Results**
> The relationship between reading comprehension and verbal language skills was examined using the Spearman rank correlation coefficient. We hypothesized that there would be a positive relationship and performed a one-tailed test. There was a strong

significant correlation ($r_s = .92$, $p < .001$), supporting the research hypothesis.

Kendall's Tau-b

Kendall's tau, τ, is similar to the Spearman correlation, appropriate for use with ranked data. Unlike Spearman, however, tau can be used as an unbiased estimate of a population parameter.[11] It is based on the concept of *concordance*, which is the probability that a pair of X,Y scores occur in similar order within the distribution. The statistic can range from -1.0 (where all pairs are *discordant*) to $+1.0$ (where all pairs are concordant).

There are actually three versions of Kendall's correlation: tau-a, tau-b, and tau-c. Versions a and b are similar, but b adjusts for ties and is used more often. Version c is used less often with data that are not symmetrical in the number of possible rankings.

Kendall's tau-b will typically be slightly smaller than the Spearman correlation for the same data, as shown in Table 29-2, although the significance of the two tests will usually be similar.[11] The Spearman correlation has historically been used more often, but that is likely

---

Table 29-2 Rank Correlations Using Spearman and Kendall's tau-b: Verbal and Reading Comprehension Scores ($N = 16$)

A. Data: Scatterplot

Scatterplot with Verbal on the x-axis (40–100) and Reading on the y-axis (40–100). ① The scatterplot reveals a strong positive linear pattern.

B. SPSS Output: Nonparametric Correlations

Correlations

			Verbal	Reading
Kendall's tau-b	Verbal	Correlation Coefficient	1.000	❷ .802**
		Sig. (2-tailed)	.	❷ .000
		N	16	16
	Reading	Correlation Coefficient	.802**	1.000
		Sig. (2-tailed)	.000	.
		N	16	16
Spearman's rho	Verbal	Correlation Coefficient	1.000	❸ .920**
		Sig. (2-tailed)	.	❸ .000
		N	16	16
	Reading	Correlation Coefficient	.920**	1.000
		Sig. (2-tailed)	.000	.
		N	16	16

**Correlation is significant at the 0.01 level (1-tailed).

---

❶ The scatterplot reveals a strong positive linear pattern.

❷ Kendall's tau-b results in a correlation of .802, which is significant ($p < .001$). The tau correlation is a more conservative test, accounting for tied ranks in the data.

❸ Spearman's rho results in a correlation of .920, which is significant ($p < .001$).

Table 29-3	Critical Values of Spearman's Rank Correlation Coefficient, r_s				
	α_2	.10	.05	.02	.01
n	α_1	.05	.025	.01	.005
10		.564	.648	.745	.794
11		.536	.618	.709	.755
12		.503	.587	.671	.727
13		.484	.560	.648	.703
14		.464	.538	.622	.675
15		.443	.521	.604	.654
16		.429	.503	.582	.635

This is an abridged version of this table for purposes of illustration. Refer to the Chapter 29 Supplement for the full table.

because it is much easier to calculate by hand than τ, which is more complex and arduous—an issue that is no longer relevant with statistical packages.

 See the *Chapter 29 Supplement* for data and calculations for Spearman's rho.

Correlation of Dichotomies

Measures of association are also useful with dichotomous variables on the nominal or ordinal scale. The integers 0 and 1 are usually assigned to represent the levels of a dichotomous variable. When either X or Y (or both) is a dichotomy, specialized correlation coefficients are used to test associations.

- The **phi coefficient, ϕ**, is used when both X and Y are dichotomous variables. Phi is a special case of the product–moment correlation coefficient, given only two values of X and Y arranged in a 2×2 contingency table. Phi can be calculated using the chi-square statistic, described in Chapter 28, or it can be run as a Pearson correlation with the same result.
- The **point biserial correlation coefficient, r_{pb}**, is used when one dichotomous variable (X) is correlated with one continuous variable (Y). It, too, is a special case of the product–moment coefficient, given that scores on Y are classified into two series: those who scored 0 and those who scored 1 on X. The point biserial coefficient reflects the degree to which the continuous variable discriminates between the two categories of the dichotomous variable. It is statistically equivalent to an independent t-test where the dichotomous variable identifies two groups.
- The **rank biserial correlation, r_{rb}** is a variant of the point biserial procedure, used when a dichotomy is

correlated with a continuous variable on the ordinal scale.[12] Like other nonparametric tests, the total sample is ranked, and then the average rank of each X category is computed. If there is an association between the variables, the higher ranks will be associated with the category labeled 1, and lower ranks will be associated with the category labeled 0. This analysis is analogous to the Mann-Whitney U test, where the dichotomous variable identifies two groups.

 See the *Chapter 29 Supplement* for illustrations and calculations of phi, point biserial and rank biserial correlations.

Interpreting Correlation Coefficients

Correlation Versus Comparison

The interpretation of correlation is based on the concept of *covariance*. If two distributions vary directly, so that a change in X is proportional to a change in Y, then X and Y are said to covary. With great consistency in X and Y scores, covariance is high. This is reflected in a coefficient close to 1.00. This concept must be distinguished from the determination of *differences between* two distributions.

To illustrate this point, suppose you were told that exam scores for courses in anatomy and physiology were highly correlated. Would it be reasonable to infer, then, that a student with a 90 in anatomy would be expected to attain a score close to 90 in physiology?

Consider the paired distributions of exam grades listed in Table 29-4. Obviously, the scores are decidedly different. The anatomy scores range from 47 to 65 and the physiology scores from 63 to 76. The mean anatomy grade is 55.3, whereas the mean physiology grade is 69.6. Each student's scores have a proportional relationship, resulting in a high correlation coefficient (r = .87), but the values do not agree with each other. Correlation, therefore, will not necessarily provide information about the difference between sets of data, only about the relative order of scores, whatever their magnitude. The t-test is required to examine differences. It is inappropriate to make inferences about similarities or differences between distributions based on correlation coefficients.

Correlation and Causation

It is also important to distinguish the concepts of causation and correlation. The presence of a statistical association between two variables does not necessarily imply the presence of a causal relationship. In many situations a strong relationship between variables X and Y may

Table 29-4	Anatomy and Physiology Grades ($r = .87$)	
STUDENT	**ANATOMY**	**PHYSIOLOGY**
1	50	60
2	56	72
3	52	7
4	57	71
5	47	63
6	65	75
7	60	76
Mean	55 ± 6.2	69 ± 5.9

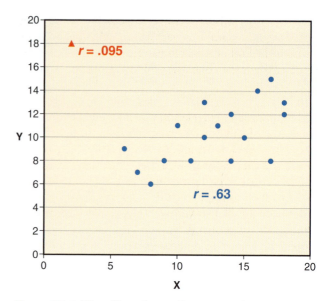

Figure 29–4 The effect of an outlier on correlation. Without the outlier, the original distribution has a linear correlation of $r = .63$, $p = .007$. With the single outlier included (red triangle), the correlation is $r = .095$, $p = .707$.

actually be a function of some third variable, or a set of variables, that is related to both X and Y.

For example, researchers have shown that weak grip strength and slowed hand reaction time are associated with falling in elderly persons.[13] Certainly, we would not infer that decreased hand function causes falls. However, weak hand musculature may be associated with general deconditioning and is related to balance and motor recovery deficits. These associated factors are more likely to be the contributory factors to falls. Therefore, a study that examined the correlation between falls and hand function would not be able to make any valid assumptions about causative factors (see Fig. 29-3).

Outliers

If a set of data points represents a distribution of related scores, the points will tend to cluster in a pattern. But sometimes, one or two deviant scores are separated from the cluster, so that they distort the statistical association. For example, the blue data points in Figure 29-4 show some variability, but most of the points fall within a definite linear pattern ($r = .63$). With the addition of one point that does not fit with the rest of the pattern, the correlation reduces to $r = .10$. This point is called an **outlier,** because it lies outside the obvious cluster of scores. This point has an unusual XY value and has significantly altered the statistical description of the data.

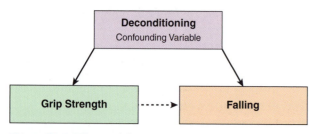

Figure 29–3 The need for caution in assigning cause to a correlation. The relationship between grip strength and falls is actually a function of their mutual relationship with deconditioning.

Why Outliers Occur

Researchers must consider several possibilities regarding outliers. The score may, indeed, be a true score but an extreme one, because the sample is too small to generate a full range of observations. If more subjects were tested, there might be less of a discrepancy between the outlier and the rest of the scores.

There may be also be circumstances peculiar to this data point that are responsible for the large deviation. For example, the score may be a function of error in measurement or recording, equipment malfunction, or some miscalculation. It may be possible to go back to the original data to find and correct this type of error. Other extraneous factors may also contribute to the aberrant score, some of which are correctable, others that are not. For instance, the data point may have been collected by a different tester who is not reliable. Or the researcher may find that the subject was inappropriately included in the sample.

Outliers can have serious effects on the outcome and should always be examined using a scatter plot. Some researchers consider scores beyond three standard deviations from the mean to be outliers.

The researcher must determine if outliers should be retained or discarded in the analysis. This decision should be made only after a thorough evaluation of the experimental conditions, the data collection procedures, and the data themselves. As a general rule, there is no statistical rationale for discarding an outlier. However, if a causal factor can be identified, the point may be omitted, provided that the causal factor is unique to the outlier.[14] It is helpful to perform the analysis with and without the outlier, to demonstrate how inclusion of the score changes the conclusions drawn from the data.

Range of Test Values

Generalization of correlation values should be limited to the range of values used to obtain the correlation. For example, if age and strength were correlated for subjects between 2 and 15 years old, a strong positive relationship would probably be found. It would not, however, be legitimate to extrapolate this relationship to subjects older than 15, as the sample data are not sufficient to know if the relationship holds beyond that age. Therefore, it is not safe to assume that correlation values for a total sample validly represent any subgroup of the sample, and vice versa.

Restricting the Range of Scores

The magnitude of the correlation coefficient is a function of how closely a cluster of scores resembles a straight line. When the range of X or Y scores is limited, correlation will not adequately reflect the extent of their relationship. For instance, if the range of X values is only at the lower end of the scale, it would not be possible to see the true linear relationship between the two variables. Such a correlation may be close to zero, even though the true correlation between variables may be quite high. It is advisable to include as wide a range of values as possible for correlation analysis.

Scores must also show variance to be able to demonstrate correlation. If all scores cluster around the same values, a linear relationship cannot be demonstrated. If correlation studies include subjects with similar scores, the correlation may appear artificially low. When recruiting subjects for a correlation study, researchers should make sure there is a range of scores.

■ Partial Correlation

The product–moment correlation coefficient, r, offers the researcher a simple and easily understood measure of the association between X and Y. The interpretation of r is limited, however, because it cannot account for the possible influence of other variables on that relationship.

➤ **CASE IN POINT #3**

Clinicians and researchers are often interested in identifying factors that influence rehabilitation hospital length of stay (LOS). Age has been recognized as an influential factor. We can design a study to look at the relationship between age and LOS. However, studies have also shown that physical function can impact

LOS.[15] If we were interested in studying the relationship between age and length of hospital stay, we might need to consider the additional effect of mobility.

Assume that we have found a strong correlation between age and LOS, $r = .70$. This relationship is illustrated by the shaded overlapped portion in Figure 29-5A. If, however, older patients also tend to have greater functional limitations, then the observed relationship between hospital stay and age may actually be the result of their mutual relationship with function; that is, the hospital stay may actually be better explained by the patient's functional status.

We can resolve this dilemma by looking at the relationship between hospital stay and age with the effect of functional status controlled, using a process called **partial correlation**.

The *partial correlation coefficient* is the correlation between X and Y, with the effect of a third variable, Z, statistically removed. For instance, in the preceding example, assume X is age, Y is hospital stay, and Z is functional status. We would want to know how much of the observed relationship between age and hospital stay (r_{XY}) can be attributed to the confounding influence of function, and how much is purely the relationship between age and hospital stay. The term $r_{XY \cdot Z}$ is used to represent the correlation of X and Y, with the effect of Z eliminated.

For example, suppose we are given the following correlations for a sample of 50 patients:

$$r_{XY} = .70 \text{ (hospital stay with age)}$$
$$r_{XZ} = -.82 \text{ (hospital stay with function)}$$
$$r_{YZ} = -.68 \text{ (function with age)}$$

We "remove" the effect of function from r_{XY} by first determining how much of the variance in both hospital stay and age is explained by function, as shown in Figure 29-5B and C. The overlapped, shaded portions represent the shared variance between the two variables. Panel D shows how these relationships intersect. Once we remove the effect of function, the remaining overlap between hospital stay and age is reduced (the white area). This area represents the relationship between hospital stay and age with the effect of function canceled out. This is the partial correlation.

🔑 The measure of shared variance is best defined by squaring the correlation coefficient. For example, for a correlation of .70 for hospital stay and age, $r^2 = .49$. Therefore, approximately 50% of the variance in hospital stay can be accounted by age. This concept will be revisited in Chapter 30.

For the data in our example, $r_{XY \cdot Z} = .34$. When we compare this partial correlation to the original correlation

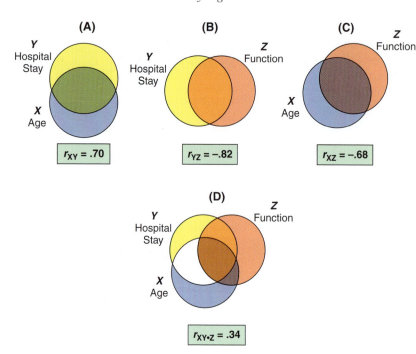

Figure 29–5 Representation of partial correlation between hospital stay (Y) and age (X), with the effect of function (Z) removed. In A, B, and C, the simple correlations between each pair of variables are illustrated. The overlapping areas represent their shared variance. In D, the shaded areas represent those parts of hospital stay and age that are explained by function. The white area shows the common variance in hospital stay and age that is not related to function, or their partial correlation.

of X and Y ($r_{XY} = .70$), we can see that age and hospital stay no longer demonstrate as strong a relationship. A large part of the observed association between them could be accounted for by their common relationship with functional status.

The simple correlation between X and Y is called a *zero-order correlation*. The term $r_{XY \cdot Z}$ is called a *first-order partial correlation*, because it represents a correlation with the effect of one variable eliminated. The significance of a first-order partial correlation can be determined by referring to critical values of r using $n - 3$ degrees of freedom. Partial correlation can be expanded to control for more than one variable at a time.

Partial correlation is a useful analytic tool for eliminating competing explanations for an association, thereby providing a clearer explanation of the true nature of an observed relationship and ruling out extraneous factors. This discussion will be expanded in Chapter 30 in relation to regression analysis.

COMMENTARY

Smoking is one of the leading causes of statistics.

—*Fletcher Knebel (1911-1993)*

American author

Correlation is a statistic that is generally understood, yet often misinterpreted or misused. Researchers, practitioners, and consumers must be aware of the potential danger of using statistical correlation as evidence of a clinical association simply on the basis of numbers, recognizing that any two quantitative variables can be correlated, whether or not they are based on a logical framework. Most importantly, the interpretation must be able to support what the correlation means, or why the two variables are related—which often translates to

trying to establish a causal relationship. All statistical analysis is limited by the clinical significance of the data being analyzed.

There are many examples of spurious correlations that illustrate this point. For example, Snedecor and Cochran[7] cite a correlation of –.98 between the annual birth rate in Great Britain from 1875 to 1920 and the annual production of pig iron in the United States. Maybe we can view these variables as related to some general socioeconomic trends, but surely, neither one could seriously be considered a function of the other. Willoughby[16] really puts this into perspective, arguing that a high positive correlation between a boy's height and the length of his trousers would not mean that lengthening trousers would produce taller boys! Researchers are often tempted to draw conclusions about relationships without considering the potential relevance of a third variable that might actually be the cause for both. This important caveat will be addressed further in different contexts in several upcoming chapters.

REFERENCES

1. Hinkle DE, Wiersma W, Jurs SG. *Applied Statistics for the Behavioral Sciences*. 5th ed. Boston: Houghton Mifflin; 2003.
2. Taylor RR. Deciding on an approach to data analysis. In: R.R. Taylor, ed. *Kielhofner's Research in Occupational Therapy: Methods of Inquiry for Enhancing Practice*. 2nd ed. Philadelphia: FA Davis; 2017:330-341.
3. Dumas HM, Haley SM, Ludlow LH, Carey TM. Recovery of ambulation during inpatient rehabilitation: physical therapist prognosis for children and adolescents with traumatic brain injury. *Phys Ther* 2004;84(3):232-242.
4. Field A. *Discovering Statistics Using IBM SPSS Statistics*. 5th ed. Thousand Oaks, CA: Sage; 2018.
5. Confidence interval online calculators. Available at https://www.sdmproject.com/utilities/?show=Conf.%20intervals. Accessed January 7, 2019.
6. The confidence interval of rho. VassarStats: Website for Statistical Computation. Available at http://vassarstats.net/rho.html. Accessed January 7, 2019.
7. Cohen J. *Statistical Power Analysis for the Behavioral Sciences*. 2nd ed. Hillsdale, NJ: Lawrence Erlbaum; 1988.
8. Hulme C, Snowling MJ. The interface between spoken and written language: developmental disorders. *Philos Trans R Soc Lond B Biol Sci*;369(1634):20120395.
9. Scholes S, Coombs N, Pedisic Z, et al. Age- and sex-specific criterion validity of the Health Survey for England Physical Activity and Sedentary Behavior Assessment Questionnaire as compared with accelerometry. *Am J Epidemiol* 2014;179(12):1493-1502.
10. Busschaert C, De Bourdeaudhuij I, Van Holle V, Chastin SF, Cardon G, De Cocker K. Reliability and validity of three questionnaires measuring context-specific sedentary behaviour and associated correlates in adolescents, adults and older adults. *Int J Behav Nutr Phys Act* 2015;12:117.
11. Daniel WW. *Applied Nonparametric Statistics*. 2nd ed. Independence, KY: Cengage Learning; 2000.
12. Glass GV. Note on rank-biserial correlation. *Educ Psychol Measur* 1966;26:623-631.
13. Nevitt MC, Cummings SR, Hudes ES. Risk factors for injurious falls: a prospective study. *J Gerontol* 1991;46:M164-170.
14. Snedecor GW, Cochran WG. *Statistical Methods*. 8th ed. Ames, IA: Iowa State University Press; 1989.
15. Graham JE, Radice-Neumann DM, Reistetter TA, Hammond FM, Dijkers MP, Granger CV. Influence of sex and age on inpatient rehabilitation outcomes among older adults with traumatic brain injury. *Arch Phys Med Rehabil* 2010;91(1):43-50.
16. Willoughby RR. Cum hoc ergo propter hoc. *School and Society* 1940;51:485.

CHAPTER 30

Regression

Correlation statistics are useful for describing the relative strength of a relationship between variables. However, when a researcher wants to predict an outcome or to explain the nature of that relationship, a **regression** procedure is used. These functions are crucial to effective clinical decision making, helping to explain empirical clinical observations and providing information that can be used to set realistic goals for our patients. They also have important implications for prognosis, efficiency, and quality of patient care, especially in situations where resources are limited.

The purpose of this chapter is to describe the foundations of regression and how it can be used to interpret clinical data. Discussions include techniques for simple linear regression, multiple regression, logistic regression, and analysis of covariance.

■ The Basics of Regression

The value of a correlation coefficient, r, is an indicator of the degree of a relationship between two variables. The value of r is limited in its interpretation, however, because it represents only the strength of an association, not its predictive accuracy.

Coefficient of Determination (r^2)

To understand how relationships can be explained, we must go back to the concepts of variance and correlation,

illustrated in Figure 30-1. In panel A there is almost total overlap of variance for two variables, X and Y. These variables would be highly correlated. By knowing values of X, we could accurately predict Y. In panel B, there is almost no overlap. These variables have very little variance in common and X would not be predictive of Y. In panel C, two variables have substantial, but not complete, overlap. In this case, some other

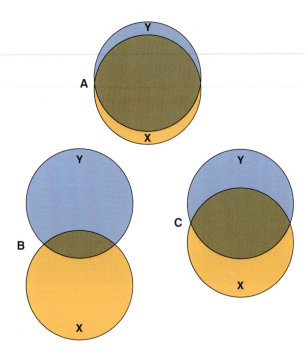

Figure 30–1 Conceptual illustrations of shared variance in the prediction of Y by knowing X. **A)** Almost total overlap of variance between X and Y, so X would be highly predictive of Y with shared variance. **B)** Very little overlap, indicating that X does not help explain Y. **C)** Moderate overlap, some prediction accuracy, but there is still a portion of variance in Y that is not explained by X.

unknown or unidentified factors must account for the remaining variance.

Statisticians have shown that the square of the correlation coefficient, r^2, indicates the proportion of variance that is shared by two variables, or that portion of variance in Y that can be *explained* by knowing the variance in X. Therefore, r^2 is a measure of the accuracy of prediction of Y based on X. This term is called the **coefficient of determination**, but you will typically only see it referred to as "R squared." Values of r^2 will range from 0.00 to 1.00. No negative ratios are possible because it is a squared value.

■ Simple Linear Regression

The primary goal of regression is to develop an equation to calculate a predicted value based on a related variable. In its simplest form, *linear regression* involves the examination of two variables that are linearly related, to determine how well an *independent variable* X predicts values of a *dependent variable* Y. Both X and Y variables are expected to be continuous.

> 📌 Dependent variables may also be called *response* or *outcome* variables. Independent variables may also be referred to as *predictor* variables, *explanatory* variables, or **covariates**.

> ➤ **CASE IN POINT #1**
> Research has shown that there is a high positive correlation between body mass index (BMI) and systolic blood pressure (SBP).[1] Let's consider hypothetical data from a sample of 10 women, to determine if we can predict their SBP by knowing their BMI. These variables have a correlation of $r = .87$.

In this example, we want to predict values of SBP (Y) by knowing values of BMI (X). The scatterplot in Figure 30-2A illustrates the unlikely situation where X and Y are perfectly correlated, $r = 1.00$. Therefore, the line that connects the dots would allow us to predict an exact value of Y for each value of X simply by finding the coordinates along the line. That means that if we know the value of X, we wouldn't even have to measure Y, because we could accurately predict it.

With correlations less than 1.00, however, we can't be as accurate, and we would only be able to estimate Y values. So let's consider a more realistic scenario, as shown in Figure 30-2B. We can see that the data fall in a linear pattern, with larger values of BMI associated with larger values of SBP, but it's not perfect ($r = .87$).

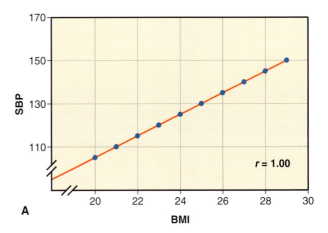

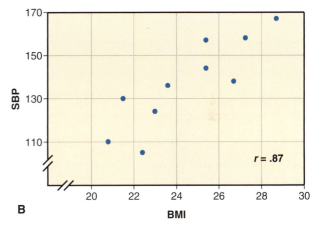

Figure 30–2 Scatter plots of BMI (X) and systolic blood pressure (Y) for 10 women. **A)** Perfect correlation with regression line, **B)** Plot with strong correlation.

> 🔑 Scatterplots for correlation analysis do not specify independent and dependent variables, and it does not matter which variable is designated as X or Y. In regression, however, these designations are relevant. The independent variable (the predictor) is always plotted along the X axis, and the dependent variable (the response) is plotted along the Y axis.

The Regression Line

Even if correlation is not perfect, we can still use the distribution to predict Y scores. We want to draw a line to fit the data, but the line would not go through all the points, making it only an estimate. Because some points would fall above and below the line, its prediction would not be exact, and there will be some error. The process of regression identifies the one line that "best" describes the orientation of all data points in the scatter plot. This is called the **linear regression line** or the **line of best fit**.

The Regression Equation

The algebraic representation of the regression line is given by

$$\hat{Y} = a + bX$$

The quantity $\hat{Y}$ (Y-hat) is the predicted value of Y. The term a is the **regression constant**. It is the Y-intercept, representing the value of Y when $X = 0$. This can be a positive or negative value. The term b is the **regression coefficient**. It is the slope of the line, which is the rate of change in Y for each one-unit change in X. If $b = 0$, the slope of the line is horizontal, indicating no relationship between X and Y, where Y is constant for all values of X. The positive or negative direction of the slope will correspond to a positive or negative correlation between X and Y.

> 📌 You may remember learning the equation for a straight line a little differently from algebra as $Y = mX + b$, or some version of that. It all means the same thing, just a little change in terminology and letters.

The Regression Model

Figure 30-3A shows the regression of SBP (Y) on BMI (X) for the sample of 10 women. The values that fall on the regression line are the predicted values, $\hat{Y}$, for any given value of X. However, we can see that most data points fall above or below the line. Therefore, if we substitute any X value in the regression equation and solve for $\hat{Y}$, we will obtain a predicted value that will probably be somewhat different from the actual value of Y, some with more error than others.

We can visualize this error component in Figure 30-3B. The actual Y value for each data point is some positive or negative vertical distance from $\hat{Y}$ on the regression line. These distances $(Y - \hat{Y})$ are called **residuals**, which represent the degree of error in the regression line.

The line of best fit for a set of data points is the unique line that will minimize these error components and yield the smallest total residuals, $\Sigma(Y-\hat{Y})$. However, to get the sum of the residuals, we must first square these values to get rid of minus signs $[\Sigma(Y-\hat{Y})^2]$ because the sum of the residuals will always equal zero (remember calculating sums of squares in Chapter 22). Therefore, this method of "fitting" the regression line is called **least squares method**. The sum of the squared residuals will reflect the total error.

The Regression Line and Residuals

Table 30-1A shows the SBP and BMI data for 10 women. Values for the regression coefficient, B, for BMI and the

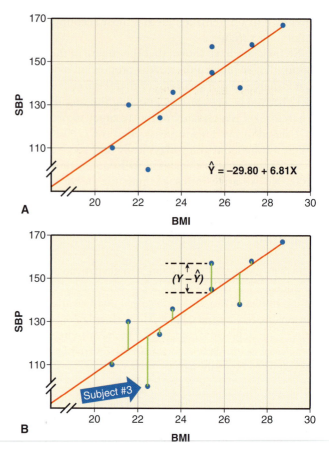

A

B

Figure 30–3 **A)** Least squares regression line for the linear regression of SBP on BMI. **B)** Deviation of scores from the regression line. Vertical distances represent residuals, $Y-\hat{Y}$. The value for subject #3 is located at $X=22.45$, $Y = 105$, with a residual of -18.08.

regression constant are reported in Table 30-1 ❺, yielding the regression equation

$$SBP = -29.80 + 6.81(BMI)$$

The sign of the regression coefficient indicates the direction of the relationship between X and Y, which will also match the sign of the correlation coefficient.

> 📌 If you like the math, the regression coefficients can be determined by:
>
> $$b = \frac{\Sigma XY - (\Sigma X)(\Sigma Y)}{n\Sigma X^2 - (\Sigma X)^2}$$
>
> $$a = \bar{X} - b\bar{Y}$$

> See the *Chapter 30 Supplement* for illustration of calculation of terms for the regression line.

A. Data

$$\hat{Y} = -29.80 + 6.81X \quad \textbf{❶}$$

Subject	BMI(X)	SBP(Y)	$\hat{Y}$	$Y-\hat{Y}$
1	20.80	110	111.85	−1.85
2	21.55	130	116.96	13.04
3	22.45	105	123.08	−18.08
4	23.00	124	126.83	−2.83
5	23.60	136	130.92	5.08
6	25.40	145	143.17	1.83
7	25.40	157	143.17	13.83
8	26.70	138	152.03	−14.03
9	27.25	158	155.77	2.23
10	28.70	167	165.65	1.35

Based on data shown in Figure 30-3

B. Residual Plot

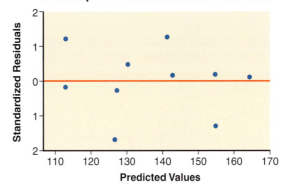

Scatterplot of Standardized Residuals

C. SPSS Output: Linear Regression

Descriptive Statistics ❷

	Mean	Std. Deviation	N
SBP	137.0000	20.48848	10
BMI	24.4850	2.61014	10

Model Summary ❸

Model	R	R Square	Adjusted R Square	Std. Error of the Estimate
1	.868[a]	.753	.722	10.79634

a. Predictors: (Constant), BMI

Correlations ❷

		SBP	BMI
Pearson Correlation	SBP	1.000	.868
	BMI	.868	1.000
Sig. (1-tailed)	SBP	.	.001
	BMI	.001	.

ANOVA[a] ❹

Model		Sum of Squares	df	Mean Square	F	Sig.
1	Regression	2845.512	1	2845.512	24.412	.001[b]
	Residual	932.488	8	116.561		
	Total	3778.000	9			

a. Dependent Variable: SBP
b. Predictors: (Constant), BMI

Coefficients[a]

Model		Unstandardized Coefficients ❺ B	Std. Error	Standardized Coefficients Beta	❻ t	Sig.	95% Confidence Interval for B Lower Bound	Upper Bound
1	(Constant)	−29.800	33.931		−.878	.405	−108.046	48.446
	BMI	6.812	1.379	.868	4.941	.001	3.633	9.992

a. Dependent Variable: SBP

---

❶ The data show raw scores, predicted values of SBP ($\hat{Y}$) and residual scores ($Y-\hat{Y}$).

❷ Descriptive statistics for each variable and their correlation. BMI and SBP have a strong positive correlation ($r = .868$).

❸ R-square and SEE reflect the degree of accuracy in the regression equation.

❹ The analysis of variance of regression demonstrates that there is a significant relationship ($p = .001$) between the independent and dependent variables (matches correlation). The *df* associated with SS_{reg} equal the number of predictor variables, in this case $k = 1$. The total *df* will equal $N-1$. The df for the residual variance, df_{res}, will be $N - k - 1$.

❺ The regression equation is: $\hat{Y} = -29.80 + 6.81(BMI)$.

❻ A *t*-test is used to test the significance of the regression coefficient for BMI. This *p* value will equal the probability identified in the ANOVA and correlation, as they are all essentially testing the same thing. A significance test for the constant is run, but it is not meaningful, and is ignored.

Portions of the output have been omitted for clarity.

We can use these values to calculate the predicted score ($\hat{Y}$) for any individual using the regression equation. For example, if we were presented with a woman with a BMI of 22.45 (subject #3), we would predict that her SBP would be

$$SBP = -29.80 + 6.81\,(22.45) = 123.08$$

The actual blood pressure value for this subject, however, was 105. Therefore, the residual or error component of prediction is

$$(Y - \hat{Y}) = 105 - 123.08 = -18.08$$

The data point for this subject falls below the regression line. Therefore, the regression equation overestimates SBP for this subject, and the residual is negative.

Residuals are shown under the column labeled ($Y - \hat{Y}$) in Table 30-1A. Most of the errors of prediction in this example are relatively small, because the correlation for these data is strong, and the points cluster close to the regression line. Note that six of the subjects have residuals of 5 points or less, as these points rest very close to the regression line.

Prediction Accuracy

In the section labeled Model Summary in Table 30-1 ❸ we get several pieces of information related to prediction accuracy.

- The value for R is the correlation coefficient between the two variables ($R = .868$). Regression analysis uses the uppercase R instead of r.
- The value for R^2 indicates the proportion of variance in the dependent variable that is explained by the independent variable. In this example, $R^2 = .753$. This would generally be considered a strong relationship, with BMI accounting for more than 75% of the variance in SBP.
- The **adjusted R Square** is slightly smaller than R^2. Because we can always expect some degree of error when explaining variance, this represents a chance-corrected value of R^2. Some researchers prefer to report the adjusted value as a more accurate reflection of the strength of the regression. This value becomes more relevant when there are several predictor variables.
- The **standard error of the estimate (SEE)** reflects the variance of errors on either side of the regression line, or the residuals. The SEE can be thought of as an indicator of the average error of prediction for the regression equation. Therefore, the SEE is helpful for interpreting the usefulness of a regression equation where reliance on a correlation coefficient can be misleading.

Tests of Significance

The regression analysis tests the null hypothesis H_0: $b = 0$ and is analogous to testing the significance of the correlation between X and Y. If H_0 is true, the slope of the regression line would essentially be horizontal. If H_0 is false, b is significantly different from zero.

This hypothesis is tested in three ways. First, we can see the significance of the correlation coefficient (see Table 30-1 ❷). Second, an **analysis of variance of regression** tests how much of the variance in scores is explained by the regression line. The sum of squares for the regression reflects the variance that is explained by the relationship between SBP and BMI (see Table 30-1 ❹). Third, the slope (regression coefficient) is tested using a t-test (see Table 30-1 ❻). These analyses are all essentially testing the same thing, resulting in $p = .001$. Therefore, we reject H_0 and conclude that there is a significant relationship between SBP and BMI. These p values do not indicate how strong the association is, just that it is not likely to have occurred by chance.

📌 There is a direct relationship between R^2 and the analysis of variance of regression, as both are measures of shared variance:

$$R^2 = \frac{SS_{reg}}{SS_{total}} = \frac{2845.512}{3778.000} = .753$$

▶ **Results**

Linear regression was used to examine the strength of the relationship between BMI and SBP. The correlation between these variables was strong ($r = .868$, $p = .001$). The regression resulted in $R^2 = .753$, fitting the regression line $Y = -29.80 + 6.81(BMI)$. These data suggest that BMI is a strong predictor of SBP.

Assumptions for Regression Analysis

In any regression procedure, we recognize that the straight line we fit to sample data is only an approximation of the true regression line that exists for the underlying population. To make inferences about population parameters from sample data, we must consider the statistical assumptions that affect the validity of the regression equation.

For any given value of X, we can assume that a normal distribution of Y scores exists in the population; that is, the observed value of Y in a sample for a given X is actually one random score from the larger distribution of possible Y scores at that value of X. This means that if we had studied many subjects at each level of BMI, we would see a range of blood pressure scores for the same value of X.

Some of these Y values would be above the regression line, some would be below it, and some might be right on it. For instance, subjects #6 and #7 both had a BMI of 25.40, but different blood pressure scores. As shown in Table 30-1A, subject #6 has a predicted score very close to the actual score, and subject #7 has a larger residual. Theoretically, if we took measurements for many women with a BMI of 25.40, we would get varied SBP scores that would form a normal distribution, and the mean of the Y scores would fall on the regression line (equal to $\hat{Y}$). Therefore, the least-squares line is actually an estimate of the population regression line, and each point on the line is an estimate of the population mean $\bar{Y}$ at each value of X. Having several measures for each value of X reduces standard error, and improves the accuracy of prediction.

Analysis of Residuals

One way to determine if the normality assumption for regression analysis has been met is to examine a plot of residuals, as shown in Figure 30-4. By plotting the residuals on the Y-axis against the predicted scores on the X-axis, we can appreciate the magnitude and distribution of the residual scores. The central horizontal axis represents the mean of the residuals, or zero deviation from the regression line. When the linear regression model is a good fit, the residual scores will be randomly dispersed close to zero, as in panel A. The wider the distribution of residuals around the zero axis, the greater the error.

Other patterns illustrate problematic residual distributions. The pattern in panel B indicates that the variance of the residuals is not consistent but is dependent on the value of the predicted variable. Residual error increases as the predicted value gets larger. Therefore, the assumptions of normality and equality of variance are not met. A curvilinear pattern, shown in panel C, reflects a nonlinear relationship, negating the validity of the linear model. Other deviant residual patterns may be observed, such as diagonal patterns or a run of positive or negative residuals, all indicating some problem in the interpretation of the regression model.

Standardized residuals can be obtained by dividing each residual score by the standard deviation of the residual distribution. These values are often used instead of observed residuals to normalize the scale of measurement, analogous to z-scores, allowing the residuals to be expressed in standard deviation units. The residual plot in Table 30-1 ❷ shows these values for the SBP study. The standardized residuals are on the Y axis, ranging from –2 to +2 SD (a 95% confidence interval). We can see that the residuals are distributed around the center line, none going beyond ±2 SD, and the horizontal pattern suggests no bias. This approach is especially useful when different distributions are compared.

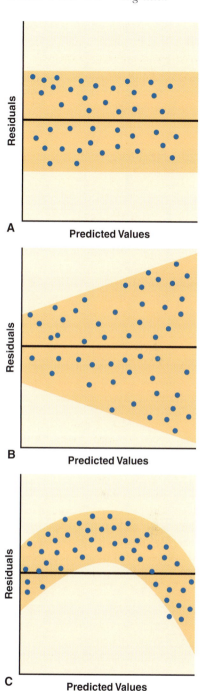

Figure 30–4 Patterns of residuals (Y-axis) against predicted scores (X-axis). **A)** Horizontal band demonstrates that assumptions for linear regression have been met. **B)** Residuals increase as predicted values increase. **C)** Curvilinear pattern indicates nonlinear relationship.

Transforming Data

When residual data do not fall into the horizontal pattern, the researcher may choose to transform one or both sets of data to more closely satisfy the necessary assumptions.

Such transformations may stabilize the variance in the data, normalize the distributions, or create a more linear relationship (see Appendix C). When curvilinear tendencies are observed, polynomial regression models may be used to better represent the data. This approach is discussed later in this chapter.

■ Multiple Regression

Multiple regression is an extension of simple linear regression analysis, allowing for prediction of Y using a set of several independent X variables. The intent is to explain more of the variance in Y than one predictor can do alone. Like simple linear regression, multiple regression is also based on the concept of least squares, so that the model minimizes error in predicting Y. However, we can no longer visualize regression as a single line, but conceptually as a linear relationship in a multidimensional space.

Multiple regression can accommodate continuous and categorical independent variables, which may be naturally occurring or experimentally manipulated. The dependent variable, Y, must be a continuous measure.

➤ CASE IN POINT #2

Consider again the question of BMI as a predictor of SBP, but this time we'll expand it with a hypothetical sample of 145 men and women. In this group, the correlation of BMI and SBP is $r = .68$ and $r^2 = .46$. Based on this relationship, we would expect that the remaining variance in SBP (54%) must be a function of other factors. For this example, we will look at the potential additional contributions of diet (daily grams of fat intake), cholesterol (CHOL), age, and gender.

Table 30-2 **①** shows the correlations among these variables. We can see that BMI, diet, and CHOL have significant correlations with SBP. In Table 30-2B, the results of a multiple regression are presented. This looks like the simple linear regression output, with a few important differences.

Prediction Accuracy

The model summary shows the value of R^2, which tells us that together this set of 5 predictor variables accounts for 53% of the total variance in SBP (see Table 30-2 **②**). The adjusted R^2 is a slightly lower value. With more variables in the equation, there is more error variance, which is reflected in this value. The ANOVA confirms a significant model ($p < .001$) (see Table 30-2 **③**).

The Regression Equation

The multiple regression equation now accommodates several predictor variables:

$$\hat{Y} = a + b_1 X_1 + b_2 X_2 + ... \, b_k X_k$$

The subscript k denotes the number of independent variables in the equation. The equation includes the regression constant, a, and regression coefficients, b_1 through b_k, for each independent variable.

Regression Coefficients

The regression coefficients are interpreted as *weights* that identify how much each variable contributes to the explanation of Y. As part of the analysis, a test of significance is performed on each regression coefficient, to test the null hypothesis, H_0: $b = 0$ for that independent variable (see Table 30-2 **⑥**). In this example, only the coefficients for diet and CHOL are significant, while BMI, age, and gender are not. Therefore, these variables are not making a significant contribution to the prediction of SBP.

📌 The p value for BMI is .054, arguably a significant outcome. The decision to consider BMI important may be justified by the researcher within the clinical context of these variables. However, as we shall see shortly, the strict demarcation of .05 to indicate significance may influence further analysis of the data.

In Table 30-2 **④**, the coefficients for the regression equation are shown:

$$\text{SBP} = 75.130 + .673(\text{BMI}) + .110(\text{diet}) + .092(\text{CHOL}) + -.029(\text{age}) - .047(\text{gender})$$

Based on this equation, for a 27-year-old male subject with BMI = 24, diet = 45.0 g, CHOL = 155, gender = 1 (coded for male), we can predict SBP as follows:

$$\text{SBP} = 75.130 + .673(24) + .110(45) + .092(155) - .029(27) - .047(1) = 109.662$$

Assume this person's true SBP was 95. Therefore, the residual would be $95 - 109.662 = -14.662$. The negative residual indicates that the predicted value is higher than the actual value.

🔑 Equations derived in a regression study are specific to the sample used. Prediction accuracy is often reduced when applied to different subjects.[2] *Cross-validation studies* involve collection of data from a new sample to evaluate how well the formula predicts outcomes with different individuals. This is not just a replication study, but rather a way to validate results from the original study for clinical use.

Table 30-2   Multiple Regression Analysis: Prediction of Systolic Blood Pressure from BMI, Diet, Cholesterol, Age, and Gender (N=145)

A. SPSS Output: Correlations

Correlations ❶

		SBP	BMI	DIET	CHOL	AGE	GENDER
Pearson Correlation	SBP	1.000	.679**	.696**	.601**	−.004	−.025
	BMI	.679**	1.000	.865**	.674**	.012	−.008
	DIET	.696**	.865**	1.000	.674**	−.009	−.055
	CHOL	.601**	.674**	.674**	1.000	.140*	−.033
	AGE	−.004	.012	−.009	.140*	1.000	−.042
	GENDER	−.025	−.008	−.055	−.033	−.042	1.000

**Correlation is significant at the 0.01 level (2-tailed). *Correlation significant at the 0.05 level (2-tailed).
SBP = Systolic blood pressure, BMI = body mass index, DIET = daily fat intake, CHOL= Cholesterol

B. SPSS Output: Multiple Regression

Model Summary ❷

Model	R	R Square	Adjusted R Square	SEE
1	.728ᵃ	.530	.513	8.42354

a. Predictors: (Constant), GENDER, BMI, AGE, CHOL, DIET

ANOVAᵃ

Model		Sum of Squares	df	Mean Square	F	Sig. ❸
1	Regression	11105.773	5	221.155	31.303	.000ᵇ
	Residual	9862.889	139	70.956		
	Total	20968.662	144			

a. Dependent Variable: SBP
b. Predictors: (Constant), GENDER, BMI, AGE, CHOL, DIET

Coefficientsᵃ

Model		Unstandardized Coefficients ❹ B	Std. Error	Standardized Coefficients ❺ Beta	t	Sig. ❻	95% Confidence Interval for B Lower Bound	Upper Bound	Collinearity Statistics ❼ Tolerance	VIF
1	(Constant)	75.130	7.775		9.663	.000	59.757	90.503		
	BMI	.673	.347	.233	1.941	.054	−.013	1.359	.236	4.240
	DIET	.110	.038	.352	2.922	.004	.036	.185	.233	4.286
	CHOL	.092	.036	.211	2.552	.012	.021	.163	.493	2.027
	AGE	−.029	.053	−.033	−.547	.585	−.135	.076	.959	1.043
	GENDER	.047	1.407	.002	.034	.973	−2.735	2.829	.989	1.011

a. Dependent Variable: SBP

---

❶ The correlation matrix provides an overview of correlations among all variables in the equation. It is redundant, and only the top triangular portion needs to be considered.

❷ R^2 and adjusted R^2 are shown. The value of R is reported, but it is not meaningful with multiple independent variables and is ignored.

❸ The ANOVA shows a significant relationship between SBP and the set of independent variables.

❹ B = regression coefficients for each variable in the equation:
Y = 75.13 + .673(BMI) + .110(Diet) + .092(CHOL) − .029(Age) − .047(Gender)

❺ Standardized regression coefficients (beta weights). These values allow comparison of weights across variables.

❻ Tests of significance of regression coefficients for each independent variable. Values for the constant are ignored.

❼ Tolerance and VIF reflect the degree of collinearity with other variables. Lower values for tolerance and higher values for VIF indicate greater collinearity.

Portions of the output have been omitted for clarity.

Standardized Regression Coefficients

Researchers often want to establish the relative importance of specific variables within a multiple regression equation. For example, we might be tempted to consider BMI most influential because its coefficient is higher than any others. However, the regression coefficients cannot be directly compared in this way because they are based on different units of measurement. When it is of interest to determine which variables are more heavily weighted, coefficients are converted to *z* scores or standardized **beta weights** (see Table 30-2 **5**).

For example, the beta weights show that diet has the greatest influence on the regression, followed by BMI and CHOL. The sign of the beta weight indicates the positive or negative relationship between each variable and *Y*, but only the absolute value is considered in determining the relative weight. Many authors present beta weights in addition to regression coefficients in a research report to provide the reader with a full and practical interpretation of the comparable importance of each variable.

Collinearity

A problem can occur in the interpretation of beta weights if the independent variables in the regression equation are correlated with each other. This concern is called **collinearity** or *multicollinearity*. The coefficients assigned to variables within the equation are based on the assumption that each variable provides independent information, contributing a unique part of the total explanation of the variance in *Y*, as depicted in Figure 30-5A. If independent variables are related to each other, however, the information they provide to the model is partially redundant, as in Figure 30-5B.

In that case, one variable may be seen as contributing a lot of information with a larger beta weight, and the second variable may be seen as contributing little. Each variable may be highly predictive of *Y* when used alone, but they are redundant when used together. This situation can be avoided by determining the intercorrelations among predictor variables prior to running a regression analysis and selecting independent variables that are not highly correlated with each other.

Partial Correlation

The interpretation of collinearity is based on the concept of **partial correlation** (see Chapter 29). Each regression coefficient represents the contribution of a single variable after having accounted for the effect of all other variables in the equation. Importantly, therefore, the value of a regression coefficient is dependent on which other independent variables are in the equation.

In our example, we can see that BMI and CHOL both have a high correlation with diet, which will influence

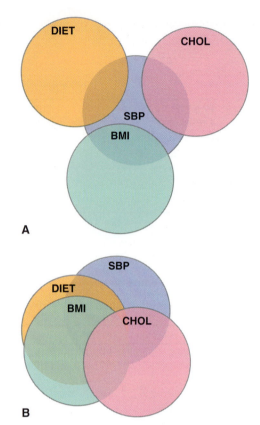

A

B

Figure 30–5 Illustration of collinearity. **A)** DIET, BMI and CHOL have independent associations with SBP, each contributing unique variance to explain SBP. **B)** DIET, BMI and CHOL have strong associations with each other, and therefore present redundant information in the explanation of SBP.

their partial correlation with SBP, even though independently they both have high correlations with SBP (see Table 30-2 **1**).

Collinearity Statistics

The degree of collinearity in the data is expressed in two ways (see Table 30-2 **7**). One criterion is **tolerance level**, which ranges from 0.00, indicating that the variable is perfectly correlated with other entered variables, to 1.00 which means that the other variables are not related. The higher the tolerance, the more new information a variable will contribute to the equation. The **variance inflation factor (VIF)** also measures collinearity, and is equal to 1/tolerance. It is always ≥ 1.0 and the higher the value, the greater the collinearity.

There is no consensus on thresholds to indicate acceptable limits of collinearity. Some suggest that VIF factors above 4 or 5 or tolerance levels less than .25 are cause for concern, while others suggest a VIF of 10 or tolerance as low as .20 as a cutoff. For these data, given their correlations, BMI and diet are probably redundant of each other.

Some computer programs will automatically generate tolerance levels for each variable. Others offer options that must be specifically requested to include collinearity statistics in the output.

 It is important to recognize that, in this type of regression, all five variables are included in the regression equation, regardless of whether they are significant. The coefficients in a regression equation are dependent on which other variables are included and can change substantially if the analysis was repeated with a different combination of independent variables with different levels of collinearity. Therefore, regression coefficients do not provide absolute estimates of the importance of any independent variable. The interpretation must be made within the context of the set of variables used and characteristics of the sample.

▶ Results

The multiple regression examined the association between SBP and BMI, diet, cholesterol, age, and gender, resulting in a total R^2 of .530 ($p < .001$) and a final equation of $Y = 75.130 + .673(BMI) + .110(diet) + .092(cholesterol) − .029(age) − .047$ (gender). Significant coefficients were obtained for BMI ($p = .054$), diet ($p = .004$), and cholesterol ($p = .012$). These three variables had high correlations with each other ($r \geq .674$) and BMI and diet have low tolerance levels, indicating collinearity with other variables. Standardized beta coefficients were highest for diet ($\beta = .352$), BMI ($\beta = .233$), and cholesterol ($\beta = .211$). Age and gender did not provide significant contributions to predicting SBP within this model.

■ Power and Effect Size for Regression

The value of R^2 is often used as an effect size index for regression, like r is used for correlation. However, for power analyses this value is converted to f^2. For the SBP example,

$$f^2 = \frac{R^2}{1-R^2} = \frac{.53}{1-.53} = 1.128$$

Cohen[3] proposed the following conventional effect sizes and corresponding R^2 values:

Small	$f^2 = .02$	$R^2 = .02$
Medium	$f^2 = .15$	$R^2 = .13$
Large	$f^2 = .35$	$R^2 = .26$

See Box 30-1 for description of power analysis and sample size estimates for regression.

Power is important to the interpretation of regression. Like correlation, regression can be sensitive to sample size, often finding significance with low values of R^2

Box 30-1 Power and Sample Size Estimates for Regression

Post Hoc Analysis: Determining Power

Using G*Power to determine power requires entering the effect size f^2, level of significance, total sample size, and the number of independent variables. For this analysis, $f^2 = 1.128$, $\alpha = .05$, $N = 145$, with 5 independent variables. This results in power of 1.00 (*see chapter supplement*)—you can't do better than that!

A Priori Analysis: Estimating Sample Size

To estimate sample size we need to know how many predictor variables will be included, the desired level of f^2 and power, and the estimated effect size. For this example, assume that we are expecting $R^2 = .25$ which converts to $f^2 = .33$. Using $\alpha = .05$ and 80% power with 5 independent variables, the estimated sample size is 45 (*see chapter supplement*).

This outcome illustrates two important considerations in regression analysis. First, we can see that our sample of 145 subjects contributed marked power to the analysis. Also, the greater the number of independent variables, the larger the needed sample.

when samples are large. It is the value of R^2 that must be considered in context, not solely a p value (see Focus on Evidence 30-1)

 See the *Chapter 30 Supplement* for illustration of power and sample size calculations using G*Power for regression analysis.

■ Stepwise Multiple Regression

Multiple regression can be run by "forcing" or "entering" a set of variables into the equation, as we have done in the SBP example. With all five variables included, the equation accounted for 53% of the variance in SBP values, although the results demonstrated that the independent variables did not all make significant contributions to that estimate and there was some collinearity. We might ask then, can we establish a more efficient model, to achieve this level of prediction accuracy with fewer variables?

To answer this question, we use a procedure called **stepwise multiple regression**, which applies specific statistical criteria to retain or eliminate variables to maximize prediction accuracy with the smallest number of predictors. It is not unusual to find that only a few independent variables will explain almost as much of the variation in the dependent variable as can be explained by a larger number of variables. This approach is useful for honing in on those variables that make the most valuable contribution to a given relationship, thereby creating an economical model.

Focus on Evidence 30–1
Statistical Danger!

In 1986, a *New York Times* report cited a study of intelligence tests, with the headline "Children's Height Linked to Test Scores."[26] The story was based on an article published in the journal *Pediatrics*, which involved the analysis of data from the National Health Examination Survey on more than 16,000 children from 6 to 17 years old.[27] Intellectual ability was measured using the Wechsler Intelligence Scale for Children, yielding an IQ score. The Pearson product-moment correlation was used to detect the relationship between IQ and height, and multiple regression was used to examine the influence of other related variables, including family income, race, birth order, and family size.

The results showed a significant positive correlation, indicating a direct relationship between height and IQ, with $r = .18$, $p < .001$. The regression model showed that taken together, the other related variables accounted for 30% of the variance, and height only contributed another 2% ($p < .001$). In a separate longitudinal analysis of a subset of 2,177 children from 8 to 13 years of age, the researchers found no relationship between change in height and change in IQ over 2 to 5 years.

In their discussion, the authors cited several studies that showed significant correlations between height and intellectual performance dating from 1893 to 1975, with correlations between .12 and .36. They stated that their results of a small but statistically significant association supported these findings. However, given that they found no association between change in height and IQ in their sample, they suggested that any processes responsible for the relationship must occur early in childhood, before the age of 8. They also suggested that any therapies designed to facilitate physical growth were unlikely to promote intellectual growth.

But back to the *New York Times*—the report that would be more likely seen by the public. Imagine the impact of such a "significant" finding—especially for parents of shorter children! Of course, the newspaper article did not mention the actual correlation, just its significance, and offered the public no understanding of the meaning of a correlation versus R^2, the power of the test with such a large sample, or the difference between correlation and causation to put the predictive relationship in perspective. The primary author is quoted as saying, "We feel that it may well be possible that short children are treated somewhat different, and might be thought of as younger or less intellectually mature."

Studies continue to show some relationship between height and intelligence, generally with low correlations, offering many potential explanations for other contributing factors, including prenatal conditions and genetics.[28-30] Understanding the impact of these types of findings, without understanding the statistical implications, requires considerable caution.

The Steps

Stepwise regression is accomplished in "steps" by evaluating the contribution of each independent variable in sequential fashion based on an inclusion criterion, usually set at $p \leq .05$. First, all proposed independent variables are correlated with the dependent variable, and the one variable with the highest significant correlation is entered into the equation at step 1. For our example, referring back to Table 30-2A, we can see that diet has the highest correlation with SBP ($r = .699$, $p < .001$). Therefore, we expect diet to be entered in the first step.

After the first variable is entered, the variables that were excluded are examined to see if any have a partial correlation that is significant; that is, do they have any important information to add? If so, the variable with the highest partial correlation will be entered in the next step. This process continues until, at some point, either all variables have been entered or the addition of more variables will not significantly improve the prediction accuracy of the model, ending the analysis.

The Stepwise Models

Table 30-3 shows the output for the stepwise regression for the SBP study. In each section the number of steps is identified under the column labeled Model. Data for the first step are shown in Table 30-3 ❷. As expected, diet was entered, resulting in $R^2 = .484$. The regression equation for this first step is:

$$SBP = 100.163 + .218(\text{diet})$$

Next we examine the remaining "excluded" variables for their partial correlation with Y, that is, their correlation with SBP with the effect of diet removed (see Table 30-3 ❸). The variable with the highest significant partial correlation coefficient is then added to the equation in step 2, in this case, cholesterol (partial $r = .248$ $p = .003$). Data for the second step are shown in Table 30-3 ❹. With the addition of cholesterol, we have increased R^2 to .516.

At this point we look again at the excluded variables. None of the partial correlations of the remaining three variables are significant, indicating that they have no new information to add to the explanation of SBP (see Table 30-4 ❺). Therefore, no further variables were entered after step 2, and the final model for the stepwise regression is

$$SBP = 81.918 + .167 \text{ (diet)} + .105 \text{ (CHOL)}$$

Note that the coefficient for diet has changed from step 1 to step 2 with the addition of cholesterol into the equation. Note, too, that for this analysis, an

Table 30-3   Stepwise Multiple Regression: Prediction of SBP

SPSS Output: Stepwise Multiple Regression

Variables Entered/Removed[a]

Model	Variables Entered	Variables Removed	Method
1	DIET	.	Stepwise
2	CHOL	.	Stepwise

a. Dependent Variable: SBP

Model Summary

Model	R	R Square	Adjusted R Square	Std. Error of the Estimate	R Square Change
1	.696[a]	❷ .484	.480	8.69951	.484
2	.718[b]	❹ .516	.509	8.45685	.032

a. Predictors: (Constant), DIET
b. Predictors: (Constant), DIET, CHOL

ANOVA[a]

Model		Sum of Squares	df	Mean Square	F	Sig.
1	Regression	10146.209	1	10146.209	134.065	❷ .000[b]
	Residual	10822.453	143	75.681		
	Total	20968.662	144			
2	Regression	10813.067	2	5406.533	75.597	❹ .000[c]
	Residual	10155.595	142	71.518		
	Total	20968.662	144			

a. Dependent Variable: SBP
b. Predictors: (Constant), DIET
c. Predictors: (Constant), DIET, CHOL

Coefficients[a]

Model		Unstandardized Coefficients B	Std. Error	Standardized Coefficients Beta	t	Sig.	95% Confidence Interval for B Lower Bound	Upper Bound	Collinearity Statistics Tolerance	VIF
1	(Constant)	❷ 100.163	2.024		49.500	.000	96.163	104.163		
	DIET	.218	.019	.696	11.579	.000	.181	.255	1.000	1.000
2	(Constant)	❹ 81.918	6.290		13.022	.000	69.483	94.353		
	DIET	.167	.025	.533	6.737	.000	.118	.216	.545	1.834
	CHOL	.105	.034	.241	3.054	.000	.037	.172	.545	1.834

a. Dependent Variable: SBP

Excluded Variables[a]

Model		Beta In	t	Sig.	Partial Correlation	Collinearity Tolerance	Statistics VIF
1	BMI	.306[b]	2.615	.010	.214	.253	3.960
	CHOL	.241[b]	3.054	.003	❸ .248	.545	1.834
	AGE	.003[b]	.049	.961	.004	1.000	1.000
	GENDER	.013[b]	.223	.824	.019	.997	1.003
2	BMI	.233[c]	1.967	.051	❺ .163	.237	4.213
	AGE	−.034[c]	−.564	.574	−.047	.961	1.041
	GENDER	.012[c]	.212	.832	.018	.997	1.003

a. Dependent Variable: SBP
b. Predictors: (Constant), DIET
c. Predictors: (Constant), DIET, CHOL

Continued

Table 30-3   Stepwise Multiple Regression: Prediction of SBP—cont'd

1 The derived model has two steps, entering DIET on the first step and CHOL on the second step.

2 DIET enters on the first step with R^2 = .484 ($p < .001$ from ANOVA). The regression equation for the first step:
$\hat{Y}$ = 100.063 + .218(DIET).

3 Of the remaining variables after DIET is entered, partial correlations for both CHOL and BMI are significant, but CHOL has the higher partial correlation, and therefore will be the next variable entered.

4 The second step includes DIET and CHOL, increasing R^2 to .516, which is also significant. The regression equation for the second step: $\hat{Y}$ = 81.918 + .167(DIET) + .105(CHOL).

5 In step 2, after DIET and CHOL are entered, none of the remaining variables have significant partial correlations, and the regression stops at step 2. BMI is no longer significant (using a strict .05 cutoff). BMI has a low tolerance and high VIF, indicating it is correlated with other variable already in the equation.

additional value has been requested in the model summary, labelled *R Square Change*. This value will tell us how much more variance is being explained as we progress from step to step. In this case, by adding cholesterol in step 2, the regression explains 3.2% more variance in SBP.

The final R^2 of .516, generated in the stepwise regression with two independent variables, is only slightly less than the R^2 of .530 obtained with the full model in Table 30-2. The adjusted R^2 values are even closer. With fewer variables we have accounted for comparable variance, with a decreased probability that chance is operating.

We might argue that p = .051 for BMI should still be considered significant and should enter in a third step, but it does not enter because the strict statistical criterion of ≤.05 is not met. However, we can also see that BMI has a low tolerance, indicating that it is redundant to other variables already entered.

> **Results**

Stepwise multiple regression was performed to examine the contributions of BMI, diet, cholesterol, age and gender to prediction of SBP. Diet entered in step 1, with R^2 = .484, p <.001). Adding cholesterol in step 2 increased R^2 to .516 (p <.001), a change of .032. The remaining variables were not entered. The final regression model was Y = 81.918 + .167(diet) + .105 (cholesterol). Beta weights showed that diet had a stronger contribution (β = .533) than cholesterol (β = .241). These data suggest that diet and cholesterol are important predictors of systolic blood pressure. BMI had a strong relationship with SBP (r = .679), but did not enter the equation because of collinearity (VIF = 4.213), likely related to its high correlation with diet (r = .865) and cholesterol (r = .674).

The results of this analysis demonstrate an important caveat in interpreting results of stepwise regression. BMI may not have entered the equation because of its collinearity with other variables, but that does not mean that it has no predictive relationship with SBP. If the purpose of the study is to establish the most efficient statistical model to predict SBP, then data are only needed for diet and cholesterol. But, when considering relevant clinical variables (according to these hypothetical data), the importance of BMI should not be ignored. The fact that a variable does not enter in a stepwise analysis does not necessarily indicate that it is unimportant or unrelated to the dependent variable.

Inclusion Procedures

Variables can be entered into a regression using three types of inclusion strategies. *Forward inclusion* means that the model starts with no variables and adds variables one by one until no further variables meet the inclusion criterion. This procedure is differentiated from *stepwise* regression in many statistical programs. While both proceed using a forward selection method, adding a new variable at each step, the stepwise procedure can also remove a variable at any step, if that variable no longer contributes significantly to the model, once other variables have been added to the equation. The *removal criterion* is usually set at p = .10.

In the *backward deletion* method, the model starts with all variables in the equation. Using criteria for removal, variables that do not contribute to the solution are removed one at a time. The variable with the smallest partial correlation is taken out first. Steps proceed until no remaining variables are qualified for removal.

There are times when a researcher collects data on several variables, and regression results in no variables being entered if none of them satisfy the minimal inclusion criteria. In that situation, the researcher must search for a new set of independent variables to explain the dependent variable. It usually helps to look at correlations among variables first, to determine if relationships are worth analyzing. Sometimes backwards inclusion may find relationships that are missed with forward selection methods. Because the analysis starts with all variables entered, their relationships are more easily identified, as compared to bringing one variable into the equation at a time.

Hierarchical Regression

Another approach to multiple regression involves entering sets of variables in sequential stages or "blocks." Independent variables entered in the first block are often those the researcher wants to control, such as demographic data. After these effects are tested, other variables can be entered in subsequent blocks to see what they add. Each stage can be run with all variables entered or using other methods of inclusion.

For example, we might enter age and gender in the first block to account for these characteristics, thereby removing their effect from further analysis. In a second block, we can enter all of the remaining variables, or we might have a rationale for grouping subsets further. These results will vary from other methods because of the effect of entry order.

> See online data files for Table 30-3 at www.davisplus.com for examples of output with enter, stepwise, forward, backward, and hierarchical inclusion methods using the SBP data.

■ Dummy Variables

One of the general assumptions for regression analysis is that variables are continuous. However, many of the variables that may be useful predictors for a regression analysis, such as gender, occupation, education, and race, are measured on a categorical scale. We can also look at group membership in an experimental study as a categorical variable. It is possible to include such variables in a regression equation, although the numbers assigned to categories cannot be treated as quantitative scores. One way to do this is to create a set of coded variables called **dummy variables**.

Coding

In statistics, *coding* is the process of assigning numerals to represent categorical or group membership. For regression analysis we use 0 and 1 to code for the absence and presence of a dichotomous variable, respectively. All dummy variables are dichotomous. For example, for a variable like gender, we might arbitrarily code male = 0 and female = 1. In essence, then, we are coding 1 for

female and 0 for anyone who is not female. We can use these codes as scores in a regression equation and treat them as interval data. For instance, gender was included as a predictor of SBP in the multiple regression (see Table 30-2). Assume we tested only the effect of gender (X), getting the following regression equation:

$$\hat{Y} = 150 - 27.5X$$

Using the dummy code for Males,

$$SBP = 150 - 27.5 (1) = 122.5$$

and for Females,

$$SBP = 150 - 27.5 (0) = 150$$

With only this one dummy variable, these predicted values are actually the means for SBP for females and males. The regression coefficient for X is the difference between the means for the groups coded 0 and 1.

Coding with More than Two Categories

When a categorical variable has more than two levels, more than one dummy variable is required to represent it. For example, let's assume we had information on smoker status from our subjects. We could assess smoking in three categories: never smoked, former smoker, current smoker. If we coded these categories with numbers 1 through 3, it would represent an apparent ordinal scale, but this would make no sense in a regression because the numbers have no quantitative meaning. A current smoker is not three times more of something than someone who never smoked.

Therefore, we must create a dichotomous dummy variable for each category, as follows:

$$X_1 = 1 \text{ if "current smoker"}$$
$$0 \text{ if not "current smoker"}$$

$$X_2 = 1 \text{ if "former smoker"}$$
$$0 \text{ if not "former smoker"}$$

Each variable codes for the presence or absence of a specific class membership. We do not need to create a third variable for "never smoked" because anyone who has zero for X_1 and X_2 will be in that category. We can show how this works by defining each group with a unique combination of values for X_1 and X_2:

	X_1	X_2
Current Smoker	1	0
Former Smoker	0	1
Never Smoked	0	0

The number of dummy variables needed to define a categorical variable will always be one less than the number of categories.

The variables X_1 and X_2 are entered as variables in a regression equation, and an individual's score on each one will be based on the coding scheme. Suppose we wanted to predict an individual's blood pressure based on their smoking status. Assume the following equation was derived:

$$\hat{Y} = 120 + 30X_1 + 20X_2$$

Therefore, the predicted values for a current smoker would be:

$$SBP = 120 + 30(1) + 20(0) = 150$$

For a former smoker:

$$SBP = 120 + 30(0) + 20(1) = 140$$

For someone who never smoked:

$$SBP = 120 + 30(0) + 20(0) = 120$$

Several dummy variables can be combined with quantitative variables in a regression equation. Because many variables of interest are measured as categories, the use of dummy variables provides an important mechanism for creating a fuller explanation of clinical phenomena. Some computer programs will automatically generate dummy codes for nominal variables. For others, the researcher must specify the coding scheme.

Regression and Significant Differences

Regression is often thought of only as a prediction process. However, it can also serve the same purpose as a *t*-test or ANOVA, to determine if there are significant differences across groups. Statistically, these tests are actually forms of regression—they just come at the question a little differently.

For instance, in a regression using gender as an independent variable, we are asking if there is a relationship between gender and SBP. For the smoking example, we are asking if there is a relationship between smoking status and SBP. If we performed *t*-tests or ANOVAs, these variables would represent groups (levels of the independent variable), and we would analyze differences across these groups in SBP based on their variance components. Regression is essentially doing the same thing. The ANOVA that is generated as part of the regression analysis would examine how much variance in the data can be explained by gender or smoking status. This would be identical to a regular ANOVA looking at group means. Therefore, a regression technique is feasible with an experimental design with group membership as an independent variable.

🔖 Another type of regression procedure, called *discriminant analysis*, also looks at the relationship between group membership as the outcome variable and measured independent variables. This test will be described further in Chapter 31.

■ Nonlinear Regression

Another consideration in the interpretation of regression data is the adequacy of a linear fit. Just as with correlation, linear regression procedures are useful only if the distribution of scores demonstrates a linear association between Y and a set of X scores. The lack of a significant slope does not necessarily mean that X and Y are unrelated but may indicate that the relationship does not follow a straight line.

> ### ➤ CASE IN POINT #3
> Research has shown a decline in psychomotor performance with age.[4] Consider a hypothetical study to examine the relationship between psychomotor ability (scored 0-15) and age for a sample of 30 individuals aged 10 to 50 years.

Hypothetical data for this study are shown in Figure 30-6. Using linear techniques to analyze the data, the correlation is weak, resulting in $R^2 = .125$.

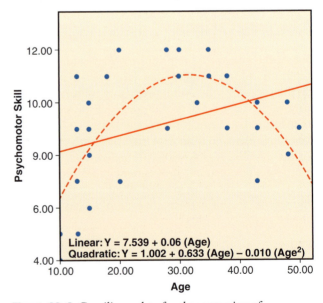

Figure 30–6 Curvilinear data for the regression of psychomotor skill on age. The solid line represents the linear regression ($R^2 = .125$), and the curve (dashed line) is derived through a second-order polynomial regression.

Based on this information alone, one would assume that X and Y were not related.

However, examination of the scatter plot reveals that the data form a distinctly curved pattern with an increase in psychomotor ability through early years and then a decline in later years. Therefore, it makes sense to draw a "line," or more precisely a curve, that accurately reflects the relationship between X and Y. We can express this curve statistically in the form of a quadratic equation:

$$\hat{Y} = a + b_1X + b_2X^2$$

This type of equation is considered a *second order regression equation*. It defines a parabolic or **quadratic curve** with one turn (see Chapter 26). The process of deriving its equation is called **polynomial regression**. Clearly, this fitted curve is more representative of the data points than the linear regression line, with $R^2 = .449$. Polynomial regression is also based on the concept of least squares, so that the vertical distance of each point from the curve is minimized. Therefore, the curve can be used for predicting Y scores in the same way as a linear regression line (See Focus on Evidence 30-2).

Table 30-4 shows the analysis of variance for both a linear and quadratic regression of psychomotor ability on age. The *F*-ratio for the linear regression is not significant ($p = .279$), and R^2 is quite weak at $.042$, as we might expect from looking at the data (see Table 30-4 ❶).

The quadratic regression is significant ($p = .007$), indicating that the quadratic curve is a good fit for these data (see Table 30-4 ❷). The equation for the curve is

$$\text{Score} = 1.261 + .686(\text{Age}) - .011(\text{Age}^2)$$

Therefore, a person who is 43 years old could be expected to have a psychomotor score of

$$\text{Score} = 1.261 + .686(43) - .011(1849) = 10.42$$

If you look at the curve in Figure 30-6 and draw a vertical line from age 43 on the X axis, it should hit the curve around this point. However, you will also notice that there were three people in the sample who were 43 years old, and only one got a score close to its predicted value.

A closer look at the analysis of variance helps us see how differently these two approaches explain the data. Note that the total sum of squares for both analyses is the same ($SS_t = 223.367$); that is, the total variability in the sample is the same, regardless of which type of regression is performed. What is different is the amount of that variance that is explained by each of the regression models. The sum of squares attributable to the linear regression is 9.33, whereas for the quadratic regression it is 68.11 (see Table 30-4 ❸). This indicates that a greater proportion of the total variability is explained by the curve. We can also see that the residual error represents a smaller portion of the total variance in the quadratic regression.

> ➤ **Results**
>
> The scatterplot of data shows a distinctly nonlinear relationship between psychomotor ability and age. Therefore, linear and polynomial regressions were performed. The linear regression was not significant ($R^2 = .042$, $p = .279$). Using a curve estimate, we found a significant quadratic function ($R^2 = .305$, $p = .007$), with a final equation of $Y = 1.261 + .686 (\text{AGE}) - .011 (\text{AGE}^2)$. These data suggest that there is a strong curvilinear relationship between psychomotor ability and age.

Focus on Evidence 30–2
If Only They Could Talk

The Glasgow Coma Scale (GSC) is used to assess the level of consciousness in patients following trauma. Rutledge et al[31] identified problems in using the GCS in intubated patients because the scale requires verbal responses that are blocked by intubation. The purpose of their study was to develop a basis for predicting the verbal score using only the motor and eye responses of the scale. The authors designed a prospective study to assess 2,521 patients in an intensive care unit who could provide verbal responses. They used a multiple regression procedure to determine if the motor and eye variables were strong predictors of the verbal score, resulting in the following second order regression equation:

$$\text{Verbal Score} = 2.3976 - .9253(\text{GCS motor}) - .9214(\text{GCS eye}) + .2208 (\text{GCSmotor}^2) + .2318(\text{GCS eye}^2)$$

The accuracy of the model was extremely high, predicting 83% of the variance in the verbal score. To confirm the equation, the authors compared the predicted verbal score to the actual verbal score for a test sample of 736 patients, with $R^2 = .85$, $p = .0001$.

Of course, the ultimate purpose of developing such a model is to extend its use to a different set of subjects. Therefore, the model must be cross-validated by testing it on different groups. For example, Meredith et al[32] tested the equation using a retrospective sample of over 14,000 patients taken from a trauma registry by comparing their predicted and actual GCS scores. Cheung et al[33] also compared the equation with other estimates and found it provided adequate scores. Both findings supported the predictive validity of the model, confirming the ability to determine an accurate GCS score in the absence of a verbal component. Based on these findings, the equation could be used with some confidence with patients who are intubated to predict their verbal response, thereby allowing a reasonable estimate of the GCS score.

Table 30-4   Linear and Polynomial Regression of Psychomotor Ability on Age (*N* = 30)

A. SPSS Output: Linear Regression Model

Model Summary

R	① R Square	Adjusted R Square	Std. Error of the Estimate
.204	.042	.008	2.765

The independent variable is age.

ANOVA

		Sum of Squares	df	Mean Square	F	① Sig.
Regression	③	9.330	1	9.330	1.221	.279
Residual		214.037	28	7.644		
Total		223.367	29			

The independent variable is age.

Coefficients

	Unstandardized Coefficients B	Std. Error	Standardized Coefficients Beta	t	① Sig.
Age	.043	.039	.204	1.105	.279
(Constant)	8.594	1.175		7.315	.000

B. SPSS Output: Polynomial Regression- Quadratic Model

Model Summary

R	② R Square	Adjusted R Square	Std. Error of the Estimate
.552	.305	.253	2.398

The independent variable is age.

ANOVA

		Sum of Squares	df	Mean Square	F	Sig.
Regression	③	68.105	2	34.052	5.922	.007
Residual		155.262	27	5.750		
Total		223.367	29			

The independent variable is age.

Coefficients

	Unstandardized Coefficients ⑤ B	Std. Error	Standardized Coefficients Beta	t	② Sig.
Age	.686	.204	3.242	3.364	.002
Age**2 ④	−.011	.004	−3.081	−3.197	.004
(Constant)	1.261	2.510		.502	.619

① The value of R-square shows that linear prediction is quite weak. The ANOVA and regression show that the linear model is not significant ($p = .279$).

② The value of R-square is substantially increased with the quadratic curve, indicating that the curve is a better fit to the data. The ANOVA and regression show that the quadratic function is significant ($p = .004$).

③ The regression variance is larger and the error variance lower with the quadratic function, indicating that the curve explains more variance than the linear regression.

④ The symbol for exponent is a double asterisk. This term is Age squared.

⑤ The polynomial equation for the quadratic curve is: $\hat{Y} = 1.231 + .686(Age) - .011(Age^2)$

Portions of the output have been omitted for clarity. Data are shown in Figure 30-6.

■ Logistic Regression

Is there a relationship between prematurity and the occurrence of sudden unexpected infant death (SUID)?[13] Does intensity of physical activity predict the incidence of depression in adults?[14] Are musculoskeletal disorders predictive of the occurrence of deficits in activities of daily living (ADLs)?[15]

These questions require estimating the relationship between two measured variables—one a predictor variable and the other an outcome, and therefore lend themselves to a regression analysis. However, unlike linear regression that applies to continuous outcomes, these questions incorporate dichotomous dependent variables that represent the occurrence or nonoccurrence of a particular event, or the presence or absence of a condition—SUID or survival, depression or no depression, ADL deficit or no deficit. For this purpose, we use a process of **logistic regression**. This approach is helpful for clinical decision-making and is especially suited to epidemiologic study (see Chapter 34).

The Regression Equation

Logistic regression is analogous to multiple regression in that it is used to explain or predict an outcome (dependent) variable using one or more predictor (independent) variables. The result is a best-fitting equation with coefficients, predicted values, and residuals that reflect the contribution of each independent variable. Predictors may be a combination of continuous or dummy-coded categorical variables, and logistic regression can be run with all variables entered or in a stepwise or hierarchical fashion.

Although similar in purpose, there are several important differences that distinguish logistic regression. First, because the outcome is dichotomous, rather than predicting a continuous value of an outcome variable, the logistic regression equation predicts the *probability* of an event occurring.

Another important distinction is the method used to develop the regression equation. Where multiple regression uses the least squares method to find the best-fitting line, logistic regression uses the process of **maximum likelihood estimation**.[16] This is an iterative process whereby equations are generated and revised until a best fitting model is obtained. This results in the "most likely" solution that demonstrates the best odds of the equation accurately predicting who did and did not meet the outcome event.

> ## ► CASE IN POINT #4
>
> Many studies have examined the impact of patient characteristics on discharge status following rehabilitation.[17] Suppose we wanted to predict discharge disposition following rehabilitation for patients who had a stroke. For the sake of illustration, we will look at two possible outcomes: whether patients return home or go to a facility for long-term care (LTC). If we could determine the probability that a patient will or will not go home, we would have data to help us set appropriate goals and begin suitable discharge planning as soon as possible.
>
> In this study, we will examine hypothetical data for 100 patients, 56 who went home and 44 who went to LTC. We will consider four variables to determine if they will be useful predictors of discharge status: functional status at admission, age, marital status, and gender.

Coding Variables

The dependent variable in logistic regression is a dichotomous outcome that is coded 0 for the *reference group* and 1 for the *target group*. The target is typically considered the group with the adverse outcome. Therefore, for this example, we would code 0 for going home (reference), and 1 for going to LTC (target). Only codes of 0 and 1 are used, to represent the absence or presence of the outcome event.

> 📌 With a dichotomous outcome, this test is termed *logistic regression*, which will be the focus here. With more than two categories, the process involves *multinomial logistic regression*, which is beyond the scope of this text. Useful references are available.[18-20] Help from a statistician is recommended.

In logistic regression, the independent predictor variables may be dichotomous or continuous. In this example, age is a continuous variable. The others are dichotomous and can be assigned the codes 0 and 1, with 1 representing potential risk factors. These variables are also called *indicator variables*. For variables like gender, with no obvious adverse condition, the codes may be arbitrary (although in some situations gender may be a risk factor). Categorical variables with more than two levels must be defined using dummy coding.

> ► For the discharge study, the following codes were assigned:
>
> | | |
> |---|---|
> | Function (ADL) | 0 = independent; 1 = limited |
> | Age | Continuous |
> | Marital status | 0 = married; 1 = not married |
> | Gender | 0 = male; 1 = female |

The research question is: What is the likelihood that an individual will be discharged to LTC given this combination of factors? Table 30-5 shows the distribution of data for discharge destination (44 went to LTC, 56 went home) and function (56 were limited in ADL, 44 were independent).

Understanding Odds

The outcome of logistic regression is based on the probability of a given event, which can take values between 0 and 1. Because of this value restriction and to make outcomes more interpretable, the probabilities are converted to **odds** (see Box 30-2). Odds tell us how much more likely it is that an individual belongs to the target group than to the reference group, or the proportion of people with the adverse outcome in relation to those

Table 30-5   Relationship Between Level of Independence and Discharge Destination

		1 LTC		0 Home	Total
1 Limited ADL	*a*	31	*b*	25	56
0 Independent	*c*	13	*d*	31	44
Total		44		56	100

Box 30-2   Probabilities and Odds

The probability of an event reflects the number of times you expect to see an outcome out of all possible trials, ranging between 0 and 1 (see Chapter 23). Odds represent the probability that the event will occur divided by the probability that the event will not occur.

If the probability of occurrence is X, then the probability of nonoccurrence is 1–X. Therefore,

Odds = probability/1–probability
Probability = odds/1 + odds

For example, if a horse runs 100 races and wins 50, the probability of winning is 50%. The odds are .50/.50 = 1 (even odds). If the horse runs 100 races and wins 25, the probability of winning is 25%, but the odds are .25/.75 = 0.33, or 1 win to 3 losses.

In the discharge study, for those with limitations in ADL, the odds of being discharged to LTC are 2.96 (Table 31-1). Therefore,

Probability = 2.96/3.96 = .75

There is a 75% probability that someone with limited ADL will be discharged to LTC. A patient with limited ADL is almost 3 times more likely to go to LTC than someone without limitation.

---

without it. For example, for the 56 people who were limited in ADL, the odds of going to LTC are

$$\frac{31(\text{went to LTC})}{25(\text{went home})} = 1.24$$

For the 44 people who were independent, the odds of going to LTC are

$$\frac{13(\text{went to LTC})}{31(\text{went home})} = .419$$

The ratio of these two values is the **odds ratio (OR)**—the odds of going to LTC for those limited in ADL versus odds of going to LTC for those who were independent:

$$\text{OR} = \frac{1.24}{.419} = 2.96$$

Therefore, the odds of going to LTC are 2.96 times higher for those who are limited in ADL than for those who are functionally independent.

If the proportions of individuals who go to LTC and home are the same, the OR will be 1.0, considered the null value. An OR less than 1.0 means that there is a decreased risk, and greater than 1.0 indicates an increased risk.

To make this process easier, the odds ratio can be calculated from the data in Table 30-5 as *ad/bc*, using the cell designations in the table. For these data,

$$\text{OR} = \frac{(31)(31)}{(25)(13)} = 2.96$$

Applications of the odds ratio will be discussed further in Chapter 34.

 See the *Chapter 30 Supplement* for calculation of and interpretation of probabilities associated with logistic regression.

Strength of Logistic Regression

Like multiple regression, several statistics are used to indicate the degree to which the logistic regression accurately predicts membership of cases to the categories of the dependent variable. We cannot use an R^2 estimate, like we do for multiple regression, because it doesn't work with a dichotomous outcome.

One of the most useful measures is a classification table, providing data on how well the regression has correctly predicted each patient's true outcome (see Table 30-6 ❺). In this case, the overall correct prediction is 73%. We can see that prediction accuracy was higher for those discharged home (78.6% correctly classified) than for those who went to LTC (65.9% correctly classified).

Other statistics used to indicate the strength of a logistic regression equation are shown in Table 30-6A. An *omnibus test* (❷) is an overall estimate of the significance of the full set of regression coefficients. Likened to an overall *F* test in multiple regression, this significant result ($p < .001$) indicates that the regression equation provides meaningful coefficients that are significantly different from zero.

Two "pseudo-R^2" values are reported in the model summary (❸). The *Cox & Snell R Square* has a theoretical maximum less than 1, even for a "perfect" model.[21] The *Nagelkerke R Square* is an adjusted version of the Cox & Snell value that allows the scale to cover the full range from 0 to 1.[22] These can be interpreted like R^2.

The –2 log likelihood index (–2LL) is based on the concept of *deviance*, or *lack of fit* to the regression

Table 30-6   Logistic Regression Analysis: Risk Factors Associated with Discharge Disposition Following Rehabilitation (N=100)

A. SPSS Output: Strength of Regression

Block 1: Method = Enter ❶

Omnibus Tests of Model Coefficients

		Chi-square	df	Sig.
Step 1	Step ❷	26.855	4	.000
	Block	26.855	4	.000
	Model	26.855	4	.000

Model Summary ❸

Step	−2 Log likelihood	Cox & Snell R Square	Nagelkerke R Square
1	110.381[a]	.236	.315

a. Estimation terminated at iteration number 5 because parameter estimates change by less than .001.

Hosmer and Lemeshow Test ❹

Step	Chi-square	df	Sig.
1	11.228	8	.189

Classification Table[a] ❺

Observed			Predicted Discharge Home	Discharge LTC	Percentage Correct
Step 1	Discharge	Home	44	12	78.6
		LTC	15	29	65.9
	Overall Percentage				73.0

a. The cut value is .500

B. SPSS Output: Regression Coefficients and Odds Ratios

Variables in the Equation

		❼ B	S.E.	❼ Wald	df	❼ Sig.	❽ Exp(B)	❾ 95% CI for EXP(B) Lower	Upper
Step 1[a]	Age	.117	0.37	10.106	1	.001	1.125	1.046	1.209
	ADL(1) ❻	.965	.481	4.031	1	.045	2.625	1.023	6.736
	Marital(1)	1.019	.480	4.499	1	.034	2.770	1.081	7.103
	Gender(1)	−.592	.474	1.561	1	.212	.553	.218	1.401
	Constant	−10.274	2.935	12.252	1	.000	.000		

❶ The independent variables are entered into the equation simultaneously (as opposed to stepwise procedures).

❷ Chi-square is used to test the null hypothesis that the regression coefficients equal zero. Because all variables were entered simultaneously, this analysis includes only one block and one step, which is why values are redundant. These would be different if a stepwise or hierarchical procedure was run. The *df* equal the number of predictor variables.

❸ The Model Summary provides information on the degree to which the model accurately predicts group membership, similar to the use of R^2 in multiple regression.

❹ The Hosmer and Lemeshow test is a measure of goodness of fit to the logistic model using a chi-square distribution.

❺ A classification table compares predicted outcomes to observed results. Overall, 73% of the subjects were correctly classified.

❻ The (1) after each categorical variable name indicates the code for the target category.

❼ Regression coefficients (B) and the constant are listed for each variable in the logistic regression equation. Each coefficient is tested for significance using the Wald statistic. Gender is the only variable that is not significant.

❽ The exponent of the regression coefficient (Exp(B)) is the adjusted odds ratio associated with each independent variable. Data for the constant is ignored.

❾ Confidence intervals for the odds ratios show that ADL, age and marital status do not contain the null value of 1.0. Only the interval for gender contains 1.0, which is consistent with the associated probability.

Portions of the output have been omitted for clarity.

model (❸), analogous to looking at error sums of squares in linear regression (smaller value means better fit). This value is not useful by itself, but is used to calculate chi-square for the *Hosmer-Lemeshow test* (❹), which is a goodness of fit test that indicates if the observed proportions match the expected proportions of event rates generated by the model. If this test is *not* significant, it indicates a good fit, as it does here (p = .189).

Regression Coefficients and Odds Ratios

The essential part of the logistic regression is the derivation of regression coefficients (B) for predictor variables (see Table 30-6 ❼). An OR is computed for each variable by taking the exponent of B (❽). For example, for a subject who is limited in ADL (ADL = 1), the odds of going to LTC are $e^{.965}$ = 2.625 (Use the e^x key on your scientific calculator). This number represents the odds of going to LTC with a one-unit change in the value of X. With a dichotomous variable, this means that an individual who is limited in ADL is 2.6 times more likely to go LTC as compared to one who is independent (a change from 0 to 1 for ADL).

The coefficients are tested to determine if they are significantly different from zero using the *Wald statistic* (❼), which is analogous to the t-test used in linear regression. Confidence intervals can also be determined for each OR (❾). A significant OR will not contain the null value 1.0 within the confidence interval. We can see that this is true for the odds ratios associated with ADL, age, and marital status.

Adjusted Odds Ratios

When the logistic regression equation includes several independent variables, as in our example, each odds ratio is actually corrected for the influence of the other variables, called **adjusted odds ratios** (sometimes abbreviated aOR). Just as independent variables in multiple regression can exhibit collinearity, independent variables in logistic regression will affect each other. This is an important consideration for prediction models. For instance, for the simple association between discharge status and ADL, we found an odds ratio of 2.96, but the adjusted odds ratio is 2.63 when other variables are included.

Continuous Variables

When an independent variable is continuous, interpretation is more complex. Consider the effect of age on discharge status, with an adjusted OR of 1.125. Because the OR relates to the relative increase in odds with a one-unit increase in X, we can interpret this value as the odds associated with any 1-year difference in age. For instance, from 70 to 71 the odds of going to LTC have increased by .125.

To account for larger unit differences, we multiply the regression coefficient by the unit difference and then take the exponent to obtain the odds ratio. For age (B = .117), with a 2-year difference, we determine the odds ratio by $e^{(2 \times .117)}$ =1.264. Someone who is 72 is 1.264 times more likely to go to LTC than someone who is 70—a little increase. However, for a 10-year difference in age, we find $e^{(10 \times .117)}$ = 3.222. The odds of going to LTC are more than 3 times greater for someone who is 80 as compared to someone who is 70. Many researchers choose to categorize continuous variables into subgroups to simplify this interpretation.

Interpretation of Results

The interpretation of logistic regression depends on the research question. In many research situations, the investigator is interested in one particular variable but wants to control for potential confounders. Using the discharge study, for example, we might be specifically interested in the effect of function on discharge status, but we would want to account for the influence of demographic factors as covariates. In that case we might report that the odds ratio for ADL was 2.63, adjusted for age, marital status and gender. Adjusted odds ratios are often based on these types of demographic variables.

Alternatively, we could approach this analysis using a broader question, wanting to understand how these four factors are related to discharge status. In that case, we would summarize results, suggesting that ADL, marital status, and age are most influential in predicting discharge status. In addition to the increased likelihood of going to LTC if the patient is functionally limited, those who are not married are almost 2.77 times more likely to be sent to LTC than those who are married. The actual regression analysis is the same for both of these purposes. The difference lies only in the interpretation.

> ➤ **Results**
> Results of the logistic regression showed that 73% of the sample was correctly classified by the final model. ADL, age, and marital status provided significant contributions to prediction of discharge status. The adjusted OR for ADL was 2.63 (95% CI, 1.02 to 6.74) and for marital status was 2.77 (95% CI, 1.08 to 7.10). Both are significant but with wide confidence intervals. The adjusted OR associated with age was 1.13 (95% CI, 1.05 to 1.21). There was an increased risk of discharge to LTC with limited function, being unmarried, or being older. The Hosmer & Lemeshow Test (X^2(4) = 11.23, p = .189) indicates that the regression model is a good fit to the observed data. The Cox & Snell R^2 = .235 and the Nagelkerke R^2 = .315.

These data will often be provided in tabular form to show ORs, confidence intervals, and probability values for each independent variable.

Sample Size Estimates

A commonly used "rule of thumb" in logistic regression is based on a minimum ratio of 10 cases per predictor variable (subjects per variable, SPV). There is, however, some debate that this approach might be too conservative, with simulation studies showing the regression can be stable with fewer subjects.[23] Long[24] suggests that the minimum number should be 100.

Peduzzi et al[25] offer the following guideline for a minimum number of cases, based on knowing the proportion of positive cases in the population (*p*) and the number of independent variables in the equation (*k*):

$$N = 10 * \frac{k}{p}$$

For example, for the rehabilitation discharge study, we have four covariates in the model (*k* = 4). Assume that information from the literature indicates that the proportion of stroke survivors who are discharged to LTC is approximately 20%.[26] The minimum number of cases required would be

$$N = 10 * \frac{4}{.20} = 200$$

Sample size estimates are important when using logistic regression to create predictive models, such as in the development of clinical prediction rules (see Chapter 33). If samples are too small, the predictive validity of the model will be limited.

 Calculations for power and sample size for logistic regression in G*Power are complex. See the *Chapter 30 Supplement* for illustration of this process.

Propensity Scores

In observational studies, it is often relevant to balance characteristics of exposed and unexposed groups when trying to ascertain causal relationships. In the design of randomized trials, it is important to balance the baseline characteristics of comparison groups. However, even with random assignment, participants in each group may vary sufficiently to confound comparisons. Matching techniques are often used to "equate" groups on specific traits, such as age or gender. However, when there are several potential confounders, this process can become untenable. A procedure called **propensity score** matching can be used to minimize group differences.

Propensity scores are based on a binary logistic regression, with group membership as the dependent variable and the possible confounders as the independent predictor variables. This results in a single propensity score, regardless of the number of covariates. The score will range from 0 to 1, reflecting the probability that the subject belongs to one group or the other.[27] By matching subjects on the basis of their propensity scores, baseline differences can be controlled and researchers can have greater confidence in drawing conclusions about group differences.[28,29] Although this approach cannot completely replace the RCT, it can reduce bias and provide some guidance in situations where random assignment is not tenable.

Importantly, propensity scores are only as good as the variables used to define them. They cannot provide adjustment for unmeasured variables, known or unknown—which is what random assignment is intended to do. The scores will also vary depending on which covariates are used. For these reasons, there is considerable debate on whether propensity scores should be used.[30]

Statisticians can provide advice for use of propensity scores with specific designs. Many statistical programs will match participants by calculating propensity scores, including SPSS, Stata, and SAS.

◼ Analysis of Covariance

Matching is one design technique to equate groups on particular characteristics. A different statistical approach, called the **analysis of covariance (ANCOVA)** involves adjusting scores on the dependent variable to account for the effect of covariates in group comparisons. This procedure is a combination of ANOVA and regression.

➤ CASE IN POINT #5

Suppose we wanted to compare the effect of two teaching strategies on the clinical performance of students in their first year of clinical training. We hypothesize that there will be a difference in clinical performance after training with videotaped cases (Strategy 1) or discussion groups (Strategy 2). We randomly assign 24 students to two groups (*n* = 12 per group) and compare their clinical scores at the end of their training period.

The issue of concern is the ability to equate groups at baseline, so that observed differences following intervention can be attributed to the intervention and not to other unexplained factors. For example, we may be concerned that a student's academic performance could confound the effect of teaching strategy on clinical performance. If there is a correlation between academic and clinical performance, we would want to know if the grade point average (GPA) in the two groups was evenly distributed. If one group happens to have a higher GPA than the other, our results could be misleading (assuming GPA does reflect academic performance).

In this posttest-only design, teaching strategy is the independent variable, clinical performance is the dependent variable, and GPA is a **covariate**, a potentially confounding variable that we want to control. For instance, if one group has a higher GPA, then that group's mean for the dependent variable is adjusted downward. A lower group mean on the covariate results in the clinical score being raised. The degree of adjustment depends on the difference between groups on GPA. Essentially, ANCOVA estimates what the group clinical performance means *would have been* had the groups been equal on their average GPA.

The null hypothesis for the ANCOVA is based on adjusted means:

$$H_0: \bar{X}_1' - \bar{X}_2' = 0$$

where $\bar{X}'$ is an adjusted mean

> Think of this analogy—you want to compare the heights of three people, each one standing on a different step. It will be hard to know who is taller or shorter because they are on different levels. The step height is the covariate. If we could "adjust" the steps, lowering the higher step and raising the lower step, so that everyone would be on the "same level," we would eliminate the effect of step level, and we can then observe how different their heights are.

The Research Question

To illustrate how the ANCOVA offers this control, let's first look at the hypothetical comparison between the two teaching strategies without considering GPA. Suppose we obtain the following means for clinical performance on a standardized test:

Strategy 1: Video 49.3 (± 18.5)
Strategy 2: Discussion 44.2 (± 24.1)

An ANOVA shows that the group means are not significantly different ($p = .562$) (see Table 30-7 ❷). Based on this result, we would conclude that the teaching strategies are not different.

However, because we know that there is a strong correlation ($r = .83$) between academic and clinical performance (see Table 30-7 ❶), we might want to be sure that the two groups were equivalent on GPA before drawing

that conclusion. Our question then becomes, "Is there a difference in clinical performance using video sessions or discussion groups when taking GPA into account?"

> Typically, we would test the difference between two groups using an unpaired *t*-test. In this case, the ANOVA is used so that the results can be compared to the results of the ANCOVA. However, the outcome of a *t*-test would be identical.

Using Regression

Figure 30-7A shows the distribution of GPA and clinical performance scores for Strategy 1 (Video) and Strategy 2 (Discussion) with their respective regression lines. The dependent variable, clinical performance score, is plotted along the *Y*-axis, and the covariate, GPA, is plotted along the *X*-axis. We can see from this scatterplot that these variables are highly correlated within each group.

We can also see that the regression line for Strategy 1 is higher than Strategy 2, indicating that Group 1 had higher values of clinical performance for any given GPA, even though the sample means for clinical score are not significantly different.

There is, however, another important difference. If we look at the mean GPA for each group, we can see that the Strategy 1 group has a lower average GPA than those using Strategy 2. Because GPA is a correlate of clinical performance, it is reasonable to believe that this difference could have confounded the comparison of teaching strategies.

Adjusted Means

To eliminate the differential effect of GPA, we want to *artificially equate* the two groups on GPA, using the GPA *grand mean* for the total sample as the best estimate for both groups. The means for GPA are

Strategy 1	2.73
Strategy 2	3.10
Grand mean	2.92

We now want to know what average clinical score we would expect for Strategy 1 and Strategy 2 if the groups had the same mean GPA. If we assign a mean GPA of 2.92 to both groups, we can use the regression lines to predict what the mean clinical score (Y) would be. As shown in Figure 30-7B, by drawing a vertical line at $\bar{X} = 2.92$, we would intersect the regression lines at $\bar{Y}_1' = 57.4$ and $\bar{Y}_2' = 36.1$. These are the **adjusted means** for each group.

Note that the adjusted mean for Strategy 1 is higher than the observed mean, and for Strategy 2 it is lower. These differences reflect variation in the covariate.

Table 30-7 Analysis of Covariance for Comparison of Clinical Performance Following Two Teaching Strategies ($N = 24$)

A. SPSS Output: Descriptive Statistics

Group Statistics ❶

	Strategy	N	Mean	Std. Deviation
ClinicalPerf	Video	12	49.3333	18.50962
	Discussion	12	44.1667	24.11651
GPA	Video	12	2.7317	.4372
	Descussion	12	3.1000	.4991

Correlations

		ClinicalPerf
GPA	Pearson Correlation	❶ .833**
	Sig. (2-tailed)	.000
	N	24

**Correlation is significant at the 0.01 level (2-tailed).

B. SPSS Output: One-Way ANOVA

ANOVA

Dependent Variable: ClinicalPerf

Source	Sum of Squares	df	Mean Square	F	Sig.	Partial Eta Squared	Observed Power[b]
Strategy ❷	160.167	1	160.167	.347	❷ .562	.016	.087
Error	10166.333	22	462.106				
Total	10326.500	23					

C. SPSS Output: Analysis of Covariance

Tests of Between-Subjects Effects ❸

Dependent Variable: ClinicalPerf

Source	Sum of Squares	df	Mean Square	F	Sig.	Partial Eta Squared	Observed Power[b]
Strategy ❹	232.949	1	232.949	6.140	❹ .022	.235	.655
GPA ❺	9004.537	1	9004.537	237.328	❺ .000	.922	1.000
Strategy* GPA ❻	55.024	1	55.024	1.450	❻ .243	.068	.209
Error	758.825	20	37.941				
Total	10326.500	23					

Estimates

Dependent Variable: Clinical Perf

Strategy	❼ Mean	Std. Error	95% Confidence Interval Lower Bound	95% Confidence Interval Upper Bound
Video	56.718[a]	1.943	52.666	60.770
Discussion	35.530[a]	1.906	31.555	39.505

❼ a. Covariates appearing in the model are evaluated at the following values: GPA = 2.9158.

❶ Observed means and correlation are presented for Clinical Performance and GPA for each group.

❷ The ANOVA shows no significant difference in clinical performance between the two teaching strategies ($p = .562$).

❸ The ANCOVA is run with GPA as the covariate.

❹ There is a significant difference between the two strategies based on the adjusted means ($p = .022$).

❺ The effect of GPA is significant. This is a necessary condition for validity of the ANCOVA, indicating a significant correlation with the dependent variable, clinical performance (see ❶). The df equal the number of covariates.

❻ The interaction between GPA and Strategy is not significant, indicating homogeneity of slopes. This is also a necessary condition for the validity of the ANCOVA. The df is the product of df for strategy and GPA.

❼ These are the adjusted means based on the average GPA for both groups of 2.92. Note that the adjusted mean for Video is larger and the mean for Discussion is smaller than the observed means (see ❶).

Portions of the output have been omitted for clarity.

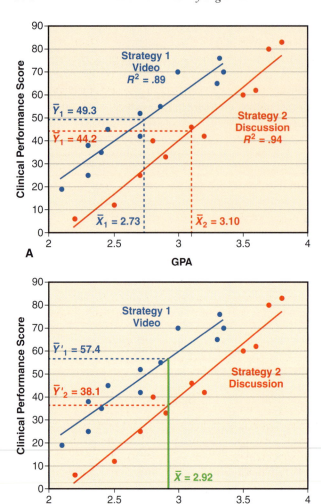

Figure 30–7 Comparison of the effectiveness of two teaching strategies on clinical performance with GPA as a covariate. **A)** Regression lines (dashed lines) define the relationship between clinical performance score and GPA for each group. The R^2 values show that this relationship is strong in each group. Solid blue and red lines intersect the regression lines at the means for each group on clinical performance ($\bar{Y}$) and GPA ($\bar{X}$). **B)** The solid green line is the combined mean for GPA and the dotted blue and red lines are adjusted mean scores ($\bar{Y}'_1$ and $\bar{Y}'_2$) for clinical performance for each group.

Therefore, we have adjusted scores by removing the effect of GPA—as if they were now standing on the same step! This process can also work in the opposite direction, where group means initially appear significantly different, but are no longer different once adjusted.

Computer Output

An analysis of variance is run on the adjusted values. Table 30-7 ❸ shows the results of this analysis for the teaching strategy data. Recall that the ANOVA showed

no significant difference between these strategies. In the summary table for the ANCOVA, the first line represents the variance attributable to the difference between groups based on the adjusted means (see Table 30-7 ❹). Now we find that the difference between the strategy groups is significant ($p = .022$), and we can reject the null hypothesis. We conclude that clinical performance does differ between those exposed to videotaped cases and discussion groups when *adjusted* for their grade point average, with better clinical performance following video sessions.

We have increased the power of our test by decreasing the unexplained variance. We have accounted for more of the variance in clinical performance by knowing GPA than we did by knowing teaching strategy alone.

 Power and sample size estimates for the ANCOVA are similar to the ANOVA. See the *Chapter 30 Supplement* for illustration of power analysis with the ANCOVA using G*Power.

A criticism of the ANCOVA is that the adjusted means are not real scores, impeding generalization of data from an ANCOVA. Interpretation of findings, including estimates of effect size, must take these adjustments into account.

Linearity of the Covariate

For an ANCOVA to be valid, the covariate must be correlated with the dependent variable. This is reflected in the second line of the ANCOVA. More precisely, it tests the hypothesis that the slope of the regression line is different from zero (see Table 30-7 ❺). If this test is not significant, the covariate is not linearly related to the dependent variable, and therefore, there will be no basis for adjusting means. In this example, we can see that the covariate of GPA is significant ($p < .001$). This value should always be examined to determine that the ANCOVA is an appropriate test.

Homogeneity of Slopes

The ANCOVA requires that the slopes of the regression lines for each group be parallel. Unequal slopes indicate that the relationship between the covariate and dependent variable is different for each group. Therefore, the adjusted means will be based on different proportional relationships, and their comparison will be meaningless. A test for **homogeneity of slopes** can be performed by looking at the interaction between the independent variable and the covariate, in this case between Strategy and GPA. As shown in Table 30.7 ❻, the interaction is not significant ($p = .243$)—a good thing—indicating that the slopes of the regression lines are not significantly different. This property is illustrated in Figure 30-7. This is a necessary condition for the validity of the ANCOVA.

Additional Assumptions

Two other assumptions are important considerations for running an ANCOVA. First, the variable chosen as the covariate must be related to the dependent variable but must also be independent of the independent variable, that is, the independent variable should not influence the value of the covariate. For example, we would not want to measure GPA after the clinical performance test, as it is possible that the clinical experience could influence future academic performance. To avoid this situation, covariates should always be measured prior to introduction of the independent variable.

Second, the validity of the ANCOVA is also influenced by the reliability of the covariate. Any error found in the covariate is compounded when the regression coefficients and adjusted means are calculated. Therefore, justification for using the adjusted scores is based on accuracy of the covariate.

> ### ▶ Results
> An analysis of variance was used to compare the clinical performance means for video ($\overline{X}$ = 49.33 ± 18.5) and discussion groups ($\overline{X}$ = 44.17 ± 24.1), showing no significant difference ($F(1,22)$ = .347, p = .562, n_p^2 = .016). Based on a high correlation between clinical performance and GPA (r = .833, $p <$ .001), an analysis of covariance was run using GPA as a covariate. The mean GPA for the video group ($\overline{X}$ = 2.73) was lower than for the discussion group ($\overline{X}$ = 3.10). The ANCOVA showed a significant difference between groups ($F(1,20)$ = 6.14, p = .022, n_p^2 = .235), based on adjusted means for video ($\overline{X}'$ = 57.43) and discussion ($\overline{X}'$ = 36.07) groups. The video strategy was superior to the discussion strategy with GPA taken into account.

 The ANCOVA can incorporate varied designs, including a 2-way analysis and repeated measures. Multiple comparisons can also be run on the adjusted means to confirm mean differences.

Using Multiple Covariates

There may be instances where one covariate is not sufficient to account for group baseline differences. Several characteristics may be relevant to understanding the dependent variable. For example, we might want to include prior clinical experience as another covariate in addition to GPA. The analysis of covariance can be extended to accommodate any number of covariates.

When several covariates are used, the precision of the analysis can be greatly enhanced, as long as the covariates are all *highly correlated with the dependent variable* and *not*

correlated with each other. If the covariates are correlated with each other, they provide redundant information and no additional benefit is gained by including them. In fact, using a large number of interrelated covariates can be a disadvantage because it will decrease statistical power. It is important, therefore, to make educated choices about the use of covariates. Previous research and pilot studies may be able to document which variables are most highly correlated with the dependent variable and which are least likely to be related to each other. Like regression, the outcome of an ANCOVA can also be significantly altered if a different combination of covariates are used. Researchers must decide which covariates will be most meaningful and decide early so that data are collected on the proper variables.

Pretest–Posttest Adjustments

The ANCOVA is often used to control for initial differences between groups in a pretest-posttest design. Even with randomization, initial measurements on the dependent variable are often different enough across groups to be of concern in further comparison. Therefore, the pretest score can be used as a covariate.

Differences between pretest and posttest scores are frequently analyzed as change scores, but the use of the pretest as a covariate in an ANCOVA is often preferred because of the potential for compounded measurement error (see Chapter 9). However, the ANCOVA is not a remedy for a study with poor reliability. Although some research questions may be more readily answered by the use of change scores, the researcher should consider what type of data will best serve the analysis.

Intact Groups

Because of its "correction" function, the ANCOVA is widely used. However, there are limitations to its application. When studies involve groups that are not formed randomly, such as intact groups, there is often a concern about whether the groups are balanced on important variables. Many researchers use the ANCOVA as a way of controlling these differences in quasi-experimental studies, thinking that this approach can substitute for randomization. Ironically, in this type of situation, where such control is most needed, the ANCOVA does not work well.[31,32] The problem is that baseline means from intact groups cannot be considered to come from a common underlying population, an assumption that is made with randomly assigned groups. This situation can bias the adjusted means, making them inaccurate estimates. Although a common strategy, readers should be cautious about interpretation of results when this approach is used.

COMMENTARY

Life is like a sewer — what you get out of it depends on what you put into it.

—*Tom Lehrer (1928-)*

American mathematician and satirist

Regression procedures are ubiquitous in healthcare literature, and therefore understanding how data can be interpreted is important to valid application. One of the most important lessons is that such analyses are dependent on the variables that are entered in the equation. With different combinations of variables, individual regression coefficients will vary, potentially changing the overall R^2 – and conclusions.

From an evidence-based practice perspective, we need to be sure that we do not discount important variables because of collinearity. Different combinations of input variables can produce results that may suggest one variable is not relevant, when it is important, but related to another variable. The results of such an analysis could be interpreted as saying that a variable is unimportant to a decision, but this may not be the case at all. This is especially true with stepwise procedures. It is essential to remember, therefore, that the relationships defined by a regression equation can be interpreted only within the context of the specific variables included in that equation.

Criticisms of regression, especially stepwise procedures, suggest that because computers have improved our ability to produce complex analyses, we have come to rely more on statistical outcomes than on our own judgments about what variables are important in the context of a study or clinical practice.[33] This point emphasizes the need to evaluate data based on logical and theoretical rationales—not just *p* values.

REFERENCES

1. Dua S, Bhuker M, Sharma P, Dhall M, Kapoor S. Body mass index relates to blood pressure among adults. *N Am J Med Sci* 2014;6(2):89-95.
2. Grimm LG, Yarnold PR, eds. *Reading and Understanding Multivariate Statistics*. Washington, D.C.: American Pyschological Association, 1995.
3. Cohen J. *Statistical Power Analysis for the Behavioral Sciences*. 2nd ed. Hillsdale, NJ: Lawrence Erlbaum; 1988.
4. UPI Dispatch, Science Desk. Children's height linked to test scores. *New York Times* October 8, 1986.
5. Wilson DM, Hammer LD, Duncan PM, Dornbusch SM, Ritter PL, Hintz RL, Gross RT, Rosenfeld RG. Growth and intellectual development. *Pediatrics* 1986;78(4):646-650.
6. Keller MC, Garver-Apgar CE, Wright MJ, Martin NG, Corley RP, Stallings MC, Hewitt JK, Zietsch BP. The genetic correlation between height and IQ: shared genes or assortative mating? *PLoS Genet* 2013;9(4):e1003451.
7. Beauchamp JP, Cesarini D, Johannesson M, Lindqvist E, Apicella C. On the sources of the height-intelligence correlation: new insights from a bivariate ACE model with assortative mating. *Behav Genet* 2011;41(2):242-252.
8. Silventoinen K, Posthuma D, van Beijsterveldt T, Bartels M, Boomsma DI. Genetic contributions to the association between height and intelligence: Evidence from Dutch twin data from childhood to middle age. *Genes Brain Behav* 2006;5(8):585-595.
9. Houx PJ, Jolles J. Age-related decline of psychomotor speed: effects of age, brain health, sex, and education. *Percept Mot Skills* 1993;76(1):195-211.
10. Rutledge R, Lentz CW, Fakhry S, Hunt J. Appropriate use of the Glasgow Coma Scale in intubated patients: a linear regression prediction of the Glasgow verbal score from the Glasgow eye and motor scores. *J Trauma* 1996;41(3):514-522.
11. Meredith W, Rutledge R, Fakhry SM, Emery S, Kromhout-Schiro S. The conundrum of the Glasgow Coma Scale in intubated patients: a linear regression prediction of the Glasgow verbal score from the Glasgow eye and motor scores. *J Trauma* 1998;44(5):839-844; discussion 844-835.
12. Cheng K, Bassil R, Carandang R, Hall W, Muehlschlegel S. The estimated verbal GCS subscore in intubated traumatic brain injury patients: is it really better? *J Neurotrauma* 2017;34(8):1603-1609.
13. Ostfeld BM, Schwartz-Soicher O, Reichman NE, Teitler JO, Hegyi T. Prematurity and sudden unexpecte infant deaths in the United States. *Pediatrics* 2017;140(1).
14. Noh JW, Lee SA, Choi HJ, Hong JH, Kim MH, Kwon YD. Relationship between the intensity of physical activity and depressive symptoms among Korean adults: analysis of Korea Health Panel data. *J Phys Ther Sci* 2015;27(4):1233-1237.
15. Stamm TA, Pieber K, Crevenna R, Dorner TE. Impairment in the activities of daily living in older adults with and without osteoporosis, osteoarthritis and chronic back pain: a secondary analysis of population-based health survey data. *BMC Musculoskelet Disord* 2016;17:139.
16. Menard S. *Logistic Regression: From Introductory to Advanced Concepts and Applications*. Thousand Oaks, CA: SAGE Publications; 2010.
17. Pinedo S, Erazo P, Tejada P, Lizarraga N, Aycart J, Miranda M, Zaldibar B, Gamio A, Gomez I, Sanmartin V, et al. Rehabilitation efficiency and destination on discharge after stroke. *Eur J Phys Rehabil Med* 2014;50(3):323-333.
18. Field A. *Discovering Statistics Using IBM SPSS Statistics*. 5th ed. Thousand Oaks, CA: Sage; 2018.
19. Kwak C, Clayton-Matthews A. Multinomial logistic regression. *Nurs Res* 2002;51(6):404-410.
20. Laerd Statistics. Multinomial logistic regression using SPSS statistics. Available at https://statistics.laerd.com/spss-tutorials/multinomial-logistic-regression-using-spss-statistics.php. Accessed January 12, 2019.
21. Cox DR, Snell EJ. *The Analysis of Binary Data*. 2nd ed. Boca Raton, FL: Chapman & Hall; 1989.
22. Nagelkerke NJD. A note on the general definition of the coefficient of determination. *Biometrika* 1991;78(3):691-692.

23. Vittinghoff E, McCulloch CE. Relaxing the rule of ten events per variable in logistic and Cox regression. *Am J Epidemiol* 2007;165(6):710-718.

24. Long JS. *Regression Models for Categorical and Limited Dependent Variables* Thousand Oaks, CA: Sage; 1997.

25. Peduzzi P, Concato J, Kemper E, Holford TR, Feinstein AR. A simulation study of the number of events per variable in logistic regression analysis. *J Clin Epidemiol* 1996;49(12):1373-1379.

26. Bejot Y, Troisgros O, Gremeaux V, Lucas B, Jacquin A, Khoumri C, Aboa-Eboule C, Benaim C, Casillas JM, Giroud M. Poststroke disposition and associated factors in a population-based study: the Dijon Stroke Registry. *Stroke* 2012;43(8):2071-2077.

27. Andrade C. Propensity score matching in nonrandomized studies: a concept simply explained using antidepressant treatment during pregnancy as an example. *J Clin Psychiatry* 2017;78(2): e162-e165.

28. Streiner DL, Norman GR. The pros and cons of propensity scores. *Chest* 2012;142(6):1380-1382.

29. Staffa SJ, Zurakowski D. Five steps to successfully implement and evaluate propensity score matching in clinical research studies. *Anesth Analg* 2018;127(4):1066-1073.

30. King G, R. N. Why propensity scores should not be used for matching. Political Analysis. Available at http://j.mp/2ovYGsW. Accessed February 9, 2019.

31. Henson RK. ANCOVA with intact groups: don't do it! Presentation at the Annual Meeting of the Mid-South Educational Research Association. New Orleans, LA. Available at https://archive.org/stream/ERIC_ED426086/ERIC_ED426086_djvu.txt. Accessed January 11, 2019.

32. Huck SW. *Reading Statistics and Research*. 6th ed. Boston: Pearson; 2012.

33. Dallal GE. Simplifying a multiple regression equation. *The Little Handbook of Statistical Practice*. Available at http://www.jerrydallal.com/lhsp/simplify.htm. Accessed January 8, 2019.

Multivariate Analysis

Multivariate analysis refers to a set of statistical procedures that are distinguished by the ability to examine several response variables within a single study and to account for their potential interrelationships in the analysis of the data. These tests are distinguished from *univariate analysis* procedures, such as the *t*-test and analysis of variance, which accommodate only one measured variable.

In a brief introduction such as this, it is not possible to cover the full scope of these complex statistical procedures. The purpose of this chapter is to present concepts related to commonly used procedures including factor analysis, sequential equation modeling, cluster analysis, multivariate analysis of variance, and survival analysis.

■ Exploratory Factor Analysis

The technique of **factor analysis** is quite different from any of the statistical procedures we have examined thus far. Rather than using data for comparison or prediction, factor analysis examines the structure within a large number of variables, to reflect how they cluster to represent different dimensions of a construct.

Factor analysis is more controversial than other analytic methods because it leaves room for subjectivity and judgment. However, it makes an important contribution to multivariate methods because it can provide insights into the nature of abstract constructs and allows us to superimpose order on complex phenomena. A statistician

should be consulted to make decisions about using particular methods under specific research conditions. Those interested in greater detail should refer to several useful resources.[1-5]

The overarching term "factor analysis" is actually used to refer to several approaches with different goals. **Exploratory factor analysis (EFA)** is used to examine linear combinations of underlying **factors** that explain a latent variable or construct. **Confirmatory factor analysis (CFA)** is used to confirm hypotheses about the structure of underlying constructs. These two approaches will be discussed in the following sections. A third technique called **principal components analysis (PCA)** attempts to reduce data to a smaller set of summary variables or *components* that account for most of the variance in a set of observed variables. Although many of the statistical techniques used for these analyses are similar, there are important differences in assumptions and purpose.

 -See the *Chapter 31 Supplement* for further discussion of principal components analysis.

Exploratory Factor Analysis

The concept of EFA is illustrated in Figure 31-1. The set of "variables" at the top are part of an overarching construct of "green." We assume that there is some relationship among circles that have similar hues of green, that light green circles are related to other light green circles, but not to darker green circles, but together all the hues explain "green." Through factor analysis, these variables are reorganized into three relatively independent factors, each one representing a unique cluster of variables that are highly correlated among themselves but poorly correlated with items on other factors. Not all factors are equal, however. For instance, factor 1 accounts for more of the variance in the data than the others, with factors 2 and 3 accounting for successively less variance.

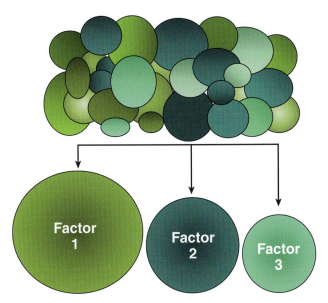

Figure 31–1 Conceptual representation of exploratory factor analysis, showing how multiple "green" items are grouped into three independent factors that explain the structure in a latent trait of "greenness."

Latent traits are constructs that cannot be directly measured, but that influence behavior (see Chapter 10). The purpose of EFA is to determine how different variables relate to each other to contribute to an understanding of a latent trait. This approach is often used in the development and validation of health questionnaires that focus on a behavioral construct.

➤ CASE IN POINT #1

Consider a hypothetical study of behaviors related to chronic low back pain (LBP). Through a review of literature we have identified relevant variables and have constructed a questionnaire with

seven items, each measured on a 5-point Likert scale, based on the frequency with which each behavior is observed, from 1 = "never exhibited" to 5 = "almost always exhibited."

How often do you exhibit these behaviors related to your low back pain?

1. Complaining about pain
2. Changing position frequently while sitting
3. Groaning or moaning
4. Rubbing my back
5. Isolating myself
6. Moving stiffly
7. Walking stiffly

The questionnaire is distributed to a sample of 150 patients. We are interested in determining how these variables are related to each other and if they represent different theoretical elements of the latent trait of pain behavior.

The process of EFA begins by considering the inter-correlations among all the variables (see Table 31-1).

➤ The highest correlations among the seven variables are:
- "Complains of pain" and "Groans" ($r = .719$)
- "Changes position" and "Rubs back" ($r = .876$)
- "Moves stiffly" and "Walks stiffly" ($r = .816$)

The variable "Isolates oneself" does not have a strong correlation with any other items, Its highest correlations are with "Changes position" and "Rubs back" ($r = .176$, $r = .133$, respectively).

Several tests are used to determine how well the correlations help to explain the variance among these variables—all with big and confusing names. The *Kaiser-Meyer-Olkin (KMO) Measure of Sampling Adequacy* assesses the proportion of variance among the variables that can be considered *common variance* (see Table 31-2 ❶).

Table 31-1	Correlations of Chronic Low Back Pain Behaviors						
	COMPLAINS ABOUT PAIN	**CHANGES POSITION**	**GROANS**	**RUBS BACK**	**ISOLATES ONESELF**	**MOVES STIFFLY**	**WALKS STIFFLY**
Complains About Pain	1.000	–.566	**.719*****	–.586	–.013	.249	.257
Changes Position		1.000	–.474	**.876*****	**–.176****	–.237	–.272
Groans			1.000	–.479	.094	.038	.115
Rubs Back				1.000	**–.133***	–.243	–.265
Isolates Oneself					1.000	–.020	.086
Moves Stiffly						1.000	**.816*****
Walks Stiffly							1.000

Bolded values represent the largest correlations for each pair of variables.
*$p = .053$, **$p = .016$, *** $p<.001$

SPSS Output: Exploratory Factor Analysis

KMO and Bartlett's Test

Kaiser-Meyer-Olkin Measure of Sampling Adequacy.	❶	.651
Bartlett's Test of Sphericity	Approx. Chi-Square	582.054
	df	21
	Sig. ❷	.000

Communalities ❸

	Initial	Extraction
Complains about pain	.629	.982
Changes position	.778	.968
Groans	.557	.550
Rubs back	.780	.795
Isolates oneself	.087	.041
Moves stiffly	.689	.933
Walks stiffly	.683	.719

Extraction Method: Principal Axis Factoring.

Total Variance Explained

Initial Eigenvalues

Factor	Total	% of Variance	Cumulative %
1	3.152	45.033	45.033
2	1.572	22.463	67.496
3	1.029	14.705	❺ 82.201
4	.706	10.081	92.282
5	.250	3.574	95.856
6	.168	2.400	98.256
7 ❹	.122	1.744	100.000

Extraction Method: Principal Axis Factoring.

Factor Matrix[a] ❻

	Factor 1	Factor 2	Factor 3
Complains about pain	.823	−.241	.497
Changes position	−.864	.225	.414
Groans	.608	−.324	.274
Rubs back	−.820	.202	.284
Isolates oneself	.116	−.039	−.162
Moves stiffly	.506	.821	.050
Walks stiffly	.509	.677	.016

Extraction Method: Principal Axis Factoring.
a. Attempted to extract 3 factors. More than 25 iterations required. (Convergence=.008). Extraction was terminated.

Rotated Factor Matrix[a] ❼

	Factor 1	Factor 2	Factor 3
Complains about pain	.965	.181	−.133
Changes position	−.430	−.157	.871
Groans	.712	−.002	−.205
Rubs back	−.470	−.167	.739
Isolates oneself	−.004	.007	−.202
Moves stiffly	.062	.962	−.062
Walks stiffly	.099	.833	−.123

Extraction Method: Principal Axis Factoring.
Rotation Method: Varimax with Kaiser Normalization.
a. Rotation converged in 4 iterations.

---

❶ The KMO value is above the minimal acceptable value of 0.6, indicating that the pattern of correlations is sufficiently tight to make the factor analysis meaningful.

❷ The test of sphericity is significant, indicating that the correlations among variables are significantly different from zero.

❸ Communalities indicate the extent to which each variable correlates with the rest of the data. Only the variable "isolates oneself" shows a low communality, indicating that its variance is not likely to contribute to any factor.

❹ Seven factors are initially identified in the data, corresponding to the number of variables entered. The eigenvalues reflect the amount of common variance accounted for by each factor. Using the 1.0 cutoff for the eigenvalue, the analysis stopped at 3 factors

❺ The three factors initially account for a cumulative 82.2% of the variance in the data.

❻ The factor loadings in the unrotated factor matrix do not clearly distinguish the factors.

❼ The loadings from the rotated factor matrix show a clearer picture. Highlighted cells identify variables assigned to each factor. The variable "Isolates oneself" loads highest on factor 3, but does not meet the 0.4 standard.

Portions of the output have been omitted for clarity.

The lower the proportion, the more suited the data are to factor analysis—variables will likely break out into separate factors. The KMO statistic takes values between 0 and 1, with stronger values closer to 1, and 0.6 considered a minimal acceptable level.[6] For the pain behavior data, the KMO test = 0.651, which just passes the minimal standard.

Bartlett's Test of Sphericity uses the chi-square distribution to test the null hypothesis that intercorrelations equal zero (Table 31-2 ➋). We want this to be a significant value, that is, we want to reject the null hypothesis. This value is significant for the pain behavior data ($p < .001$). Because sample sizes are usually large in factor analysis, this test has high power and is rarely nonsignificant.

Communalities give us a measure of the proportion of each variable's variance that can be explained by factors (Table 31-2 ➌). Higher communalities, above 0.4, indicate that variables will contribute to the factor structure. Values less than 0.4 reflect variables that may not be a significant part of any factor. For example, we may be concerned that the variable "Isolates oneself" will be problematic.

Extraction of Factors

Through a complex series of manipulations, the analysis derives factors through a process called **extraction**. The number of factors that are extracted depends on how much of the total variance in the data can be explained by a factor, and the extent to which factors are independent of each other. Several methods are available for this process. The most commonly used method for EFA is called **principal axis factoring**. This method defines factors based on their intercorrelations.

📌 Although used less often, other methods of extraction include *maximum likelihood method, alpha factoring, image factoring, ordinary least squares,* and *generalized least squares methods.*[7] These methods differ in how variance is used to determine factors.[8]

Determining the Number of Factors

The first factor that is "extracted" from the data will account for as much of the variance in the data as possible. The second factor represents the extraction of the next highest possible amount of variance from the remaining variance. Each successive factor that is identified "uses up" another portion of the total variance, until all the variance within the test items has been accounted for. The number of factors derived from a set of variables will always equal the number of variables.

As shown in Table 31-2 ➍, this analysis has extracted seven factors (because there are seven variables). However, several factors account for small amounts of variance and do not really contribute to an understanding of the

structure of the data. The data are usually characterized most efficiently using only the first few components. Therefore, we need to establish a cutoff point to limit the number of factors for further analysis.

The statistic used to set this cutoff is called an **eigenvalue**. Eigenvalues tell us how much of the total variance is explained by a factor. Factor 1 will always account for more variance than the other factors (in this example 45.0%). The most common approach restricts retaining factors to those with an eigenvalue of at least 1.00 (Table 31-2 ➎). Some statisticians recommend retaining factors that account for at least 70% of the total variance.[9]

➤ Using the criteria of eigenvalues above 1.00, three factors were identified for the pain behavior data, accounting for 82.2% of the variance in the original data.

 These factors are not "real" yet—they are only statistical entities at this point—and do not indicate which variables are related to which factors. Up to this point the analysis is simply relying on variance to identify factors. It will not be until the end of the analysis that the "factors" will make sense.

The Factor Matrix

The result of the factor analysis is a **factor matrix** for the three factors that have been extracted (Table 31.2 ➏). The coefficients listed in the table are called **factor loadings**, which are measures of the correlation between the individual item and the overall factor. Loadings are interpreted like correlation coefficients, ranging from 0.00 to ±1.00. Generally, loadings above .40 are considered meaningful, although some researchers use .30 as the minimum. Only the absolute value is considered in this interpretation. The sign indicates if the variable is positively or negatively correlated with the factor.

Ideally, each variable will have a loading close to 1.00 on one factor and loadings close to 0.00 on all other factors. These would be considered "pure" factors. This rarely happens, however, and so we look at the highest loadings for each variable. When one variable loads heavily on more than one factor, those factors do not represent unique concepts, and there is some correlation between them. The researcher must then reconsider the nature of the variables included in the analysis and how they relate to the construct that is being studied.

Unfortunately, this factor matrix is often difficult to interpret because it does not provide the most unique structure possible; that is, several variables may be "loaded" on more than one factor. For instance, if we look across the rows for "Moves stiffly" and "Walks stiffly," we can see that factor loadings are moderately strong for both Factors 1 and 2. Therefore, the next step is to develop a unique statistical solution so that each variable relates highly to only one factor.

Factor Rotation

This concept can be illustrated more simply using a two-dimensional example. Assume we have identified only two factors, Factor 1 and Factor 2. We could plot each of the seven variables against these two axes, as shown in Figure 31-2A. The vertical axis represents Factor 1 and the horizontal axis represents Factor 2. As we can see, variables sit in the geometric space somewhere between the two factors, not directly on either of the axes. Therefore, this plot does not present a clear "structure" in the data in terms of specific factor assignments. If, however, we could rearrange the orientation of axes and variables without altering the underlying relationships, we might be able to create a structure that will help us interpret these relationships.

We do this by a process of **factor rotation**, turning the axes in such a way as to maximize the orientation of variables near one of the axes. There are actually several ways that factor axes can be statistically rotated to arrive at this solution (see Box 31-1). This example uses the most common approach, called **varimax rotation**, which tries to minimize the number of variables that have high loadings on each factor, simplifying interpretation.[10]

This rotation is illustrated in Figure 31-2B. The rotation improves the spatial structure of the variables so that distinct factors are now visible; that is, several of the variables lie directly on or close to one of the axes. The higher the loading, the more the variable appears at the extremes of the axes. We find that variables 2, 6, and 7 now have the closest orientation to Factor 1, and variables 1 and 5 have the closest orientation to Factor 2. Variables 3 and 4, clustered around the origin (loadings close to zero), show little or no relationship to either factor.

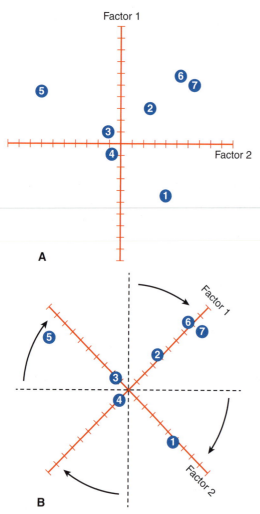

A

B

Figure 31–2 Factor axes showing loadings of 7 variables on two factors. **(A)** Unrotated solution. **(B)** Rotated solution, showing how variables are now loaded closely on one of the two factors. For this illustration, the factor loadings are hypothetical. We cannot use the factor loadings given in Table 31-2, as those represent coordinates in a three-dimensional space.

Box 31-1   Types of Rotation

There are actually several forms of factor rotation that can be used under different circumstances. Varimax rotation is considered **orthogonal rotation** because the axes stay perpendicular to each other as they are rotated. This means that the two factors are independent of each other (orthogonal means independent); that is, they maintain maximal separation. **Oblique rotation** allows the axes to change their orientation to each other. Therefore, some variables could be close to two factors, and the factors would be correlated. This might lead to a more realistic solution in some cases. However, the orthogonal solution will typically be easier to interpret, and in many cases will provide a comparable solution to oblique rotation.

Although varimax rotation is used most often because it generally presents the clearest factor structure, there are several other forms of orthogonal rotation.[10] The two most commonly found in the literature include:

- *Quartimax rotation* minimizes the number of factors needed to explain each variable, simplifying row loadings.
- *Equamax rotation*, a combination of varimax and quartimax methods, minimizes the number of variables that load highly on a factor, and the number of factors needed to explain a variable.

Each of these methods will result in a slightly different positioning of the axes. For some analyses it may be necessary to try different solutions to develop the one that best differentiates factors. Fortunately, these processes are easily requested in a computer analysis. See Tabachnick and Fiddell[8] and other references for more detailed discussion of these rotation strategies.

In the actual factor analysis, we have to think of a three-dimensional space with three axes. It is difficult to conceive of this type of analysis without a computer. We must visualize a spatial solution that provides the one best linear combination where each of the variables would be located directly on or near one of the axes, which would indicate that the variable was "loaded" on that factor. We would then be able to identify which variables "belonged" to each factor.

The Rotated Factor Matrix

This process results in the creation of a *rotated factor matrix* that should provide a clearer statistical picture (Table 31-2 ❼). We interpret this information by looking across each row of the matrix to determine which factor has the highest loading for that variable. Highlighted values show the one loading for each variable that has the strongest relationship to one of the factors. The factors are starting to take on meaning.

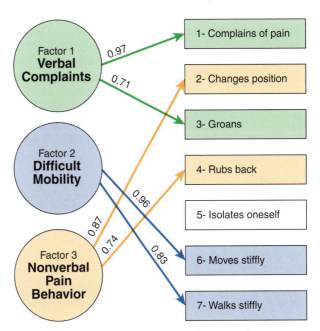

➤ • "Complains of pain" and "Groans" load highest on factor 1.
 • "Moves stiffly" and "Walks stiffly" load highest on factor 2.
 • "Changes position" and "Rubs back" load highest on factor 3.
 • The item for "Isolates oneself" does not have a sufficiently high loading on any factor.

Figure 31–3 Names assigned to three factors in the pain behavior study. Numbers on arrows are the factor loadings. Item 5 did not load on any factor and may not be appropriately included as part of pain behavior based on this analysis.

Naming Factors

The final step in a factor analysis is the naming of factors according to a common theme or theoretical construct that characterizes the variables in the factor. This is a subjective and sometimes difficult task, especially in situations when the variables within a factor do not have obvious ties. The researcher must look for commonalties and theoretical relationships that will explain the latent trait being studied and come up with a factor name that reflects it. Figure 31-3 shows how the seven variables have been organized into three factors, and the names that have been assigned to describe them.

Sometimes certain combinations of variables don't easily suggest a factor name, and it may be necessary to reexamine the nature of the construct being studied and the variables included. We must also recognize that similar analyses on different samples or with a different combination of variables may organize data differently, as will different methods of extraction or rotation.

Note that item 5, "Isolates oneself," does not appear to be a meaningful variable for understanding these pain behaviors. Its low communality and factor loadings suggest that it is not part of the larger construct. Two approaches may be taken to handle this situation. One would be to eliminate this item in future studies. But it

is still possible that it has some importance to the overall construct of pain behavior. It may also be reasonable, then, to consider other items that should be included in the analysis that would better explicate the theoretical foundations of pain behavior.

What we have now is a set of variables that contribute to a construct we are calling "chronic pain behavior." We can begin to understand the structure of pain behavior by focusing on three elements that we have labelled mobility, verbal complaints, and nonverbal complaints. As we move forward in this research, we can explore how each of these elements contributes to a patient's reactions to treatment, interactions with family, participation in work or social activities, and so on. The factor analysis has provided a framework from which we can better understand these types of theoretical relationships.

 Note that although "Changes position" and "Rubs back" have been assigned to factor 3 (nonverbal behavior), they both have loadings >.40 on factor 1, indicating that there may be a correlation between verbal and nonverbal behaviors.

➤ **Results**
Factor analysis, using principal axis factoring and varimax rotation, was conducted to determine the structure underlying

behaviors related to chronic LBP. We confirmed the suitability of the data using the Kaiser-Meyer-Olkin test, which was .651, and Bartlett's test of sphericity, which was significant (χ^2 (21) = 582.05, p < .001), both meeting minimal standards. Communalities for the 7 items were between .55 and .98, except for item 5 (Isolates oneself), which had a communality of .041.

The analysis derived three factors, retaining factors with an eigenvalue greater than 1.0, representing 82.2% of the original variance. Factor loadings above .40 were used to assign variables to factors. Factor 1 corresponded to verbal complaints (Complaints of pain and Groaning). Factor 2 represented difficult mobility (Moves stiffly and Walks stiffly). Factor 3 described nonverbal pain behaviors (Rubs back and Changes position). Item 5 (Isolates onself) did not meet the .40 threshold for any factor and does not contribute to an understanding of the behaviors in this construct.

A table containing values in the rotated factor matrix is usually provided in the results section of a research report.

Factor Scores

An interesting use of factor analysis is the creation of a smaller set of composite scores that can be used in further statistical analysis. Scores can be created for each factor by multiplying each variable value by a weighting, and then summing the weighted scores for all variables within that factor. This results in a **factor score**. Factor scores can be calculated for each subject for each factor, and those scores can then be used for further statistical testing. This process decreases the total number of variables used, which improves variance estimates for analyses such as regression. By using factor scores, large data sets became much more manageable.

Sample Size for Factor Analysis

Because of the exploratory nature of factor analysis, there is an expectation of stability within the data for an EFA. One common approach to setting sample size is based on the subject-to-variables (STV) ratio. However, there is really no consensus regarding the "rules of thumb" that are recommended. One guideline is to have at least 300 cases for any study,[11] although solutions that have the majority of factor loadings >.80 do not require as large a sample and may be sufficient with about 150 cases.[8] Others have recommended a minimum number of observations at least five times the number of variables (a STV ratio of at least 5),[11] with a minimum of 100 observations regardless of the STV ratio.[12] Still others have argued that a STV of 10 to 1 should be used. Because we are not dealing with probabilities, power is not an issue per se, but larger samples will provide a better estimate of variance components within the data.

Confirmatory Factor Analysis

Confirmatory factor analysis is similar to EFA in many ways, but with a distinctly different purpose. The main differences are related to hypothesis testing and the final fit of a model. EFA is run with no prior assumptions about how factors will be manifested. It explores the variance structure and factors are then identified. For CFA, however, a model is proposed at the outset, and a hypothesis is set forth to assess how well sample data support the theorized factor model. The model is often based on findings from an EFA or it may be developed to represent a theory (see Focus on Evidence 31-1). The criteria for variable inclusion are usually more stringent in CFA, with a rule of thumb that variables with factor loadings <0.7 are dropped.

CFA is a measurement approach based on the assumption that you enter the factor analysis with a firm idea about the theoretical foundation of the model, the number of factors you will encounter, and which variables should load onto each factor. Therefore, it is reasonable to think of EFA as *theory-generating* and CFA as *theory-testing* techniques.[13] This approach is often used to establish construct validity for items in a questionnaire or scale (see Chapter 10).

Take a look back at the discussion of factor analysis in the continued development of the Arthritis Impact Measurement Scale (AIMS) in Chapter 10, which also illustrated exploratory and confirmatory approaches.

■ Structural Equation Modeling

Previous discussions of regression and factor analysis procedures have emphasized exploring relationships, a process in which we have been careful to avoid an assumption of causation. However, a different approach called **causal modeling** can be used to illustrate possible causal relationships. These procedures examine whether a pattern of intercorrelations among variables "fits" an underlying theory of how constructs are linked and the directionality of those relationships.[17,18]

Models are studied using a process of **structural equation modeling (SEM)**, which is a confirmatory approach for hypothesis testing, combining elements of factor analysis and multiple regression. The process for SEM is quite complex, and this discussion will focus on a conceptual understanding of how results are reported and interpreted. Several useful references are available for those who are looking for greater detail.[8,19-23]

Focus on Evidence 31–1
The Whole Is More Than the Sum of Its Parts

The Minnesota Living with Heart Failure Questionnaire (MLHFQ) is the most widely used measure of health-related quality of life (QOL) in patients with heart failure (HF).[14] The MLHFQ is a self-administered tool consisting of 21 items with responses on a 6-point scale (0-5), ranging from "no impairment" to "very much impaired." Three summary scores are used: a total score as well as two subscales, physical and emotional. Only eight items are used in the total score. The MLHRQ has shown good responsiveness, sensitivity to change, and reliability.[15]

The MLHRQ is often used as a basis for evaluating changes in QOL, as a foundation for clinical decision-making, intervention, and monitoring progress or decline in patients with heart failure (HF). Therefore, it is important to recognize the underlying premise for each subscale to understand how the scores can influence these judgments. Because the dimensions of the test had not been verified, Garin et al[38] explored the components of the MLHFQ using data for 3,847 patients with HF from 21 countries. The factorial structure of the MLHFQ was assessed by randomly dividing the sample into two subsamples, the first used to conduct an EFA, which was then tested on the second subsample using a CFA.

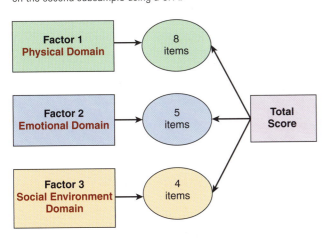

The EFA resulted in a three-factor solution, which was composed of physical and emotional items, but a third factor related to social environment was also identified. These factors were used for the CFA model, which also included a general factor based on the full 21-items scale, as well as the three specific factors. The CFA confirmed factors for physical, emotional, and social domains, and also confirmed that the total score represented a singular construct of QOL.

There are two important concepts illustrated by this type of study. One is the value of an initial EFA to develop a theoretical framework for a scale, which revealed a third domain related to the social environment that was not considered part of the original scale. Given the chronic nature of HF, this finding highlights the relevance of social issues for evidence-based practice, considerations that could change decision-making regarding the long-term impact of the disease. The second is confirmation of the construct validity of the total score as a representation of the overall effect of HF on QOL. By studying the scale in this way, the researchers demonstrated that individual items could load directly onto the total score as well as onto one of the three specific domains. This was pertinent because not all of the items loaded onto one of the three subscales.

An added benefit of using a large international sample was the cross-cultural validation of the MLHFQ, which has been translated into many languages. Because most of the validation work was based on the original English version, these data support the use of the tool across settings and countries, providing essential clarification for using the tool in clinical trials.

Source: Garin O, Ferrer M, Pont A, et al. Evidence on the global measurement model of the Minnesota Living with Heart Failure Questionnaire. *Qual Life Res* 2013;22(10):2675-2684.

Yes, another meaning for the acronym SEM! It has been used for standard error of the mean (Chapter 22), standard error of measurement (Chapter 9), and now structural equation modeling. A popular set of letters!

Confirmatory factor analysis is actually a special case of SEM and is often used as a precursor to define how variables are related within factors that fit a theory, but CFA is not used to explore causal connections. Structural models are designed to assess latent trait variables but may also include observed or measured variables as well (see Chapter 10).

➤ CASE IN POINT #2

Wang and Geng[24] were interested in exploring the relationship between socioeconomic status (SES) and health, which has been documented in many countries. Research has also shown a growing understanding that lifestyle also has significant effect on physical and psychological health.[25] They used data from the 2015 Chinese General Social Survey to assess if these theoretical relationships were manifested in Chinese culture.

The Path Diagram

SEM begins with the proposal of a theoretical premise, a researcher's conceptualization of possible causal relationships based on prior research, theory, empirical observations and experiences, expert opinion, and, most importantly, logical explanations. The model shows designated pathways that the researcher believes best describe the underlying theory. The analysis then examines variance and correlations (covariance) in the data to see how well the model explains observed findings in a given sample, deriving a *structural equation*, analogous to a multiple regression equation. Researchers often work in an iterative fashion, proposing an initial model that is tested and revised several times until a good fit is determined. The final model may be revised by taking out variables or changing paths.

The hypothesized model is depicted in a **path diagram**, illustrated in Figure 31-4 for the SES study. In the context of SEM, the independent predictor variable is SES, which is called an **exogenous variable**, indicating that its causes are *external* to the model and not included in the theory. The dependent outcome variables of lifestyle, physical health, and psychological health are called **endogenous variables**. These variables are assumed to be "caused by" SES conditions. The authors provided operational definitions for each of these variables, which were measured using self-report scales.

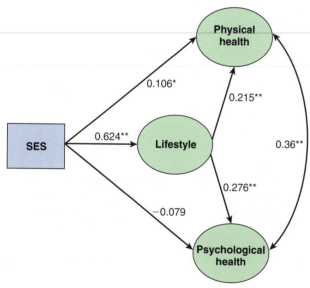

Figure 31–4 Structural model showing theorized influence of socioeconomic status on physical and psychological health, with lifestyle as a mediating variable. Coefficients represent the relative strength of the relationship between variables (*indicates *p* < .05; ** indicates *p* < .01). Adapted from Wang J, Geng L. Effects of socioeconomic status on physical and psychological health: lifestyle as a mediator. *Int J Environ Res Public Health* 2019;16(2). pii:E281. Figure 2. Used under the terms and conditions of the Creative Commons Attribution (CC-BY) license (http://creativecommons.org/licenses/by/4.0/).

You may read studies that use *path analysis*, which is a form of SEM. SEM is intended to be used when latent variables are being tested, whereas path analysis is meant to be used with variables that are directly observed or measured, called *manifest* variables. Path analysis is based on a set of restrictive assumptions that make its application less useful. Both methods use comparable statistics and diagrams and can be interpreted in a similar way.

Direct and Indirect Effects

Variables are connected in the path diagram by a series of arrows going towards or away from each variable, showing the theorized causal relationships. Curved bidirectional arrows indicate a noncausal correlation between variables. In this example, the curved arrow indicates the correlation between physical and psychological health disability.

SEM distinguishes three types of effects. The *direct effect* of the exogenous variable on the endogenous variables is shown with straight unidirectional arrows, sometimes called *causal paths*. This is illustrated by the direct path from SES to lifestyle, physical heath, and psychological health.

Indirect effects are identified by a chain of two or more straight arrows, all going in the same direction through a *mediating variable*. The mediating variable essentially serves as both a cause and effect. In our example, lifestyle is a mediating variable. The *total effect* is the sum of direct and indirect effects.

> In the SES study, researchers hypothesized that people with higher SES would be in better physical and psychological health and that a healthier lifestyle would mediate these relationships, also resulting in better physical and psychological health.

Arrows in the path diagram are labeled with *path coefficients*, which represent weights for the effect of one variable on another, similar to standardized beta weights in multiple regression (see Chapter 30). Therefore, they indicate the relative importance of the variables in predicting the outcomes. We can see the effect of SES on lifestyle is the strongest. The significance of these coefficients is also indicated in the diagram.

 See the *Chapter 31 Supplement* for calculations of indirect and total effects for the SES study.

Goodness of Fit

Several indices are used to test for "goodness of fit," assessing how well the model represents the structure of the sample data. Some indices reflect the degree to which the model and data coincide, and others reflecting the degree to which they differ.[26] Those reported most often in the literature include the *comparative fit index (CFI)*, the *goodness of fit index (GFI)* and the *adjusted goodness of fit index (AGFI)*. These values range from 0 to 1.0, with values above .90 considered a good fit.[27] Another commonly used index is the *root mean square error of approximation (RMSEA)*, which reflects the discrepancy between the model and data. Therefore, values closer to zero indicate a good fit. The chi-square statistic can also be used to test the hypothesis of a good fit (see Chapter 28). Typically, researchers will calculate several goodness of fit measures to demonstrate the stability of the final model. For instance, in the SES study, the RMSEA = 0.046 and the CFI = 0.941, both indicating that the model is appropriate.

Interpretation of SEM

It is important to appreciate that structural equations modeling does not "prove" cause-and-effect relationships. A model that shows a good fit to the data can only "support" the relevant theory. It can, however, allow inferences about causal effects if the data can show that the causal factors precede the outcomes. Interpretations must be made in context. It is always possible that other untested models could provide stronger explanations or that other variables need to be tapped to make the model clearer. It is also important to demonstrate logical connections and to rule out competing explanations—often a difficult task.[13] Results should always be interpreted with the understanding that they cannot establish cause and effect in the same way as a randomized trial.

> ### Results
> Results showed that SES had a significant positive impact on physical health, but the impact on psychological health was not significant. Lifestyle had positive effects on both physical and psychological health and it played a mediating role between SES and both health domains. The authors suggest that these findings support these relationships across cultures, as the model reflects outcomes of studies from other countries.

📌 Specialized software is necessary to generate structural equations.[20] LISREL (*LInear Structural RELations*) is a proprietary software package that is commonly used.[28] SPSS can be used with an add-on program called AMOS (*Analysis of MOvement Structure*).[29] Statistical help is recommended for those who want to run these complex analyses.

■ Cluster Analysis

When researchers are interested in the underlying structures in a set of data, factor analysis is one approach to determine how groups of correlated *variables* contribute to that structure. In an analogous process, **cluster analysis** looks for groupings of *people* that demonstrate similar characteristics. Rather than generating factors, this analysis generates *clusters* of subjects that must be examined to determine how they relate to each other.

> ### ➤ CASE IN POINT #3
> Michel et al[30] studied the prognosis of functional recovery in patients who had experienced a hip fracture. Data were collected from 207 patients through structured questionnaires administered in an interview to assess demographic, psychosocial, medical, mobility, and functional characteristics pre-fracture and 1-year post surgery. The purpose of the study was to establish homogeneous clusters that would describe groupings of patients with similar profiles.

Figure 31-5 shows the hierarchical structure, or *cluster tree*, for this analysis. The cluster analysis goes through successive iterations to reorganize the data to determine how the patients' characteristics relate to each other. Starting with 207 patients, the first iteration created two clusters, with 79 and 128 subjects. These groupings were further differentiated in successive steps.

Like factor analysis, this statistical technique requires judgment in establishing a cluster solution. In this analysis, the researchers determined a solution of four clusters of patients with similar profiles in terms of 13 predictor variables and 7 outcome variables. Beyond four clusters, the groupings became too small to allow meaningful descriptions. Once clusters are statistically determined, researchers must then consider how the clusters are differentiated, describing the patient characteristics that distinguish the groupings, and how those profiles can be used in clinical practice. Figure 31-6 illustrates how selected characteristics were distributed across the four clusters identified in the hip fracture study.

> ### Results
> Cluster 1 was the largest group (n = 79), demonstrating the highest level of walking and ADL function. Few members of this group had comorbidities or had experienced falls, and were generally independent. Those in cluster 2 (n = 62) had poorer outcomes. Not one patient regained prefracture function or ability to walk without difficulty. More of these patients had comorbidities and had experienced falls.

Cluster 3 was the smallest cluster ($n = 27$). Close to 40% lived in nursing homes, tended to have more comorbidities, and experienced falls. Most could not walk without difficulty, although close to half had regained walking function.

Those in cluster 4 ($n = 39$) exhibited the poorest performance, with few being independent in walking or ADL. They were more likely to live in a nursing home, be disoriented, have comorbid problems, and be confined to a wheelchair or bed.

Clinicians can examine the characteristics within each cluster to understand how these profiles emerge, allowing for development of specific management strategies that are appropriate for patients with similar combinations of characteristics.

Multivariate Analysis of Variance

Many clinical research designs incorporate tests for more than one dependent variable. For example, if we were interested in the physiological effects of exercise, we might measure heart rate, systolic and diastolic blood pressure, respiration, oxygen consumption, and other related variables on each subject at the same time. It makes sense to do this because it is efficient to collect data on as many relevant variables as possible at one time and because it is useful to see how one person's responses vary on all these parameters concurrently. These types of data are usually analyzed using *t*-tests or analyses of variance, with each dependent variable being tested in a separate comparison.

This approach to data analysis presents two major problems. First, the use of multiple tests of significance within a single study can increase the probability of a Type I error (see Chapter 26). The second problem relates to the assumption that each test represents an independent event. However, if we measure heart rate, blood pressure, and respiration on one person, we cannot assume that the responses are unrelated. Most likely, changes in one variable will influence the others. Therefore, these responses are not independent events and should not be analyzed as if they were.

The purpose of a **multivariate analysis of variance (MANOVA)** is to account for the relationship among several dependent variables when comparing groups or conditions. It addresses a research question that purposefully includes multiple outcome measures that have related effects. In many situations, a MANOVA can be more powerful than multiple analyses of variance if the dependent variables are correlated because it can account for multicollinearity that would not be evident with separate ANOVAs. In addition, it is possible that individual tests would not show a significant effect, but when the variables are tested as a composite defining a theoretical construct, significant relationships may become evident.

This test can be applied to all types of experimental designs, including repeated measures, factorial designs, and analyses of covariance. Like the ANOVA, the MANOVA is subject to assumptions of normality, homogeneity of variance, and use of continuous interval/ratio measures for dependent variables. It may be useful to review concepts presented in Chapter 25, as they will apply to the MANOVA as well.

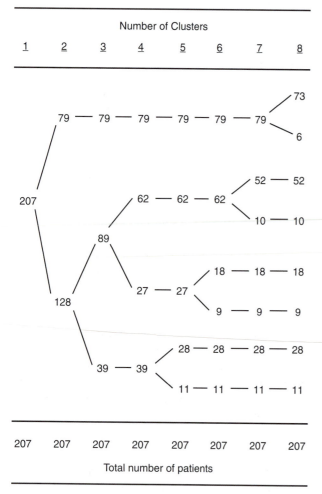

Figure 31–5 Cluster analysis in a study of functional recovery following hip fracture. The authors determined that the solution with four clusters best described the characteristics of the sample. From Michel JP, Hoffmeyer P, Klopfenstein C, et al. Prognosis of functional recovery 1 year after hip fracture typical patient profiles through cluster analysis. *J Gerontol: Med Sci* 2000;55A(9):M508-515, Figure 1, p. 511. Used with permission of the Gerontological Society of America.

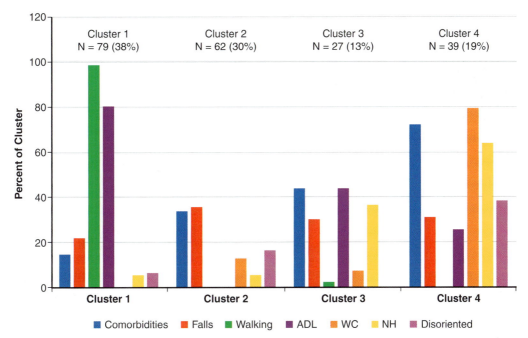

Figure 31–6 Four clusters showing characteristics of patients who suffered a hip fracture. These clusters describe percentages for having one or more comorbidities, falls in previous 3 months, walking without difficulty, regaining prior ADL level, being confined to a wheelchair (WC), living in a nursing home (NH), or being disoriented. Blank spaces indicate 0.0%. Data source: Michel JP, Hoffmeyer P Klopfenstein C, et al. Prognosis of functional recovery 1 year after hip fracture: typical patient profiles through cluster analysis. *J Gerontol: Med Sci* 2000;55A(9):M508-515.

▶ CASE IN POINT #4

Rahman et al[31] used a cross-sectional study design to evaluate gait in patients who had a total knee arthroplasty (TKA). Using accelerometry, they evaluated seven gait parameters, including joint angles and temporal stride characteristics. Three patient groups were tested: patients who were pre-op, those who were 8 weeks post-op, a third group that was 52 weeks post-op, and a fourth group of age-matched controls. The researchers wanted to test the hypothesis that pre-op patients would exhibit poorer gait characteristics than post-op patients or normal controls.

If we were to use a standard analysis of variance for this study, we would have to perform seven separate analyses, one for each gait variable, comparing means for each variable across the four groups. That number of comparisons would also contribute to substantial inflation of the α level of significance.

Vectors

In a multivariate model we no longer look at a single value for each group, but rather we are concerned with the overall effect on all dependent variables. We conceptualize this effect as a multidimensional value, called a *vector*. The mean vector, $\overline{V}$, for each group represents the means of all dependent variables for that group. The null hypothesis states that there is no difference between these vectors. In statistical terms, a vector can be thought of as a set of group means. In the gait study, each vector would represent seven means.

The center point of the vector is considered the *group centroid*. The purpose of the MANOVA is to determine if there is a significant difference among the group centroids. Like the ANOVA, the total variance in the sample is partitioned into parts that represent between-groups and within-groups error effects, although in the multivariate case, variability is measured against centroids rather than individual group means.

Multivariate Test Statistics

The MANOVA produces several statistics that represent the degree of difference between groups, each partitioning the variance in a slightly different way. These include *Wilk's lambda*, *the Hotelling–Lawley trace*, the *Pillai–Bartlett trace*, and *Roy's largest characteristic root (MCR)*. For the sake of consistency in generating critical values for these statistics, most programs convert these to *F*-values.

Unfortunately, statisticians are not in agreement as to which one of these procedures should be used, although in most cases the tests yield similar results.[32] The rationale for choosing one test over the others is based on a complex consideration of statistical power and how well the assumptions underlying each test are met, concepts well beyond the scope of this discussion. Readers are encouraged to consult with a statistician to make these decisions based on the specific research situation.

> ▶ **Results**
> A MANOVA was used to compare the three patient groups and the control group on several gait parameters. The MANOVA showed a significant difference in gait variables across the four groups (Roy's Largest Root = 2.95, $F(8,94) = 34.66$, $p<.001$).

Follow-Up Tests

The MANOVA is an omnibus test like the analysis of variance. Therefore, because this analysis demonstrates a significant effect, follow-up *post hoc* analyses are necessary. There are two common ways to do this. The first is to run univariate ANOVAs on each dependent variable, followed by multiple comparison tests (see Chapter 26). However, this strategy negates the purpose of looking at the dependent variables together to account for their correlation, and ignores the potential for Type I error. A preferred method uses a procedure called discriminant analysis.

Discriminant Analysis

Discriminant analysis is a form of multiple regression, used when the dependent variable is categorical. It is a technique for distinguishing between two or more groups based on a set of characteristics that are predictors of group membership. An equation is generated that classifies subjects according to their scores, and the model is then examined to see if the classifications were correct.

> 📌 Discriminant analysis has an important distinction from logistic regression, which is also based on a categorical dependent variable. In discriminant analysis, the independent variables are assumed to be normally distributed, and variances are assumed to be equal across groups. Logistic regression is best applied when independent variables are dichotomous.

The discriminant analysis generates a statistical model called a *discriminant function*, an equation that represents the linear combination of variables that makes the groups as statistically distinct as possible. When more than two groups are involved, the analysis becomes more complex, necessitating the development of more than one discriminant function. The analysis can be performed using a fixed set of variables or in a stepwise manner to reduce the discriminant function to a minimum number of relevant variables.

Functions are generated according to an eigenvalue, which you recall from our discussion of factor analysis, indicates the amount of variance explained by that function. In this case the eigenvalue represents the between-groups/within-groups variance. The first function will account for the most variance, and the second function will account for variance that is not explained in the first. The number of functions will be the lesser of the number of groups minus 1, or the number of independent variables. In the TKA study, with four groups, three discriminant functions were generated.

The accuracy of the discriminant analysis is based on **canonical correlation**, which expresses the relationship of group membership with variables in the discriminant function. This is tested in two ways. The first method uses chi-square to test significance of the correlation. The second is Wilk's lambda, λ, which estimates the proportion of total variance that is NOT explained by the group effect, or the error variance. Therefore, $1-\lambda$ is an index of explained variance, which can be interpreted as R^2.

> 🔑 Although discriminant analysis is multivariate, it is actually analogous to an ANOVA or *t*-test, just turned around. With an ANOVA, means are compared across groups (the independent variable) to see if they are significantly different on the dependent variable. With discriminant analysis, the group membership becomes the dependent variable (to be predicted), and the outcome measures become the independent variables (predictors). If there is only one measured variable, the results of an ANOVA and discriminant analysis will be the same. If there are several measured variables, the discriminant analysis can be more useful, accounting for their interdependence and controlling for potential Type I error.

Post-Hoc Test for MANOVA

Discriminant analysis is often used as a *post-hoc* procedure for a MANOVA, preferable to multiple ANOVAs because it maintains the integrity of the multivariate research question. This approach was used in the TKA study following a significant MANOVA.

> ▶ **Results**
> For the TKA study, with four groups, three discriminant functions were generated. The first explained 95.5% of the variance. The second and third functions did not contribute significantly to the outcome, with 3.7% and 0.8% of the variance, respectively. Together these functions differentiated between the healthy age-matched controls and all three patient groups

($\lambda = 0.222$, χ^2 (24) = 144.50, $p<.001$). The three patient groups all showed a continued deficit in gait, with no significant improvement in the post-op groups.

The results using the first two discriminant functions are plotted in Fig. 31.7. Each point in the graph represents the vector for each subject on the combined independent variables. There is a clear separation between the three patient groups and the controls. Further analysis of these data includes looking at coefficients in the discriminant function equations for each of the measured variables to determine which have contributed most to the group differentiation. For example, in the TKA study, researchers could determine which of the gait parameters were most effective in differentiating between patients and controls.

■ Survival Analysis

Many research questions focus on the effectiveness of intervention or prognoses, with measurement of short-term effects. Long-term outcomes, however, may be of greater

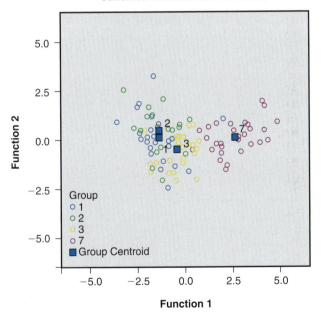

Canonical Discriminant Functions

Figure 31–7 Plot of discriminant functions showing separation between TKA patient groups and healthy age-matched controls (group 7). Group 1: pre-op; Group 2: 8 weeks post-op; Group 3: 52 weeks post-op. Large squares represent group centroids. Adapted from Rahman J, Tang Q, Monda M, et al. Gait assessment as a functional outcome measure in total knee arthroplasty: A cross-sectional study. *BMC Musculoskeletal Disord* 2015;16:66. Figure 3. Used under terms of the Creative Commons Attribution International License (http://creativecommons.org/licenses/by/4.0/).

interest in relation to survival or prevention because they better reflect the true impact of interventions. Long-term effects are typically evaluated with reference to survival time to an identified "event." The concept of **survival analysis** is important to understanding prognosis and treatment effectiveness. It answers questions relating to time, such as: "How long will it be before I am better?" "How long am I going to live?" "When in the future will the risk of recurrence of a disorder increase or decrease?"

Survival analysis is based on the documentation of a *terminal event.* The most common use is in the estimate of life expectancy. For many diseases, such as cancer or cardiovascular disease, the terminal event of interest may be death. Life expectancy can also be examined in relation to functional conditions. For example, Strauss et al[33] looked at decline in function and life expectancy in older persons with cerebral palsy (CP). They were able to demonstrate that survival rates of ambulatory older adults with CP were only moderately worse than the general population but were much poorer for those who had lost mobility.

Survival time can also refer to other events, such as time to relapse, injury, or loss of function. For instance, Ruland et al[34] used survival analysis to examine time to recurrence of stroke. Grossman and Moore[35] followed the longitudinal course of aphasia and decline of sentence comprehension. Verghese et al[36] documented that the incidence and prevalence of gait disorders were high in community-residing older adults and that gait disorders were associated with greater risk of institutionalization and death over a 5-year period.

> **► CASE IN POINT #5**
>
> Infectious gangrene of the foot is a serious complication of diabetes, often leading to amputation. Huang et al[37] studied the association between several risk factors and mortality in 157 patients with type 2 diabetes who had received treatment for foot gangrene between 2002 and 2009. Within the sample, 90 patients had a major amputation (above the ankle), and 67 had a minor amputation (below the ankle).

Methods of Analysis for Survival Data

Estimates of survival present a special dilemma for analysis because it is not possible to follow all subjects to the terminal event. Even in long-term studies, data collection has to stop at some point, and some individuals will not have reached the terminal event at that point. Therefore, we could not know how long those subjects would survive. Individuals may drop out of a study or be lost to follow-up, leaving their end point undocumented. There may also be a variation in the onset of disease or treatment, often resulting in patients entering a study at different times.

Censored Observations

When individuals are followed for this type of analysis, those who have not yet reached the terminal event by the end of the study are considered **censored observations**. These censored survival times will underestimate the true (but unknown) time to the event because it will occur beyond the end of the study.[38] Therefore, special methods of analysis are needed to account for censored data.

Although techniques such as analysis of variance and regression are often used to follow responses over time, censored observations make them inappropriate for survival analysis. Taking a mean survival time for a cohort of patients will be misleading because the mean will continually change as different individuals reach the terminal event. A mean survival time can only be accurate when all cases in the cohort have reached that end point.

Kaplan-Meier Estimates

The most common method of determining survival time is the **Kaplan-Meier estimate**, which does not depend on grouping data into specific time intervals. This approach generates a step function, changing the survival estimate each time a subject reaches the terminal event. Graphic displays of survival functions computed with this technique provide a useful visual understanding of the survival function as a series of steps of decreasing magnitude. The *survival curve* is based on the successive probabilities of occurrence of the terminal event at a certain point of time. The *log rank test* is used to test the null hypothesis that two survival curves are not different.

The advantage of this approach is the ability to compare different groups based on individual characteristics, circumstances, or interventions. It can account for censored data from withdrawal, loss to follow-up, or not yet reaching the terminal event. Each subject's data includes the event status (occurrence or censored) and the time to the event (or censoring). Figure 31-8 shows survival curves over a 9-year period for patients in the diabetes study, comparing survival time for those experiencing minor or major amputations. Years of follow-up are shown on the X-axis and the probability of survival is on the Y-axis.

> ➤ At the start of the study, both groups of patients had the same probability of survival. This probability decreased over time in both groups, but rate of decline was steeper for patients with a major amputation. We can see that the distinction between the groups became evident within the first year of follow-up. After 3 years, the probability of survival for those with minor amputation was around 70%, whereas it was closer to 45% for those with a major amputation.

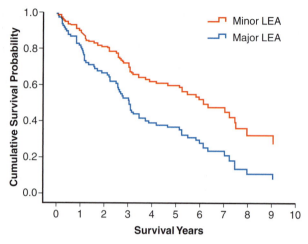

Figure 31–8 Kaplan-Meier survival curve comparing risk of death following minor and major amputation in patients with diabetes and foot infections. By drawing a line at the .50 mark, you can determine the median survival time for both groups. Adapted from Huang YY, Lin CW, Yang HM, et al. Survival and associated risk factors in patients with diabetes and amputations caused by infectious foot gangrene. *J Foot Ankle Res* 2018; 11:1. Figure 1. Used under terms of the Creative Commons Attribution International License (http://creativecommons.org/licenses/by/4.0/).

⊘ FUN FACT

If you were a fan of the classic series *Game of Thrones*, you know there was a high probability of mortality for many of the characters. Using Kaplan-Meier survival analysis, Lystad and Brown[39] studied death rates for seasons 1 through 7. They documented that of 330 characters, 186 (56.4%) had suffered violent deaths within that time period. Survival time ranged from 11 seconds to 57 hours/15 minutes, with a median survival time of 28 hours/48 minutes. The probability of dying within the first hour was 14%. Survival was worse for characters who were male, lowborn, or who had switched allegiance. The authors concluded that there is great potential for preventing violent deaths in the *Game of Thrones* world by instituting a stable government, expanding commerce, and investment in public health!

Even if you weren't a fan, this paper is a fun and comprehensive illustration of the analysis of survival curves for different groups within this "population."

Cox Proportional Hazards Model

Survival time is often dependent on many interrelated factors that can contribute to increased or decreased probabilities of survival or failure. A regression model can be used to adjust survival estimates on the basis of several independent variables. Standard multiple regression methods cannot be used because survival times are typically not normally distributed and because of censored observations. The most commonly used method is the **Cox proportional hazards model**, which is conceptually similar to multiple regression but without assumptions about the shape of distributions. For this reason, this analysis is often considered a nonparametric technique.

The proportional hazards model is based on the *hazard function*, which is related to the survival curve. This function represents the risk of dying (or the terminal event) at a given point in time, assuming that one has survived up to that point. The dependent variable is the hazard (risk), and the independent variables, or covariates, are those factors thought to explain or influence the outcome. Variables may be continuous, dichotomous or ordinal.[40] For example, in the amputation study, associated risk factors included age, diabetes duration, HbAlc, level of hypertension, renal function, and ankle-brachial index.

Survival curves allow for comparison of the hazard risk, and therefore survival time, associated with the different groups. In the amputation example, level of amputation is the intervention, and we can determine if the different levels contribute to a different survival risk.

Like odds ratios generated from a logistic regression, a **hazard ratio (HR)** can be generated from coefficients in the hazard function. A HR of 1.0 indicates that there is no excess risk associated with the covariates. A value greater than 1.0 indicates that a covariate is positively associated with the probability of the terminal event—thereby decreasing survival. A HR less than 1.0 indicates that the covariate is protective, decreasing the probability of the terminal event, and thereby increasing survival time. Confidence intervals can be expressed for the hazard ratio to indicate significance, with a null value of 1.0.

> ### ▶ Results
>
> For the 5 years of the amputation study, 109 of the 157 patients died, with a median survival time of 3.12 years and a 5-year survival rate of 40%. Patients with a minor amputation had a better median survival rate (5.5 years) than those with a major amputation (1.9 years) ($p < .001$). Cox regression analysis demonstrated that age [HR 1.04 (95% CI, 1.01-1.06)] and major amputation [HR 1.80 (95% CI, 1.05-3.09)] were independent factors associated with mortality.

The confidence intervals for these hazard ratios do not contain 1.0 and therefore are significant. The authors concluded that efforts to limit amputations to the below-ankle level resulted in better survival. They suggested that this outcome could be due to other related disabilities with higher amputation level, such as limited mobility or higher risk for falls. Survival curves do not tell us why the groups are different. Separate curves can be generated for subgroups to determine how other covariates affect the outcome. For example, in the amputation study, separate hazard ratios were obtained for several covariates, including age and renal function.

COMMENTARY

Life is really simple, but we insist on making it complicated.

—Confucius (551-479 BC)

Chinese teacher and philosopher

Multivariate analyses have become popular in behavioral research because of the increased availability of computer programs to implement them. Their applications are, however, not well understood by many clinical researchers, and many studies using multivariate designs are still analyzed using univariate statistical methods.

Multivariate techniques can accommodate a wide variety of data and are able to account for the complex interaction and associations that exist in most clinical phenomena. Many research questions could be investigated more thoroughly if investigators considered multivariate models when planning their studies. This chapter has been limited to a discussion of the conceptual elements of multivariate analysis but with enough of an introduction to terminology and application that the beginning researcher should be able to understand research reports and follow computer output. Statisticians can be extremely helpful in sorting through the different methods, many of which provide different approaches to the same question.

Although there is great potential for improving explanation of clinical data using multivariate methods, an important caveat is that clinical research need not be complicated to be meaningful. A problem is not necessarily better solved by a complex analysis, nor should such an approach be taken just because computer programs are available. The indiscriminate use of multiple measurements is not a useful substitute for a well-defined study with a select number of variables. To be sure, the results of multivariate analyses are harder to interpret and involve some risk of judgmental error, such as in factor analysis or cluster analysis. Many important and concise research questions can be answered using simpler

methods and designs, and many clinical variables can be studied effectively using a single criterion measure. On the other hand, simple analysis is not necessarily better just because the interpretation of results will be easier and clearer. The choice of analytic method must be based on the research question and theoretical foundations behind it.

REFERENCES

1. Pett MA, Lackey NR, Sullivan JJ. *Making Sense of Factor Analysis: The Use of Factor Analysis for Instrument Development in Health Care Research.* Thousand Oaks, CA: Sage; 2003.
2. Fabrigar LR, Wegener DT. *Exploratory Factor Analysis.* New York: Oxford University Press; 2012.
3. Kachigan SK. *Mutlivariate Statistical Analysis: A Conceptual Introduction.* 2nd ed. New York: Radius Press; 1991.
4. Grimm LG, Yarnold PR, eds. *Reading and Understanding Multivariate Statistics.* Washington, D.C.: American Pyschological Association; 1995.
5. Field A. *Discovering Statistics Using IBM SPSS Statistics.* 5th ed. Thousand Oaks, CA: Sage; 2018.
6. Kaiser H. An index of factorial simplicity. *Psychometrika* 1974;39(1):31-36.
7. IBM Knowledge Center. Factor Analysis Extraction. Available at https://www.ibm.com/support/knowledgecenter/en/SSLVMB_24.0.0/spss/base/idh_fact_ext.html. Accessed February 13, 2019.
8. Tabachnick BG, Fidell LS. *Using Multivariate Statistics.* 7th ed. New York: Pearson; 2018.
9. Pituch KA, Stevens JP. *Applied Multivariate Statistics for the Social Sciences: Analyses with SAS and IBM's SPSS.* 6th ed. New York: Routledge; 2016.
10. IBM Knowledge Center. IBM SPSS Statistics V23.0 documentation. Factor Analysis Rotation. Available at https://www.ibm.com/support/knowledgecenter/en/SSLVMB_23.0.0/spss/base/idh_fact_rot.html. Accessed February 13, 2019.
11. Bryant FB, Yarnold PR. Principal-components analysis and exploratory and confirmatory factor analysis. In: Grimm LG, Yarnold PR, eds. *Reading and Understanding Mulivariatte Statistics.* Washington, DC: American Psychological Association; 1995:99-136.
12. Gorsuch RL. *Factor Analysis.* 2nd ed. Hillsdale, NJ: Lawrence Erlbaum; 1983.
13. Huck SW. *Reading Statistics and Research.* 6th ed. Boston: Pearson; 2012.
14. Rector TS, Cohn JN. Assessment of patient outcome with the Minnesota Living with Heart Failure Questionnaire: reliability and validity during a randomized, double-blind, placebo-controlled trial of pimobendan. Pimobendan Multicenter Research Group. *Am Heart J* 1992;124(4):1017-1025.
15. Garin O, Ferrer M, Pont A, Rue M, Kotzeva A, Wiklund I, Van Ganse E, Alonso J. Disease-specific health-related quality of life questionnaires for heart failure: a systematic review with meta-analyses. *Qual Life Res* 2009;18(1):71-85.
16. Garin O, Ferrer M, Pont A, et al. Evidence on the global measurement model of the Minnesota Living with Heart Failure Questionnaire. *Qual Life Res* 2013;22(10):2675-2684.
17. Aron A, Coups EJ, Aron EN. *Statistics for the Behavioral and Social Sciences: A Brief Course.* 6th ed. Boston: Pearson; 2019.
18. Schreiber JB, Nora A, Stage FK, Barlow EA, King J. Reporting structural equation modeling and confirmatory factor analysis results: a review. *J Educ Res* 2006;99(6):323-337.
19. Hox JJ, Bechger TM. An introduction to structural equation modeling. *Fam Sci Rev* 1998;11(4):354-373.
20. Blunch NJ. *Introduction to Structural Equation Modeling Using IBM SPSS Statistics and AMOS.* 2nd ed. Los Angeles, CA: Sage; 2013.
21. Schumacker RE, Lomax RG. *A Beginner's Guide to Structural Equation Modeling.* 4th ed. New York: Routledge; 2016.
22. Raykov T, Marcoulides GA. *A First Course in Structural Equation Modeling.* 2nd ed. Mahwah, NJ: Lawrence Erlbaum Associates; 2006.
23. Klem L. Structural Equation Modeling. In: Grimm LG, Yarnold PR, eds. *Reading and Understanding More Multivariate Statistics.* Washington, DC: American Psychological Association; 2000:227-260.
24. Wang J, Geng L. Effects of socioeconomic status on physical and psychological health: lifestyle as a mediator. *Int J Environ Res Public Health* 2019;16(281).
25. Simandan D. Rethinking the health consequences of social class and social mobility. *Soc Sci Med* 2018;200:258-261.
26. Hooper D, Coughlan J, Mullen MR. Structural equation modelling: guidelines for determining model fit. *Electronic J Bus Res Meth* 2008;6(1):53-60.
27. Hu L, Bentler PM. Cutoff criteria for fit indexes in covariance structure analysis: conventional criteria versus new alternatives. *Structural Equation Modeling* 1999;6(1):1-55.
28. SSI Scientific Software. LISREL 10.1 Release notes. Available at http://www.ssicentral.com/lisrel/lisrel10.pdf. Accessed February 2, 2019.
29. IBM SPSS Amos. Available at https://www.ibm.com/us-en/marketplace/structural-equation-modeling-sem. Accessed February 4, 2019.
30. Michel JP, Hoffmeyer P, Klopfenstein C, Bruchez M, Grab B, d'Epinay CL. Prognosis of functional recovery 1 year after hip fracture: typical patient profiles through cluster analysis. *J Gerontol A Biol Sci Med Sci* 2000;55(9):M508-515.
31. Rahman J, Tang Q, Monda M, Miles J, McCarthy I. Gait assessment as a functional outcome measure in total knee arthroplasty: a cross-sectional study. *BMC Musculoskelet Disord* 2015;16:66.
32. Warne RT. A primer on multivariate analysis of variance (MANOVA) for behavioral scientists. *Pract Assess Res Eval* 2014;19(17):1-10.
33. Strauss D, Ojdana K, Shavelle R, Rosenbloom L. Decline in function and life expectancy of older persons with cerebral palsy. *NeuroRehabilitation* 2004;19(1):69-78.
34. Ruland S, Richardson D, Hung E, et al. Predictors of recurrent stroke in African Americans. *Neurology* 2006;67(4):567-571.
35. Grossman M, Moore P. A longitudinal study of sentence comprehension difficulty in primary progressive aphasia. *J Neurol Neurosurg Psychiatry* 2005;76(5):644-649.

36. Verghese J, LeValley A, Hall CB, Katz MJ, Ambrose AF, Lipton RB. Epidemiology of gait disorders in community-residing older adults. *J Am Geriatr Soc* 2006;54(2): 255-261.

37. Huang YY, Lin CW, Yang HM, Hung SY, Chen IW. Survival and associated risk factors in patients with diabetes and amputations caused by infectious foot gangrene. *J Foot Ankle Res* 2018;11:1.

38. Clark TG, Bradburn MJ, Love SB, Altman DG. Survival analysis part I: basic concepts and first analyses. *Br J Cancer* 2003;89(2):232-238.

39. Lystad RP, Brown BT. "Death is certain, the time is not": mortality and survival in *Game of Thrones. Inj Epidemiol* 2018;5(1):44.

40. Bradburn MJ, Clark TG, Love SB, Altman DG. Survival analysis part II: multivariate data analysis—an introduction to concepts and methods. *Br J Cancer* 2003;89(3):431-436.

Measurement Revisited: Reliability and Validity Statistics

—with K. Douglas Gross

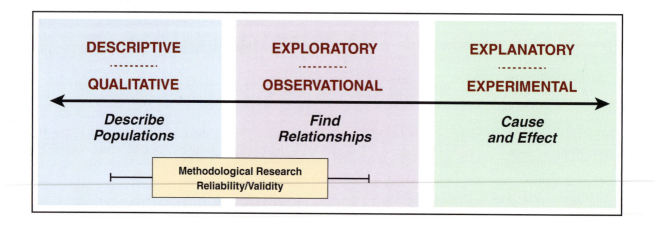

Reliability and validity are foundational concepts for evidence-based practice, as we strive to measure bodily impairments, activity limitations, quality of life, and other outcomes in a meaningful way. Sound clinical decision-making depends on having confidence in our measurements to accurately determine when an intervention is effective, when changes in patient status have occurred, or when test results are diagnostic.

It would be misleading to suggest that any statistic should be used exclusively for a single purpose. Some statistics, commonly used to assess the reliability of a clinical test, are also well-suited for assessment of criterion-referenced validity, depending on the nature of the question being asked. Recognizing this versatility, the purpose of this chapter is to expand on the

concepts presented in Chapters 9 and 10 by describing statistical procedures commonly used to assess the reliability or validity of a clinical test or measure, including the intraclass correlation coefficient, standard error of measurement, measures of agreement, internal consistency, and estimates of effect size and change. It will be helpful to review earlier material in preparation for understanding the statistical procedures described here.

■ Intraclass Correlation Coefficient

A **relative reliability** coefficient reflects true variance in a set of continuous scores as a proportion of the total variance (see Chapter 9). One of the most commonly used relative reliability indices is the **intraclass correlation coefficient (ICC)**. The ICC is primarily used to assess the test-retest or rater reliability of a quantitative (interval or ratio) measure. Possible ICC values range from 0.00 to 1.00, with higher values indicating greater reliability. Because the ICC is a unitless index, it is permissible to compare the ICCs of alternative testing methods to determine which is the more reliable test. This is possible even when scores are assigned using different units of measurement.

The ICC has the advantage of being able to assess reliability across two, three, or more sets of scores, giving it broad applicability for assessment of test-retest reliability across multiple test administrations, interrater reliability across multiple raters, or intrarater reliability over repeated trials. This applicability is one of several advantages that distinguishes the ICC from other correlation coefficients, such as Pearson's *r*, which can only register correlation between two sets of scores, and does not assess agreement.

> ### ➤ CASE IN POINT #1
>
> The Timed 10-Meter Walk Test (10mWT) is often used as a measure of functional mobility and gait speed in patients with neurological disorders and mobility limitations.[1] The patient walks without assistance for 10 meters. To account for initial acceleration and terminal deceleration, time is measured with a stopwatch during the intermediate 6 meters. The test can be performed at a comfortable walking pace or at the patient's fastest speed. To illustrate application of the ICC, we will use hypothetical 10mWT data from eight patients and four raters who acquired concurrent measurements of each patient's performance (see Table 32-1).

The ICC is calculated using variance estimates obtained from a repeated measures analysis of variance (ANOVA) that compares scores across raters. From

Table 32-1   Hypothetical Data for the 10mWT (seconds)

ID	RATER 1 (Trial 1)	RATER 2 (Trial 2)	RATER 3 (Trial 3)	RATER 4 (Trial 4)
1	5.0	6.0	9.0	4.5
2	9.0	13.0	10.0	8.5
3	9.5	12.0	18.5	12.5
4	18.0	15.0	12.5	20.0
5	12.0	15.0	18.5	10.0
6	20.0	25.0	22.5	18.0
7	32.0	30.5	28.0	40.0
8	42.0	38.0	50.0	42.5
$\bar{X}$ (sd)	18.4 (12.7)	19.3 (10.8)	21.1 (13.3)	19.5 (14.3)

these variance estimates, there are different equations that can be used to calculate an ICC value depending on the type of measurements that are obtained (ICC form), and the intended purpose and design of the reliability study (ICC model).[2]

Forms of the ICC

The ICC coefficient can be expressed in one of two *forms*, depending on whether the assigned scores are derived from single ratings or from mean ratings across several trials. Commonly, reliability studies are designed so that a single rating is acquired from each subject—this is *form 1*. In some studies, however, each subject's score is calculated as a mean value across several trials—called *form k*. If, for example, it is known ahead of time that measurements tend to be unstable, it may be necessary to record a mean of several trials in order to ensure more satisfactory reliability. Recording mean scores has the effect of improving reliability since random error is reduced whenever overestimates and underestimates are "averaged out." Note, however, that a calculated reliability coefficient based on mean scores should only be generalized to other settings in which a mean score is also recorded. It should never be used to estimate reliability in acquiring a single measured score.

Models of the ICC

The *model* of the ICC depends on whether the results of the reliability analysis are to be generalized beyond the particular testing situation of the study. Assume, for example, that we wish to establish the inter-rater reliability for four clinicians scoring the 10mWT. We must first decide whether these raters can be regarded as having been "randomly selected" from among a much larger population of clinicians with a similar background and training. If so, then our ultimate purpose in calculating the reliability of these raters would be to generalize the findings to other clinicians who comprise the larger population of raters. Since it would be exceedingly rare for investigators to have access to all members of the target population from which to make a truly random selection, our use of the term "random" in this context is theoretical. The essential point is that we intend to generalize the outcome to other similar raters. Therefore, these raters would represent a **random effect**.

Alternatively, the four raters in our study could represent a **fixed effect**, indicating that these are the only raters of interest. Perhaps we are planning a future investigation in which we will train these raters to administer the 10mWT to measure the effects of an experimental intervention. In that instance, our sole objective in a preliminary reliability study may be to establish that these particular raters can reliably administer the 10mWT in accordance with the upcoming study protocol. We would not care about generalizing our reliability findings to any larger population of clinicians outside of the current study.

In addition to identifying raters as either a "random" or "fixed" effect, we must also clarify the role of the subjects. Typically, subjects in clinical research are considered a random effect since investigators usually intend to generalize the findings from their study to a larger population of similar individuals to whom the test may be administered. The distinction between random and fixed effects helps us choose an appropriate ICC model.

> 📌 A way to think about random or fixed effects has been called the *"replaceability test."*[3] Subjects are generally considered random because you can theoretically replace them with other similar subjects. For raters, the question is whether you can replace these raters with others like them, or are they the only ones of interest?

There are three *models* of the ICC, as defined by Shrout and Fleiss.[2] These models are distinguished according to how the subjects are assigned to different raters and whether the raters and subjects are random or fixed effects.[4]

Model 1

In model 1, raters are considered randomly chosen from a larger population, but some subjects are assessed by different sets of raters. This model is rarely applied. While it may occasionally be appropriate, for example, in large multisite studies where different raters work with different sets of subjects, this model makes it difficult to derive meaningful estimates of rater variance.[5] Because model 1 is seldom used, it will not be discussed further. For specific information on model 1, refer to references at the end of this chapter.[2,6]

Model 2

Model 2 is the most commonly used model of the ICC for assessing inter-rater reliability. In this model, each subject is assessed by the same set of raters who are considered "randomly" chosen from the larger population of potential raters or clinicians. Study participants are similarly regarded as representative of a larger population of potential test subjects or patients. Using model 2, therefore, both subject and rater are considered random effects. Model 2 also works well for test-retest reliability assessments because each test administration is considered representative of the larger population of all possible test administrations.

> ➤ Consider the data from Table 32-1. Assume we want to assess inter-rater reliability of the 10mWT, with four raters observing a set of eight patients. Assume that each patient performs the test three times and the patient's score is recorded as the mean of the three trials. Consider the values in the table as the mean scores. These raters are typical of the larger population of clinicians that use the 10mWT, and so the results from this reliability study may be generalizable to other clinicians. In this setting, model 2 is appropriate using form *k* because the recorded scores are means of three trials (k = 3).

Model 3

In model 3, each subject is assessed by the same set of raters, but the raters represent the only raters of interest. With no intention to generalize findings to other clinicians, rater is considered a fixed effect. Subjects, however, are still considered a random effect. Therefore, model 3 is a *mixed model*. Model 3 is also the appropriate statistic to measure intra-rater reliability, as the measurements of a single rater are rarely considered representative of a larger population of potential raters.[2]

> ➤ We can design a study to determine intra-rater reliability of a single clinician in assessing the 10mWT across four trials. Using data from Table 32-1, assume that each column represents a different trial with each trial tested by the same rater who records a single score from each subject. We can look at the consistency of this one rater's scores across the trials. The results of our analysis would only apply to the one rater being studied. In this setting, model 3, form 1 is appropriate.

Classifications of the ICC

The ICC is classified using two numbers in parentheses. The first number designates the *model* (1, 2, or 3). The second number signifies the *form*, using either a single measurement (1) or the mean of several measurements (*k*). Accordingly, we can designate six types of ICCs:

- Model 1: ICC(1,1) or ICC(1,*k*)
- Model 2: ICC(2,1) or ICC(2,*k*)
- Model 3: ICC(3,1) or ICC(3,*k*)

The *k* represents the number of scores used to obtain a mean, and can be replaced with the actual number of scores when notating the ICC. For the above examples:

- In the inter-rater reliability study, ICC (2,3) would be used to indicate a random model with the mean of three trials recorded as scores.
- In the intra-rater reliability study, the rater takes a single measurement at each trial. Therefore, ICC(3,1) would be used to indicate a mixed model with single scores.

Analysis of Variance

The ICC is based on variance estimates obtained from a repeated measures ANOVA, shown in Table 32-2. The results for the 10mWT data include values obtained from the ANOVA along with ICC output for model 2 and model 3.

In the ANOVA, the *between items* variance reflects differences across raters' scores. The *residual* variance is an error term. The associated *F* statistic (see Table 32-2 ❸) is determined by the ratio of these two sources of variance. If the *F* ratio is significant, it suggests that the variance across scores assigned by the different raters is large in comparison to residual error, indicating that the raters' scores are markedly different from one another and may not be reliable. In this example, the *F* ratio is not statistically significant (*p* =.554), suggesting high interrater reliability.

The *between people* variance reflects differences between study participants' scores (see Table 32-2 ❶). Heterogeneity among participants is an important characteristic of samples for reliability testing, and this heterogeneity is reflected in a high *between people* mean square value. An *F* ratio comparing between people variance to residual error is not included in the ANOVA table but is reported later in the ICC output (see Table 32-2 ❻). In this example, the *between people* effect is significant (*p* <.001). This is an expected and necessary condition for reliability testing. The validity of the ICC will be suspect if this *F* test is not significant.

> 📌 If this were a study of test-retest reliability, the "between items" variance would be indicative of the consistency of scoring across different test administrations, rather than across different raters.

> 🌐 See the *Chapter 32 Supplement* for calculations of ICCs for models 2 and 3, and instructions for using SPSS to generate ICCs for the output shown in Table 32-2.

Confidence Intervals

Because ICC values are obtained using data from a sample of study subjects, confidence intervals can be generated to indicate a range of values within which the ICC in the target population is likely to be found. As shown in Table 32-2 ❼, ICC(2,1) is .918, with the 95% CI = .787 to .980. In contrast, ICC(2,*k*) is .978, with the 95% CI = .937 to .995. As expected, by recording a mean score rather than a single measured value for each participant, random error has decreased and reliability improved when calculating ICC(2,*k*). The surrounding confidence interval provides a context for interpreting an ICC value that is calculated using study sample data (see Focus on Evidence 32-1).

Interpretation of the ICC

Like other forms of reliability, there are no standard values for acceptable reliability using the ICC. The savvy evidence-based practice clinician must determine "how much" reliability is needed to justify use of a particular tool for a designated purpose (see Box 32-1).

Explaining Low ICC Values

There are two major reasons for finding low ICC values. The first explanation is obvious: the raters or test-retest scores do not agree. This is not a straightforward interpretation, however, with more than two raters or trials. For instance, the ICC is an average based on variance across all raters, and disagreement may involve all raters, some raters, or only one rater. Looking at means for each rater or graphing their scores can be helpful in pinpointing specific sources of disagreement.

A second reason is related to insufficient variance among study subjects. A lack of variability can occur when study subjects are homogeneous on the measured attribute, or when the rating system itself restricts possible scores to only a very narrow range. The ICC value indicates the proportion of the total variance across a set of scores that is attributable to heterogeneity among study participants (after other sources of variance have been taken into account). If subject scores are very similar to one another, the relative contribution of other sources of variance (including variance across raters) to the total variance observed in the dataset will be increased, resulting in a deflated ICC value. This effect can be checked by looking at the magnitude and significance of the *between people* source of variance in the ANOVA table (see Table 32-2 ❶ ❻). If subjects' scores are excessively homogeneous, this value will not be significant, and the derived ICC value will be deflated.

> 🔑 Although statistical programs report multiple values of the ICC using the same data, it should be clear that only one value will be appropriate for a given study. The selection of an ICC model and form should be made as part of the data collection plan based on appropriate design considerations. Generally, for the same set of data, model 2 will yield smaller values than model 3, although they are often close. Within each model, ICC form 1 based on single ratings will yield lower values than ICC form *k* based on mean ratings (see Table 32-2 ❺). Given these potential differences, the specific model and form of the ICC should always be reported.

Table 32-2   ICC for Models 2 and 3 Based on Repeated Measures ANOVA (*N* = 8)

A. SPSS Output: ANOVA

ANOVA

Source		Sum of Squares	df	Mean Square	F	Sig.
Between People **①**		4330.719	7	618.674	**②**	
Within People	Between Items	30.156	3	10.052	.715 **③**	.554
	Residual	295.344	21	14.064		
	Total	325.500	24	13.563		
Total		4656.219	31	150.201		

B. SPSS Output: ICC Model 2

Intraclass Correlation Coefficient

⑤	Intraclass Correlation[a]	**⑦** 95% Confidence Interval Lower Bound	Upper Bound	**⑥** F Test with True Value 0 Value	df1	df2	Sig
Single Measures	.918	.787	.980	43.990	7	21	.000
Average Measures	.978	.937	.995	43.990	7	21	.000

Two-way random effects model where both people effects and measures are random. **④**
a. Type A intraclass correlation coefficients using an absolute agreement definition. **⑧**

C. SPSS Output: ICC Model 3

Intraclass Correlation Coefficient

⑤	Intraclass Correlation[a]	**⑦** 95% Confidence Interval Lower Bound	Upper Bound	**⑥** F Test with True Value 0 Value	df1	df2	Sig
Single Measures	.915	.776	.980	43.990	7	21	.000
Average Measures	.977	.933	.995	43.990	7	21	.000

Two-way mixed effects model where people effects are random and measures effects are fixed. **④**
a. Type C intraclass correlation coefficients using a consistency definition. **⑧**

① "Between People" is the between-subjects effect. "Between Items" is the effect of rater. "Residual" is the error term.

② The *F* test for the between-subjects effect is not printed as part of the ANOVA. It can be computed using MS between people divided by MS residual. This value is reported with the ICC (see **⑥**).

③ There is no significant difference between raters (*p* = .554). This is a good thing when you are looking for reliability! This is a test of significance across the four raters.

④ The ICC for model 2 is based on a two-way random model, and for model 3 it is based on a two-way mixed model.

⑤ Each model is run for both single measures (form 1) and average measures (form *k*). The researcher must determine which value to use, based on the study design. Single measures = ICC(2,1) or ICC(3,1). Average measures = ICC(2,k) or ICC(3,k).

⑥ This is the *F* test for the between-subjects effect, which was not reported with the ANOVA (*F* = 43.99). This effect is significant (*p* < .001), which tells us that the subjects are different from each other.

⑦ The 95% confidence intervals are shown for both forms of the ICC in each model.

⑧ In SPSS, model 2 is run using type A ICC (absolute agreement). Model 3 is run using type C ICC (consistency). This parameter is specified by the researcher when the test is run.

Portions of the output have been omitted for clarity.

Focus on Evidence 32–1
Reliability, Evidence, and Confidence

Several inventories have been developed to assess disability associated with chronic low back pain. The Roland Morris Disability Questionnaire (RMDQ)[7] is a commonly used tool that has been subjected to reliability testing over several decades, including many versions in languages other than English. Several systematic reviews have shown that the questionnaire has strong reliability, with varying ICC values generally above .85.[8]

In 2002, however, Davidson and Keating[9] compared the RMDQ with several other disability measures to determine differences in their reliability, finding that the RMDQ had a substantially lower ICC of .53 (95% CI = .29 to .71), and .42 (95% CI = -.07 to .75) in a subgroup of patients. Based on these values, the authors suggested that the RMDQ did not have sufficient reliability for clinical application.

As we consider evidence to help us with clinical decisions about choosing measurement tools, Riddle and Stratford[10] suggest caution with this type of conclusion for two reasons. One stems from the need to consider the volume of evidence reported in the literature. Many articles published before and after the 2002 study showed very different results with much higher reliability values. We know that research is always subject to error, and it is possible that the Davidson study had a unique cohort of patients or raters, or other design elements that contributed to their findings.

The second concern is statistical. When we express indices like the ICC as a single value, it is considered a *point estimate*, a single statistic obtained from the sample that is used to estimate an uncertain population parameter. Such estimates are subject to sampling error, and therefore, may not be closely consistent with population scores. That is why we need to look at confidence intervals. In the 2002 study, the confidence intervals were quite wide, with upper bounds that did, in fact, approach acceptable levels of reliability. In one of the confidence intervals, the lower bound contained a negative value, which suggests that the *between subjects* variance would not be significant.[11] Obviously, the point estimate from this study included a great deal of uncertainty, and results should be viewed in this light.

Results can vary from study to study for many different reasons. As evidence-based clinicians, we must face the challenge of considering design issues, statistical approaches, and the overall state of knowledge in making clinical decisions. We want to have confidence in those decisions—not using tests that are unreliable, and just as importantly, not dismissing a test that could provide strong clinical data. Referring to systematic reviews and meta-analyses can be a useful way to look for consistency across studies (see Chapter 37).

Box 32-1 Close Only Counts in Horseshoes

Reliability cannot be interpreted as an all-or-none condition. It is a measurement property that is attained to varying degrees. So "how much" reliability is acceptable?

The amount of tolerable error depends on how a measured value will be used in decision making. Wainner[12] uses the example of a field goal in football, where passing through the uprights allows a certain margin of error for success. In the clinic, we must determine what margin of error is acceptable. For instance, clinicians generally consider 5 degrees of error for range of motion measurements acceptable. But does it matter if we are assessing range of motion in the shoulder or in the distal phalanx of the finger? If we performed a 6-minute walk test, how precise must we be in measuring distance walked? If we were off by 3 cm, would that change how we used the test score? But what if we were measuring leg length? Or performing a surgical procedure? In some scenarios, a difference of millimeters could dramatically change how we manage a patient, while in other scenarios this margin of error is trivial.

Several recommendations have been published for acceptable ranges of reliability, all with a common proviso that "acceptable" depends on the purpose of the measurement and the type of reliability being considered. With relative indices such as the ICC for test-retest or rater reliability, there appears to be agreement that for most clinical purposes, .70 is considered a minimal standard for a test to be useful. Distinctions can be made when using reliability to judge individual clinical performance, which may require higher reliability than when judging group performance.[13] Some suggest that slightly lower values can be acceptable for softer variables, such as sociological and psychological measures, or during the early stages of scale development in research.[14,15] As measurement of a variable matures, expectations may increase to .80.[16,17] When scales are used for clinical decision making, however, the minimum standard may be as high as .90 for measurements requiring great precision.[18]

Bottom line: As a starting point for clinical applications, excellent relative reliability implies an ICC above .90, with good reliability above .75 and moderate reliability between .50 and .75. Anything lower would be considered poor—***BUT "acceptable reliability" is a judgment call by the researcher or clinician who understands the nature of the measured variable and whether the measurements are precise enough to be used meaningfully.*** Those who cite references (including this one!) to stipulate the acceptable reliability of a tool should provide a rationale as to why a particular level of reliability is appropriate for their measures.

> ➤ **Results**
> The 10mWT was assessed for inter-rater reliability among four raters, and for intra-rater reliability for one clinician over four trials. For inter-rater reliability, ICC(2,3) was .978 (95%CI: .937 to .995) with scores based on the mean of three trials. For intra-rater reliability ICC(3,1) was .915 (95%CI: .776 to .980). Both measures reflect strong relative reliability.

■ Standard Error of Measurement

In addition to comparing the relative reliability of different instruments, clinicians are interested in anticipating the stability of an instrument's scores over time as a practical application of reliability for clinical measures. This is best assessed using an **absolute reliability** index of test-retest reliability. The statistic most commonly used for this purpose is the **standard error of measurement (SEM)**. The advantage of this approach is that it is in the original unit of measurement, and therefore, has direct clinical application.

Theoretically, if we were to repeatedly administer a test to one individual under constant conditions with no true change in performance, responses might still vary somewhat from trial to trial as a result of random error. If we could plot an individual's responses over an infinite number of test administrations, it would reveal a distribution of scores resembling a normal curve, with the mean value approximating the individual's true score and random error causing other scores to fall above or below the mean with similar frequency. The standard deviation of this theoretical distribution is the SEM. Using an instrument that demonstrates strong test-retest reliability, errors would be minimal, and the theoretical distribution of all possible scores would be less variable, resulting in a smaller SEM. If a test is perfectly reliable, the SEM would be zero.

Obviously, collecting data on an infinite number of trials for any one individual is impossible. Therefore, we need another way to estimate the true score and the variability of repeated trials. We do this by considering the test-retest reliability of the measurement within a group of individuals.[18]

Calculating the SEM

> ➤ **CASE IN POINT #2**
> Clinical manifestation of carpal tunnel syndrome (CTS) often includes hand weakness, which can be assessed as grip strength to indicate severity or improvement following intervention.[19] Suppose we are interested in determining test-retest reliability of grip strength, measured in pounds, among 50 patients with CTS. Each patient performs two trials separated by a rest period. Assume that each patient's true strength is stable and that the group is representative of a larger population of similar patients with CTS.

The results of this hypothetical reliability study are shown in Table 32-3A. Descriptive data show the means and standard deviations for each trial, as well as the mean difference across trials. The means for each trial are close, and the mean difference is only .46 pounds. The ANOVA and ICC data are also reported, suggesting high test-retest relative reliability, with ICC(2,1) = .905 (see Table 32-3).

To calculate an SEM value for absolute reliability in the measure of grip strength within this group, we can use any of three methods of estimating variance, illustrated in Table 32-3B.[20] Each of these methods is based on variance within the distribution of scores.

- **Method ❶** uses the standard deviation of the difference scores.
- **Method ❷** uses the MS error term from the ANOVA.
- **Method ❸** uses the pooled standard deviation of trials 1 and 2 with the ICC test-retest reliability coefficient. The pooled standard deviation is essentially the average of the two trials.

Disregarding small rounding errors, the SEM = 4.38 pounds, regardless of which method is used to calculate it. Since this value was calculated using data from a representative sample of patients, it can now be used to estimate the extent of expected measurement error when administering the same test to a different individual from the same patient population.

🔑 Riddle and Stratford[20] caution that the distribution of difference scores in a test-retest reliability study must be normal. If the distribution differs from the normal distribution, it may indicate that systematic error is present. Using the Shapiro-Wilk test of normality (see Chapter 23), the distribution of difference scores for the CTS study was not significantly different from normal ($p = .401$).

Clinical Application of the SEM

Knowing the SEM and ICC from a reliability study provides a basis for making judgments about the usefulness of a measuring tool for individuals in practice. We have previously discussed the interpretation of relative reliability (see Box 32-1), and we can consider the ICC(2,1) of .905 for the CTS study to be strong. We do not, however, have similar standards for absolute measures of reliability like the SEM.

When we take a single clinical measurement and use it to judge a patient's condition or progress, we are assuming that the value represents the individual's true score. But knowing that there is potential error within that value, it is more accurate to consider the degree of confidence we can have that the true score is contained within a certain range

Table 32-3　Test-Retest Reliability Results for Grip Strength in Patients with Carpal Tunnel Syndrome (*N*=50)

A. SPSS Output: ICC (2,1) for Test-Retest Reliability

Item Statistics

	Mean	Std. Deviation	N
trial1	66.0800	③ 15.03715	50
trial2	66.5400	③ 13.19432	50
Difference	−.4600	① 6.19812	50

ANOVA

		Sum of Squares	df	Mean Square	F	Sig.
Between People		18668.890	49	380.998		
Within People	Between Items	5.290	1	5.290	.275	.602
	Residual	941.210	49	② 19.208		
	Total	946.500	50	18.930		
Total		19615.390	99	198.135		

Intraclass Correlation Coefficient

	Intraclass Correlation[a]	95% Confidence Interval Lower Bound	95% Confidence Interval Upper Bound	F Test with True Value 0 Value	df1	df2	Sig
Single Measures	.905	.839	.945	19.835	49	49	.000
Average Measures	.950	.912	.972	19.835	49	49	.000

Two-way random effects model where both people effects and measures effects are random.
a. Type A intraclass correlation coefficients using an absolute agreement definition.

B. Calculation of SEM

① **Using the standard deviation of difference scores:**　$SEM = \dfrac{s_d}{\sqrt{2}} = \dfrac{6.198}{\sqrt{2}} = 4.383$

② **Using the MS error term:**　$SEM = \sqrt{MS_E} = \sqrt{19.208} = 4.383$

③ **Using pooled standard deviations (s_p) of test-retest trials:**

$SEM = s_p \sqrt{1 - ICC} = \sqrt{(s_1^2 + s_2^2)/2} \times \sqrt{1 - ICC} = \sqrt{(15.037^2 + 13.194^2)/2} \times \sqrt{1 - .905} = 4.357$

Differences in calculations are due to rounding. Portions of the output have been omitted for clarity.

---

of values. We do this by creating a confidence interval around an observed clinical measure, based on the SEM.

$$CI = X \pm z \,(SEM)$$

where X is the individual's observed score.

Assume we record a single measure of 60 pounds for a patient's grip strength.

95% CI = 60 ± 1.96 (4.38)

= 60 ±8.58

95% CI = 51.42 to 68.58

> Based on an SEM of 4.38 pounds from the previous reliability study, we can estimate with 95% confidence that this patient's true grip strength is somewhere within the interval 51.42 to 68.58 pounds, a range of 17 pounds.

Some clinicians prefer using the 90% CI:

90% CI = 60 ± 1.645(4.38)

= 60 ± 7.21

90% CI = 52.79 to 67.21

▶ The 90% confidence interval creates an error range of 14.42 pounds. The 90% confidence interval is narrower, but we are also less confident that this individual's true score is contained within that interval.

The SEM and the ICC provide a benchmark for evaluating individual patient performance over time. To be confident in a measured score, we want the relative test-retest reliability coefficient (ICC) to be high and the absolute reliability (SEM) to reflect a limited range. What constitutes a "low" SEM value, however, must be based on a clinical judgment about how the measurement will be applied to decision making. It is also important to recognize that the SEM is population specific. Characteristics of study samples should be clearly described so that the results can be applied appropriately. Performance may be different for people with various disorders or in different settings. The SEM also has implications for interpreting change, which will be discussed later in this chapter.

▶ **Results**

The means for trial 1 (66.08 ± 15.04) and trial 2 (66.54 ± 13.19) were not significantly different ($p = .602$). The mean difference was .46 pounds (± 6.19). ICC(2,1) was used to evaluate the test-retest reliability of grip strength, which demonstrated strong reliability (ICC(2,1) = .905 (95% CI: .830 to .945). The SEM was 4.38, indicating that this test should be able to develop reasonable estimates of patient performance.

📌 We can obtain the SEM from published reliability studies even when they do not include it in their analysis. It is possible to calculate the SEM from the reported ICC, means, and standard deviations for test-retest trials or the standard deviation of the difference scores (see Table 32-3B).

Two additional measures of absolute reliability, the **coefficient of variation** and **method error**, can be used to analyze response stability, although they are used less often. The coefficient of variation was described in Chapter 22. The *Chapter 32 supplement* includes a description of method error.

■ Agreement

When the unit of measurement is categorical (nominal or ordinal) rather than quantitative (ratio or interval), it is not appropriate to estimate reliability using the ICC. In that case, relative reliability is assessed using a measure of agreement. The simplest index is **percent agreement**. This is a measure of how frequently raters agree

on categorical scores, or how frequently test–retest scores agree. Percent agreement is the proportion of observations for which agreement is achieved (P_o):

$$P_O = \frac{\text{number of observed agreements}}{\text{number of possible agreements}}$$

▶ **CASE IN POINT #3**

Suppose two clinicians wanted to establish their interrater agreement for evaluating level of function for self-care on a 3-point scale. They evaluate 100 patients who have had a spinal cord injury to determine if they are independent (IND), need some assistance (ASST), or are dependent (DEP). We'll assume they've created operational definitions to guide their grading.

We can summarize these functional data to show agreements and disagreements by arranging them in a frequency table, or a **crosstabulation**, with output shown in Table 32-4A (see Chapter 28). The gold highlighted quantities along the diagonal (extending from the upper left to the bottom right) represent the number of times raters agreed on their ratings. (Ignore values highlighted in green for now.) All values off the diagonal represent disagreements.

Of 100 possible agreements, the raters agreed on 66 patients, and did not agree on 34 patients. Therefore, the proportion of observed agreements (P_o) is

$$P_o = 66/100 = .66$$

The two clinicians agreed on their ratings 66% of the time.

There is a limitation to this interpretation, however. To truly determine reliability of categorical assignment, we must consider the possibility that some portion of the observed agreements could have occurred merely by chance. Like playing the game "Rock, Paper, Scissors." if two raters were to assign subjects to categories completely at random, some degree of agreement would still be expected. Because of this tendency, percent agreement will often be an overestimate of a test's true reliability. A different statistic is needed that will discount the proportion of agreement that is expected due to chance alone.

Kappa Statistic

Kappa, κ, is a *chance-corrected* measure of agreement. In addition to looking at the proportion of observed agreements (P_o), kappa also considers the proportion of agreements expected by chance (P_c):

$$P_C = \frac{\text{number of expected chance agreements}}{\text{number of possible agreements}}$$

We can illustrate this application using the frequency data for functional assessment shown in Table 32-4 ❶.

Table 32-4   Percent Agreement and Kappa: Ratings of Functional Assessment for Two Raters (N = 100)

A. Data

Rater2 * Rater1 Crosstabulation

			Rater1 IND	ASST	DEP	Total	
Rater2	IND	Count	① 25	5	7	37	Observed agreements =
		Expected Count	① 15.5	11.1	10.4	37.0	25 + 24 + 17 = 66
	ASST	Count	6	24	4	34	$P_0 = \dfrac{66}{100} = .66$
		Expected Count	14.3	10.2	9.5	34.0	
	DEP	Count	11	1	17	29	Expected agreements =
		Expected Count	12.2	8.7	8.1	29.0	15.5 + 10.2 + 8.1 = 33.8
Total		Count	42	30	28	100	$P_c = \dfrac{33.8}{100} = .34$
		Expected Count	42.0	30.0	30.0	100.0	

B. SPSS Output: Kappa

Symmetric Measures

		Value	Standard Error	Approximate Significance
Measure of Agreement	Kappa	② .486	③ .072	④ .000
N of Valid Cases		100		

$$\kappa = \frac{P_0 - P_C}{1 - P_C} = \frac{.66 - .34}{1 - .34} = .485 \quad ②$$

C. Calculating Confidence Intervals

95% CI = $\kappa \pm 1.96$ (SEκ)

   = .486 ± 1.96 (.072) = .486 ± .141

95% CI = .345 to .627

---

① Crosstabulation table shows observed and expected frequencies in each cell. Along the diagonal, agreements are highlighted in gold and expected frequencies in green.

② Kappa = .486.

③ This is the standard error of kappa (SEκ) that can be used to calculate confidence intervals.

④ The probability associated with kappa is $p < .001$.

Calculations vary due to rounding differences. Portions of the output have been omitted for clarity.

The expected frequency of agreement by chance alone is highlighted in green in each of the cells along the diagonal. These values are calculated for each cell as the product of the column sum and row sum, divided by the total number of subjects scored. Therefore, for example, the expected chance frequency for the IND cell is $(42 \times 37)/100 = 15.5$ (see Chapter 28).

As shown, the sum of expected chance agreements = 33.8, resulting in a proportion of agreement expected by chance alone of .338 or 34%. This tells us that even if these two raters were just guessing, we could expect agreement between them 34% of the time.

Calculating Kappa

The proportion of observations that can be attributed to reliable measurement is defined as the proportion of observed agreements less the contribution of chance.

$$P_o - P_c$$

The maximum available non-chance agreements would be $1 - P_c$. Kappa represents percent agreement based on these correction factors:

$$\kappa = \frac{P_O - P_C}{1 - P_C}$$

Kappa indicates the proportion of the available *non-chance agreements* that is attained by the raters. In this example, we find that with the effects of chance eliminated, kappa is .49, indicating that 49% of the available non-chance agreement was attained. This "chance-corrected" percentage is a more meaningful reliability estimate for categorical assignments.

Like other statistics, kappa is a point estimate. Confidence intervals can be calculated, as shown in Table 32-4C.

Strength of Association

Landis and Koch[21] have suggested the following criteria for interpreting kappa:

- Excellent agreement- above .80
- Substantial agreement- .60 to .80
- Moderate agreement- .40 to .60
- Poor to fair agreement- below .40

For the functional assessment example, then, we have achieved only a moderate degree of reliability. However, the interpretation of this outcome, like any other reliability coefficient, must depend on how the data will be used and the degree of precision required for making rational clinical decisions. It is also helpful to consider confidence intervals to appreciate the application of these values. For example, the confidence interval for the functional assessment data shows a lower boundary in the poor to fair range.

> ▶ **Results**
>
> The percent agreement for the two raters was 66% for identification of level of independence, assistance, or dependence in 100 participants. The kappa statistic resulted in a chance-corrected agreement of .49 (95% CI: .345 to .627). Using the criteria from Landis and Koch, this is considered a fair to moderate level of agreement.

Weighted Kappa

For some applications, kappa is limited in that it does not differentiate among disagreements of greater or lesser severity. Because it is calculated using only the frequencies along the agreement diagonal, kappa assumes that all disagreements (off the diagonal) are of equal seriousness. There may be instances, however, when a researcher wants to assign greater weight to some disagreements in order to account for differential risks.

For example, rating patients as IND when they are really DEP would mean they would be left without needed assistance, creating a potentially unsafe environment. By comparison, assigning ASST to a patient who is actually IND, while it could result in providing unneeded help, would not be as serious in terms of the patient's safety.

When disagreements can be differentiated in this way, a modified version of the kappa statistic, called **weighted kappa, κ_w**, can be used to estimate reliability.[22] Weighted kappa allows the researcher to specify differential weights to the off-diagonal cells, thereby assigning a greater penalty for some disagreements than for others. Different weighting schemes can be applied when calculating κ_w to accommodate desired levels of adjustment for particular instances of disagreement. Weighted kappa can only be used when the grades represent ordinal ranks, however. It cannot be used with nominal categories, whereas unweighted kappa can be used with nominal or ordinal categories.

 See the *Chapter 32 Supplement* for further discussion of weighted kappa, including examples of calculations with different weighting schemes.

Limitations of Kappa

Average Agreement

It is important to recognize that kappa represents an *average rate of agreement* across a set of scores. It will not indicate if most of the disagreement is accounted for by one specific category or rater. It is useful to examine the data when discussing results, to see where the major discrepancies may lie.

Variance

As with other reliability measures, variance among study subjects is required for kappa to be meaningful. In a group of subjects with homogeneous characteristics, expected agreement by chance alone will necessarily be high, leaving little room for substantial non-chance agreement, thereby deflating kappa. This is also a relevant consideration when assessing the reliability of a diagnostic test to detect the presence or absence of a health condition. If the prevalence of the target condition is either very high or very low in the study sample, the calculated kappa may be depressed.

Number of Categories

Kappa is also influenced by the number of categories used. As the number of categories increases, the extent of agreement will generally decrease. This is logical, as with more possibilities of assignment, there is room for greater discrepancy between raters. Therefore, if values of kappa are to be compared across alternative testing methods, these tests should assign scores using the same number of possible categories. It may also be necessary to collapse categories to better reflect agreement within a set of data.

🖈 With data rated as a dichotomy (the presence or absence of a trait), the ICC can be used as an alternative to kappa for estimating relative reliability using scores of 0 and 1. The ICC has been shown to be equivalent to measures of nominal agreement, simplifying computation in cases where more than two raters are involved.[23,24]

> **▶ CASE IN POINT #4**
> Consider a hypothetical functional assessment composed of six items: walking, climbing stairs, carrying 5 pounds, reaching for a phone, dressing, and getting in and out of a car. Each item is scored on an ordinal scale from 1 to 5, with 5 reflecting complete independence. The maximum possible total score is 30, which would indicate that an individual was fully independent in all items. We collect data on 14 patients.

■ Internal Consistency

Some measuring instruments, including many questionnaires and physical performance batteries, are composed of multiple items that in total provide a comprehensive reflection of the broader construct being measured. For instance, the quantitative portion of the Graduate Record Examination (QGRE) includes numerous items to test a student's overall mathematical ability. Similarly, scales measuring overall functional capacity typically consist of multiple items corresponding to different functional tasks. In each of these examples, we want to draw conclusions about an individual's performance based on the total score across all contributing items (see Chapter 12).

One assumption that is inherent in the use of such scales is the **internal consistency** of the items. A good scale is one that assesses different aspects of the same overarching construct. For example, each item comprising a multi-item scale of physical function should reflect an aspect of physical performance and not an aspect of emotional function or some other distinct construct. Statistically, if the multiple items comprising a scale are truly measuring the same overarching attribute, then individual item scores should be moderately correlated with one other and with the total summative score on the scale.

🔑 The concept of internal consistency should not be confused with content or construct validity (see Chapter 10). Internal consistency is a measure of reliability, indicating if item scores are correlated and thereby measuring the same thing. However, even if the items in a scale are measuring the same thing, the scale may not be measuring what it is intended to measure, which is a validity issue.

Cronbach's Alpha (α)

The most commonly applied statistical index of internal consistency is **Cronbach's alpha (α)**.[25] Alpha can be used when item scores are dichotomous or when there are more than two response choices (such as ordinal multiple choice scores).

Internal consistency is a function of the correlation among these six item scores as well as the correlation of each individual item score with the total score. Hypothetical output for this analysis shows that $\alpha = .894$ (see Table 32-5 ❶). Like other correlation coefficients, α is a proportion, with possible values ranging from 0.00 to 1.00. A value that approaches .90 is considered strong, so the scale can be considered to have high internal consistency.

🖈 In a bit of a twist, Cronbach's α should show moderate correlations among items, between .70 and .90.[16,26,27] If items have too low a correlation, they are possibly measuring different traits, but if the items have too high a correlation, they are probably redundant, and some items could be removed without jeopardizing the reliability of the scale.

Item-to-Total Correlations

Using results of the analysis for Cronbach's α, we also examine individual items to determine how well they fit the overall scale. In Table 32-5 ❷, the means and standard deviations for each item are displayed. We can see that walking had the highest mean functional score and car transfer the lowest. The scale totals averaged 16.00, indicating that this sample was only moderately functional (see Table 32-5 ❸). We can also look at correlations among items. All 6 item-pairs have correlations above .60 except for car transfer, which has consistently low correlations with all other items (see Table 32-5 ❹). Perhaps this one variable should not be part of the scale, possibly representing a unique component of function that is distinct from the other items.

To investigate this possibility, we can compute α repeatedly, each time eliminating one item from the analysis. In Table 32-5C, we see what happens to the total score when each item is deleted. In the first column, the mean total score is higher when car transfer is deleted, whereas these values remain fairly stable for all other items. The third column in this panel shows the correlation of each item with the sum of the remaining items, or the **item-to-total correlation**. Only car transfer has a low correlation of .19, suggesting that this item is not related to the total

Table 32-5   Output for Internal Consistency of a Functional Scale with 6 Items Using Cronbach's Alpha (*N*=14)

A. Item Statistics

Reliability Statistics

Cronbach's Alpha	Cronbach's Alpha Based on Standardized Items	N of Items
① .894	.881	6

Item Statistics ②

	Mean	Std. Deviation	N
Car	1.86	.770	14
Carry	2.79	1.251	14
Dressing	2.57	1.089	14
Reach	3.00	1.240	14
Stairs	2.36	1.336	14
Walk	3.43	1.089	14

Scale Statistics ③

Mean	Variance	Std. Deviation	N of Items
16.00	30.769	5.547	6

B. Correlations

Inter-Item Correlation Matrix ④

	Car	Carry	Dressing	Reach	Stairs	Walk
Car	1.000	.125	.196	−.081	.278	.354
Carry	.125	1.000	.830	.843	.739	.637
Dressing	.196	.830	1.000	.797	.694	.750
Reach	−.081	.843	.797	1.000	.603	.740
Stairs	.278	.739	.694	.603	1.000	.785
Walk	.354	.637	.750	.740	.785	1.000

C. Item-Total Statistics

Item-Total Statistics

	Scale Mean if Item Deleted	Scale Variance if Item Deleted	Corrected Item-Total Correlation	Squared Multiple Correlation	Cronbach's Alpha if Item Deleted
Car	14.14	28.593	.192	.566	⑤ .932
Carry	13.21	19.874	.836	.904	.854
Dressing	13.43	21.033	.856	.777	.854
Reach	13.00	20.615	.765	.916	.867
Stairs	13.64	19.632	.790	.817	.863
Walk	12.57	21.187	.837	.893	.856

① Cronbach's alpha is .894.

② The means for each of the variables are shown with standard deviations.

③ The mean total score was 16.00. With a maximum score of 30, this reflects patients who were only moderately functional.

④ Inter-item correlations show moderately strong relationships among all items except for car transfers.

⑤ Item-total statistics show how alpha changes with each item omitted from the scale. Alpha stays consistent except for an increase when car transfer is omitted.

test score derived from all other items. In contrast, each of the other 5 items has a correlation of approximately .80 or higher with the total score. These results can be interpreted in two ways. The initial α = .894 is considered strong, even though it increases when car transfer is removed. A Cronbach's α as high as .932 (without car transfer) suggests that items in the scale may be redundant (see Table 32-5 **5**).

> **Results**
>
> The function scale was composed of six items, scored 1 to 5, with 5 representing full independence. The average total score was 16.00, indicating that this sample was composed of individuals with moderate function. Cronbach's alpha was .89. Correlations among the six items were generally strong (>.603) except for car transfer which had correlations <.36 with all other items. Item-total statistics showed that when car transfer was removed, alpha increased to .932. The item-total correlations ranged from .82 to .92 for all items except car transfer which was .19. These scores suggest that car transfer does not fit with other items on this scale. Without the car transfer item, the rest of the scale shows strong internal consistency.

■ Limits of Agreement

Reliability is an essential property when measurements are taken with alternate forms of an instrument. For example, we might want to compare different types of dynamometers for measuring strength,[28] different types of spirometers for assessing pulmonary function,[29] or different types of monitoring devices for measuring blood glucose.[30] Although different in design and mechanics, we would expect these different methods to record similar values.

The analysis of reliability in this situation focuses on the agreement between alternative methods based on their difference scores. We can consider two methods in agreement when the difference between measurements is small enough for the methods to be considered interchangeable.[31] This property is an important practical concern as we strive for effective and efficient clinical measurement across settings, where different types of instruments are used for similar purposes.[32]

Analyzing Difference Scores

Two analysis procedures have historically been applied to evaluate consistency of measurements using alternative methods. The correlation coefficient, r, has been used to demonstrate covariance among methods. However, we know this is a poor estimate of reliability, as it does not necessarily reflect the extent of agreement in the data and does not provide an absolute index using the same unit of measurement as the tool itself. The second procedure is the paired *t*-test, (or repeated measures ANOVA) which is used to show that mean scores for two (or more) methods are not significantly different from one another. This approach is also problematic, however, as two group distributions may show no statistical difference but still be composed of pairs of observations that are in poor agreement. A pragmatic alternative for examining agreement across methods is an index called **limits of agreement (LoA)**.[32]

> ### ▶ CASE IN POINT #5
>
> Accurate measurement of blood pressure (BP) is important for detection and monitoring of hypertension. Automated and manual methods are often used interchangeably. Several studies have compared the two methods to determine their reliability, with varied results.[33] We will consider hypothetical data for systolic blood pressure (SBP) measures on 50 patients using both devices.

The differences between these alternate methods was calculated by subtracting the values obtained using the automated device from the values obtained using the manual sphygmomanometer (this direction is arbitrary but must be consistent) (see Table 32-6). Therefore, a positive difference score reflects a higher reading for the manual system. The mean of the difference scores was .90 mmHg. On average, then, the manual measurement was higher, but the average difference between the methods was quite small.

Patterns of Difference Scores

A visual analysis can help to clarify this relationship. The scatterplot in Figure 32-1 demonstrates a relatively strong correlation between values obtained using the two methods (r = .82), although scores are not in complete agreement.

Bland-Altman Plots

A further understanding of this relationship can be achieved by examining the spread of difference scores. When differences between methods vary widely from a shared mean, poorer agreement is evident. Assuming a normal distribution and random variation, we would expect 95% of the difference scores to fall within ±1.96 SD

Table 32-6	Systolic Blood Pressure (mmHg) Taken With Manual and Automated Methods (*N* = 50)			
	MEAN	**SD**	**MIN.**	**MAX.**
Manual	135.16	19.47	90.0	172.0
Automated	134.26	18.12	85.0	175.0
Difference	.90	11.40	−17.0	24.0

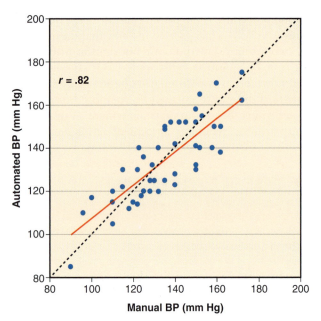

Figure 32–1 Correlation of manual and automatic BP measures. The red line is the regression line. The black dashed line is the line of identity, which emerges from the origin. Points along the line of identity would indicate perfect agreement.

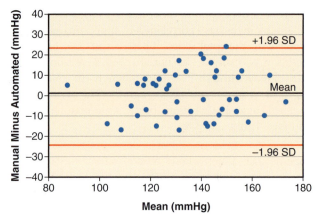

Figure 32–2 A Bland-Altman plot showing agreement of manual and automated BP devices. The mean difference score is .09 mmHg. The 95% limits of agreement are at +22.34 and –22.52 mmHg. All but one point falls within the 95% limits, with scores evenly spread across low and high BP values.

from the mean difference score ($\bar{d}$). This would set the 95% **limits of agreement**. Scores beyond these limits would indicate outliers, suggesting poor reliability. The mean difference score was .90 ± 11.40 (see Table 32-6).

$$95\% \text{ LoA} = \bar{d} \pm 1.96 \text{ (SD)}$$

$$= .90 \pm 1.96 \text{ (11.40)}$$

$$95\% \text{ LoA} = -22.25 \text{ to } 22.43$$

Figure 32-2 shows how difference scores are interpreted using a **Bland-Altman plot**, named for those who developed this strategy.[32,34] The *Y*-axis shows the difference scores (manual – automated) for each subject. Values at zero indicate no difference. Values on the *X*-axis represent the mean of the two measures for each subject. For instance, for the leftmost point in Figure 32-2, the difference between the two measures for this individual was 5.0 mmHg, and the average of the manual and automated scores for that person was 87.5.

A line is drawn at the mean difference score for the total sample on the *Y*-axis. The closer the mean difference score is to zero, the more closely the two measurement methods agree. The 95% limits of agreement are shown at 1.96 SD above and below this mean. This is a range of almost 45 mmHg. Our question, then, is would we be comfortable using either method to measure SBP if we knew that the measured values might disagree by this much?

In a perfect scenario, there would be no difference between the two methods, and we should see all the

difference scores equal zero. As this is unlikely, we would hope to see an unbiased pattern, with difference scores clustering above and below the zero line in a random distribution within the limits of agreement. The spread of scores above and below zero difference helps us decide if the disagreement is acceptable when we substitute one measurement method for the other. For instance, if most scores fall above the zero line, one method would be consistently measuring a higher score than the other, indicating that disagreement is systematic rather than random.

Because the difference scores are plotted for each subject against the mean of that subject's two measured scores, we can also determine if different patterns of disagreement exist for subjects with high or low mean scores. For example, we might see lower difference scores for those with low mean scores, and higher difference scores for those with high mean scores. Such a pattern would suggest that disagreement between the two methods would depend on whether a patient had a high or low SBP level. For example, in Figure 32-2, we can see larger difference scores (approaching the upper limit) for some individuals who had higher mean SBP values. Individuals with lower mean scores did not show as wide a spread.

> ▶ **Results**
> The mean difference score between manual and automated measures was .90 mm Hg (SD = 11.40), with a range from −17.0 to 24.0 mmHg. The scores on both methods were highly correlated (*r* = .82). The Bland-Altman plot shows most difference scores were within the limits of agreement, with a range both above and below the mean difference. However, several larger difference scores were found in some patients with high mean

blood pressure scores. In these patients, manual measurements exceeded automated measurements. Generally, the two instruments show good reliability, but it may be advisable to use the same method for monitoring individuals with higher blood pressure.

In addition to assessing the reliability of alternative instruments, the Bland-Altman plot can also be used to test criterion validity when a new instrument is measured against an established measure that derives scores in the same units. The same process can be used to establish test-retest or rater reliability, looking at the differences between the two test scores. With highly reliable tests, there should be only small variability around the center line and narrow limits of agreement.

■ Measuring Change

A central objective of clinical care is the promotion of positive change or prevention of decline in our clients. Accurate documentation of this change is the cornerstone of successful decision-making, goal-setting, and reimbursement. Clinicians may use terms like "better," "improved," "worse," or "declined" to indicate when a patient's condition appears to have changed, yet these general descriptors are insufficient for making valid and reliable judgments based on measured values.

Responsiveness is the ability of a measuring instrument to register a change in score whenever an actual change in status has occurred.[35] We can understand responsiveness indices as a ratio of signal (true change) to noise (random error variability).

Two concerns guide our interpretation of measured change scores. We first ask whether the recorded change score might be due entirely to measurement error, or whether we can have confidence that some real improvement or decline has occurred. Our second concern is whether the documented change is sufficient to have meaningful impact on a patient's care or an individual's behavior. When we think about measuring a difference in response from one time to another, we can conceptualize the amount of change along a continuum, as shown in Figure 32-3. Measured change scores are first evaluated against a threshold for measurement error, and second to a threshold that distinguishes impactful change. The first concern is a reliability issue, while the second is a validity issue.

Minimal Detectable Change

The **minimal detectable change (MDC)** is the minimal amount of measured change required before we

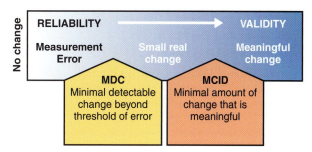

Figure 32–3 Along a continuum of change, MDC = minimal detectable change, and MCID = minimal clinically important difference. Determining the threshold of error is a matter of reliability, while characterizing meaningful change is a matter of validity.

can eliminate the possibility that measurement error is solely responsible. If measured change exceeds the MDC value for that instrument, we can confidently conclude that at least a portion of the measured change was due to real improvement (or decline) in performance.[36]

Calculating the MDC
The MDC is based on the SEM, obtained from a sample of stable persons who are not expected to change.

$$MDC = z * SEM * \sqrt{2}$$

The MDC establishes a threshold value that is linked to either the 90% ($z = 1.65$) or 95% ($z = 1.96$) confidence interval. MDC_{95} means that 95% of stable persons demonstrate random variation of less than this amount when tested on multiple occasions. When a measured change score exceeds the MDC_{95} value, we can have 95% confidence in ruling out random measurement error as solely responsible for the observed change.

MDC is dependent on the size of the reliability coefficient used to calculate the SEM. With a less reliable measure, both SEM and MDC values will increase (see Focus on Evidence 32-2). Instruments that do not demonstrate good test-retest stability will have larger MDCs, indicating that even greater change scores are required before measurement error can be ruled out as the sole source.

 To test a sample of patients who are considered stable, researchers will often look at the scores for patients in a control group. Since these patients did not receive intervention, they are not expected to change.

Focus on Evidence 32–2
Reliability and Change

Many tools are available to provide ratings of pain. Chuang and colleagues[37] studied a combination of a numerical pain rating scale (NPRS) and a faces pain scale (FPS) to establish test-retest reliability in patients who had had a stroke (see Chapter 12). They believed that the combination of scales would provide a useful approach to account for potential language, visual, and perceptual problems associated with stroke.

They studied 50 patients who participated in an outpatient occupational therapy program, 29 with left-sided lesions, and 21 with right-sided lesions. The patients continued to receive routine occupational therapy focused on functional training during the study. The patients were asked to rate current pain intensity in their involved arm using both scales on two occasions with a one-week interval. Ratings were taken at the same time of day to minimize diurnal variation.

Relative test-retest reliability was reflected by an ICC of .82, which is considered good. Absolute reliability was assessed using the SEM, which was .81. They used this value to calculate an MDC$_{90}$ of 1.87, which means that a measured change exceeding 1.87 points on the combined scale should (at a 90% confidence level) indicate that true change had occurred. Using limits of agreement, they were also able to show that there was strong test-retest agreement, with most scores falling within 95% limits. However, they did not account for the outliers and for the fact that differences between the measures were more variable for those with lower pain ratings.

The authors concluded that the combined NPRS-FPS is a reliable pain measure for people with stroke but acknowledged that further work is needed to determine its responsiveness to change with specific interventions, to examine its use with broader populations, and to establish reliability over different timeframes. Remember that reliability is not an absolute characteristic of a measurement, and how these scales function can differ across settings and samples. Every study adds more information to support further research, and to add to the body of knowledge that can inform our decisions. We have to use the information wisely, knowing there is still uncertainty in these conclusions.

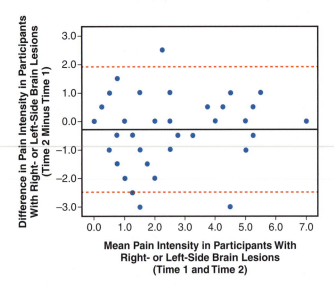

From Chuang L, Wu C, Lin K, Hsieh C. Relative and absolute reliability of a vertical numerical pain rating scale supplemented with a faces pain scale after stroke. *Phys Ther.* 2014;94:129-138, Figure 2A, p.134. Used with permission.

▶ CASE IN POINT #6

The Western Ontario and McMaster Universities Osteoarthritis Index (WOMAC) is a widely used health questionnaire that evaluates pain, stiffness, and functional limitation in patients with osteoarthritis of the knee and hip. Each of the three subscales contains items using a 5-point Likert scale (0-4) representing intensity: none, mild, moderate, severe, or extreme. The final score for each subscale is summed and standardized to a range of values from 0-100, where 0 represents best health status. Quintana et al[36] were interested in studying the responsiveness of the WOMAC in a group of patients following total hip replacement (THR). They tested 469 patients at baseline and 6 months following surgery.

For the functional limitation subscale of the WOMAC, the investigators obtained an SEM of 4.30. Using this SEM value, they calculated the MDC$_{95}$:

$$MDC_{95} = 1.96 * 4.30 * \sqrt{2} = 11.92$$

This result tells us that we can expect 95% of stable patients in this population to demonstrate random variation of less than 11.92 points on the 0-100 function scale with repeated testing.[36] Therefore, if before and after THR we measure a change greater than 11.92 points, this would allow us to conclude that some true change (in excess of expected measurement error) had occurred. The importance of this value is a matter of clinical judgment.

Minimal Clinically Important Difference (MCID)

In clinical care, short-term treatment goals may be written with the MDC in mind. However, beyond simply determining whether measured changes are minimally "real," the clinician also wants to have confidence that measured improvement is indicative of progress towards meeting longer-term treatment objectives, and that measured changes are important. This determination can depend on the variable being measured, the type of patient or health condition, the severity of disability, and cultural norms.[38] The most common threshold for meaningful change is the **minimal clinically important difference (MCID)** (see Fig. 32-3). This has been defined as

> *... the smallest change in an outcome measure that is perceived as beneficial by the patient, and that would lead to a change in the patient's medical management, assuming an absence of excessive side effects and costs.*[39]

This definition of MCID inherently reflects an element of judgment, and several perspectives must be considered.[38] For the patient, it may mean that a change has resulted in noticeable improvement in function or a substantive reduction in symptoms. We may find, however, that different patients assign different value to the same amount of measured improvement. To what extent does quality of life impact this perception?[40] What amount of change in a score will correspond to a perception of trivial, small but important, moderate to large improvement, or deterioration?[41] From the clinician's perspective, the critical determination may be whether or not the change is sufficient to warrant a revision of the treatment plan or the prognosis for recovery. At an institutional level, change may be viewed as important only when it is sufficient to influence healthcare policy.[42]

Two basic approaches have been used to define important change and to characterize the responsiveness of an instrument to detect these changes when they occur. Distribution-based indices provide estimates of responsiveness based on variance within a sample of patients. Anchor-based statistics seek to establish a threshold for determining when change is of sufficient magnitude to have meaningful impact.

Distribution-Based Approach

Distribution-based measures determine the responsiveness of an instrument based on statistical characteristics of an observed sample, such as differences between group means and variance across subjects. The MDC is considered a distribution-based index. These indices do not account for the patient's perception of change but do account for variation within a group. Several distribution-based methods have been proposed to assess the responsiveness of an instrument.

Pretest-Posttest Data

One approach has been to analyze change scores using a pretest-posttest study design. Repeated measures *t*-tests or analyses of variance are used to establish significant differences from time 1 to time 2.[43] Measurements may be taken once before and once after intervention, or there may be multiple measures while the individual is followed over time.[44] This approach can involve only one group of subjects studied before and after treatment or it may incorporate two or more treatment groups. The assumption is made that substantial changes in status will occur as a result of treatment. Therefore, a responsive instrument should be able to record significant differences when comparing scores before and after treatment in the same group, or across different groups of treated and untreated subjects. A statistically significant difference would demonstrate that the instrument was sufficiently responsive to the changes brought about by treatment.

> 🔑 It is important, in this context, to distinguish between a *statistically significant difference* and a *clinically important change*. Statistically significant differences may or may not reflect changes that have meaningful impact or that will direct clinical care. The absolute magnitude of a measured effect may be more relevant than its statistical significance when attempting to determine relevant impact.

Effect Size

Looking at **effect size** is generally considered more appropriate to determine if meaningful change has occurred, because it does take group variability into account. We have looked at effect size in many previous chapters related to the context of power of a test. Although all effect size indices are based on change and variance, in the current context it is a standardized measure of change from baseline to final measurement. Several effect size indices have been used (see Table 32-7).

The **effect size index (ES)** is a ratio of the mean change score (signal) divided by the standard deviation of the baseline scores (noise). Therefore, a measure that has high variability in initial scores will tend to have a smaller effect size. Conventional effect sizes are used to reflect the degree of change, with .20 or less representing a small change; .50 representing moderate change; and .80 representing a large change.[46] This index is the one used to determine power with the *t*-test, and these conventional effect sizes are the same criteria used in that power analysis (see Chapter 24).

The **standardized response mean (SRM)** is a ratio of change from pretest to posttest divided by the standard

Table 32-7	Effect Size Indices Used to Assess Responsiveness to Change	
STATISTIC	**FORMULA**	**APPLICATION**
Effect Size[44,47]	$$ES = \frac{\bar{X}_{post} - \bar{X}_{pre}}{S_{pre}}$$	• Difference between pretest and posttest means, divided by standard deviation of pretest scores • Provides information on magnitude of change in standardized units relative to baseline standard deviation • Not affected by sample size but may vary among samples with different baseline variability.
Standardized Response Mean[45]	$$SRM = \frac{\bar{X}_{post} - \bar{X}_{pre}}{S_{change}}$$	• Provides information on magnitude of change in standardized units relative to variability of change. • Will vary as a function of effectiveness of treatment.
Guyatt's Responsiveness Index[34,46]	$$GRI = \frac{MCID}{\sqrt{2 * MS_E}}$$	• Provides a measure of impactful change relative to variability in scores among patients who are clinically stable. • Denominator includes MS_E term from ANOVA, which may be obtained for test-retest reliability or repeated observations in clinically stable patients.

deviation of the change scores.[47] Therefore, a distribution that has high variability in the degree of change will tend to have a small SRM.

Guyatt's responsiveness index (GRI) uses an anchor-based MCID for the measure being studied, or the smallest difference between baseline and posttest that would represent a meaningful benefit in a group of patients.[48] We will discuss various methods to determine an anchor-based MCID shortly. When the MCID is not known, the difference between baseline and posttest can be used.[35] The denominator for this index is obtained from an ANOVA of repeated observations in a group of subjects who are clinically stable, which is a measure of test-retest reliability. Therefore, the denominator reflects the intrinsic variability of the instrument.

> ▶ Researchers in the WOMAC study used the ES, SRM, and GRI indices to explore responsiveness, shown in Table 32-8. All values were greater than .80 and are therefore considered quite large, indicating that the WOMAC is a responsive instrument that is capable of detecting change over time.

It is of interest to note the consistently higher values derived from the ES index and lower values derived from the GRI. The different denominators used for these indices contribute to the different calculated estimates.

Anchor-Based Approaches

Anchor-based approaches are focused on estimation of impactful change. The MCID is anchored to an external criterion that indicates when important change has occurred according to the patient, clinician, or other stakeholder. In an anchor-based approach, the magnitude

Table 32-8	Effect Size Measures of Responsiveness for the WOMAC in Patients Following Total Hip Replacement					
	AT 6 MONTHS			**AT 2 YEARS**		
Subscale	**ES**	**SRM**	**GRI**	**ES**	**SRM**	**GRI**
Pain	2.10	1.86	1.10	2.24	1.98	2.18
Function	2.34	1.80	1.45	2.56	1.97	1.79
Stiffness	1.61	1.39	.81	1.81	1.53	1.12

Data taken from Quintana et al[36], adapted from Table III, p. 1080. Used with permission.
ES = effect size index; SRM = standardized response mean; GRI = Guyatt's Responsiveness Index.

of a measured change score obtained using a clinical test is compared to an external "anchor" that characterizes the patient or stakeholder's perception of whether they are "better," "worse," or "no different." The MCID value for an instrument can be helpful when setting long-term treatment objectives in the clinic since it provides a threshold for determining how much measured change is needed before meaningful impact is likely to be reported.

 The disadvantage of anchor-based methods is that they do not take into account the variability or potential measurement error in an instrument. Therefore, it is important to establish the reliability and MDC of an instrument when using it to estimate important change.

Global Rating of Change

The determination of important difference from the patient or clinician's perspective has most often been evaluated using an ordinal scale. Scales generally range from "a great deal worse" to "a great deal better," with as few as 5 to as many as 15 ordinal rankings (see Table 32-9). A score of zero indicates that no change has been perceived.[39,49] In studies that derive an MCID value, rankings of "somewhat better" or "somewhat worse" have usually been used to establish the threshold indicating when minimally important change was perceived.

> ▶ **Results**
>
> In the WOMAC study, patients were asked to rate their perceived improvement following intervention based on a 5-point scale. Possible responses were "a great deal better," "somewhat better," "equal," "somewhat worse," or "a great deal worse." The MCID was based on the WOMAC scores for those who rated themselves at least "somewhat better," which corresponded to a change of at least 25 points for all three WOMAC subscales.[36] Therefore, changes beyond 25 points were considered to reflect meaningful improvement.

When assessing meaningful change, anchor-based methods are generally preferred over distribution-based methods because they reflect a definition of what is considered important.[50] However, using both distribution-based and anchor-based approaches should provide a strong foundation for understanding how best to interpret measured change in the context of imperfect test-retest reliability and differing perceptions of value for the patient.[51,52]

Interpreting the MCID

Several considerations are important for interpreting the MCID.

Going beyond MDC.

The MCID sets a threshold for meaningful change, while the MDC only sets a threshold for substantive change, whether or not that substantive change is perceived as having real impact or value. Interestingly, in some studies, researchers find an MDC value that is larger than the MCID.[53-56] This may seem illogical—in theory, it makes little sense that an MDC would ever be greater than an MCID. We would expect important differences to always be greater than measurement error. This is not an investigative error, however. It is merely a consequence of the fact that these two statistics quantify distinct constructs and are derived from different data.

The MDC is a reliability statistic and is calculated using test-retest data based on group values. In contrast, the MCID is a validity measure, based on individual patient perceptions about whether change was meaningful.[57] When MDC and MCID values fail to align in the expected way, clinicians will typically use the larger of the two values as the threshold for most evidence-based applications, recognizing that these values provide guidelines and not absolute limits.

Baseline Scores.

A second consideration is the potential effect of a patient's baseline score. Patients who have lower initial scores may have greater incentive to recognize and appreciate even small improvements in their status.[58] A patient's perception of important change can vary depending on where they start.[59,60]

Recall Bias.

A third concern is related to *recall bias*, which can influence how a patient remembers what has happened most recently but may have less clear memory of their status in the more distant past.[61] This is most relevant when asking patients to reflect on changes during a longer episode of care, as some patients may underestimate the extent of their improvement if they cannot accurately remember their status at baseline.

Inconsistent Methodology.

Perhaps the greatest challenge for evidence-based practice is the lack of consistency in the MCID obtained in different studies for the same instrument.[57] Unfortunately for clinical decision making, this means that we cannot view the MCID as a universal fixed attribute of a test, but must consider the method of calculation and the specific context within which it was obtained, including the population and setting.

Table 32-9	15-Point Global Rating Scale to Assess Magnitude of Change	
	RATING	**DESCRIPTION OF CHANGE**
Feeling Better →	7	A very great deal better
	6	A great deal better
	5	Quite a bit better
	4	Moderately better
	3	Somewhat better
	2	A little bit better
	1	A tiny bit better, almost the same
	0	No change
Feeling Worse ↓	–1	A tiny bit worse, almost the same
	–2	A little bit worse
	–3	Somewhat worse
	–4	Moderately worse
	–5	Quite a bit worse
	–6	A great deal worse
	–7	A very great deal worse

Lack of Confidence Intervals. Because the MCID is typically reported as a single value without confidence intervals, we don't have a good sense of an applicable range of possible scores and therefore run the risk of misclassifying patients whose scores do not meet the threshold, but for whom impactful change may still have occurred.

> In addition to making judgments about a patient's degree of improvement, the MCID can be used to estimate how much of a change would be considered important in a research study. The MCID value for the primary outcome can be used to estimate needed sample size as part of *a priori* power analysis. Results from clinical trials can be compared to the MCID as a way of determining whether measured treatment effects are likely to have meaningful impact.[62] The MCID can also be used to establish the margin in a non-inferiority study (see Chapter 14).

MDC and MCID Proportion

Group values must be interpreted with reference to their sample size and variability. We know that power is greatly influenced by the number of subjects in a sample. Therefore, with a large sample, small differences may turn out to be significant even when they are clinically meaningless. We also recognize that a mean is a measure of central tendency and that individuals in the sample do not all experience that amount of change—some will have achieved more and some less. Therefore, any conclusions about an individual patient's response based on a mean may be flawed. Without looking at variability within the sample, we may be missing important information.

When studying a dichotomous variable, decisions about improvement or decline are straightforward—the patient has either gotten better or not, cured or not cured. When dealing with a continuous measure, however, it is necessary to determine how much change is meaningful. Therefore, the proportion of individuals in a group that achieve minimal change can be considered another important benchmark to evaluate an intervention's effectiveness. **MDC** or **MCID proportion** is the percentage of patients whose measured change scores exceed the minimal threshold, either for detectable change or for clinically meaningful change. These values can be especially useful for examining group data during program evaluation or quality assurance reviews.[51]

> In the study of responsiveness for the WOMAC, the MDC proportion was greater than 80% for pain and function subscales, and the MCID proportion was between 70% to 80% after 2 years following hip joint replacement. These values demonstrate that a large majority of patients in this population perceive themselves as "better" following intervention.

COMMENTARY

If you can't measure something, you can't understand it. If you can't understand it, you can't control it. If you can't control it, you can't improve it.

—*H. James Harrington (1929-)*

Leader in performance improvement methodologies

Measurement is essential to the care of patients, design of studies, management of systems, and decision making. Because there are so many approaches to measuring clinical or organizational phenomena, we must be clear in reporting and knowledgeable in the consumption of data. What we learn from looking through professional literature, however, is that preferred methods for analyzing reliability and validity seem to vary with different researchers and within different disciplines, with little consensus.

As evidence-based practitioners, we should be aware of the intended application of the data and the degree of precision needed to make safe and meaningful clinical decisions. When considering reliability or validity, we cannot allow ourselves to fall into the trap of using specific standards just because they have been used or recommended by others. Guidelines are just that—not gold standards. Researchers and clinicians are obligated to justify their interpretation of acceptable measurement characteristics.

Researchers should address each of these relevant issues in their reports, so that others can interpret their work properly. Many articles are published with no such discussion, leaving the reader to guess why a particular statistic was used or a standard applied. Because statistics can be applied in so many ways, it is important to maintain an exchange of ideas that promotes such accountability. By having to justify our choices, we are forced to consider what a statistic can really tell us about a variable and what conclusions are warranted.

Clinical judgments regarding validity of measurements must be based on some criterion that is relevant for a particular patient. Any given study will present data from a sample that has specific properties and that has been studied in a specific context over a given time period. Clinicians must appraise that information to determine if it is appropriately applied to their patients. Published values may provide an estimate that can be used to predict our own patients' responses, but it is essential that we remain cognizant of the limits of statistics as we apply them to our own decision making.

As our understanding of validity grows, we will continue to struggle with the definitions of clinical significance. The evidence-based practitioner will benefit from complete reporting of effect sizes and change values in clinical studies. Estimates are needed for different settings, conditions, age groups, and baselines. Clinicians, patients, and health policy analysts all want to appreciate how much better is truly "better."

REFERENCES

1. Tyson S, Connell L. The psychometric properties and clinical utility of measures of walking and mobility in neurological conditions: a systematic review. *Clin Rehabil* 2009;23(11): 1018-1033.
2. Shrout PE, Fleiss JL. Intraclass correlation: uses in assessing rater reliability. *Psychol Bull* 1979;86:420-428.
3. Jackson SE, Brashers DE. *Random Factors in ANOVA*. Thousand Oaks, CA: Sage Publications; 1994.
4. McGraw KO, Wong SP. Forming inferences about some intraclass correlation coefficients. *Psychol Methods* 1996;1(1):30-46.
5. Nichols DP. SPSS Library: Choosing an intraclass correlation coefficient. UCLA Institute for Digital Research and Education. Available at http://stats.idre.ucla.edu/spss/library/spss-library-choosing-an-intraclass-correlation-coefficient/. Accessed March 4, 2017.
6. Weir JP. Quantifying test-retest reliability using the intraclass correlation coefficient and the SEM. *J Strength Cond Res* 2005; 19(1):231-240.
7. Roland M, Morris R. A study of the natural history of back pain. Part I: development of a reliable and sensitive measure of disability in low-back pain. *Spine* 1983;8(2):141-144.
8. Chiarotto A, Maxwell LJ, Terwee CB, Wells GA, Tugwell P, Ostelo RW. Roland-Morris Disability Questionnaire and Oswestry Disability Index: Which has better measurement properties for measuring physical functioning in nonspecific low back pain? Systematic review and meta-analysis. *Phys Ther* 2016;96(10):1620-1637.
9. Davidson M, Keating JL. A comparison of five low back disability questionnaires: reliability and responsiveness. *Phys Ther* 2002;82(1):8-24.
10. Riddle DL, Stratford PW. Roland-Morris scale reliability. *Phys Ther* 2002;82(5):512-515.
11. Lahey MA, Downey RG, Saal FE. Intraclass correlations: there's more there than meets the eye. *Psych Bull* 1983;93(3): 586-595.
12. Wainner RS. Reliability of the clinical examination: how close is "close enough"? *J Orthop Sports Phys Ther* 2003;33(9): 488-491.
13. Streiner DL, Norman GR. *Health Measurement Scales: A Practical Guide to Their Development and Use.* 5 ed. Oxford: Oxford Press 2015.
14. Chinn S. Statistics in respiratory medicine. 2. Repeatability and method comparison. *Thorax* 1991;46(6):454-456.
15. Cicchetti DV. Guidelines, criteria, and rules of thumb for evaluating normed and standardized assessment instruments in psychology. *Psychol Assessment* 1994;6(4):284-290.
16. Nunnally J, Bernstein IH. *Psychometric Theory.* 3rd ed. New York: McGraw-Hill; 1994.
17. Salkind NJ. *Tests & Measurement for People Who (Think They) Hate Tests & Measurement.* Thousand Oaks, CA: Sage Publications; 2006.
18. Nunnally JC. Psychometric theory— 25 years ago and now. *Educ Res* 1975;4(10):7-14, 19-21.
19. Baker NA, Moehling KK, Desai AR, Gustafson NP. Effect of carpal tunnel syndrome on grip and pinch strength compared with sex- and age-matched normative data. *Arthritis Care Res (Hoboken)* 2013;65(12):2041-2045.
20. Riddle DL, Stratford PW. *Is This a Real Change? Interpreting Patient Outcomes in Physical Therapy.* Philadelphia: F.A. Davis; 2013.
21. Landis JR, Koch GG. The measurement of observer agreement for categorical data. *Biometrics* 1977;33(1):159-174.
22. Cohen J. Weighted kappa: Nominal scale agreement with provisions for scale disagreement or partial credit. *Psychol Bull* 1968; 70:313.
23. Fleiss JL, Cohen J. The equivalence of weighted kappa on the intraclass correlation coefficient as measures of reliablity. *Educ Psychol Meas* 1973;33:613-619.
24. Bartko JJ, Carpenter WT, Jr. On the methods and theory of reliability. *J Nerv Ment Dis* 1976;163(5):307-317.
25. Cronbach LJ. Coefficient alpha and the internal structure of tests. *Psychometrika* 1951;16:297-334.
26. Boyle GJ. Does item homogeneity indicate internal consistency or item redundancy in psychometric scales? *Personality Individ Differences* 1991;12:291-294.
27. Hattie J. Methodology review: assessing unidimensionality of tests and items. *Applied Psycholog Meas* 1985;9(2):139-164.
28. Chamorro C, Armijo-Olivo S, De la Fuente C, Fuentes J, Javier Chirosa L. Absolute reliability and concurrent validity of hand held dynamometry and isokinetic dynamometry in the hip, knee and ankle joint: systematic review and meta-analysis. *Open Med (Wars)* 2017;12:359-375.
29. Joo S, Lee K, Song C. A comparative study of smartphone game with spirometry for pulmonary function assessment in stroke patients. *Biomed Res Int* 2018;2018:2439312.
30. Rodbard D. Characterizing accuracy and precision of glucose sensors and meters. *J Diabetes Sci Technol* 2014;8(5):980-985.
31. Ottenbacher KJ, Stull GA. The analysis and interpretation of method comparison studies in rehabilitation research. *Am J Phys Med Rehabil* 1993;72:266-271.
32. Bland JM, Altman DG. Statistical methods for assessing agreement between two methods of clinical measurement. *Lancet* 1986;1(8476):307-310.
33. Skirton H, Chamberlain W, Lawson C, Ryan H, Young E. A systematic review of variability and reliability of manual and automated blood pressure readings. *J Clin Nurs* 2011;20(5-6): 602-614.
34. Giavarina D. Understanding Bland Altman analysis. *Biochem Med (Zagreb)* 2015;25(2):141-151.
35. Wright JG, Young NL. A comparison of different indices of responsiveness. *J Clin Epidemiol* 1997;50(3):239-246.
36. Quintana JM, Escobar A, Bilbao A, Arostegui I, Lafuente I, Vidaurreta I. Responsiveness and clinically important differences for the WOMAC and SF-36 after hip joint replacement. *Osteoarthritis Cartilage* 2005;13(12):1076-1083.

37. Chuang LL, Wu CY, Lin KC, Hsieh CJ. Relative and absolute reliability of a vertical numerical pain rating scale supplemented with a faces pain scale after stroke. *Phys Ther* 2014;94(1):129-138.

38. Crosby RD, Kolotkin RL, Williams GR. Defining clinically meaningful change in health-related quality of life. *J Clin Epidemiol* 2003;56(5):395-407.

39. Jaeschke R, Singer J, Guyatt GH. Measurement of health status. Ascertaining the minimal clinically important difference. *Control Clin Trials* 1989;10(4):407-415.

40. Beaton DE, Tarasuk V, Katz JN, Wright JG, Bombardier C. "Are you better?" A qualitative study of the meaning of recovery. *Arthritis Rheum* 2001;45(3):270-279.

41. Guyatt GH, Feeny DH, Patrick DL. Measuring health-related quality of life. *Ann Intern Med* 1993;118(8):622-629.

42. Osoba D, Rodrigues G, Myles J, Zee B, Pater J. Interpreting the significance of changes in health-related quality-of-life scores. *J Clin Oncol* 1998;16(1):139-144.

43. Stratford PW, Binkley JM, Riddle DL. Health status measures: strategies and analytic methods for assessing change scores. *Phys Ther* 1996;76:1109-1123.

44. Stratford PW, Binkley J, Solomon P, Gill C, Finch E. Assessing change over time in patients with low back pain. *Phys Ther* 1994; 74(6):528-533.

45. Kazis LE, Anderson JJ, Meenan RF. Effect sizes for interpreting changes in health status. *Med Care* 1989;27(3):S178-S189.

46. Cohen J. *Statistical Power Analysis for the Behavioral Sciences.* 2nd ed. Hillsdale, NJ: Lawrence Erlbaum; 1988.

47. Liang MH, Fossel AH, Larson MG. Comparisons of five health status instruments for orthopedic evaluation. *Med Care* 1990; 28(7):632-642.

48. Guyatt G, Walter S, Norman G. Measuring change over time: Assessing the usefulness of evaluative instruments. *J Chronic Dis* 1987;40(2):171-178.

49. Guyatt GH, Osoba D, Wu AW, Wyrwich KW, Norman GR. Methods to explain the clinical significance of health status measures. *Mayo Clin Proc* 2002;77(4):371-383.

50. de Vet HC, Terwee CB, Ostelo RW, Beckerman H, Knol DL, Bouter LM. Minimal changes in health status questionnaires: Distinction between minimally detectable change and minimally important change. *Health Qual Life Outcomes* 2006;4:54.

51. Haley SM, Fragala-Pinkham MA. Interpreting change scores of tests and measures used in physical therapy. *Phys Ther* 2006; 86(5):735-743.

52. Eton DT, Cella D, Yost KJ, Yount SE, Peterman AH, Neuberg DS, Sledge GW, Wood WC. A combination of distribution- and anchor-based approaches determined minimally important differences (MIDs) for four endpoints in a breast cancer scale. *J Clin Epidemiol* 2004;57(9):898-910.

53. Young BA, Walker MJ, Strunce JB, Boyles RE, Whitman JM, Childs JD. Responsiveness of the Neck Disability Index in patients with mechanical neck disorders. *Spine J* 2009;9(10): 802-808.

54. Dawson J, Doll H, Boller I, Fitzpatrick R, Little C, Rees J, Carr A. Comparative responsiveness and minimal change for the Oxford Elbow Score following surgery. *Qual Life Res* 2008; 17(10):1257-1267.

55. Kocks JW, Tuinenga MG, Uil SM, van den Berg JW, Stahl E, van der Molen T. Health status measurement in COPD: the minimal clinically important difference of the clinical COPD questionnaire. *Respir Res* 2006;7:62.

56. Carey H, Martin K, Combs-Miller S, Heathcock JC. Reliability and responsiveness of the Timed Up and Go Test in children with cerebral palsy. *Pediatr Phys Ther* 2016;28(4): 401-408.

57. Wright A, Hannon J, Hegedus EJ, Kavchak AE. Clinimetrics corner: a closer look at the minimal clinically important difference (MCID). *J Man Manip Ther* 2012;20(3):160-166.

58. Beaton DE, Boers M, Wells GA. Many faces of the minimal clinically important difference (MCID): a literature review and directions for future research. *Curr Opin Rheumatol* 2002;14(2): 109-114.

59. Wang YC, Hart DL, Stratford PW, Mioduski JE. Baseline dependency of minimal clinically important improvement. *Phys Ther* 2011;91(5):675-688.

60. Terwee CB, Roorda LD, Dekker J, Bierma-Zeinstra SM, Peat G, Jordan KP, Croft P, de Vet HC. Mind the MIC: large variation among populations and methods. *J Clin Epidemiol* 2010;63(5):524-534.

61. Norman GR, Stratford P, Regehr G. Methodological problems in the retrospective computation of responsiveness to change: the lesson of Cronbach. *J Clin Epidemiol* 1997;50(8): 869-879.

62. Revicki D, Hays RD, Cella D, Sloan J. Recommended methods for determining responsiveness and minimally important differences for patient-reported outcomes. *J Clin Epidemiol* 2008; 61(2):102-109.

Diagnostic Accuracy

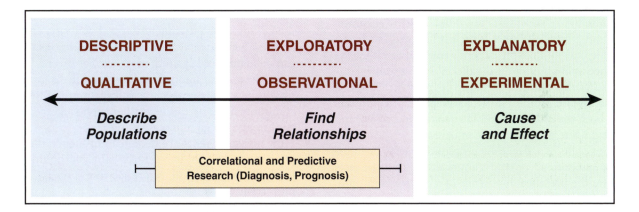

One of the essential purposes of measurement is to distinguish people based on a criterion, distinctions that can influence how we proceed with a patient's care. Clinicians face uncertainty in many aspects of patient management and often apply their expertise, intuition, and judgment to make decisions about appropriate treatment or prevention. Given our focus on evidence-based practice, however, we are better prepared for decision-making when we can apply explicit criteria that help to reduce uncertainty.

An essential component of decision-making is the ability to diagnose a condition, to determine its presence or absence, to apply screening procedures to identify those at risk for certain disorders, and to classify patients who are likely to benefit from specific intervention strategies or further diagnostic tests. Because these procedures involve allocation of resources, influence patient management decisions, and present potential risks to patients, it is important to verify their validity and to understand how results are appropriately applied to clinical practice. The purpose of this chapter is to present statistical procedures related to accuracy of diagnostic and screening tools, making judgments regarding diagnostic probability, choosing cutoff scores, and the application of clinical prediction rules.

■ Validity of Diagnostic Tests

The term "diagnosis" can be used in different ways, depending on its context. It is literally the act of making a judgment about the exact character of a condition, situation or problem.[1] In healthcare, the traditional usage focuses on identification of a disease or systemic disorder through lab tests or other procedures. It can also be used to mean identification of impairments, functional limitation, or disability to make judgments about an individual's ability to participate in life roles. A diagnosis can be based on a score from a health scale, used to indicate the presence of a latent trait that impacts an individual's life, such as depression, dementia, risk for falls, or quality of life. In each of these instances, the diagnosis will lead to a clinical decision regarding therapy, medication, surgery or other strategy to improve the condition or prevent an adverse outcome. Therefore, sound decisions depend on the validity of the test, to assure that these actions are warranted.

The purpose of a study of diagnostic accuracy is to determine if a "new" test, the **index test**, is accurate, based on a **gold standard** which is "known" to be an accurate indication of the patient's true status, either the presence or absence of the condition. These studies usually use a cohort design, enrolling people who are at risk for the disease of interest. All participants are administered both the index test and the gold standard test, and the diagnostic outcomes are compared.

The results of a diagnostic procedure may be dichotomous, categorical, or continuous, although most tests indicate the presence or absence of a certain condition. Ordinal and continuous scales are often converted to dichotomous outcomes using cutoff scores to indicate a "normal" or "abnormal" state.

► CASE IN POINT #1

Vertebral fractures (VFx) are associated with various comorbidities and mortality, particularly in older individuals. However, many individuals with such fractures do not present overt symptoms, and more than two-thirds go undetected.[2] Height loss has been used as a screening measure, although studies are not clear as to how much height loss is indicative of VFx.

Yoh et al[3] studied the relationship between height loss and presence of VFx in 151 postmenopausal women to determine the best cutoff score for screening. Radiographic data were used to define the diagnosis of vertebral fracture. A cutoff of height loss ≥ 4 cm was considered the criterion for identifying potential VFx.

Assessing Validity

The ideal diagnostic test, of course, would always be accurate in discriminating between those with and without the disease or condition—it would always have a positive result for someone with the condition, whether a mild or severe case, and a negative result for everyone else. But we know that tests are not perfect. They may miss identifying some individuals with a particular disorder, or they may indicate illness in those without the disorder. Validity will depend on several criteria:

- Determination of accuracy is based on the validity of the gold standard. However, for many clinical variables there is no true "gold standard" and a **reference standard** must be operationally defined that is "assumed" to be an accurate outcome. This can be especially challenging with measurement of constructs such as balance, function, or pain. Clearly, the validity of the index test will depend on the validity of the standard used.

- Validity is dependent on the sample used to verify the test. Selection of participants will often be purposive, to assure that they adequately represent the target population for which the test would be used. This means that inclusion and exclusion criteria must be specified. Because many conditions can be manifested as mild, moderate, or severe, generalization of findings depends on the extent to which the sample reflects the full spectrum of the condition. Validity can be further supported by confirmation on a separate sample.

- How measurements are taken can influence the assessment of an index test. All subjects should get both the index and reference test. This is important to assure that the decision to use a test is not based on other clinical information, or an *a priori* opinion of whether the patient has the condition. Blinding those who take the measurements will reduce potential bias. Operational definitions should be clear, and testers should be evaluated for their reliability so that measurement error is minimized.

- Because many conditions will change over time, the timing of the index and reference test can be important, to be sure that they are measuring the same thing. For diagnosis, this should be concurrent.

- Clinicians should be able to evaluate the methodologic quality of diagnostic validity studies. Studies with poor quality of design or analysis may overestimate the accuracy of diagnostic tests.[4-6] The *Standards for Reporting of Diagnostic Accuracy (STARD)* provide a checklist for inclusion of all relevant information that comprise essential elements of design, analysis, and interpretation of diagnostic test studies (see Chapter 38).[8]

► Radiographic data were considered a gold standard in the diagnosis of VFx. The index test was determination of height loss, calculated as maximum height recalled by the patient minus the current height. Although this method has potential for inaccurate recall, it has been shown to be a useful measure for purposes of identifying VFx.[8]

Participants were invited to participate in the VFx study through outpatient clinics in one community. Exclusion criteria included pre-existing metabolic bone disease or severe skeletal deformity. The participants had a range of scores, with median height loss of 3.2 cm with an interquartile range of 1.5 to 7 cm. The x-rays and height measures occurred at the same session, controlling for any changes in condition.

Positive and Negative Tests

The validity of a diagnostic test is evaluated in terms of its ability to accurately detect the true presence or absence of the target condition. Our challenge is to determine how likely it is that someone who tests positive actually has the disorder and someone who tests negative does not.

If we compare the positive and negative results of a diagnostic test to the reference standard diagnosis, there are four possible scenarios, which are summarized in a familiar 2×2 arrangement (see Table 33-1). The columns indicate the true presence or absence of the disease (Dx+ or Dx–), as determined by the reference standard. The rows indicate whether positive or negative results were obtained using the index test. The cells labeled *a* and *d* represent **true positive** and **true negative** test results, respectively. Individuals who have the target condition are accurately detected by a positive test (cell *a*) and individuals who do not have the target condition are accurately detected by a negative test (cell *d*). The overall **diagnostic accuracy** of a test is the proportion of all correct tests in the sample, $(a+d)/N$.

Cell *b* represents the **false positives**, those who are incorrectly assigned a positive test result despite not having the target condition, and cell *c* represents the **false negatives**, individuals who are incorrectly assigned

a negative test result despite the presence of the target disease.

Sensitivity and Specificity

To analyze these values, we can calculate two proportions which indicate the accuracy of the height loss test in detecting the true presence or absence of vertebral fractures (see Table 33-2A and B). Proportions can range from 0.0 to 1.0. The closer to 1.0, the stronger the association.

Sensitivity is the test's ability to obtain a positive test when the target condition is really present, or the *true positive rate* (also called the *hit rate*).

$$\text{Sensitivity} = \frac{a}{a + c}$$

This value is the proportion of individuals who test positive for the condition out of all those who actually have it, or the probability of obtaining a correct positive test in patients who have the target condition. *A highly sensitive test will correctly classify those who have the condition of interest.*

Specificity is the test's ability to obtain a negative test when the condition is really absent, or the *true negative rate*.

$$\text{Specificity} = \frac{d}{b + d}$$

This value is the proportion of individuals who test negative for the condition out of all those who are truly normal, or the probability of a correct negative test in those who do not have the target condition. *A highly specific test will rarely test positive when a person does not have the disease.*

> ➤ Using ≥ 4 cm as the cutoff results in sensitivity of the height loss test of 79%. Of the 62 patients identified as having VFx, 49 tested positive using this criterion. The specificity of the test was also 79%. Of the 89 patients who did not have a VFx, 70 were considered negative. These statistics indicate that the height loss criterion of ≥ 4 cm is fairly accurate for identifying both those with and without fractures.

The complement of sensitivity (1 – sensitivity) is the **false negative rate**, or the probability of obtaining an incorrect negative test in patients who do have the target disorder. The complement of specificity (1 – specificity) is the **false positive rate**, sometimes called the *false alarm* rate. This is the probability of an incorrect positive test in those who do not have the target condition.

Table 33-1	**Summary of Diagnostic Test Results**		
	Reference Standard True Diagnosis		
	Dx+	**Dx–**	Total
Positive Test	*a* True positive	*b* False positive	*a+b*
Negative Test	*c* False negative	*d* True negative	*c+d*
Total	*a+c*	*b+d*	*N*

Table 33-2   Results of Screening for Vertebral Fracture (VFx) Based on ≥ 4 cm Height Loss (*N* = 151)

A. Data

	Reference Standard		
	VFx	No VFx	Total
Height Loss ≥4 cm	49 *a*	19 *b*	68 *a + b*
Height Loss <4 cm	13 *c*	70 *d*	83 *c + d*
Total	62 *a + c*	89 *b + d*	*N* 151

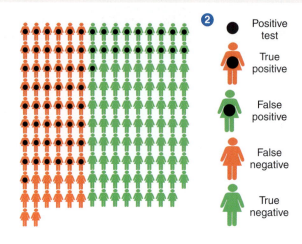

B. Diagnostic Statistics

Diagnostic accuracy	(*a* + *d*)/*N*	(49 + 70)/151 = .788 (79%) ❸
Sensitivity	*a*/(*a* + *c*)	49/62 = .790 (79%)
Specificity	*d*/(*b* + *d*)	70/89 = .787 (79%)
False positive rate (1−specificity)	*b*/(*b* + *d*)	19/89 = .213 (21%)
False negative rate (1−sensitivity)	*c*/(*a* + *c*)	13/62 = .210 (21%)
Positive predictive value (PV+)	*a*/(*a* + *b*)	49/68 = .721 (72%)
Negative predictive value (PV−)	*d*/(*c* + *d*)	70/83 = .843 (84%)
Prevalence	(*a* + *c*)/*N*	62/151 = .411 (41%)
Positive likelihood ratio (LR+)	sensitivity/1-specificity	.790/.213 = 3.71 ❹
Negative likelihood ratio (LR−)	1-sensitivity/specificity	.21/.79 = .27

C. Confidence Intervals

Sensitivity	95% CI: 0.69 to 0.89	**Specficity**	95% CI: 0.70 to 0.87
PV+	95% CI: 0.61 to 0.83	**PV−**	95% CI: 0.77 to 0.92
LR+	95% CI: 2.44 to 5.63	**LR−**	95% CI: 0.16 to 0.44

❶ The distribution of positive and negative tests VFx for 151 patients based on x-rays (reference standard) and height loss of ≥4cm. Cell a = true positives; cell b = false positives; cell c = false negatives; cell d = true negatives.

❷ Visualization of distribution of positive and negative tests. Each patient is represented by an icon, red indicating those who do have a VFx and green indicating those who do not. The black dot indicates an individual who tested positive.

❸ Diagnostic tests are typically reported as percentages or ❹ taken to 2 decimal places.

Confidence intervals were obtained using the CCRB CI Calculator: Diagnostic Statistics.[9] Calculations vary due to rounding differences.

Based on data from Yoh K, Kuwahara A, Tanaka K. Detective value of historical height loss and current height/knee height ratio for prevalent vertebral fracture in Japanese postmenopausal women. *J Bone Miner Metab* 2014;32(5):533-538.

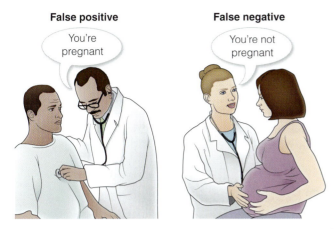

False positive You're pregnant

False negative You're not pregnant

From Raffensperger, Orthopedic Interventions for the Physical Therapist Assistant, FA Davis, Philadelphia, 2020, with permission.

Predictive Value

In addition to sensitivity and specificity, the usefulness of a diagnostic tool can be assessed by its feasibility. A test must demonstrate that it is an efficient use of time and resources and that it yields a sufficient number of accurate responses to be clinically useful. This characteristic is assessed by the test's **predictive value**. A *positive predictive value* (PV+) estimates the likelihood that a person who tests positive actually has the disease:

$$PV+ = \frac{a}{a+b}$$

which represents the proportion of those who tested positive who were true positives. *A test with a high positive predictive value will provide a strong estimate of the actual number of patients who have the target condition.*

Similarly, a *negative predictive value* (PV–) indicates the probability that a person who tests negative is actually disease free. Therefore,

$$PV- = \frac{d}{c+d}$$

which is the proportion of all those who tested negative who were true negatives. *A test with a high negative predictive value will provide a strong estimate of the number of people who do not have the target condition.*

▶ For the VFx study, a PV+ of 72% tells us that almost three-quarters of those who tested positive actually had a VFx. Nineteen patients who tested positive were not diagnosed

with a fracture. The PV– was higher at 84%. Therefore, a high proportion of patients who tested negative were actually negative.

Predictive value may be of greatest importance in deciding whether to implement a screening program to identify individuals who at risk for developing a disease or who may be in an early stage. The utility of the test is based on how many cases are identified as a result of early detection. Outcomes must be balanced against cost as well as the impact of results, which may lead to the application of treatments that have inherent risks. When the positive predictive value is low, only a small portion of those who test positive actually have the target condition. Therefore, considerable resources will probably be needed to evaluate these people further to separate false positives, or unnecessary treatments will be applied. Policy decisions are often based on a balance between the use of available resources and the potential harmful effects resulting from not identifying those with the target condition (see further discussion in Focus on Evidence 33-1).

The Effect of Prevalence

Sensitivity, specificity, and predictive value are influenced by the **prevalence** of the target condition in the population. Prevalence refers to the number of cases of a condition existing in a given population at any one time. These data are typically collected using a cross-sectional design within a defined time period. For a test with a given sensitivity and specificity, the likelihood of identifying cases with the condition is increased when prevalence is high—when the condition is common. Therefore, when prevalence is high, a test will tend to have a higher positive predictive value. Sensitivity and specificity can be biased when the study sample does not reflect the prevalence in the overall population. This situation may inflate or deflate these values.

When prevalence is low—the condition is rare—one can expect many more false positives, just by chance. A positive predictive value can be increased either by increasing the specificity of the test (changing the criterion) or by targeting a subgroup of the population that is at high risk for the target condition. We will discuss shortly how prevalence can influence clinical diagnoses.

Ruling In and Ruling Out

When we consider the diagnostic accuracy of a test, very high values of sensitivity and specificity provide a certain level of confidence in interpretation. If a test has high sensitivity, it will properly identify most of those who have the disorder. If the test has high specificity, it will properly identify most of those without the condition. But how do these definitions relate to confidence in diagnostic decisions? Consider these two questions:

- If a patient has a positive test, can we be confident in ruling **IN** the diagnosis?
- If a patient has a negative test, can we be confident in ruling **OUT** the diagnosis?

Sensitivity and specificity help us answer these questions but probably not the way you would expect. When a test has *high specificity*, a positive test *rules in* the diagnosis. When a test has *high sensitivity*, a negative test *rules out* the diagnosis. Straus and colleagues[10] offer two mnemonics to remember these relationships (see Fig. 33-1). Unfortunately, there is no consensus on what a "high" value is. Mostly, it refers to values closer to 1.0—not a big help. Sensitivity and specificity values above .90 will generally result in "few" false negatives and false positives. The impact of these values will depend on the test and the risks associated with misdiagnosis.

> Ruling in and out can get confusing, so think of it this way. A highly specific test will accurately identify most of the patients who do **NOT** have the disorder. If the test is so good at finding those who are normal, we can be pretty sure that someone with a positive test **DOES** have the disorder (ruling **IN** the diagnosis)—because if he didn't have the disorder, the test would have correctly identified him as normal!
>
> Conversely, a highly sensitive test will identify most of those who **DO** have the disorder. Therefore, we can be pretty sure that someone with a negative test does **NOT** have the disorder (ruling **OUT** the diagnosis)—because if he did have the disorder, the test would have correctly diagnosed him!

These concepts are also related to predictive value. With a more specific test, negative cases are identified more readily. Therefore, it is less likely that an individual with a positive test will actually be normal. This results in a high positive predictive value. With a more sensitive test, positive cases are identified more readily; that is, we will not miss many true cases. Therefore, it is less likely that an individual with a negative test will have the disease. This leads to a high negative predictive value.

If we use the example of the VFx study (see Table 33-2), with specificity of 79% (and a PV- of 84%), we can be confident that someone with a positive test is at risk for VFx. Similarly, with sensitivity of 79% (and a PV+ of 72%), if someone has a negative test, we can be fairly sure that person is really not at risk. The height loss test seems to be a reasonable procedure to identify both those with and without risk for VFx, helping us reasonably rule the risk in or out.

■ Pretest and Posttest Probabilities

The validity of a diagnostic test is based on how strongly it can support a decision to rule the disorder in or out. Therefore, a test is considered a good one if it can help to increase our certainty about a patient's diagnosis (see Box 33-1).

Pretest Probabilities

When we begin to evaluate a patient by taking a history and using screening or other subjective procedures, we begin to rule in and rule out certain conditions and eventually generate one or more hypotheses about the likely diagnosis. A hypothesis can be translated into a measure of probability or confidence, indicating the clinician's estimate of how likely a particular disorder is present. This has been termed the **pretest probability** or *prior probability* of the disorder—what we think might be the problem *before* we perform any formal testing.[13]

The concept of a pretest probability is related to differential diagnosis. Conceptually, it represents a "best guess" or clinical impression, which can be determined in different ways. Following initial examination, clinicians may exercise judgment based on experience with certain types of patients to estimate the probability of a diagnosis,[14] although such estimates are not always reliable.[15,16] In our example, for instance, a clinician who has a lot of experience with patients with vertebral fractures may be able to generate an initial hypothesis about a patient's condition just based on initial observation and complaints.

Information from the literature can also be used to help with this estimate by referring to prevalence of the disorder using population data. For instance, some studies have shown that the prevalence of vertebral fractures

| **SpPin** | With high **S**pecificity, a **P**ositive test rules **in** the diagnosis |
| **SnNout** | With high **S**e**n**sitivity, a **N**egative test rules **out** the diagnosis |

Figure 33–1 Mnemonics to remember the relationship of sensitivity and specificity for ruling in and ruling out a diagnosis based on a test result.

Box 33-1   Quantifying Uncertainty: Bayes' Theorem

In the late 1700s, a British mathematician and minister named Thomas Bayes (1701-1761) put forth a basic premise in *An Essay towards solving a Problem in the Doctrine of Chances.* His thesis was that by updating initial beliefs with objective new information, we get a new and improved belief. Over time, this idea has become a major strategy for solving crises of uncertainty, even breaking Germany's Enigma code during World War II, being used for DNA decoding, and in Homeland Security.[11] And of course, it has become a major premise for diagnosis and clinical decision-making.

Bayes' theorem (also called formula, law, or rule), describes the probability of an event based on prior knowledge of conditions related to the event. It is a way of looking at

probability theory—how we revise probabilities when we are presented with new information. It allows us to put a quantitative value on our uncertainty, estimating how much we should change our "belief" and how confident we should be in making that change.[12] The theorem has contributed to statistical inference and provides an essential philosophical foundation for evidence-based practice.

From Price R. An Essay towards solving a Problem in the Doctrine of Chances. By the Late Rev. Mr. Bayes, F. R. S. Communicated by Mr. Price, in a Letter to John Canton, A. M. F. R. S. *Philos Transactions (1683-1775)* 1763;53: 370-418.

---

among older women and men is about 20%.[16] It would be important to determine if the characteristics of the samples used in these studies were sufficiently similar to your patient's profile to make them applicable. Data from a study sample can also be used to indicate the prevalence within the accessible population.

> ➤ The height loss study demonstrated a 41% prevalence of vertebral fractures (*n*=62) in its sample of 151 patients.[3] Knowing this, before any further testing, our best estimate is that the pretest probability of a patient being at risk for VFx is 41%.

With no other information, this value gives us our best initial guess of likelihood that a patient could have this condition.

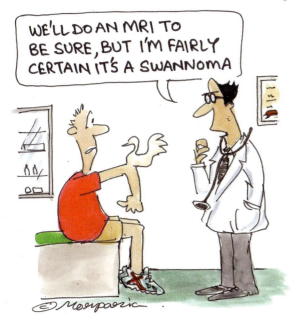

From Hemant Morparia.

Posttest Probabilities

A diagnostic test allows a clinician to revise the pretest probability estimate of the disorder, to be more confident in the diagnosis, to improve certainty. The revised likelihood of the diagnosis based on the outcome of a test is the **posttest probability**, or *posterior probability*— what we think the problem is (or is not) once we know the test result. A good test will allow us to have a high posttest probability, confirming the diagnosis, or a low posttest probability, causing us to abandon it.

Decision-Making Thresholds

Being able to estimate a pretest probability is central to deciding if a condition is present and if further testing or treatment is warranted. Based on the initial hypothesis and pretest probability of a condition, the clinician must decide if a diagnostic test is necessary or useful to confirm the actual diagnosis. Straus et al[11] suggest that two thresholds should be considered, as illustrated in Figure 33-2A. With a very low pretest probability, the diagnosis is so unlikely that testing is not useful—it will provide little additional information to improve certainty. Even with a positive test, results are likely to be false positives. Therefore, treatment should not be initiated and other diagnoses should be considered.

In contrast, with a very high pretest probability, the likelihood of the diagnosis is so strong that testing may be unnecessary for the same reason—results are unlikely to offer any additional useful information. Therefore, treatment should just be initiated without taking time for testing. Even with a negative test, results are likely to be false negatives. Perhaps more common, however, the pretest probability is not definitive, and testing is necessary to pursue the diagnosis.

This approach must also take into consideration other factors such as the relative severity of the disorder, the test's cost, or the discomfort or risk. Therefore, the

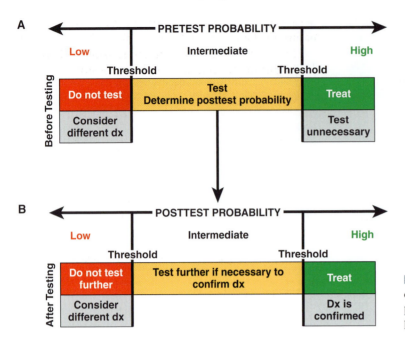

Figure 33–2 Thresholds for deciding to test or treat. **(A)** Thresholds based on pretest probabilities, **(B)** thresholds based on posttest probabilities.

threshold for testing may vary for different conditions. A test that requires a potentially harmful procedure may not be worthwhile if the condition has little consequence. However, when considering the possibility of a dangerous condition, the risk may be reasonable. For instance, lumbar puncture may be needed to rule out life-threatening conditions but may not be a first test to rule out less severe conditions. In contrast, a patient may exhibit symptoms that could mean the presence of a deep venous thrombosis (DVT), which is potentially life threatening. Even if the symptoms are minimal and the pretest probability is low, the clinician may feel compelled to test for the condition to safely rule it out before continuing with other tests or interventions.

> If sensitivity and specificity add up to 100%, (sensitivity = 1-specificity), the test will not contribute to a change in pretest to posttest probabilities. For a test to be useful, the difference between sensitivity and 1 − specificity (true positive rate − true negative rate) should be greater than zero, preferably at least 50%, and ideally 100%.[13]

Once a test is performed, we still face decision-making thresholds. With a high posttest probability, the diagnosis is confirmed, and treatment can be initiated with confidence. With a low posttest probability, a different diagnosis should be considered. When the posttest probability is not definitive, further testing may be necessary. In that case, the posttest probability associated with the first test becomes the pretest probability for the next test. In this way, sequential testing continues to refine the decision-making process.

Likelihood Ratios

Once we have established an initial hypothesis that the patient may have a particular diagnosis, we want to determine if a test can make us more confident in that diagnosis. A measure called the **likelihood ratio (LR)** tells us *how much more likely it is that a person has the diagnosis after the test is done*; that is, it will help us determine the posttest probability. We can determine a LR for a positive or negative test.

The LR indicates the value of the test for increasing certainty about a positive diagnosis, or its "confirming power."[18] Likelihood ratios are being reported more often in the literature as an important standard for evidence-based practice. The LR has an advantage over sensitivity, specificity, and predictive values because it is independent of disease prevalence and therefore can be applied across settings and patients.

Positive Likelihood Ratio

To understand this statistic, let us assume that a patient tests positive on the height loss test. If this were a perfect test, we would be certain that the patient has a VFx (true positive). But we hesitate to draw this conclusion definitively because we know that some patients who are not at risk will also test positive (false positive). Therefore, to determine if this test improves our diagnostic conclusion, we must correct the true positive rate by the false positive rate. This is our **positive likelihood ratio (LR+)**:

$$LR+ = \frac{\text{true positive rate}}{\text{false positive rate}} = \frac{\text{sensitivity}}{1 - \text{specificity}}$$

The LR+ will tell us how many times more likely a positive test will be seen in those with the disorder than in those without the disorder. *A good test will have a high positive likelihood ratio.*

Negative Likelihood Ratio

Now let's assume the patient has a negative test. With a perfect test we would be sure this patient did not have a fracture. But because we are concerned about the possibility of a false negative, we need to determine if a negative test improves our diagnostic conclusion by looking at the ratio of the false negative rate to the true negative rate. This is our **negative likelihood ratio (LR–)**:

$$LR- = \frac{\text{false positive rate}}{\text{true positive rate}} = \frac{1 - \text{sensitivity}}{\text{specificity}}$$

The LR– will tell us how many times more likely a negative test will be seen in those with the disorder than in those without the disorder. *A good test will have a low negative likelihood ratio.*

 Likelihood ratios *always refer to the likelihood of the disorder being present.*[19] That's why we would like to see a high LR+ to indicate that the disorder is likely to be present with a positive test. A very low LR– means that the disorder has a small probability of being present with a negative test.

Interpreting Likelihood Ratios

The value of the likelihood ratio is somewhat intuitive, in that a larger LR+ indicates a greater likelihood of the disease, and a smaller LR– indicates a smaller likelihood of the disease. These values have been interpreted according to the scale shown in Figure 33-3.[20] A LR+ over 5 and a LR– lower than .2 represent relatively important effects. Likelihood ratios between .2 to .5 and

between 2 to 5 may be important, depending on the nature of the diagnosis being studied. Values close to 1.0 represent unimportant effects. A likelihood ratio of 1.0 means the true-positive and false positive (or true-negative and false negative) rates are the same, making the results of the test useless.

> ▶ For the height loss data, the LR+ = 3.71. Therefore, with a positive test, the likelihood of a patient having a VFx is increased by almost four times. This represents a potentially important value. The LR– = .27, which represents a less important value. Based on these data, height loss should help to improve our confidence with a positive test.

 Going back to the concepts of **SpPin** and **SnNout**:[13]

- A large LR+ (>10) indicates that a positive test is good at ruling the disorder **IN**.
- A low LR– (<.01) indicates that a negative test is good at ruling the disorder **OUT**.
- A LR close to 1.0 does not contribute to the probability that a person has or does not have the disorder.

We can confirm these guidelines by looking at posttest probabilities.

A Nomogram to Determine Posttest Probabilities

A nomogram has been developed based on Bayes' theorem that can be used to determine posttest probabilities using pretest probabilities and likelihood ratios for positive and negative tests (see Fig. 33-4).[21] To use the nomogram, we start on the left by marking the pretest probability, based on the known prevalence of the condition. For our example, we will use the sample prevalence to get a pretest probability of 41%. The positive and negative likelihood ratios are identified on the center line. If we draw lines from the pretest probability through these points, extending them to the right margin, we can estimate the posttest probabilities associated with a positive and negative test. The posttest probability is about 72% for a positive test and 16% for a negative test.

Therefore, if we obtain a positive test we have substantially improved our confidence in the patient being at risk for VFx, going from 41% to 72%. If we obtain a

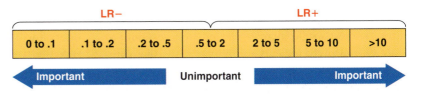

Figure 33–3 Scale for interpreting the relative importance of positive and negative likelihood ratios.

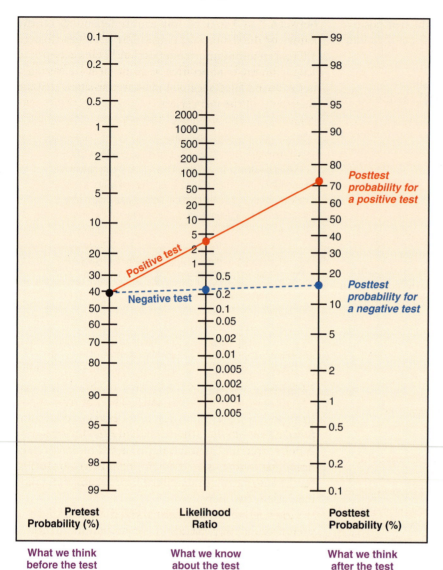

Figure 33–4 A nomogram used to determine the posttest probability for the VFx study, based on 41% pretest probability with LR+ = 3.71 and LR– = .27. The posttest probability for a positive test is 72%, and for a negative test 16%. Based on Fagan TJ. Letter: Nomogram for Bayes Theorem. *N Engl J Med* 1975;293(5):257.

negative test, however, there is only a 16% chance the patient has a VFx.

The posttest probability is dependent on the sensitivity and specificity of the diagnostic test (translated to a likelihood ratio) as well as the clinician's estimate of the pretest probability for an individual patient. Using the nomogram, for example, with a positive test for height loss, if we had started with a pretest probability of 20%, we would get a posttest probability of about 50% for a positive test. But if the pretest probability was only 5%, a positive test would increase our posttest certainty to only 15%. Where we start will influence the degree to which our certainty can be improved by the test. When greater precision is desired, posttest probabilities can be calculated using the pretest probability and likelihood ratios (see Box 33-2).

Confidence Intervals

Sensitivity, specificity, predictive values, and likelihood ratios are all point estimates, and should also be expressed in terms of confidence intervals (see Table 33-2C). Although these values are often not reported, they are important to understanding the true nature of these estimates. Given a sample of scores, the confidence interval will indicate the range within which we can be sure the true population value will fall. Although not interpreted in terms of significance testing, confidence intervals for these measures of diagnostic accuracy will

Posttest probabilities can be calculated directly by converting pretest probabilities to odds. For the vertebral fracture example, with prevalence of 41% and LR+ = 3.71, LR− = .27:

Step 1: Convert pretest probability (prevalence) to pretest odds:

$$Pretest\ odds = \frac{pretest\ probability}{1-pretest\ probability} = \frac{.41}{1-.41} = .695$$

Step 2: Multiply pretest odds by LR+ and LR− to get posttest odds:

$$Posttest\ odds = pretest\ odds \times LR$$
$$For\ positive\ test = .695 \times 3.71 = 2.578$$
$$For\ negative\ test = .695 \times .27 = .188$$

Step 3: Convert posttest odds to posttest probability:

$$Posttest\ probability = \frac{posttest\ odds}{posttest\ odds +1}$$
$$For\ positive\ test: = \frac{2.578}{3.578} = .721$$
$$For\ negative\ test: = \frac{.188}{1.188} = .158$$

Compare these values with the results estimated from the nomogram. The calculations will typically be more exact.

indicate the relative stability of the test's results; that is, with a wide confidence interval we would be less likely to consider the value a good estimate. The process for calculating confidence intervals for diagnostic tests is complex,[22] and more easily carried out by a confidence interval calculator.

See the *Chapter 33 Supplement* for a clean copy of the nomogram for your use and formulas for calculation of confidence intervals. Links are also provided for Web-based programs that provide interactive nomograms, as well as calculators for posttest probabilities, sample size, and confidence intervals for diagnostic tests.[9,23,24]

■ Receiver Operating Characteristic (ROC) Curves

Although continuous scales are considered preferable for screening because they are more precise, they are often converted to a dichotomous outcome for diagnostic purposes. This requires establishing a **cutoff score** to demarcate a positive or negative test. For example, in the VFx study, a height loss of more than 4 cm was considered indicative of vertebral fracture. However, if a cutoff

score of 3 cm was used, the sensitivity and specificity would be different, influencing posttest probabilities. The problem, then, is to determine what cutoff score should be used. This decision point must be based on the relative importance of and desired balance between sensitivity and specificity, or the cost of incorrect outcomes versus the benefits of correct outcomes.

In weighing sensitivity and specificity, consider this analogy: Although there may be costs associated with unnecessary preparations for a predicted storm that does not occur (*false positive*), these costs would probably be considered minor relative to the danger of failing to prepare for a storm that does occur (*false negative*). There are criteria, for instance, for a storm "warning" versus a storm "watch." The point at which the alert moves to the more severe warning would be the cutoff point. There will often be an inverse relationship between these estimates.

Cutoff Scores

Suppose we use the 4-cm height loss criterion to predict risk for vertebral fracture, and an individual with only 1 cm height loss is referred for an x-ray to determine if a fracture is present. If the individual is not truly at risk (false positive), the test may be considered low cost, compared to the situation where an individual who is at risk is not correctly diagnosed (false negative) and not referred for testing. Therefore, it might be reasonable to set the cutoff score low to avoid false negatives, thereby increasing sensitivity.

Conversely, consider a scenario where a test is used to determine the presence of a condition that requires potentially life-threatening surgery. A physician would want to avoid the procedure for a patient who does not truly have the condition. For that situation, the threshold might be set high to avoid false positives, increasing specificity. We would not want to perform this procedure unless we knew for certain that it was warranted.

Obviously, it is desirable for a screening test to be both sensitive and specific. Unfortunately, there is often a trade-off between these two characteristics. One way to evaluate this decision point would be to look at several cutoff points to determine the sensitivity and specificity at each point. We could then consider the relative trade-off to determine the most appropriate cutoff score based on the consequences of false negatives versus false positives. It is often necessary to combine the results of several tests to minimize the trade-off. The decision about the relative importance of false positives versus false negatives should be a collaborative one between clinician and patient (see Focus on Evidence 33-1).

Focus on Evidence 33–1
Moving the Goal Posts: Statistics Versus Meaningful Conversation

Prostate cancer is one of the most common forms of cancer in men, with estimates of 165.000 new cases and 29,000 deaths in 2018.[25] Tests of prostate-specific antigen (PSA) levels may indicate prostate cancer, with a traditional cutoff of 4.0 ng/mL.[26] At that level, sensitivity has been estimated at 21% and specificity at 91%.[27] These values suggest that a high PSA test can "rule in" cancer (SpPin), but with such low sensitivity, the test cannot rule it out (SnNout). Therefore, as a screening test, it is likely to result in many false positives, with many other factors that can also result in an elevated PSA count, including urinary tract infection, recent ejaculation, prostatitis, prostate enlargement, and changes occurring after age 40.[28] The estimated prevalence of prostate cancer is 25% for those with PSA between 4.0 and 10.0 ng/mL,[29] with a LR− of .87 and LR+ of 2.33. These ratios are relatively uninformative (in the "unimportant" range). This was confirmed in one study that analyzed results with different PSA cutoff points, resulting in an ROC curve with AUC of only .678.[30] The PV+ has been estimated at 30%, indicating that less than one in three men with an abnormal test will have cancer on biopsy.[31]

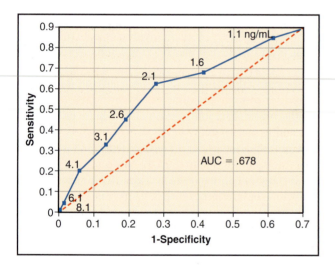

In 2008, the U.S. Preventive Services Task Force (USPSTF) issued guidelines that stated that there was insufficient evidence to make a recommendation on PSA-based screening, particularly in men younger than 75 years, but they did recommend against use of the test for men older than 75. Even though prevalence of prostate cancer is higher among older men, the slow progression of the disease indicates that testing is unlikely to affect mortality.

In 2012, based on results of a clinical trial, recommendations were revised, discouraging the use of PSA screening for all men, regardless of age, race, or family history, concluding that the benefits of such testing did not outweigh harms.[32,33] The harms stem from treatment or further testing following a false-positive test, including infection and hospitalization from prostate biopsy, surgery or radiation therapy causing bowel problems, urinary incontinence, or erectile dysfunction—all issues that can seriously impact quality of life.

In 2018, evidence was reexamined and recommendations were revised again. Now guidelines suggest that PSA testing could be selectively beneficial for men between 55-69 but still recommend against testing for men 70 years and older.[34] The recommendation for men aged 55 to 69 states that the decision to undergo screening should be an individual one in consultation between patient and healthcare provider, considering the risks, benefits, and personal preferences of the patient—which fits well with the concept of evidence-based practice.[35]

This story provides two significant and related lessons. The first is the important consideration of numbers as guidelines, not absolute values to dictate decisions. As with all research findings, clinicians must work with patients to interpret risks and benefits and account for their preferences, acknowledging that statistics have inherent uncertainty. And the second is the recognition that evidence isn't stagnant, and revisions are common as research studies are reexamined or new information becomes available. Bayes would be pleased that the system is able to reconsider findings, allowing new information to change recommendations!

Curve derived from data from Thompson JM, Ankerst DP, Chi C, et al. Operating characteristics of prostate-specific antigen in men with an initial PSA of 3.0 ng/mL or lower. *JAMA* 2005;294(1):66-70, from Table 3, p. 69.

The ROC Curve

The balance between sensitivity and specificity can be examined using a graphic representation called a **receiver operating characteristic (ROC) curve**—a way to examine the ratio of signal to noise.

Suppose we were listening to a radio station that has a weak signal. We turn the volume up so we can hear better, but as we do so, we not only pick up the desired signal but also background noise. Initially, the signal will increase faster than the noise, but there will come a point, as we increase volume,

that the noise will grow faster than the signal. If we set the volume to its maximum, we may claim that the signal is strong, but the noise will be so great that the signal will be indecipherable. Therefore, the optimal setting will be that point where we detect the largest ratio of signal to noise.

This is what we are trying to do with a diagnostic test. We want to detect the "signal" (the true positive and true negative) with the least amount of interference possible (false positive and false negative). The ROC curve diagrams this relationship. It allows us to answer the question: How well can a test discriminate between signal and noise—can it discriminate between the presence or absence of disease?

Coordinates of the ROC Curve

The process of constructing an ROC curve involves setting several cutoff points for a test and calculating sensitivity and specificity at each one. The curve is then created by plotting a point for each cutoff score that represents the proportion of patients correctly identified as having the condition on the Y axis (true positives or sensitivity) against the proportion of patients incorrectly identified as having the condition (false positives or 1– specificity) on the X axis.

To illustrate this process, consider again the example of vertebral fracture using a hypothetical dataset for the sample of 151 patients. Table 33-3A shows the distribution of scores for the patients who did and did not have a VFx, with height loss values from 1 cm to ≥ 6 cm.

Table 33-3B shows the sensitivity and specificity at six cutoff points based on the number of true-positive and true-negative scores. It is generally recommended that at least five to six points be used to plot an ROC curve. For example, if we use a cutoff score of 1 cm, then all those with a height loss of 1 cm or more will be identified as having a fracture. At that level, all those with a VFx have been correctly identified but all those without a VFx have been incorrectly identified. This cutoff point is so low that everyone meets it, leading to sensitivity of 1.0 but specificity of zero (and 1– specificity of 1.0).

Alternatively, using a cutoff of 6 cm, we have correctly identified all those who do not have a VFx but have missed all but 11 who do have a fracture. This leads to a corresponding sensitivity of .18 and specificity of 1.00, which results in 1– specificity of 0.00. Similarly, with a cutoff score of 3 cm, all those who had a height loss of less than 3 cm will be considered negative. Those with height loss ≥3 cm will be diagnosed positive. When this cutoff score is used, 53 individuals are correctly diagnosed and 26 are incorrectly diagnosed. This leads to a corresponding sensitivity of .86 and 1– specificity of .29.

These values are plotted to create the ROC curve (see Table 33-3 ❺). The curve is completed at the origin and the upper right hand corners, reflecting cutoff points above and below the highest and lowest scores.

Interpreting the ROC Curve

The ROC curve is plotted on a square with values of 1.0 for sensitivity and 1– specificity at the upper left and lower right corners, respectively. A perfect test instrument will have a true positive rate of 1.0 and a false positive rate of zero, resulting in a curve that essentially fills the square from the origin to the upper left corner to the upper right hand corner. A noninformative curve occurs when the true-positive and false-positive rates are equal, which means that the test provides no better information than 50:50 chance. Such a "curve" starts at the origin and moves diagonally to the upper right hand corner (shown as the broken line).

Area Under the Curve

If we want to get a sense of the quality of the ROC curve, we can look to see how closely it approximates the perfect curve. Although this provides a visual approximation, a quantitative standard is more definitive. The best index for this purpose is a measure of the **area under the curve (AUC)**. This value equals the probability of correctly choosing between normal and abnormal signals.

> ➤ As shown in Table 33-3 ❸, the AUC = .815 for the height loss data, which is generally considered a good curve. This means that presented with a randomly chosen pair of patients, one with VFx and one without, the clinician would correctly identify the patient with a VFx 82% of the time.

Therefore, the area represents the ability of the test to discriminate between those with and without the test condition. A perfect test has an AUC of 1.00—allowing 100% identification of individuals who have the disorder. The AUC can also be used to compare curves from two tests to determine which is a better diagnostic tool.

Choosing a Cutoff Point

In addition to making comparisons or describing the relative effectiveness of a test for identifying a disorder, we can also use the ROC curve to decide which cutoff point would be most useful. Most ROC curves have a steep initial section, which reflects a large increase in sensitivity with little change in the false positive rate. A relatively flat region across the top is also typical. Neither of these sections of the curve make sense for choosing a cutoff point, as they represent little change in one component of the curve.

The best cutoff point will typically be at the point where the curve turns.[36] This will be the point at which there is a maximal difference between the true positive rate and the false positive rate—the difference between sensitivity and 1– specificity, known as the *Youden index*.[37]

> ➤ Yoh et al[3] used the Youden index to determine the best cutoff point at ≥4.0 cm. In Table 33-3 ❺ we can see a marked turn at that point, suggesting that this cutoff would provide the best balance between sensitivity and specificity for this test (79% and 79%, respectively). At that point we would miss diagnosing a VFx for 13 out of 62 individuals with a fracture and would incorrectly diagnose 19 out of the 89 individuals without fracture.

A. Data

Height Loss	Known Group 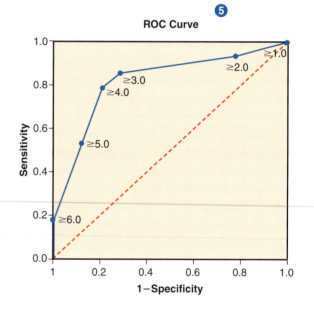	
	Fracture n = 62	No Fracture n = 89
1.0–1.9 cm	4	19
2.0–2.9 cm	5	44
3.0–3.9 cm	4	7
4.0–4.9 cm	17	8
5.0–5.9 cm	21	11
≥6.0 cm	11	0

B. Cutoff Points

Cutoff Point	True Positives	True Negatives	Coordinates of the ROC Curve ❷			Youden Index
			Sensitivity	Specificity	1−Specificity	
≥1.0 cm	62	0	1.00	0.00	1.00	0.0
≥2.0 cm	58	19	.94	.21	.79	.15
≥3.0 cm	53	63	.86	.71	.29	.57
≥4.0 cm	49	70	.79	.79	.21	.58
≥5.0 cm	32	78	.52	.88	.12	.40
≥6.0 cm	11	89	.18	1.00	0.00	.18

An Individual has a positive test if height loss is equal to or greater than the cutoff point.

C. SPSS Output: ROC Curve

Area Under the Curve

Test Result Variables(s): HL

❸ Area	Std. Error	Asymptotic Sig.	95% Confidence Interval	
			Lower Bound	Upper Bound
.815	.037	.000	.743	.888

The test result variable(s): HL has at least one tie between the positive actual state group and the negative actual state group. Statistics may be biased.

Coordinates of the Curve ❹

Test Result Variables(s): HL

Positive if Greater Than or Equal To[a]	Sensitivity	1−Specificity
.0000	1.000	1.000
1.5000	.935	.787
2.5000	.855	.292
3.5000	.790	.213
4.5000	.516	.124
5.5000	.177	.000
7.0000	.000	.000

The test result variable(s): HL has at least one tie between the positive actual state group and the negative actual state group.
a. The smallest cutoff value is the minimum observed test value minus 1, and the largest cutoff value is the maximum observed test value plus 1. All the other cutoff values are the averages of two consecutive ordered observed test values.

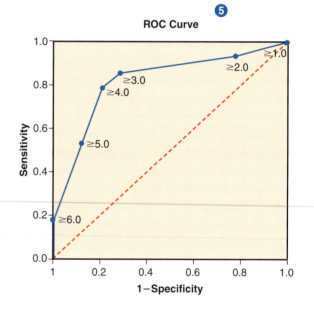

ROC Curve ❺

❶ Data show the amount of height loss experienced by patients with and without diagnosed fractures.

❷ The number of true positives and negatives at each cutoff point are shown, with the associated sensitivity, specificity, and 1−specificity values. Sensitivity is the true positive rate, and 1−specificity is the false positive rate. These provide coordinates for the ROC curve. The Youden Index is the difference between sensitivity and 1−specificity.

❸ The area under the curve is .815, which is significant ($p < .001$) with a narrow confidence interval. We are 95% confident that the true area under the curve will fall between 74% and 89%.

❹ The coordinates of the curve are listed, although SPSS calculates the cutoff values a little differently (see footnote). The values for sensitivity and 1-specificity may vary slightly from hand calculations shown in (B), but these will not change the overall shape of the curve.

❺ The ROC curve is presented, showing its relationship to the null curve at 50% (dashed line). The curve could be interpreted as turning at either ≥3 cm or ≥4.0 cm, depending on the relative importance of sensitivity and specificity. The study by Yoh et al[3] used the 4 cm cutoff point.

Portions of output have been omitted for clarity. Values may vary due to rounding.

The highest values for the Youden index are .58 for the cutoff at ≥4.0, and .57 at ≥3.0, suggesting that there is little difference between these points in terms of how they would contribute to determination of posttest probabilities. Therefore, we might also consider the turn of the curve at ≥3 cm to indicate a meaningful cutoff point. Using this criterion, we would have a higher sensitivity at 86% and slightly lower specificity at 71%. The final choice of a cutoff must be based on how the clinician and patient see the impact of an incorrect identification in a positive or negative direction. For instance, one might consider it more important to identify those with a potential VFx using a more sensitive test, as opposed to taking an x-ray of someone who is suspected of having a VFx and find out she does not. The ROC curve should act as a guide for that decision.

> ➤ **Results**
>
> In a sample of 151 postmenopausal women, radiographic diagnosis of VFx was present in 41% of the subjects. Using a cutoff value of ≥4 cm of height loss, sensitivity was 79% (95% CI: .69 to .88), specificity was 79% (95% CI: .70 to .87), PV+ was 72% (95% CI: .61 to .83), PV− was 84% (95% CI: .77 to .92), LR+ was 3.71 (95% CI: 2.44 to 5.63), and LR− was .27 (95% CI: .16 to .44). ROC curve analysis showed AUC = .815 (95% CI: .743 to .888). These values show that height loss of ≥4 cm is a good cutoff value for screening women for vertebral fracture.
>
> ---
>
> *Note: These values will often be presented in a table to avoid having to express this much data in a narrative form.*

> ✒ **HISTORICAL NOTE**
> The ROC curve has its roots in World War II, with tests of the ability of radar operators to determine whether a blip on a radar screen represented an object or noise.[38] Following the attack on Pearl Harbor, the U.S. Army began research to increase the accuracy of correctly detecting Japanese aircraft from radar signals. For this purpose, they measured the ability of radar receiver operators to make these important distinctions, which was called "receiver operating characteristics." This process later formed the basis for signal detection theory.

■ Clinical Prediction Rules

A **clinical prediction rule (CPR)** is a tool that quantifies the contributions of different variables to the diagnosis, prognosis, or likely response to treatment for an individual patient.[39] It may include information derived from the history, physical exam, lab tests, or patient complaints. These "rules" are intended to simplify and increase accuracy of diagnostic and prognostic assessments by demonstrating how specific clusters of clinical findings can be used to efficiently predict outcomes.[40,41]

> 📌 You may also see CPRs referred to as *clinical decision rules, clinical decision guidelines,* or *clinical prediction guides.* And of course, don't confuse this acronym with cardiopulmonary resuscitation!

Diagnosis

Perhaps the most obvious application of a CPR is to assist in the diagnosis of a disorder based on clinical signs.

> *Stiell et al[42] developed clinical prediction rules for the use of radiography with suspected acute ankle injuries. They noted that many patients with ankle injuries did not have a fracture, and yet the typical response to emergency care was to order an x-ray. Estimates had shown that the prevalence of fractures with ankle injuries was less than 15%.*

This study addressed an interest in efficiency and cost-savings as well as a desire for diagnostic accuracy. The prediction rules that were developed through this process have come to be known as the *Ottawa Ankle Rules (OARs)* (based on Stiell's affiliation with Ottawa Civic Hospital), which include rules for both ankle and midfoot injuries. The indicators for ruling out a fracture are based on a lack of tenderness in specific areas of the foot or ankle and the patient's ability to bear weight on the affected limb, even with a limp. Figure 33-5 shows these guidelines, which have been validated in different countries[43-47] in different populations,[48,49] and in various settings.[50,51]

Systematic reviews of the OARs have shown that they are 95% to 100% sensitive, with a negative likelihood ratio of .08.[52-54] If we apply the LR− to a pretest probability of 15% (prevalence estimate), the posttest probability is approximately 1.5%, indicating that a fracture is not likely (try it out on the nomogram).

Using the logic of SnNout, with a test that is highly sensitive, a negative test will effectively rule out the disorder. Therefore, a negative result using the OARs will consistently and accurately rule out fractures after ankle or foot injury, making an x-ray unnecessary. This rule has effectively and substantially reduced the number of radiographs taken.[55]

Reviews have also shown that the OARs have much lower specificity, ranging from 40% to 50%, translating to a positive likelihood ratio around 1.5. With low specificity, a positive test does not necessarily mean a fracture is present, requiring an x-ray to confirm a fracture. For example, a LR+ of 1.5 translates to about 20% posttest probability, barely different from the pretest probability.

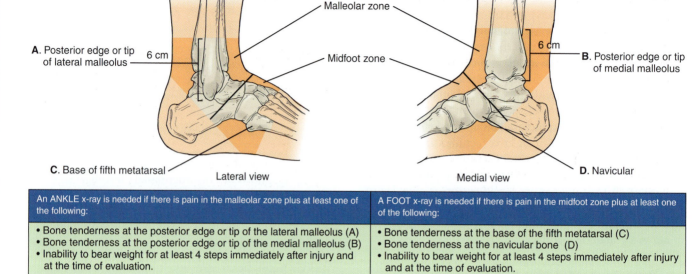

Figure 33–5 The Ottawa Ankle Rules. (*From Starkey, Examination of Orthopedic & Athletic Injuries 4th Ed., FA Davis, Philadelphia, 2015, with permission.*)

Other examples of diagnostic prediction rules include guidelines for detecting deep venous thrombosis,[56] pulmonary embolism,[57] coronary artery disease,[58] and sleep apnea.[59] Guidelines have also been developed for ordering x-rays for knee injuries, called the Ottawa Knee Rules,[60,61] and cervical spine injuries, called the Canadian C-Spine Rule.[62]

Prognosis

Clinical predication rules can also be established to determine the degree to which certain outcomes can be expected.

> *Dionne and colleagues[63] developed a CPR to predict the 2-year work disability status of people who were treated for back pain in primary care settings. Based on data from 337 patients, they derived a model based on seven predictors to identify those who did not return to work (failure is a positive test) versus those who could be expected to return to work (success is a negative test). Predictors included patient expectations, radiating pain, previous back surgery, pain intensity, changing position, irritable temper, and difficulty sleeping. They found 16.9% prevalence of an adverse outcome, with 57 patients failing to return to work, and 280 returning to work—indicating 79% sensitivity and 64% specificity.*

These data translated to a PV+ of 31% and a PV– of 94%. The high PV– indicates a high probability that a person who tests negative on the prediction rule is able to return to work. The authors suggest that although decision rules often focus on positive predictive values to confirm a diagnosis, the nature of the outcome must determine the more relevant measure of diagnostic validity. In this case, considering the frequency of back pain and the resources spent on its care even with benign cases, an instrument that allows identification of those at low risk of adverse outcome is quite useful.

Other examples of prognostic clinical prediction rules include identifying risk for functional decline in older community-dwelling women,[64] identifying patients at risk of complications following cardiac surgery,[65] and identifying factors that lead to hospitalization with asthma.[66]

Response to Intervention

Clinical prediction rules have also been developed to determine the likelihood that a patient will respond positively to a specific intervention.

> *Margolis et al[67] used a retrospective cohort design to develop a prediction model to determine in which patients' venous leg ulcers will heal within 24 weeks with standard limb compression bandages. Data confirmed a simple prognostic model including two variables: wound area >5 cm² (1 point) and duration > 6 months (1 point). A score of 0 (negative test) was predictive of healing with compression bandages. They validated the data in another sample, confirming these findings.*

Their data resulted in sensitivity of 65% and specificity of 91%, with PV+ = 59% and PV– = 93%. Therefore, healthcare providers can be reasonably certain that using compression bandages will be effective in patients with a score of 0. Patients with scores of 1 or 2 are less likely to heal and should be considered for other therapies. This model was supported through construction of a ROC curve with area under the curve of .87, indicating that the model correctly discriminated between ulcers that healed as compared to those that did not heal 87% of the time.

It is important to note that CPRs are often misunderstood in this context, as providing evidence of treatment effectiveness. Because there are no control subjects in a prediction rule study that did not receive the treatment, it is impossible to infer whether treatment was more or less effective than an alternative. For instance, in the leg ulcer study, all subjects got the compression bandages, and we can say that those with certain characteristics got better with that intervention. However, we cannot say what might have happened had they not received the intervention.

Other examples of CPRs for intervention response include identifying patients who will benefit from cervical manipulation for neck pain,[68] from spinal manipulation for low back pain,[69] from patellar taping for anterior knee pain,[70] and prediction of the need for hospitalization of children with acute asthma exacerbations using predictors available upon admission to the emergency department.[71]

Validating Clinical Prediction Rules

The development of a clinical prediction rule is a three-step process, involving creation of the rule, validation, and assessment of the impact on clinical practice.[40,72] Some studies may include all three steps, but most will be published separately.

Deriving the Model

First, the factors that potentially contribute to prediction of the outcome are identified in a cohort of patients. This allows for *derivation* of the rule, establishing which variables are most predictive. This requires identification of a set of predictors and the relevant outcome, specified as a reference standard for those with and without the condition of interest. Data collection may include questionnaires, interviews, or examination of medical records. The adequacy of a prediction rule is dependent on which variables are included in the derivation and how the outcome is assessed.

CPRs are usually analyzed using logistic regression, often with stepwise procedures to delimit the predictors to the smallest number that can most accurately predict the outcome. This was illustrated in the study of limb compression bandages, which started with a complex model including 10 variables, such as race, wound area, inability to walk one block, and other wound characteristics. The final equation needed only wound area and duration to create a strong prediction model.[67] The area under the ROC curve was 89% for the 10-item rule versus 87% for the 2-item model.

Validation of the Rule

The second step requires *validation* of the rule in several cohorts in different settings to demonstrate that the model continues to work for other individuals besides those used to derive it. This is an essential step to assure that chance was not a factor in the initial study and to verify that the study sample was not unique. This step may require several studies to fully assess how well the rule works in a variety of settings.

In the study of return to work status, Dionne et al[63] randomly divided their total sample into two subgroups, the first used to derive the model and the second to validate it. This is called a *split sample.* They found strong confirmation, noting that 37% of subjects were correctly classified in the initial sample and 40% in the validation sample.

This technique of using a split sample is useful for early validation, but further validation studies should be run on different samples taken from other settings with characteristics that are different from the original sample, as well as with other investigators. Unfortunately, many prediction rules are adopted without the benefit of this validation.

Impact Analysis

Finally, an *impact analysis* will demonstrate if the rule has changed clinician behavior and resulted in beneficial outcomes. A CPR is only effective if it is widely implemented, if it can be applied accurately, and if it can be shown to reduce costs or risk. The Ottawa Ankle Rules, for example, have been studied in many countries and settings, and with different populations, all reporting significant decreases in the number of unnecessary ankle radiographs.[47,73] Even with the widespread acceptance of this CPR, however, researchers and clinicians continue to test its validity, with varying degrees of success.[52]

Impact analyses are best performed using a randomized design, whereby patients are managed with usual care or the CPR. For example, the OARs have been tested against usual care and other prediction rules, consistently showing that the number of x-rays is reduced and that negative tests are accurate.[74-77]

Levels of Evidence for CPRs

McGinn et al[38] have proposed a hierarchy of evidence to judge the applicability of a clinical decision rule, based on its having gone through the full process of validation (see Fig. 33-6). Widespread use of a CPR is not recommended until it has been validated in at least one prospective study in a variety of settings, and an impact analysis has demonstrated its clinical utility.

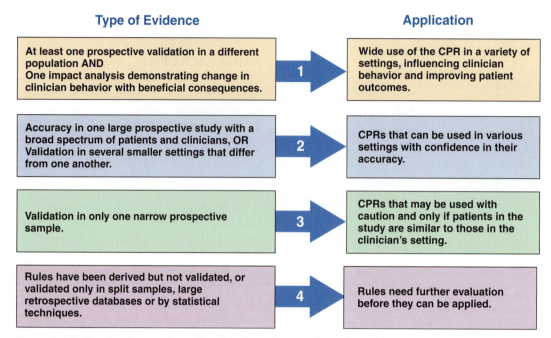

Type of Evidence		Application
At least one prospective validation in a different population AND One impact analysis demonstrating change in clinician behavior with beneficial consequences.	1	Wide use of the CPR in a variety of settings, influencing clinician behavior and improving patient outcomes.
Accuracy in one large prospective study with a broad spectrum of patients and clinicians, OR Validation in several smaller settings that differ from one another.	2	CPRs that can be used in various settings with confidence in their accuracy.
Validation in only one narrow prospective sample.	3	CPRs that may be used with caution and only if patients in the study are similar to those in the clinician's setting.
Rules have been derived but not validated, or validated only in split samples, large retrospective databases or by statistical techniques.	4	Rules need further evaluation before they can be applied.

Figure 33–6 Four levels of evidence for clinical prediction rules. Adapted from McGinn TG, Guyatt GH, Wyer PC, et al. User's guides to the medical literature: XXII: how to use articles about clinical decision rules. *JAMA* 2000;284:79-84, Table 1, p. 81.

COMMENTARY

Medicine is a science of uncertainty and an art of probability.

—*Sir William Osler (1849-1919)*

Canadian physician

Author of *The Principles and Practice of Medicine*, 1892

A diagnostic decision can be consequential, depending on the seriousness of the condition, as it will generally direct decisions regarding further management. If the diagnosis is incorrect (a false positive or false negative), then the intervention path (or lack of one) may be useless at best or harmful at worst. The cognitive process of clinical reasoning is not black and white, and how we proceed through it can be influenced by many factors.

Bayes' theorem suggests that we stay open to new information in decision-making but does not tell us how to revise our opinions, or how to reconcile quantitative findings with conflicting clinical intuition—emphasizing the need to improve our skills in critically appraising evidence.[14] Bordage[78] offers three types of potential diagnostic errors:

- *Data gathering errors* such as ineffective history taking (too little or too much information), missing symptoms, overreliance on someone else's history, or failure to validate findings with the patient

- *Data integration errors* such as failing to consider findings, faulty estimate of prevalence, misconceptions about causal factors, or over- or underestimating meaning of information.
- *Situational factors* such as not enough time to pursue needed information or consultation.

Elstein and Schwarz[14] also suggest that we are influenced by recalling recent diagnostic experiences, being overwhelmed by the complexity of a case, looking for more common conditions, and our own clinical experience. Data have also shown that the order in which we gather evidence can be a factor, as we tend to put more weight on more recent information.[79]

The use of evidence to improve diagnostic certainty is essential. At any point, we may seek new evidence, always recognizing that our current evidence may be insufficient or will be outdated in the future. Using evidence provides no guarantees—and diagnostic measures should not dictate decisions but only inform them.

REFERENCES

1. *Cambridge Dictionary.* Available at https://dictionary.cambridge. org/us/. Accessed August 5, 2019.

2. Schousboe JT. Epidemiology of vertebral fractures. *J Clin Densitom* 2016;19(1):8-22.

3. Yoh K, Kuwabara A, Tanaka K. Detective value of historical height loss and current height/knee height ratio for prevalent vertebral fracture in Japanese postmenopausal women. *J Bone Miner Metab* 2014;32(5):533-538.

4. Gatsonis C, Paliwal P. Meta-analysis of diagnostic and screening test accuracy evaluations: methodologic primer. *AJR Am J Roentgenol* 2006;187(2):271-281.

5. Deeks JJ. Systematic reviews in health care: Systematic reviews of evaluations of diagnostic and screening tests. *BMJ* 2001; 323(7305):157-162.

6. Tatsioni A, Zarin DA, Aronson N, Samson DJ, Flamm CR, Schmid C, Lau J. Challenges in systematic reviews of diagnostic technologies. *Ann Intern Med* 2005;142(12 Pt 2):1048-1055.

7. Bossuyt PM, Reitsma JB, Bruns DE, Gatsonis CA, Glasziou PP, Irwig LM, Lijmer JG, Moher D, Rennie D, de Vet HC. Towards complete and accurate reporting of studies of diagnostic accuracy: the STARD initiative. *BMJ* 2003;326(7379):41-44.

8. Siminoski K, Warshawski RS, Jen H, Lee K. The accuracy of historical height loss for the detection of vertebral fractures in postmenopausal women. *Osteoporos Int* 2006;17(2):290-296.

9. Centre for Clinical Research and Biostatistics (CCRB). C.I. Calculator: Diagnostic Statistics. Available at https://www2. ccrb.cuhk.edu.hk/stat/confidence%20interval/Diagnostic% 20Statistic.htm. Accessed February 20, 2019.

10. Straus SE, Glasziou P, Richardson WS, Haynes RB, Pattani R, Veroniki AA. *Evidence-Based Medicine: How to Practice and Teach EBM.* 5th ed. London: Elsevier; 2019.

11. Price R. An Essay towards solving a Problem in the Doctrine of Chances. By the Late Rev. Mr. Bayes, F. R. S. Communicated by Mr. Price, in a Letter to John Canton, A. M. F. R. S. *Philos Transactions (1683-1775)* 1763;53:370-418.

12. McGrayne SB. *The Theory That Would Not Die: How Bayes' Rule Cracked the Enigma Code, Hunted Down Russian Submarines & Emerged Triumphant from Two Centuries of Controversy.* New Haven, CT: Yale University Press; 2011.

13. Davidson M. The interpretation of diagnostic test: a primer for physiotherapists. *Aust J Physiother* 2002;48(3):227-232.

14. Elstein AS, Schwartz A. Clinical problem solving and diagnostic decision making: selective review of the cognitive literature. *BMJ* 2002;324(7339):729-732.

15. Cahan A, Gilon D, Manor O, Paltiel O. Clinical experience did not reduce the variance in physicians' estimates of pretest probability in a cross-sectional survey. *J Clin Epidemiol* 2005; 58(11):1211-1216.

16. Phelps MA, Levitt MA. Pretest probability estimates: a pitfall to the clinical utility of evidence-based medicine? *Acad Emerg Med* 2004;11(6):692-694.

17. Waterloo S, Ahmed LA, Center JR, Eisman JA, Morseth B, Nguyen ND, Nguyen T, Sogaard AJ, Emaus N. Prevalence of vertebral fractures in women and men in the population-based Tromsø Study. *BMC Musculoskelet Disord* 2012;13:3-3.

18. Van den Ende J, Moreira J, Basinga P, Bisoffi Z. The trouble with likelihood ratios. *Lancet* 2005;366(9485):548.

19. Attia J. Moving beyond sensitivity and specificity: using likelihood ratios to help interpret diagnostic tests. *Aust Prescr* 2003;26(3):111-13.

20. Geyman JP, Deyo RA, Ramsey SD. *Evidence-Based Clinical Practice: Concepts and Approaches.* Boston: Butterworth Heinemann; 2000.

21. Fagan TJ. Letter: Nomogram for Bayes theorem. *N Engl J Med* 1975;293(5):257.

22. Mercaldo ND, Lau KF, Zhou XH. Confidence intervals for predictive values with an emphasis to case-control studies. *Stat Med* 2007;26(10):2170-2183.

23. Center for Evidence Based Medicine. Likelihood Ratio nomogram. Available at http://www.cebm.net/shockwave/nomogram. html. Accessed February 20, 2019.

24. Schwartz A. Diagnostic Test Calculator. Available at http:// araw.mede.uic.edu/cgi-bin/testcalc.pl. Accessed February 20, 2019. (*Plots the nomogram from raw data.*)

25. Siegel RL, Miller KD, Jemal A. Cancer statistics, 2018. *CA Cancer J Clin* 2018;68(1):7-30.

26. Mettlin C, Lee F, Drago J, Murphy GP. The American Cancer Society National Prostate Cancer Detection Project. Findings on the detection of early prostate cancer in 2425 men. *Cancer* 1991;67(12):2949-2958.

27. Wolf AM, Wender RC, Etzioni RB, Thompson IM, D'Amico AV, Volk RJ, Brooks DD, Dash C, Guessous I, Andrews K, DeSantis C, Smith RA. American Cancer Society guideline for the early detection of prostate cancer: update 2010. *CA Cancer J Clin* 2010;60(2):70-98.

28. Carter HB. Prostate-specific antigen (PSA) screening for prostate cancer: Revisiting the evidence. *JAMA* 2018;319(18):1866-1868.

29. Hoffman RM, Clanon DL, Littenberg B, Frank JJ, Peirce JC. Using the free-to-total prostate-specific antigen ratio to detect prostate cancer in men with nonspecific elevations of prostate-specific antigen levels. *J Gen Intern Med* 2000;15(10):739-748.

30. Thompson IM, Ankerst DP, Chi C, Lucia MS, Goodman PJ, Crowley JJ, Parnes HL, Coltman CA, Jr. Operating characteristics of prostate-specific antigen in men with an initial PSA level of 3.0 ng/ml or lower. *JAMA* 2005;294(1):66-70.

31. Wilbur J. Prostate cancer screening: the continuing controversy. *Am Fam Physician* 2008;78(12):1377-1384.

32. Barocas DA, Mallin K, Graves AJ, Penson DF, Palis B, Winchester DP, Chang SS. Effect of the USPSTF Grade D recommendation against screening for prostate cancer on incident prostate cancer diagnoses in the United States. *J Urol* 2015;194(6):1587-1593.

33. Moyer VA. Screening for prostate cancer: U.S. Preventive Services Task Force recommendation statement. *Ann Intern Med* 2012;157(2):120-134.

34. US Preventive Services Task Force. Screening for prostate cancer: US Preventive Services Task Force recommendation statement [published online May 8, 2018]. *JAMA* doi:101001/ jama20183710.

35. US Preventive Services Task Force. Grade definitions, 2012. Available at https://www.uspreventiveservicestaskforce.org/ Page/Name/grade-definitions. Accessed June 20, 2017.

36. Centor RM. Signal detectability: the use of ROC curves and their analyses. *Med Decis Making* 1991;11(2):102-106.

37. Akobeng AK. Understanding diagnostic tests 3: Receiver operating characteristic curves. *Acta Paediatr* 2007;96(5):644-647.

38. Fan J, Upadhye S, Worster A. Understanding receiver operating characteristic (ROC) curves. *Cjem* 2006;8(1):19-20.

39. Laupacis A, Sekar N, Stiell IG. Clinical prediction rules. A review and suggested modifications of methodological standards. *JAMA* 1997;277(6):488-494.

40. McGinn TG, Guyatt GH, Wyer PC, Naylor CD, Stiell IG, Richardson WS. Users' guides to the medical literature: XXII: how to use articles about clinical decision rules. Evidence-Based Medicine Working Group. *JAMA* 2000;284(1):79-84.

41. Wasson JH, Sox HC, Neff RK, Goldman L. Clinical prediction rules. Applications and methodological standards. *N Engl J Med* 1985;313(13):793-799.

42. Stiell IG, McKnight RD, Greenberg GH, McDowell I, Nair RC, Wells GA, Johns C, Worthington JR. Implementation of the Ottawa ankle rules. *JAMA* 1994;271(11):827-832.

43. Emparanza JI, Aginaga JR. Validation of the Ottawa Knee Rules. *Ann Emerg Med* 2001;38(4):364-368.

44. Broomhead A, Stuart P. Validation of the Ottawa Ankle Rules in Australia. *Emerg Med (Fremantle)* 2003;15(2):126-132.

45. Yazdani S, Jahandideh H, Ghofrani H. Validation of the Ottawa Ankle Rules in Iran: A prospective survey. *BMC Emerg Med* 2006;6:3.

46. Meena S, Gangary SK. Validation of the Ottawa Ankle Rules in Indian scenario. *Arch Trauma Res* 2015;4(2):e20969.

47. Can U, Ruckert R, Held U, Buchmann P, Platz A, Bachmann LM. Safety and efficiency of the Ottawa Ankle Rule in a Swiss population with ankle sprains. *Swiss Med Wkly* 2008;138 (19-20):292-296.

48. Leisey J. Prospective validation of the Ottawa Ankle Rules in a deployed military population. *Mil Med* 2004;169(10):804-806.

49. Gravel J, Hedrei P, Grimard G, Gouin S. Prospective validation and head-to-head comparison of 3 ankle rules in a pediatric population. *Ann Emerg Med* 2009;54(4):534-540.e1.

50. Stiell IG, Bennett C. Implementation of clinical decision rules in the emergency department. *Acad Emerg Med* 2007; 14(11):955-959.

51. McBride KL. Validation of the Ottawa Ankle Rules. Experience at a community hospital. *Can Fam Physician* 1997;43:459-465.

52. Bachmann LM, Kolb E, Koller MT, Steurer J, ter Riet G. Accuracy of Ottawa Ankle Rules to exclude fractures of the ankle and mid-foot: Systematic review. *BMJ* 2003;326(7386):417.

53. Beckenkamp PR, Lin CC, Macaskill P, Michaleff ZA, Maher CG, Moseley AM. Diagnostic accuracy of the Ottawa Ankle and Midfoot Rules: a systematic review with meta-analysis. *Br J Sports Med* 2017;51(6):504-510.

54. Jenkin M, Sitler MR, Kelly JD. Clinical usefulness of the Ottawa Ankle Rules for detecting fractures of the ankle and midfoot. *J Athl Train* 2010;45(5):480-82.

55. Gwilym SE, Aslam N, Ribbans WJ, Holloway V. The impact of implementing the Ottawa Ankle Rules on ankle radiography requests in A&E. *Int J Clin Pract* 2003;57(7):625-627.

56. Goodacre S, Sutton AJ, Sampson FC. Meta-analysis: The value of clinical assessment in the diagnosis of deep venous thrombosis. *Ann Intern Med* 2005;143(2):129-139.

57. Righini M, Bounameaux H. External validation and comparison of recently described prediction rules for suspected pulmonary embolism. *Curr Opin Pulm Med* 2004;10(5):345-349.

58. Genders TS, Steyerberg EW, Alkadhi H, Leschka S, Desbiolles L, Nieman K, et al. A clinical prediction rule for the diagnosis of coronary artery disease: Validation, updating, and extension. *Eur Heart J* 2011;32(11):1316-1330.

59. Miranda Serrano E, Lopez-Picado A, Etxagibel A, Casi A, Cancelo K, Aguirregomoscorta JI, et al. Derivation and validation of a clinical prediction rule for sleep apnoea syndrome for use in primary care. *BJGP Open* 2018;2(2):bjgpopen18X101481.

60. Stiell IG, Greenberg GH, Wells GA, McDowell I, Cwinn AA, Smith NA, Cacciotti TF, Sivilotti ML. Prospective validation of a decision rule for the use of radiography in acute knee injuries. *JAMA* 1996;275(8):611-5.

61. Stiell IG, Wells GA, Hoag RH, Sivilotti ML, Cacciotti TF, Verbeek PR, Greenway KT, McDowell I, Cwinn AA, Greenberg GH, Nichol G, Michael JA. Implementation of the Ottawa Knee Rule for the use of radiography in acute knee injuries. *JAMA* 1997;278(23):2075-9.

62 Stiell IG, Wells GA, Vandemheen KL, Clement CM, Lesiuk H, De Maio VJ, Laupacis A, Schull M, McKnight RD, Verbeek R, Brison R, Cass D, Dreyer J, Eisenhauer MA, Greenberg GH, MacPhail I, Morrison L, Reardon M, Worthington J. The Canadian C-spine rule for radiography in alert and stable trauma patients. *JAMA* 2001;286(15):1841-8.

63. Dionne CE, Bourbonnais R, Fremont P, Rossignol M, Stock SR, Larocque I. A clinical return-to-work rule for patients with back pain. *CMAJ* 2005;172(12):1559-1567.

64. Sarkisian CA, Liu H, Gutierrez PR, Seeley DG, Cummings SR, Mangione CM. Modifiable risk factors predict functional decline among older women: a prospectively validated clinical prediction tool. The Study of Osteoporotic Fractures Research Group. *J Am Geriatr Soc* 2000;48(2):170-178.

65. Fortescue EB, Kahn K, Bates DW. Prediction rules for complications in coronary bypass surgery: a comparison and methodological critique. *Med Care* 2000;38(8):820-835.

66. Schatz M, Cook EF, Joshua A, Petitti D. Risk factors for asthma hospitalizations in a managed care organization: development of a clinical prediction rule. *Am J Manag Care* 2003;9(8):538-547.

67. Margolis DJ, Berlin JA, Strom BL. Which venous leg ulcers will heal with limb compression bandages? *Am J Med* 2000; 109(1):15-19.

68. Tseng YL, Wang WT, Chen WY, Hou TJ, Chen TC, Lieu FK. Predictors for the immediate responders to cervical manipulation in patients with neck pain. *Man Ther* 2006; 11(4):306-315.

69. Fritz JM, Childs JD, Flynn TW. Pragmatic application of a clinical prediction rule in primary care to identify patients with low back pain with a good prognosis following a brief spinal manipulation intervention. *BMC Fam Pract* 2005;6(1):29.

70. Lesher JD, Sutlive TG, Miller GA, Chine NJ, Garber MB, Wainner RS. Development of a clinical prediction rule for classifying patients with patellofemoral pain syndrome who respond to patellar taping. *J Orthop Sports Phys Ther* 2006; 36(11):854-866.

71. Arnold DH, Gebretsadik T, Moons KG, Harrell FE, Hartert TV. Development and internal validation of a pediatric acute asthma prediction rule for hospitalization. *J Allergy Clin Immunol Pract* 2015;3(2):228-235.

72. Childs JD, Cleland JA. Development and application of clinical prediction rules to improve decision making in physical therapist practice. *Phys Ther* 2006;86(1):122-131.

73. Nugent PJ. Ottawa Ankle Rules accurately assess injuries and reduce reliance on radiographs. *J Fam Pract* 2004;53(10): 785-788.

74. Derksen RJ, Knijnenberg LM, Fransen G, Breederveld RS, Heymans MW, Schipper IB. Diagnostic performance of the Bernese versus Ottawa Ankle Rules: Results of a randomised controlled trial. *Injury* 2015;46(8):1645-1649.

75. Ho JK, Chau JP, Chan JT, Yau CH. Nurse-initiated radiographic-test protocol for ankle injuries: A randomized controlled trial. *Int Emerg Nurs* 2018;41:1-6.

76. Auleley GR, Ravaud P, Giraudeau B, Kerboull L, Nizard R, Massin P, Garreau de Loubresse C, Vallee C, Durieux P. Implementation of the Ottawa Ankle Rules in France. A multicenter randomized controlled trial. *JAMA* 1997; 277(24):1935-1939.

77. Tajmir S, Raja AS, Ip IK, Andruchow J, Silveira P, Smith S, Khorasani R. Impact of clinical decision support on radiography for acute ankle injuries: randomized trial. *West J Emerg Med* 2017;18(3):487-495.

78. Bordage G. Why did I miss the diagnosis? Some cognitive explanations and educational implications. *Acad Med* 1999; 74(10 Suppl):S138-143.

79. Bergus GR, Chapman GB, Gjerde C, Elstein AS. Clinical reasoning about new symptoms despite preexisting disease: sources of error and order effects. *Fam Med* 1995;27(5): 314-320.

Epidemiology: Measuring Risk

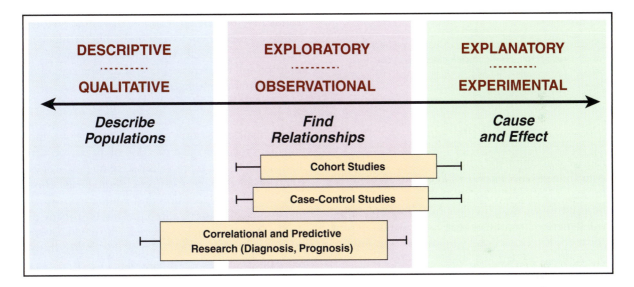

An important perspective in healthcare research is based on principles of **epidemiology**, which focus on the distribution and determinants of health outcomes in different populations. This information can be used to understand patterns of disease in different groups, to evaluate causative and preventive factors, and to understand the effectiveness of health policy and resource allocation. Research findings can have direct influence on decision-making related to diagnosis, prognosis, or intervention. Epidemiology involves descriptive and analytic approaches, which are appropriate for both observational and experimental designs (see Chapters 16 and 19). The purpose of this chapter is to present statistical methods for measures of disease frequency, estimates of health risks for cohort and case-control studies, and the evaluation of treatment effects in randomized trials.

■ The Scope of Epidemiology

Epidemiology literally began as the study of "epidemics," concerned primarily with mortality and morbidity from acute infectious diseases. Many of the health standards we take for granted today, such as clean water supplies, treatment of sewage, and food refrigeration, can be credited to discoveries made through epidemiological investigations. Epidemiologists try to identify those who have a specific disorder, when and where the disorder developed, and what exposures are associated with its presence. Epidemiologic questions often arise out of clinical experience, laboratory findings, or public health concerns about the relationship between societal practices and disease outcomes. Through the analysis of health status indicators and population characteristics, epidemiologists try to identify and explain the causal factors in disease patterns.

As medical cures and treatments have been developed to control many of these problems, and as patterns of disease have changed, the scope of epidemiology has broadened. Today clinical epidemiology includes the study of chronic disease, disability, and health status. This approach fits with the World Health Organization's definition of health which encompasses social, psychological and physical well-being.[1]

> The terms *disease, disorder,* and *disability* will be used interchangeably to represent health outcomes, recognizing the variety of conditions of interest, including illness, injury, and physical, psychological, or social dysfunction.

■ Descriptive Epidemiology

Descriptive epidemiologic studies are done when little is known about the occurrence or determinant of health conditions. They will often provide information that can be used to set priorities for healthcare planning and will generate hypotheses that can be studied using analytic methods. Descriptive studies may be presented as case reports, correlational studies, or cross-sectional surveys.

Person, Place, and Time

The purpose of descriptive epidemiologic studies is to describe patterns of health, disease, and disability in terms of person, place, and time.

WHO Experiences this Disorder?
Relevant characteristics might include age, sex, religion, race, cultural background, education, socioeconomic status, occupation, and so on. This is the *demography* of the disorder. Epidemiologists try to determine if individuals with certain characteristics are more at risk for a particular disorder than others. For example, researchers have studied the increasing prevalence of type 2 diabetes in adolescents,[2] the incidence of incontinence in women over age 45,[3] and more recently the outbreak of measles among school-aged children.[4]

WHERE is the Frequency of Disorder Highest or Lowest?
Epidemiologists are concerned with identifying restricted areas within a city or large geographic areas in which disease or exposures are commonly found. They

look at environmental factors such as weather, local industry, water and food sources, and lifestyle as potential causative factors. For instance, the early studies in AIDS documented high incidence in San Francisco and New York.[5] Legionnaire's disease[6] and severe acute respiratory syndrome (SARS)[7] are other examples of diseases that had specific geographic origins (See Box 34-1).

WHEN does the Disorder Occur Most or Least Frequently?
The epidemiologist will compare the present frequency of a disorder with that of different time periods. When the frequency of occurrence varies significantly at one point in time, some specific time-related causative factor is sought. Seasonal variations may become obvious, or trends may be related to other historical factors. For example, researchers have found a higher incidence of hip fractures in elderly individuals during winter months[8] and an increased rate of hospitalization due to adult asthma symptoms in spring months.[9]

Disease Frequency

The statistical measures used to describe epidemiologic outcomes focus on quantification of disease occurrence. The simplest measure of disease frequency would be a count of the number of affected individuals. However, meaningful interpretation and comparisons of such a measure would also require knowing how many people there were in the total population who could have gotten the disease and the length of time over which the occurrence of the disease was monitored. Therefore, measures of disease frequency will always include reference to population size and time period of observation.

For example, we might document 35 cases of a disease within 1 year in a population of 3,200 people, or 35/3,200/year. Typically, population size is expressed in terms of thousands, such as 1,000 (10^3), 10,000 (10^4), and 100,000 (10^5). For instance, the preceding values could be expressed as 109.4 cases per 10,000 per year. To make estimates more useful, such rates are usually calculated in whole numbers, such as 1,094/100,000/year.

The number of cases of a disease that exist in a population reflects the risk of disease for that group. It describes the relative importance of the disease and can provide a basis for comparison with other groups who may have different exposure histories. The two most common measures of disease frequency are prevalence and incidence.

Prevalence
Prevalence is a proportion reflecting the number of *existing* cases of a disorder relative to the total population at a given point in time. It provides an estimate of the probability that an individual will have a particular disorder at

Box 34-1   The London Cholera Epidemic of 1854

The pioneering work of John Snow, a London physician in the mid-18th century, serves as the classic example of descriptive epidemiology. The era saw a cholera pandemic that caused many deaths in Europe, rivaling the plague. Following an epidemic in London in the late 1840's, Snow argued that an infectious microbe was the causal factor, not an airborne gas as most believed. Because vomiting and diarrhea were the primary symptoms of the disease, he reasoned that cholera was a pathology of the gastrointestinal tract, suggesting that something had to be ingested.[10] His hypothesis was not well accepted, however, and it was actually not until 1883 that the cholera organism was finally accepted as the causative agent.

Snow noted that between 1849 and 1853, the incidence of cholera had lessened, and that during this interval an important change had taken place in the water supply of several districts in south London, which was serviced by two companies. The *Lambeth Company* had noted that water from the Thames River had become polluted and in 1852 moved their waterworks upriver where the water was cleaner, thereby "obtaining a supply of water quite free from the sewage of London."[11] These districts were also supplied by the *Southwark and Vauxhall Company*, which continued to draw its water from the London section of the river which was just downstream from a sewer outlet.

In the summer of 1854 cholera reappeared in London. Snow recognized the potential for a "Grand Experiment" that involved thousands of people "of both sexes, of every age and occupation, and of every rank and station…" who were naturally divided into two groups, based on the origin of their water supply.[11] Through meticulous investigation over 7 weeks, Snow's data showed that mortality was much higher for homes supplied by the contaminated *Southwark and Vauxhall Company*.

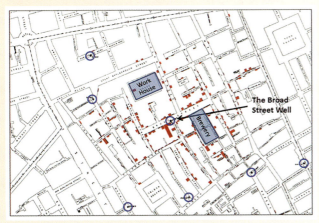

Adapted from Peter Gleick via ScienceBlogs.com.

Snow's most important investigation, however, occurred later in the summer in the Soho section of London, where a devastating outbreak of cholera killed almost 600 people within a few days at the end of August, 1854. Through door-to-door interviews, he noted that many of the deaths occurred in homes near the intersection of Broad Street and Cambridge Street, which was the location of the Broad Street water pump—supplied by *Southwark and Vauxhall*. He also found that in a workhouse on an adjacent street, surrounded by houses in which deaths had occurred, only five cholera deaths were seen among 535 inmates. It turned out that the workhouse had its own well. Snow also visited a brewery on Broad Street and found that no deaths had occurred. The owner said the men never drank water—only beer! Snow also found that individuals who had visited the Broad Street area and others who had purposely obtained water from that pump had died.

In his detailed map, Snow indicated each death by a bar at each address (in red), clearly demonstrating how the deaths clustered around the Broad Street pump. On September 7, 1854, Snow convinced the Board of Guardians of his hypothesis, and on the next day the pump handle was removed. The epidemic ended almost immediately (although it must also be noted that by then most of the residents had left the area). An investigation of the pump revealed that its well was about 28 feet deep, and that a sewer flowed within yards of the well at 22 feet down.[12]

What is most noteworthy about this history is the manner in which John Snow mounted his investigations. Brody et al[10] point out the significance of the fact that Snow did not use his map to generate his hypothesis. Rather, he developed his hypothesis from his observations and then gathered data and anecdotal information that provided cumulative evidence to support his theory that the contaminated water was the problem. The map only illustrated his data. What is all the more remarkable is that Snow formed his conclusions nearly 30 years before Louis Pasteur's work with germ theory. He called the agents that caused diseases like cholera "special animal poisons," and understood that even if scientists were unable to identify the "thing" that caused cholera, they could still have enough information to prevent further spreading of the disease.[13] These lessons were the foundation for contemporary geographic investigations into disease patterns.

---

that time. *Prevalent cases* are all persons with a particular health outcome within a specified time period, regardless of when they developed or were diagnosed with the disorder. Prevalence (P) is calculated as

$$P = \frac{\text{number of existing cases at a given point}}{\text{total population at risk}}$$

We know that obesity has become a national concern. The 2000 National Health Interview Survey data showed that the number of adults with self-reported obesity was 7,058 out of a sample of 32,375.[14]

The prevalence of obesity in this population is 7,058/32,375 = .22, or 22%. Because this value reflects the cross-sectional status of the population at a single point in time, it is also called *point prevalence*.

Period prevalence can be established for a specified period in time. For example, data obtained from a random sample of 973 newspaper employees found that the number of individuals categorized as having upper limb musculoskeletal complaints after one year was 395.[15] Therefore, this estimate, combining existing with new cases of musculoskeletal complaints during the period of 1 year, is 41%.

> 📌 Prevalence was also discussed in Chapter 33 in reference to establishing estimates of pretest probability for diagnostic testing.

Prevalence is most useful as an indicator for planning health services, because it reflects the impact of a disease on the population. Therefore, a measure of prevalence can be used to project requirements such as healthcare personnel, community services, specialized medical equipment, or number of hospital beds. Prevalence should not, however, be used as a basis for examining etiology of a disease because it is influenced by the length of survival of those with the disorder; that is, prevalence is a function of both the number of individuals who develop the disease and the duration or severity of the illness. Because this estimate looks at the total number of individuals who have the disease at a given time, that number will be large if the disease tends to be of long duration.

Incidence

The measure of **incidence** quantifies the number of *new* cases of a disorder or disease in the population during a specified time period and, therefore, represents an estimate of the risk of developing the disease during that time. Incidence discounts the effect of duration of illness that is present in prevalence measures. By examining incidence rates for subgroups of the population, such as age groups, ethnic groups, and geographic locations, the researcher can identify those groups that demonstrate higher disease rates and target them to investigate specific exposures. Incidence can be expressed as cumulative incidence or incidence rate.

Cumulative incidence (CI) quantifies the number of individuals who develop a disorder during a specified time period in a population that is at risk for the health outcome:

$$CI = \frac{\text{number of new cases at a given time}}{\text{total population at risk}}$$

> *Burdorf et al[16] studied the onset of low back pain in 196 novice golfers. In their initial assessment, they found that 80 subjects (41% of the sample) had experienced back pain before the study or at the time of entry (these were prevalent cases). They followed the sample over a 1-year period, and identified 16 new cases.*

Therefore, the 1-year cumulative incidence of first-time back pain for this cohort was 16/196 = .08, or 8%. The specification of the time period of observation is essential to the interpretation of this value. The number of cases would be perceived differently if subjects were followed for 1 or 10 years. Other issues that require consideration in interpreting a measure of cumulative incidence include the possibility that the number of individuals at risk in the cohort will vary over time and the possibility that the condition under study is caused by other, competing risks.

Person-Time

Measuring the total population at risk for cumulative incidence assumes that all subjects were followed for the entire observation period. However, some individuals in the population may enter the study at different times, some may drop out, and others who acquire the disease are no longer at risk. Therefore, the length of the follow-up period is not uniform for all participants. To account for these differences, *incidence rate* (IR) can be calculated:

$$IR = \frac{\text{number of new cases during a given period}}{\text{total person-time}}$$

As in cumulative incidence, the numerator for this estimate represents the number of new cases of the disorder. However, the denominator is the sum of the time periods of observation for all individuals in the population at risk during the study time frame, or **person-time**.

> *In the 1976 Nurses' Health Study, 121,700 female nurses were enrolled. During the period of 1976 to 1992, investigators identified 3,603 new cases of breast cancer.[17] Of the women originally enrolled, some left the study as a result of death or loss to follow-up at various times during the period, and some developed breast cancer after different amounts of time, contributing different amounts of time to the denominator.*

In other words, a woman who died in 1977 would have contributed 1 person-year to the denominator, whereas two women who developed breast cancer in 1990 would have contributed a total of 28 person-years to the denominator. Researchers totaled the amount of time each subject was *known to be at risk* between 1976 and 1992, and obtained the total *person-years* observed, in this case 1,794,565 person-years of observation. The incidence rate was, therefore, 3,606/1,794,565 = .002 or 2 cases per 1,000 person-years (2×10^{-3} years). Incidence rate is often a more efficient measure than cumulative incidence, as it allows for inclusion of all subjects, regardless of the amount of time they were able to participate. Cumulative incidence would only account for those subjects who were available for the entire study period.

The Relationship Between Prevalence and Incidence

The relationship between prevalence and incidence is a function of the average duration of the outcome of interest. If the incidence of the disorder is low (few new cases occur), but the duration of the disorder is long, then the prevalence or proportion of the population that has the disease at a given point in time may be large. If, however, incidence is high (many new cases of the disease occur), but the disorder is manifest for a short duration (either by quick recovery or death), the prevalence may be low. For example, a chronic disease such as arthritis may have a low incidence but high prevalence. A short-duration condition like a common cold may have a high incidence but low prevalence, because lots of people get colds but few actually have colds at any one point in time.

Vital Statistics

Epidemiologists often use incidence measures to describe the health status of populations in terms of birth and death rates that inform us about the consequences of disease. The *birth rate* is obtained by dividing the number of live births during the year by the total population at midyear. The *mortality rate* quantifies the incidence of death in a population by dividing the number of deaths during a specific time period by the total population at the midpoint of the time period. These data are generally available through records of state vital statistics reports, census data, and birth and death certificates.

When a rate is a summary value for a total population it is considered a *crude* rate. For instance, a crude mortality rate can reflect total mortality for the population from all causes of death, obtained by dividing the total number of deaths during the year by the average midyear population. This value is usually expressed as the number of deaths per 100,000 population. However, when different categories within the population differentially contribute to this rate, it may be more meaningful to look at category-specific rates. A *cause-specific rate* looks only at the number of deaths from a particular disease or condition within a year divided by the average midyear population. For instance, rates may reflect

mortality specifically resulting from diseases such as cancer and heart disease or from motor vehicle accidents. The *case-fatality rate* is the number of deaths from a disease relative to the number of individuals who had the disease during a given time period.

Other commonly used categories are age, sex, and race. *Age-specific rates* are probably most common because of the differential effect of many diseases across the life span. For example, if one looks at the death rate for cancer across age groups, we would find that mortality was higher for older age categories. Therefore, it may be more meaningful to present age-specific mortality rates for each decade of life, rather than a crude mortality rate. However, this results in a long list of rates that may not be useful for certain comparisons. An overall rate would be more practical, but it would have to account for the variation in rates across age categories. For instance, if we compare the crude cancer mortality rate for today versus the crude rate from 50 years ago, we would have to account for the fact that a larger proportion of the total population now falls in the older age range. Therefore, epidemiologists will often report *age-adjusted mortality rates* that reflect different weightings for the uneven categories. Methods for calculating adjusted rates are described in most epidemiology texts.

■ Analytic Epidemiology: Measures of Risk

Analytic epidemiology is concerned with testing hypotheses. Measures of association are typically derived for case-control and cohort studies to assess the relationship between specific **exposures** and health outcomes (see Chapter 19). These tests will establish if an association exists and the strength of that association. If an association does exist, we say that the specific exposure represents a **risk factor** for the outcome.

The focus on exposures takes a broad view that reflects contemporary concerns including lifestyle practices such as smoking, substance abuse, drinking alcohol or coffee, and eating foods high in cholesterol or salt; occupational hazards, such as repetitive tasks or heavy lifting; environmental influences, such as second-hand smoke, toxic waste, and sunlight; and specific interventions, such as exercise, medications, or other treatment modalities. These exposures may increase or decrease the likelihood of developing certain disorders or influence the ultimate outcome of a disorder.

This is a fundamental process in the determination of prognosis, as we attempt to predict outcomes based on patient characteristics. As with all measures of association, risk does not necessarily mean that the exposure causes the outcome. Criteria for evaluating causation were described in Chapter 19.

Relative vs Absolute Effects

Analyses of association are based on a measure of effect that looks at the frequency of disease among those who were and were not exposed to the risk factor. A *relative effect* is a ratio that describes the risks associated with the exposed group as compared to those who were not exposed. An *absolute effect* is the actual difference between the rate of disease in the exposed and unexposed groups, or the difference in the risk of developing the disease between these two groups. To illustrate the concepts of relative and absolute effect, suppose we purchased two books, one costing $3 and the other $6. The absolute difference is $3, whereas the relative difference is that the second book is twice as expensive as the first. If two other books cost $10 and $20, the absolute difference would be $10, but the relative difference would also be twice the cost of the first book. Therefore, the relative effect is based on the absolute effect, but takes into account the baseline value. Analogously, we can use measures of incidence of disease in exposed and unexposed groups to determine both relative and absolute effects of particular exposures.

Relative Risk

To analyze risk, data are typically organized in a 2×2 contingency table, a format that should be familiar by now (see Table 34-1). The columns represent the classification of disorder status (the outcome), and the rows represent exposure status. For consistency in presentation and calculation, the cells in the table are designated *a*, *b*, *c*, and *d*, as shown. Therefore, cell *a* represents those who have the disorder and were exposed, cell *b* represents those who do not have the disorder and were exposed, and so on. The marginal totals are the number of individuals who were exposed ($a + b$) and not exposed

($c + d$), and the number of individuals who have the disorder ($a + c$) and do not have the disorder ($b + d$). The sum of all four cells is the total sample size (N).

The incidence of a health outcome represents its **absolute risk (AR)**, which can be calculated for the exposed (AR_E) and unexposed (AR_0) groups. The AR_E is the number of cases of the disorder among the total exposed sample, or $a/(a+b)$. The AR_0 is the number of cases of the disorder among the total unexposed sample, or $c/(c+d)$. Each of these estimates reflects the probability of the health outcome for the exposed or unexposed groups.

Although these measures are informative, it is usually more relevant to ask how many times more likely are exposed persons to develop the disorder, relative to those who were not exposed. **Relative risk (RR)** (also called *risk ratio*) is the ratio of these two probabilities:

$$RR = \frac{AR_E}{AR_0} = \frac{a/(a+b)}{c/(c+d)}$$

This value indicates the likelihood that someone who has been exposed to a risk factor will develop the disorder, as compared with one who has not been exposed. Measures of relative risk are appropriate for use with cohort or experimental studies.

If the incidence rates of the outcome are the same for the exposed and unexposed groups, the RR is 1.0, indicating that risk is the same for exposed and unexposed persons. This represents the null value for relative risk. A RR greater than 1.0 indicates that exposed persons have a greater risk of developing the health outcome than unexposed. A RR less than 1.0 means that the exposure decreases the risk of developing the disorder.

 The calculation for relative risk is based on the assumption that all subjects in the cohort were followed for the same amount of time. When follow-up time differs, it is the person-time for exposed and nonexposed groups that should be used for marginal totals, rather than just the total number of subjects in each category.

▶ CASE IN POINT #1

Many studies have shown an inverse relationship between physical activity and risk of hip fracture. Hoidrup et al[18] used a cohort design to test the hypothesis that leisure physical activity would decrease the risk of hip fracture in community-dwelling adults. Data were taken from longitudinal studies over 6 birth cohorts.

For this example, we will consider a hypothetical subsample of 130 women (see Table 34–2). The research

Table 34-1   Summary of Diagnostic Test Results

		Disorder		
		Yes	**No**	**Total**
Exposure	**Yes**	*a*	*b*	*a+b*
	No	*c*	*d*	*c+d*
	Total	*a+c*	*b+d*	*N*

Table 34-2   Relative Risk: Physical Activity and Risk of Hip Fracture (*N* = 130)

A. Crosstabulation

Activity level * Hip Fx Crosstabulation ①

Count		Hip Fx Yes	Hip Fx No	Total
Activity level	> 2hr/wk	48	50	98
	Sedentary ①	20	12	32
Total		68	62	130

②

$$RR = \frac{a/(a+b)}{c/(c+d)} = \frac{48/98}{20/32} = 0.78$$

B. SPSS Output: Relative Risk and Chi-Square

Risk Estimate

	Value	95% CI Lower	95% CI Upper
Odds Ratio for Activity level (>2hr/wk / Sedentary) ④	.576	.254	1.305
For cohort Hip Fx = Yes ②	.784	.560	③ 1.097
For cohort Hip Fx = No ④	1.361	.836	2.215
N of Valid Cases	130		

Chi-Square Tests ⑤

	Value	df	Sig. (2-sided)
Chi-Square	1.768ᵃ	1	.184
N of Valid Cases	130		

a. 0 cells (0.0%) have expected count less than 5. The minimum expected count is 15.26.

① The crosstabulation shows the relationship between activity level (exposure) and hip fracture (disorder).

② The relative risk is calculated for the risk of hip fracture, with the presence of hip fracture as the reference value (Hip Fx = Yes). Therefore, with >2hr/wk of physical activity, the risk of hip fracture is reduced (less than 1.0).

③ The confidence interval for RR contains the null value 1.0.

④ These two values are ignored. SPSS automatically generates the OR, which is not relevant for a cohort study. The cohort value of RR will depend on which of the outcomes is considered the reference. If Hip Fx = No was the reference, the columns in the contingency table would be reversed.

⑤ The chi-square test indicates there is no significant difference (*p* = .184) between observed frequencies and what would be expected by chance.

Portions of the output have been omitted for clarity.

Data source: Høidrup S, Sørensen T, Strøger U, et al. Leisure-time physical activity levels and changes in relation to risk of hip fracture in men and women. *Am J Epidemiol* 2001; 154:60-68.

question is: Does physical activity reduce the risk of hip fracture in elderly women? Physical activity is the exposure (2hr/week compared to sedentary), and the occurrence of hip fracture is the health outcome.

Our first step is to determine the proportion of patients who exercised (the exposed group) who also sustained a hip fracture. This is the AR_E of hip fracture among exercisers, 48 out of 98, or 49%. Then we determine what proportion of sedentary patients (the unexposed group) sustained a hip fracture. This is the AR_0 of hip fracture for those who did not exercise, 20 out of 32, or 63%. Therefore, the RR = .78 for the hip fracture

study (see Table 34-2 ②). Because the RR is less than 1.0, physical activity would be considered a preventive factor, decreasing the risk of hip fracture compared to individuals who do not exercise. Those who were active at least 2 hours/week were .78 times as likely (~25% less likely) to suffer a hip fracture as compared with those who were sedentary.

Confidence Intervals for Relative Risk

An important assumption in any research study is that we can draw reasonable inferences about population characteristics based on sample data. This assumption holds true for epidemiologic studies as well. When a risk estimate is derived from a particular set of subjects, the researcher will use that estimate to make generalizations about expected behaviors or outcomes in others who have similar exposure histories. Therefore, it is important to determine a measure of true effect using a confidence interval. For the hip fracture study, 95% CI: .56 to 1.097 (Table 34-2 ❸). This interval contains the null value of 1.0 and therefore does not represent a significant risk estimate.

Chi-square can be used as a test of significance, to determine if the proportions differ across categories in a crosstabulation (see Chapter 28). In this example, the value of chi-square results in $p = .184$ (see Table 34-2 ❺), which is not significant. This confirms the conclusion drawn from the confidence interval. Chi-square tells us that the proportion of individuals with and without hip fracture who did or did not exercise was not different from what would be expected by chance.

> **➤ Results**
> Relative risk of hip fracture associated with physical activity was 0.78 (95% CI: 0.560 to 1.097). Although the RR shows a reduced risk for hip fracture with physical activity, this value is not significant ($\chi^2(1) = 1.768$, $p = .184$).

Odds Ratio

A case-control study differs from a cohort study in that subjects are purposefully chosen based on the presence or absence of disease (cases or controls) and therefore, we cannot determine the incidence rate of the disorder. Relative risk cannot be established because we cannot calculate absolute risk. The relative risk can be estimated, however, using an **odds ratio (OR)**, which is calculated using the formula

$$OR = \frac{a/c}{b/d} = \frac{ad}{bc}$$

The odds ratio is interpreted in the same way as relative risk, with a null value of 1.0.

> **➤ CASE IN POINT #2**
> Plantar fasciitis is a localized inflammatory condition leading to heel pain. Riddle et al[19] conducted a case-control study to identify risk factors for the disorder, including body mass index (BMI). The researchers assembled a sample of 50 cases and 100 controls, with a 1:2 match on age and gender. Among the cases, 29 individuals had a BMI over 30 (considered obese); among the controls, 17 subjects had a BMI over 30.

Table 34-3 shows the distribution of scores for subjects with lower and high BMI (exposure) and those with and without plantar fasciitis (outcome), with a crude odds ratio of 6.74. This means that the odds of developing plantar fasciitis are almost 7 times as much for those who are obese than for those who are not. The confidence interval has a wide range, but does not contain the null value, and therefore this estimate is significant, confirmed with a chi-square analysis ($p < .001$).

📌 Please refer to Chapter 31 for a full explanation of the concept of odds and the derivation of odds ratios. Adjusted odds ratios can be generated as part of logistic regression analysis to account for the effect of multiple exposures on an outcome.

> **➤ Results**
> The odds ratio for the relationship between plantar fasciitis and BMI was 6.74 (95% CI: 3.13 to 14.51), which was significant $p < .001$. Those with BMI above 30 were almost 7 times more likely to develop plantar fasciitis than those with BMI ≤30.

Power and Sample Size

Like other statistics, RR and OR are subject to Type I and Type II errors. To determine adequate sample size in planning, RR and OR are considered the effect size. Consider, for example, the study of physical activity and hip fracture (see Table 34-2), which resulted in RR = .78 ($p = .184$). It would be of interest to determine if this result could be an issue of a small sample. To solve for sample size, we must estimate RR or OR and the expected proportion of exposure among cases and controls. Rather than being concerned about power, for this analysis we must specify the degree of *precision* we want in our estimate. For instance, we could specify that we would like our results to be within 10% or 20% of the true risk. The greater the precision (lower percentage), the larger the needed sample size will be.

 Estimating sample size for RR and OR requires working with proportions. See the *Chapter 34 Supplement* for illustration of these analyses for relative risk and odds ratios.

Effect Modification and Confounding

Quite often, in the analysis of the association between a risk factor and exposure, clinicians recognize the potential influence of one or more extraneous factors that may obscure the association. In some cases, these extraneous variables provide important information to understand how the association varies across different

Table 34-3   Odds Ratio: Body Mass Index and Plantar Fasciitis (*N*=150)

A. Crosstabulation

BMI * Plantar fasciitis Crosstabulation

Count		Plantar fasciitis		
		Yes	No	Total
BMI	> 30	29	17	46
	<=30	21	83	104
Total		50	100	150

$$OR = \frac{ad}{bc} = \frac{(29)(83)}{(21)(17)} = 6.74$$ ❷

B. SPSS Output: Odds Ratio and Chi-Square

Risk Estimate

	Value	95% CI	
		Lower	Upper
Odds Ratio for BMI (>30 / <=30)	❷ 6.742	3.132	❸ 14.512
For cohort Plantar fasciitis = Yes ❺	3.122	2.008	4.855
For cohort Plantar fasciitis = No	.463	.314	.684
N of Valid Cases	150		

Chi-Square Tests ❹

	Value	df	Sig. (2-sided)
Chi-Square	26.353[a]	1	.000
N of Valid Cases	150		

a. 0 cells (0.0%) have expected count less than 5. The minimum expected count is 15.33.

❶ The crosstabulation shows the relationship between BMI (exposure) and plantar fasciitis (disorder).

❷ The odds ratio is calculated for the risk of plantar fasciitis, with the presence of plantar fasciitis as the reference value. Therefore, with BMI >30, the risk of plantar fasciitis is increased 6.74 times.

❸ The confidence interval for OR does not contain 1.0.

❹ The chi-square test indicates there is a significant effect (*p* <.000).

❺ SPSS automatically generates relative risk, which can be ignored for a case-control study.

Portions of the output have been omitted for clarity.

Data source: Riddle DL, Pulisic M, Pidcoe P, Johnson RE. Risk factors for plantar fasciitis: a matched case-control study. *J Bone Joint Surg Am* 2003; 85A: 872-7.

---

subgroups, such as age or gender. In other situations, such variables create a bias in the interpretation, interfering with the true association being studied. These two complications of analysis are called effect modification and confounding.

The simplest type of analyses are based on *crude* data. These are data concerning the exposure and outcome status of all subjects regardless of any other risks or characteristics. Although analyses based on crude data are often reported in the literature, many studies require more complicated analyses to evaluate the role

of other factors in the relationship of exposure and outcome. These analyses are accomplished through stratification or multivariate methods such as logistic regression, to provide *adjusted* measures of association (see Chapter 31).

Effect Modification

Effect modification refers to a difference in the magnitude of an effect measure across levels of another variable. An effect modifier will change the relative risk associated with the exposure for different subgroups in the population. Researchers study and report effect modification by stratifying the sample to explain why the subgroups respond differently. An effect modifier will interact with the exposure and disease variables in such a way as to present a constant effect. It is a natural phenomenon that exists independent of the study design and will always be a factor in interpretation of risk. Effect modifiers tend to be biologically related to the variables being studied.

> ### ➤ CASE IN POINT #3
> Researchers have studied the association between diabetes and risk of endometrial cancer, with many conflicting results. Friberg et al[20] hypothesized that this relationship could be misunderstood because of major modifiers such as physical activity. They studied a cohort of over 36,000 women over 7 years and stratified the sample by high or low physical activity.

Data for this study are shown in Table 34-4, showing how the distributions varied across strata.

> ➤ For the total sample, RR = 2.37, indicating that those with diabetes had more than two times the risk of cancer compared to those without diabetes. However, for those who were physically active, RR = 1.06, indicating that those with diabetes had no increased risk as compared to those without diabetes who were active. For those with low activity, the RR = 2.67. The risk associated with endometrial cancer increased by more than two times for those who had diabetes who did not exercise.

The fact that the risk estimates are different for each stratum indicates that the association between diabetes and endometrial cancer is significantly modified by physical activity.

Confounding

Confounding variables can be thought of as nuisance variables. They may or may not be present, depending on the source population and how subjects are chosen. Measures of association must be interpreted in terms of the potential for confounding effects of extraneous variables in the design. Confounding is introduced when extraneous variables interfere with the observed association between the exposure and outcome.

A *confounder* is a variable that is (1) associated with the exposure, (2) is a risk factor for the disease independent of the exposure, and (3) is not part of the causal link between the exposure and the disease. When confounding is present, the statistical outcome may not be documenting the true causal factor. A commonly used method to adjust for a potential confounder is stratification in which the comparison between exposure and disease is done at specific levels of the potential confounder. When a study mentions that they controlled for a factor in the analysis, they have tried to remove the effect of that variable (see Focus on Evidence 34-1).

> ### ➤ CASE IN POINT #4
> Jackson and coworkers[24] examined the association between risk of mortality and receiving influenza vaccine in elders over 65 year. They studied 252 cases who died during an influenza season and 576 age-matched controls. The crude odds ratio was .76 (95% CI: .47 to 1.06), indicating that receiving the vaccine decreased the risk of death.

The confidence interval for the odds ratio contains 1.0, indicating that the difference in mortality between those who do and do not get the vaccine is not significant. The researchers were interested, however, in the potentially confounding effect of limited functional status, which would be associated with not getting the vaccine, would be a risk factor for mortality, and is not a causal link between the vaccine and mortality. Because older individuals who have functional limitations would be less likely to visit a clinic to get the vaccine, and mortality is also related to functional decline, the crude odds ratio may be an underestimate of the protective nature of the vaccine on mortality.

> ➤ When rates were adjusted for the effect of functional limitations, the odds ratio was lowered to .59 (95% CI: .41 to .83), and was now significant.

If there was no discrepancy between the crude and adjusted estimates, there would be no confounding. The degree of discrepancy is indicative of the extent to which function confounded the original data. By eliminating the effect of functional status, a stronger and significant relationship was seen between getting the vaccine and decreased mortality.

Table 34-4	Association of Diabetes and Endometrial Cancer Stratified by Physical Activity		
		N	**RR(95% CI)**
Total	No diabetes	203	2.37
	Diabetes	22	(1.51 -3.74)
High Physical Activity	No diabetes	103	1.06
	Diabetes	5	(.43-2.60)
Low Physical Activity	No diabetes	100	2.67
	Diabetes	17	(1.58-4.53)

Data source: Friberg E, Mantzoros CS, Wolk A. Diabetes and risk of endometrial cancer: a population-based prospective cohort study. *Cancer Epidemiol Biomarkers Prev* 2007;16(2):276-280.

Focus on Evidence 34–1
Confounding and Simpson's Paradox

Because confounding is a common problem, understanding its potential for influencing interpretation of data is important, especially when looking for causal explanations. An extreme form of confounding occurs when results for subgroups are the opposite of the crude result—a phenomenon popularly known as *Simpson's Paradox*.[21,22]

To illustrate this problem, Charig et al[23] conducted a study to evaluate the success rates of different treatments for kidney stones. They studied 700 patients with kidney stones and classified them according to stones being <2 cm or ≥2 cm. Two treatment approaches were used based on clinical evaluation: open surgical procedures (SURG) and percutaneous nephrolithotomy (PN). Success was defined as no stones at 3 months or stones reduced to particles <2 mm in size. In comparing success rates, here is what they found:

Combined Sample			
	Successful	Not Successful	Success Rate
SURG	273	77	273/350 = 78%
PN	289	6	289/350 = 83%

Small Stones (<2 cm)			
	Successful	Not Successful	Success Rate
SURG	81	6	81/87 = 93%
PN	234	36	234/270 = 87%

Large Stones (≥2 cm)			
	Successful	Not Successful	Success Rate
SURG	192	71	192/263 = 73%
PN	55	25	55/80 = 69%

If we look at the data for the total sample, we would conclude that PN is the more effective treatment (83% vs. 78% success). However, if we look separately at the data for patients with small or large stones, we can see that the SURG procedures had a higher success rate in both instances.

How does this paradoxical result happen? The confounding variable in this case relates to how the decision to use one treatment or the other is determined. Open SURG procedures were generally used for stones > 2 cm, whereas the closed procedures (PN) were performed for smaller stones. The combined data ignores the fact that success is influenced by stone size more strongly than by treatment.

Charig et al[23] did not do statistical analyses to determine if the values within the contingency tables represented significant effects, but if you are so inclined, you can calculate chi-square—you will find that no significant effects exist. Simpson's paradox has nothing to do with the significance of these findings, but it illustrates how numbers can be misleading without considering confounding variables.

Data from Charig CR, Webb DR, Payne SR, Wickham JEA. Comparison of treatment of renal calculi by open surgery, percutaneous nephrolithotomy, and extracorporeal shockwave lithotripsy. *BMJ* 1986;292(6524):879-882

To evaluate the effect of confounding in an analysis, the researcher must collect information on the potentially confounding variable. If the investigators in the vaccine study did not collect data on the subjects' functional status, the preceding analysis would not have been possible. Therefore, the researcher must be able to predict what variables are possible confounders. It is conceivable that several confounding factors will be operating in one study. Age and gender are often considered potential confounders because of their common association with disease or disability as well as being related to the presence of many exposures. In addition to controlling for confounding in the analysis, researchers can use design strategies, such as matching or homogeneous subjects, to control for these effects.

Researchers attempt to cancel the effect of a confounding variable in the design or analysis of a study. In contrast, effect modifiers are studied so they can be reported. Data are stratified to evaluate and *remove* confounders. They are stratified to *explain* effect modification. Researchers must consider the potential influence of confounding and effect modification in all analyses and account for them in the design or analysis of data as much as possible.

■ Analytic Epidemiology: Measures of Treatment Effect

When making clinical decisions regarding the effectiveness of interventions, we will generally be concerned with three questions: (1) Does the treatment work? (2) If it works, how does it compare with other treatments? (3) Is the treatment safe? We want to know if the treatment will improve the patient's condition, or we may want to know if it will prevent or decrease the risk of an adverse event.

Randomized controlled trials (RCT) are the most effective approach for answering these questions. For many research questions, measurements of a dependent variable are taken before and after an intervention, and the degree of change is subjected to a statistical test to determine if there is a significant difference. This often becomes the basis for deciding whether to use the intervention. Such a conclusion is limited, however, because it does not tell us if the difference is clinically important, nor does it help us estimate the likelihood that our own patient will respond favorably. We know that even with a well-established intervention, patients do not all respond the same way, so how can we weigh the risks and benefits for a particular patient?

We can consider the outcome of treatment in terms of an "event," which is classified as a success or failure. The success of a treatment may be indicated by whether an *adverse event* is prevented, or if there is a beneficial outcome based on a specific threshold. In an RCT, then, the success of the intervention is determined by the difference in beneficial or adverse outcomes between treatment and control groups. The concept of relative risk (RR) can be used here in reference to treatment effect (the exposure), indicating if the risk of a particular outcome for the control group is higher or lower than for the treatment group.

> ### ▶ CASE IN POINT #5
>
> Headaches arising from cervical musculoskeletal disorders are common. Jull et al[25] designed a multicenter RCT that studied the effectiveness of a combination of exercise and manipulative therapy for reducing cervicogenic headaches, as compared to a control group that received no therapy. A primary outcome was the frequency of headaches over a 7-week treatment period.

By setting a threshold that identifies a successful or unsuccessful outcome, we can appreciate the effect of treatment based on clinically important change. In this study, the authors set a standard of less than 50% reduction in headache frequency as a benchmark for "failure" of treatment, or an adverse event. If the reduction in recurrence of headache was greater than 50%, it was considered a success.

Table 34-5A shows results for the comparison of combined manipulative therapy and exercise with the control group. We can see that of the 49 patients who received the experimental intervention, 9 had recurring headaches (<50% reduction). Of the 48 patients in the control group, 34 had recurring headaches.

Event Rates

We can examine differences between group responses in terms of "event rates," or the proportion of subjects in the experimental and control groups that achieved an adverse outcome. We calculate two values:

- The **experimental event rate (EER)**, which is the proportion of people in the treatment group who experienced the adverse outcome, $a/(a+b)$.

- The **control event rate (CER)**, which is the proportion of people in the control group who experienced the adverse outcome, $c/(c+d)$.

The calculations of these values are shown in Table 34-5B. For this study, the EER is 18% and the CER is 71%. These values indicate the risk of headaches recurring for each group. But how do they compare?

The ratio of these two values is the **relative risk (RR)** associated with the intervention:

$$RR = \frac{EER}{CER} = \frac{.18}{.71} = .25$$

> ▶ The RR associated with the exercise and manipulative therapy is .25. This means that the intervention group was only one-quarter as likely (75% less likely) to experience a recurrence of headache as the control group.

> 📌 EER and CER are actually the same as the estimate of absolute risk and incidence, described earlier in defining RR. The term "event rate" is used in the context of a clinical trial, where the outcome is a comparison of proportions for those who experience the adverse event in treatment and control groups. When the outcome is continuous, as in the frequency of headaches, it must be converted to a dichotomous outcome to determine when an event has or has not occurred.

Risk Reduction

This effect can be understood as a relative value that reflects how much the risk of an adverse event is reduced in the treatment group compared with the control group, called **relative risk reduction (RRR)**. The RRR is the difference in event rates between the two study groups, expressed as a proportion of the event rate in the untreated group:

$$RRR = \frac{CER - EER}{CER} = \frac{.71 - .18}{.71} = .75$$

This value is also equal to 1 − RR (1 − .25). This estimate is a measure of efficacy of the intervention and can provide information to assess clinical significance of findings.

> ▶ RRR = .75 for the headache study. This tells us that the chance of developing a headache is reduced by 75% in the intervention group as compared to the control.

As we have discussed before, the disadvantage of a relative value is that it does not tell us anything about the actual size of the effect. Figure 34-1 illustrates this

| **Table 34-5** | **Measures of Treatment Effect: RCT Comparing Exercise and Manipulative Therapy for Cervicogenic Headaches With a Control Condition ($N = 97$)** |

A. Data

	Treatment Outcome		
	FAILURE <50% reduction in headaches	SUCCESS ≥50% reduction in headaches	Total
Manipulation + Exercise	9	40	49 *a + b*
Control	34	14	83 *c + d*
Total	43 *a + c*	54 *b + d*	97

B. RISK MEASURES

Experimental Event Rate (EER)	EER = *a/a + b* ❶	EER = 9/49 = .18
Control Event Rate (CER)	CER = *c/c + d* ❶	CER = 34/48 = .71
Relative Risk (RR)	RR = EER/CER	RR = .18/.71 = .25
Relative Risk Reduction (RRR)	RRR = (CER − EER)/CER	RRR = .53/.71 = .75
Absolute Risk Reduction (ARR)	ARR = CER-EER	ARR = .71 − .18 = .53
Number Needed to Treat (NNT)	NNT = 1/ARR	NNT = 1/.53 = 1.9

C. CONFIDENCE INTERVALS FOR ARR AND NNT

$$95\% \text{ CI} = \text{ARR} \pm 1.96 \text{ (SE)}$$

$$SE = \sqrt{\frac{EER(1 - EER)}{n_{exp}} + \frac{CER(1 - CER)}{n_{control}}} = \sqrt{\frac{.18(1 - .18)}{49} + \frac{.71(1 - .71)}{48}} = .085$$

❷ **For ARR:** 95% CI = .53 ± 1.96 (.085) = .53 ± 1.67   95% CI = .363 to .697

For NNT: 95% CI = $\frac{1}{.697}$ to $\frac{1}{.363}$ 95% CI = 1.43 to 2.75

---

❶ The EER is the proportion of treated people who had the adverse outcome (absolute risk for the experimental group). The CER is the proportion of the control group who had the adverse outcome (absolute risk for the control group). The calculation of CER and EER will depend on which column is designated as the adverse event.

❷ Confidence intervals for NNT are based on the inverse of values used to get the CI for ARR. Calculation of NNH is based on absolute risk increase (ARI) which equals EER − CER. Calculations proceed in the same way as NNT.

Data source: Jull G, Trott P, Potter H, et al. A randomized controlled trial of exercise and manipulative therapy for cervicogenic headache. *Spine* 2002;27 (17):1835-184

---

limitation. Study A represents the headache study. Study B is a hypothetical study with different results, where the EER was 8% and the CER was 2%. These effects are substantially lower than in study A and may not be clinically meaningful, and yet the RRR would also be .75. Importantly, then, a high value for RRR may or may not indicate a large treatment effect.

A more clinically useful measure is the **absolute risk reduction (ARR)**, which indicates the actual difference in

event rate between the control and experimental groups, simply calculated by:

$$\text{ARR} = \text{CER} - \text{EER} = .71 - .18 = .53$$

For the headache study, there is a 53% reduction in event rate associated with the intervention. For study B, we can see that there is only a 6% reduction. Therefore, the ARR is a better reflection of the true difference in the studies' outcomes, or the magnitude of the treatment effectiveness.

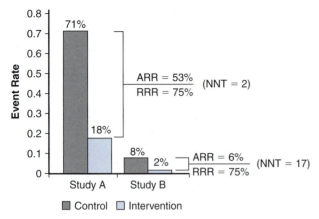

Figure 34–1 Results from two studies of treatment for cervicogenic headache, illustrating the important difference in absolute and relative risk measures. Bars represent the event rates for the intervention and control groups, indicating the number of patients who did NOT benefit from treatment. Both studies show a reduced risk with intervention. Although the relative risk reduction (RRR) is the same for both studies, the absolute risk reduction (ARR) and number needed to treat (NNT) are substantially different. Data source for Study A: Jull G, Trott P, Potter H, et al. A randomized controlled trial of exercise and manipulative therapy for cervicogenic headache. *Spine* 2002;27(17):1835-1843.

This example illustrates the importance of considering baseline risk when interpreting risk reduction.[26] The control event rate can be used as an estimate of the risk for all subjects at the start of the study, before intervention is applied. Although an RRR of 75% would be considered impressive, we can see that this value is not meaningful when the baseline risk is only 8%. The ARR indicates that the treatment will be of minor benefit in study B. Compare that to a baseline risk of 71% for study A, and we can see that treatment can be of greater benefit.

Number Needed to Treat

The degree of risk reduction should help us decide whether a treatment is worth pursuing, based on the likelihood that the outcome will be successful. The ARR, however, does not provide the clinician with a clinical value that is easily interpreted. A more useful statistic is the **number needed to treat (NNT)**, which provides information about effectiveness in terms of patient numbers.[27] For an intervention focused on prevention, such as medication to prevent a heart attack, it is defined as the number of patients that would need to be treated to prevent one adverse outcome. For an intervention used to improve performance, such as exercise to recover function, it is the number of patients needed to achieve one beneficial outcome. The larger the treatment effect, the smaller the NNT. It can be calculated for any trial that reports a binary outcome.

The NNT is easily calculated as the reciprocal of the ARR (expressed as a decimal). For the headache data:

$$NNT = \frac{1}{ARR} = \frac{1}{.53} = 1.9$$

The NNT is always *rounded up* to the nearest whole number. A large treatment effect will translate to a small number needed to treat.

> ➤ For the headache example, the NNT is 1.9, which is rounded up to 2.0. Therefore, we would need to treat two patients with manipulative therapy and exercise to prevent a recurrence of headaches in one patient. This result means one out of two patients is likely to experience a successful outcome, an outcome that would be considered clinically meaningful.

If the NNT is 1.0, this means that we would need to treat 1 patient to avoid 1 adverse outcome; that is, every patient will benefit from treatment. This is, of course, the ideal, although not often the case. The closer to 1.0, the better the NNT. If an NNT was 30, it would mean that 30 patients would need to be treated to prevent one adverse event. If the ARR is zero (no difference between CER and EER), the treatment has had no effect, and the NNT will be infinity. We would need to treat an infinite number of people to see any benefit. Because the NNT is based on the ARR, it is always interpreted in reference to the control condition, whether placebo or usual care.

Confidence Intervals for NNT

The NNT is a point estimate, and therefore, should be presented with a confidence interval for accurate interpretation. The confidence limits for NNT are the reciprocals of the confidence limits for ARR, in reverse order (see Table 34-5C). The null value for ARR is zero, which converts to infinity for the NNT.

> ➤ **Results**
> In the study of cervicogenic headache, the absolute risk reduction was .53 (95% CI: .36 to .70), which translated to NNT of 1.9 (95% CI: 1.43 to 2.75), which was rounded up to 2.0. Therefore, we would need to treat 2 patients with manipulative therapy and exercise to prevent a recurrence of headaches in 1 patient. Therefore, overall, 1 out of 2 patients should experience a successful outcome.

Number Needed to Harm (NNH)

The NNT reflects the *prevention* of an adverse event or *improvement* in performance, which is considered a successful outcome. These values must also be considered in the context of potential harms. We can apply this same concept to evaluate serious side-effects, risks, or complications that occur from treatment outside of the intended effects. Unfortunately, many treatments that have strong therapeutic effects (low NNT) also tend to have more serious side effects.[28] When an intervention poses excess risk to the patient, we want to assess the absolute risk increase (ARI) associated with it, or the magnitude of a detrimental treatment effect. This is the opposite of NNT, when the control group does better than the experimental group—the treatment causes an adverse outcome. Therefore, ARI = EER – CER. The reciprocal of this value is called the number needed to harm (NNH), which indicates the number of patients who would need to be treated to *cause* one adverse outcome.

Opposite to the interpretation of NNT, a larger NNH means a patient is less likely to experience an adverse outcome. The NNH is always *rounded down* to the nearest whole number. An NNH of 100 would mean that we would need to treat 100 patients to cause one adverse event. An NNH of 1.0, however, would mean that every patient would experience an adverse event. The NNH should be considered along with the

NNT to evaluate the balance between benefit and harm of an intervention (see Focus on Evidence 34-2). The NNH may involve a different outcome than used to evaluate the success of treatment, such as a dangerous side effect.

> It is important to understand that NNT and NNH are calculated based on binary outcomes. Outcomes based on continuous measures can be used by setting particular thresholds, such as minimal clinically important change.[29]

Interpretation of NNT and NNH

In terms of clinical decision making, NNT and NNH provide a useful number to help a clinician and patient decide if one or alternative treatments are worth pursuing, weighing their potential benefit or harm. These values are particularly useful for expressing the relative effectiveness or safety of different interventions. It quantifies the effort required to obtain a beneficial outcome. Several factors must be considered, however,

---

Focus on Evidence 34–2
Weighing Benefits and Harms

Bipolar depression (BD) is a common disorder with several evidence-based interventions, many of which present risks of substantial side effects. Ketter and colleagues[28] examined data from more than 100 randomized, double-blind, placebo-controlled trials to evaluate potential benefits and risks of a variety of pharmacotherapies that are used for acute BD. Their approach focused on clinical effectiveness, basing NNT on at least 50% improvement in mood rating compared with a placebo. Incidence of adverse events was based on the typical side effects for each drug, including sedation, restlessness (akasthisia), and anxiety. The advantage of using NNT and NNH can be illustrated by or a portion of their findings:

TREATMENT	NNT (95%CI)	SIDE EFFECT	NNH (95%CI)
Lurasidone monotherapy	5 (4–8)	Akathisia	15 (10–33)
Quetiapine	6 (5–9)	Sedation	5 (4–5)
Lamotrigine	12 (8–41)	Sedation	37 (Not Sig)
Armodafinil (adjunctive)	9 (4–43)	Anxiety	29 (17–107)

Here's what we can take from this.

- Lurasidone had a relatively low NNT and a higher value for NNH. Therefore, the benefit of this treatment was greater than the risk of akathisia, indicating it is more likely to be effective than to cause harm. This distinction is further supported by the

fact that the confidence intervals are narrow and do not overlap for NNT and NNH.
- Quetiapine's effectiveness is supported by a relatively low NNT, but the NNH was even lower, indicating that while this treatment may be effective, it is also likely to cause sedation in many patients.
- Lamotrigine had a favorably high NNH, indicating that it was more tolerable than other medications, but that is offset by a double-digit NNT, suggesting that it is less effective.
- Adjunctive armodafinil therapy had a somewhat higher NNT (but still single digit) and a much higher NNH for anxiety, suggesting that it is more likely to yield a good response than it is to present harm. However, because the confidence intervals for NNT and NNH show a large overlap, these effects may not be as obvious in practice.

Using the data presented here (there were several other treatments described in the study), the authors concluded that lurasidone and lamotrigine presented the best balance between effectiveness and tolerability compared with other treatments. These types of findings may seem frustrating, as they do not provide a definitive answer, the way a test of significance would. But because these treatments have different benefits and risks, and can affect patients differently, these data give providers and patients information that can help them personalize benefits versus harm and weigh the options.

Data source: Ketter TA, Miller S, Dell'Osso B, et al. Balancing benefits and harms of treatments for acute bipolar depression. *J Affect Disord* 2014; 169 Suppl 1: S24-S33.

when comparing values of NNT or NNH across different interventions or studies.

(1) **NNT and NNH must be interpreted in terms of a time period for treatment and follow-up.**   The duration of the treatment may make a difference in the frequency of expected positive or negative outcomes. Generally, the NNT will be smaller for an intervention of longer duration.[30] The comparison of values for different treatments is only valid when the outcome is measured within the same time period. For instance, for the headache study the report should read: The NNT equals 2 based on treatment over 7 weeks.

(2) **The interpretation of NNT and NNH will depend on baseline risk.**   Because some patients will have a greater risk of an adverse outcome before treatment begins, the NNT or NNH must be adjusted to account for low and high baseline risks. It may not be reasonable to assume that the same relative risk applies to all patients.[31] The patient's age, gender or initial severity of disease may alter the relative risk associated with the intervention. Therefore, when extrapolating NNT or NNH measures from the literature, the baseline risk must be taken into account. The control event rate can be used as an indicator of the baseline risk without treatment.

(3) **To compare values across studies, the outcomes of interest must be the same.**   For example, in the evaluation of exercise programs, an NNT of 20 for preventing falls in the elderly may be interpreted differently from an NNT of 20 for preventing hip fracture. The NNT for a drug treatment to reduce hypertension will be different if the adverse event is stroke, heart attack, or death. In the study of cervicogenic headache, the threshold for success was set at 50%. If this threshold were changed, the resulting NNTs would not be comparable.

The same holds true for NNH, as specific side effects will be of varied interest across patients.[28]

(4) **The validity of the clinical trial must be taken into account.**   Because NNTs are used to make individual patient decisions and to support reimbursement policies, the degree to which research studies represent actual clinical expectations will influence the application of effective treatments. Both internal and external validity must be considered. Replication is important to determine if results stand up to different samples. Patients seen in a practice setting may differ substantially from those used in studies.

(5) **There are no standard limits for NNT or NNH that dictate a decision.**   Like all research results, NNT or NNH should be incorporated into decision-making along with the clinician's experience and judgment, the patient's preferences, and the nature of the disorder that is being treated.[31] For some interventions an NNT of 2 or 3 would be considered good, whereas for others an NNT of 20 or 40 may still be considered clinically effective. The application of both NNT and NNH must be based on an understanding of the severity of the disease and its consequences, balanced with the probable benefit. If dealing with a disease that has a high mortality rate, for example, an intervention with an NNT of 40 may still be worth considering. An NNT of 100 may be acceptable if the treatment is easy to take and has few side effects, but an NNT of 5 may be too high for an expensive drug that carries substantial risk of side effects. Therefore, the value of NNT and NNH should always be interpreted within the context of a specific disorder, treatment, outcome, disease severity, and time period. Because treatments should be more likely to help than harm, we strive for interventions with lower NNTs and higher NNHs.

COMMENTARY

The work of epidemiology is related to unanswered questions, but also to unquestioned answers.

—*Patricia Buffler (1938-2013)*

American epidemiologist

A traditional biomedical model defines health narrowly as the absence of *disease*. Based on this definition, epidemiologists collect data to determine frequency of occurrence

of and risk factors for disease. Under this model, we open ourselves to looking at risk factors which have an effect at the biological level of the individual. Using a more complete model of health, epidemiology is able to focus on the occurrence of health-related states and risk factors related to physical, social, and psychological health status as well. The ICF model provides an excellent framework for this approach (see Chapter 1). In addition to disease, we can begin to look at the concept of risk in terms of impairments that lead to physical disability and use measures of risk to help us set priorities and evaluate functional outcomes.

As healthcare professionals strive to embrace evidence-based decision-making, our questions must take on a variety of forms, dealing with interventions or screening tools, as well as larger policy issues that have direct application to practice. Decisions regarding choice of intervention, who gets intervention (including prevention), and the intensity and frequency of intervention may be aided by an understanding of the risk reduction associated with specific patient characteristics, activities or treatments. We may understand the physiological rationale for applying specific exercises for reducing pain or improving mobility, but do we know what factors may alter the success of our treatments, or which patients are more likely to improve? Such information can provide new insight into the rationales we use for making treatment decisions.

REFERENCES

1. World Health Organization. Constitution. *WHO Chronicle* 1947;1:29.
2. Molnar D. The prevalence of the metabolic syndrome and type 2 diabetes mellitus in children and adolescents. *Int J Obes Relat Metab Disord* 2004;28 Suppl 3:S70-74.
3. Swanson JG, Kaczorowski J, Skelly J, Finkelstein M. Urinary incontinence: Common problem among women over 45. *Can Fam Physician* 2005;51:84-85.
4. Gibney KB, Brahmi A, O'Hara M, Morey R, Franklin L. Challenges in managing a school-based measles outbreak in Melbourne, Australia, 2014. *Aust N Z J Public Health* 2017; 41(1):80-84.
5. Hardy AM, Allen JR, Morgan WM, Curran JW. The incidence rate of acquired immunodeficiency syndrome in selected populations. *JAMA* 1985;253(2):215-220.
6. Fraser DW, Tsai TR, Orenstein W, Parkin WE, Beecham HJ, Sharrar RG, Harris J, Mallison GF, Martin SM, McDade JE, Shepard CC, Brachman PS. Legionnaires' disease: Description of an epidemic of pneumonia. *N Engl J Med* 1977;297(22): 1189-1197.
7. Tsang KW, Ho PL, Ooi GC, Yee WK, Wang T, Chan-Yeung M, Lam WK, Seto WH, Yam LY, Cheung TM, Wong PC, Lam B, Ip MS, Chan J, Yuen KY, Lai KN. A cluster of cases of severe acute respiratory syndrome in Hong Kong. *N Engl J Med* 2003;348(20):1977-1985.
8. Jacobsen SJ, Goldberg J, Miles TP, Brody JA, Stiers W, Rimm AA. Seasonal variation in the incidence of hip fracture among white persons aged 65 years and older in the United States, 1984-1987. *Am J Epidemiol* 1991;133(10):996-1004.
9. Chen CH, Xirasagar S, Lin HC. Seasonality in adult asthma admissions, air pollutant levels, and climate: A population-based study. *J Asthma* 2006;43(4):287-292.
10. Brody H, Rip MR, Vinten-Johansen P, Paneth N, Rachman S. Map-making and myth-making in Broad Street: the London cholera epidemic, 1854. *Lancet* 2000;356(9223):64-68.
11. Snow J. *On the Mode of Communication of Cholera*. 2nd ed. London: John Churchill; 1855.
12. John Snow 1813-1858. From BBC Online, 2001. Available at https://www.ph.ucla.edu/epi/snow/bbc_snow.htm. Accessed March 14, 2019.
13. One-hundred-fifty year old lessons of John Snow still relevant today. *MSU Today*, August 26, 2004. Available at https://msutoday.msu.edu/news/2004/one-hundred-fifty-year-old-lessons-of-john-snow-still-relevant-today/. Accessed March 14, 2019.
14. National Center for Health Statistics. Centers for Disease Control and Prevention (CDC). Early release of selected estimates from the 2000 and early 2001 National Health Interview Surveys (9/20/01). Available at https://www.cdc.gov/nchs/data/nhis/combined0901.pdf. Accessed March 14, 2019.
15. Bernard B, Sauter S, Fine L, Petersen M, Hales T. Job task and psychosocial risk factors for work-related musculoskeletal disorders among newspaper employees. *Scand J Work Environ Health* 1994;20(6):417-426.
16. Burdorf A, Van Der Steenhoven GA, Tromp-Klaren EG. A one-year prospective study on back pain among novice golfers. *Am J Sports Med* 1996;24(5):659-664.
17. Laden F, Spiegelman D, Neas LM, Colditz GA, Hankinson SE, Manson JE, Byrne C, Rosner BA, Speizer FE, Hunter DJ. Geographic variation in breast cancer incidence rates in a cohort of U.S. women. *J Natl Cancer Inst* 1997;89(18): 1373-1378.
18. Høidrup S, Sorensen TI, Stroger U, Lauritzen JB, Schroll M, Gronbaek M. Leisure-time physical activity levels and changes in relation to risk of hip fracture in men and women. *Am J Epidemiol* 2001;154(1):60-8.
19. Riddle DL, Pulisic M, Pidcoe P, Johnson RE. Risk factors for plantar fasciitis: a matched case-control study. *J Bone Joint Surg Am* 2003;85-A(5):872-877.
20. Friberg E, Mantzoros CS, Wolk A. Diabetes and risk of endometrial cancer: a population-based prospective cohort study. *Cancer Epidemiol Biomarkers Prev* 2007;16(2): 276-280.
21. Simpson EH. The interpretation of interaction in contingency tables. *J Royal Stat Soc Series B* 1951;13:238-41.
22. Colin RB. On Simpson's Paradox and the Sure-Thing Principle. *J Am Stat Assoc* 1972;67(338):364-366.
23. Charig CR, Webb DR, Payne SR, Wickham JEA. Comparison of treatment of renal calculi by open surgery, percutaneous nephrolithotomy, and extracorporeal shockwave lithotripsy. *BMJ* 1986;292(6524):879-882.
24. Jackson LA, Nelson JC, Benson P, Neuzil KM, Reid RJ, Psaty BM, Heckbert SR, Larson EB, Weiss NS. Functional status is a confounder of the association of influenza vaccine and risk of all cause mortality in seniors. *Int J Epidemiol* 2006;35(2): 345-352.
25. Jull G, Trott P, Potter H, Zito G, Niere K, Shirley D, Emberson J, Marschner I, Richardson C. A randomized controlled trial of exercise and manipulative therapy for cervicogenic headache. *Spine* 2002;27(17):1835-1843.
26. Akobeng AK. Understanding measures of treatment effect in clinical trials. *Arch Dis Child* 2005;90(1):54-56.
27. Weeks DL, Noteboom JT. Using the number needed to treat in clinical practice. *Arch Phys Med Rehabil* 2004;85(10): 1729-1731.

28. Ketter TA, Miller S, Dell'Osso B, Calabrese JR, Frye MA, Citrome L. Balancing benefits and harms of treatments for acute bipolar depression. *J Affect Disord* 2014;169 Suppl 1:S24-33.

29. Froud R, Eldridge S, Lall R, Underwood M. Estimating the number needed to treat from continuous outcomes in randomised controlled trials: methodological challenges and worked example using data from the UK Back Pain Exercise and Manipulation (BEAM) trial. *BMC Med Res Methodol* 2009;9:35.

30. Osiri M, Suarez-Almazor ME, Wells GA, Robinson V, Tugwell P. Number needed to treat (NNT): implication in rheumatology clinical practice. *Ann Rheum Dis* 2003;62(4):316-321.

31. McQuay HJ, Moore RA. Using numerical results from systematic reviews in clinical practice. *Ann Intern Med* 1997; 126(9):712-720.

Putting It All Together

CHAPTER 35 **Writing a Research Proposal** 548

CHAPTER 36 **Critical Appraisal: Evaluating Research Reports** 557

CHAPTER 37 **Synthesizing Literature: Systematic Reviews and Meta-Analyses** 574

CHAPTER 38 **Disseminating Research** 597

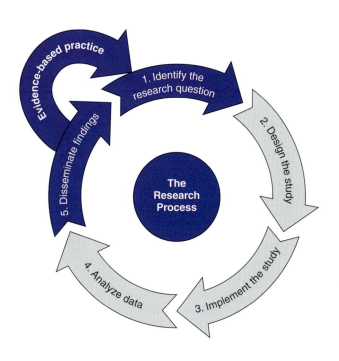

Writing a Research Proposal

The initial stages of the research process include development of the research question and delineation of methods of data collection. The success of the project depends on how well these elements have been defined in advance, so that the proper resources are gathered and methods proceed with reliability and validity. The plan that describes all these preparatory elements is the **research proposal**. The proposal describes the purpose of the study, the importance of the research question, the research protocol, and justifies the feasibility of the project. A proposal can be likened to a blueprint for a building—providing a foundation to guide the work to its conclusion. Proposals are necessary for both quantitative and qualitative studies.

Whether you are preparing a proposal for a funding agency, a thesis or dissertation, or a non-funded project, proposal guidelines are quite similar. The purpose of this chapter is to describe the process of developing and writing a research proposal.

the research question is refined enough to be studied, that the assumptions and theoretical rationale on which the study is based are logical, and that the method is appropriate for answering the question.
- The well-prepared proposal constitutes the body of a grant application when external funding is required.
- The proposal will provide details about the project so that ethical issues can be addressed, the needed expertise and competence of researchers and supportive personnel can be documented, and the feasibility of the project can be substantiated.
- The proposal serves as an application for review by peer or administrative committees. This is the document that will be carefully scrutinized by the Institutional Review Board (IRB) (see Chapter 7).
- The proposal enhances communication among colleagues who may be co-investigators and with consultants whose advice may be needed.
- The careful, detailed account of the study procedures serves as a guide throughout the data collection phase to ensure that the researchers follow the outlined protocol.

The research proposal, therefore, is an indispensable instrument in initiating and implementing a project. The exact format depends on the requirements of the institution, funding agency, or academic committee that will review and approve the project. The order of presentation of material may vary, as may the extent of the information that is required.

■ Purposes of the Research Proposal

A research proposal serves several purposes.

- It represents the synthesis of the researcher's critical thinking and the scientific literature to ensure that

■ The Research Team

Research projects are not solo endeavors. As the planning begins, a research team should be recruited to help frame the research question and methods. The team is led by the *principal investigator (PI)*, who has ultimate responsibility for the project, providing leadership for the planning effort and eventual implementation. The PI is typically an experienced investigator with a track record of prior research. In some instances, a co-PI can be designated to strengthen the team leadership. Other members of the team may include other investigators, a statistician, project manager, research assistants, staff support, and other collaborators.

📌 Although working on a thesis or dissertation may feel like you are on your own, even these projects benefit from collaboration, perhaps with a statistician or with colleagues who can assist with data collection—and of course, your advisor.

■ Components of a Proposal

A research proposal has two basic parts, as shown in Table 35-1. The first part provides details of the research plan, and the other describes the administrative support required to carry out the project. The body of the research proposal is the narrative portion that will explain the purpose and importance of the study and describe the design and procedures in detail.

Before the proposal is written, the researcher must review guidelines and required formats specified by funding agencies or academic institutions. As the project proceeds, it is helpful to follow an organized working plan that focuses the important elements of the project. Although this outline will vary for some agencies, the following sections reflect the basic components required for most research proposals.

Title and Abstract

The title of a research proposal will become the project's introduction to all potential reviewers and should compel their interest. It should be concise but informative, describing what you will do, how you will do it, and what outcome you are looking for. For example, a title such as "Meniscal surgery and exercise" is certainly concise, but the reader is likely to say, "what about it?" With a few more words, this title will say much more: "A randomized controlled trial of meniscal surgery compared with exercise and patient education for treatment of meniscal tears in young adults."[1] This summarizes the research question, the study design, the interventions, and the intended population.

A summary or **abstract** of the project, often limited to one page, is required by most funding agencies and institutional review boards. Specific headings may be required to organize content. The abstract should highlight the purpose and importance of the proposed

Table 35-1 General Format of a Research Proposal

The Research Plan

Title

Abstract

Statement of Purpose
1. Statement of the research problem
2. Specific aims or objectives
3. Research hypotheses or guiding questions
4. Rationale and significance of the study

Background
1. Review of literature related to:
   - Theory and supportive rationale
   - Related studies
   - Methods
2. Previous work by the investigator that supports the project

Methods
1. Design:
   - Type of study and appropriate design (randomized trial, cohort, case-control)
   - Interventions and outcomes
   - Explanation of potential confounders to be assessed
2. Participants: Characteristics, sampling method, recruitment and selection strategy, sample size estimates
3. Procedures
   - Data collection methods
   - Measurement: Instrumentation, plans to establish reliability and validity
   - Operational definitions
   - Timetable and organizational chart
4. Data management
   - Analysis: statistics
   - Expected outcomes

References

Appendices/ Letters of support

Documentation of informed consent

The Administrative Plan

Personnel: Qualifications, job descriptions, time commitment

Facilities and Resources: Space, equipment, technical support

Budget: *Direct Costs-* Salaries, equipment, facilities, supplies, and travel; *Indirect Costs-* Overhead

project. A brief description of the method should identify the study subjects, procedures, and methods for data analysis. The proposed duration of the study and overall projected costs may be stated. Because the summary is likely to be read before the detailed proposal, it must make a positive impression, conveying specifically what is to be done and why the study is important.

Although they form the first part of the proposal, it is actually a good idea to write your title and abstract last, after you've completed all the planning, when you have finalized your question, aims, and rationale.

Statement of Purpose

The opening section of the proposal identifies the subject area to be studied. As an introduction, this statement should convey a clear sense of the importance of the problem in terms of applicability of potential findings to clinical practice, patient care, or health policy. It may begin as a broad definition but should lead the reader logically toward a definition of the specific delimited topic, which will become the focus of the present project (see Chapter 3). The proposal should show how the current work contributes to what is already known. Reviewers will look at the likelihood that the project can exert a sustained, powerful influence on the research field involved.[2] Researchers will often include data on the prevalence and societal costs associated with the disorder being studied as part of the justification for the study.

The problem statement, therefore, presents a rationale for the specific question being addressed by the project. No single project can be expected to solve a problem in its entirety. On the other hand, each project should clearly contribute to the solution. Each study expands the evidence that can be used to support the body of knowledge related to the research problem. The content of the opening section of the proposal should clearly demonstrate this contribution.

When seeking funding, researchers must match their projects to an agency's goals and priorities. Some agencies require a letter of intent prior to submission and will accept applications only from appropriate institutions for projects that will fit their mission. NIH publishes *funding opportunity announcements (FOA)* that specify current areas of interest, and applications must relate to an FOA.[3]

Purpose, Hypothesis, and Specific Aims

In a brief statement, the researcher must state precisely what the project is expected to accomplish. The *purpose* of the study should follow clearly from the justification presented earlier. If the research is quantitative, the purpose is translated here into research hypotheses stated in positive terms so they reflect the expectations of outcome. "Null" hypotheses that serve a statistical function do not belong in the text, unless the purpose of the research is specifically to show no difference, as in a non-inferiority study (see Chapter 14). If the research is descriptive in nature, the author will state the characteristics or behaviors that will be documented in this work and what questions the data will answer about the target population.

Many granting agencies require a statement of *specific aims or objectives* for a project (see Chapter 3). For instance, a study's objectives might be to add to the body of knowledge in a certain content area, to test a theoretical proposition, to demonstrate differences between certain treatments to develop more effective and efficient intervention strategies, to document the reliability of an instrument, or to establish the relationship between specific variables as a basis for making treatment planning decisions. These objectives are derived from the research hypotheses or descriptive questions. Objectives help reviewers focus the description of methods and will often help the researcher guide the discussion of results when the study is completed.

Background

The presentation of background information will expand on the theoretical rationale presented in the introduction, adding pertinent facts, observations, or claims that have led the investigator to the proposed research question. The review may include relevant epidemiological factors, demographics, or the impact of the research issue on healthcare policy or practice and the potential impact on patients. This information is derived from a full literature review, describing the state of knowledge on the topic. The content of this section should show the logic for selecting subjects, selecting the variables to be studied and the methods of measurement.

This review of literature should acknowledge consistencies and conflicts found in prior reports. The possible reasons for inconsistencies and identifiable limitations of previous studies should be elucidated to provide further evidence that more study is needed. This section should end with a summary of the facts, problems, or controversies found in the literature and the relevant perspectives of the researcher that lead directly back to the specific need and stated purpose of the proposed study.

Background information can be strengthened when investigators have run pilot studies and obtained preliminary data that demonstrate the viability of the methods and promise of what the data might show.

Methods

The methods section is probably the most important part of the proposal and should be both concise and clear. The author should include enough detailed information so that reviewers can judge the soundness of the work, members of the institutional review board (IRB) can determine how subjects are being protected from harm, and the researcher can support the feasibility of the study.

Design

The opening section identifies the overall study design that will be employed to test the research hypothesis or answer the research question. This section should clarify the type of research being done, connecting the design to the aims of the study. The project may address intervention, diagnosis, or prognosis questions. The reviewer should have a clear idea of what test or intervention will be applied, what outcomes will be assessed, and what variables may be measured as potential confounders. For an intervention study, the methods of randomization should be described. Potential confounders should also be identified, as they will need to be measured.

Qualitative proposals address different types of questions that do not fit neatly into quantitative research designs. Several references provide useful guidelines for developing qualitative proposals, including strategies for improving the acceptance of qualitative methods by review committees.[4-9]

Participants

The description of participants in human studies is extremely important because of the inherent variability among them and the vast number of extraneous factors that may affect human behavior or performance. The researcher must describe who the participants will be in terms of *inclusion* and *exclusion* criteria, how many and from where they will be recruited, how they are to be selected, and the method by which they will be assigned to groups for an experimental study. For observational studies, case definitions must be provided. For qualitative studies, the process of identification of relevant participants should be described. Characteristics such as age, sex, height, weight, disability, diagnosis, and duration of hospitalization should be defined if they are relevant to the study. NIH and other agencies will assess the adequacy of plans to include subjects from both genders, all racial and ethnic groups, and young and older age groups, as appropriate for the goals of the research.[10]

Plans to foster adherence to the study's activities should be described. Participants may drop out for various reasons, and there are many strategies that can be used to follow up and maintain contact, with the intent to keep subjects interested and compliant.

 Funding agencies and institutional review boards will likely require a power analysis to demonstrate the appropriateness of the proposed sample size.

Procedures

The procedures section describes precisely what is to be done from beginning to end of the investigation, in chronological sequence. Procedures also include how, and by whom data are to be collected. Operational definitions should be provided for independent and dependent variables. If these procedures are extensive and lengthy, they may be briefly described in the text with references to appendixes that will present the details in full. The researcher should include strategies for controlling extraneous variables.

Equipment that will be used for intervention or outcome measurement must be fully explained. Devices should be described with explicit information such as brand name and model and should be documented for reliability and validity. If measurement tools are new, relatively unknown, or developed by the researcher, they should be defined in sufficient detail and a figure should be included. If the measurement tool is a questionnaire, the entire document may be presented as an appendix to the proposal or a set of sample questions may be included in the narrative.

A timeline chart or flow sheet will also serve to summarize the procedural sequence. Table 35-2 is a hypothetical sample, showing the sequence of events over 20 months, starting with lab construction and ending with preparing a manuscript. The written description of methods should be consistent with the timeline. Such a display of the "work schedule" will assist reviewers in evaluating the feasibility of the investigation in terms of time and available funding.

FUN FACT

In 1949, Capt. Edward A. Murphy, an aerospace engineer at Edwards Air Force Base, was researching how much sudden deceleration a person could tolerate in a crash. One day, after finding that a transducer was wired wrong, he admonished the technician responsible and said, "If there is any way to do it wrong, he'll find it" — and Murphy's Law was born.[11] At least that's the story. Since then, hundreds of "laws" and "corollaries" have been published in many fields, all reflecting the ironic nature of reality in science, business, education—even love! One important purpose of a proposal is to try to avoid as many of Murphy's prophecies as possible. Unfortunately, you can expect them to pop up to some extent in every study!

Data Management

The plan for data analysis should outline specific procedures for recording, storing, and reducing data and for statistically analyzing the data. Reviewers will examine both descriptive and analytical methods to determine their appropriateness for the design of the study and the type of measurement. It is often helpful to obtain the services of a statistician to be sure that this section is

Table 35-2   Sample Research Timeline

Activity	\\ MONTHS \\ 1	2	3	4	5	6	7	8	9	10	11	12	13	14	15	16	17	18	19	20
Lab construction	▓	▓	▓																	
Pilot testing				▓	▓															
IRB submission						▓														
Budget office review						▓														
Submission to agency							▓													
Expected approval								▓												
Recruitment									▓											
Data collection										▓	▓	▓	▓	▓	▓					
Data analysis																▓	▓	▓		
Prepare manuscript																			▓	▓

accurate and complete. The funding agency will probably have a statistician review it.

References

The final part of the narrative portion of the proposal should be a listing of literature cited in the paper. Some agencies require the use of a specific bibliographic style, but often this is left to the discretion of the researcher. Whatever style is used, it should be consistent throughout the document.

Appendices

Appendices may include supplementary material such as sample surveys, equipment details, or letters of support to confirm resources that are needed to carry out the project. For example, letters may confirm the commitment of various sites or leaders to provide resources for the project by allowing data collection to occur in their institution. Consultants will clarify their expertise and contributions to the study.

Documentation of Informed Consent

All proposals should document the process for protection of human subjects. A copy of the informed consent form must accompany the proposal when subjects will be directly involved in the study. Researchers should be familiar with the *Common Rule* and should document their training in ethical principles (see Chapter 7).[12] Reviewers will assess the potential risks for subjects associated with involvement in the research.

Most funding agencies and sponsoring institutions require IRB approval before a proposal is submitted and reviewed. The time delays inherent in obtaining this approval must be built into the timetable for submitting the proposal. Documentation of IRB approval must accompany the proposal.

■ Plan for Administrative Support

Personnel

Identification of the investigators and their qualifications is an important element of a proposal, especially when external funding is being sought. This will probably not be a factor in student research, except where expert assistance is required for carrying out parts of the project. Funding agencies will examine investigators' education, experience, track record of research, and prior publications to determine that they have appropriate experience.

Qualifications are evaluated through a *biosketch*, a concise summary of each investigator's background and expertise relevant to the project, including education, employment history, and selected publications or prior grants. A common format has been developed by NIH, which has been adopted by many other granting agencies. NIH restricts this document to five pages, so being concise is important. Some agencies will require that the PI is someone with an MD or PhD, others may accept professional doctorates. Because of these kinds of criteria, the inclusion of information about the investigators in a proposed study is essential to the process of evaluation by an agency or foundation.

 A biosketch should be written specifically for each proposal, to emphasize activities and accomplishments of the researcher that are relevant to the project. For example, particular publications may be listed that demonstrate the researcher's prior work in the area of study. A personal statement should also be directed to the aims of the project and the agency's priorities.

See the *Chapter 35 Supplement* for the NIH biosketch format.

Resources and Environment

Many funding agencies and academic or clinical institutions will also ask for information regarding existing resources for carrying out the proposed project to assess the organizational resources available to support the research. The investigator will be asked to describe available laboratory facilities, equipment, clinical sites, computer capability, office space, and so on, to demonstrate that the project is feasible within the institution's environment. The areas in which data collection will take place should be described, as should the areas where equipment will be housed.

In addition, administrative support services may need to be described. Documentation of staff support and technical assistance will be evaluated by reviewers in regard to the feasibility and justification of the applicant's budget request.

Budget

Every proposal, even those written for student research, should include an estimate of projected expenses, to demonstrate the feasibility of the project. For a grant application, the budget is an extremely important part of the proposal and must be complete and detailed according to the instructions of the funding agency. Students may need to show how resources will be made available to them if there is no funding associated with the project. Many schools provide small seed grants for faculty to run pilot studies. Some will also provide assistance to students for their thesis or dissertation projects.

The format and content of the budget will vary depending on the type of research proposal. Generally, the budget is presented by category as a summary of totals and as an itemized budget. For grant applications, a narrative section, the *budget justification*, must explain the projected costs in each category. For grants that are

expected to run more than 1 year, many agencies require only the first year's budget to be itemized, with summaries of projected expenses for additional years.

The NIH now uses *modular budgets* for new, renewal, and revised applications. This approach uses "modules" or increments for direct costs rather than line items. Modules may represent from $25,000 up to $250,000 a year.[13] A typical modular budget will request the same modules in each year, although there may be exceptions for expenses that will only exist in the first year, such as equipment costs.

Direct Costs

Direct costs are those associated with carrying out the project, including salaries, equipment, facilities, supplies, and travel. If study participants will be given honoraria, this should be described and budgeted (see Chapter 7).

Salaries. Salaries typically represent the largest part of the budget. The itemized personnel budget identifies the names of each individual who will participate in the study, their proposed title (such as principal investigator, consultant, statistician, project manager, research assistant), the salary for each individual, and the percentage of full-time or number of hours that will be devoted to the project. Dollar amounts may be based on percentage of the individual's full-time salary or an hourly wage for a specified time period. Some personnel may be asked to participate in the project with no remuneration. These individuals should also be listed, showing no salary request. Associated fringe benefit amounts are listed separately based on the total amount of projected salaries and wages.

Reviewers will scrutinize the personnel budget particularly to evaluate the appropriateness of the time commitment of each participant. The budget justification should explain the responsibilities of each participant and should show that participants will realistically be able to achieve the desired outcomes. It is undesirable to have too few investigators to carry out the work, but it is equally undesirable to have too many, each with very small percentages of effort.

Equipment. Equipment costs are given for all equipment that will be purchased with grant funds, if such purchases would be covered. Costs should reflect reasonable current prices and any charges related to installation, calibration, and maintenance. Most granting agencies define "equipment" as items costing at least $300 and having an extended life expectancy of at least 3 to 5 years. The narrative should provide details of equipment, such as manufacturer, model, and special accessories that are needed.

Facilities. The budget may include a request for funds for alteration or renovations to facilities. If space must be altered to accommodate equipment or to provide a work area, the contractors' estimates should be confirmed before specifying those costs in the budget. Explanations of all construction costs should be provided in detail, justifying why they are necessary for the study.

> 📌 Many agencies will not fund equipment or construction costs, with an expectation that the institution will provide the infrastructure for carrying out the project.

Supplies.   The category of supplies refers to consumable materials, as opposed to capital equipment. Questionnaires and survey instruments, office supplies, supplies for running research tests, and equipment items costing less than $300 are examples of "supply" items. Specific quantities of these supplies should be given with justification. A category of "other expenses" may also be included to account for miscellaneous items, such as telephone costs and photocopying.

Travel.   Depending on the nature of the project and the regulations of the funding agency, *travel expenses* may be budgeted. Travel to and from the institutional "home base" to collect data is certainly part of conducting a project and is likely to be an acceptable expense. Travel to meetings where data may be presented is more indirectly related to the project but can often be justified. Travel costs may also be applied to patients who must be transported for purposes of the research.

Indirect Costs

Indirect costs relate principally to the overhead charged by the sponsoring institution for administrative activities, facility maintenance, and any other support services. Funding agencies usually limit the amount of support that may be used for indirect costs based on a defined percentage of the total budget. These rates will differ across agencies and may be negotiated. In cases where the customary institutional charge exceeds the set limit, the budget narrative should specify the manner in which such a discrepancy will be handled. The total budget for the project is the sum of all direct and indirect costs.

> 🔑 In every institution where funded research is conducted, an administrative officer responsible for grants and contracts will be able to assist researchers with the general "anatomy" of a proposal budget and will provide information about fringe benefits, indirect cost rates, and institutional support. Consultation with this individual is essential and should begin early in the process of developing a research proposal budget. The administrative officer must sign off on the proposal before it is submitted reflecting institutional approval of the proposed project. This can take some time and should be factored into planning so that grant submission is on time.

■ Writing the Proposal

Whether you are writing a proposal for academic requirements or funding, attention must be paid to formatting and writing style. It is helpful to read other proposals that were submitted to and funded by the agencies that are being considered, many of which can be found online or colleagues may be willing to share their successful or rejected attempts. Maintaining a checklist of all the details required in the proposal allows the investigators to keep tabs on their own progress in completing the document.

> 📌 The research proposal is a forward-looking document. The researcher's thinking begins with the present, acknowledges and draws from the past, but primarily leads to the future. Therefore, the statement of the problem is written in the present tense, the background is written in the past tense, and the method (which is the proposed research) is written in the future tense.

Format

The format required for a proposal varies among agencies and academic institutions. The researcher must follow the specific instructions provided by the sponsoring agency, including seemingly trivial details such as pagination, page limits, line spacing, fonts, and margins. The method of citing references should be consistent throughout, and tables and appendices should be clearly labeled and cited in the text. Some formats require tables and figures to be embedded with text, while others require that they be placed at the end of the document.

> 📌 Agencies have little tolerance for applications that are not well organized, have typographical errors, grammatical mistakes, sloppy formatting, or that do not adhere to format requirements.[14] Details are important.

Be Concise, Logical, and Convincing

Writing in clear and concise language is essential (see Chapter 38). Starting with an outline can be helpful to facilitate organization of the proposal. The use of headings and subheadings is recommended to help reviewers follow the logic of the material and locate material quickly. Use of bullets and bolded terms can help to highlight important points.

The tone of the document should be positive, persuasive, and scholarly. The researcher must convince reviewers that the proposed research question is important, that there is a need to conduct the proposed research, and that the research team has the knowledge, ability, and resources to accomplish the study objectives.

Becoming familiar with review criteria can be helpful to maximize the potential for your proposal to be scored successfully. As much as possible, use the same terminology as in the criteria so that the reviewer can readily find all the information needed to satisfy each criterion.

If several team members have been involved in writing sections of the proposal, one editor should do a final pass to assure consistency in writing style as well as formatting. A proposal that is sensible, factual, and realistic will receive the attention it deserves.

■ Funding

When seeking financial support, one of the first decisions that will be made in the preparation of a proposal will be identification of a funding agency. Researchers must focus proposals to address the agency's priorities. There are essentially four types of funding sources.

- Many government agencies, like the NIH, are dedicated to supporting research in different areas. Web resources are available that list grant opportunities.[15,16]
- Foundations and professional societies offer many opportunities for funding, often at lower levels than governmental agencies. A good source of information is the *Foundation Center*, which lists foundations and their funding priorities.[17]

- Industry support of research comes primarily from pharmaceutical companies and device manufacturers, typically with the intent to show their product's effectiveness. Conflicts of interest should be addressed up front under these circumstances.
- Intramural funding is often available from academic or clinical institutions. These are usually "seed grants," providing minimal funding to support pilot studies.

■ Submitting the Proposal

Some submissions are still required in hard copy, some with multiple copies, but most use electronic submission. These often include forms that need to be completed online, especially around budget.

Take deadlines seriously. Electronic submission portals will cut off at the deadline. Best advice—don't leave things to the last minute. Build in time to get the approvals you need from the IRB, your budget office, or trial registries (see Chapter 14). Make sure the application is complete, including all necessary forms.

Don't be discouraged if your application is not accepted. Submitting proposals for small non-funded projects will often be successful, as they are intended to be initial efforts, but rejections are not unexpected with larger grants because of the competition for limited funds. Remember that most successful researchers paid their dues too! Rejections come with feedback that can be used constructively to improve the proposal for resubmission to the same or a different agency.

COMMENTARY

Murphy's Laws
If anything can go wrong, it will.
Nothing is as easy as it looks.
Everything takes longer than you think.

—Said to be named for Edward Murphy, Jr. (1918-1990)

American aerospace engineer

For those who have not developed proposals before, getting advice from colleagues who have been successful is a great place to start. They may be willing to share their successes and rejections, which can be invaluable. Researchers should expect to edit and revise the proposal several times through the development process. Indeed, the original draft may be substantially changed when the process is finished.

Writers should seek three kinds of individuals to provide feedback on the proposal. First, a person who is knowledgeable about the topic and the relevance of the project should be asked to evaluate the appropriateness, accuracy, and thoroughness of the presentation. Another who understands research design and methodology will concentrate on the validity of the research methods relative to the research question and specific aims. The third should be someone who is unfamiliar with the subject matter and who will react to the readability of the paper with "fresh eyes." All three may notice inconsistencies, instances of unnecessary professional jargon, or redundancy. This kind of preliminary review by colleagues is valuable for inspiring the researcher's confidence that the proposal is ready for formal review and subsequent successful implementation.

But Murphy's law is always looming. Researchers need to keep track of what works and doesn't work along the way. Subjects drop out or don't respond, equipment fails, schedules don't work, measurements are less reliable than planned, data collection takes longer than planned, and problems may arise in safety of subjects. These problems don't surface until after data collection is started, and it is helpful to brainstorm in the planning stage as to how such issues will be handled, should they arise. Murphy probably never understood how much his initial observation strikes a true chord every day!

REFERENCES

1. Skou ST, Lind M, Holmich P, Jensen HP, Jensen C, Afzal M, Jorgensen U, Thorlund JB. Study protocol for a randomised controlled trial of meniscal surgery compared with exercise and patient education for treatment of meniscal tears in young adults. *BMJ Open* 2017;7(8):e017436.
2. National Institutes of Health. Center for Scientific Review. Available at https://public.csr.nih.gov/. Accessed April 6, 2019.
3. National Institutes of Health. NIH Guide to Grants and Contracts. Available at https://grants.nih.gov/funding/searchguide/index.html#/. Accessed April 6, 2019.
4. Heath AW. The proposal in qualitative research. *Qual Report* 1997;3(1). Available at https://nsuworks.nova.edu/tqr/vol3/iss1/1/. Accessed April 6, 2019.
5. Morse JM. The adjudication of qualitative proposals. *Qual Health Res* 2003;13(6):739-742.
6. Morse JM. A review committee's guide for evaluating qualitative proposals. *Qual Health Res* 2003;13(6):833-851.
7. Penrod J. Getting funded: writing a successful qualitative small-project proposal. *Qual Health Res* 2003;13(6):821-832.
8. Sandelowski M, Barroso J. Writing the proposal for a qualitative research methodology project. *Qual Health Res* 2003;13(6):781-820.
9. Knafl KA, Deatrick JA. Top 10 tips for successful qualitative grantsmanship. *Res Nurs Health* 2005;28(6):441-443.
10. National Institutes of Health. Inclusion of Women and Minorities as Participants in Research Involving Human Subjects–Policy Implementation Page. Available at https://grants.nih.gov/grants/funding/women_min/women_min.htm. Accessed April 6, 2019.
11. Murphy's laws site: All the laws of Murphy in one place. Available at http://www.murphys-laws.com/murphy/murphy-laws.html. Accessed January 30, 2019.
12. Office of Human Research Protections. Federal policy for the protection of human subjects ('Common Rule'). Available at https://www.hhs.gov/ohrp/regulations-and-policy/regulations/common-rule/index.html. Accessed January 27, 2018.
13. National Institutes of Health. NIH Modular Research Grant Applications. Available at https://grants.nih.gov/grants/how-to-apply-application-guide/format-and-write/develop-your-budget/modular.htm. Accessed April 6, 2019.
14. National Institutes of Health. How to Apply—Application Guide. Available at https://grants.nih.gov/grants/how-to-apply-application-guide.html. Accessed April 6, 2019.
15. National Institutes of Health. Clinical research and the HIPAA privacy rule. Available at https://privacyruleandresearch.nih.gov/clin_research.asp. Accessed January 21, 2018.
16. National Science Foundation (NSF). Available at https://www.nsf.gov/awardsearch/. Accessed August 12, 2019.
17. Foundation Center. Available at https://foundationcenter.org/. Accessed April 6, 2019.

Critical Appraisal: Evaluating Research Reports

The success of evidence-based practice will depend on how well we incorporate research findings into our clinical judgments and treatment decisions. We have a responsibility to evaluate research reports to determine whether the findings provide sufficient evidence to support the effectiveness of current practices or offer alternatives that will improve patient care.

The purpose of **critical appraisal** is to determine the scientific merit of a research report and its applicability to clinical decision making. Whether a published paper or conference presentation, we can evaluate a study for the general purpose of understanding current information in our areas of practice, or we may be focused on its application to a particular patient problem. In the latter case, the clinician will pose a clinical question using the PICO format to direct a search and identify appropriate research reports (see Chapter 5).

Clinicians often express that one of the foremost barriers to evidence-based practice is a lack of skill in searching for and appraising the literature.[1-3] To be a critical consumer, those who seek evidence must be able to retrieve and read published studies and make judgments about the validity and relevance of the information. The search process was covered in Chapter 6. The purpose of this chapter is to take the mystique out of appraisal by providing a structured framework to guide critical evaluation of individual published studies, and to foster informed judgments about the quality and usefulness of the research. This discussion will focus on studies for intervention, diagnosis, prognosis, and qualitative research, but concepts can be readily applied to most types of research. You can refer to appropriate chapters indicated in each section for background on relevant design and analysis elements.

■ Levels of Evidence

Published studies come in all shapes and sizes— with stronger and weaker designs, with well-controlled or biased procedures, using statistics appropriately or not, and drawing conclusions that may or may not be warranted. As we strive to use the literature to support clinical decisions, our goal is to identify studies with sufficient validity so that we can be confident in the application of results to our own practice.

The classification of **levels of evidence** can be used as an initial criterion to judge the rigor of a study's design. Criteria reflect the degree of confidence one *should have* by considering the type of study.[4] It will help to refer back to Chapter 5 to review these classifications for both quantitative and qualitative studies, which are broadly summarized in Table 36-1.[5] Different criteria are used for different types of studies within each level. These criteria are not hard and fast, however, and any

Table 36-1	Summary of Levels of Evidence
Quantitative Studies	
Level 1	Systematic review/Meta-analysis
Level 2	Individual study with strong design
Level 3	Study with less rigorous design
Level 4	Case series
Level 5	Mechanistic reasoning
Grade up	Strong effect size, strong design
Grade down	Poor design, lack of consistency with other studies, small effect
Qualitative Studies	
Level 1	Generalizable studies
Level 2	Conceptual studies
Level 3	Descriptive studies
Level 4	Case studies

See Chapter 5 for a full description of levels of evidence.

study may be judged stronger or weaker depending on its implementation and precision.

When we think about questions that can help us sort through all the information in research reports, it is reasonable to seek the highest level of evidence that is available. For most categories, this will involve a systematic review or meta-analysis, which will synthesize literature on a topic. But no study is perfect and ascribing a high level of evidence to a study by virtue of its design does not mean that the study will provide a valid or definitive result to answer your clinical question. Criteria have been developed to judge the quality of a study, allowing for "grading up" or "grading down," based on rigor of design and strength of effect.[6] For instance, a well-designed observational study may be more relevant than a randomized trial that has design flaws. That's where critical appraisal comes in.

Criteria for grading evidence and assessing systematic reviews and meta-analyses will be addressed in Chapter 37.

■ The Appraisal Process

Appraisal begins, of course, with finding a relevant study. Search strategies must be applied to identify articles that are relevant to the clinical question. The initial impression of an article can influence how willing a reader will be to examine it further. The first pass is reading the abstract to determine if the study addresses the clinical question. Be aware, however, that there may inconsistency between the information reported in an abstract versus the full text report.[7,8] Therefore, abstracts may not include all relevant information, or they may mischaracterize the results of the study.[7,9] If the relevance

of the study is not clear from the abstract, reading full-text is important to make such a judgment. Without studying the details of the report, there is no way to truly understand the study's validity.

Although appraisal tends to focus on design and analysis, we can also pay attention to the clarity of the writing—the logical presentation of literature and background theory, development of the research question, description of methods and analysis procedures, and the depth of discussion. We should not have to wade through excessive jargon or try to decipher exactly what was done. We should not have to search for information that will allow us to judge the quality of the study. The contribution of a good study can be obscured if it is not presented in an understandable way.

To avoid being overwhelmed with this process, we need a systematic way of reviewing an article step by step, asking specific questions for each section and for each type of study, to make the process more straightforward. In the end, if and how the evidence is applied will be the reader's critical judgment.

 The Equator Network (**E**nhancing the **QUA**lity and **T**ransparency **O**f health **R**esearch) is an international initiative that seeks to improve the quality of published research by promoting transparent and accurate reporting through the use of robust reporting guidelines.[10] These guidelines are intended to help authors include appropriate information in published studies but are often used to guide critical appraisal as well, particularly to identify if appropriate information is included. Guidelines are available for a wide variety of study types, including randomized trials, observational studies, diagnostic and prognostic studies, clinical practice guidelines, and qualitative research. These reporting guidelines will be discussed in greater detail in Chapter 38.

 See the *Chapter 36 Supplement* for links to EQUATOR guidelines, appraisal worksheets for several types of studies, and other critical appraisal resources.

■ Core Questions

Clinicians and researchers will evaluate literature from three perspectives. First, the assessment will help to determine if the study has validity in terms of design and analysis. Second, the results of the study are examined to determine if findings are meaningful—the importance of an intervention effect, the accuracy of diagnostic tests, the degree of risk associated with prognostic variables, or the implications of qualitative interpretations. Finally, the clinician may consider the relevance of results to general practice or to a particular patient's management.

Although methodological criteria for assessing validity do vary for different designs, there are several core questions that frame the evaluation of any research article. Table 36-2 lists suggested questions according to where the information should be found in an article: introduction, methods, results, discussion, and conclusions. There is no standard format for critical appraisal, and this template should be used only as a guide to the evaluation process. Some studies may require different questions that address issues specific to that study. Although most questions can be answered using "yes" or "no" responses, the intent is to provide justification for that answer—*why is it yes or no* and what are the implications of the answer? These answers are not black and white, and readers must apply principles of design and analysis procedures to judge a study's value.

Is the Study Valid?

Introduction: What Is the Study About?

Before we can assess the validity of a study, we must first understand its intent. Readers begin with the abstract, which will include fairly concise information about the purpose, participants, methods, results, and major conclusions of the presented work. If results and conclusions seem applicable, the next step is to read the full article to confirm methods and findings.

Establishing the Question

In the opening paragraphs of an article, the author should establish the general problem being investigated and its importance. The background material should demonstrate that the researchers have thoughtfully and thoroughly synthesized the literature and related theoretical models. This synthesis should provide a rationale for pursuing this particular line of research, establishing what it will contribute to what is already known on the topic (see Chapter 3). Readers should understand the context of the question and be convinced that the study was needed.

By the end of the introduction, the study's specific purpose, aims or hypotheses should be apparent. Depending on the scope of the study, more than one question may be proposed. From these statements, readers should know whether the study is designed to be descriptive, observational, explanatory, qualitative, or mixed methods research. Questions should follow the PICO standard (see Chapter 5). They should clearly identify to whom the study applies, the methods used, how measurements were taken, what comparisons were made, and what outcomes were expected.

 A research "question" is not always phrased as a question. Authors may state the *purpose* of the study, the study's *aims*, or specific *hypotheses*. Qualitative studies may state a general goal to explore certain characteristics or experiences of participants. Regardless of how it is stated, however, the reader should be able to discern what the researcher intended to study.

Methods: How Was the Study Designed and Implemented?

The method section of a research report is the heart of the study, giving us details about what the investigation involved. This is where we learn enough to decide if the results and conclusions of the study are valid. Flaws or omissions detected in the methods section affect the usefulness of interpretations derived from the study. The method section is typically divided into several parts.

Table 36-2	Core Questions for Evaluating Research Studies

Is the Study Valid?

Introduction: What is the study about?
- Is the research question clearly stated?
- What type of research is being done?

Methods: How was the study designed and implemented?
- Who were the participants and how were they selected?
- How does the design control for potential confounding variables to support validity of findings?
- Were data collection procedures clearly defined with documentation of reliability and validity?
- Was data analysis appropriate to the research question and the data?

Are the Results Meaningful?

Results: What were the outcomes?
- Were results presented clearly in text, tables or figures?
- Were the data analyzed appropriately?
- How large was the effect, and is it large enough to be clinically meaningful?

Discussion: How are the results interpreted?
- Is the author's interpretation of results supported by the data?
- Does the author acknowledge limitations that could impact how the results can be applied?

Are the Results Relevant to My Patient?

Conclusions: Are the findings useful?
- Does the author discuss the clinical relevance of findings?
- Were the participants in the study sufficiently similar to my patient?
- Is the approach feasible in my setting, and will it be acceptable to my patient?
- Is this approach worth the effort to incorporate it into my treatment plan?

Participants

Readers must know who is being studied to interpret the validity of conclusions and to understand the extent to which the findings can be applied to clinical situations.

- How were participants recruited?
- What were inclusion and exclusion criteria?
- How were participants selected, and from what accessible population were they chosen?
- How many participants were studied? Is the sample size adequate?

This information helps to characterize the target population and establish the accessible population, essential information to determine how the results of the study can be generalized. Sample size is an issue related to statistical power, which may impact the significance of outcomes, and authors should describe how they estimated how many subjects were needed.

Design

The researchers will have chosen from a number of experimental, quasi-experimental, observational, descriptive, or qualitative designs and should clearly describe their choice. Based on the stated purpose of the project, readers should be able to judge the appropriateness of the choice that the researchers made.

- What is the research design, and is it appropriate for answering the research question?
- How does the design control for potential confounders?
- Do the authors provide a rationale for their choice of interventions and measurements?
- Was the time frame of the study adequate?

Information on study design will allow the reader to determine if the study is free of bias and how well it controls for threats to internal validity. It will also provide a framework for understanding points of data collection, the extent to which subjects are followed over time, and the validity of the measurements.

Data Collection

Much of the validity of a study is dependent on data collection methods.

- How were variables operationally defined?
- Were measurements assessed for reliability?
- Are data collection procedures described clearly and in sufficient detail to allow replication?

Reliability should be documented, preferably by assessment within the study, but it is often referenced from previous studies. Validity of measurement methods should also be documented based on prior research. It is essential to establish that measures are appropriate to the research question, and that results will provide accurate and meaningful information.

Procedures should be reported as a sequence of events from beginning to end. Description should include who was involved in data collection, what the participants were asked to do, and when and how often assessments were taken. Whether data are collected via electronic instrumentation, questionnaires or interviews, or by physical or observational measures, authors should provide sufficient detail so that readers could, in a similar setting with similar subjects, replicate the study procedures.

Data Analysis

The last part of the method section is typically focused on analysis. The author should present the plan for data management, tying it directly to the research question and the study design.

- Are appropriate statistics used to analyze the data?
- Has the author addressed each research question in the analysis?
- Have quantitative outcomes been expressed in terms of effect size, confidence intervals, or levels of significance?
- Are qualitative findings described to demonstrate how participants' experiences address the research question?

This section should list the type of statistics or analytic procedures that were used. For qualitative studies, there should be a rich description of how narrative information has been transcribed, coded, and interpreted.

Unfortunately, this is the part of an article that can be intimidating, especially if it is complex—and yet it can be vital to the interpretation of outcomes. While it is not necessary to have a statistician's background or be an experienced qualitative researcher, it is important to have a general understanding to adequately interpret results. By default, we often accept that the author applied the correct methods, but that is not always the case—*caveat emptor*! The use or misuse of statistics should be judged on the basis of two major factors: the nature of measurements (scale, reliability, linearity, normality) and the study design (explanatory or observational). Improper application of statistical tests violates statistical conclusion validity and detracts from the meaningful interpretation of data.

Are the Results Meaningful?

Results: What Were the Outcomes?

The results section of a research report should contain the findings of the study without interpretation or commentary.

- Did participants complete the protocol as originally designed?

- Were all participants accounted for in the final measurements?
- Do the results address the research question?
- Do the results support or refute the proposed hypotheses or aims?
- How large an effect was noted?

Results should provide a clear picture of whether data do or do not support the expected outcomes. If hypotheses were proposed, the author should indicate if each one is accepted or rejected based on the data. When statistics are used, data should be presented as descriptive values to characterize the sample, and test results should be tied to significance levels, effect size indices, and confidence intervals. When expected differences or effects are not obtained, the author should describe a power analysis to determine the likelihood of Type II error. Figures and tables are often a more efficient way to present detailed information. For qualitative studies, results will be in narrative form.

Authors should report the degree of follow-up that was achieved and if attrition was present in the study sample, providing a flowchart that indicates the number of participants involved at each stage of the process. Reasons for attrition should be provided to help determine if bias was present. The format of the flowchart will vary with the type of study, which can be found in reporting guidelines.

> When a study has potential importance for your clinical decision-making, and you find that the design or analysis presented is beyond your experience, refer to your textbook or Web resources. Hopefully they will provide reasonable explanation for you to get through it. When that is not sufficient, take advantage of connections with clinical and academic colleagues to find resources that can help you sort through the relevant data.

Discussion: How Are the Results Interpreted?

A research report culminates in the author's discussion and conclusions, putting the results of the study in context. This is where the author will present interpretation of results. The discussion section of an article should address each of the research questions, all results, and should show how prior research supports or conflicts with the study's findings. The author should suggest the clinical importance of the findings, and whether the outcomes do or do not fit expectations.

- Do the stated conclusions flow logically from the obtained results?
- What alternative explanations does the author consider for the obtained findings?
- How are the findings related to prior research?

- Are limitations addressed?
- Are the results clinically important?

Readers must determine if the evidence is strong enough to support a change in some aspect of practice or how we think about an approach to patient management. When statistical analyses are done, authors should reflect on the relative clinical versus statistical significance. Sometimes the results do not provide a definitive conclusion but do suggest how the findings contribute to continued understanding of the variables that were studied. Data are strengthened by a cross-validation approach, where results are replicated on a separate but comparable sample. This is rarely done, however, and authors should provide evidence from prior research to support their findings. As critical consumers of the products of clinical research, readers should study the discussion and conclusion sections of the research report to decide whether the authors' conclusions are warranted.

 Many journals require that authors declare *conflicts of interest* (COI), often in a statement at the beginning or end of the article. COI refers to situations in which financial or other personal considerations may compromise, or have the appearance of compromising, a researcher's judgment in conducting and reporting research. When conflicts occur, researchers must be vigilant to assure that they do not introduce bias.[11] For instance, researchers funded by drug companies or equipment manufacturers must show that these connections do not influence outcomes. Readers should be aware of COIs and judge the degree to which bias has been prevented.

Are the Results Relevant to My Patient?

Conclusions: Are the Findings Useful?

Finally, we get to the bottom line. A conclusion section may be incorporated into the end of the discussion, or it may be a separate section. The author should summarize interpretation of the results and describe how results pertain to practice or to basic knowledge.

- Are the findings of sufficient strength to inform management of particular patients?
- Were the participants sufficiently similar to my patient to allow generalization of findings?
- If the study does provide potentially useful findings, will the patient find the treatment or test acceptable?
- Is the treatment or test feasible, given my clinical setting and available resources?

This last part of the evaluative process is based on the reader's perspective. When the intent is to inform a clinical decision for a particular patient, practitioners should consider the four elements of evidence-based practice (see Fig. 36-1). First, we look for the best available evidence. After evaluating a study, we should have an idea of its scientific merit. The clinician's expertise and judgment will then be important as the results are weighed to determine if the findings are relevant. Knowing that no study will include participants exactly like your patient, a good question to ask is: How different would my patient have to be from the patients in the study before this evidence was of no use to me?"

The patient's preferences will dictate the acceptability of a treatment or test. The ultimate decision rests on judgment by the clinician and patient based on relevant information—is the treatment or test worth adopting with consideration of its benefits and harms? Finally, it is worth considering if the methods used are feasible in your own setting, or if special equipment or training is needed for implementation.

■ Intervention Studies

The core questions described thus far provide a general foundation for understanding research studies. There are, however, several additional questions that need to be addressed depending on the type of study. This section will focus on intervention studies, which may address efficacy in randomized controlled trials (RCTs), or effectiveness in pragmatic trials, quasi-experimental studies, single-subject designs or N-of-1 trials. The question should clearly state the population being studied, the intervention, the

comparison treatment, and the outcomes that will be measured. Because intervention studies are intended to look for cause-and-effect relationships, issues of internal validity and generalizability should be scrutinized. Additional questions specific to intervention studies are listed in Table 36-3.

See content related to the design of intervention studies in Chapters 13-18. Relevant statistical tests are described in Chapters 22-34.

Are the Results of the Study Valid?

Participants: Authors should specify how participants were recruited using probability or nonprobability methods. Inclusion and exclusion criteria should be provided, and sample size estimates described, including how the effect size was determined. This is where external validity of the study will be established. When nonprobability samples are used (as is often the case), it is important to ask if it affects the relevance of the study population.

Design: Description of the study should indicate the type of experimental design that is being used, including the number of groups, the number or levels of independent variables (the intervention), the number of dependent variables (the outcomes), and the frequency of measurements. The validity of an intervention study will depend in large part on how randomization was achieved, including concealed allocation, to create comparison groups that are balanced in terms of known and unknown confounding variables. It should be clear if repeated measures are used and how order or carryover effects are controlled. The author should document the extent to which groups were treated equally, except for the experimental treatment. When the design does not allow for random assignment, researchers should address how they controlled for potential bias.

Data Collection: Operational definitions should be provided so that all intervention and measurement procedures could be replicated. Researchers should provide evidence of validity for the chosen measurement tools, especially if they are not standard measures. As much as possible, bias should be controlled by blinding researchers, participants, and assessors to group assignment. Groups should be treated equally except for the intervention. Therefore, differences between groups observed at the end of the study should be attributable to the treatment. When designs do not adhere to these standards, authors should explain why and discuss how they controlled for potential biases. Information in this section, combined with information about design, will help you determine the internal validity of the study.

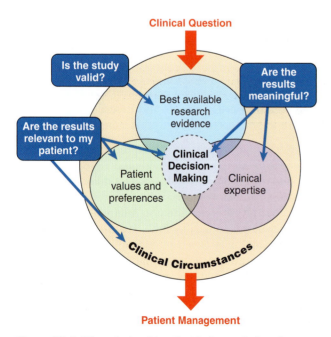

Figure 36-1 The relationship of critical appraisal to the components of evidence-based practice.

Table 36-3	Questions Specific to Validity of an Intervention Study
Are the Results of the Study Valid?	
Question	• Does the question clearly state the population being studied, the treatments being compared, and the outcome measures (PICO)?
Participants	• What type of sampling procedure was used? • How were participants recruited and selected? • Was a power analysis done to determine sample size?
Design	• Does the study design address efficacy or effectiveness? • Were research hypotheses proposed to indicate expected relationships? • Have the independent and dependent variables been clearly described? • Was random assignment used to form study groups or to systematically vary the order of repeated measurements? • Was allocation concealment used? • Was the study internally valid? Were other factors present that could have affected the outcome?
Data Collection	• Were outcome measurements taken at reasonable time intervals, and were participants followed for a sufficient time period? • Were all relevant outcomes evaluated? • Were the groups treated equally, aside from the intervention? • Were investigators, participants, and those involved in data collection blinded to group assignment?
Data Analysis	• Were groups similar at baseline on relevant characteristics? • Were all participants who entered the trial properly accounted for at its conclusion? • Were participants analyzed in the groups to which they were initially assigned (intention to treat analysis)? • Were effect sizes determined? • Were confidence intervals provided? • Were research hypotheses accepted or rejected?
Are the Results Meaningful?	
	• Are the results both statistically and clinically significant? • Did the authors consider alternative explanations for outcomes? • If outcomes were not significant, was a power analysis done?
Are the Results Relevant to My Patient?	
	• Are values of NNT and NNH included to put the intervention's benefits or harms in context? • Are the outcomes of the intervention consistent with my patient's preferences? • Are the treatment benefits worth the potential harm or costs?

See related content on design of intervention studies in Chapters 13-18.

Data Analysis: The study design will influence the selection of statistical analysis procedures. Mean differences may be used to determine the effect of the experimental treatment with statistics such as *t*-tests or analysis of variance. These values should include confidence intervals as measures of precision. Analysis of covariance may be used if there the researcher can justify appropriate covariates. When looking at the benefit of an intervention, researchers may look at effect size, relative risk reduction (RRR), attributable risk reduction (ARR), and number needed to treat (NNT) or number needed to harm (NNH).

Researchers should provide data to confirm that groups are similar at baseline on relevant characteristics. If significant differences are observed before treatment is initiated, authors should indicate how they handled data to account for those differences. Validity will also depend on the extent to which participants are adherent to the protocol, and the degree of attrition that occurs during the study. To maintain the benefit of randomized groups, investigators should account for all participants at the end of the study, including those who "dropped out," and should analyze subject data according to the groups they were assigned to, even if they did not maintain that group membership. Authors should confirm that an *intention-to-treat analysis* was done. A flow diagram should be included to demonstrate how subjects were recruited and assigned to groups. Researchers should account for differential attrition in treatment groups.

Are the Results Meaningful?

The intent of an intervention study is to demonstrate the benefit of a treatment as compared to a control condition. The author should clearly state if hypotheses were supported or not and propose reasons based on previous research. Despite the pervasive use of *p* values to indicate significant differences, confidence intervals and effect sizes provide more relevant information to judge the importance of the findings. Researchers should present data that reflects the amount of change or difference and its relative importance. If differences are not significant, the author should address the potential for Type II error.

Are the Results Relevant to My Patient?

The relevance of findings will depend on how well the participants represent your patient, the feasibility of the intervention in your setting, and the acceptability of a decision to use it. Even a study that shows a large effect may not be realistic or affordable. When the results of a study are not clear cut, which is probably more often than not, values of NNT and NNH can be directly applied to decisions in consultation with the patient, especially when weighing the relative benefits and risks associated with an intervention. Even if researchers do not express their results using these values, it is often possible to calculate them based on presented data.

■ Studies of Diagnostic Accuracy

This category of studies relates to the validity of a test and how meaningful the results will be for determining a patient's condition or disease state. It should be clear if the intent is to compare two tests, to estimate the accuracy of one test, or to examine a test's utility across participant groups. Additional questions for diagnostic accuracy studies are listed in Table 36-4.

> See content related to design and analysis of diagnostic accuracy studies and studies of clinical measurement in Chapter 33.

Table 36-4 Questions Specific to Validity of a Diagnostic Accuracy Study

Are the Results of the Study Valid?

Participants	• Was the sample representative of the full spectrum of patients who are affected by the disorder?
Design	• Was there an independent comparison with an appropriate reference standard? • How was validity of the reference standard established? • Were all participants given the reference standard and index tests regardless of the test result?
Data Collection	• Were the methods for performing the test and reference standard described in sufficient detail to allow replication? • Were those performing the index test blinded to the patient's reference standard results?
Data Analysis	• Were measures of diagnostic accuracy calculated, including sensitivity, specificity, predictive values, and likelihood ratios, including confidence intervals? • If the index test was continuous, how was a cutoff point determined? • Were tests interpreted independently of clinical information about the patient?

Are the Results Meaningful?

	• For diagnostic tests, do values of sensitivity, specificity, and likelihood ratios improve posttest probabilities of diagnosing the disorder? • Is there a reasonable balance between the risk of false positives versus false negatives? • Are the authors' conclusions justified within a clinical context?

Are the Results Relevant to My Patient?

	• What are the relative benefits of performing the test versus risk or cost? • Do the results of the test provide meaningful information that contributes to informed choices in management of my patient?

See Chapter 33 for content related to design of studies of diagnostic accuracy.

Are the Results of the Study Valid?

Participants: In order to judge the validity of a test, the sample must be representative of the spectrum of patients to whom the test would apply, and inclusion and exclusion criteria should be specified. Some measurements may simply be judged present or absent, others may be assessed for different levels of severity or magnitude. The sample must reflect the full range of the condition. Without such variance, it will not be possible to accurately determine how well the test reflects true scores. Therefore, samples are usually purposive, to assure a diversity of subject characteristics. This information is usually described in a table.

Design: The meaningfulness of a test is based on criterion validity, in which the measure being assessed for accuracy (the index test) is tested against a criterion (the reference standard). The validity of the reference standard, therefore, must be documented. Sometimes there is a gold standard which is well-established as a known criterion, but an accepted reference standard must be defined for more abstract measures. Authors should be able to justify the reference standard through prior research. The index test and reference standard should be independent of each other, so that interpretation of findings is not biased.

Data Collection: Both index and reference tests should be given to all participants, even if the reference standard indicates the absence of the target condition. Methods of measurement should be well documented, including a full description of how bias was controlled by blinding those who administer and score tests to the subject's true diagnosis or condition.

> Studies that assess clinical measurements can be appraised using questions similar to those for diagnostic accuracy, but with a focus on reliability and content, criterion-related, or construct validity for the measurement of impairments and activity or participation restrictions. See Chapters 9, 10 and 32 for further discussion of this form of methodological research.

Data Analysis: Statistics for diagnostic accuracy should include sensitivity, specificity, predictive values, and likelihood ratios, with an indication of the benefit of the test for determining posttest probabilities. Confidence intervals should be included. Because readers may want to handle results for different purposes, authors should report data in a way that will allow readers to make calculations.

For tests on a continuous scale, an ROC curve should be generated, the area under the curve included, and the method for determining the cutoff point described. A flow diagram should be included to show how subjects were recruited and how attrition affected ratios.

Are the Results Meaningful?

Authors should include their interpretation of data by discussing if the obtained statistics represent strong or weak effects. These are subjective determinations and should be made within a clinical context. Although literature should be cited, authors should not rely solely on a standard range of values to indicate when a relationship is considered weak or strong. Clinicians should judge the relative risks associated with false positives versus false negatives. Results should be discussed in terms of costs and clinical consequences related to the index test.

Are the Results Relevant to My Patient?

Results should be considered within the context of the patients to whom they will apply to determine if they will impact patient management decisions. The research should lead to greater confidence in diagnostic accuracy and decisions to use a specific measure. When more than one test is available for a given purpose or when there are different risks or costs associated with them, the clinician and patient may weigh these considerations in deciding how to proceed.

■ Studies of Prognosis

Studies of prognosis are based on observational designs, involving the determination of the predictive value of exposures and patient characteristics on eventual health outcomes. The research question should clearly state the expected associations based on prior research as well as biologic mechanisms. Additional questions for prognostic studies are listed in Table 36-5.

> See content related to the design of prognosis studies in Chapters 19 and 34. Relevant statistics are described in Chapters 30, 31, and 34.

Is the Study Valid?

Participants: The sample should represent the population of interest, composed of patients who are at a similar time in the course of the disorder so that prognosis can be monitored over time. Participants' characteristics must be comprehensively described as well as how and from where they were recruited. The method for recruiting cases and controls should be clearly explained.

Table 36-5 Questions Specific to Validity of a Prognosis Study	
Are the Results of the Study Valid?	
Participants	• Was the sample composed of a representative group of participants at a similar point in their disorder? • Were participants recruited in an appropriate way?
Design	• Was the study prospective or retrospective? • Were the prognostic indicators appropriate for predicting outcomes? • Were cases and controls appropriately defined? What are the risks for misclassification? • Were exposures adequately defined and measured for all participants? • Was follow-up sufficiently long and complete? • Were the individuals collecting data blinded to the participant's prognostic status? • Were objective and unbiased outcome measures used?
Data Collection	• Were evaluators blinded to the patient's prognosis? • Were outcome data collected from all participants? • Were assessments reliable? • Were potential confounders identified and measured?
Data Analysis	• Were appropriate prognostic estimates derived? • Were subgroups of participants examined for differences in prognostic estimates? • Were confounders accounted for in the analysis? • Did the investigators account for missing data?
Are the Results Meaningful?	
	• How likely are the outcomes within a given period of time? • How precise are the prognostic estimates?
Are the Results Relevant to My Patient?	
	• Are the participants in the study sufficiently similar to my patient? • Will results lead to selecting or avoiding certain intervention or prevention approaches? • Will the results affect what I tell my patient?

See Chapters 19 and 34 for content on design of prognosis studies.

Design: Prognosis can be assessed using cross-sectional, cohort, or case-control designs in retrospective or prospective ways. Each of these designs has strengths and limitations in terms of being able to document a temporal sequence. When trying to determine factors that will impact a long-term outcome, the duration of follow-up must be described, as interpretations can only be made within that timeframe, and there must be sufficient time for the outcome to develop.

Data Collection: The outcome of interest must be operationally defined and measured at the beginning of the study as well as in follow-up. The method for determining exposures should also be defined, including strategies for reducing bias. Reliability and validity should be documented for all measurements. Potential confounders must be identified at the outset so that data can be collected. These often include demographic factors such as age and gender, but will also include health conditions, personal and lifestyle characteristics, and comorbidities that could be connected to the outcome. Those who take

measurements should be blinded to the subject's prior status. Data must be documented throughout the study, as it is not uncommon for attrition to occur for various reasons. As much as possible, all participants should be followed to the study's end point, even if they did not complete all measurement sessions.

Data Analysis: Depending on how the research question is stated, analysis may include statistics such as relative risk (RR) and odd ratios (OR), sensitivity and specificity, or regression analyses that will adjust values for covariates. When predicting continuous outcomes, multiple regression and R^2 may be used to demonstrate the strength of predictive relationships. Survival analysis may be appropriate when comparing two or more subgroups on long-term outcomes with hazard ratios (HR).

A flow diagram should be included to account for subjects who dropped out and describe how they handled missing data. Researchers should also establish that those who drop out are not significantly different on important covariates from those who remain.

Are the Results Meaningful?

Authors should be able to discuss how their findings are supported by previous research. Researchers should be able to discuss the clinical context and application of the findings. Effect sizes should be reported, typically as RR, OR, or HR estimates, with appropriate confidence intervals. When appropriate, adjusted values should be presented that account for the contributions of potentially confounding variables.

 If the research question in an observational study addresses a potentially causative relationship between exposure and outcome, the authors should describe how results meet the criteria to support causation. Although they do not provide the level of control inherent in explanatory designs, these designs are essential to study the effects of conditions when it is not feasible to assign individuals to groups (see Chapter 19).

Are the Results Relevant to My Patient?

The application of prognostic findings requires substantial judgment on the part of the clinician and patient. Prognosis is a risk measure, not an absolute value like we obtain when comparing interventions. Therefore, by looking at the risk estimates associated with the predictive factors, the provider and patient should discuss the meaning of prognostic implications. Because there are often several covariates that are potential confounders in establishing risk, it is important to consider just how well the sample resembles the patient's profile—recognizing that there will never be a study with the exact characteristics of the patient. Understanding the concept of risk, and being able to explain it to a patient, is essential to using data for decision-making.

■ Qualitative Studies

Although qualitative inquiry is fundamentally different from quantitative study, the core questions for critique can still be applied. However, these questions will be answered from a different perspective, as there will not be specific variables or statistics to organize data.[12,13] Additional questions for qualitative studies are listed in Table 36-6.

Research questions for qualitative study are usually broad but should provide a clear context for the study and the behaviors or experiences that it will explore. Literature review should provide a foundation for understanding the phenomenon being studied and methods that will be used to study it.

Table 36-6 **Questions Specific to Validity of a Qualitative Study**	
Are the Results of the Study Valid?	
Participants	• What sampling strategy was used to recruit participants? • How did the researchers justify the choice of participants?
Design	• What approach did the authors use to frame the research question? • Did the authors justify the qualitative method chosen?
Data Collection	• Were methods of data collection described in sufficient detail?
Data Analysis	• Did authors make analysis procedures explicit? • Did the authors describe how they derived emerging theory and themes? • Did the investigators document the trustworthiness of the study through triangulation and other indicators of quality? • Did investigators demonstrate reflexivity through confirmation of findings with others?
Are the Results Meaningful?	
	• Did the discussion include a description of contexts that are relevant to the question? • Did the authors discuss how emergent theory fit within the context of the study? • Were new insights presented that increase understanding of the findings?
Are the Results Relevant to My Patient?	
	• Did the authors provide sufficient information to address transferability of the study findings? • Will results lead to new considerations as part intervention or prevention approaches? • Will the results affect what I tell my patient?

See Chapter 21 for content related to design and analysis of qualitative research.

See content related to design of qualitative studies and mixed methods research in Chapter 21.

Are the Results of the Study Valid?

Participants: In qualitative study, participants are recruited purposefully to identify individuals who can provide insights relevant to the research question. Characteristics of participants should be fully documented. Samples may be small, but the number of participants will depend on the nature of the question. Readers should judge adequate sample size and characteristics of participants relative to how well a topic is understood and how diverse a sample is needed to meaningfully represent the concepts being studied.[14] Authors should make this rationale clear based on previous research. If theoretical sampling is used, wherein participants are continually recruited until no new perspectives emerge, the author should provide a full description so that readers can understand who has been studied.

Design: Authors should justify why they have chosen a particular approach, such as ethnography, grounded theory, or phenomenology. Although there may be some overlap, each perspective drives a different approach to data collection that should fit the research question.[13]

Data Collection: Authors should be comprehensive in their description of data collection methods, such as narrative text from interviews, focus groups, observation, or field notes. These methods can vary widely from study to study and must be geared toward the specific question being asked. For instance, the structure of questions for interviews and an interview guide should be described. Readers should be able to discern how observational data are obtained, and how the investigator was inserted into the setting for that observation.

 Mixed methods research incorporates elements of both quantitative and qualitative research. Therefore, criteria for critical appraisal will take both approaches into account.

Data Analysis: Because of the voluminous amounts of data typically obtained in qualitative studies, it is imperative that authors provide details about how data were coded, how themes were developed, and how theory was derived.

The rigor of qualitative data is considered its *trustworthiness*. Criteria focus on how well the narrative data have been confirmed for reliability. Authors should be explicit in how they have assessed the qualities of credibility, transferability, dependability, and confirmability

using techniques such as triangulation of data and member checking. Researcher *reflexivity* should also be described, indicating how others were engaged in confirmation of data interpretation.[15]

Are the Results Meaningful?

Findings from qualitative studies are reported in narrative form, describing themes, presenting quotes, or explaining the derivation of theory. Because of their subjective nature, results must provide a context for how findings can be interpreted and how they fit with what is already known from previous research. Authors must be careful to put their findings in perspective, and not to claim implications that go beyond the study's context.[12] They should, however, offer insights into how results expand understanding of the issues under study, and how further study can improve that understanding.

Are the Results Relevant to My Patient?

The application of findings from qualitative research can be challenging because of the limited samples and the individual perspectives that comprise the data. The *transferability* or generalizability of the study requires "thick description" of participant characteristics, setting, data collection methods, analysis strategies, and interpretation of findings, so that clinicians can determine if there is a connection to their setting or patient. The findings of a qualitative study should present an opportunity for providers to consider how a patient's experiences and values can impact their care.

■ Critically Appraised Topics

As we search for information to apply to our clinical decision-making, we all benefit from applying evidence to patient care in a timely way. Many questions arise out of daily clinical practice. A systematic review is intended to provide a critical understanding of the quality of evidence on a topic, but is based on an overview of the topic, not its application to a specific patient situation (see Chapter 37). An alternative format, called a **critically appraised topic (CAT)**, has become popular to provide a brief summary of a search and critical appraisal of literature related to a focused clinical question.[16-20]

A CAT is an evidence-based and patient-based tool, typically initiated because of a patient encounter that reveals a knowledge gap.[21] The process of developing a CAT follows the five steps for evidence-based practice: Ask a question, acquire relevant literature, appraise the quality of the study, apply findings to patient care, and assess the success of the clinical application (see

Chapter 5) The author of a CAT searches for and appraises "current best evidence" from the literature, summarizes the evidence, integrates it with clinical expertise and finally suggests how the information can be applied to a patient scenario.[17] The critique will address internal, external, construct, and statistical conclusion validity.

Format of a CAT

A CAT provides a standardized format to present a critique of one or more articles and a statement of the clinical relevance of the results. Although the format of a CAT can vary, the essential elements remain fairly standard. It is intended to be a concise document, typically one to two pages. Table 36-7 shows one common layout. At minimum, a CAT should contain the following information:

- **Title:** A concise statement that will be used to catalogue the CAT.

- **Author and Date:** The author of the CAT should be specified as well as the date the search was executed. CATs are often revised as new evidence becomes available. Some authors will include an "expiration date" that suggests when the review should be revised to account for more recent literature. This could be as short as 1 year or as long as 5 years, depending on the depth of research on the topic.

- **Clinical scenario:** A brief description of the patient case that prompted the question.

- **Clinical question:** This is the question that was developed from the patient case. It includes the elements of PICO: The patient population, the intervention that is being considered (or diagnostic test or prognostic variables), a comparison (if relevant), and the outcomes of interest. This structure helps to refine the question and identifies key elements of an efficient database search.

- **Clinical bottom line:** A concise summary of how the results can be applied, including a description of how results will affect clinical decisions or actions.

- **Search history:** Description of the search strategy used to obtain the studies that are being appraised. This includes databases used and terms entered at each step. Relevant studies are selected, often based on achieving highest levels of evidence.

- **Citations:** Full bibliographic citations of studies selected for review.

- **Summary of the study:** Is the evidence in this study valid? This section should provide a description of the study based on the questions shown in Tables 34-3 through 34-6, including the type of study participants, procedures, and design and analysis elements.

- **Summary of the evidence:** The results of the study should be summarized in narrative and/or tabular format. Specific effect size estimates should be provided as appropriate, such as means and mean differences, confidence intervals, odds ratios, likelihood ratios, sensitivity and specificity, and NNT or NNH. If these estimates are not included in the research report, the CAT author may be able to calculate them if sufficient data are provided in the report. Results of qualitative studies will be presented in narrative form, organized around themes or theoretical propositions.

- **Additional Comments:** Provide critical comments on the study using appraisal guidelines, including issues related to sampling, methods, data analysis, quality of discussion, and interpretation of results. This section should address internal, external, construct, and statistical validity, with comments on positive and negative aspects of the study.

The Centre for Evidence-Based Medicine (CEBM) offers a *CATMaker and EBM Calculators,* that assist with creation of the CAT as well as calculating outcomes such as risk and NNT.[22]

A CAT plays an important role in fostering evidence-based practice. First, it is based on a specific clinical question, prompted by a clinician's need to clarify an aspect of patient care related to intervention, diagnosis, prognosis, or harm.[19] This question is developed using the PICO format, as shown in Table 36-7. The clinician searches the literature explicitly to provide an answer to this question, with the intent of influencing management of the patient.

The second unique feature of a CAT is the inclusion of a *clinical bottom line*, or a conclusion by the CAT author as to the value of the findings. The usefulness of the bottom line depends on the ability of the CAT author to accurately assess the validity of the literature, and to grasp the relevance of findings for a particular patient's management.[17] This information is then useful to others who may encounter similar patients, who can take advantage of the summary for efficient decision-making.

Table 36-7	Format for a Critically Appraised Topic on Intervention

Title: Community-based occupational therapy improves functioning in older adults with dementia
Appraiser: Leslie Portney
Date of Appraisal: August, 2017

Clinical Scenario: AR is an 85-year-old female who experiences mild Alzheimer's dementia. She lives with her daughter and her daughter's family (husband and two teenage children). AR is able to function with supervision but has exhibited increasing problems with activities of daily living. She has also exhibited some agitation in her interactions with the family. Her daughter works from home and is able to supervise her mother around the house. Her daughter has expressed concern for her own ability to handle her mother's functional limitations. She has asked if community occupational therapy services would be beneficial for improving her mother's function.

Clinical Question: In older adults with dementia, does community-based occupational therapy improve daily functioning?
   Patient/Problem: Community-dwelling elders with mild to moderate dementia
   Intervention: Community-based occupational therapy
   Comparison: No therapy
   Outcome: Functional performance

Clinical Bottom Line: Community-based occupational therapy improves daily functioning in older adults with dementia and increases caregiver feelings of competence.

Search History:
Databases: CINAHL, MEDLINE
Search terms: Occupational therapy
 Dementia
 Community

Citation: Graff MJ, Vernooij-Dassen MJ, Thijsson M, et al. Community based occupational therapy for patients with dementia and their care givers: randomized controlled trial. *BMJ* 2006;333(7580):1196-1201 (PMID 17114212)

Summary of Study:
Design: Randomized controlled trial
Sample: Patients were recruited from memory clinics and day clinics of a geriatrics department in one region of the Netherlands. A total of 135 patients ≥ 65 years of age who had mild-to-moderate dementia were living in the community and were visited by caregivers at least once weekly. Exclusion criteria included depression, severe behavioral symptoms, severe illness, and < 3 months of treatment with the same dose of a cholinesterase inhibitor or memantine.
Intervention: Patients were randomly assigned to 10 1-hour sessions of OT at home over 5 weeks (n=68) or no OT (n=67), stratified by mild or moderate dementia. Assessors were blind to group allocation. First four sessions focused on evaluation of options and goal setting. In remaining sessions, patients were taught to optimize strategies to improve ADLs, and caregivers were trained in supervisory, problem solving, and coping strategies. OTs were experienced in the use of client-centered guidelines for patients with dementia.
Outcome Measures: Patients were assessed for motor and process skills and deterioration of ADLs. Caregivers were assessed for sense of competence. All measurements utilized standardized tools. Assessments were made at baseline, 6 weeks, and 12 weeks.
Data Analysis: Intention to treat analysis was applied at 12 weeks (78% retention), with last observation carried forward. Analysis of covariance was applied with age, sex, and baseline scores as covariates.
The Evidence
At 6 and 212 weeks, patients in the OT group had better motor and process skills and less deterioration in ADL, and caregivers in the OT group had higher competence scores than the non-OT group.

% Improved	Process skills		Motor skills		Caregiver competence	
	6 weeks	12 weeks	6 weeks	12 weeks	6 weeks	12 weeks
OT Group	84%	75%	78%	82%	58%	48%
Control Group	9%	9%	12%	10%	18%	24%
NNT (95% CI)	1.3 (1.2 to 1.4)	1.5 (1.4 to 1.6)	1.5 (1.4 to 1.6)	1.4 (1.3 to 1.5)	2.5 (1.3 to 2.7)	4.2 (4.0 to 4.4)

Table 36-7	**Format for a Critically Appraised Topic on Intervention—cont'd**

Comments

- Randomized block design provided good control over bias, including assessor blinding.
- Sample may have limited generalizability because of recruitment from specific outpatient clinics, eliminating general practice and other institutions.
- Outcomes were based on selected tasks and goals developed with the OT. It is not clear if these tasks were measured at baseline, which could inflate the beneficial effects. However, targeting goals that are personalized and important to the patient and caregiver makes the difference in effect sizes more meaningful.
- Inclusion of caregiver perceptions of confidence provide an important context for evaluating the success of the program.
- Results can be generalized only to patients who are already stable on cholinesterase inhibitors at the outset. The benefits of intervention are, therefore, in addition to those of the medication. It is not known how these strategies will work in the absence of such medication.
- NNTs are quite low with narrow confidence intervals, indicating this should be an effective intervention.
- OTs trained in providing community-based support can effectively improve function of those with dementia and confidence of their caregivers following a 10-week program.

Using CATs for Clinical Decision-Making

The utility of CATs will depend on the clinician's ability to readily access the information within the clinical setting. Wyer[16] suggests that CATs may serve to make the results of journal clubs or case conferences available to clinical staff to improve the care of subsequent patients (see Box 36-1). He offers the perspective that building such bridges and making them available at the point of care should be an essential part of evidence-based practice. Many institutions have established online "CAT Banks" that provide ready access to summaries of articles on specific topics.[23-26]

Links to several CAT databases are provided in the *Chapter 36 Supplement* under Critical Appraisal Resources. By the way, be careful when searching for "CAT banks," as you will undoubtedly find lots of ceramic banks in the shape of felines!

Limitations of CATs

CATs do have limitations as a source of clinical information. They have a short shelf life as new evidence becomes available, which is why revision dates may be included. Clinicians must recognize that CATs may not represent a rigorous search of the literature, as in a systematic review. CATs are often based on only one or two references and may not represent the full scope of literature on a topic. Their usefulness is conditional on the critical appraisal skills and accuracy of the author. It is therefore the reader's responsibility to determine the relevance of the clinical question, the logic of the search strategy, and the application of validity criteria in the review. It is also important to assess the strength of the CAT

Box 36-1   Join the Club!
Journal clubs have been around since the late 1850s when William Osler, then at McGill University, wanted to keep up with progress in European journals.[27] Today journal clubs are quite common in clinical settings, presenting an opportunity for colleagues to meet regularly to discuss published research that is relevant to their professional interests.[28] Journal clubs are useful for teaching practitioners how to search for articles relevant to their clinical practice. It also encourages clinicians to read and critically appraise articles with colleagues, sharing perspectives and knowledge, and discussing how the research can impact practice. These discussions may focus on a single patient problem, or they may relate to a general area of practice for the group. Although formats can vary greatly, typically the group will choose an article to review, which is made available to all participants who will read it and come prepared with questions or comments. A clinician is identified as the leader of the session, with the responsibility to present the study, reviewing the background to the question, describing methods and their validity, focusing on results and summarizing key findings. The presentation leads to robust discussion by the group regarding the study's quality and the impact of the findings for practice. The journal club provides a nonthreatening way for colleagues to develop skills in critical appraisal and to expand their appreciation for evidence-based practice. Several good references discuss how to develop and run journals clubs, including onsite and online versions.[29-33]

author's conclusions in relation to the evidence provided. Notwithstanding these limitations, however, in the hands of a discerning reader, CATs provide a practical method for sharing evidence to inform clinical decisions.

COMMENTARY

Knowledge is knowing a tomato is a fruit. Wisdom is not putting it in a fruit salad.

—Miles Kington (1941-2008)

British journalist

Being a critical consumer of the literature means that we can make judgements about how we can apply the results of published studies to our patient care. Critical appraisal may not result in a firm decision about the quality of a study. The checklists don't provide a score that tells us which study to use—they only provide the means for us to consider a study's findings, and to determine whether to accept them based on evaluation of validity and relevance. This is a skill that must be developed and practiced. No study is perfect, but that does not mean that we should "tear apart" every study we read—that could lead us to discard important contributions. Sometimes in critical appraisal there is a tendency to be overly critical, finding many flaws, major and minor, real and potential. Most importantly, although we can use guidelines to address the components of a study, it will still come down to the reader's ability to make judgments about the study's validity, and to apply findings within a clinical context.

Because of the nature of clinical research, there will always be some aspects of the design that could have been tighter or cleaner. The important element is whether the limitations in the design are "fatal flaws," making the findings useless. In refereed journals, the articles that make it to the publication stage have been screened, but this does not guarantee the results will be clinically useful. Regardless of the imperfections that exist in the clinical research process, it is our job as evidence-based practitioners to find the merits of the study and decide whether to accept them for our use.

The next step in EBP is integration of the evidence into clinical decision-making, which must then be followed by assessment of the process. Was the best evidence obtained, were articles sufficiently appraised, and did the evidence foster a successful outcome with my patient?

The task of critical appraisal can be fostered by reading systematic reviews, in which studies have been appraised and summarized by others in a "systematic" way to reflect the state of knowledge on a particular topic. Reviews may not be comprehensive, however, and it is not unusual to find that many of the reviewed studies are not methodologically sound for various reasons. We cannot blindly depend on systematic reviews to offer those judgments, making critical appraisal skills that much more important for our own evidence-based practice. We head there next, to discuss systematic reviews and how we can use them most effectively.

REFERENCES

1. Dysart AM, Tomlin GS. Factors related to evidence-based practice among U.S. occupational therapy clinicians. *Am J Occup Ther* 2002;56(3):275-284.
2. Sadeghi-Bazargani H, Tabrizi JS, Azami-Aghdash S. Barriers to evidence-based medicine: a systematic review. *J Eval Clin Pract* 2014;20(6):793-802.
3. Scurlock-Evans L, Upton P, Upton D. Evidence-based practice in physiotherapy: a systematic review of barriers, enablers and interventions. *Physiotherapy* 2014;100(3):208-219.
4. Centre for Evidence-Based Medicine. OCEBM Levels of Evidence. Available at http://www.cebm.net/ocebm-levels-of-evidence/. Accessed April 28, 2017.
5. Daly J, Willis K, Small R, Green J, Welch N, Kealy M, Hughes E. A hierarchy of evidence for assessing qualitative health research. *J Clin Epidemiol* 2007;60(1):43-49.
6. Kavanagh BP. The GRADE system for rating clinical guidelines. *PLoS medicine* 2009;6(9):e1000094-e1000094.
7. Li G, Abbade LPF, Nwosu I, Jin Y, Leenus A, Maaz M, Wang M, Bhatt M, Zielinski L, Sanger N, et al. A scoping review of comparisons between abstracts and full reports in primary biomedical research. *BMC Med Res Methodol* 2017;17(1):181.
8. Jellison S, Roberts W, Bowers A, Combs T, Beaman J, Wayant C, Vassar M. Evaluation of spin in abstracts of papers in psychiatry and psychology journals. *BMJ Evid Based Med* 2019:10.1136/bmjebm-2019-111176.
9. Assem Y, Adie S, Tang J, Harris IA. The over-representation of significant p values in abstracts compared to corresponding full texts: A systematic review of surgical randomized trials. *Contemp Clin Trials Commun* 2017;7:194-199.
10. Equator Network. Enhancing the Quality and Transparency of Health Research. Available at http://www.equator-network.org/. Accessed April 3, 2019.
11. Romain PL. Conflicts of interest in research: looking out for number one means keeping the primary interest front and center. *Curr Rev Musculoskelet Med* 2015;8(2):122-127.
12. Ryan F, Coughlan M, Cronin P. Step-by-step guide to critiquing research. Part 2: Qualitative research. *Br J Nurs* 2007;16(12):738-744.
13. Walsh D, Downe S. Appraising the quality of qualitative research. *Midwifery* 2006;22(2):108-119.

14. Sandelowski M. Sample size in qualitative research. *Res Nurs Health* 1995;18(2):179-183.

15. Palaganas EC, Sanchez MC, Molintas MP, Caricativo RD. Reflexivity in qualitative research: A journey of learning. *Qual Report* 2017;22(2):426-438. Available at https://nsuworks. nova.edu/tqr/vol422/iss422/425. Accessed March 4, 2019.

16. Wyer PC. The critically appraised topic: closing the evidence-transfer gap. *Ann Emerg Med* 1997;30(5):639-640.

17. Fetters L, Figueiredo EM, Keane-Miller D, McSweeney DJ, Tsao CC. Critically appraised topics. *Pediatr Phys Ther* 2004;16(1):19-21.

18. Johnson CJ. Getting started in evidence-based practice for childhood speech-language disorders. *Am J Speech Lang Pathol* 2006;15(1):20-35.

19. Straus SE, Glasziou P, Richardson WS, Haynes RB, Pattani R, Veroniki AA. *Evidence-Based Medicine: How to Practice and Teach EBM*. 5th ed. London: Elsevier; 2019.

20. Sadigh G, Parker R, Kelly AM, Cronin P. How to write a critically appraised topic (CAT). *Acad Radiol* 2012;19(7):872-888.

21. Kelly AM, Cronin P. How to perform a critically appraised topic: part 1, ask, search, and apply. *AJR Am J Roentgenol* 2011; 197(5):1039-1047.

22. Centre for Evidence-Based Medicine. CATMaker and EBMN calculators. Available at https://www.cebm.net/2014/06/catmaker-ebm-calculators/. Accessed March 27, 2019.

23. University of British Columbia. Critically appraised topics (CATs). Rehabilitation Science Online Programs. Available at http://www.mrsc.ubc.ca/site_page.asp?pageid=98. Accessed March 27, 2019.

24. University of Texas Health Science Center. Welcome to CATs library. Available at https://cats.uthscsa.edu/. Accessed August 20, 2019.

25. University of Oklahoma Health Sciences Center College of Allied Health. Crtically appraised topic. Available at https://alliedhealth.ouhsc.edu/Departments/Rehabilitation-Sciences/Critically-Appraised-Topics-CAT. Accessed August 20, 2019.

26. Pacific University. School of Occupational Therapy CATS. Available at https://commons.pacificu.edu/otcats/. Accessed March 27, 2019.

27. Cushing H. *The Life of Sir William Osler*. Oxford: Clarendon Press; 1925.

28. Aronson JK. Journal Clubs: 1. Origins. *Evid Based Med* 2017; 22(6):231.

29. Johnson A, Thornby KA, Ferrill M. Critical appraisal of biomedical literature with a succinct journal club template: the ROOTs format. *Hosp Pharm* 2017;52(7):488-495.

30. Ellington AL. Insights gained from an online journal club for fieldwork educators. *Occup Ther Health Care* 2018;32(1):72-78.

31. Szucs KA, Benson JD, Haneman B. Using a guided journal club as a teaching strategy to enhance learning skills for evidence-based practice. *Occup Ther Health Care* 2017;31(2):143-149.

32. Chan TM, Thoma B, Radecki R, Topf J, Woo HH, Kao LS, Cochran A, Hiremath S, Lin M. Ten steps for setting up an online journal club. *J Contin Educ Health Prof* 2015;35(2):148-154.

33. Bowles P, Marenah K, Ricketts D, Rogers B. How to prepare for and present at a journal club. *Br J Hosp Med (Lond)* 2013;74 Suppl 10:C150-152.

Synthesizing Literature: Systematic Reviews and Meta-Analyses

—with David Scalzitti

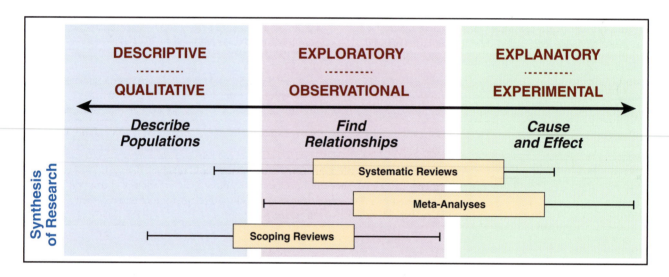

In seeking the evidence on which to base clinical practice, we are faced with myriad published papers and websites, often offering unclear or conflicting information regarding the choice of interventions, diagnostic tools, or expectations of outcomes. We also face the need to critically appraise these studies to determine how well they support clinical decisions—a potentially overwhelming task when the number of studies is large (see Chapter 36). Any single study, even if well-designed, is essentially a form of tentative evidence, which needs confirmation by additional research. Therefore, researchers and practitioners benefit from syntheses of literature that summarize and critique published studies.

Systematic reviews present comprehensive information regarding findings from several sources with an analysis of the methodological quality of the studies. Reviews can be extended by pooling data from several studies in a process of meta-analysis, which presents collective statistical measures of effect size. A more recent contribution to synthesis is the scoping review, which is a broader and less structured approach that offers assessment of emerging evidence.

The purpose of this chapter is to describe the process of synthesizing literature, how reviews are developed and written, and how data can be presented and interpreted. Because searching for published studies is an important part of synthesis, reviewing the content in Chapter 6 will be useful.

■ Purpose of Systematic Reviews

Systematic reviews are a form of research using a rigorous process of searching, appraising, and summarizing existing information on a selected topic. The procedures for conducting the review are intended to be inclusive of the body of research evidence at the time the review is undertaken. Varied types of reviews can serve different purposes (see Table 37-1). Reviews are most commonly focused on the effectiveness of interventions but can be used to address the accuracy of diagnostic and measurement tools, to identify prognostic or risk factors, and to develop recommendations for clinical practice guidelines.[1,2] Results provide a structured approach

Table 37-1 Types of Evidence Synthesis	
SYSTEMATIC REVIEWS/META-ANALYSES	
Systematic Review	A summary of the medical literature that uses explicit methods to perform a thorough literature search and critical appraisal of individual studies.
Meta-Analysis	A statistical technique to pool results of valid studies within a systematic review. Analysis of intervention studies involves differences between treatment and comparison intervention. Analysis of diagnostic or prognostic factors can include risk estimates.
Overview	A systematic review that synthesizes systematic reviews on the same topic. Does not appraise individual trials.[8]
Network Meta-Analysis	A systematic review with meta-analysis that assesses the relative effectiveness of two treatments when they have not been compared directly in a randomized trial but have each been compared to other treatments. Allows for estimation of heterogeneity in evidence from different pairs of treatments.[9]
Rapid Review	A form of evidence synthesis that may provide more timely information for decision making compared with standard systematic reviews.[10]
Living Systematic Review	A systematic review which is continuously updated to incorporate evidence as it becomes available. Generally lives online.[11]
Mixed Methods Review	A systematic review that combines findings from both quantitative and qualitative studies.
Scoping Review	Exploratory assessments of available literature on a broad topic.
GUIDELINES	
Clinical Practice Guideline	Statements that include recommendations to optimize patient care, informed by a systematic review of evidence and an assessment of the benefits and harms of alternative care options. Also called an evidence-based practice guideline.[1]
Outcome-Based Practice Guideline	An evidence-based clinical practice guideline that includes a measure of the effectiveness of the guideline to determine if the recommendation has improved the quality of care.[12]
Preference-Based Practice Guideline	An evidence-based clinical practice guideline that combines patient preferences for possible outcomes of the intervention.[13]
Expert-Based Practice Guideline	A practice guideline that is based primarily on the opinion of experts in the field, which may or may not be evidence-based. Also called a consensus-based guideline.

to examining data to inform practitioners in their decisions to maintain, alter, or discard methods of clinical practice and to aid researchers in designing further research.

The key word "systematic" differentiates this process from the time-honored "review" article. Traditional narrative literature reviews are a good source of background information, but they do not include a comprehensive search, detailed description of review methods, criteria used to select articles, or documented evaluation of study validity. They can also be subject to bias because authors may use their own clinical perspective that may not represent the breadth of information available.

Methods for conducting systematic reviews have been standardized through the efforts of the international Cochrane Collaboration (see Box 37-1).[3] Guidelines for reporting systematic reviews and meta-analyses are included in the *Preferred Reporting Items for Systematic Reviews and Meta-Analyses* (PRISMA) checklist.[4]

 See the *Chapter 37 Supplement* for the full PRISMA checklist and links to its extensions.

Box 37-1   The Cochrane Legacy

The impetus for developing the current procedures for systematic reviews in healthcare can be traced to a 1979 letter written by Archie Cochrane (1908-1988), a British physician who suggested that a critical summary of randomized clinical trials was needed in medical specialties to provide a reliable source of evidence for medical care.[5] In 1993, The *Cochrane Collaboration* was initiated in his honor, creating an international not-for-profit organization dedicated to dissemination of systematic reviews to ensure quality of evidence through critical analysis. Twelve Cochrane Centres, located in countries around the world, take responsibility for supporting members through training and coordinating review activities.

Rigorous standards have been developed to ensure that these reviews provide accurate and thorough appraisals of the literature with frequent updates. The *Cochrane Handbook for Systematic Reviews of Interventions* is a detailed reference for writing systematic reviews that can be accessed online.[3] The Collaboration also provides a software program, *RevMan*, for users to create systematic reviews as well as tables, graphs, and figures for meta-analysis.[6] The Cochrane Library includes a number of other databases, including information on methodologic studies, technology assessment, and economic evaluations.[7] One specialized database, the Cochrane Central Register of Controlled Trials, is an inventory of high quality clinical trials that are likely to be eligible for inclusion in a systematic review.

Archie Cochrane's legacy will continue to have far-reaching effects on the quality of evidence-based practice around the world.

 Systematic reviews are team efforts, and at minimum should include persons with relevant expertise in the clinical content and research methodology. A research librarian is an invaluable resource. This team should be organized early in the process of developing a systematic review and may undergo training to ensure reliability of their critical appraisal skills.

■ The Research Question

A systematic review includes the same sections as other research reports, with an introduction followed by methods, results, and discussion (see Fig. 37-1). Like any other research study, it begins with the statement of and rationale for the research question. This question serves as the foundation for locating relevant references for the review, and as a guide to drawing conclusions.

Types of Research Questions

Systematic reviews can focus on several types of clinical questions. The PICO format helps to frame the questions, just as it does for individual studies (see Chapter 5). For interventions, the question should include population characteristics, intervention and comparisons, and outcome measures.

> *Spinal manipulative therapy (SMT) is a common treatment option for patients with acute low back pain. However, results of RCTs have not provided consistent findings about the effectiveness of SMT. Paige et al[14] did a systematic review to evaluate the effectiveness and harms of SMT compared with sham or usual care to reduce pain in patients with acute (≤ 6 weeks) low back pain.*

A question about diagnostic accuracy should specify the target condition, index test(s), reference standard, and outcomes.

> *Ankle decision rules have been developed to reduce the number of radiographs of the ankle and foot. Although three systematic reviews have examined the accuracy of the Ottawa Ankle and Foot Rules, none had yet compared several available tests. Barelds et al[15] did a systematic review to compare the accuracy of six clinical decision rules intended to exclude ankle fractures in the emergency department.*

Questions about prognosis require identifying the population, prognostic factors, and outcomes of interest.

> *With rising incidence and decreased mortality associated with breast cancer, more survivors are faced with pain as a sequela of treatment. Leysen et al[16] conducted a systematic review to investigate which risk factors were associated*

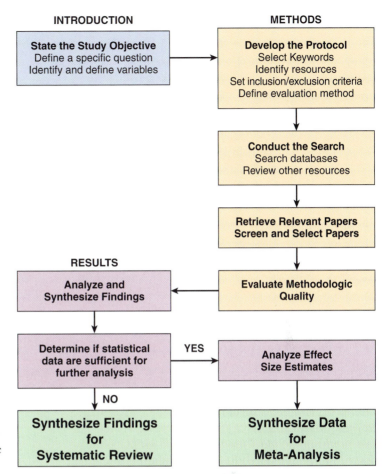

Figure 37–1 Components of the systematic review process, showing the distinction between systematic reviews and meta-analyses.

with the development of chronic pain in breast cancer survivors who were at least 6 months post-treatment.

Systematic reviews can also address qualitative research, to explore patient experiences related to their care.[17] One Cochrane Review Group is dedicated to developing methods for critical analysis of qualitative studies as well as an appreciation for the role of qualitative studies in evidence-based practice.

Traumatic spinal cord injury (SCI) impacts an individual's return to the community and to paid employment. Hilton et al[18] published a systematic review to answer the question, "What are the barriers and facilitators influencing peoples experience of return to work following SCI?" They reviewed qualitative studies that investigated themes related to personal and environmental factors.

Background and Research Rationale

The justification for a systematic review is based on a review of literature to examine the current state of knowledge in an area of interest. This background typically includes epidemiologic or demographic data to demonstrate the prevalence of the condition being studied and its health impact. Information on etiology, pathophysiology, variations in treatment options and their effectiveness, and conflicting ideas about patient management provide a rationale for the review question. The background should also include findings of any existing systematic reviews and make a valid case as to why a new or updated review is needed.

▶ **CASE IN POINT #1**

Motor skills are fundamental to childhood development. However, the effectiveness of treatment options for children with mild to moderate movement disorders is not clear. Lucas et al[20] conducted a systematic review to investigate the effectiveness of conservative interventions to improve gross motor skills in children with a range of neurodevelopmental disorders.

See the *Chapter 37 Supplement* for the full article by Lucas et al[20] along with their supplemental materials including search strategy, lists of included and excluded studies, forms for data collection, and forest and funnel plots.

■ Methods

The methods section of a systematic review specifies criteria for choosing studies to include in the review, describes the process of searching for references, and how these studies were evaluated. Whereas in primary studies, researchers specify characteristics of subjects that will determine who will be chosen to participate in a study, in a systematic review, the "subjects" are the studies themselves. Therefore, "selection" criteria specify inclusion and exclusion requirements for studies to be eligible for the review. These include study design, description of participants, and definitions of interventions and outcomes. These requirements must be clearly stipulated prior to searching the literature to facilitate transparency and consistency in the selection process.

Selection Criteria

Study Design

The classification of levels of evidence for research delineates the types of studies that are considered strongest for drawing conclusions about interventions, diagnostic tools, prognosis, harm, and screening (see Chapter 5, Table 5-4). These levels act as a guide to decide which studies should be included in a systematic review. Many authors restrict systematic reviews of interventions to the "gold standard" of RCTs published in peer-reviewed journals. When the literature is replete with RCTs on a particular topic, this may be an effective strategy. However, when published work is less robust or when randomized trials on the topic are not feasible, the researcher may find that using studies at lower levels of evidence is necessary. Quasi-experimental studies, observational cohort or case-control studies, and case series can also be valuable for understanding the scope of knowledge about an intervention. The decision to broaden the scope to include nonrandomized designs into a systematic review of an intervention should be determined in advance of conducting the search.

> ▶ The motor skills study restricted the systematic review to RCTs, quasi-randomized controlled trials, and randomized crossover trials. They also included conference abstracts and clinical trials registered with international registries.

Selection criteria for studies of prognosis or diagnosis will focus on observational designs, and would have to specify inclusion criteria such as prospective or retrospective studies, including case-control, cohort, or cross-sectional designs.

Participants

The population of interest must be specified to identify the types of participants or patients recruited in the chosen studies. Characteristics may include age range, gender, or specific diagnostic categories. Case definitions should be specified. Settings from which participants are recruited should be described if relevant. Because participant characteristics can vary widely across studies, systematic reviews should set reasonably broad criteria that can reflect the type of individuals to whom the intervention would apply.

> ▶ In the study of gross motor skills, researchers included studies with participants between 3 to 18 years who had neurological conditions that affect coordinated movement such as fetal alcohol syndrome, cerebral palsy, low birth weight, and acquired brain injury, among others. They excluded studies that included participants with genetic disorders, hearing or visual impairments, or intellectual disability.

Interventions

Selection criteria must include definitions of the interventions and comparison treatments. It is virtually impossible to find studies that applied interventions in exactly the same way, so these definitions are generally broad enough to allow a reasonable match.

> ▶ The motor skills study defined intervention as any nonpharmacological or non-surgical therapy that had the intent of improving gross motor performance. Treatment could be carried out in home, community, or school-based settings and had to be delivered by a trained healthcare professional such as a physical or occupational therapist. Comparison treatments could include no treatment, placebo, waiting list or usual therapy.

If relevant to conclusions, interventions can be restricted to a certain duration of treatment or length of follow-up. This will limit the number of acceptable studies but may be important for considering the optimal dose of the intervention and the duration of the treatment effect. For systematic reviews of diagnosis and prognosis, criteria for inclusion of the index tests and risk factors need to be defined.

Outcome Measures

Outcomes include measurements or endpoints, including improvement in condition or reduction of symptoms. In studies of risk, outcomes may relate to onset or prevention of disease or other conditions. Reviewers may specify that studies use particular instruments, such as a health status questionnaire or a diagnostic test. Researchers may require specific primary outcomes and allow for a variety of secondary outcomes. The actual tools used to measure outcomes may be different across studies, but they should all be assessing the same construct. When doing a review for a meta-analysis, researchers may also restrict studies to those that report results using specific statistical outcomes, such as means and confidence intervals, number needed to treat (NNT), risk ratios, or measures of diagnostic accuracy.

▶ Lucas et al[20] specified the primary outcome as gross motor performance measured with a standardized assessment tool. Secondary outcomes could include compliance, parental and child satisfaction, or cost.

📌 After the methods for the systematic review have been developed, it is recommended that the protocol be registered. This helps to minimize duplication of reviews and to reduce bias by providing the opportunity to check the completed review against the protocol. For example, the protocol for the study by Lucas et al[20] was registered with PROSPERO, a prospective registry for health-related topics, available through the UK National Health Service.[21]

The Search Strategy

A major component of the methods section is the description of the search strategy, guided by the selection criteria. The goal is to amass a comprehensive list of relevant references that can be considered for the review. Before beginning a systematic review, it is important to locate other reviews on the same topic to be sure your review will contribute new information. Depending on the rate of reporting research on a particular topic, systematic reviews may need updating every 3 to 5 years.

The first step of the search is to specify which databases and search terms will be used. The strategy should include any restrictions on language or dates of publication. For practical purposes, many reviewers only include articles written in English. However, such a restriction may introduce bias, as studies with positive findings are more likely to be published in larger English-language journals.[22]

Commonly used databases include MEDLINE, EMBASE, SCOPUS, CINAHL, and the Cochrane Collaboration, among many others (see Chapter 6). Authors should provide a detailed description of the search strategy and search terms as a useful reference and to allow for replication of the process. For this purpose, the search strategy should have high *sensitivity* to find all relevant references, although it will also retrieve some irrelevant studies. The intent, however, is to be as comprehensive as possible. More than one database should be employed to provide the most thorough search possible. In addition to online resources, hand searching through pertinent journals and reference lists of published papers can help to ensure that the search is complete. It is often helpful to identify a small number of exemplar articles on the topic that can assist in the selection of keywords that can trigger "similar articles" in a search.

▶ Investigators in the motor skills study performed searches of eight electronic databases. They restricted references to publications in English that were published from January 1980 to June 2015. They also performed hand searches of the reference lists of relevant articles, conference abstracts, and registries of clinical trials. A supplement to their article provides details of the search terms used for each of the electronic searches.

📌 Because systematic reviews often take many months to complete, researchers may need to update the search periodically, especially as the final paper is being prepared, to ensure the most recent evidence is included.

Unpublished Findings

Systematic reviews are obviously influenced by the literature that is available at the time the search is performed. Therefore, results can be impacted if relevant data are not published, limiting their access, and potentially affecting clinical decisions (see Focus on Evidence 37-1).

One source of concern is **publication bias**, the situation when researchers fail to submit studies with results that are not statistically significant, or editors decline to publish such studies.[23] Therefore, a systematic review will not reflect the true nature of evidence. This practice has created bias against studies with "negative" or inconclusive results. These studies may still have strong designs and important outcomes but may be underpowered. Because the value of a systematic review is to broaden the evidence *for or against* a proposed outcome, evidence of no effect must be part of the picture. Authors of systematic reviews should make a concerted effort to find these studies by contacting authors directly or by looking at entries in clinical trials registries.

Another concern is the accessibility of **grey literature**, research information that is only available through formats other than customary journals, such as conference proceedings, abstracts, agency reports, websites, theses, or dissertations.[24-26] It is important to balance the desire for higher levels of evidence with the

Focus on Evidence 37–1
Many Shades of Grey

Research has shown that meta-analyses that exclude unpublished data or grey literature can exaggerate estimates of intervention effect, positively and negatively.[27] For example, Turner et al[28] reviewed 74 studies of 12 antidepressant drugs that were registered with the Food and Drug Administration (FDA) between 1987 and 2004. They found that 31% were not published. With four exceptions, they found that all positive studies were published, and of 35 non-significant studies, 22 were not published and 11 were published in a way that implied a positive outcome. In another study, Hart et al[29] investigated the effect of including grey literature, including clinical guidelines and conference proceedings, in 42 meta-analyses that studied nine different drugs. They found that incorporating

unpublished FDA data resulted in lower efficacy of the drug in 46% of the trials compared to results using only published data; 7% had identical efficacy, and 46% showed greater efficacy. One study that estimated harm showed more harm from the drug after inclusion of unpublished data. They concluded that the effect of including unpublished outcome data varies by the drug and measured outcome. However, it was clear that when grey literature was included, the majority of studies in their analysis resulted in substantially different outcomes, potentially leading to serious bias in the conclusions, one way or the other. This influence of grey literature has been supported by the results of several other studies.[24,25] Clearly, the impact of these omissions in the literature can be widespread, as it influences credibility of hypotheses and clinical conclusions.[30]

---

need to find the "best evidence available." Although there is no true consensus, many advocates have recommended considering grey literature to assure that a systematic review is truly comprehensive. Benzies et al[26] have published a checklist to use as an aid in deciding whether to include the grey literature in a systematic review. Items that should trigger its use include complex interventions and outcomes, lack of consensus about outcomes, and low volume or quality of evidence. Many reference sources have emerged to help with this type of search (see Chapter 6).

Screening References

The initial search will yield numerous articles that need to be screened to determine if they fit the selection criteria. The screening process should be clearly described in the review. The first task is to remove duplicate titles, especially important when multiple databases are used. This task may be accomplished by hand but is greatly facilitated by the use of reference management databases.

Even with a careful search strategy, one should not expect that all identified papers will meet the pre-established criteria. Therefore, one or more authors must sort through the titles and abstracts of the remaining articles to eliminate any that are clearly not related to the search criteria. The reviewers should err on the side of caution during this initial step and not eliminate any article where the title and abstract does not provide adequate information to make a determination.

Abstracts may not contain sufficient detail to know if an article meets selection criteria. Therefore, once the list is honed to potentially relevant studies, the next step requires locating the full text. Many articles will be freely available online, but this may also require use of

inter-library loan, purchasing full-text articles, or requesting full text by contacting study.

> Although it may be tempting to filter a search by only references that are available in full-text, this is counterproductive as it will result in less than a comprehensive search and is likely to bias the conclusions of the review authors.

At least two authors should review the full-text citations to determine which articles meet the inclusion criteria. Multiple reviewers are needed to improve the trustworthiness of the screening process. Reasons for exclusion of articles at this stage should be documented and reported in the published review. Titles can be stored in bibliographic databases or in a spreadsheet to facilitate tracking and management of the citations retrieved.

Data Extraction

With a list of appropriate references, the process continues with critical review of the selected studies. As a rule, a minimum of two primary reviewers should independently assess content and rate the quality and applicability of each selected paper or information source, a process called *data extraction*. This information is usually recorded on a *data extraction form*, which includes all of the elements that will be assessed for study quality. Using a consistent and independent process allows reviewers to gather the same information on each study, so that comparisons can be readily made with minimal bias.

Extraction forms include sections for the citation of the study, eligibility criteria, and characteristics related to the PICO question. They also include sections for assessing study quality and extracting data for the study's results. The extraction form should be designed and pilot-tested prior to extracting information from the articles for the systematic review. Sample data extraction forms for intervention studies are available from the Cochrane website.[31] Extraction forms for systematic reviews of diagnosis and prognosis should include the appropriate fields related to these types of clinical questions.

> 📌 Because many interventions are complex, reviewers may consider utilizing the *Template for Intervention Description and Replication* (TIDieR) checklist to standardize the evaluation of interventions.[32-34] This 12-item checklist is intended to improve the quality of description of interventions and comparison procedures in publications. Although the emphasis is on trials, the guidelines can be applied across all types of studies.

Reliability

As we do for all research studies, we want to establish the reliability of our "measurements," in this case the ability of reviewers to be consistent in the evaluation of articles. It is useful for reviewers to assess a few sample papers in a training process to judge their reliability. When disagreements occur, they should be resolved by consensus, by resolution from a third party, or by clarifying the evaluation criteria. A reliability coefficient, such as kappa, can be calculated to demonstrate how often the reviewers were in agreement for each item on the extraction form (see Chapter 32).

> 🜍 See the *Chapter 37 Supplement* for sample extraction forms and a link to the TIDieR template.

◼ Results

The results section of the systematic review will report the outcome of the search and screening process.

The PRISMA Flow Diagram

Clinical trials use a flow diagram to demonstrate how subjects are recruited for a study, indicating those who are eligible, those who drop out, and those who remain in the study (see Chapter 15). In a similar way, a systematic review needs to document the process of identifying or excluding relevant studies using the PRISMA flow diagram.[4] Figure 37-2 illustrates the flow of articles though the steps of selection in the systematic review of gross motor skills.

In order to complete the diagram, accurate records need to be maintained during each step of the article selection process. It should include the number of articles retrieved from the search, the number of abstracts screened, the number of full-text articles assessed, the final number selected for the systematic review, and the

number of full-text articles excluded. When possible, reasons should be reported for the exclusion of full-text articles that were initially assessed for eligibility.

> ➤ In the motor skills study, a total of 3,092 citations were identified through the electronic and hand searches. After duplicate and ineligible citations were removed, 190 full-text articles were screened for eligibility requirements. A standard form was used for reviewers to assess study eligibility (available as a supplement). The final synthesis was based on nine papers.

It is not uncommon to see this degree of elimination of citations because many false positives may be retrieved by the search in order to ensure all the true positives were identified. It is important to have a systematic process for this screening process to facilitate getting through such a large number of studies.

Assessing Methodological Quality

Studies will differ in quality based on their design and analysis, affecting the validity of their findings. Therefore, it is important to consider *methodological quality* when synthesizing several studies, to determine if forms of bias affect the value of results for answering the research question. Whether the designs are RCTs or observational, authors often neglect to provide important information in the research report that is necessary to determine validity. As part of a systematic review, quality assessment will provide possible explanations for differences in study results.

Several tools have been developed to assess study quality for interventions, diagnostic tools, or prognostic factors. These tools are checklists that contain a series of items reflecting essential information needed to judge quality and bias, typically requiring a "yes" or "no" response (some include an option for "unclear"). Some scales provide a total score based on summing the "yes" responses for each study, and may suggest values that indicate poor, medium, or high quality.

There is no gold standard for this process, and many tools and scoring systems have not been validated.[35] Nonetheless, these various tools generally focus on a number of relevant concepts to assess the internal validity of a study and risk of bias. The criteria used to judge quality and the resultant ratings must be described in a systematic review so that readers can evaluate the strength of the reviewer's conclusions. Those conducting the review must be familiar with the operational definitions for each criterion and reliability of their assessments should be established.

We will illustrate this process using two of the more commonly used methods for RCTs, the PEDro scale and the Cochrane Risk of Bias Tool. Assessments for

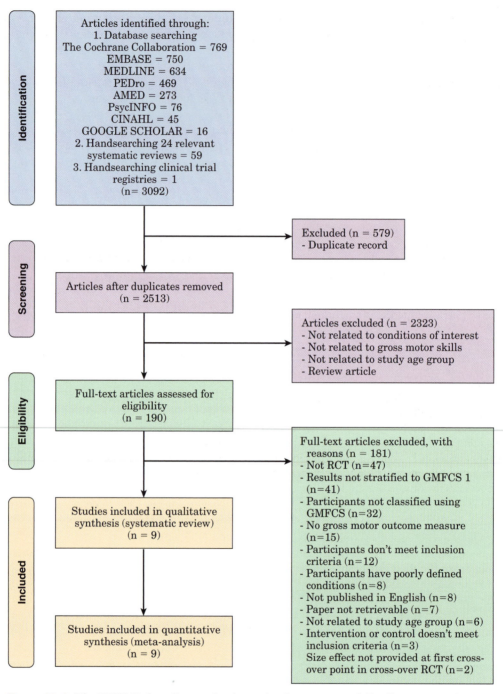

Figure 37–2 The PRISMA flow diagram for the study of gross motor skills, illustrating each step in the process to identify the final selection of studies to be reviewed. Adapted from Lucas BR, Elliott EJ, Coggan S, et al. Interventions to improve gross motor performance in children with neurodevelopmental disorders: a meta-analysis. *BMC Pediatrics* 2016;16:193, Figure 1. Used under Creative Commons license (BY/4.0) (http://creativecommons.org/publicdomain/zero/1.0/).

other types of designs will be described, including diagnostic accuracy, prognosis, case-control and cohort studies, and measurement studies.

> The EQUATOR (*Enhancing the QUAlity and Transparency Of health Research*) Network provides a database of reporting guidelines for many different trial types.[36] Although these are primarily for use by authors to standardize content, these guidelines may also be helpful as checklists in judging study quality (see Chapter 38).

The PEDro Scale

The *Physiotherapy Evidence Database* (PEDro) scale has been widely used in medical and rehabilitation literature to provide a summary score for study quality of clinical trials. Developed by physiotherapists at the University of Sydney, it is based on information reported from the methods and results sections. In addition to items related to randomization, blinding and attrition, the scale also includes items related to analysis of design and statistics (see Table 37-2). Each of 10 items (items 2 through 11) is graded "yes" if the criterion is met or "no" if it is not met or unclear. The number of items marked "yes" are summed, with a maximum total score of 10. The first item listed on the scale relates to external validity and is not scored. The PEDro scale and individual items on the scale have demonstrated reasonable reliability.[37,38] The scale scores may be considered interval level measurement for parametric analysis.[39]

Systematic reviews that use the PEDro scale usually provide the overall score for each study and often show scores for each individual item on the scale. Table 37-3

Table 37-2   Items in the PEDro Scale

1. Eligibility criteria were specified.[a]
2. Subjects were randomly allocated to groups (in a crossover study, subjects were randomly allocated an order in which treatments were received).
3. Allocation was concealed.
4. The groups were similar at baseline regarding the most important prognostic indicators.
5. There was blinding of all subjects.
6. There was blinding of all those who administered the intervention.
7. There was blinding of all assessors who measured at least one key outcome.
8. Measures of at least one key outcome were obtained from more than 85% of the subjects initially allocated to groups.
9. All subjects for whom outcome measures were available received the treatment or control condition as allocated or, where this was not the case, data for at least one key outcome was analyzed by "intention to treat."
10. The results of between-group statistical comparisons are reported for at least one key outcome.
11. The study provides both point measures and measures of variability for at least one key unbecome.

[a] This first item refers to external validity and is not included in the total PEDro score.

Available at www.pedro.org.au. Used with permission. Accessed 17, 2019. Full explanation of each criterion is included in the *Chapter 37 Supplement* and can be found on the PEDro website.

Table 37-3   PEDro Ratings for Eligible Studies in the Systematic Review by Lucas et al[20]

Study	PEDro CRITERION SCORE										
	2	3	4	5	6	7	8	9	10	11	Total
Chysagis 2012	Y	Y	Y	Y	N	N	Y	Y	Y	Y	8
Fong 2012	Y	N	Y	N	N	Y	N	Y	Y	Y	6
Fong 2013	Y	N	Y	N	N	Y	N	Y	Y	Y	6
Hammond 2013	Y	N	Y	N	N	N	Y	N	Y	Y	5
Hiller 2010	Y	Y	Y	N	N	Y	Y	N	Y	Y	7
Ledebt 2005	Y	N	Y	N	N	N	N	N	Y	N	3
Peens 2008	Y	N	Y	N	N	N	N	N	Y	Y	4
Polatajko 1995	Y	N	Y	N	N	Y	Y	N	Y	Y	6
Tsai 2009	N	N	Y	N	N	N	N	N	Y	Y	3
Total Yes Ratings	**8/9**	**2/9**	**9/9**	**1/9**	**0/9**	**4/9**	**4/9**	**3/9**	**9/9**	**8/9**	

Adapted from Lucas BR, Elliott EJ, Coggan S, et al. Interventions to improve gross motor performance in children with neurodevelopmental disorders: a meta-analysis. *BMC Pediatrics* 2016;16:193, Table 4. Used under Creative Commons license (BY/4.0) (http://creativecommons.org/publicdomain/zero/1.0/).

is an example of such a table using the PEDro scores for the studies in the systematic review by Lucas et al.[20]

Cutoff Scores

Some systematic reviews have used a cutoff threshold for the total PEDro score to demarcate high quality clinical trials or to assign ratings of high, fair, or poor quality. However, there is little agreement as to how PEDro summary scores should be used, what score constitutes "high quality," and whether including only those trials in a systematic review will increase or reduce biased results.[40,41]

We must also be cognizant of the differences among scales, understanding that a study judged to be of high quality on the PEDro scale may not be similarly assessed with other methods. It is essential, therefore, that authors of systematic reviews provide an explicit rationale if using a specific cut-off to include studies in a systematic review.

> ➤ Lucas et al[20] used the PEDro scale to assess the nine studies in the motor skills systematic review, Scores indicate that six of the studies achieved a total rating of 5 or higher. The majority of studies did not conceal allocation (item 3), did not blind subjects or testers (items 5, 6, 7), and did not account for missing data or did not perform an intention-to-treat analysis (items 8 and 9).

Cochrane Risk of Bias Tool

Another approach to rating study quality has been developed by the Cochrane Collaboration. The *Cochrane Risk of Bias Tool* explores the risk of bias in each study included in a systematic review, focusing on how the design and conduct of a trial contributes to the believability of the results.[3] The tool includes seven items with defined criteria, allowing the reviewer to provide a judgment of "low risk" or "high risk" of bias, or "unclear." Rather than serving as a checklist or a scale, this domain-based tool presents a visual overview of quality related to seven categories. This image is generally included in each Cochrane systematic review.[6] Using the data from the motor skills systematic review by Lucas et al,[20] Figure 37-3 illustrates how the tool would present their results.

The categories that define risk include five addressing internal validity, one addressing reporting bias (such as publication bias), and a final category representing a judgment regarding other sources of bias such as early stopping of the study, severe baseline imbalances, or claims of fraud. The assessment of internal validity is based on four threats:

- **Selection bias** can distort treatment effects because of the way comparison groups are formed and can be controlled with random assignment and concealment of allocation.

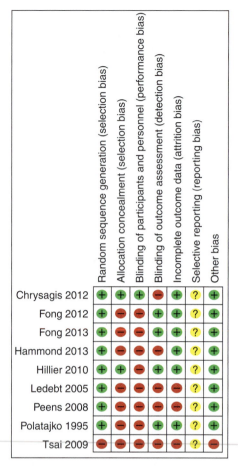

Figure 37–3 Cochrane Risk of Bias domains completed using the data from the studies included in the systematic review by Lucas et al.[20] ⊕ = low risk of bias, ⊖ = high risk of bias and ? = unclear. This figure was generated using *RevMan* software available through the Cochrane Collaboration.

- **Performance bias** refers to differences in the provision of care to experimental and control groups. This is most effectively controlled through blinding of those who receive and give care.
- **Attrition bias** is related to the differential loss of subjects across comparison groups. This becomes especially relevant for studies with follow-up periods and is addressed through intention-to-treat analysis.
- **Detection bias** occurs if outcome assessment differs across comparison groups. Control is achieved by documenting reliability of measurements.

> ➤ The risk of bias tool indicates that allocation concealment and blinding were not used in the majority of studies in the motor skills systematic review. Given the information included

in the reports, reporting bias could not be determined, but other sources of bias were not identified. This approach confirms the same important methodological flaws identified by the PEDro scale.

Methodological Assessments for Other Designs

Studies of Diagnostic Accuracy

The *Quality Assessment of Diagnostic Accuracy Studies* (QUADAS and QUADAS-2) checklist has been developed to assess methodological quality of diagnostic accuracy studies in systematic reviews. The QUADAS-2 consists of 10 signaling questions in four key domains: patient selection, the index test, the reference standard, and flow and timing. This tool does not provide a total score. Instead, reviewers provide judgments of the risk of bias in each domain (high, low, or unclear) and concerns regarding applicability (high, low, or unclear).[42]

The original QUADAS was published in 2004 as a 14-item scale that generates a numeric score based on a sum of items with "yes" answers.[43] The revised QUADAS-2 was developed in 2011, changing the assessment format, but the original scale is still in use.

Studies of Prognosis

The *Quality in Prognosis Studies* (QUIPS) checklist addresses six potential sources of bias in studies that look at predictive prognostic models.[44] The six areas relate to participants and the risk of selection bias, attrition and handling of missing data, prognostic factor measurement, outcome measurement, risk of study confounding, and statistical analysis.

Observational Studies

The *Newcastle-Ottawa Scale Quality Assessment Form* (NOS) has been used to assess quality in systematic reviews of cohort and case-control studies, such as in epidemiologic studies of risk factors.[45] The NOS includes eight items that assess three dimensions: selection of the study groups, comparability, and outcome assessment. Each of the eight items is rated, and receives one star if it receives the highest rating, with the exception of the comparability item which can receive two stars. This results in a maximum score of nine stars for the NOS.[46]

Studies of Clinical Measurement

The *COnsensus-based Standards for the selection of health Measurement INstruments* (COSMIN) is a checklist that considers properties of reliability, validity, and responsiveness to assess the quality of studies included in a systematic review of clinical measurements.[47] A COSMIN Risk of Bias checklist has been developed specifically for assessing the methodological quality of studies of patient-reported outcome measures (PROM).[48] Standards refer to design and statistical methods based on classical test theory and item response theory (see Chapter 12).

 See the *Chapter 37 Supplement* for links to methodological assessment tools used with a variety of research designs.

Data Synthesis

Once the articles of interest have been critically reviewed and data extracted, the researchers must then determine if and how the results of the studies can be summarized and synthesized. This is the final part of the results section. The process is facilitated by using a table to summarize the information obtained from data extraction, including design, description of participants, the interventions, and outcomes. Table 37-4 shows a small portion of such a table from the motor skills systematic review. The specific columns and included data can vary depending on the nature of the question. These tables can be extensive if the systematic review incorporates many studies. Many authors choose to include the score for methodological quality as well.

This summary leads to a judgement about the strength of the body of evidence. How much agreement is there among study findings? This is an assessment of the degree to which studies have similar or dissimilar findings—an indication of *clinical homogeneity* or *heterogeneity*.[49] Relevant factors to consider are:

- Composition of groups, including different inclusion and exclusion criteria, different baseline levels, and the presence of complications or comorbid conditions.
- Differences in timing or dose of intervention or exposure.
- Design of the study, including length of follow-up and proportion of subjects who dropped out.
- Management of patients, including how treatments were delivered.

If papers have published conflicting or inconclusive findings, it can be difficult to interpret the results of the systematic review. It can be helpful to cluster studies that focused on similar outcomes or those that show agreement, to better understand the extent of consistency. Studies with small sample sizes or small effect sizes may show no significant effect of the intervention, leaving the possibility of a Type II error. The choice of measurement scale or tool may affect the sensitivity or responsiveness of measurement.

	STUDY DESIGN	PARTICIPANTS	INTERVENTION	INTERVENTION DOSE	OUTCOMES	INTERVENTION APPROACH	PEDro SCORE
Table 37-4		Excerpt					

Table 37-4   Excerpt of Study Summaries From the Systematic Review by Lucas et al[20]

	STUDY DESIGN	PARTICIPANTS	INTERVENTION	INTERVENTION DOSE	OUTCOMES	INTERVENTION APPROACH	PEDro SCORE
Tsai et al 2009	RCT	From classrooms in southern Taiwan Age: 9-10 yrs DX: DCD $N = 27$ Gender not reported	Table tennis vs regular classroom activities	Intervention ($n = 3$) Three 50 min training sessions per week Control ($n = 14$) No treatment	Primary: gross motor skills (M-ABC, Ball skills, Static/ dynamic balance Secondary: none reported	Task-oriented	3
Hiller et al 2010	RCT	From Minimal Motor Disorder Unit of hospital in Adelaide, Australia Age: 5-8 yrs Dx: DCD $N = 13$ Gender not reported	Aquatic therapy vs waiting list	Intervention ($n = 6$), weekly 30- min sessions over 8 weeks in 1:1 format Control ($n = 6$) Waiting list	Primary: gross motor skills (M-ABC, ball skills, static/ dynamic balance Secondary: self-concept, parent's perception of change	Traditional	7

Adapted from Lucas BR, Elliott EJ, Coggan S, et al. Interventions to improve gross motor performance in children with neurodevelopmental disorders: a meta-analysis. *BMC Pediatrics* 2016;16:193, Table 3. Used under Creative Commons license (BY/4.0) (http://creativecommons.org/publicdomain/zero/1.0/).

■ Discussion and Conclusions

The final section of the systematic review is a discussion of findings and the reviewer's overall conclusions based on the quality and consistency of evidence that was obtained. This can be a complex process if studies have varying methods and results, as is often the case. The reviewer has the responsibility to integrate the findings to clarify the state of knowledge in a clinical context. By comparing studies in terms of their quality and procedures, the discussion will put the results in context with what was previously known on the topic, including other systematic reviews.

The *Cochrane Handbook*[3] recommends the following organization to the discussion section:

- Summary of main results (benefits and harms)
- Overall completeness and applicability of evidence
- Description of overall quality of the evidence
- Potential biases in the review process
- Agreements and disagreements with other studies or reviews.

The focus of the discussion should be on the reporting of overall results across studies and should avoid being a summary of each individual study. Conclusions of a systematic review should propose implications for

practice and research. They may also include recommendations for updating and identification of conclusions which are likely to change with additional evidence. The discussion by Lucas et al[20] illustrates this organization nicely.

Unfortunately, all too often systematic reviews do not come to a definitive conclusion. This may be related to the comprehensiveness of the search and screening process, but is also likely to be a limitation of the available evidence at the time the review is conducted. In that circumstance, systematic reviews play a vital role as a precursor to well-designed studies. A conclusion that additional research is needed may include specific recommendations related to improving study quality, including standardization of interventions and outcome measures.

> ➤ In their systematic review, Lucas et al[20] concluded that their evidence did support the effectiveness of some interventions, but the low quality of the evidence reduced their confidence to adopt these intervention. They were able to identify some forms of treatment that appeared most successful but acknowledged that high-quality intervention trials are urgently needed to determine which treatments and dosages will be most effective. This information is needed to inform management decisions and to guide allocation of treatment resources.

Although rare, a systematic review will sometimes identify findings that are unlikely to change with additional study. For example, a Cochrane review that included data from 1,106 participants in eight trials demonstrated the effectiveness of antibiotics to reduce the incidence of infections after an open fracture of a limb.[50] The review concluded that in middle- and high-income countries further placebo-controlled randomized trials are unlikely to be justified, except in the specific case of open fractures of the fingers. The review did identify there may still be a need for additional research in countries where antibiotics are not in routine use. This example illustrates why many journals require that systematic reviews be cited in the introduction to clinical trials to document that the trial is warranted (see Chapter 3, Focus on Evidence 3-1).

■ Meta-Analysis

Because we are faced with massive amounts of information from primary studies, the ability to apply statistical methods to calculate combined estimates of effects can provide more confidence in the interpretation of outcomes. **Meta-analysis** is an extension of a systematic review that incorporates a statistical pooling of data from several studies that have related research hypotheses. The term was coined by psychologist Gene Glass in 1976, which he defined as the "analysis of analyses."[51] This approach can be used with clinical trials, diagnostic or prognostic studies, and in the assessment of clinical practice guidelines. When studies meet criteria for clinical homogeneity, the synthesis of results can go beyond the descriptive systematic analysis to include a meta-analysis (see Fig. 37-1). When measurements are inconsistent or comparisons do not make sense, systematic review may have to be sufficient to qualitatively synthesize the information.

Meta-analytic methods have also been described for qualitative studies.[52] These studies focus on theory building and synthesis of different methods to explore the conceptual basis for the phenomenon being studied.[53]

Advantages of Meta-Analysis

Meta-analysis requires that selected studies provide common estimates of the outcome variable so that the separate samples in each study can be viewed as part of one larger target population. The major advantage of meta-analysis is increased power obtained by pooling data from several samples, thereby improving estimates of effect size and generalization of findings. Individual studies may have nonsignificant findings because of small sample

size. Therefore, aggregating and pooling data from several studies has the potential effect of increasing the ability to detect important differences. This quantitative approach can also resolve uncertainty when conflicting results occur by showing how different studies contribute to the overall effect.

Effect Size

The concept of **effect size** is central to meta-analysis. For intervention studies this will usually include the **standardized mean difference (SMD)**, which is the difference between group means divided by their pooled standard deviation. This value is the same as Cohen's *d*, which is used as the effect size for a *t*-test (see Chapter 24). Lucas et al [20] performed a meta-analysis on the studies of interventions to improve gross motor skill using the SMD. For observational studies, the effect size may be a risk ratio or a measure of diagnostic accuracy.

Estimates from individual studies are combined to reflect the overall size of the effect of the independent variable. Meta-analysis does not pool subjects into a single sample; rather each study adds to the estimate of the population parameter (the measured variable) by contributing its sample effect size index. The result is usually a more precise overall estimate.

Weighting Effect Size

Because sample sizes vary across studies, their contributions to the overall meta-analysis effect are not equal. A study with a larger sample will contribute a more precise estimate of effect than one with fewer subjects. Therefore, adjustments in the calculation of the effect size are used to differentially weight the contribution of each individual study. The methods for calculating weights are specific to the index used and can be carried out using various software programs, several of which are in the public domain. The Cochrane Collaboration supports the use of *RevMan* software to perform these analyses.[6]

 See the *Chapter 37 Supplement* for a link to more information on weightings for effect size.

Forest Plots

The results of a meta-analysis are usually reported in a **forest plot** that illustrates the weighted effect sizes of individual studies and a cumulative summary (see Fig. 37-4). In this example, the plot lists each study with its intervention and outcomes, and the sample size for intervention and control groups. The result for each individual study is represented by a *tree plot*, which

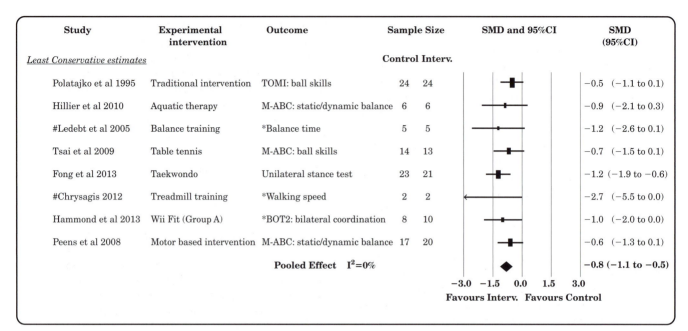

Study	Experimental intervention	Outcome	Sample Size		SMD and 95%CI	SMD (95%CI)
Least Conservative estimates			Control	Interv.		
Polatajko et al 1995	Traditional intervention	TOMI: ball skills	24	24		−0.5 (−1.1 to 0.1)
Hillier et al 2010	Aquatic therapy	M-ABC: static/dynamic balance	6	6		−0.9 (−2.1 to 0.3)
#Ledebt et al 2005	Balance training	*Balance time	5	5		−1.2 (−2.6 to 0.1)
Tsai et al 2009	Table tennis	M-ABC: ball skills	14	13		−0.7 (−1.5 to 0.1)
Fong et al 2013	Taekwondo	Unilateral stance test	23	21		−1.2 (−1.9 to −0.6)
#Chrysagis 2012	Treadmill training	*Walking speed	2	2		−2.7 (−5.5 to 0.0)
Hammond et al 2013	Wii Fit (Group A)	*BOT2: bilateral coordination	8	10		−1.0 (−2.0 to 0.0)
Peens et al 2008	Motor based intervention	M-ABC: static/dynamic balance	17	20		−0.6 (−1.3 to 0.1)
	Pooled Effect I^2=0%					−0.8 (−1.1 to −0.5)

−3.0 −1.5   0.0   1.5   3.0
Favours Interv.   Favours Control

Figure 37–4 Forest plot illustrating the results of the meta-analysis of studies of interventions to improve gross motor performance using the least conservative estimates of group differences. In the final meta-analysis one reference that had used the same cohort as another study was eliminated, leaving eight studies. The # denotes studies with only one outcome measure. The * denotes an outcome where a lower score is better. From Lucas BR, Elliott EJ, Coggan S, et al. Interventions to improve gross motor performance in children with neurodevelopmental disorders: a meta-analysis. *BMC Pediatrics* 2016;16:193, Figure 4. Used under Creative Commons license (BY/4.0) (http://creativecommons.org/publicdomain/zero/1.0/).

includes a small square icon, in this case representing the SMD between groups, and a horizontal line representing the 95% confidence interval for the SMD. The size of the square icon corresponds to the weight of the study based on sample size. The exact values for the tree plot are listed to the right. The center vertical line of the plot represents the null hypothesis, in this case indicating no difference between group means, or an SMD of 0.0. Effect sizes that fall to the left of the null value favor the intervention. The pooled effect size is shown at the bottom of the forest plot as a diamond shape. The width of the diamond reflects the confidence interval for the pooled value.

 When studies involve dichotomous outcomes, effect sizes are usually reported as risk ratios or odds ratios. The central vertical line in a forest plot would represent the null value of 1.0, indicating no increased risk (see Chapter 34). Effect sizes to the left would indicate a decreased risk, and effect sizes to the right would indicate increased risk.

➤ For the meta-analysis of interventions to improve gross motor skills, all SMDs are left of the center line, which favors the intervention. However, all confidence intervals but one cross or meet the center line (they contain zero), indicating differences that would not be considered significant. Only the effectiveness of Taekwondo in the study by Fong et al[54] showed a significant treatment effect. However, the pooled effect size, also left of the center line, does not contain the null value, demonstrating an overall significant effect in favor of the intervention.

HISTORICAL NOTE

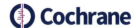

Many will recognize this figure as the symbol of the Cochrane Collaboration. If you look carefully, you will see that the graph between the forward and backward facing Cs is actually a forest plot from a meta-analysis in a Cochrane systematic review.[55] A number of studies had demonstrated that giving corticosteroids to women who are about to give birth to a premature infant could save the life of the newborn. Adoption of this treatment was slow, however, until after the publication of this meta-analysis, which demonstrated a reduced risk in favor of the corticosteroid treatment. Updates to this systematic review continue to support the beneficial effect of this treatment.[56]

Used with permission from Cochrane.

Evaluating Statistical Heterogeneity

Because the interpretation of meta-analysis is based on a pooled sample, it is important to assess the degree to which studies are similar in design and treatment effect. If results are inconsistent or conflicting, it will be difficult to draw conclusions and generalize findings. Measures of **heterogeneity** can be applied to test the null hypothesis that all studies are measuring the same effect based on the similarity of patient populations, types of intervention or exposure, and the outcomes that were measured. One sign of consistency can be visualized in the forest plot by seeing that point estimates and confidence intervals have some overlap.

You will see two statistics reported for this purpose. **Cochran's *Q*** is a weighted sum of squares for study effect sizes.[57] It is tested using χ^2 with *k*-1 degrees of freedom, where *k* is the number of studies. A nonsignificant test indicates that there is a common treatment effect across studies, and therefore the observed differences are what would be expected by chance. A large chi-square value indicates that a common treatment effect is unlikely. Unfortunately, this test is not considered rigorous, as it is sensitive to the number of studies involved.[58]

The *I*[2] **statistic** is used more often and is based on *Q*. It represents the percentage of total variance across studies that is due to true differences in treatment effect rather than due to chance.[57] A value of 0% indicates no heterogeneity, and higher percentages suggest greater heterogeneity. An advantage of this approach is that it focuses on variability rather than statistical significance, and therefore allows comparison across studies that have used different methods or outcome measures and will not be affected by the number of studies being analyzed.

> ➤ The value of *I*[2] for the meta-analysis by Lucas et al[20] was 0%, indicating that heterogeneity was unlikely to be present and that the data were appropriate for pooling. This value is reported in the forest plot at the bottom of the column for outcomes (see Fig. 37-4).

Various software packages will calculate these values and generate forest plots.[59,60] When high heterogeneity exists, authors should consider if it can be explained as a random effect or if the meta-analysis should not be performed.[3]

Sensitivity Analysis

Because there are so many differences in study designs and methods of data synthesis, there is always a question regarding the sensitivity of results of a systematic review; that is, would the conclusion of the review be different if the method of analysis was changed?[3] **Sensitivity analysis** is a technique that assesses if findings change when key assumptions differ, such as examining subgroups of studies that meet different inclusion and exclusion criteria. For meta-analysis this process also involves reanalyzing data using different statistical approaches or accounting for inconsistencies in reporting of results in individual studies.

> ➤ Since a number of different gross motor outcome measures were reported in the studies in the systematic review by Lucas et al,[20] they presented their meta-analysis results in two ways. The *most conservative estimate* was based on the gross motor outcome that demonstrated the smallest difference between the intervention and the comparison group. The *least conservative estimate* was based on the outcome with the largest difference. If only one gross motor outcome was present in a study, it was used for both meta-analyses. The forest plot in Figure 37-4 shows results for the least conservative estimates with a pooled effect size for the SMD of −.8 (95% CI, −1.1 to −.5). However, when the most conservative outcome measures were used, the overall SMD decreased to -.1 (95% CI, −.3 to .2) and no longer indicated a significant difference between the intervention and the comparison interventions. This difference is a potentially important factor in judging the true effectiveness of the interventions.

If the sensitivity analysis does not show substantially changed results, it strengthens findings of the meta-analysis. When the sensitivity analysis leads to a different conclusion, the interpretation should be more guarded. Authors should clarify potential reasons for this discrepancy. In this example, the difference in the outcome measures selected was a potentially important factor in judging intervention effectiveness.

Funnel Plots

While meta-analysis can yield a statistically accurate estimate of an effect of the studies included in the analysis, if these studies are a biased sample of the literature, the calculated effect will reflect that bias. The problem of publication bias, discussed earlier, is especially problematic for meta-analysis because studies that report large effects for a given variable are more likely to be published.

Researchers can examine results of a meta-analysis for this possibility using a **funnel plot**, which is a scatterplot of treatment effect against a measure of precision or variability for each study. Figure 37-5 is a funnel plot from the meta-analysis by Lucas et al[20] based on the least conservative effect size values from each study.

The X-axis represents the treatment effect for each study, the SMD in this example. A vertical line is drawn at the mean effect size, the mean SMD. The Y-axis represents a measure of variance, such as standard error for mean differences, or log(odds) for risk measures. The scale is reversed so that smaller values are at the top (studies with less variance).[3,61] In the absence of publication bias, differences between studies should be a matter of random error, and we would expect to see studies with large and small variance showing up with high and low SMDs, creating a symmetrical plot. In the presence of publication bias, however, we would expect to see an asymmetrical pattern, resulting in a gap in one corner of the funnel.[3]

Visual analysis of the plot in Figure 37-5 suggests a publication bias may be present. While most studies cluster around the mean at the top, there is one data point in the lower left corner, far to the left of the vertical line, resulting in a more asymmetrical appearance. Although funnel plots are more informative with a larger number of studies, we can see that most of the studies had small variability (near the top) with SMDs clustered around the mean. Only one study had substantially larger variability and a lower SMD (lower left). This pattern suggests that other studies may be missing from this analysis. This interpretation is a matter of judgment. There are statistical procedures that can be used to estimate the degree of bias, most requiring specialized software.[61]

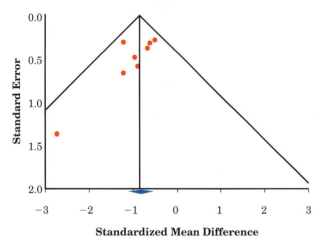

Figure 37–5 Funnel plot showing potential publication bias based on outlier in lower left corner. The red dots represent the individual studies, and the blue diamond at the bottom represents the pooled effect size and its 95% confidence interval. Adapted from Lucas BR, Elliott EJ, Coggan S, et al. Interventions to improve gross motor performance in children with neurodevelopmental disorders: a meta-analysis. *BMC Pediatrics* 2016;16:193, Additional file 5. Used under Creative Commons license (BY/4.0) (http://creativecommons.org/publicdomain/zero/1.0/).

For illustrative purposes, we have focused primarily on data using the *least conservative estimates* for most of this discussion. Refer to the *Chapter 37 Supplement* to see the full-text of the article by Lucas et al,[20] including forest plots and funnel plots for both least and most conservative values, as well as the additional files that are available online. Their discussion does a good job of explaining the rationale behind their analysis.

Grading the Body of Evidence

Authors of systematic reviews and meta-analyses can assess the quality of the body of evidence using the *Grade of Recommendation, Assessment, Development and Evaluation* (GRADE) system.[62-64] Four levels of quality have been defined for studies of interventions, associated with types of study designs (see Table 37-5). Reviews based on randomized trials or strong observational studies are rated high. This rating can be downgraded one or more levels, however, by the presence of one or more of the following factors:

- High likelihood of bias from study design and implementation
- Indirectness of population, intervention, control, or outcomes
- Unexplained heterogeneity or inconsistency of the findings
- Imprecision or very wide confidence intervals
- Publication bias

In rare cases, observational studies with sound methods, large treatment effects, and no bias may be upgraded one or two levels.

> Using the GRADE criteria, Lucas et al[20] downgraded the overall quality of the evidence for their meta-analyses. Even though they included only RCTs, the ratings of methodological quality showed several design flaws, including that few studies used blinding or intention-to-treat analyses, both important controls for RCTs. In addition, the funnel plot showed potential publication bias. Therefore, for the meta-analysis using the least conservative data they downgraded findings to "very low quality."

 Clinical practice guidelines, which provide recommendations to optimize patient care based on systematic reviews and a comparison of benefits and harms of different options, may utilize the GRADE approach in their summarizing a body of evidence for each clinical question.[63] A database of current clinical practice guidelines for healthcare is maintained by the ECRI Guidelines trust.[65] This resource continues the work previously done by the National Guideline Clearinghouse.

Table 37-5	GRADE Levels of Quality of a Body of Evidence for Interventions
QUALITY	**STUDY DESIGN**
• **High**	Randomized trials or double-upgraded observational studies
• **Moderate**	Downgraded randomized trials or upgraded observational studies
• **Low**	Double-downgraded randomized trials or observational studies
• **Very low**	Triple-downgraded randomized trials, downgraded observational studies, or case series/case reports

See the *Chapter 37 Supplement* for links to additional discussion on evaluating clinical practice guidelines and using the GRADE approach to rate the quality of studies of diagnostic accuracy and prognosis.[66-68]

■ Appraisal of Systematic Reviews and Meta-Analyses

Because systematic reviews and meta-analyses are typically seen as the highest form of evidence in a literature search, clinicians must take responsibility for critical appraisal of reviews, to determine if they are valid in their presentation of findings (see Chapter 36). We have to assure ourselves that the authors of the review have done an adequate job of locating, summarizing, evaluating, and synthesizing the information that we will use for our clinical decisions. In deciding to apply evidence from a systematic review to patient care, a clinician should be able to address three primary questions (see Table 37-6), the same questions used to critique all other types of studies: 1) Are the results of the study valid? 2) What are the results? 3) Are the results meaningful to my patient?

A MeaSurement Tool to Assess systematic Reviews (AMSTAR) was developed to provide a more formal appraisal of a systematic review. The original AMSTAR was a checklist with 11 items to critically appraise a systematic review. A new version, the AMSTAR-2, was recently developed and has undergone psychometric testing.[69]

The AMSTAR-2 includes 16 items that are each answered as yes or no but does not generate a total score. This checklist refers to adequacy of reporting in each component of the review, including a clear research question, criteria for selection of studies, a comprehensive search, reliability of reviewers, and assessing risk of bias. For a meta-analysis, it will also include use of appropriate statistical estimates, and evaluation of heterogeneity and publication bias. The appraiser is expected to make a judgment regarding the overall confidence in the results of the systematic review (high, moderate, low, and critically low) based on the number of noncritical weaknesses and critical flaws in the systematic review identified by the checklist.

See Chapter 36 for discussion of critical appraisal. The *Chapter 37 Supplement* contains links to methods for appraising systematic reviews and information on AMSTAR-2.

Table 37-6	Core Questions for Appraising Systematic Reviews and Meta-Analyses

ARE THE RESULTS OF THE STUDY VALID?

- Was the research question clearly stated using components of PICO?
- Were inclusion criteria specified for design, participants, treatment and comparisons, and outcomes?
- Was a thorough search strategy detailed?
- Were reviews and data extraction performed by at least two reviewers using consistent criteria?
- Was the assessment of methodological quality or bias described?
- If a meta-analysis was done, were appropriate statistical procedures used?

ARE THE RESULTS MEANINGFUL?

- Was the result of screening presented as a PRISMA diagram, detailing included and excluded studies (with reasons)?
- What were the results of assessment of risk of bias, and how will these findings influence interpretation of results?
- How was heterogeneity evaluated?
- Were results of a meta-analysis presented as effect sizes in a forest plot?
- Was a funnel plot used to document publication bias?
- Did the authors interpret results?

ARE THE RESULTS RELEVANT TO MY PATIENT?

- Were included studies relevant to my patient in terms of participants, interventions and outcomes?
- Were results consistent with a meaningful effect that will influence clinical decisions?

■ Scoping Reviews

Systematic reviews typically address very specific clinical questions. However, not every topic in healthcare is appropriate for a systematic review. For example, background clinical questions on more general topics and foreground clinical questions with a paucity of supporting evidence cannot be answered by a systematic review. A scoping review plays a different role, mapping the body of knowledge on a topic for which the body of literature has not been comprehensively reviewed.[70,71] It is an exploratory method that is especially useful when an area of inquiry exhibits a complex or heterogeneous nature that would preclude a formal systematic review. Scoping reviews summarize evidence on a topic to describe consistencies or inconsistencies in current practice, to identify gaps in the literature, clarify concepts, and can serve as a precursor to systematic reviews.[72]

> ➤ **CASE IN POINT #2**
>
> Despite an increased focus on patient and family involvement in healthcare, these concepts remain poorly defined in the literature. Olding et al[73] completed a scoping review to investigate the range of literature on patient and family involvement in critical and intensive care settings.

Scoping Review Methods

Although conducted for a different purpose than systematic reviews, scoping reviews do require rigorous and transparent methods to establish the trustworthiness of the findings.[72] Much of the processes associated with scoping reviews are similar to those in systematic reviews, including stating a question and providing background to support the rationale, specifying inclusion criteria for references, describing a comprehensive search strategy, screening citations, and extraction of study characteristics. The *PRISMA Extension for Scoping Reviews* (PRISMA-ScR) includes a 22-item checklist that defines standard reporting items to guide the development and implementation of scoping reviews.[74]

The Research Question

There are some important differences between scoping reviews and systematic reviews, however. One distinction is how the research question is developed. Rather than using a framework like PICO, which is too specific, a broader approach is needed that identifies a context for the study's objectives, which will guide study selection criteria.[75] These may be expressed as a question or statement of purpose.

> ➤ Olding et al[69] set the following objective for their study on patient involvement in healthcare:
>
> *This scoping review investigates the extent and range of literature on patient and family involvement in critical and intensive care settings. The aim was to identify methodological and empirical gaps within the existing literature in order to inform an emerging research agenda in this topic area.*

> See the *Chapter 37 Supplement* for references on scoping reviews, including the full-text article by Olding et al[69] and the PRISMA-ScR statement for reporting guidelines for scoping reviews.

A unique feature of scoping reviews is a recommendation for consultation with stakeholders as another form of input.[70,76] This can include expert researchers, practitioners, and information scientists, as well as patients, policy makers, or health services professionals. These individuals can help to clarify relevant information, propose directions for the search, prioritize research questions, and put findings in context.

> ➤ The research questions that guided the review of patient and family involvement were developed in collaboration with an international group of researchers, physicians, nurses, policy directors, and health services analysts who served on an advisory board for a larger study of interprofessional collaboration and patient/family involvement in intensive care settings.

Methods

Even though questions are broad, scoping reviews must still be focused and precise in terms of their objectives so that criteria for searching can be defined.[75] Scoping reviews use a more comprehensive approach to the search for sources, incorporating clinical trials, observational studies, and qualitative and case studies and may include grey literature. The search can be applied using an iterative process that allows new sources to be continually identified based on obtained information—which is why scoping reviews can take longer to complete. They also provide an overview of existing evidence regardless of quality, providing a map of evidence that has been generated rather than seeking information on a specific practice or policy.[77] Therefore, scoping reviews do not involve methodological appraisal. Findings are generally organized along a thematic analysis.

> ➤ Olding et al[73] established three criteria for study selection. Studies had to be set in an intensive or critical care setting,

address the topic of patient/family involvement, and include a sample of adult patients, their families, and care providers. They searched four databases for English-language literature published between 2003-2014. This time period was purposefully chosen to provide insight into the expansion of literature on the topic. The search strategy included an extensive list of MeSH terms, developed in consultation with a health information scientist. They also examined reference lists of existing literature and consulted with experts in the field to find eligible articles not identified in the search.

The articles identified in the search should be screened by multiple reviewers to determine which citations meet the inclusion criteria. Records should be kept and the screening process summarized using a PRISMA flow diagram.[74] The data extraction process is referred to as charting the results in a table that aligns with the research question. The authors should define the process for collating this information.

▶ In the study of patient/family involvement, two reviewers charted articles by extracting information on study aim, setting, design, and population. They then applied a content analysis to inductively identify patterns in the ways patient and family involvement were described (see Chapter 21). The process allowed them to comment on general trends, address gaps, and thematically describe the components of patient and family involvement.

Results

The results section of a scoping review will report the results of the search and the number of articles selected. This section may be organized according to main conceptual categories that relate to the purpose and to the information charted. A map or diagram may be presented regarding the number of studies that relate to each of these categories, but results are generally described narratively. Results will include a rich description of the major concepts and themes that were identified through the review.

▶ The search resulted in a total of 892 articles. After screening, 124 studies were reviewed: 61 quantitative, 61 qualitative, and 2 mixed methods. The researchers identified components of patient involvement and family involvement involving

participation in care and communication. They also noted that "patient involvement" was not a well-defined concept.

Discussion

The discussion section of a scoping review will be similar to a systematic review in that the results and limitations of the review are discussed. The results are placed in context of current literature, practice, and healthcare policy. Unlike a systematic review, however, the quality of the body of literature cannot be graded. As the body of literature used is more varied, the limitations in the sources should be highlighted. The conclusion of a scoping review may include recommendations for primary research in areas where gaps have been identified or for systematic reviews. Direct recommendations for practice are limited by the lack of formal methodological assessment. Therefore, practice implications should relate specifically to the objectives of the review.[73]

▶ Olding et al[73] discussed knowledge gaps related to patients and families and socio-cultural issues that affected involvement. They identified study limitations related to the time frame of their search and not having looked into grey literature. They also suggested that future research focus on the nature of patient involvement, examination of contextual factors, and interprofessional dynamics that shape patient and family involvement in intensive care settings.

📌 Several useful references are available for those who want to explore scoping reviews further. [70, 71,75,76] The Joanna Briggs Institute in Australia has developed a comprehensive resource manual.[77]

Although scoping reviews are a more recent contribution than systematic reviews, they are quickly becoming more common in the healthcare literature. They are not intended to provide a specific answer to a focused clinical question, but they support evidence-based practice by providing clinicians and researchers with information about the current state of knowledge on a topic. These studies typically focus on areas that are not well understood, creating an opportunity for practitioners to explore how they relate to their practice, and where further research is needed.

COMMENTARY

We are drowning in information but starved for knowledge.

—John Naisbitt (1929–)

American author, Megatrends: Ten New Directions Transforming Our Lives, 1982

The value of conducting and reading systematic reviews, meta-analyses, or scoping reviews cannot be overestimated. It is reassuring that others are taking the time to carry out and share rigorous analyses of the existing literature.

A cautionary note is important, however, as these reviews are not panaceas and may not offer definitive treatment options for practice as much they will help to clarify areas of practice that require further research. In a review of 2,535 reviews from the Cochrane Library, Clarke et al[78] found that 82% of them indicated a need for further evaluation of the interventions studied.

To be useful as clinical references for evidence-based practice, systematic reviews should include transparent high-quality methods and be updated regularly as new data become available. For instance, the review groups for the Cochrane Collaboration are responsible for updates on a regular schedule depending on the currency of the question and availability of additional sources.[3] Sometimes the update will include more recent studies, or it may indicate that no further research has been done since the original review was published. Both types of information are important.

Most importantly, as with any research report, systematic reviews are valuable tools to help us integrate information from many studies—but they are only tools. We must recognize that the results are only as good as the decisions that were made in developing and interpreting the review—which studies were included, how they were analyzed, and the degree to which the information is up to date. The results of reviews with only a small number of references should be viewed with some caution. In addition, descriptions of studies used in reviews are necessarily brief overviews, and do not provide details about interventions or measurements that may be important to a clinician for application to a particular patient. Strong statistical outcomes do not necessarily translate to clinically important ones.

Concerns have been raised that results of systematic reviews and meta-analyses may be misinterpreted or misused by the public and policy makers when the methods are questionable, including the pooling of studies with different populations and interventions that should not be combined.[79] Systematic reviews and meta-analyses represent a vital component of evidence-based practice but will not replace sound clinical decision making.

REFERENCES

1. Institute of Medicine. *Clinical Practice Guidelines We Can Trust.* Washington, D.C.: National Acadamies Press; 2011:266.
2. Scalzitti DA. Evidence-based guidelines: application to clinical practice. *Phys Ther* 2001;81(10):1622-1628.
3. Cochrane Training. Cochrane Handbook for Systematic Reviews of Interventions. Available at https://training.cochrane.org/handbook. Accessed February 8, 2019.
4. Preferred Reporting Items for Systematic Reviews and Meta-Analyses (PRISMA). Available at http://www.prisma-statement.org/. Accessed February 8, 2019.
5. Chalmers I. Archie Cochrane (1909-1988). *J R Soc Med* 2008;101(1):41-44.
6. Review Manager (RevMan) [Computer Program]. Version 5.3. Copenhagen: The Nordic Cochrane Centre, The Cochrane Collaboration, 2014.
7. Cochrane Library. Cochrane Database of Systematic Reviews. Available at https://www.cochranelibrary.com/cdsr/about-cdsr. Accessed February 8, 2019.
8. Smith V, Devane D, Begley CM, Clarke M. Methodology in conducting a systematic review of systematic reviews of healthcare interventions. *BMC Med Res Methodol* 2011; 11(1):15.
9. Lumley T. Network meta-analysis for indirect treatment comparisons. *Stat Med* 2002;21(16):2313-2324.
10. Hartling L, Guise JM, Hempel S, Featherstone R, Mitchell MD, Motu'apuaka ML, Robinson KA, Schoelles K, Totten A, Whitlock E, et al. *EPC Methods: AHRQ End-User Perspectives of Rapid Reviews.* Rockville, MD: Agency for Healthcare Research and Quality; 2016. Available at https://www.ncbi.nlm.nih.gov/books/NBK362006. Accessed April 20, 2019.
11. Elliott JH, Synnot A, Turner T, Simmonds M, Akl EA, McDonald S, Salanti G, Meerpohl J, MacLehose H, Hilton J, et al. Living systematic review: 1. Introduction-the why, what, when, and how. *J Clin Epidemiol* 2017;91:23-30.
12. Owens DK, Nease RF, Jr. Development of outcome-based practice guidelines: a method for structuring problems and synthesizing evidence. *Jt Comm J Qual Improv* 1993;19(7): 248-263.
13. Zhang Y, Coello PA, Brozek J, Wiercioch W, Etxeandia-Ikobaltzeta I, Akl EA, Meerpohl JJ, Alhazzani W, Carrasco-Labra A, Morgan RL, et al. Using patient values and preferences to inform the importance of health outcomes in practice guideline development following the GRADE approach. *Health Qual Life Outcomes* 2017;15(1):52.
14. Paige NM, Miake-Lye IM, Booth MS, Beroes JM, Mardian AS, Dougherty P, Branson R, Tang B, Morton SC, Shekelle PG. Association of spinal manipulative therapy with clinical benefit and harm for acute low back pain: systematic review and meta-analysis. *JAMA* 2017;317(14):1451-1460.

15. Barelds I, Krijnen WP, van de Leur JP, van der Schans CP, Goddard RJ. Diagnostic accuracy of clinical decision rules to exclude fractures in acute ankle injuries: systematic review and meta-analysis. *J Emerg Med* 2017;53(3):353-368.

16. Leysen L, Beckwee D, Nijs J, Pas R, Bilterys T, Vermeir S, Adriaenssens N. Risk factors of pain in breast cancer survivors: a systematic review and meta-analysis. *Support Care Cancer* 2017;25(12):3607-3643.

17. Dixon-Woods M, Fitzpatrick R. Qualitative research in systematic reviews. *BMJ* 2001;323(7316):765-766.

18. Hilton G, Unsworth C, Murphy G. The experience of attempting to return to work following spinal cord injury: a systematic review of the qualitative literature. *Disabil Rehabil* 2018;40(15):1745-1753.

19. Agency for Healthcare Research and Quality. Research tools and data. Available at https://www.ahrq.gov/research/index.html. Accessed February 8, 2019.

20. Lucas BR, Elliott EJ, Coggan S, Pinto RZ, Jirikowic T, McCoy SW, Latimer J. Interventions to improve gross motor performance in children with neurodevelopmental disorders: a meta-analysis. *BMC pediatrics* 2016;16(1):193-193.

21. PROSPERO. International Prospective Register of Systematic Reviews. National Institute for Health Research, National Health Service. Available at https://www.crd.york.ac.uk/prospero/. Accessed February 8, 2019.

22. Moher D, Pham B, Lawson ML, Klassen TP. The inclusion of reports of randomised trials published in languages other than English in systematic reviews. *Health Technol Assess* 2003;7(41):1-90.

23. Pickar JH. Do journals have a publication bias? *Maturitas* 2007;57(1):16-19.

24. Hopewell S, McDonald S, Clarke M, Egger M. Grey literature in meta-analyses of randomized trials of health care interventions. *Cochrane Database Syst Rev* 2007(2):Mr000010.

25. Mahood Q, Van Eerd D, Irvin E. Searching for grey literature for systematic reviews: challenges and benefits. *Res Synth Methods* 2014;5(3):221-234.

26. Benzies KM, Premji S, Hayden KA, Serrett K. State-of-the-evidence reviews: advantages and challenges of including grey literature. *Worldviews Evid Based Nurs* 2006;3(2):55-61.

27. McAuley L, Pham B, Tugwell P, Moher D. Does the inclusion of grey literature influence estimates of intervention effectiveness reported in meta-analyses? *Lancet* 2000;356(9237):1228-1231.

28. Turner EH, Matthews AM, Linardatos E, Tell RA, Rosenthal R. Selective publication of antidepressant trials and its influence on apparent efficacy. *N Engl J Med* 2008;358(3):252-260.

29. Hart B, Lundh A, Bero L. Effect of reporting bias on meta-analyses of drug trials: reanalysis of meta-analyses. *BMJ* 2012;344:d7202.

30. Porter RJ, Boden JM, Miskowiak K, Malhi GS. Failure to publish negative results: A systematic bias in psychiatric literature. *Aust N Z J Psychiatry* 2017;51(3):212-214.

31. Cochrane Collaboration. Available at https://community.cochrane.org/organizational-info/resources/resources-groups/managing-editors-portal/editorialpolicy/editorial-resources-committee. Accessed March 28, 2019.

32. Hoffmann TC, Walker MF, Langhorne P, Eames S, Thomas E, Glasziou P. What's in a name? The challenge of describing interventions in systematic reviews: analysis of a random sample of reviews of non-pharmacological stroke interventions. *BMJ Open* 2015;5(11):e009051.

33. Hoffmann TC, Glasziou PP, Boutron I, Milne R, Perera R, Moher D, Altman DG, Barbour V, Macdonald H, Johnston M, et al. Better reporting of interventions: template for intervention description and replication (TIDieR) checklist and guide. *BMJ* 2014;348:g1687.

34. van Vliet P, Hunter SM, Donaldson C, Pomeroy V. Using the TIDieR Checklist to standardize the description of a functional strength training intervention for the upper limb after stroke. *J Neurol Phys Ther* 2016;40(3):203-208.

35. Olivo SA, Macedo LG, Gadotti IC, Fuentes J, Stanton T, Magee DJ. Scales to assess the quality of randomized controlled trials: a systematic review. *Phys Ther* 2008;88(2):156-175.

36. Equator Network. Enhancing the Quality and Transparency of Health Research. Available at http://www.equator-network.org/. Accessed, April 3, 2019.

37. Tooth L, Bennett S, McCluskey A, Hoffmann T, McKenna K, Lovarini M. Appraising the quality of randomized controlled trials: inter-rater reliability for the OTseeker evidence database. *J Eval Clin Pract* 2005;11(6):547-555.

38. Maher CG, Sherrington C, Herbert RD, Moseley AM, Elkins M. Reliability of the PEDro scale for rating quality of randomized controlled trials. *Phys Ther* 2003;83(8):713-721.

39. de Morton NA. The PEDro scale is a valid measure of the methodological quality of clinical trials: a demographic study. *Aust J Physiother* 2009;55(2):129-133.

40. da Costa BR, Hilfiker R, Egger M. PEDro's bias: summary quality scores should not be used in meta-analysis. *J Clin Epidemiol* 2013;66(1):75-77.

41. Costa LO, Maher CG, Moseley AM, Elkins MR, Shiwa SR, Herbert RD, Sherrington C. da Costa and colleagues' criticism of PEDro scores is not supported by the data. *J Clin Epidemiol* 2013;66(10):1192-1193.

42. Whiting PF, Rutjes AW, Westwood ME, Mallett S, Deeks JJ, Reitsma JB, Leeflang MM, Sterne JA, Bossuyt PM. QUADAS-2: a revised tool for the quality assessment of diagnostic accuracy studies. *Ann Intern Med* 2011;155(8):529-536.

43. Whiting PF, Weswood ME, Rutjes AW, Reitsma JB, Bossuyt PN, Kleijnen J. Evaluation of QUADAS, a tool for the quality assessment of diagnostic accuracy studies. *BMC medical research methodology* 2006;6:9.

44. Hayden JA, van der Windt DA, Cartwright JL, Cote P, Bombardier C. Assessing bias in studies of prognostic factors. *Ann Intern Med* 2013;158(4):280-286.

45. Luchini C, Stubbs B, Solmi M, Veronese N. Assessing the quality of studies in meta-analyses: Advantages and limitations of the Newcastle Ottawa Scale. *World J Meta-Anal* 2017;5(4):80-84.

46. Wells G, Shea B, O'Connell O, et al. The Newcastle-Ottawa Scale (NOS) for assessing the quality of nonrandomized studies in meta-analysis. Ottawa Hospital, Our Research. Available at http://www.ohri.ca/programs/clinical_epidemiology/oxford.asp Accessed August 18, 2019.

47. COSMIN. Available at https://www.cosmin.nl/. Accessed April 17, 2019.

48. Mokkink LB, de Vet HCW, Prinsen CAC, Patrick DL, Alonso J, Bouter LM, Terwee CB. COSMIN Risk of Bias checklist for systematic reviews of Patient-Reported Outcome Measures. *Qual Life Res* 2018;27(5):1171-1179.

49. Simon S. Do the pieces fit together? Systematic reviews and meta-analysis. In: Simon SD, ed. *Statistical Evidence in Medical Trials: What Do the Data Really Tell Us?* New York: Oxford University Press; 2006:101-136.

50. Gosselin RA, Roberts I, Gillespie WJ. Antibiotics for preventing infection in open limb fractures. *Cochrane Database Syst Rev* 2004(1):Cd003764.

51. Glass GV. Primary, secondary and meta-analysis of research. *Educ Res* 1976(5):3-8.

52. Sandelowski M, Barroso J. Creating metasummaries of qualitative findings. *Nurs Res* 2003;52(4):226-233.

53. Timulak L. Meta-analysis of qualitative studies: a tool for reviewing qualitative research findings in psychotherapy. *Psychother Res* 2009;19(4-5):591-600.

54. Fong SS, Chung JW, Chow LP, Ma AW, Tsang WW. Differential effect of Taekwondo training on knee muscle strength and reactive and static balance control in children with developmental coordination disorder: a randomized controlled trial. *Res Dev Disabil* 2013;34(5):1446-1455.

55. Farquhar C, Marjoribanks J. A short history of systematic reviews. *BJOG* 2019.

56. Roberts D, Brown J, Medley N, Dalziel SR. Antenatal corticosteroids for accelerating fetal lung maturation for women at risk of preterm birth. *Cochrane Database Syst Rev* 2017;3:CD004454.

57. Higgins JP, Thompson SG, Deeks JJ, Altman DG. Measuring inconsistency in meta-analyses. *BMJ* 2003;327(7414):557-560.

58. Hardy RJ, Thompson SG. Detecting and describing heterogeneity in meta-analysis. *Stat Med* 1998;17(8):841-856.

59. Chapter 9.5.4. Incorporating heterogeneity into random-effects models. Cochrane Handbook for Systematic Reviews of Interventions. Version 5.1.0 [updated March 2011]. The Cochrane Collaboration, 2011. Available at: http://handbook.cochrane.org/chapter_9/9_5_4_incorporating_heterogeneity_into_random_effectsmodels.htm. Accessed April 21, 2019.

60. MEDCALC. Meta-analysis: introduction. Available at https://www.medcalc.org/manual/meta-analysis-introduction.php. Accessed April 19, 2019.

61. Borenstein M, Hedges LV, Higgins JPT, Rothstein HR. *Introduction to Meta-Analysis.* West Sussex, UK: John Wiley & Sons; 2009.

62. Atkins D, Best D, Briss PA, Eccles M, Falck-Ytter Y, Flottorp S, Guyatt GH, Harbour RT, Haugh MC, Henry D, et al. Grading quality of evidence and strength of recommendations. *BMJ* 2004;328(7454):1490.

63. GRADEpro. Available at https://gradepro.org/. Accessed March 28, 2019.

64. Guyatt GH, Oxman AD, Vist GE, Kunz R, Falck-Ytter Y, Alonso-Coello P, Schunemann HJ. GRADE: an emerging consensus on rating quality of evidence and strength of recommendations. *BMJ* 2008;336(7650):924-926.

65. ECRI Guidelines Trust. Available at https://guidelines.ecri.org/. Accessed April 12, 2019.

66. Brożek JL, Akl EA, Jaeschke R, Lang DM, Bossuyt P, Glasziou P, Helfand M, Ueffing E, Alonso-Coello P, Meerpohl J, et al. Grading quality of evidence and strength of recommendations in clinical practice guidelines. Part 2 of 3. The GRADE approach to grading quality of evidence about diagnostic tests and strategies. *Allergy* 2009;64(8):1109-1116.

67. Brożek JL, Akl EA, Alonso-Coello P, Lang D, Jaeschke R, Williams JW, Phillips B, Lelgemann M, Lethaby A, Bousquet J, et al. Grading quality of evidence and strength of recommendations in clinical practice guidelines. Part 1 of 3. An overview of the GRADE approach and grading quality of evidence about interventions. *Allergy* 2009;64(5):669-677.

68. Huguet A, Hayden JA, Stinson J, McGrath PJ, Chambers CT, Tougas ME, Wozney L. Judging the quality of evidence in reviews of prognostic factor research: adapting the GRADE framework. *Syst Rev* 2013;2:71.

69. Shea BJ, Reeves BC, Wells G, Thuku M, Hamel C, Moran J, Moher D, Tugwell P, Welch V, Kristjansson E, et al. AMSTAR 2: a critical appraisal tool for systematic reviews that include randomised or non-randomised studies of healthcare interventions, or both. *BMJ* 2017;358:j4008.

70. Arksey H, O'Malley L. Scoping studies: towards a methodological framework. *Int J Soc Res Methodol* 2005;8:19-32.

71. Peters MD, Godfrey CM, Khalil H, McInerney P, Parker D, Soares CB. Guidance for conducting systematic scoping reviews. *Int J Evid Based Healthc* 2015;13(3):141-146.

72. Munn Z, Peters MDJ, Stern C, Tufanaru C, McArthur A, Aromataris E. Systematic review or scoping review? Guidance for authors when choosing between a systematic or scoping review approach. *BMC Med Res Methodol* 2018;18(1):143.

73. Olding M, McMillan SE, Reeves S, Schmitt MH, Puntillo K, Kitto S. Patient and family involvement in adult critical and intensive care settings: a scoping review. *Health Expect* 2016; 19(6):1183-1202.

74. Tricco AC, Lillie E, Zarin W, O'Brien KK, Colquhoun H, Levac D, Moher D, Peters MDJ, Horsley T, Weeks L, et al. PRISMA Extension for Scoping Reviews (PRISMA-ScR): Checklist and Explanation. *Ann Intern Med* 2018;169(7): 467-473.

75. Peters MD. In no uncertain terms: the importance of a defined objective in scoping reviews. *JBI Database System Rev Implement Rep* 2016;14(2):1-4.

76. Levac D, Colquhoun H, O'Brien KK. Scoping studies: advancing the methodology. *Implement Sci* 2010;5:69.

77. Peters MDJ, Godfrey C, McInerney P, Soares CB, Khalil H, Parker D. Chapter 11: Scoping reviews. In: Aromataris E, Munn Z, eds. *Joanna Briggs Institute Reviewer's Manual*: The Joanna Briggs Institute; 2017. Available from https://reviewersmanual.joannabriggs.org/. Accessed April 20, 2019.

78. Clarke L, Clarke M, Clarke T. How useful are Cochrane reviews in identifying research needs? *J Health Serv Res Policy* 2007;12(2):101-103.

79. Barnard ND, Willett WC, Ding EL. The misuse of meta-analysis in nutrition research. *JAMA* 2017;318(15): 1435-1436.

CHAPTER
38

Disseminating Research

—with Peter S. Cahn

The culmination of the research process comes when you can share your findings with the clinical and scientific communities. Only shared information can clarify, amplify, and expand the professional body of knowledge. This is the important link between the research process and practice. Without dissemination, evidence-based practice cannot be realized.

Determining the most appropriate format to present your research will depend on the project and your intended audience. Research findings can be developed into a written article, which provides a permanent record that a broad range of professionals may access. Oral reports and poster presentations at professional meetings serve to disseminate research information in a timely fashion, although the audience is limited, and the record of research findings will be found only in abstract form. Graduate students may be required to document their work in the form of a thesis or dissertation but may be given the option of writing it in the form of a journal article. In the digital era, scholarly communication may also occur in nontraditional media. The purpose of this chapter is to describe the process of deciding the appropriate venue for your research study and preparing and submitting the results for publication or presentation.

■ Choosing a Journal

The typical place to disseminate a completed research study is through a peer-reviewed journal. This venue not only assures the widest audience of interested readers but also carries weight in the professional community. With over 28,000 peer-reviewed journals, you will likely face more than one possible choice of where to submit your work.[1] To winnow the universe of possible publication channels, review the journals' aim and scope. Editors reveal that one of the most common reasons for rejecting a manuscript is that it does not fit the editorial mission of the journal. You can search for recently published articles to gain a sense of a journal's mission.

 The *Journal/Author Name Estimator (JANE)* is a free online tool that will suggest possible journals based on a title or abstract.[2] Some journals require subscription while others are online open access. Many print journals also provide options for online or open access publication.

Journal Impact

Despite all the considerations in selecting a target journal, one factor often outweighs the others—reputation, for which several indices have been developed. The most common index is the **impact factor**, also called the *journal impact factor (JIF)*, which measures how frequently a journal's articles have been cited elsewhere in the previous 2 years. *Web of Science*, a subscription-based service, calculates impact factors for thousands of journals. It is considered a reflection of the relative importance of a journal and often influences where certain researchers choose to publish their work. Some journals also report a 5-year impact factor.

The impact factor, however, does not necessarily reflect the importance of a journal within a defined field of study. The 2-year window for citation favors disciplines where discoveries occur frequently and consensus changes rapidly. For example, professional journals in rehabilitation fields often have ratings between 1.0 and 4.0, whereas the impact factor for some the flagship medical journals can be over 50. Lower scores do not imply that those journals are lower quality or less influential. Articles that appear in specialty journals tend to receive fewer citations, but they are more likely to reach an appropriate specialized audience.

The use of the impact factor has become a point of controversy.[3] Its original intention was to support budgetary decisions of libraries, not to serve as a measure of scientific worth for individual studies. In response, editors and authors have introduced several other indicators of scholarly impact (see Box 38-1).

Open Access Journals

The diminished viability of traditional publishing models and the desire to make research findings widely available have triggered the development of **open access** journals, which are distributed online free at no cost to the reader. In exchange for rapid publication of manuscripts for free,

authors bear some of the cost, typically ranging from $1,000 to $3,000 (see Box 38-2).

There are three types of open access:

- *Green open access* means that after an article is published in a traditional subscription journal, the author makes a copy available in a separate repository.
- *Gold open access* refers to journals that make all articles freely available on their website without restrictions.
- *Hybrid gold access* refers to traditional subscription journals that provide an option to an author to publish articles with free access immediately on the journal's website by paying a fee.

There are several types of licenses for open access articles, usually obtained through *Creative Commons (CC)* licensing.[7] Two types are used most often. *Noncommercial open access* (CC-BY-NC) permits only noncommercial reuse, distribution, and reproduction of an article, provided the original work is properly cited and unchanged. *Unrestricted open access* (CC-BY) allows others to use the article for any purpose, including

---

Box 38-1   Making an Impact

In addition to impact factor, journal home pages may also display additional metrics. These are all intended to provide more nuanced data about a journal's reach.

- The *source normalized impact per paper (SNIP)* measures the average citation impact for a journal. It includes all journals indexed in the Scopus database (see Chapter 6). It differs from impact factor in that SNIP corrects for differences in citation practices between scientific fields, allowing for more accurate between-field comparisons.[4]
- The *systematic impact factor (SIF)* is designed to reflect quality of a journal based on criteria such as citations, editorial board, and online resources.[5] Indexing is free but there is a fee for an evaluation to obtain the SIF score. This index is used extensively by international journals.
- The *SCImago Journal Rank (SJR)* is a measure of the number of times an average article in a particular journal is cited. It differs from the impact factor in that each citation is weighted by the rank of the citing journal, thereby reflecting the average prestige per journal article.[6]

Be careful about how you use these scores, however. New indices seem to pop up quite often, being developed by analytic companies or publishers interested in marketing their products. None of them actually provides a quality assessment of the research being published. These factors may be most important for researchers seeking funding and faculty seeking promotion, but depending on the context of the research, they may have less "impact" for evidence-based practice.

Box 38-2   Eyes Open About Open Access

Unfortunately, the benefits of open access and internet publishing have spawned some exploitive practices. "Predatory publishers" or "pseudojournals" are so named because they are aggressive about recruiting research manuscripts and then charging publication fees to authors without providing the editorial and publishing services associated with legitimate journals. They lure authors with lists of prestigious editorial board members (who may not know their names are being used), accept almost all submissions, and mislead authors about impact and readership.[10] Many of these journals have titles and logos that are deceptively similar to reputable journals, easily misleading authors and clinicians seeking sound evidence.[11]

Readers need to be aware of these practices, so they can make judgments about the reliability of evidence. Researchers must be especially aware, as publishing in such journals can compromise the credibility of one's work, and articles may not be accessible through established databases like PubMed or CINAHL.[12] Searching in only online journals for full-text may limit your view of the available literature.

One caveat—some reputable journals do require payment to defray the cost of open access publishing without being predatory. Checklists have been published to help readers discern the validity of a journal, including *Think. Check. Submit,* an initiative that was launched in 2015 to raise awareness and to distinguish disreputable journals from quality, open access journals.[12,13] Guidance is available to help identify the characteristics of reputable peer-reviewed journals.[14,15]

commercial use, as long as it is properly cited with a link to the Creative Commons license and description of what changes were made.

Other useful resources regarding open access include the *Directory of Open Access Journals (DOAJ)*[8] and *Unpaywall*,[9] both of which maintain a database of full-text open access journals.

> 📌 See the *Chapter 38 Supplement* for an example of an open access article. Other examples can also be found in the supplements for Chapters 37 and 38. The terms of the license are noted at the bottom of the first page of each article.

Authorship

Authorship credit is an important element of research publication. It implies responsibility and accountability for the published work. To avoid conflicts late in the process, collaborators should decide authorship before a project begins, including the order in which authors will be credited. As interprofessional research expands, articles are increasingly attributed to multiple authors.[16] The names should be listed in order of contributions. The first author is typically designated as the *primary author*, and the last author often represents a senior researcher who provided oversight to the project.

Most journals require all authors to provide a signed copyright release that includes a statement of their contributions to the article. These may include:

- Conception and design of the study
- Participation in data collection
- Carrying out data analysis
- Writing the article
- Project management
- Obtaining funding
- Reviewing the final paper or other consultation.

Journals may include these disclosures on the first page or at the end of the article.

Criteria for Authorship

The *International Committee of Medical Journal Editors* (ICMJE) has established four criteria for authorship, all of which should be met for someone to be included as an author[17]:

1. Substantial contributions to the conception and design of the work or the acquisition, analysis or interpretation of data; AND
2. Drafting the work or revising it critically for important intellectual content; AND
3. Final approval of the version to be published; AND

4. Agreement to be accountable for all aspects of the work in ensuring that questions related to the accuracy or integrity of any part of the work are appropriately investigated and resolved.

All authors should meet these four criteria, and anyone who meets these criteria should be included as an author (see Box 38-3). The definition of "substantial contribution" may be open to interpretation, but items 2 and 4 have been considered minimum thresholds.[18] Other contributors who do not qualify for authorship should be recognized in an acknowledgment at the end of the document.

The primary author is also usually designated as the *corresponding author*, who will take responsibility for communication with the journal during manuscript submission, peer review, and any other administrative requirements, including IRB approval, clinical trial registration, and obtaining author statements of contributions and conflict of interest information. This person will also be identified on the first page of the article with an email address as a contact for readers.

Standards for Reporting

Replicability is an essential component of evidence-based practice. For scientists to validate and build on the work of others, the research process must be communicated

---

Box 38-3 Taking Credit Where Credit Is Not Due

In 1981, John Darsee was a physician and researcher at Brigham & Women's Hospital in Boston, leading NIH-funded research in cardiology. He had published several studies in prestigious medical journals, studies that had been cited in more than 300 subsequent articles. When it was uncovered that he had fabricated data, nine published studies were retracted as well as many abstracts.[19]

But this isn't solely about one researcher's scientific misconduct. Many of Darsee's colleagues were coauthors on these studies and were unaware of his manipulations of data because they had little or no direct contact with the work that was reported. In some cases they were not even aware that the studies using their names had actually been performed—sometimes not knowing that their names were on an abstract until after it had been published.[20]

Although Darsee avowed that his coauthors had no responsibility for what happened, it isn't that simple. There are inherent responsibilities in assuming authorship, even if one is not directly involved in data collection. Coauthors should be able to defend the research and be confident of its integrity. That is why journals require signed statements with all authors testifying to their level of involvement, assuring that they have had meaningful participation in the planning, design, interpretation, and writing of the article.

with sufficient detail and clarity. To support best practice in publishing scientific studies, many journal editors and researchers have agreed to unified standards for reporting each type of research. The standards provide guidelines for authors so that they will include appropriate sections and information in their manuscripts in a way that can be understood by readers, replicated by researchers, used by clinicians for evidence-based practice, and included in a systematic review (see Table 38-1). These guidelines have been brought together under the "umbrella" of the *EQUATOR* network (*Enhancing the QUAlity and Transparency Of health Research)*, which is an international collaboration that promotes quality and consistency in research publications.[21]

This effort grew out of original work that focused solely on randomized controlled trials (RCT), with the development of the *Consolidated Standards of Reporting Trials* (CONSORT) (see Table 38-2). These guidelines

consist of a checklist and template for a flow diagram to document the selection and attrition of subjects (refer to Figs. 13-2 and 15-2). Several extensions have since been developed that address unique features of specific designs, such as repeated measures, noninferiority, N-of-1, or pragmatic trials. The TIDieR (*Template for Intervention Description and Replication*) checklist complements CONSORT, with guidelines specific to describing intervention.[22] Standards have also been developed for other forms of health-related research, including observational designs, diagnostic and prognostic studies, clinical practice guidelines, qualitative research, case reports, and systematic reviews. These checklists have many items in common with the CONSORT statement. All of these guidelines can be accessed on the EQUATOR website.[21] *Elaboration and Explanation Papers* have been written to clarify each item on these checklists.

Table 38-1	Standards for Reporting Various Types of Studies
Randomized Trials	
CONSORT	*Consolidated Standards of Reporting Trials:* Randomized trials, N-of-1 trials, reporting of harms, pragmatic trials, non-inferiority trials
Observational Studies	
STROBE	*Strengthening the Reporting of Observational Studies in Epidemiology:* Cohort studies, case-control studies, cross-sectional studies
Systematic Reviews and Meta-Analyses	
PRISMA	*Preferred Reporting Items for Systematic Reviews and Meta-Analyses:* Systematic reviews and meta-analyses, scoping reviews, improving harms
Diagnostic Accuracy and Prognostic Studies	
STARD	*Standards for Reporting of Diagnostic Accuracy:* Diagnostic/prognostic studies
TRIPOD	*Transparent Reporting of a multivariable Prediction model for individual Prognosis Or Diagnosis:* Checklist for prediction model development and validation
Qualitative Research	
SRQR	*Standards for Reporting Qualitative Research*
COREQ	*Consolidated criteria for Reporting Qualitative research:* Qualitative research interviews and focus groups
Case Reports	
CARE	*Consensus-based Clinical Case Reporting*
Clinical Guidelines	
AGREE	*Appraisal of Guidelines, Research and Evaluation*
RIGHT	*Reporting Tool for Practice Guidelines in Health Care*
Study Protocols	
SPIRIT	*Standard Protocol Items: Recommendations for Intervention Trials*
PRISMA-P	*Preferred Reporting Items for Systematic Review and Meta-Analysis Protocols*
Quality and Economic Guidelines	
SQUIRE	*Standards for Quality Improvement Reporting Excellence*
CHEERS	*Consolidated Health Economic Evaluation Reporting Standards*

Links to guidelines and extensions can be found at http://www.equator-network.org/.

Table 38-2 CONSORT 2010 Checklist of Information to Include When Reporting a Randomized Trial

SECTION/TOPIC	ITEM #	CHECKLIST ITEM
Title and Abstract	1a	Identification as a randomized trial in the title
	1b	Structured summary of trial design, methods, results, and conclusions (see CONSORT for abstracts)
Introduction		
Background and Objectives	2a	Scientific background and explanation of rationale
	2b	Specific objectives or hypotheses
Methods		
Trial Design	3a	Description of trial design (such as parallel, factorial) including allocation ratio
	3b	Important changes to methods after trial commencement (such as eligibility criteria), with reasons
Participants	4a	Eligibility criteria for participants
	4b	Settings and locations where the data were collected
Interventions	5	The interventions for each group with sufficient details to allow replication, including how and when they were actually administered
Outcomes	6a	Completely defined prespecified primary and secondary outcome measures, including how and when they were assessed
	6b	Any changes to trial outcomes after the trial commenced, with reasons
Sample Size	7a	How sample size was determined
	7b	When applicable, explanation of any interim analyses and stopping guidelines
Random Sequence Generation	8a	Method used to generate the random allocation sequence
	8b	Type of randomization; details of any restriction (such as blocking and block size)
Random Allocation Concealment Mechanism	9	Mechanism used to implement the random allocation sequence (such as sequentially numbered containers), describing any steps taken to conceal the sequence until interventions were assigned
Implementation of Randomization	10	Who generated the random allocation sequence, who enrolled participants, and who assigned participants to interventions
Blinding	11a	If done, who was blinded after assignment to interventions (for example, participants, care providers, those assessing outcomes) and how
	11b	If relevant, description of the similarity of interventions
Statistical Methods	12a	Statistical methods used to compare groups for primary and secondary outcomes
	12b	Methods for additional analyses, such as subgroup analyses and adjusted analyses
Results		
Participant Flow (Flowchart)	13a	For each group, the numbers of participants who were randomly assigned, received intended treatment, and were analyzed for the primary outcome
	13b	For each group, losses and exclusions after randomization, together with reasons
Recruitment	14a	Dates defining the periods of recruitment and follow-up
	14b	Why the trial ended or was stopped
Baseline Data	15	A table showing baseline demographic and clinical characteristics for each group
Numbers Analyzed	16	For each group, number of participants (denominator) included in each analysis and whether the analysis was by original assigned groups
Outcomes and Estimation	17a	For each primary and secondary outcome, results for each group, and the estimated effect size and its precision (such as 95% confidence interval)
	17b	For binary outcomes, presentation of both absolute and relative effect sizes is recommended
Ancillary Analyses	18	Results of any other analyses performed, including subgroup analyses and adjusted analyses, distinguishing prespecified from exploratory

Continued

Table 38-2   CONSORT 2010 Checklist of Information to Include When Reporting a Randomized Trial—cont'd

SECTION/TOPIC	ITEM #	CHECKLIST ITEM
Harms	19	All important harms or unintended effects in each group (for specific guidance see CONSORT for harms)
Discussions **Limitations**	20	Trial limitations, addressing sources of potential bias, imprecision, and, if relevant, multiplicity of analyses
Generalizability	21	Generalizability (external validity, applicability) of the trial findings
Interpretation	22	Interpretation consistent with results, balancing benefits and harms, and considering other relevant evidence
Other Information **Registration**	23	Registration number and name of trial registry
Protocol	24	Where the full trial protocol can be accessed, if available
Funding	25	Sources of funding and other support (such as supply of drugs), role of funders

Source: Moher D, Hopewell S, Schulz KF, et al. CONSORT 2010 explanation and elaboration: updated guidelines for reporting parallel group randomised trials. *BMJ* 2010;340:c869. Available at http://www.consort-statement.org/downloads.

For purposes of illustration, this discussion will focus on standards for RCTs using the CONSORT statement as a guide. However, this checklist serves as reasonable guidance for all types of studies. See the *Chapter 38 Supplement* for links to checklists and extensions for intervention, observational and qualitative designs.

■ Structure of the Written Research Report

Journal articles typically follow the IMRAD format (introduction, methods, results, discussion). As the CONSORT statement illustrates, the elements of a research report require substantive detail. Whichever reporting guidelines you follow, each section should be indicated by headings and subheadings within the article. The introduction provides the rationale for the study, the methods and results describe what you did and what you found, and the discussion shapes the "story," where you situate the research question in a larger context. Together, the sections of the report make the case for the significance of your research and how it advances the scholarly conversation.[23]

The items in the CONSORT statement represents guidelines for the inclusion of needed information. The actual order in which specific information is presented may vary in different articles. The important message is that the information is there and is easy to find.

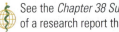 See the *Chapter 38 Supplement* for an annotated example of a research report that follows the CONSORT guidelines.

Title and Abstract

Most readers will encounter the *title* of your study first, so it should be appropriately descriptive. It should include the population or condition, the specific intervention or predictive factors, the outcome, and the type of research or design. Many readers will choose to read an article based solely on the title, so you want to make sure it provides adequate information. One journal estimates that 50% of its website traffic comes from Google, so including keywords in the title that might be used in a literature search will allow more readers to find your study.[24] Limiting acronyms in the title will also attract a wider range of readers. Some journals will restrict the length of the title to a number of characters or words. A good guideline is to limit the title to 15 words.

Research reports include an *abstract* that summarizes the content of the article. The structure of the abstract will be defined by the journal, including such categories as purpose or background, description of subjects, procedures used, summary of the results, and major conclusions. The journal will also indicate a limit on words for the abstract, usually between 250 to 500 words, which means providing a complete but condensed description of the study. To engage the reader's interest in reading further, the abstract should be clearly written and include the key information needed to understand the study.[25] To assure that it accurately reflects the finalized report, abstracts should be written after the paper is completed.

The title and abstract play an important role in electronic searches. Therefore, they must be able to stand alone, despite their brevity. Many journals ask authors to include four to eight *keywords* that will be listed at the end of the abstract, words that can be used as search terms, and may include MeSH terms (see Chapter 6). Keywords also help editors identify appropriate peer reviewers for the manuscript.

> 📌 Studies that have been submitted to a clinical trials registry are required to provide their identification number and date of registration.

Introduction

The body of the article begins with the *introduction*, which usually does not have a subheading. It provides a description of the research question and the specific motivation for the author to answer it. A compelling justification will point to gaps or conflicts in the literature and may include demographics, incidence, or costs associated with the condition of interest. After reading the first paragraph of the introduction, the reader should understand the problem being studied and why it is important (see Chapter 3). A review of literature will follow with a concise description of the current state of knowledge on the topic, referencing recent findings as well as classic studies. Systematic reviews can be helpful in the introduction to provide a comprehensive perspective.

> 🔑 Many journals now require that a systematic review be cited to demonstrate that the author has considered the full range of available information on the topic and that the research is warranted. If the search for a systematic review was unsuccessful, a statement to that effect should be included.

The literature review should reflect the relevant background that is necessary to support the theoretical rationale for the study without providing the equivalent of an annotated bibliography. Citing literature selectively will keep the focus on your research question. The introduction should logically end with a statement of the specific purpose of the study, delineating the variables that were studied and the research hypotheses or guiding questions that have been investigated in the study.

Methods

The *methods* section is the map you followed when conducting your research. The details should be clear enough that someone else could recreate the steps you took in conducting your research. Although the methods section comes second in the study, many authors write it first because it is the most straightforward.

Methods are composed of several subsections, each labeled with its own subheading. The first subsection is

often a description of the *study design*, although this may be included at the end of the introduction.

The next section is typically labeled *subjects* or *participants*. It should begin by explaining how participants were recruited, the setting or accessible population from which they were drawn, and the timeframe for data collection. Observational studies should include how cases and controls were defined. This will be important information to establish external validity. Eligibility should be defined by inclusion and exclusion criteria. Most journals require a statement documenting that subjects read and signed an informed consent form and that the appropriate Institutional Review Board (IRB) approved the project.

The methods section continues with a description of the study *procedures*, the number of groups, the randomization procedure if applicable, and how blinding was incorporated. This section explains how data were obtained, through direct measurement, interview, or observation, or by accessing data from other sources such as medical records or questionnaires. The variables being studied should be clearly spelled out, including the independent and dependent variables, as well as potential confounders that were measured.

Operational definitions of interventions and outcome measurements should be included with sufficient detail to allow replication. If follow-up data are obtained, the methods for contacting participants should be explained. If appropriate, primary and secondary outcomes should be delineated. If the measurement or treatment procedures are standardized and well known, they can be described briefly and you can refer the reader to the original sources for a more detailed description. Description of equipment should include manufacturer and model.

Many researchers develop a written protocol that is used as a guide during data collection to be sure that all procedures are followed properly. This protocol can easily serve as an outline for this section of the report. Presenting procedures in chronological order also helps to create a logical presentation. Diagrams, photographs, and tables can clarify how data were collected. Be sure to get permission for any material taken from other sources and for the use of photographs from patients or participants.

The methods section ends with a full description of the procedures used for *data analysis*, including specific statistical procedures and the accepted level of significance. For intervention studies, a statement should clarify if an intention-to-treat analysis was done (see Chapter 15). This section should include a description of the method used to determine the needed sample size, including level of significance, desired power, estimated effect size and how this value was determined. Procedures for handling missing data should be described. If unique statistical methods are used, they should be explained and referenced. Analysis plans should be clear for each of the specified outcomes.

Results

The *results* section contains a report of results without commentary or interpretation. It is a description of all findings, usually accompanied by a visual depiction of how data do or do not support the specific aims or hypotheses of the study. The narrative should present general descriptions of findings, and the tables and figures will present the details.

The results should begin with the description of the final sample, including a flow diagram showing how many participants were part of the final analysis and reasons for attrition (see Chapter 14). The results usually include a table that shows baseline measures for demographic and clinical variables for each group. Baseline characteristics should be examined and statistical comparison reported to indicate if groups were equivalent at the start. The flow diagram should indicate why attrition occurred, loss to follow-up, and to what extent participants remained in their assigned groups. The results of an intention-to-treat analysis should be described, including how missing data affected outcomes.

Statistical results should be presented for primary and secondary outcomes. Descriptive statistics should be included for each group and the total sample. Means should be expressed with standard deviations (or medians with ranges for non-normal distributions). The outcomes of statistical tests for group differences should include values for test statistics, degrees of freedom, *p* values, and effect size. Observational and correlational studies should include measures of risk or diagnostic accuracy, results of regression analyses, and, if appropriate, present the number needed to treat (NNT) or number needed to harm (NNH) (see Chapter 34). All point estimates should also be expressed with confidence intervals. If expected findings are not significant, the possibility of Type II error should be addressed through a power analysis.

> Sometimes nonsignificant outcomes are referred to as "negative results," which is really a misrepresentation of findings. It means that the study hypothesis was not supported, but this can be useful information! Because this is a statistical issue, it is more appropriate to refer to such studies as having "nonsignificant" findings.

Two major principles guide the writing of the results section. One is that tables and figures should not duplicate the narrative. Refer to the tables and figures for details, but only summarize the details in the text. The reader should be able to understand the results without referring to the tables and should be able to understand the tables without referring to the text. Second, the author should not discuss how this information could be applied to practice or interpret the outcomes—that will come in the discussion section.

Discussion

The *discussion* section is where you will establish the take-home message of the research report. It reflects your interpretation of the results in terms of the purpose of the study and its relation to clinical practice. This part of the article is the least formulaic in format, but it must be logical and focused. It will include comments on the importance of the results, immediate or potential applicability of results to clinical practice, generalizability of findings, limitations of the study, suggestions for future research, and clinical implications.

The discussion may begin with an overview of findings. It should describe the importance of these findings, not simply reiterate the results, with a focus on explanations and interpretations of the observed outcomes, emphasizing how they either support or refute previous work or clinical theories. All results should be addressed, including those that were not statistically significant, explaining how effect size and clinical significance should be interpreted. It is helpful to develop and outline for the discussion, reflecting important points that you want to make about your findings, which can then be compared to the results of previous studies.

The limitations of the study, including possible extraneous variables that could have affected the outcomes, should be identified and their effect on internal validity explained. Some of these factors may have been identified before the study began and others will have become evident during the course of data collection or analysis. These may include a small sample size, attrition of subjects, or lack of subject adherence to the protocol. It is essential to delineate extraneous factors so that the reader can examine the results realistically. External validity may also present a limitation if the sample came from one setting or particular geographic area or if sample characteristics affect generalizability of findings.

Every research endeavor leads to further questions. Sometimes, these questions arise out of the expressed limitations of a study and the need to clarify extraneous factors, design issues, or the effect of specific treatment procedures. Given the results of a study, you may want to reconsider a particular theory and how it may be applied. Suggestions for future research will develop from these ideas and should be proposed.

Conclusion

The *conclusion* is a brief restatement of the purpose of the study and its principal findings. It is often written to state the deductions made from the results. Phrases like "the results of this study indicate" and "this study demonstrates" serve to link the summary of results and the meaning of those results. This section may be a subheading or it may be the final paragraph in the discussion.

References

There are two common formats for citing references throughout the text and in the listing of references at the end of the manuscript. One method uses superscripts in the order of citation, using the format defined by the National Library of Medicine (NLM) or the American Medical Association (AMA) style guides.[26-28] Others follow recommendations of the American Psychological Association (APA), which requires references to be cited by author and year within parentheses in the text and alphabetical in the reference list.[29] The format required for a particular journal will be detailed in the *Instructions to Authors* and should be followed carefully.

Supplementary Materials

Many journals will allow inclusion of material in an appendix that is important for understanding the study but may be too large for tables or figures within the article, such as the questions on a survey instrument. The appendix will be placed at the end of the article, following references. Journals may limit the number of pages for appendices.

Journals may also support inclusion of supplementary materials or additional files that readers can access online. These can include the dataset used, additional analyses or figures, full copies of surveys, or videos and photos. These should be relevant to content and referenced within the body of the text.

Additional Information

Many journals will list additional information at the beginning or end of the article. Open access journals will describe the type of license for the publication, usually at the bottom of the first page. Other common elements include a statement regarding authors' conflicts of interest, the authors' individual contributions to the study, and acknowledgments of others who contributed to the study. Registration numbers should be included for studies and protocols that have been included in a registry. Specific funding information should also be given.

■ Submitting the Manuscript

Once you have prepared the manuscript and selected an appropriate journal, the next step is submission. This will usually occur through an online portal. Although the general format of a research report is fairly consistent in medical and scientific writing, each journal has its own particular rules about organization, length of a manuscript, preparation of tables and figures, and the method of reference citation. For example, many journals want figures and tables to be submitted separately or at the end of the paper. There will likely be strict requirements for reproducing figures. Consult the journal's *Instructions to Authors* for detailed guidelines about formatting. Failure to follow the instructions is a reason for rejection.

 Standard policy for scientific journals states that authors can submit an article to only one journal at a time. This protects journals from conflicts in copyright. If an article is rejected, the author can then submit it to a different journal. Submitting the same article to two journals at the same time is considered a violation of research integrity.

Peer Review

Upon submission of a manuscript, the journal's editorial team will review it and determine if it meets their criteria for **peer review**. If a manuscript passes the initial screen, editors will send it to at least two reviewers who are content experts who volunteer their time to assure quality in journal submissions. Many journals conduct double-blind peer review, meaning that neither you nor the reviewers know each other's identity. In a single-blind review the reviewer will know the authors' names.

After review, you will receive the reviewers' comments along with a summary by a member of the editorial team. This can take several weeks or longer, depending on the journal's turn-around-time. Peer reviewers will comment on the importance of the study and may make suggestions to clarify content, explain gaps, or highlight problems with the study design or analysis. The editors' recommendations will include their decision to accept with minor revisions, revise and resubmit, or reject.

If you have the opportunity to revise and resubmit a manuscript, take the reviewers' comments seriously. For the resubmission, follow the journal's instructions carefully. Some request highlighted changes, some prefer use of track changes, and others may require a table detailing how you addressed each comment and where the edits appear. The back and forth of the editorial process can feel tedious but almost always results in a clearer, more impactful article.

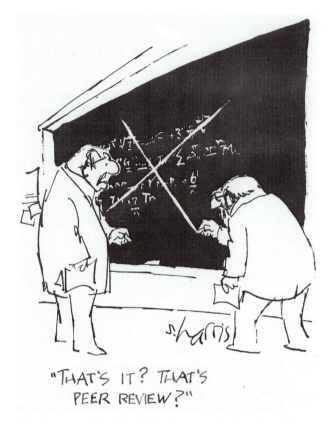

"THAT'S IT? THAT'S PEER REVIEW?"

Illustration courtesy of Sidney Harris. Used with permission from ScienceCartoonsPlus.com.

Understanding the structure of a research report is important for writing an article and for appraising it. The processes described in Chapters 36 and 37 for critical appraisal and systematic reviews are useful considerations, as they both reflect how others would appraise your work. CONSORT and other guidelines can also be used to focus critical appraisal. It is helpful to use this same approach when critiquing your own work for clarity and quality as your writing progresses.

Writing Style

The goal of scientific writing is to convey research studies clearly so that readers can evaluate and apply the findings. Scientific writing is not the creative process we learned in school. The standard article template leaves little room for metaphors or colorful language, although this does not mean writing needs to be stilted. Pinker[30] has identified "the curse of knowledge" as a primary source of the impenetrable prose that characterizes some journal articles. So steeped are researchers in their scholarly enterprise, they may not see the importance of communicating their work for a wider audience. Abbreviations and jargon creep in when authors write only for other specialists.

Writing with the reader in mind requires that you design a logical structure for the manuscript, explain technical terms, and avoid abstraction. An abundance of style manuals attest to the widespread need for guidance in writing clearly. You can sidestep some common pitfalls by following these principles:

- Each paragraph should start with a topic sentence and make one main point. If you have come to the end of a page on the computer screen without a paragraph break, you probably have included more than one main point.
- Present points logically, following an intentional sequence of ideas that will be obvious to the reader.
- Don't worry about using the same words repetitively— if certain terms are used often, stay consistent to avoid any confusion.
- Use "people first" language, rather than describing people by their disease or disability. "*Stroke patients*" are "*Persons who have had a stroke.*"
- Avoid excess verbiage that serves only to sound fancier or overemphasize. For example, say "*use*" instead of "*utilize.*" There is no need to say an outcome is "*very practical*;" just being "*practical*" is sufficient.
- Use active rather than passive voice as much as possible, saying "*we applied the intervention,*" not "*the intervention was applied.*" An exception is avoiding the first-person active voice. It is better to say, "*The subjects were asked to complete the questionnaire,*" rather than "*I asked the subjects to complete the questionnaire.*"

Other Types of Written Submissions

Several types of journal submissions other than a full-length research article can provide an opportunity for being published. Each may have different limitations on words, references, or other material. Some will be peer-reviewed, and others will not. Depending on the stage of research completed or complexity of your methods, a briefer format may be appropriate to convey your findings.

- **Case reports** provide an in-depth description of a unique or novel case or clinical approaches to care (see Chapter 20).

- **Reviews** can be a good option for those newer to the research process, working with a team on a systematic review, meta-analysis, or scoping review summarizing major research (see Chapter 37). Reviews may also be submitted as clinical guidelines based on literature review. These will be treated like other research studies and will be peer-reviewed.

- **Perspectives/Commentaries/Expert views** are all different forms of overview in an area of contemporary interest, a description of a new approach to patient care, or presenting a point of view regarding issues of current concern in the discipline.

- **Short reports** are used in some journals as brief articles about research projects featuring preliminary data.

- **Letters to the editor** can provide an opportunity to comment on a published study or address a contemporary professional issue. Letters should include references to support critical statements. If published, the author of the original article or other experts will be asked to provide a response.

> 📌 In Chapter 19, Focus on Evidence 19-1 described the contributions of Alice Stewart and the many *letters to the editor* she wrote to inform the medical community about her findings related to x-rays and childhood leukemia.[31]

- **Trial protocols** present a full description of a study protocol that has not yet been implemented. These are primarily focused on studies that are prospectively registered with a clinical trials registry.

- **Book reviews** are critical and unbiased evaluations of a recently published book. Some journals include these by invitation only.

- **Editorials** comment on a professional issue, often related to content of specific articles included in that journal issue. These may be written by one of the journal's editors or by someone who is invited to write a guest editorial.

Each journal will provide detailed guidelines for these types of acceptable publications in their *Instructions to Authors*.

■ Presentations

Presentations at conferences are an important form of dissemination, allowing new information to be shared in a timely way. They encourage direct interchange of ideas and stimulate consideration of new directions in research. They also provide an opportunity for researchers to receive valuable feedback from colleagues on work in progress, especially useful as one prepares to submit for publication. Research presentations may be offered as an oral presentation or poster. Several useful references provide suggestions for developing abstracts and effective platform and poster presentations.[32-35]

> 📌 Other types of conference presentations include educational sessions, symposia, or workshops, which may be 90 minutes or longer. Abstracts for these types of sessions usually require objectives, outcomes, and references.

Submitting Abstracts

Professional organizations typically put out a *call for abstracts* to solicit submissions, which must follow specific guidelines, including subheadings and number of words. Abstracts are usually submitted online and deadlines may be 9 months to a year before the actual conference, with strict enforcement. The abstracts are evaluated by a committee of expert reviewers who will decide which ones to accept based on quality, importance and, often, relevance to the conference's theme.[25]

> 📌 When submitting an abstract, you may be asked to choose a preference for a poster or oral presentation. However, because of limitations of time or space, your abstract may be accepted for a different format. You may be asked to indicate with your submission if you would be willing to change formats.

Oral Presentations

Oral presentations, also called *concurrent sessions* or *platform presentations*, are an important form of communication that occurs in an open forum at a conference. These presentations usually have a time limit of 10 to 20 minutes followed by 5 minutes of questions. This means you must be concise in delivery of content, as moderators will strictly adhere to time limits. It is very disappointing when presenters are cut off when they still have not covered their discussion or conclusions. Experienced speakers may be comfortable speaking informally, using slides as a guide, and are able to judge their timing. For those with less experience, it is often helpful for the talk to be written out. In either case, rehearsal to establish timing is a good idea. Only one person should do the presentation. Coauthors can participate in question and answer periods.

Format of an Oral Presentation

The content of an oral presentation follows the general format of a journal article, albeit much briefer. It includes an introduction, methods, data analysis, results, discussion, and conclusions. However, you don't have to stick to the "rules" about what goes into each section the way you do for an article. You can use abbreviations or acronyms that are familiar to your audience, and you can combine information from different sections, as long as it logically conveys your message. Know your audience, their background, and level of knowledge. Are you presenting to a general clinical audience, an interprofessional group, or to expert researchers? Tailor your focus and depth of content.

The introduction and method sections should be as brief as possible. The question should be stated clearly, with just enough background to justify the study and establish what it will contribute to current knowledge. Audiences appreciate your stating hypotheses or aims that will allow them to follow the logic of the presentation. The methods section should describe the research in sufficient detail for the audience to understand what was done. There is no time to include comprehensive descriptions, so important decisions have to be made about what information is necessary.

The most important parts of the presentation are the results and discussion. Keep to the key points. You want these sections to focus on the "take home" message. Include discussion of important limitations. The presentation should end with a clear statement of conclusions and implications for practice and further research.

Visual Presentation

Because oral presentations typically present a lot of information in a short amount of time, the use of slides is essential for the audience to be able to follow along. Slides should emphasize and illustrate content to focus the audience's attention on important details. Although some recommendations suggest having no more than 15-20 slides, the number of slides should be determined by identifying the key points of the written text—but keep it as minimal as possible.

People generally find it difficult to listen to one thing and read another at the same time. Slides should follow the language used in the presentation but should not contain every word. The slides should serve as an outline of the work, and the speaker should not read the slides. Use of bullets is helpful to avoid long sentences. Most importantly, the audience should be able to read the slides easily from a distance. Limit the verbiage on the slide to phrases or terms that will guide the listener to the important points.

The adage "a picture is worth a thousand words" applies here. Photographs and graphs greatly facilitate the audience's understanding of methods and results. Videos may be informative but should not last more than a minute or two. Don't put up a graphic and expect the audience to interpret it on the spot—guide them through the information.

When a study has generated a lot of data, you may have to be selective in what to include because listeners cannot absorb mounds of data in such a short time span. Tables may be useful when actual data are relevant—but they are often so busy that the audience cannot read them. Is every p value important, or can you show which variables are significantly different in a chart? Don't apologize for busy or unreadable slides—just don't include them! Graphics are usually more informative.

Many conferences request that you submit your slides in advance so they can be uploaded for participants to access them before they attend your session (avoiding the need for handouts). This timing needs to be built into your planning. Some will also request your slide deck in advance so that it can be loaded onto the computer in the presentation room. This allows for a smooth transition between successive speakers.

Some other hints: If you are not a seasoned speaker, it is a good idea to rehearse your presentation for timing and clarity. Ask colleagues to listen and give you feedback. Remember your public speaking lessons—speak slowly and clearly, don't sway at the podium, look up from your paper if you are reading it. Get to the room where you will be presenting with good lead time so you can load your slides onto the computer and you can become familiar with the set-up and surroundings. You will be able to see your slides on the computer at the podium, so you do not have to keep looking backwards at the screen to know what is being projected. Mostly, relax and enjoy the experience! Remember people are there because they are interested in your work.

Presentation programs like PowerPoint provide a lot of creative options—ornate backgrounds, fancy fonts, animations, colors, clip art. Keep it simple. The purpose of a professional presentation is to get the information across, not to entertain. You want the audience to be engaged, not distracted by watching words fly in and fade out or slides with novel transitions. Keep colors to a minimum and use a consistent theme. Some people like dark backgrounds, others like lighter backgrounds. Both work well—just make sure the backgrounds work with your graphics.

Poster Presentations

A poster presentation is a report of research that is displayed so that it can be read and viewed by large groups in a casual atmosphere. Posters afford a special opportunity for researchers and their colleagues to exchange ideas in conference settings. Poster sessions are organized so that each poster is available for several hours, although the author may be required to stand with it for only 1 or 2 hours. Posters are usually displayed in an open area where interested participants view the posters in a less formal manner. In this case, the researcher is available to answer questions or engage in discussion. The advantage of the poster presentation is that interested members of the audience can study the implications of a study at a comfortable pace, and the researcher has an opportunity to clarify or amplify details of the study. The disadvantage is that most posters are viewed by a small number of people.

Content and Layout

There is no fixed format for a poster. If you take the time to view posters at a conference, you will see a wide variety, and you can judge for yourself which are more effective than others. You want a poster to look interesting, not overwhelming to those passing by. Figure 38-1 is one sample arrangement of a poster.

The poster should contain the major elements of the study in a clear, brief series of statements including title, purpose, hypothesis or specific aims, method, results and discussion, and conclusions. The poster should be self-explanatory, but "telegraphic" in style; that is, content should include key words and phrases and not necessarily complete sentences. Tables, graphs, or photographs should summarize and illustrate important findings or unique aspects of the method. The most effective posters do not contain so much written material that the observer gets lost but should be complete enough to allow the observer to understand the full intent of the study.

The conference sponsor will provide guidelines about the size and composition of the board that will be available and how the poster will be affixed (if you need to bring push pins). The customary size is 4 feet high and 4, 6, or 8 feet wide. Many free poster templates are available on the Web for different sizes. These can be designed using a single PowerPoint slide. The content elements can be moved about the template to find the best arrangement for the logical flow of information. The introductory materials should be placed at the top left and the conclusion at the bottom right. The effective poster should be legible and uncluttered with content presented in sharp contrast to its background. The size and type of the text should be readable from 4 feet away, including data in tables and figure legends. If a study is funded, you may include information about the grant and funding agency on the bottom of the poster.

Some researchers like to include references on a poster, but this may be a space issue. When the poster cannot accommodate important information, presenters may have handouts for viewers with copies of the poster and additional material.

Posters can be printed in a variety of ways. You should find out what resources are available to you through your institution. Many commercial vendors can print them, but beware of costs. Get estimates of time needed for printing to be sure the poster is ready when you need it!

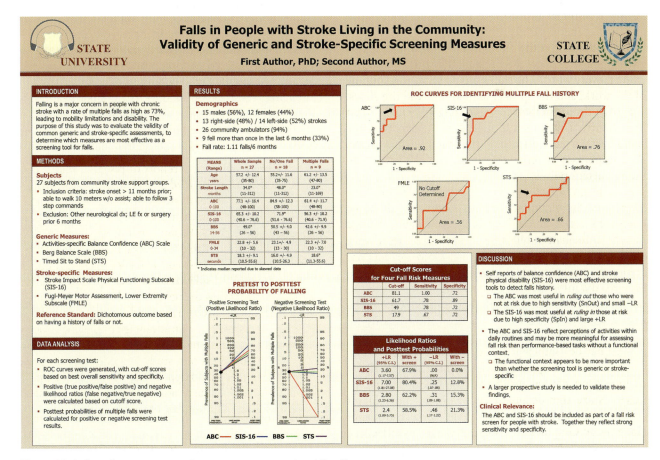

Figure 38–1 Sample arrangement for a poster presentation (4' x 6').

E-posters

Technology continues to introduce more flexibility and creativity into the presentation of posters. A recent option is the *e-poster*. Instead of displaying a printed poster on a presentation board, the e-poster appears on monitors or computers placed around the room. It is still a PowerPoint presentation, but it can include multimedia, more effectively conveying information that would not necessarily be possible with a traditional printed poster. It can include elements such as slide shows, videos, animated charts or graphs, or 3D rotation of a model. Conferences are using this model differently, some having authors stand with the monitor, as they do with a regular poster, and some are including a dedicated time for authors to actually do a short presentation of their e-poster. If the e-poster stays up at times when the author is not there, it may be on a loop that allows those passing by to see the full presentation. The conference sponsor will set requirements and limits, such as the size of the file, if it can accommodate videos, and if internet is available. It is worth searching for examples of this format on the Web.

Depending on the size of a conference, there may be dozens or even hundreds of oral presentations and poster displays. Being able to share your work with colleagues is a rewarding experience. However, it should not be the final product. It is unfortunate that so many presented studies never end up in publication, limiting the degree of dissemination. Even if you feel your study is not ready for prime time in a peer-reviewed journal, consider other opportunities that have been suggested to share your work with a larger audience.

■ Promoting Your Work

An author's role does not end with publication. Depending on the nature of your research, your field of study, and the volume of publications on the topic, your work may not be found or read by others. However, it is not arrogant to let people know about your published research. Many colleagues appreciate being alerted to relevant studies that they might have missed. One of the hallmarks of evidence-based practice is how readily we share important information that can contribute to clinical decision-making.

You can obtain the digital object identifier (DOI) for your article from the publisher (see Chapter 6). This unique link points readers to your article and remains stable even if Web pages shift. You can also obtain a DOI for posters and other research outputs using a free service like *Figshare*.[36]

Consider sharing a link to the DOI on platforms such as *Twitter* or *LinkedIn*, or in your email signature. You can also upload your work and alert followers on social media platforms like ResearchGate[37] and Academia.[38] Research communication platforms like ORCID[39] or Kudos[40] can help you find other ways to promote your research.

When an article is published, authors sign a copyright release—the journal owns the copyright, not the author. In general, copyright agreements allow you to post your published articles on personal websites and use them in presentations, but there may be other restrictions. To determine the specific permissions of your publisher, consult their policies or refer to *How Can I Share It?*[41]

Other Venues for Dissemination

Professional journals and conference presentations are not the only ways to share your research. The results of research can also be relevant to other consumers, including policy analysts, lobbying groups, local agencies offering health services, healthcare administrators, associations focused on specific conditions, and, most importantly, to consumers and patients.

Many organizations, including news outlets, will summarize published studies that would be of interest to their audiences. Research offices at many institutions can connect investigators with communications specialists to craft a press release about findings with public health significance. Even if a project may not have wide appeal, it is helpful to summarize your conclusions in plain language. *WeShareScience* is a website that allows authors to post short video abstracts of their work.[42] Consider contributing to a blog or podcast as another form of dissemination of your ideas.

Colleagues who organize educational sessions or in-service sessions at their institutions may be interested in your work and may invite you to give a presentation on a particular topic. Conferences may include workshops as part of their programming, lasting a few hours or several days before the start of the main program. These invitations are usually a recognition of your expertise, providing a wonderful opportunity to share your scholarly work and to obtain feedback from invested audiences.

Most professional organizations also publish magazines and newsletters that are disseminated to general members or to special interest groups. Although largely not peer reviewed, these venues often include summaries of research or articles that focus on specific clinical issues. Some may publish research, often smaller studies that are not ready for a professional journal, but will still be of interest to readers. These are good publications for pilot studies that inform readers of the direction of your work. They may include reports of interviews with experts in certain areas, often sparked by published research. These are excellent venues for dissemination, either for those early in their research careers, or for the purpose of targeting specific audiences.

Tracking Metrics

Increasingly, journals are tracking how often an article is viewed, downloaded, and shared. *Altmetrics* provides a score that reflects mentions of your work on social media, including bookmarks, links, blog postings, tweets, policy documents, and online reference managers.[43] The score is displayed in a ring with different colored sections that represent the various media sources. This score gauges the importance of scholarly output by authors, essentially monitoring the amount of attention the work has received.[44] Reference managers like *Mendeley* will also let you know how many users have saved your citation to their personal libraries.[45] *ResearchGate* can notify you when others cite your studies.[37]

These alternative metrics do not necessarily reflect the quality of your research, but they do indicate the breadth and variety of reactions to it. Just as journals earn impact factors, individual authors can calculate the impact of their published work using the *h index* which measures a combination of the number of articles published by a researcher and the number of citations it receives.[46] Creating a profile on *Google Scholar* will not only tabulate your *h index* score, but will also allow other researchers with similar interests to learn about your work.

COMMENTARY

Do not write merely to be understood. Write so you cannot possibly be misunderstood.

—*Robert Louis Stevenson (1850-1894)*

Scottish writer

Disseminating your work occupies this book's final chapter because it marks the culmination of the research process. Yet, the considerations that go into publishing should guide the decisions you make at all prior steps. Defining your question influences where your findings will ultimately appear. Similarly, choosing a research design and a data analysis technique will shape what kind of article you will write. Veteran researchers often map out from the beginning of a project how many manuscripts it will yield and where they will be submitted.

Writing often falls prey to procrastination. The lack of a fixed timeline allows researchers to find all sorts of excuses not to write. There are always more data to collect, more references to check, and more tests to run. Writing requires stretches of uninterrupted time that are increasingly rare in our multitasking clinical and academic careers. Setting up a schedule to write can keep you focused, and you may also find that deadlines are more compelling if you collaborate with multiple authors.

One of the hallmarks of the scientific process is a commitment to *critical examination* whereby researchers subject their findings to the scrutiny of others, providing a basis for validation of data from primary sources of information. When you publish your results, you expose your work to the scholarly community—contributing to the literature and possibly facing rejection. You should be aware of principles of academic integrity, assuring that your work is original and accurate (see Chapter 7).

Think of this process as one that contributes to your growth as a scholar. When we see a journal's tables of contents or the extensive resumes of senior scholars, it is not evident how many articles required multiple submissions before they were accepted, or how many projects never received funding or were never published. You will pay your dues just as they did, so don't be discouraged.

The process of publishing your work has tangible benefits for evidence-based practice. By adding your voice—backed by evidence—to the scholarly conversation, you allow others to build on your findings in the pursuit of scientific knowledge. Through this ongoing process, clinical practices improve so that we can fulfill our professional commitment to improve health and quality of life.

REFERENCES

1. Boon S. 21st century science overload. Canadian Science Publishing, January 7, 2017. Available at http://blog.cdnsciencepub.com/21st-century-science-overload/. Accessed April 15, 2019.
2. Journal/Author Name Estimator (JANE). Available at http://jane.biosemantics.org/. Accessed April 15, 2019.
3. Ogden TL, Bartley DL. The ups and downs of journal impact factors. *Ann Occup Hyg* 2008;52(2):73-82.
4. CWTS Journal Indicators. Available at http://www.journalindicators.com/. Accessed April 7, 2019.
5. Systematic Impact Factor. Available at http://sifactor.org/. Accessed April 7, 2019.
6. Scimago Journal and Country Rank (SJR). Available at https://www.scimagojr.com/journalrank.php. Accessed April 7, 2019.
7. Creative Commons. About the licenses. Available at https://creativecommons.org/licenses/. Accessed April 13, 2019.
8. Directory of Open Access Journals (DOAJ). Available at https://doaj.org/. Accessed April 13, 2019.
9. Unpaywall. Available at https://unpaywall.org/. Accessed April 15, 2019.
10. Natarajan S, Nair AG. "FakeBooks" — predatory journals: The dark side of publishing. *Indian J Ophthalmol* 2016;64(2):107-108.
11. Stratford M. Predatory online journals lure scholars who are eager to publish. *The Chronicle of Higher Education*, March 4, 2012. Available at https://www.chronicle.com/article/Predatory-Online-Journals/131047. Accessed April 16, 2019.
12. Yucha C. Predatory publishing: what authors, reviewers, and editors need to know. *Biol Res Nurs* 2015;17(1):5-7.
13. Think. Check. Submit. Reference this list for your chosen journal to check if it is trusted. Available at http://thinkchecksubmit.org/check/. Accessed April 13, 2019.
14. Laine C, Winker MA. Identifying predatory or pseudo-journals. World Association of Medical Editors, 2017. Available at http://www.wame.org/identifying-predatory-or-pseudo-journals. Accessed April 13, 2019.
15. Sharma H, Verma S. Predatory journals: The rise of worthless biomedical science. *J Postgrad Med* 2018;64(4):226-231.
16. Greene M. The demise of the lone author. *Nature* 2007;450(7173):1165.
17. International Committee of Medical Journal Editors. Recommendations for the conduct, reporting, editing and publication of scholarly work in medical journals. Updated 2016. Available at http://www.icmje.org/icmje-recommendations/. Accessed April 13, 2019.
18. Strange K. Authorship: why not just toss a coin? *Am J Physiol Cell Physiol* 2008;295(3):C567-575.
19. Kochan CA, Budd JM. The persistence of fraud in the literature: the Darsee case. *J Am Soc Inf Sci Technol* 1992;43(7):488-493.
20. Relman AS. Lessons from the Darsee affair. *N Engl J Med* 1983;308(23):1415-1417.
21. Equator Network. Enhancing the Quality and Transparency of Health Research. Available at http://www.equator-network.org/. Accessed, April 3, 2019.
22. Hoffman TC, Glasziou PP, Boutron I, Milne R, Perera R, Moher D, et al. Better reporting of interventions: template for intervention description and replication (TIDieR) checklist and guide. *BMJ* 2014;348:g1687.
23. Lingard L, Watling C. It's a story, not a study: writing an effective research paper. *Acad Med* 2016;91(12):e12.
24. Academic Medicine. Strategies for writing effective titles: part 1. Available at http://academicmedicineblog.org/strategies-for-writing-effective-titles-part-1/. Accessed, April 25, 2019.
25. Pearce PF, Ferguson LA. How to write abstracts for manuscripts, presentations, and grants: Maximizing information in a 30-s sound bite world. *J Am Assoc Nurse Pract* 2017:452-460.
26. Patrias K, Wending D. *Citing Medicine*. Bethesda, MD: National Library of Medicine; 2007.
27. Geneva Foundation for Medical Education and Research. Comparison of citation styles: American Medical Association (AMA) and National Library of Medicine (NLM) styles. Available at https://www.gfmer.ch/writing/NLM_AMA_styles.htm. Accessed June 6, 2019.
28. JAMA & Archives Journals. *AMA Manual of Style: A Guide for Authors and Editors*. 10th ed. New York: Oxford University Press; 2007.
29. American Psychological Association. *The Publication Manual of the American Psychological Association*. 6th ed. Washington, DC: American Psychological Association; 2010.
30. Pinker S. Why academics stink at writing. *The Chronicle of Higher Education*, September 26, 2014. Available at https://www.chronicle.com/article/Why-Academics-Writing/148989. Accessed April 26, 2019.
31. Stewart A, Webb JW, Giles D, Hewitt D. X-rays and leukemia. Letter to the Editor. *Lancet* 1957;269(6967):528.
32. Berg J, Hicks R. Successful design and delivery of a professional poster. *J Am Assoc Nurse Pract* 2017;29(8):461-469.
33. Erren TC, Bourne PE. Ten simple rules for a good poster presentation. *PLoS Comput Biol* 2007;3(5):e102.
34. Gundogan B, Koshy K, Kurar L, Whitehurst K. How to make an academic poster. *Ann Med Surg (Lond)* 2016;11:69-71.
35. Hardicre J, Coad J, Devitt P. Ten steps to successful conference presentations. *Br J Nurs* 2007;16(7):402-404.
36. Figshare. Available at https://figshare.com/. Accessed August 21, 2019.
37. ResearchGate. Available at https://www.researchgate.net. Accessed March 3, 2018.
38. Academia. Available at https://www.academia.edu/. Accessed August 23, 2019.
39. ORCID. Distinguish yourself in three easy steps. Available at https://orcid.org/. Accessed April 20, 2019.
40. Kudos. Kudos for researchers. Available at https://www.growkudos.com/about/researchers. Accessed April 30, 2019.
41. How can I share it? Available at https://www.howcanishareit.com/. Accessed April 30, 2019.
42. We Share Science. Available at http://wesharescience.com/. Accessed August 21, 2019.
43. Altmetric. Available at https://www.altmetric.com/. Accessed August 25, 2019.
44. Gumpenberger C, Glanzel W, Gorraiz J. The ecstasy and the agony of the altmetric score. *Scientometrics* 2016;108:977-982.
45. Mendeley. Available at https://www.mendeley.com/. Accessed March 4, 2018.
46. Hirsch JE. An index to quantify an individual's scientific research output. *Proc Natl Acad Sci U S A* 2005;102(46):16569-16572.

Statistical Tables

TABLE A-1   **Areas Under the Normal Curve, *z*** 614

TABLE A-2   **Critical Values of *t*** 616

TABLE A-3   **Critical Values of *F* (α = .05)** 617

TABLE A-4   **Critical Values of the Pearson correlation, *r*** 618

TABLE A-5   **Critical Values of Chi-Square, χ^2** 619

TABLE A-6   **Table of Random Numbers** 620

These tables are also available in *Appendix A Online*

Additional tables available in *Appendix A Online* and in chapter supplements:

TABLE A-7   **Critical Values of the Studentized Range Statistic, *q* (α=.05)**

Also available in the Chapter 26 Supplement

TABLE A-8   **Critical Values for the Mann-Whitney *U* Test**

Also available in the Chapter 27 Supplement

TABLE A-9   **One-Tailed Probabilities Associated with *x* in the Binomial Test**

Also available in the Chapter 18 and 27 Supplements

TABLE A-10   **Critical Values of *T* for the Wilcoxon Signed-Ranks Test**

Also available in the Chapter 27 Supplement

TABLE A-11   **Critical Values of Spearman's Rank Correlation Coefficient, r_s**

Also available in the Chapter 29 Supplement

Table A-1   Areas Under the Normal Curve (z)

Z	AREA BETWEEN 0 AND Z	AREA ABOVE Z	Z	AREA BETWEEN 0 AND Z	AREA ABOVE Z	Z	AREA BETWEEN 0 AND Z	AREA ABOVE Z
0.00	.0000	.5000	0.45	.1736	.3264	0.90	.3159	.1841
0.01	.0040	.4960	0.46	.1772	.3228	0.91	.3186	.1814
0.02	.0080	.4920	0.47	.1808	.3192	0.92	.3212	.1788
0.03	.0120	.4880	0.48	.1844	.3156	0.93	.3238	.1762
0.04	.0160	.4840	0.49	.1879	.3121	0.94	.3264	.1736
0.05	.0199	.4801	0.50	.1915	.3085	0.95	.3289	.1711
0.06	.0239	.4761	0.51	.1950	.3050	0.96	.3315	.1685
0.07	.0279	.4721	0.52	.1985	.3015	0.97	.3340	.1660
0.08	.0319	.4681	0.53	.2019	.2981	0.98	.3365	.1635
0.09	.0359	.4641	0.54	.2054	.2946	0.99	.3389	.1611
0.10	.0398	.4602	0.55	.2088	.2912	1.00	.3413	.1587
0.11	.0438	.4562	0.56	.2123	.2877	1.01	.3138	.1582
0.12	.0478	.4522	0.57	.2157	.2843	1.02	.3461	.1539
0.13	.0517	.4493	0.58	.2190	.2810	1.03	.3485	.1515
0.14	.0557	.4443	0.59	.2224	.2776	1.04	.3508	.1492
0.15	.0596	.4404	0.60	.2257	.2743	1.05	.3531	.1469
0.16	.0636	.4364	0.61	.2291	.2709	1.06	.3554	.1446
0.17	.0675	.4325	0.62	.2324	.2676	1.07	.3577	.4230
0.18	.0714	.4286	0.63	.2357	.3643	1.08	.3599	.1401
0.19	.0753	.4247	0.64	.2389	.2611	1.09	.3621	.1379
0.20	.0793	.4207	0.65	.2422	.2578	1.10	.3643	.1357
0.21	.0832	.4168	0.66	.2454	.2546	1.11	.3665	.1335
0.22	.0871	.4129	0.67	.2486	.2514	1.12	.3686	.1314
0.23	.0910	.4090	0.68	.2517	.2483	1.13	.3708	.1292
0.24	.0948	.4052	0.69	.2549	.2451	1.14	.3729	.1271
0.25	.0987	.4013	0.70	.2580	.2420	1.15	.3749	.1251
0.26	.1026	.3974	0.71	.2611	.2389	1.16	.3770	.1230
0.27	.1064	.3936	0.72	.2642	.2358	1.17	.3790	.1210
0.28	.1103	.8970	0.73	.2673	.2327	1.18	.3810	.1190
0.29	.1141	.3859	0.74	.2704	.2296	1.19	.3830	.1170
0.30	.1179	.3821	0.75	.2734	.2266	1.20	.3849	.1151
0.31	.1217	.3783	0.76	.2764	.2236	1.21	.3869	.1131
0.32	.1255	.3745	0.77	.2794	.2206	1.22	.3888	.1112
0.33	.1293	.7070	0.78	.2823	.2177	1.23	.3907	.1093
0.34	.1331	.3669	0.79	.2852	.2148	1.24	.3925	.1075
0.35	.1398	.3632	0.80	.2881	.2119	1.25	.3944	.1058
0.36	.1406	.3594	0.81	.2910	.2090	1.26	.3962	.1038
0.37	.1443	.3557	0.82	.2939	.2061	1.27	.3980	.1020
0.38	.1480	.3520	0.83	.2967	.2033	1.28	.3997	.1003
0.39	.1517	.3483	0.84	.2995	.2005	1.29	.4015	.0985
0.40	.1554	.3446	0.85	.3023	.1977	1.30	.4032	.0968
0.41	.1591	.3409	0.86	.3051	.1949	1.31	.4049	.0951
0.42	.1628	.3372	0.87	.3078	.4922	1.32	.4066	.0934
0.43	.1664	.3336	0.88	.3106	.1894	1.33	.4820	.0918
0.44	.1700	.3300	0.89	.3133	.1867	1.34	.4099	.0901

Table A-1   Areas Under the Normal Curve (z) (cont'd)

Z	AREA BETWEEN 0 AND Z	AREA ABOVE Z	Z	AREA BETWEEN 0 AND Z	AREA ABOVE Z	Z	AREA BETWEEN 0 AND Z	AREA ABOVE Z
1.35	.4115	.0885	1.80	.4641	.0359	2.25	.4878	.0122
1.36	.4131	.0869	1.81	.4649	.0651	2.26	.4881	.0119
1.37	.4147	.0853	1.82	.4656	.0344	2.27	.4884	.0116
1.38	.4162	.0838	1.83	.4664	.0336	2.28	.4887	.0113
1.39	.4177	.0523	1.84	.4671	.0329	2.29	.4890	.0110
1.40	.4192	.0808	1.85	.4678	.0322	2.30	.4893	.0102
1.41	.4207	.0793	1.86	.4686	.0314	2.31	.4896	.0104
1.42	.4222	.0778	1.87	.4693	.0307	2.32	.4898	.0102
1.43	.4236	.0764	1.88	.4699	.0301	2.326	.4900	.0100
1.44	.4251	.0749	1.89	.4706	.0294	2.33	.4901	.0099
						2.34	.4904	.0096
1.45	.4265	.0735	1.90	.4713	.0287	2.35	.4906	.0094
1.46	.4279	.0721	1.91	.4719	.0281	2.36	.4909	.0091
1.47	.4292	.0708	1.92	.4726	.0274	2.37	.4911	.0089
1.48	.4306	.0694	1.93	.4732	.0268	2.38	.4913	.0087
1.49	.4319	.0681	1.94	.4738	.0262	2.39	.4916	.0084
1.50	.4332	.0668	1.95	.4744	.0256	2.40	.4918	.0082
1.51	.4345	.0655	1.96	.4750	.0250	2.41	.4920	.0080
1.52	.4357	.0643	1.97	.4756	.0244	2.42	.4922	.0078
1.53	.4370	.0630	1.98	.4761	.0390	2.43	.4925	.0075
1.54	.4382	.0618	1.99	.4767	.0233	2.44	.4927	.0073
1.55	.4394	.0606	2.00	.4772	.0228	2.45	.4929	.0071
1.56	.4406	.0594	2.01	.4778	.0222	2.46	.4931	.0069
1.57	.4418	.0892	2.02	.4783	.0217	2.47	.4932	.0068
1.58	.4429	.0571	2.03	.4788	.0212	2.48	.4934	.0066
1.59	.4441	.0559	2.04	.4793	.0207	2.49	.4936	.0064
1.60	.4452	.0548	2.05	.4798	.0202	2.50	.4938	.0062
1.61	.4463	.0537	2.06	.4803	.0197	2.51	.4940	.0060
1.62	.4474	.0526	2.07	.4808	.0192	2.52	.4941	.0059
1.63	.4484	.0516	2.08	.4812	.0188	2.53	.4943	.0057
1.64	.4495	.0505	2.09	.4817	.0183	2.54	.4945	.0055
1.645	.4500	.0500						
1.65	.4505	.0495	2.10	.4821	.0179	2.55	.4946	.0054
1.66	.4515	.0485	2.11	.4826	.0174	2.56	.4948	.0052
1.67	.4525	.0475	2.12	.4830	.0170	2.57	.4949	.0051
1.68	.4535	.0465	2.13	.4834	.0166	2.576	.4950	.0050
1.69	.4545	.0455	2.14	.4838	.0162	2.58	.4951	.0049
						2.59	.4952	.0048
1.70	.4554	.0446	2.15	.4842	.0158	2.60	.4953	.0047
1.71	.4564	.0436	2.16	.4846	.0154	2.61	.4955	.0045
1.72	.4573	.0427	2.17	.4850	.0120	2.62	.4956	.0044
1.73	.4582	.0418	2.18	.4854	.0146	2.63	.4957	.0043
1.74	.4591	.0409	2.19	.4857	.0143	2.64	.4959	.0041
1.75	.4599	.0401	2.20	.4861	.0139	2.65	.4960	.0040
1.76	.4608	.0392	2.21	.4864	.0136	2.66	.4961	.0039
1.77	.4616	.0384	2.22	.4868	.0132	2.67	.4962	.0038
1.78	.4625	.0375	2.23	.4871	.0129	2.68	.4963	.0037
1.79	.4633	.0367	2.24	.4875	.0125	2.69	.4964	.0036

Continued

Table A-1 Areas Under the Normal Curve (*z*) (cont'd)

Z	AREA BETWEEN 0 AND Z	AREA ABOVE Z	Z	AREA BETWEEN 0 AND Z	AREA ABOVE Z	Z	AREA BETWEEN 0 AND Z	AREA ABOVE Z
2.70	.7965	.0035	2.95	.4984	.0016	3.20	.49931	.00069
2.71	.4966	.0034	2.96	.4985	.0015	3.21	.49934	.00066
2.72	.4967	.0033	2.97	.4985	.0015	3.22	.49936	.00064
2.73	.4968	.0032	2.98	.4986	.0014	3.23	.49938	.00062
2.74	.4969	.0031	2.99	.4986	.0014	3.24	.49940	.00060
2.75	.4970	.0030	3.00	.4987	.0013	3.25	.49942	.00058
2.76	.4971	.0029	3.01	.4987	.0013	3.26	.49944	.00056
2.77	.4972	.0028	3.02	.4987	.0013	3.27	.49946	.00054
2.78	.4973	.0027	3.03	.4988	.0120	3.28	.49948	.00052
2.79	.4974	.0026	3.04	.4998	.0012	3.29	.49950	.00050
2.80	.4974	.0026	3.05	.49886	.00114	3.30	.49951	.00048
2.81	.4975	.0025	3.06	.49889	.00111	3.31	.49953	.00047
2.82	.4976	.0024	3.07	.49893	.00107	3.32	.49955	.00045
2.83	.4977	.0023	3.08	.49896	.00104	3.33	.49957	.00043
2.84	.4977	.0023	3.09	.49900	.00100	3.34	.49958	.00042
2.85	.4978	.0022	3.10	.49903	.00097	3.35	.49960	.00040
2.86	.4979	.0021	3.11	.49906	.00094	3.36	.49961	.00039
2.87	.4979	.0021	3.12	.49910	.00090	3.37	.49962	.00038
2.88	.4980	.0020	3.13	.49913	.00087	3.38	.49964	.00036
2.89	.4981	.0019	3.14	.49916	.00084	3.39	.49965	.00035
2.90	.4981	.0019	3.15	.49918	.00082	3.40	.49966	.00034
2.91	.4982	.0018	3.16	.49921	.00079	3.45	.49972	.00028
2.92	.4982	.0018	3.17	.49924	.00076	3.50	.49977	.00023
2.93	.4983	.0017	3.18	.49926	.00074	3.60	.49984	.00016
2.94	.4984	.0016	3.19	.49929	.00071	3.70	.49989	.00011
						3.80	.49993	.00001
						3.90	.49995	.00005
						4.00	.49997	.00003

Table A-2   Critical Values of *t*

df	α_1 .10 α_2 .20	.05 .10	.025 .05	.01 .02	.005 .01	.0005 .001
1	3.078	6.314	12.706	31.821	63.657	636.619
2	1.886	2.920	4.303	6.955	9.925	31.598
3	1.638	2.353	3.182	4.541	5.841	12.924
4	1.533	2.132	2.776	3.747	4.604	8.610
5	1.476	2.015	2.571	3.365	4.032	6.859
6	1.440	1.943	2.447	3.143	3.707	5.959
7	1.415	1.895	2.365	2.998	3.499	5.405
8	1.397	1.860	2.306	2.896	3.355	5.041
9	1.383	1.833	2.262	2.821	3.250	4.781
10	1.372	1.812	0.228	2.764	3.169	4.587
11	1.363	1.796	2.201	2.718	3.106	4.437
12	1.356	1.782	2.179	2.681	3.055	4.318
13	1.350	1.771	2.160	2.650	3.012	4.221
14	1.345	1.761	2.145	2.624	2.977	4.140
15	1.341	1.753	2.131	2.602	2.947	4.073
16	1.337	1.746	2.120	2.583	2.921	4.015
17	1.333	1.740	2.110	2.457	2.898	3.922
18	1.330	1.734	2.101	2.552	2.878	3.922
19	1.328	1.729	2.093	2.538	2.845	3.850
20	1.325	1.725	2.086	2.528	2.845	3.850
21	1.323	1.721	2.080	2.518	2.831	3.819
22	1.321	1.717	2.074	2.508	2.819	3.792
23	1.319	1.714	2.069	2.500	2.807	3.725
24	1.318	1.711	2.064	2.492	2.797	3.745
25	1.316	1.708	2.060	2.485	2.787	3.725
26	1.315	1.706	2.056	2.479	2.779	3.707
27	1.314	1.703	2.052	2.473	2.771	3.690
28	1.313	1.701	2.048	2.457	2.763	3.674
29	1.311	1.699	2.045	2.462	2.756	3.659
30	1.310	1.694	2.042	2.457	2.750	3.646
40	1.303	1.684	2.021	2.423	2.704	3.551
60	1.296	1.671	2.000	2.390	2.660	3.460
120	1.289	1.658	1.980	2.358	2.617	3.373
∞	1.282	1.645	1.960	2.326	2.576	3.291

For unpaired *t*-test $df = (n_1 - 1) + (n_2 - 1)$. For paired *t*-test, $df - n-1$. Test statistic must be greater than or equal to critical value to reject H_0.

Table A-3 Critical Values of F (α = .05)

df_e	df_b										
	1	**2**	**3**	**4**	**5**	**6**	**7**	**8**	**9**	**10**	**∞**
1	161.40	199.50	215.70	224.60	230.20	234.00	236.80	238.90	240.50	241.90	254.30
2	18.51	19.00	19.16	19.25	19.30	19.33	19.35	19.37	19.38	19.40	19.50
3	10.13	9.55	9.28	9.12	9.01	8.64	8.89	8.85	8.81	8.79	8.53
4	7.71	6.94	6.59	6.39	6.26	6.16	6.09	6.04	6.00	5.96	5.63
5	6.61	5.79	5.41	5.19	5.05	4.95	4.88	4.82	4.77	4.74	4.36
6	5.99	5.14	4.76	4.53	4.39	4.28	4.21	4.15	4.10	4.06	3.67
7	5.59	4.74	4.35	4.12	3.97	3.87	3.79	3.73	3.68	3.64	3.23
8	5.32	4.46	4.07	3.84	3.69	3.58	3.50	3.44	3.39	3.35	2.93
9	5.12	4.26	3.86	3.63	3.48	3.37	3.29	3.23	3.18	3.14	2.71
10	4.96	4.10	3.71	3.48	3.33	3.22	3.14	3.07	3.02	2.98	2.54
11	4.84	3.98	3.59	3.36	3.20	3.09	3.01	2.95	2.90	2.85	2.40
12	4.75	3.89	3.49	3.26	3.11	3.00	2.91	2.85	2.80	2.88	2.30
13	4.67	3.81	3.41	3.18	3.03	2.92	2.83	2.77	2.71	2.67	2.21
14	4.60	3.74	3.34	3.11	2.96	2.85	2.76	2.70	2.65	2.60	2.13
15	4.54	3.68	3.29	3.06	2.90	2.79	2.71	2.64	2.59	2.54	2.07
20	4.35	3.49	3.10	2.87	2.71	2.60	2.51	2.45	2.39	2.35	1.84
30	4.17	3.32	2.92	2.69	2.53	2.42	2.33	2.27	2.21	2.16	1.62
40	4.08	3.23	2.84	2.61	2.45	2.34	2.25	2.18	2.12	2.08	1.51
60	4.00	3.15	2.76	2.53	2.37	2.25	2.17	2.10	2.04	1.99	1.39
120	3.92	3.07	2.68	2.45	2.29	2.17	2.09	2.02	1.96	1.91	1.25
∞	3.84	3.00	2.60	2.37	2.21	2.10	2.01	1.94	1.88	1.83	1.00

df_b = between groups degrees of freedom for numerator (k -1);

df_e = error (within-groups) degrees of freedom for denominator (N - k);

Test statistic must be greater than or equal to critical value to reject H_0.

Table A-4   Critical Values of the Pearson Correlation, *r*

df	α_1	.05	.025	.01	.005	.0005
	α_2	.10	.05	.02	.01	.001
1		.988	,997	.9995	.9999	.9999
2		.900	.950	.980	.990	.999
3		.805	.878	.934	.959	.991
4		.729	.811	.882	.917	.974
5		.669	.755	.833	.875	.951
6		.622	.707	.789	.834	.925
7		.582	.668	.750	.798	.898
8		.549	.632	.716	.765	.872
9		.521	.602	.685	.735	.847
10		.497	.576	.658	.708	.823
11		.476	.553	.634	.684	.801
12		.458	.532	.612	.661	.780
13		.441	.514	.592	.641	.760
14		426	.497	.574	.623	.742
15		.412	.482	.558	.606	.725
16		.400	.468	.543	.590	.708
17		.389	.456	.529	.575	.693
18		.378	.444	.516	.561	.679
19		.369	.433	.503	.549	.665
20		.360	.423	.492	.537	.652
25		.323	.381	.445	.487	.597
30		.296	.349	.409	.449	.554
35		.275	.325	.381	.418	.519
40		.257	.304	.358	.393	.490
45		.243	.288	.338	.372	.465
50		.231	.273	.322	.354	.443
60		.211	.250	.295	.325	.408
70		.195	.232	.274	.302	.380
80		.183	.217	.257	.283	.357
90		.173	.205	.242	.267	.338
100		.164	.195	.230	.254	.321

$df = n - 2$. Test statistic must be greater than or equal to critical value to reject H_0.

Table A-5   Critical Values of Chi-Square, χ^2

df	α	.05	.02	.01	.01	.00
1		3.84	5.02	6.64	7.88	10.83
2		5.99	7.38	9.21	10.60	13.82
3		7.82	9.35	11.35	12.84	16.27
4		9.49	11.14	13.28	14.86	18.47
5		11.07	12.83	15.09	16.75	20.52
6		12.59	14.45	16.81	18.55	22.46
7		14.07	16.01	18.48	20.28	24.32
8		15.51	17.53	20.09	21.96	26.13
9		16.92	19.03	21 .67	23.59	27.88
10		18.31	20.48	23.21	25.19	29.59
11		19.68	21.92	24.73	26.76	31.26
12		21.03	23.34	26.22	28.30	32.91
13		22.36	24.74	27.69	29.82	34.53
14		23.69	26.12	29.14	31.32	36.12
15		25.00	27.49	30.58	32.80	37.70
16		26.30	28.85	32.00	34.27	39.25
17		27.59	30.19	33.41	35.72	40.79
18		28.87	31.53	34.81	37.16	42.31
19		30.14	32.85	36.19	38.58	43.82
20		31.41	34.17	37.57	40.00	45.32
21		32.67	35.48	38.93	41.40	46.80
22		33.92	36.78	40.29	42.80	48.27
23		35.17	38.06	41,64	44.18	49.73
24		36.42	39.36	42.98	45.56	51.18
25		37.65	40.65	44.31	46.93	52.62
26		38.89	41.92	45.64	48.29	54.05
27		40.11	43.19	46.96	49.65	55.47
28		41.34	44.46	48.28	50.99	56.89
29		42.56	45.72,	49.59	52.34	58.30
30		43.77	46.98	50.89	53.67	59.70
40		55.76	59.34	63.69	66.77	73.40
50		67.51	71.42	76.15	79.49	86.66
60		79.08	83.30	88.38	91 .95	99.61
70		90.53	95.02	100.43	104.22	112.32
80		101.88	106.63	112.33	116.32	124.84
90		113.15	118.14	124.12	128.30	137.21
100		124.34	129.56	135.81	140.47	149.45

For one-sample test $df = k$-1. For two-sample test $df = (R$-1$)(C$-1$)$. Test statistic must be greater than or equal to critical value to reject H_0.

Table A-6   Table of Random Numbers

89747	45483	44871	40670	90134	74914	89805	31185	67635	20265	45183
69188	04296	45769	99712	46544	48816	07448	53958	90961	19106	10959
09531	04454	75490	38718	88775	13132	35221	27226	45150	03310	11782
71477	21953	31726	87557	58363	49797	07691	06171	87997	29476	87918
53060	77443	08291	97504	03345	09133	90590	43504	11659	70250	74061
54013	35297	21346	92244	36160	03332	98806	40162	76512	54956	50893
35023	74291	52037	75899	01766	25552	68788	39048	97110	10148	28109
96544	30860	77686	56636	55253	71749	28969	05937	22903	47145	92747
87888	57749	38005	21474	17105	35844	31478	82778	33021	13612	46637
28899	26189	27015	65203	72387	54343	91698	48718	14150	77126	04133
47695	36105	92109	04144	96645	27072	30756	78560	27328	98232	52652
91583	38052	04180	57939	33987	12622	00123	36150	26231	80250	89158
80859	32767	76157	42393	73219	35887	51196	89077	42761	23476	24783
42072	13550	09292	10293	86360	89695	78830	32757	50731	26296	04892
67621	85921	38877	00192	24444	20849	42907	86663	94352	48158	74869
09946	14727	03867	94743	40982	64415	51409	87297	82778	05654	52817
82759	56387	42334	57754	10461	99187	61226	84209	06708	08614	63437
28962	72338	99553	64630	72982	05928	26834	23632	98443	47148	75366
39193	46816	54359	84240	05822	01151	53685	24275	96677	20700	43694
99221	49368	17548	25892	55956	19224	12790	50739	74703	08126	35658
85100	60328	22625	65537	66142	20059	59863	29531	72034	33753	49665
57520	79952	21854	87303	61238	97336	09081	32482	30120	43424	83557
70179	51732	70983	65252	95133	61173	14756	42648	61799	89619	69092
59048	74304	54482	04860	74741	20804	59246	82782	89341	56913	36197
21675	49455	83688	22021	02670	17529	71285	08767	18825	64891	66725
98527	05293	25736	60934	09509	70027	63492	76794	99552	12033	26075
95792	51286	68149	11278	69481	25848	82572	78677	60279	99475	48629
23931	17277	37698	43810	17094	41134	81091	93734	52015	07293	94847
95128	22088	11808	24601	59115	80642	09608	35813	36636	39607	83130
20912	22832	44043	18245	25882	80991	75351	31964	86800	17014	35960
67746	46580	73793	44761	42789	09659	44932	75215	44810	48445	19029
71049	77999	74307	02662	59509	81979	79285	61972	83850	27143	14226
28512	15320	76961	19597	27767	38773	67955	87556	26060	62374	66707
12057	51665	75731	93617	13464	02158	85118	07863	68504	68703	15488
68323	47022	90949	62849	04858	99454	72545	26384	14275	96129	32740
53069	29718	50813	03149	93034	01450	85741	72998	84584	48502	04472
41853	75323	21878	35065	55702	56943	32512	61683	25287	24874	23664
76834	61882	87689	61166	06793	15488	21426	01287	87432	95567	40199
59010	29583	10657	07809	38977	46347	15367	53663	46460	13765	68508
41926	71062	09284	61481	73048	27624	14816	44227	51789	35468	84084

Relating the Research Question to the Choice of Statistical Test

RESEARCH QUESTION	CHART
Is there a difference between means (or medians)?	

1 independent variable: 2 levels
  1 independent variable: ≥ 3 levels
  2 or more independent variables
	B1
	B2
	B3

Is there a difference in proportions?	B4
Is there an association between variables?	B5
Is there a predictive relationship between variables?	B6
Are measurements reliable?	B7

B1

Is there a difference between means (or medians)?

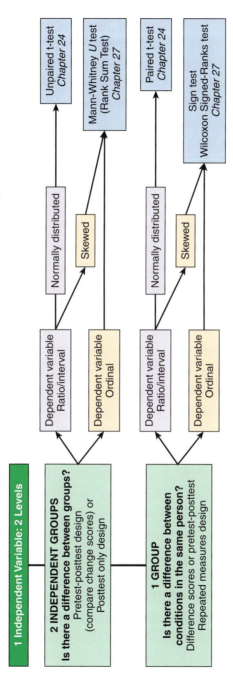

B2

Is there a difference between means (or medians)?

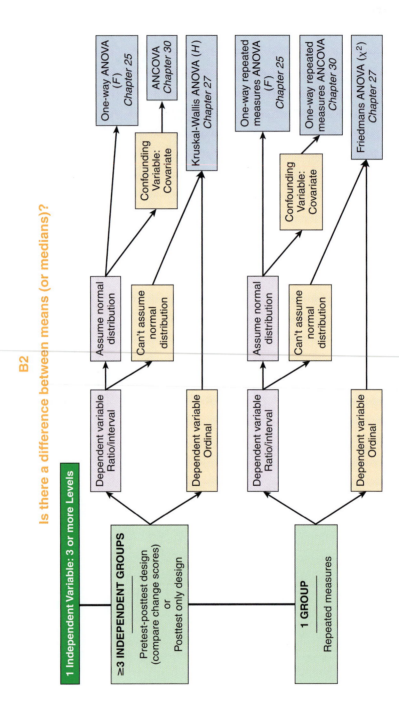

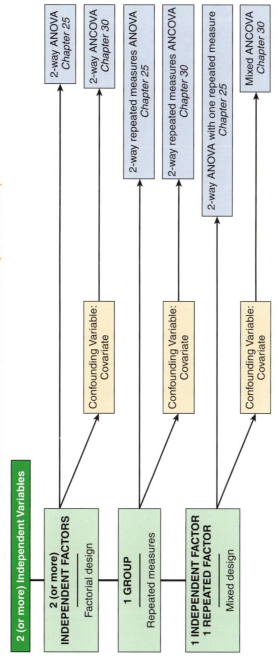

B3

Is there a difference between means (or medians)?

2 (or more) Independent Variables

2 (or more) INDEPENDENT FACTORS
Factorial design

1 GROUP
Repeated measures

1 INDEPENDENT FACTOR
1 REPEATED FACTOR
Mixed design

Confounding Variable: Covariate

Confounding Variable: Covariate

Confounding Variable: Covariate

2-way ANOVA
Chapter 25

2-way ANCOVA
Chapter 30

2-way repeated measures ANOVA
Chapter 25

2-way repeated measures ANCOVA
Chapter 30

2-way ANOVA with one repeated measure
Chapter 25

Mixed ANCOVA
Chapter 30

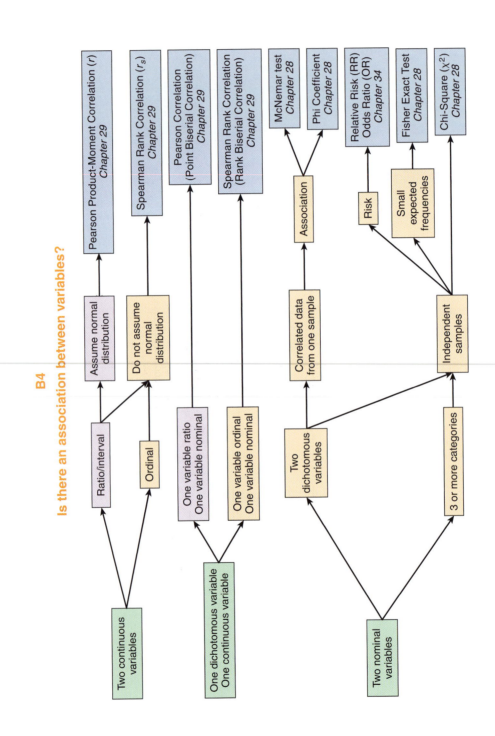

B4

Is there an association between variables?

B5

Do one (or more) independent variables predict one (or more) dependent variables?

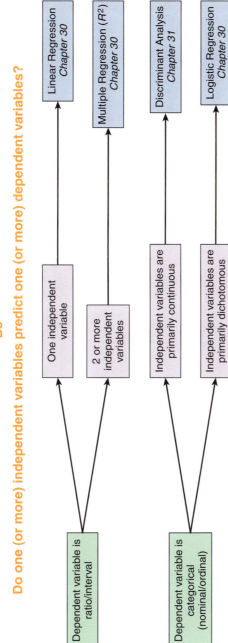

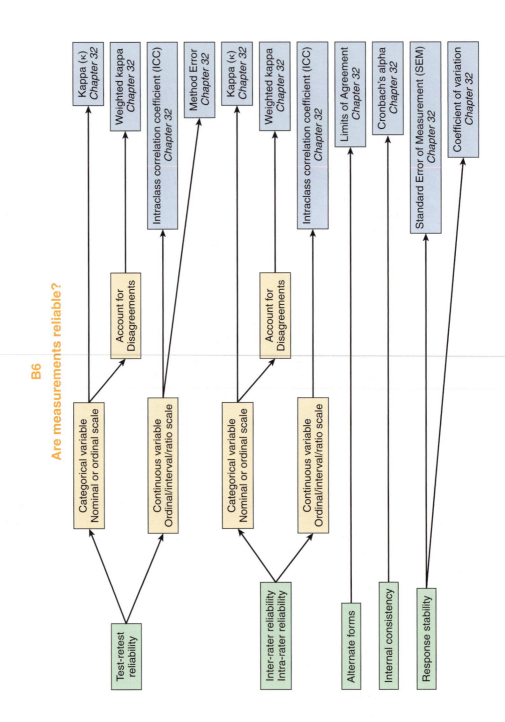

B6

Are measurements reliable?

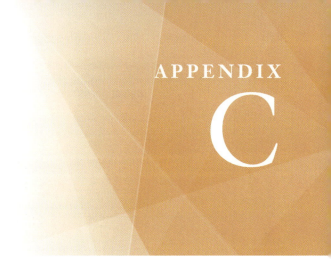

Management of Quantitative Data

An important part of the research planning process is the development of a data management plan that specifies how data will be recorded, organized, and analyzed. This plan begins with the research proposal, specifying the research question, hypotheses, and design. These plans will also translate to the data analysis section under methods in a research report. It is not unusual for these plans to change once the project is under way, but nothing should begin without a firm plan in place. This planning requires knowledge of statistical programs, data coding and format requirements. The purpose of this appendix is to describe the process of data management. SPSS will be used to illustrate the process, consistent with the presentation of statistical output throughout the text.

■ Confidentiality and Security

The research proposal will include a plan for handling data, including maintaining confidentiality of participant information. All subjects should be assigned a unique ID number that is not related to their name, medical unit number, Social Security number, or other personal identifier. Documents for data collection should include the subject ID only. A list of subject names, addresses or phone numbers and corresponding ID codes can be kept separate from other files in case participants need to be contacted.

As part of informed consent, subjects should be assured that their personal information, data from medical records, and data collected as part of the project will be accessed only as necessary for research. The institutional review board (IRB) that approves the project will want to know the type of data to be collected, the purposes for which the data will be used now and in the future, who will have access to records, and what safeguards have been put in place for security and confidentiality (see Chapter 7). Many countries have regulations in place

that define these standards. In the United States, these are part of the Privacy Rule of the Health Insurance Portability and Accountability Act (HIPAA),[1,2] and the Common Rule.[3] In Canada, they are incorporated into the Tri-Council Policy Statement: Ethical Conduct for Research Involving Humans.[4]

■ Monitoring Subject Participation

Throughout the project, researchers should have procedures in place to keep accurate and complete records of participants' involvement. Records should indicate how many participants were recruited and why some were not eligible, how many agreed to participate, and how many eventually did participate. Attrition should be monitored and reasons obtained. Initial group assignments and deviations from these assignments should be documented. This information is relevant to the validity of the project and will be important if the researcher wants to complete an intention to treat analysis. This information should also be accurately reported in a flow diagram, including reasons for drop-outs (see Chapter 15).

■ Statistical Programs

Depending on the type of data, analysis can be accomplished with a variety of sources. Spreadsheets and database systems can accommodate some analyses. Available through academic institutions, integrated Web-based platforms, such as REDCap (Research Electronic Data Capture)[5] or Survey Monkey,[6] can be useful for developing formats for secure data collection such as recording data from surveys.

A wide variety of statistical packages are available. Table C-1 lists a few of the more popular ones. Most

Table C-1	Commonly Used Statistical Packages
PROGRAM	**WEB ADDRESS**
MATLAB	*www.matlab.com*
MedCalc	*www.medcalc.org*
Minitab	*www.minitab.com*
SAS	*www.sas.com*
SPSS	*www.spss.com*
Stata	*www.stata.com*
Systat	*www.systatsoftware.com*

require licensing, but many have student versions at reduced rates. Academic and large clinical centers will often be able to support one or more of these programs. Many other programs are also on the market, and although slightly different, they adhere to certain standards that are important for data management. Most programs provide a format for data entry similar to a spreadsheet and can import spreadsheet data. Several useful references are available that detail procedures in SPSS.[7-9]

A data collection system must be carefully developed, including procedural standards and methods of recording of data. Members of the research team should understand their roles—who will take measurements, who will record data. Measurement standards should be established so there is no discrepancy in data, especially when several investigators or multiple sites are involved. When data include open-ended responses or qualitative data, the format for recording responses must be understood by all involved. If data are missing, the reason should be included. The importance of a well-organized data collection scheme becomes most evident when the researcher begins to enter and analyze data.

Data may be recorded on a separate form for each subject or may be entered directly into a computer. Many data collection methods will already involve direct entry of data, such as using online surveys. Data forms should include the subject's identification code, as well other relevant information such as the date, the individual collecting the data (if there is more than one investigator), the subject's group assignment, and demographic information such as age, gender, and diagnosis. If possible, all data should be listed in the order they will be included in the data file to facilitate data entry.

📌 Strategies for data collection and analysis for qualitative studies require unique considerations and are discussed in Chapter 21. This appendix focuses on quantitative data only.

■ Data Entry

Data may be recorded as continuous or categorical measures. Surveys and interviews may produce open-ended responses that must be coded. Figure C-1 shows data entered in SPSS for a hypothetical study that was described in Chapter 25 (see Fig 25-3). Using a 2×3 factorial design, the study examined the effect of Modality (Ice, Splint, Rest) and Medication (NSAID, no medication) on change in pain-free range of motion (ROM) for patients with lateral epicondylitis. Each subject was randomly assigned to one of six groups, each with a different combination of Modality and Medication. Measurements were taken at baseline and after 10 days and the change in ROM change calculated.

Illustration of data analysis procedures will be based on Table 25-4.

■ Data Collection

The top panel in Figure C-1 is called the *variable view*, which shows all of the variables in the data file and their characteristics. All of these values can be changed by typing in information or using drop-down menus.

Variable Names

Each variable *Name* is entered in the first column. In this example, we have six variables. Every variable in the file must have a unique name. Certain rules apply to variable names, depending on the statistical package being used. For example, in SPSS variable names cannot exceed 64 characters with no spaces, although it is advisable to keep the variable name as short as possible. The first character must be a letter. Underscores, @, #, or $ may be included in the variable name, but should not be used as the first or last character. Upper- and lower-case letters can be used and will be preserved. Researchers should be familiar with the requirements for the statistical package they use.

Type of Variable

The second column in variable view indicates the *Type* of variable. Data can be entered as numerals or characters. Quantitative data are *numeric* only, having values of single or multiple digits, and may include decimal points. Numeric values are assumed to be positive unless a minus sign is entered.

String variables are *alphanumeric*, including letters or characters, which may be combined with numbers. String variables may be letters or words that represent variable values, such as male/female or the names of states or cities. String variables can be summarized with

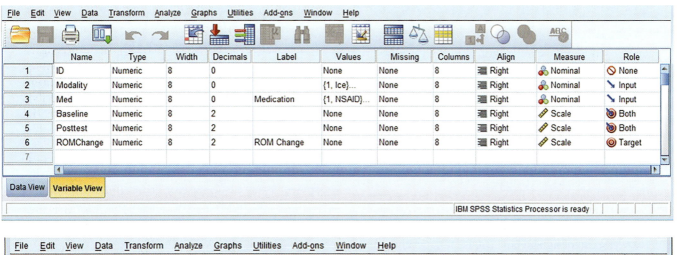

Figure C–1 SPSS screen shots of a data file, showing the variable view (top) and the data view (bottom). Data are shown only for 15 out of 60 cases. These hypothetical data are taken from Chapter 25 for a two-way study of the effect of modality and medication on change in pain-free range of motion in patients with lateral epicondylitis. Results can be found in Table 25-4. Data are available in the Chapter 25 Supplement.

frequencies, but they cannot be subject to numeric operations. Clicking on a cell under this column will bring up a list of other types of variables, including dates, which can be added or subtracted to determine length of time in days, weeks, months, or years. Other than units such as money or dates, it is advisable to code all variables as numbers rather than using letters.

Variables can also be defined according to their level of measurement. Under *Measure*, values can be designated as Scale (interval or ratio), Ordinal, or Nominal. Under the final column, *Roles*, you can choose among several options that identify the role that variable will play in your analysis, such as an independent or dependent variable. This is not a required designation, and *Input* is listed by default, allowing all variables to be used in whatever way the design warrants. For this example, the variables have been designated as independent variables (*Input*), dependent variables (*Target*), or both.

Data Format

The *Width* column lists the maximum number of characters used in a data value. For numeric variables this includes decimal places and the decimal point. This is distinguished from *Columns*, which specifies how wide the column should be for each variable. This is how much space is allocated to a variable as opposed to the actual number of characters filling the space. The default value of 8 is typically sufficient, but these values can be changed. The number of *Decimal*s in the variable value is also specified. In the example, codes for ID and group have no decimal places, but measures of ROM are taken to two places. These can be changed by the researcher to accommodate the values of each variable. Under *Align*, you can designate how you want data values to be aligned in the file: left, right, or justified.

Codes for Categorical Variables

Categorical variables are entered as codes. For example, scores of 1 through 5 can be used for responses in a Likert scale. Gender can be coded as 0 = male and 1 = female. When the research design includes group comparisons, each subject's group assignment must be identified by a code for the *grouping variable*. For instance, in the modality study there are two grouping variables, Modality and Med. When codes are used as a pure label this way, it does not matter what numbering scheme is used. However, for dichotomous variables that represent data values, such as variables used in a logistic regression, it is conventional to use 1 and 0 as codes, usually signifying the absence of a trait as zero. Many statistical procedures will only manipulate categorical data with 1 and 0 as the category codes, sometimes requiring the use of dummy variables (see Chapter 30).

Labels

Because variable names are usually kept short, it is sometimes confusing to read a printout of an analysis. It may be difficult to remember what each variable name means. For instance, items on a survey may be named Question1, Question2 and so on. To facilitate reading the output, programs allow the researcher to specify a *Label* for a variable name. These labels do not have the restrictions of variable names and can use spaces or other characters but are limited in length (256 characters in SPSS). For example, in a survey the actual question can be entered as a label. In the modality study a full label has been entered for Medication and ROM Change. Labels are not required, but with large data sets they are extremely useful.

Categorical codes can also be defined. In the *Values* column you can enter labels for codes. For instance, with a Likert scale, a score of 5 can be defined as Agree, 4 as Somewhat Agree, and so on. Although you can't see the full labels in variable view (see Fig. C-1), you can see that codes have been identified for Modality (1 = Ice, 2 = Splint, 3 = Rest) and Med (1 = NSAID, 2 = no medication). If you click on these cells in the data file, a *Value Labels* dialog box will appear where these values have been entered.

Missing Data

It is not unusual for some data points to be missing from a subject's record because of errors in recording, unavailability of information, nonresponses on surveys, noncompliance or attrition. To identify missing values, blanks are used as the default in most computer programs. Others have specific rules for identifying missing values, such as the use of a period in place of a missing datum. Zeros should not be used to represent missing values because they will be read as a value and may affect statistical calculations.

Sometimes it is useful to assign specific codes for missing values, to identify the reason for the missing information. Such distinctions can be helpful for tallying demographic data and interpretation of results, especially when there are many missing data points. Rather than just leaving a generic blank for all missing values, specific codes can be entered under *Missing*. These numeric codes should be out of range of any actual data values. For example, for an interview questionnaire, we could code 99 for a response of "Don't know" or 9 for refusal to answer a question. In this example no missing value labels have been entered.

 SPSS can perform multiple imputation to substitute values for missing data (see Chapter 15.)

Listwise and Pairwise Deletion

For some statistical procedures, you can designate one of two strategies for handling missing data under *Options*. *Listwise deletion* means that a case is dropped if it has a missing value for one or more data points. Analysis will be run only on cases with complete data, eliminating cases with any missing data from all calculations. *Pairwise deletion* can be used for some procedures when a particular comparison, descriptive value, correlation, or regression do not include every score. Cases are omitted only if they are missing any of the variables involved in the specific procedure. For instance, means can be calculated for each variable, using only cases with a value for that variable. This means that *n* could be different for each variable.

Data Entry

As shown in the bottom panel of Figure C-1, the standard structure for data entry requires that each variable is entered in a separate column. Each row of data represents a single subject's scores, called a *record* or *case*. Each individual score, or variable value, is identified as a *field*. A case is composed of several fields of data.

Data may be typed directly into a statistical program, or it may be entered in a spreadsheet first and later imported into the statistical program. If data are first saved as a spreadsheet, the same configuration of columns and rows should be used. However, the first row in each column should contain the variable name, which will then be read by the statistical program. To facilitate this transfer, the variable names should conform to the restrictions of the statistical program. Other than this first row, all other rows in the spreadsheet should contain only data. No embedded formulas or charts should be included. If formulas are used in specific cells, they should be converted to the actual data values before transferring to a statistical program.

> No matter how information is entered, the wise researcher will save the data often and back up the data file regularly. I have suffered too much, along with too many colleagues, having lost hours of work to take this advice lightly!

Code books are used to catalog the order of entry of all variables. Variable names are listed with their abbreviations and codes are listed to identify their values. Figure C-2 shows how SPSS can display all variable information. The code book is a necessary reference for all those who are involved with the study, most especially those who will analyze the data.

> The term *code book* was originally used for a book that the researcher created to list all variable names and codes. The term is still used, although it is no longer an actual book.

Data Cleaning

Once data are entered and before analyses are run, the data should be examined to detect abnormalities or errors, a process called *data cleaning*. Although it may be time consuming, it is an essential step to ensure validity of the data analysis. The process involves running a series of descriptive analyses to inspect the distribution of scores for each variable.

For instance, running a frequency distribution for categorical variables will let you see if the correct number of subjects are assigned to each code, or if there are aberrant codes entered. For continuous variables, descriptive statistics should be run to analyze means, minimums, and maximums, to be sure that the range of scores is appropriate. In this way, the researcher can ascertain if values out of the possible range have been entered. These analyses will also reveal if there are missing data. Sometimes it is useful to sort data, reordering the subjects according to the value of a particular variable, to determine if appropriate numbers have been entered.

Distributions should be examined to determine if they meet assumptions of a normal distribution using the Kolmogorov-Smirnov or Shapiro-Wilk tests (see Chapter 23, Box 23-4). Graphic analyses can be informative. Histograms, boxplots, or scatterplots can be used to identify outliers, and you can go back to determine if the value is a valid one (see Chapters 22 and 29).

Data Modification

All statistical programs include processes for *data modification* or *transformation* to create new variables or to assign new codes to existing variables. For example, we might want to compute the mean of several trials to use for data analysis. Or we might have scores for several items on a scale and want to get the sum. Continuous variables can be converted to categories by establishing codes for specific ranges of scores, such as creating age groups from a continuous measure of age. When these types of transformations are performed, a new variable is created, and must be given a new and unique variable name. These are considered linear transformations, as they apply simple arithmetic operations changes values, but does not change the shape of the distribution of scores.[10]

Computing New Variables

Computing a new variable requires that some arithmetic operations be performed on the existing data. New variables are creating using TRANSFORM > COMPUTE VARIABLE.

A new variable is defined by an arithmetic expression using various *operators*. The following symbols are used by most programs for arithmetic operations:

+ Add A + B	* Multiply A*B
− Subtract A − B	** or ^ Exponent A**2
/ Divide A/B	or A^2

These are considered *simple expressions* because they contain one operator. For instance, in the original data file for the ROM study, only baseline and posttest scores were obtained. A new variable was then defined, called

Variable Information

Variable	Position	Label	Measurement Level	Role	Column Width	Alignment	Print Format	Write Format
id	1	<none>	Scale	Input	8	Right	F8	F8
Modality	2	<none>	Nominal	Input	8	Right	F8	F8
Med	3	Medication	Nominal	Input	8	Right	F8	F8
Baseline	4	<none>	Scale	Input	8	Right	F8.2	F8.2
Posttest	5	<none>	Scale	Input	8	Right	F8.2	F8.2
ROMChange	6	ROM Change	Scale	Input	11	Right	F8.2	F8.2

Variables in the working file

Variable Values

Value		Label
Modality	1	Ice
	2	Splint
	3	Rest
Med	1	NSAID
	2	No Med

Figure C–2 Code book generated by SPSS for data from the study of the effect of modality and medication on change in pain-free elbow ROM in patients with lateral epicondylitis. The top panel shows six variables and their characteristics. This information is similar to the material in variable view. The bottom panel shows the codes used for the two categorical variables, modality group and medication group. This output is generated using FILE> Display Data File Information.

ROMChange, calculated as the difference between the baseline and posttest scores:

$$ROMChange = posttest - baseline$$

When these computations are done, the values for the new variable will appear as a new line in variable view and a new column in the data view (see Fig. C-1). These new variables can now be used in statistical procedures.

When more than one operator is used, a *compound expression* is created, such as

$$A**2*B/(C+1.0)$$

This expression is equal to

$$\frac{(A^2)(B)}{C+1.0}$$

When compound expressions are used, specific rules apply to the order in which operations take place. First, all expressions within parentheses are carried out. Second, adjacent operations are carried out in the following order: (1) exponentiation, (2) division and multiplication, and (3) addition and subtraction. Within each of these levels, operations proceed from left to right. Therefore, in the preceding expression, the first operation will be to

complete the addition (C+1.0) within the parentheses. Next, the value of *A* will be squared. This value will then be multiplied by *B*. Lastly, this product will be divided by the sum (C + 1.0). If the parentheses had been left out, the expression would be read differently. For instance, using

$$A**2*B/C+1.0$$

the expression would read

$$\frac{(A^2)(B)}{C}+1.0$$

Recoding Variables

Sometimes we want to create new codes for a categorical variable. Recodes are obtained using TRANSFORM > RECODE INTO DIFFERENT VARIABLES.

Suppose we wanted to change our design, and combine all patients in the Splint and Rest groups to compare them against the group receiving Ice. We would want to recode the group designations, creating a new variable called NewModality. We would then designate old and new values, so that all those with original codes of 2 or 3 for Modality will now have a value of 2 for NewModality.

There is an option to RECODE INTO THE SAME VARIABLE, which means the original data would be lost. Unless there are major errors that need to be corrected, it is always better to create a new variable and keep the original data intact.

Data Transformation

Many statistical procedures, like the *t*-test, analysis of variance, and linear regression, are based on assumptions about homogeneity of variance and normality that should be met to ensure the validity of the test. Although most parametric statistical procedures are considered robust to moderate violations of these assumptions, some modification to the analysis is usually necessary with striking departures. When this occurs, the researcher can choose one of two approaches to accommodate the analysis. The analytic procedure can be modified by using nonparametric statistics or nonlinear regression, or the dependent variable can be transformed to a new variable that more closely satisfies the necessary assumptions. The new variable is created by changing the scale of measurement through *data transformation*.

The three most common reasons for using data transformation are to satisfy the assumption of homogeneity of variance, to conform data to a normal distribution, or to create a more linear distribution that will fit the linear regression model. Fortunately, the same transformation will often accomplish more than one of these goals.

The most commonly used transformations are the square root, square, log, reciprocal, and arc sine transformations. The choice of which method to use will depend on characteristics of the data. It will be helpful to illustrate the transformation process using the square root transformation.

Data transformation helps in statistical calculations when the intent is to determine if groups are significantly different, or if there are significant relationships among variables. It is important, however, to remember that the transformed values are not the actual values, and units of outcomes cannot be interpreted as such.

Square Root Transformation

The square root transformation ($\sqrt{X}$) replaces each score in a distribution with its square root. This method is most appropriate when variances are roughly proportional to group means, when $s^2/\bar{X}$ is similar for all groups. The square root transformation will typically have the effect of equalizing variances.

Suppose we were given two sample distributions, A and B, shown in Table C-2. Their variances, $s_A^2 = 8.5$ and $s_B^2 = 26.5$ are quite different. We determine the applicability of the square root transformation by demonstrating that $s^2/\bar{X}$ is similar for both distributions.

Each score in both distributions is transformed to its square root for distributions A' and B'. As we can see, the effect of the transformation is a reduction in the discrepancy between the two variances. These transformed values can now be used in statistical analyses.

Square Transformation

The square transformation (X^2) is used primarily in regression analyses when the relationship between X and Y is curvilinear downward, when slope steadily decreases as X increases. This transformation will cause the relationship to appear more linear. It will also have the effect of stabilizing variances and will normalize the dependent variable when residuals are negatively skewed.

Log Transformation

The log transformation ($\log X$) is most appropriate when the standard deviations of the original data are proportional to the means, when $s/\bar{X}$ is roughly constant across distributions. In addition to equalizing variances, the log transformation is used most often to normalize a skewed distribution. In regression analyses, the log transformation can also be used to create a more linear relationship between X and Y when the regression model shows a constantly increasing slope. The effect of log transformation can be easily demonstrated by plotting scores on logarithmic or semilogarithmic graph paper.

Table C-2 Effect of Square Root Transformation

	ORIGINAL X		TRANSFORMED $\sqrt{X}$	
	A	B	A'	B'
	1	8	1.00	2.83
	3	7	1.73	2.65
	8	12	2.83	3.46
	6	5	2.45	2.24
	2	18	1.41	4.24
Σ	20	50	9.42	15.42
$\bar{X}$	4	10	1.88	3.08
s^2	8.5	26.5	0.56	0.61
$s^2/\bar{X}$	2.125	2.65		

Table C-3 Transformation Based on Largest and Smallest Scores in Two Distributions

	GROUP		$\sqrt{X}$		LOG X		1/X	
	1	2	1	2	1	2	1	2
Largest	18	40	4.24	6.32	1.26	1.60	.06	.02
Smallest	10	20	3.16	4.47	1.00	1.30	.10	.05
Range	8	20	1.08	1.85	0.26	0.30	.04	.03
Ratio	$\dfrac{\text{range}_{largest}}{\text{range}_{smallest}}$		$\dfrac{1.85}{1.08} = 1.71$		$\dfrac{.30}{.26} = 1.15$		$\dfrac{.04}{.03} = 1.33$	

Reciprocal Transformation

The reciprocal transformation (1/X) is used when the standard deviations of the original data are proportional the square of the mean, $s/\bar{X}^2$.[11] It is effective for attaining homogeneity of variance or normality. Use of this approach will minimize the skewing effect of large values of X, which will be close to zero in their reciprocal form.

Arc Sine Transformation

The arc sine transformation (arcsin $\sqrt{X}$) is also called angular transformation. It is used when data are collected in the form of proportions or percentages. The relationship $s^2 = \bar{X}(1-\bar{X})$ should be constant for all samples. This transformation is based on an angular scale, whereby each proportion, p, is replaced by the angle whose sine is $\sqrt{p}$. Angles are usually given in radians.

Choosing a Transformation

Reasons for choosing one transformation procedure may be less than obvious. Many researchers use trial and error to determine the transformation that is most successful at reorienting the data. Kirk[11] has suggested a method that may be helpful in facilitating this decision. He uses different transformations to convert the largest and smallest scores in each distribution. The difference between the largest and smallest score, or the range of the distribution, is calculated using the transformed values. The ratio of the larger to the smaller range is then calculated for each transformation. The transformation that produces the smallest ratio is selected. This process is illustrated in Table C-3, where the transformation using log X would be chosen. Ideally the transformed scores will have a nearly normal distribution without extreme outliers, and relationships between pairs of transformed variables with be linear.

REFERENCES

1. National Institutes of Health. HIPAA Resources. Available at https://privacyruleandresearch.nih.gov/. Accessed January 30, 2018.
2. Brown T. Construct validity: a unitary concept for occupational therapy assessment and measurement. *Hong Kong J Occup Ther* 2010;20(1):30-42.
3. Office of Human Research Protections. Federal policy for the protection of human subjects ('Common Rule'). Available at https://www.hhs.gov/ohrp/regulations-and-policy/regulations/common-rule/index.html. Accessed January 27, 2018.
4. Government of Canada: Panel on Research Ethics. TCPS 2 (2014). Available at http://www.pre.ethics.gc.ca/eng/policy-politique/initiatives/tcps2-eptc2/default/. Accessed March 20, 2019.
5. REDCap. Available at https://www.project-redcap.org/. Accessed April 10, 2019.
6. Survey Monkey. Available at www.surveymonkey.com. Accessed September 17, 2019.
7. Green SB, Salkind NJ. *Using SPSS for Windows and Macintosh: Analyzing and Understanding Data*. 8th ed. New York: Pearson; 2017.
8. Field A. *Discovering Statistics Using IBM SPSS Statistics*. 5th ed. Thousand Oaks, CA: Sage; 2018.
9. Huizingh E. *Applied Statistics with SPSS*. Thousand Oaks, CA: Sage Publications; 2007.
10. Warner RM. *Applied Statistics*. Thousand Oaks, CA: Sage Publications; 2013.
11. Kirk RE. *Experimental Design: Procedures for the Behavioral Sciences*. 4th ed. Thousand Oaks, CA: Sage; 2013.

Glossary

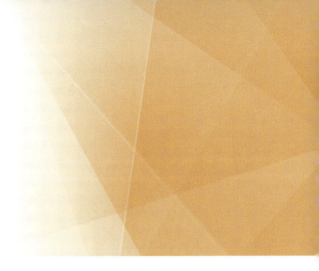

Numbers in parentheses indicate the chapter in which the term is introduced.

■ Terms

absolute reliability. Indicates how much of a measured value, expressed in the original units, is likely to be due to error. (9,32)

absolute risk increase (ARI). The increase in risk associated with an intervention as compared to the risk without the intervention (or the control condition); the absolute difference between the control event rate (CER) and the experimental event rate (EER). (34)

absolute risk reduction (ARR). The reduction in risk associated with an intervention as compared to the risk without the intervention (or the control condition); the absolute difference between the experimental event rate (EER) and the control event rate (CER). (34)

accessible population. The actual population of subjects available to be chosen for a study. This group is usually a nonrandom subset of the target population. (13)

active variable. An independent variable with levels that can be manipulated and assigned by the researcher. (14)

adjusted means. Means that have been adjusted based on the value of a covariate in an analysis of covariance. (30)

agreement. (see *percent agreement*)

allocation concealment. Implementation of a process of random assignment where those involved in the trial are shielded from knowing the upcoming participant group assignment. (14)

alpha coefficient. (see *Cronbach's alpha*)

alpha (α). Level of statistical significance, or risk of Type I error; maximum probability level that can be achieved in a statistical test to reject the null hypothesis. (23) (see also *Cronbach's alpha*)

alternate forms reliability. Reliability of two equivalent forms of a measuring instrument. (32)

alternating treatment design. A single-case design in which two (or more) treatments are compared by alternating them within a session or in alternate sessions. (18)

alternative hypothesis (H_1). Hypothesis stating the expected relationship between independent and dependent variables; considered the negation of the null hypothesis. The alternative hypothesis is accepted when the null hypothesis is rejected. (23)

analysis of covariance (ANCOVA). Statistical procedure used to compare two or more conditions while controlling for the effect of one or more covariates. (15,30)

analysis of variance (ANOVA). Statistical procedure appropriate for comparison of three or more treatment groups or conditions, or the simultaneous manipulation of two or more independent variables; based on the F statistic. (25)

a priori comparisons. (see *planned comparisons*)

arm. (see *treatment arm*)

attributable risk. An estimate used to quantify the risk of disease in an exposed group that is attributable to the exposure, by removing the risk that would have occurred as a result of other causes (risk in the unexposed group). (34)

attribute variable. An independent variable with levels that cannot be manipulated or assigned by the researcher but that represent subject characteristics (such as age and sex). (14)

attrition (experimental mortality). A threat to internal validity, referring to the differential loss of participants during the course of data collection, potentially introducing bias by changing the composition of the sample. (15)

audit trail. Comprehensive process of documenting interpretation of qualitative data. (21)

autonomy. The capacity of individuals to make decisions affecting their own lives and to act on those decisions. (7)

background question. Question related to etiology or general knowledge about a patient's condition, referring to the cause of a disease or condition, its natural history, signs and symptoms, general management, or the anatomic or physiological mechanisms that relate to pathophysiology. (5)

backward selection. Form of stepwise multiple regression. The equation starts out with all independent variables in the model, and variables are eliminated one at a time if they do not contribute significantly to the model. (30)

basic research (preclinical research). Research that contributes to basic knowledge but that does not have immediate practical goals. (2,14)

Bayes' theorem. The calculation of the probability of an event based on the prior probability of another event; used to estimate posttest probabilities based on pretest probabilities of a diagnostic outcome. (33)

beneficence. Obligation to attend to the well-being of individuals engaged as research subjects. (7)

beta (β). 1. Probability of making a Type II error. (23) 2. Used to represent coefficients for the relationship between two endogenous variables in structural equation modeling. (31)

beta weight. In a multiple regression equation, the standardized coefficient for each independent variable. (30)

between-groups variance. That portion of the total variance in a set of scores that is attributed to the difference between groups. (24,25)

between-subjects design. A design that compares independent groups. (16)

bias. Any influence that may interfere with the valid relationship between variables, potentially resulting in misleading interpretation of outcomes. (15)

binomial test. A significance test of the deviations of observations from a theoretically expected deviation for a dichotomous variable. 1. Used to evaluate data points above or below the split middle line in single-subject designs. (18) 2. Used to compare two sets of data in a repeated sample with the nonparametric sign test. (27)

Bland-Altman plot. A plot analyzing the agreement between two measurements. The mean of the two measures for each subject is plotted against the difference between the means. (see also *limits of agreement*). (32)

blinding. Techniques to reduce experimental bias by keeping participants and/or investigators ignorant of group assignments and research hypotheses. (14)

blocking variable. Attribute variable in which subjects are divided into groups or blocks that are homogeneous on a particular characteristic. (15,16)

block randomization. Distributes subjects evenly among treatment groups within small, even numbered subgroups or "blocks." (14)

Bonferroni correction (adjustment). A correction often used when multiple statistical tests are performed on the same data set to reduce Type I error. The desired level of significance (α) is divided by the number of comparisons. The resulting value is then used as the level of significance for each comparison to reject the null hypothesis. (26)

Boolean logic. In literature searches, the terms AND, NOT, and OR used to expand or narrow search terms. (6)

box plot (box-and-whisker plot). A graphic display of a distribution, showing the median, 25th and 75th percentiles (interquartile range), and highest and lowest scores. (22)

canonical correlation. A multivariate correlation procedure, whereby two sets of variables are correlated. (31)

carryover effect. A temporary or permanent change in behavior resulting from prior treatments. (10)

case-control study. A design in analytic epidemiology in which the investigator selects subjects on the basis of their having or not having a particular disease or condition and then determines their previous exposure to a risk factor. (1,19)

case report (case series). Detailed report of the symptoms, signs, diagnosis, treatment, and follow-up of one or more individual patients, usually describing interesting treatment options or uncommon conditions. (20)

case study. A qualitative research design used to study complex phenomena within their social context, investigating individuals or organizations. Can involve evaluation of interventions, policies, or theoretical premises. (21)

causal modeling. Statistical technique that examines patterns of intercorrelations among variables to determine if they fit an underlying theory of which variables cause others. (see also *structural equation modeling*) (31)

ceiling effect. A measurement limitation of an instrument whereby the scale cannot determine increased performance beyond a certain level. (10)

celeration line. (see *split middle line*)

censored observation. An observation whose value is unknown because the subject has not been in the study long enough for the outcome to have occurred; used to estimate survival curves. (31)

central tendency. Descriptive statistics that represent "averages" or scores that are representative of a distribution; includes mean, median, and mode. (22)

centroid. A point determined from the intersection of two or more means of two dependent variables (X, Y), used in multivariate analysis. (31)

chi-square (χ^2). A nonparametric test applied to categorical data, comparing observed frequencies within categories to frequencies expected by chance. (28)

classical measurement theory (CMT). Concept of measurement whereby a measured value is considered to be a function of an underlying true score and measurement error. (9, 12)

clinical practice guideline (CPG). Systematically developed statement, based on available evidence, that provide recommendations to assist practitioner and patient decisions about appropriate healthcare for specific clinical circumstances. (5,37)

clinical prediction rule. A combination of clinical findings that have been shown to predict a diagnosis, prognosis, or treatment outcome. (33)

clinical trial. (see *randomized controlled trial*)

clinical trials registry. A database that provides listing of trials in planning and implementation phases. (14)

closed-ended question. A question on a survey (interview or questionnaire) that offers a set of specific response choices that are mutually exclusive and exhaustive. (11)

cluster analysis. A multivariate statistical procedure that classifies subjects into sets based on defined characteristics. (31)

cluster random assignment. The site, representing a "cluster" of subjects, is randomly assigned to an intervention, and all individuals at that site receive that treatment. (14)

cluster sampling. A form of probability sampling in which large subgroups (clusters) are randomly selected first, and then smaller units from these clusters are successively chosen; also called multistage sampling. (13)

coefficient alpha. (see *Cronbach's alpha*)

coefficient of determination (r^2). Coefficient representing the amount of variance in one variable (Y) that can be explained (accounted for) by a second variable (X). (30)

coefficient of variation (CV). A measure of relative variation; based on the standard deviation divided by the mean, expressed as a percentage. Can be used to describe data measured on the interval or ratio scale. (22)

Cohen's d. The effect size index for comparing two groups, equals the difference between means divided by a pooled standard deviation. (see also *standardized mean difference*). (24)

cohort effects. Variations of effects of a given group as they move through time, such as individuals born in a particular era. (19,20)

cohort study. An observational study design in which a specific group is followed over time. Subjects are classified according to whether they do or do not have a particular risk factor or exposure and followed to determine disease outcomes. (19)

collinearity. The correlation between independent variables in a multiple regression equation, causing them to provide redundant information. Also called multicollinearity. (30)

Common Rule. Codification of policies related to informed consent and ethical conduct in research. (7)

communality. In factor analysis, the extent to which an item correlates with other variables. (31)

completer analysis (complete case analysis). Analysis of data in a clinical trial only for those subjects who complete the study. (15)

complex contrasts. A multiple comparison strategy in which means from two or more groups are combined as a subset and compared with other individual means or subsets of means. (26)

complex hypothesis. Contains more than one independent or dependent variable. (3)

computer adaptive testing (CAT). A computer-based test or scale in which items are adapted to the subject's ability level. (12)

concurrent validity. A form of criterion-related validity; the degree to which the outcomes of one test correlate with outcomes on a criterion test, when both tests are given at relatively the same time. (10,32)

confirmability. In qualitative research, ensuring, as much as possible, that findings are due to the experiences and ideas of the participants, rather than the characteristics and preferences of the researcher. (21)

confirmatory factor analysis (CFA). Used to support the theoretical structure of an instrument, to determine if it fits with current empirical understanding of a construct. (10, 31)

confidence interval (CI). The range of values within which a population parameter is estimated to fall, with a specific level of confidence, usually 95%. (23)

confounding. The contaminating effect of extraneous variables on interpretation of the relationship between independent and dependent variables. (15,19,34)

consecutive sampling. A form of nonprobability sampling, where subjects are recruited as they become available. (13)

constant comparison. In qualitative research, the process by which each new piece of information is compared with data already collected to determine where the data agree or conflict. (21)

construct. An abstract concept that is unobservable, that can only be measured by observing related behaviors. (see also *latent trait*) (4,8)

construct validity. 1. A type of measurement validity indicating the degree to which a theoretical construct is measured by an instrument. (10) 2. Design validity related to operational definitions of independent and dependent variables. (15)

content analysis. A procedure for analyzing and coding narrative data in a systematic way. (21)

content validity. A type of measurement validity indicating the degree to which the items in an instrument adequately reflect the content domain being measured. (10)

contingency table (crosstabulation). A two-dimensional table displaying frequencies or counts, with rows (R) and columns (C) representing categories of nominal or ordinal variables. (28)

continuity correction. (see *Yates' continuity correction*)

continuous variable. A quantitative variable that can theoretically take on values along a continuum. (8)

control event rate (CER). The number of subjects in the control group who develop the outcome of interest. (34)

control group. In an experiment, a group of subjects who resemble the experimental group but who do not receive the experimental treatment (assigned a placebo or control condition), providing a baseline of comparison to interpret effects of treatment. (14)

convenience sampling. A nonprobability sampling procedure, involving selection of the most available subjects for a study. (13)

convergent validity. An approach in construct validation, assessing the degree to which two different instruments or methods are able to measure the same construct. (10)

correlation. The tendency for variation in one variable to be related to variation in a second variable; those statistical procedures used to assess the degree of covariation between two variables. (29)

covariate. An extraneous variable that is statistically controlled in an analysis of covariance or regression analysis, so that the relationship between the independent and dependent variables is analyzed with the effect of the extraneous factor removed. (15,30)

Cox proportional hazards regression. A regression procedure used to measure the effect of one or more predictor variables on the rate (hazard) at which an outcome occurs, accounting for differing lengths of follow-up among subjects. Used in survival analysis. (31)

credibility. In qualitative research, a criterion for integrity of data, confidence in the truth or validity of findings. (21)

criterion-referenced test. A fixed standard that represents an acceptable level of performance. (10)

criterion-related validity. A type of measurement validity indicating the degree to which the outcomes of one test correlate with outcomes on a criterion test; can be assessed as concurrent validity or predictive validity. (10)

critically appraised topic (CAT). A short summary and appraisal of evidence focused on a clinical question. (36)

critical region. Area of a sample probability curve that corresponds to rejection of the null hypothesis based on the critical value of the test statistic. (23)

critical value. The value of a test statistic that must be exceeded for the null hypothesis to be rejected; the value of a statistic that defines the critical region. (23)

Cronbach's alpha (α). Reliability index of internal consistency of items on a scale. (9,32)

crossover design. A repeated measures design used to control order effects when comparing two treatments, where half of the sample receives treatment A first followed by treatment B, and the other half receives treatment B first followed by treatment A. May include a washout period. (16)

cross-sectional study. A study based on data collected at one point in time. Observations of different age or developmental groups may provide the basis for inferring trends over time. (19)

crosstabulation. (see *contingency table*)

cumulative incidence (CI). The number of new cases of a disease during a specified time period divided by the total number of people at risk; the proportion of new cases of a disease in a population. (34)

cumulative scale. A scale designed so that agreement with higher-level responses assumes agreement with all lower-level responses. Also called a Guttman scale. (12)

curvilinear relationship. The relationship between two variables that does not follow a linear proportional relationship. (29,30)

cut-off score. Score used as the demarcation of a positive or negative continuous test outcome. (12,33)

deductive reasoning. The logical process of developing specific hypotheses based on general principles. (4)

degrees of freedom (*df*). Statistical concept indicating the number of values within a distribution that are free to vary, given restrictions on the data set; usually *n*-1. (23)

Delphi survey. Survey method whereby decisions on items are based on consensus of a panel over several rounds. (11 Supplement)

dependability. In qualitative research, the stability of data over time, the degree to which the study could be repeated with similar results. (21)

dependent variable. A response variable that is assumed to depend on or be caused by another (independent) variable. (3)

descriptive research. Research studies that are designed to describe the characteristics of individuals in specific populations. (20)

descriptive statistics. Statistics that are used to characterize the shape, central tendency, and variability within a set of data, often with the intent to describe a sample or population. (22)

developmental research. A descriptive research approach designed to document how certain groups change over time on specific variables. (20)

deviation score. The distance of a single data point from the mean of the distribution. The sum of the deviation scores for a given distribution will always equal zero. (22)

dichotomy (dichotomous variable). A nominal variable having only two categories, such as yes/no and male/female; a binomial variable. (8)

difference score (*d*). The difference between two scores taken on the same individual. (19)

differential item functioning (DIF). Potential item bias in the fit of data to the Rash model, showing how an item may be measuring different abilities for subgroups. (12)

digital object identifier (DOI). A unique number assigned to scholarly articles that can be used to locate particular articles in a search. (6,38)

directional hypothesis. A research hypothesis (or alternative hypothesis) that predicts the direction of a relationship between two variables. (3)

discrete variable. A variable that can only be measured in separate units and that cannot be measured in intervals of less than 1. (8)

discriminant analysis. A multivariate statistical technique used to determine if a set of variables can predict group membership. (31)

discriminant validity. An approach in construct validation assessing the degree to which an instrument yields different results when measuring two different constructs; that is, the ability to discriminate between the constructs. (10)

disproportional sample. A sample stratified on a particular variable, when the number of subjects within a stratum is not proportional to the population size of that stratum. (13)

distribution. The total set of scores for a particular variable. (22)

divergent validity. (see *discriminant validity*)

DOI. (see *digital object identifier*)

dose-response relationship. An outcome in which risk varies, not only with the presence or absence of an exposure, but also with varying levels of the exposure's presence. (19)

double-blind study. An experiment in which both the investigator and the subject are kept ignorant of group assignment. (14)

dummy variable (coding). In regression procedures, the assignment of codes (0 and 1) to a nominal variable, reflecting the presence or absence of certain traits. (30)

ecological validity. The generalizability of study findings to real-word conditions, societal norms, and health of populations. (15)

effectiveness. Benefits of an intervention as tested under "real world" conditions. (2)

effect modification. A situation in which the strength of an association between two variables is affected by a third variable that differs across subgroups in the population. (34)

effect size. The magnitude of the difference between treatments or the magnitude of a relationship between variables. (23)

effect size index. A statistical value used to measure the effect size in standardized units based on the proportional relationship of the difference to variance. Different indices are used with various statistical tests. (23)

efficacy. Benefit of an intervention as tested under controlled experimental conditions, usually with a control group in a randomized controlled trial. (2)

eigenvalue. A measure of the proportion of the total variance accounted for by a factor in a factor analysis. (31)

endogenous variable. The variable being explained by a causal model, a dependent variable. (31)

epidemiology. That branch of research dedicated to exploring the frequency and determinants of disease or other health outcomes in populations. (34)

equipoise. The ethics of a clinical research situation in which there is genuine uncertainty regarding the comparative therapeutic merits of each arm of a trial. (14)

equivalence trial. An intervention study focused on showing that two treatments are not different, no better, no worse. (14)

error variance. That portion of the total variance in a data set that cannot be attributed to treatment effects but that is due to differences between subjects. (23)

eta squared (η^2). Effect size index for analysis of variance. (25)

ethnography. An approach to qualitative research in which the experiences of a specific cultural group are studied. (21)

exclusion criteria. Specific criteria that are used to determine who is not eligible for a study. (8,13)

exogenous variable. A variable in a causal model that is not explained by the model, with variance that is accounted for by variables outside of the model, an independent variable. (31)

expected frequencies. In a contingency table, the frequencies that would be expected if the null hypothesis is true; frequencies that are expected just by chance. (28)

experimental design. A design in which the investigator manipulates the independent variables and randomly assigns subjects to groups, and in which a control group or comparison group is used. (16)

experimental event rate (EER). The number of subjects in the experimental or treatment group who develop the outcome of interest. (34)

explained variance. Between-groups variance; that portion of the total variance in a data set that can be attributed to the differences between groups or treatment conditions. (25)

explanatory research. Utilizes various types of experimental designs to compare two or more conditions or interventions. (1,3)

exploratory factor analysis (EFA). Used to study a set of items, when the purpose is to determine how the variables cluster, or to establish what underlying concepts may be present in the construct. (10,31)

exploratory research. Observational research that has as its purpose the exploration of data to determine relationships among variables. (3,19)

exposure. An experience or condition that may be responsible for a health outcome. (19)

external criticism. Assessment of generalizability in historical research. (20)

external validity. The degree to which results of a study can be generalized to persons or settings outside the experimental situation. (15)

fabrication. Reporting data or results that have been made up. (7)

face validity. The assumption of validity of a measuring instrument based on its appearance as a reasonable measure of a given variable. (10)

factor. 1. A variable. (3) 2. An independent variable in an experimental study. (25) 3. A set of interrelated variables in a factor analysis. (31)

factor analysis. An exploratory multivariate statistical technique used to examine the structure of a latent variable within a large set of variables and to determine the underlying dimensions that exist within that set of variables. (see also *exploratory* and *confirmatory factor analysis*). (10,31)

factorial design. A design that incorporates two or more independent variables, with independent groups of subjects randomly assigned to various combinations of levels of the variables. (10)

false negative. A test result that is negative in a person who has the disease or condition of interest. (34)

falsification. Manipulating, changing, or omitting data or results such that the research is not accurately represented in the research record. (7)

false positive. A test result that is positive in a person who does not have the disease or condition of interest. (34)

familywise error rate (α_{FW}). The probability of at least one false significant finding in a series of hypothesis tests, Type I error. (26)

field notes. Notes recorded during participation or observation as part of qualitative research. (21)

Fisher's exact test. A nonparametric procedure applied to nominal data in a 2 x 2 contingency table, comparing observed frequencies within categories to frequencies expected by chance. Used when samples are too small to use the chi-square test. (28)

fixed effect. Variable levels that are nonrandom, representing the only qualities of interest. (32)

floor effect. A measurement limitation of an instrument whereby the scale cannot determine decreased performance beyond a certain level. (10)

foreground question. A clinical question that focuses on evidence to inform decisions about a particular patient's management. (5)

forest plot. Graphic display of effect sizes and confidence intervals for individual studies and pooled data in a meta-analysis. (37)

forward selection. A process used in multiple regression that enters variables one at a time into the equation based on the strength of their association with the outcome variable, until all statistically significant variables are included. (30)

frequency distribution. A table of rank ordered scores that shows the number of times each value occurs in a distribution. (22)

Friedman two-way analysis of variance by ranks (χ_r^2). A nonparametric statistical procedure for repeated measures, comparing more than two treatment conditions of one independent variable; analogous to the one-way repeated measures analysis of variance. (27)

funnel plot. Scatterplot of treatment effect size against a measure of study precision such as the standard error, used as a visual aid for detecting publication bias or study heterogeneity in a meta-analysis. (37)

gamma (γ). A coefficient representing the relationship between exogenous and endogenous variables in structural equation modeling. (31)

generalizability. 1. The quality of research that justifies application of outcomes to groups or situations other than those directly involved in the investigation, or external validity. (15) 2. The concept of reliability theory in which measurement error is viewed as multidimensional and must be interpreted under specific measurement conditions. (9)

gold standard. A measurement that defines the true value of a variable. 1. In criterion-related validity, an instrument that is considered a valid measure and that can be used as the standard for assessing validity of other instruments. (10) 2. In diagnostic testing, a procedure that accurately identifies the true disease condition (negative or positive) of the subject. (33)

goodness of fit. Use of a test to determine if an observed distribution of variables fits a given theoretical distribution. (28,31)

grand theory. A comprehensive idea that tries to explain phenomena at the societal level. (4)

Greenhouse-Geiser correction. A correction for variance differences in a repeated measures analysis of variance. (25)

grey literature. Written materials not produced by a commercial publisher, including government documents, reports of all types, fact sheets, practice guidelines, conference proceedings, and theses or dissertations. (6,37)

grounded theory. An approach to collecting and analyzing data in qualitative research, with the goal of developing theories to explain observations and experience. (21)

Guttman scale. (see *cumulative scale*)

Hawthorne effect. The effect of participants' knowledge that they are part of a study on their performance. (15)

hazard function. The probability that a subject will achieve a specific outcome in a certain time interval. (31)

hierarchical regression. Multiple regression model where sets of variables are entered in an iterative fashion. (30)

histogram. A type of bar graph, composed of a series of columns, each representing the frequency of one score or group interval. (22)

historical controls. Subjects from previous research studies that serve as controls for experimental subjects in a subsequent study. (17)

historical research. Research that seeks to examine relationships and facts based on documentation of past events. (20)

history effect. A threat to internal validity, referring to the occurrence of extraneous events prior to a posttest that can affect the dependent variable. (15)

homogeneity of slopes. Assumption in analysis of covariance that regression slopes of covariates are parallel. (30)

homogeneity of variance. An underlying assumption in parametric statistics that variances of samples are not significantly different. (23,24,25)

homogeneous sample. A sample where participants are similar on specific characteristics, such as all the same gender or age group. (15)

homoscedasticity. (see *homogeneity of variance*)

hospital-based study. An observational study that recruits cases from patients in a medical institution. (19)

Huynh-Feldt correction. A correction for variance differences in a repeated measures analysis of variance. (25)

hypothesis. A statement of the expected relationship between variables. (3)

impact factor. A rating of journal reputation based on the frequency with which articles from that journal are cited in reports in other journals. (38)

implementation science. Approach to research that focuses on understanding the influence of environment, attitudes, and resources on whether research findings are actually translated to practice. (2)

imputation. Replacement of missing data points with estimated values that are based on observed data. (15)

incidence. The proportion of people who develop a given disease or condition within a specified time period. (34)

inclusion criteria. Specific criteria that are used to determine who is eligible for a study. (13)

independent factor. An independent variable in which the levels represent independent groups of subjects. (15)

independent variable. The variable that is presumed to cause, explain, or influence a dependent variable; a variable that is manipulated or controlled by the researcher, who sets its "values" or levels. (3)

index test. A diagnostic test evaluated against a reference standard to determine if it accurately identifies those with and without the condition of interest. (33)

inductive reasoning. The logical process of developing generalizations based on specific observations or facts. (4)

inductive theories. Data-based theories that evolve through a process of inductive reasoning. (4)

inferential statistics. That branch of statistics concerned with testing hypotheses and using sample data to make generalizations concerning populations. (23)

informed consent. An ethical principle that requires obtaining the consent of the individual to participate in a study based on full prior disclosure of risks and benefits. (7)

institutional review board (IRB). That group in an institution that is responsible for reviewing research proposals that will involve human subjects to determine adherence to ethical principles. (7)

instrumentation effect. A threat to internal validity in which bias is introduced by an unreliable or inaccurate measurement system. (15)

intention-to-treat (ITT). In a randomized trial, the principle whereby data are analyzed according to original group assignments, regardless of how subjects actually received treatment. (15)

interaction effect. The differential effect of levels of one independent variable on a second independent variable. (25)

internal consistency. A form of reliability, assessing the degree to which a set of items in an instrument all measure the same trait. Typically measured using Cronbach's alpha. (9,26)

internal criticism. Assessment of the accuracy of sources in historical research. (20)

internal validity. The degree to which the relationship between the independent and dependent variables is free from the effects of extraneous factors. (15)

International Classification of Functioning, Disability and Health (ICF). A model developed by the World Health Organization that posits the relationship among a health condition, body structures/functions, activities, and participation. (1)

interprofessional. Members of multiple professions working together, contributing their various skills in an integrative fashion, sharing perspectives to inform decision making. (1)

interquartile range (IQR). The difference between the first and third quartiles in a distribution, often expressed graphically in a boxplot. (22)

inter-rater reliability. The degree to which two or more raters can obtain the same ratings for a given variable. (9,32)

interrupted time-series design (ITS). A quasi-experimental design involving a series of measurements over time, interrupted by one or more treatment occasions. (17)

interval scale. Level of measurement in which values have equal intervals, but no true zero point. (8)

intraclass correlation coefficient (ICC). A reliability coefficient used to assess test-retest and rater reliability based on an analysis of variance; a generalizability coefficient. (9,32)

intrarater reliability. The degree to which one rater can obtain the same rating on multiple occasions of measuring the same unchanging variable. (9)

item response theory (IRT). A model that examines error in a series of items that measure a latent trait, usually on a questionnaire, to determine how well the items differentiate individuals based on ability and difficulty of items. Also called *latent trait theory*. (12)

item-to-total correlation. Correlation of individual items in a scale with the total scale score; an indication of internal consistency. (9,32)

justice. Fairness in all aspects of the research process. (7)

Kaplan-Meier estimate. A nonparametric statistic used to estimate survival based on that portion of individuals living for a certain amount of time who have experienced a treatment or disease. (31)

kappa (κ). A correction factor for percent agreement measures of reliability, accounting for the potential effect of chance agreements. (9,32)

Kendall's tau (τ). A nonparametric correlation procedure for use with ordinal data. (29)

knowledge translation. Describes the process of accelerating the application of knowledge to improve outcomes and change behavior for those involved in providing care. (5)

known groups method. A technique for construct validation, in which validity is determined by the degree to which an instrument can demonstrate different scores for groups known to vary on the variable being measured. (10)

Kolmogorov-Smirnov test of normality. A test of the null hypothesis that an observed distribution does not differ from the pattern of a normal distribution. If the test is not significant ($p>.05$), the distribution does not differ from a normal distribution. (see also *Shapiro-Wilks test of normality*) (23)

Kruskal–Wallis one-way analysis of variance by ranks (*H*). A nonparametric statistical procedure for comparing more than two independent groups representing levels of one independent variable; analogous to the one-way analysis of variance. (27)

last observation carried forward (LOCF). A method of data imputation for missing scores in which a subject's last data point before dropping out is used as the outcome score. (15)

latent trait. A multidimensional construct or abstract characteristic of individuals that cannot be observed, and must be measured through a proxy. (10) (see also *item response theory*)

Latin square. A matrix of columns and rows used to assign sequences of treatments to control for order effects. (16)

least squares method. A method of fitting a regression line to a set of bivariate data so as to minimize the sum of the squared vertical deviations of *Y* values around that line. (30)

level. 1. The "value" or classification of an independent variable. (3) 2. In single-subject research, the magnitude of the target behavior; changes in level are associated with differences in magnitude between the end of one phase and the beginning of the following phase. (18)

level of measurement. The precision of a scale based on how a characteristic is measured: nominal, ordinal, interval, and ratio levels. (8)

level of significance (α). (see *alpha*).

levels of evidence. A classification system whereby the level of confidence placed in study findings is based on the type of research and control of bias in the design. (5)

Levene's test. A test of the equality of variances, used with the independent *t* test and the analysis of variance. (24,25)

likelihood ratio (LR). 1. In diagnostic testing, the ratio indicating the usefulness of the test for ruling in or ruling out a condition. A positive likelihood ratio (LR+) indicates how much the odds of a disease are increased if the test is positive. A negative likelihood ratio (LR–) indicates how much the odds of a disease are decreased if a diagnostic test is negative. (33) 2. In logistic regression, a test of the overall relationship among variables, analogous to the change in R^2 in multiple regression. (31)

Likert scale. A summative scale based on responses to a set of statements for which respondents are asked to rate their degree of agreement or disagreement. (11,12)

limits of agreement. Index of reliability between alternate forms of an instrument. (9,32)

linear regression. The process of determining a regression equation to predict values of *Y* based on a linear relationship with values of *X*. (30)

line of best fit. The regression line, representing the relationship between two variables, usually plotted on a scatter diagram. (see also *least squares method*) (30)

listwise deletion. Elimination of all cases with missing data on any variable in data analysis. (15, Appendix C)

logical positivism. Philosophical approach to inquiry based on the assumption that values can be confirmed by observation or experimentation, contrasted with naturalistic inquiry. (21)

logistic regression. Multiple regression procedure to test the effect of one or more predictor variables on a dichotomous dependent variable; predicts odds associated with presence or absence of the dependent variable based on the independent variables. (31)

logit. Standardized value that is the natural logarithm of odds. (12,31)

log rank test. A test of the null hypothesis that two survival curves are identical in a Kaplan-Meier procedure. (31)

longitudinal study. A study designed to collect data over time. (19,20)

main effect. The separate effect of one independent variable in a multifactor design. (16)

Mann–Whitney *U* test. A nonparametric statistical test for comparing two independent groups; analogous to the unpaired *t*-test. Equivalent to the Wilcoxon rank sum test. (27)

marginal means. Means for levels of main effects in a factorial design. (25)

matching. Pairing of subjects on the basis of similarities on one or more variables to make two groups more homogenous and to avoid confounding. (15)

maturation effect. A threat to internal validity, in which changes occur in the dependent variable as a result of the passing of time. (15)

Mauchley's test of sphericity. Statistical measure of sphericity in a repeated measures analysis of variance (see *sphericity*). (25)

maximum likelihood estimation. Method of estimating parameters in a statistical model that are the best fit to observed data. Used with logistic regression. (31)

McNemar test. A nonparametric statistical test to assess the relationship between correlated nominal level measures; related to the chi-square test. (28)

mean ($\bar{X}$). A measure of central tendency, computed by summing the values of several observations and dividing by the number of observations; the value that is typically called the "average." (22)

mean square (*MS*). A value representing the variance; calculated by dividing the sum of squares for a particular effect by the degrees of freedom for that effect. (22,25)

measurement error. The difference between an observed value for a measurement and the theoretical true score; may be the result of systematic or random effects. (9,32)

median. A measure of central tendency representing the 50th percentile in a ranked distribution of scores; that is, that point at which 50% of the scores fall below and 50% fall above. (22)

median survival time. In a survival analysis, the time when half the patients are expected to survive, or when the chance of surviving beyond that time is 50%. (31)

Medical Subject Headings (MeSH). Hierarchical structure of search terms developed by the National Library of Medicine. (6)

MEDLINE. Database of bibliographic references supported by the National Library of Medicine. (6)

member checking. In qualitative research, the process of sharing preliminary findings and interpretations with research participants, allowing them to offer validation, feedback, critique, and alternative explanations that ultimately contribute to the credibility of findings. (21)

meta-analysis. Use of statistical techniques to pool effect sizes from several studies with similar independent and dependent variables, resulting an overall summary effect. (5,37)

meta-theory. An overarching theory that attempts to reconcile several theoretical perspectives in the explanation of sociological, psychological, and physiological phenomena. (4)

method error. A form of reliability testing for assessing response stability based on the discrepancy between two sets of repeated scores. (32 Supplement)

methodological research. Research designed to develop or refine procedures or instruments for measuring variables, generally focusing on reliability, validity, and change. (9,10)

middle range theories. Theories that sit between basic hypotheses that guide everyday practice and the systematic efforts to develop a unified theory to explain a set of social behaviors. (4)

minimal clinically important difference (MCID). The smallest difference in a measured variable that signifies an important rather than trivial difference a measurement. (10,32)

minimal detectable change (MDC). That amount of change in a variable that must be achieved to reflect a true difference; the smallest amount of change that passes the threshold of error. (9,32)

misclassification. In cohort or case-control studies, classifying participants to an exposure or outcome category that is inaccurate. (19)

missing at random (MAR). Missing data that may be related to the methodology of the study but not to the treatment variable. (15)

missing completely at random (MCAR). Assumption that missing data are missing because of unpredictable circumstances that have no connection to the variables of interest or the study design. (15)

missing not at random (MNAR). Missing data related to group membership, creating bias in data. (15)

mixed design. A design that incorporates independent variables that are independent (between-subjects) and repeated (within-subjects) factors. Also called a split-plot design. (16)

mixed methods research. A study that incorporates both quantitative and qualitative research methods. (1,21)

mode. A measure of central tendency representing the most commonly occurring score in a distribution. (22)

model. Symbolic representation of reality delineating concepts or variables and their relationships, often demonstrating the structural components of a theory or process. (4)

multicollinearity. (see *collinearity*)

multiple baseline design. In single-subject research, a design for collecting data for more than one subject, behavior, or treatment condition wherein baseline phases are staggered to provide control. (18)

multiple comparison test. A test of differences between individual means following analysis of variance, used to control for Type I error. (26)

multiple imputation. A method of dealing with missing data by creating a random data set using the available data, predicting plausible values derived from observed data. (15)

multiple regression. A multivariate statistical technique for establishing the predictive relationship between one dependent variable and a set of independent variables. (31)

multistage sampling. (see *cluster sampling*)

multitrait-multimethod matrix (MTMM). An approach to validity testing to examine the relationship between two or more traits measured by two or more methods. (10)

multivariate analysis. A set of statistical procedures designed to analyze the relationship among three or more variables; includes techniques such as multiple regression, discriminant analysis, factor analysis, and multivariate analysis of variance. (31)

multivariate analysis of variance (MANOVA). An advanced multivariate procedure that provides a global test of significance for multiple dependent variables using an analysis of variance. (31)

N-of-1 trial. A form of single-subject investigation that applies a randomized crossover design to an individual patient. (18)

natural history. Longitudinal study of a disease or disorder, demonstrating the typical progress of the condition. (20)

naturalistic inquiry. Qualitative observation and interaction with subjects in their own natural environment. (21)

negative case analysis. In qualitative research, a method of validation by searching for concepts that do not support or may contradict themes emerging from the data. (21)

negative likelihood ratio (LR–). (see *likelihood ratio*)

negative predictive value (PV–), (see *predictive value*)

Newman-Keuls (NK) multiple comparison test. (see *Student-Newman-Keuls multiple comparison*)

nominal scale. Level of measurement for classification variables; assignment of "values" based on mutually exclusive and exhaustive categories with no inherent rank order. (8)

nondirectional hypothesis. A research hypothesis (or alternative hypothesis) that does not indicate the expected direction of the relationship between independent and dependent variables. (3)

non-inferiority margin. In a non-inferiority study, the biggest difference that would be acceptable to consider the new treatment a reasonable substitute for the standard therapy. (14)

non-inferiority trial. A clinical trial designed to show that a new treatment is no better and no worse than standard care. (14)

nonparametric statistics. A set of statistical procedures that are not based on assumptions about population parameters, or the shape of the underlying population distribution; most often used when data are measured on the nominal or ordinal scales. (8,27)

nonprobability sample. A sample that was not selected using random selection. (11,13)

normal curve. (see *normal distribution*)

normal distribution. A symmetrical bell-shaped theoretical distribution with defined properties, where most of the scores fall in the middle of the scale and progressively fewer fall at the extremes. (22)

normative research. A descriptive research approach designed to determine normal values for specific variables within a population. (20)

norm referencing. Interpretation of a score based on its value relative to a standardized score. (10)

null hypothesis (H_0). A statement of no difference or no relationship between variables; the statistical hypothesis. (3,23)

number needed to harm (NNH). The number of patients that need to be treated to observe one adverse outcome; the reciprocal of absolute risk increase (ARI). (34)

number needed to treat (NNT). The number of patients that need to be treated to prevent one adverse outcome or achieve one successful outcome; the reciprocal of absolute risk reduction (ARR). (34)

oblique rotation. In factor analysis, the rotation of factors that are correlated with each other. (31)

observational study. A study that does not involve an intervention or manipulation of an independent variable. (19)

observed frequencies. Frequencies that occur in a study of categorical variables. (28)

odds ratio (OR). An estimate of risk representing the odds that an outcome will occur given a particular exposure compared to the odds of the outcome occurring in the absence of the exposure; used as a risk estimate in case-control studies and logistic regression. (30,34)

one-tailed test. A statistical test based on a directional alternative hypothesis, in which critical values are obtained for only one tail of a distribution. (23)

one-way analysis of variance. An analysis of variance with one independent variable. (25)

one-way design. An experimental or quasi-experimental design that involves one independent variable. (16)

on-protocol analysis. Analysis of data in an experiment based only on subjects who completed the study according to assigned groups. Also called *completer analysis* or *on-treatment analysis*. (15)

open access. A term used to describe articles and journals that are free of restrictions on access. (6,38)

open-ended question. A question on a survey (interview or questionnaire) that does not restrict the respondent to specific choices but allows for a free response. (11)

open-label trial. A trial design wherein both the researchers and participants know which treatment is being administered. (14)

operational definition. Definition of a variable based on how it will be used in a particular study; how a dependent variable will be measured, how an independent variable will be manipulated. (3)

order effects. The sequential effect of one subject being exposed to several treatments in the same order; potentially manifested as carryover or practice effects. (16)

ordinal scale. Level of measurement in which scores are ranks. (8)

orthogonal. A model in which variables are independent or uncorrelated. Literally means "perpendicular" in mathematics. (26,31)

outcome variable. (see *dependent variable*)

outlier. A numeric value that does not fall within the range of most scores in a distribution. (30)

paired *t*-test. A parametric test for comparing two means for correlated samples or repeated measures; also called a correlated *t*-test. (24)

pairwise deletion. Elimination of cases with missing data on particular variables in a specific analysis only. (15, Appendix C)

paradigm shift. Fundamental transition in the way a discipline thinks about priorities and relationships, stimulating change in perspectives, and fostering preferences for varied approaches to research. (1)

parallel group design. A design comparing two independent groups that are similar on all characteristics other than the intervention. (14)

parameter. A measured characteristic of a population. (13,22)

parametric statistics. Statistical procedures for estimating population parameters and for testing hypotheses based on population parameters, with assumptions about the distribution of variables, and for use with interval or ratio measures. (8,18)

partial correlation. The correlation between two variables, with the effect of a third variable removed; also called a first-order correlation. (29)

participant observation. A method of data collection in qualitative research in which the researcher is embedded as a participant in the group that is being observed. (21)

path diagram. A flow chart that shows interconnections among variables in a causal model. (31)

patient-centered outcomes research (PCOR). An approach that has the distinct goal of engaging patients and other stakeholders in the development of questions and outcomes measures, encouraging them to become integral members of the research process. (2)

patient-oriented evidence that matters (POEM). Refers to outcomes that measure things that a patient would care about, such as symptoms, quality of life, function, cost of care, length of stay. (2)

patient-reported outcome measures (PROM). Any report of the status of a patient's health condition that comes directly from the patient, without interpretation of the patient's response by a clinician or anyone else. (2)

Pearson product–moment coefficient of correlation (*r*). A parametric statistical technique for determining the relationship between two variables. (29)

peer review. Process of review of submitted manuscripts or research proposals by subject experts to determine quality. (7,38).

percent agreement. A reliability test for categorical variables, estimating the ability of researchers to agree on category ratings. (32)

per comparison error rate (α_{PC}). Probability of making a Type I error in a single comparison. (26)

percentile. The percentage of a distribution that is below a specified value. A distribution is divided into 99 equal ranks, or percentiles, with 1% of the scores in each rank. (22)

performance bias. A source of bias related to differences in the provision of care to comparison groups. (15, 37)

per-protocol analysis. Eliminating subjects who did not get or complete their assigned treatment, and including only those subjects who sufficiently complied with the trial's protocol. (15)

person-item map. Output of a Rasch analysis that shows the distribution of persons according to ability and of items according to difficulty. (12)

person-time. The total amount of time each case in a study is at risk, used to calculate incidence rates. (34)

phase I trial. Researchers work to show that a new therapy is safe. (2,14)

phase II trial. Studies that explore efficacy and dosage effects of an intervention by measuring relevant outcomes. (2,14)

phase III trial. Builds on prior research to establish efficacy through randomized controlled studies that may include thousands of patients in multiple sites over many years. (2,14)

phase IV trial. Completed after a treatment has been approved with the purpose of gathering information on the treatment's effect in various populations or subgroups, under different clinical conditions to explore side effects associated with long-term use, and to learn about risk factors, benefits, and optimal use patterns. (2,14)

phenomenology. An approach to qualitative research involving the study of complex human experience as it is actually lived. (21)

phi coefficient (φ). A nonparametric correlation statistic for estimating the relationship between two dichotomous variables. (28,29)

PICO. An acronym used to represent identification of components of clinical and research questions: **P** = population, **I** = intervention, **C** = comparison, **O** = outcome. (3,5)

placebo. A control that is similar in every way to the experimental treatment except that it does not contain the active component that comprises the intervention's actions. (14)

plagiarism. The appropriation of another person's ideas, processes, results, or words without giving appropriate credit or attribution, and representing the work as one's own. (7)

planned comparisons. Multiple comparison tests that are designated prior to running a study. (26)

point biserial correlation (r_{pb}). A correlation statistic for estimating the relationship between a dichotomy and a continuous variable on the interval or ratio scale. (29)

point estimate. A single sample statistic that serves as an estimate of a population parameter. (22)

polynomial regression. Regression procedure for nonlinear data. (30)

polytomous. Variables that can have multiple values, such as a 5-point scale. (8,11)

population. The entire set of individuals or units to which data will be generalized. (11,13)

population-based study. A study in which participants are recruited from the general population. (19)

positive likelihood ratio (LR+). (see *likelihood ratio*)

positive predictive value (PV+). (see *predictive value*)

posterior probability. (see *posttest probability*)

post hoc comparisons. Multiple comparison tests that follow a significant analysis of variance. (26)

posttest probability (posterior probability). The probability of a condition existing after performing a diagnostic test; predictive value of a diagnostic test. Depends on the prior probability, and the test's sensitivity and specificity. (33)

power (1-β). The ability of a statistical test to find a significant difference that really does exist; the probability that a test will lead to rejection of the null hypothesis, based on sample size, variance, level of significance, and effect size. (23)

practice-based evidence (PBE). The type of evidence that is derived from real patient care problems, identifying gaps between recommended and actual practice. (2)

practice effects. The effect of learning with repeated tasks in a repeated measures design. (16)

pragmatic clinical trial (practical clinical trial) (PCT). An effectiveness trial carried out in real-world settings. Participants represent the patients who would typically receive treatment, and testing takes place in clinical practice settings. Outcomes focus on issues of importance to patients and stakeholders. (2,14)

precision. 1. The number of decimal places to which a calculation is taken. (8) 2. The acceptable degree of error in estimating sample size for relative risk. (34)

preclinical research. (see *basic research*)

predictive validity. A form of measurement validity in which an instrument is used to predict future performance. (10)

predictive value (PV). In diagnostic testing, a positive predictive value (PV+) indicates the probability that individuals with a positive test truly have the disease. A negative predictive value (PV–) indicates the probability that individuals with a negative test truly do not have the disease. (33)

predictor variable. (see *independent variable*)

pretest probability (prior probability). The probability that a condition exists prior to performing a diagnostic test. Can be estimated based on the prevalence of the condition in a specified group of subjects. (33)

prevalence. The number of cases of a disease at a given point in time, expressed as a proportion of the total population at risk. (34)

primary outcome. The measure that will be used to arrive at a decision on the overall result of the study, and which represents the greatest therapeutic benefit. (3)

primary source. Reference source that represents the original document by the original author. (6)

principal axis factoring. A method of extraction in exploratory factor analysis. (31)

principal components analysis (PCA). Multivariate analysis that converts a set of possibly correlated variables into a set of uncorrelated principal components based on variance within the data. Differentiated from factor analysis, which uses a different model to account for variance. (31)

principal investigator. That person designated as the lead investigator who will have primary responsibility for overseeing the study. (35)

prior probability. (see *pretest probability*)

probability (p). The likelihood that an event will occur, given all possible events. (23)

probability sample. A sample chosen using random selection methods. (11,13)

propensity score. A single score based on a set of characteristics generated through logistic regression that can be used in matching subjects in observational or nonrandomized studies to reduce baseline confounding. (15,31)

proportional hazards model. (see *Cox's regression*)

proposition. Statement of the relationship between variables. (4)

prospective study. A study designed to collect data following development of the research question. (19)

publication bias. Tendency for researchers and editors to publish studies finding significant effects, to the exclusion of studies finding no effect. (6,37)

purposive (purposeful) sample. A nonprobability sample in which subjects are specifically selected by the researcher on the basis of subjective judgment that they will be the most representative. (13)

Q-sort. A research methodology based on ranking variables as to their importance. (11 Supplement)

quadratic trend. A nonlinear trend, with one turn in direction. (26,30)

qualitative research. Research that derives data from observation, interviews, or verbal interactions and focuses on the meaning of experience of the participants. (1,21)

quantitative research. Measurement of outcomes using numerical data under standardized conditions. (1)

quartile (Q). Three quartiles divide a distribution of ranked data into four equal groups, each containing 25% of the scores. (22)

quasi-experimental research. Comparative research approach in which subjects cannot be randomly assigned to groups or control groups are not used. (15,17)

quota sampling. Nonprobability sampling method in which stratification is used to obtain representative proportions of specific subgroups. (13)

random assignment (random allocation). Assignment of subjects to groups using probability methods, where every subject has an equal chance of being assigned to a group. (14)

random effect. Variable levels that are chosen at random. (32)

random error. A measurement error that occurs by chance, potentially increasing or decreasing the true score value to varying degrees. (8)

random sampling. Probability method of selecting subjects for a sample, where every subject in the population has an equal chance of being chosen. (13)

random selection. (see *random sampling*)

randomization. (see *random assignment*)

randomized block design. An experimental design in which one independent variable is an attribute variable (blocking variable), creating homogeneous blocks of subjects who are then randomly assigned to levels of the other independent variable. (16)

randomized consent design (Zelen design). Involves randomizing participants to experimental treatment or standard care prior to seeking consent, and then only approaching those who will be assigned to the experimental intervention. (14)

randomized controlled trial (RCT). An experimental study in which a clinical treatment is compared with a control condition, where subjects are randomly assigned to groups. Also called a randomized clinical trial. (1,14)

range. A measure of dispersion equal to the difference between the largest and smallest scores in a distribution. (22)

rank biserial correlation (r_{rb}). A correlation procedure for estimating the degree of relationship between a dichotomy and an ordinal variable. (29)

Rasch analysis. Transformation of items on an ordinal scale to an interval scale, demonstrating the unidimensional nature of a scale. (12)

ratio scale. The highest level of measurement, in which there are equal intervals between score units and a true zero point. (8)

reactive measurement. A measurement that distorts the variable being measured, either by the subject's awareness of being measured or by influence of the measurement process. (15)

recall bias. The possible inaccuracy of participants recalling medical history or previous exposures; of particular concern in retrospective studies. (11,19)

receiver operating characteristic (ROC) curve. In diagnostic testing, a plot of sensitivity (true positive rate) against 1-specificity (false positive rate), demonstrating strength of diagnostic accuracy, used to determine the most effective cut-off score. (33)

reference standard. A value used as a standard against which to judge a criterion; may or may not be a gold standard. Used to judge criterion-related validity or diagnostic accuracy. (10)

reflexivity. In qualitative research, the critical self-examination by researchers regarding their own biases or preferences and how they might influence interpretation of data. (21)

regression analysis. A statistical procedure for examining the predictive relationship between a dependent (criterion) variable and an independent (predictor) variable. (30)

regression coefficient. In a regression equation, the weight (*b*) assigned to the independent variable; the slope of the regression line. (30)

regression line. The straight line that is drawn on a scatter plot for bivariate data from the regression equation, summarizing the relationship between variables. (see also *least squares method*). (30)

regression toward the mean (RTM). A statistical phenomenon in which scores on a pretest are likely to move toward the group mean on a posttest because of inherent positive or negative measurement error; also called statistical regression. (15)

relative reliability. Reliability measures that reflect true variance as a proportion of the total variance in a set of scores. (9)

relative risk (RR). Estimate of the magnitude of the association between an exposure and disease, indicating the likelihood that the exposed group will develop the disease relative to those who are not exposed. (34)

relative risk reduction (RRR). The reduction in risk associated with an intervention relative to the risk without the intervention (control); the absolute difference between the experimental event rate and the control event rate divided by the control event rate. (34)

reliability. The degree of consistency with which an instrument or rater measures a variable; the degree to which a measurement is free from error. (9,32)

reliability coefficient. Value used to quantify the degree of consistency in repeated measurements. (9)

repeated measure (repeated factor). An independent variable for which subjects act as their own control. Also called a within-subjects factor. (15,16)

research hypothesis. A statement of the researcher's expectations about the relationship between variables under study. (3,23)

reverse causation. A situation wherein the variable designated as the "outcome" may actually cause the "exposure." (19)

residual ($Y - \hat{Y}$). The difference between an observed value and a predicted value. (30,31)

response rate. Percentage of people who receive a survey who actually complete it. (11)

response stability. Consistency with which a response is manifested over repeated trials. (32)

responsiveness. The ability of a test to demonstrate change. (10,32)

retrospective study. A study that analyzes observations that were collected in the past. (13,19)

risk. Consideration of physical, psychological, or social harm that goes beyond expected experiences in daily life. (19,34)

risk–benefit ratio. An ethical principle that is an element of informed consent, in which the risks of a research study to the participant are evaluated in relation to the potential benefits of the study's outcomes. (7)

risk factor. A characteristic or exposure that potentially increases the likelihood of having a disease or condition. (34)

risk ratio. (see *relative risk*)

ROC curve. (see *receiver operating characteristic curve*)

run-in period. A time during which all eligible participants receive a placebo prior to implementing an intervention, and only those who are adherent to the protocol are eligible for the formal trial. (14)

sample. Subset of a population chosen for study. (13)

sampling bias. Bias that occurs when individuals who are selected for a sample overrepresent or underrepresent the underlying population characteristics. (13)

sampling distribution. A theoretical frequency distribution of a statistic based on the value of the statistic over an infinite number of samples. (18)

sampling error. The difference between an observed statistic from a sample and the population parameter. (11,13)

saturation. In the ongoing analysis of qualitative data, the point at which no new knowledge contributes to the emerging theory. (21)

scale. An ordered system based on a series of questions or items, resulting in a score that represents the degree to which a respondent possesses a particular attitude, value, or characteristic. (12)

scale of measurement. (see *level of measurement*)

scatter plot. A graphic representation of the relationship between two variables. (29)

Scheffé's multiple comparison test. A multiple comparison procedure for comparing means following a significant analysis of variance based on the *F* distribution. Considered the most conservative of the multiple comparison methods. (26)

scoping review. An exploratory review of a broad question about a clinical topic, including a comprehensive synthesis of evidence with the aim of informing practice, programs, and policy, and providing direction to future research. (5,37)

secondary analysis. An approach to research involving the use of data that were collected for another purpose. (13)

secondary outcome. Other endpoint measures, besides the primary outcome, that may be used to assess the effectiveness of the intervention, as well as side effects, costs, or other outcomes of interest. (3)

secondary source. Reference source that represents a review or report of another's work. (6)

selection bias. A threat to internal validity in which bias is introduced by initial differences between groups, when these differences are not random. (15)

self-report measures. Data based on participants' reports of their own attitudes or conditions. (12)

sensitivity. 1. A measure of validity of a screening procedure, based on the probability that someone with a disease will test positive; true positive rate. (33) 2. In a literature search, the proportion of relevant articles identified out of all relevant articles on that topic; ability to identify all pertinent citations. (6)

sensitivity analysis. A procedure in decision making to determine how decisions change as values are systematically varied. (37)

sequential analysis. In mixed methods research, the design of studies that follow each other, whereby the first study informs the second. (21)

sequential clinical trial. Experimental research design that allows consecutive entrance to a clinical trial and continuous analysis of data, permitting stopping of the trial when data are sufficient to show a significant effect. (16)

serial dependency. Correlation in a set of data collected over time, in which one observation can be predicted based on previous observations. (18)

sham treatment. Analogous to a placebo, involving a "fake" treatment as a control condition. (14)

Shapiro-Wilks test of normality. A test of the null hypothesis that states that an observed distribution does not differ from the pattern of a normal distribution. If the test is not significant ($p > .05$), the distribution does not differ from a normal distribution. (see also *Kolmogorov-Smirnov test of normality*) (23)

sign test. A nonparametric statistical procedure for comparing two correlated samples, based on comparison of positive or negative outcomes. (27)

significance. (see *statistical significance*)

significance level (α). (see *alpha level*)

simple contrast. In a multiple comparison, the contrast of two means to determine if they are significantly different from one another. (26)

simple hypothesis. A hypothesis statement that includes one independent variable and one dependent variable. (3)

single-blind study. An experiment in which either the investigator or the subject is kept ignorant of group assignment, but not both. (14)

single-subject design (SSD). An experimental design based on time-series data from one or more subjects, with data compared across baseline and intervention phases. Also called single-case design. (18)

skewed distribution. A distribution of scores that is asymmetrical, with more scores to one extreme. (22)

slope. 1. In regression analysis, the rate of change in values of Y for one unit of change in X. (30) 2. In single-study research, the rate of change in the magnitude of the target behavior over time. (18)

SnNout. Pneumonic to remember that with high sensitivity, a negative test rules out the diagnosis. (33)

snowball sampling. A nonprobability sampling method in which subjects are successively recruited by referrals from other subjects. (13)

Spearman's rank correlation coefficient (r_s). A nonparametric correlation procedure for ordinal data. Also called Spearman's rho. (29)

specificity. 1. A measure of validity of a screening procedure, based on the probability that someone who does not have a disease will test negative; true negative rate. (34) 2. In a literature search, the proportion of relevant citations retrieved, the ability to exclude irrelevant citations. (6)

sphericity. An assumption in a repeated-measures ANOVA that the variances of the differences between all possible pairs of within-subject conditions (levels of the independent variable) are equal. (25)

split-half reliability. A reliability measure of internal consistency based on dividing the items on an instrument into two halves and correlating the results. (9)

split middle line. In single-subject research, a line used to separate data points within one phase into equal halves, reflecting the trend of the data within that phase. (18)

SpPin. Pneumonic to remember that with high specificity, a positive test rules in the diagnosis. (33)

standard deviation. A descriptive statistic reflecting the variability or dispersion of scores around the mean. (22)

standard error of measurement (SEM). A reliability measure of response stability, estimating the standard error in a set of repeated scores. (9,26)

standard error of the estimate (SEE). In regression analysis, an estimate of prediction accuracy; a measure of the spread of scores around the regression line. (24)

standard error of the mean ($s_{\bar{X}}$). The standard deviation of a distribution of sample means; an estimate of the population standard deviation. (18)

standardized mean difference (SMD). Difference between group means divided by their common standard deviation (analogous to the effect size index, *d*). (24,37)

standardized residual. Difference between observed and expected values in a chi-square test divided by the expected frequency, indicating the contribution of each cell to the overall statistic. (28)

standardized response mean (SRM). One approach to evaluating effect size with change scores. Calculated as the difference between pretest and posttest scores, divided by the standard deviation of the change scores. (32)

standardized score. (see *z-score*)

statistic. A measured characteristic of a sample. (13,22)

statistical conclusion validity. The validity of conclusions drawn from statistical analyses, based on the proper application of statistical tests and principles. (15)

statistical hypothesis. (see *null hypothesis*)

statistical process control (SPC). A method of charting production outcomes over time to identify and monitor variances; can be used as a method of analysis for single-subject designs. (18)

stem-and-leaf plot. A graphic display for numerical data in a frequency distribution showing each value in the distribution. (22)

stepwise multiple regression. An approach to multiple regression that involves a sequential process of selecting variables for inclusion in the prediction equation. (30)

stopping rule. In a sequential clinical trial, the threshold for stopping a study based on crossing a boundary that indicates a difference or no difference between treatments. (16)

stratified random assignment. Accomplished by first dividing subjects into strata, and then within each stratum randomly assigning them to groups. (14)

stratified random sampling. Identifying relevant population characteristics, and partitioning members of a population into homogeneous, nonoverlapping subsets, or strata, based on these characteristics. (13)

structural equation modeling (SEM). Multivariate method of modeling theoretical causal relationships of latent variables. (31)

studentized range (*q*). Critical values used to determine significant differences in Tukey and Student-Newman-Keuls multiple comparisons.

Student-Newman-Keuls (SNK) multiple comparison. A stepwise multiple comparison procedure used to determine if means are significantly different following an analysis of variance. Also called the Newman-Keuls (NK) test. (26)

Student's *t*-test. (see *t-test*)

summative scale. A scale that results in a total score by adding values across a set of items. (12)

sum of squares (SS). A measure of variability in a set of data, equal to the sum of squared deviation scores for a distribution $[\Sigma(X - \bar{X})^2]$; the numerator in the formula for variance. Used in analysis of variance and other procedures as the basis for partitioning between-groups and within-groups variance components. (22)

superiority trials. Clinical trials that seek evidence in favor of a new treatment. (14)

survival analysis. Methods to analyze data where the variable of interest is the time until occurrence of an outcome event. (31)

systematic error. A form of measurement error, where error is constant across trials. (9)

systematic review. Review of a clearly formulated question that uses systematic and explicit methods to identify, select, and critically appraise relevant research. (1,5,37)

systematic sampling. A sampling method in which persons are randomly chosen from unordered lists using a fixed sampling interval, such as every tenth person. (13)

t-test. A parametric test for comparing two means; also called Student's *t*-test (see *paired t-test* and *unpaired t-test*). (24)

target behavior. In single-subject research, the response behavior that is monitored over time. (18)

target population. The larger population to which results of a study will be generalized, defined by clinical and demographic characteristics. (3,13)

testing effect. The effect that occurs when a test itself is responsible for observed changes in the measured variable. (15)

test–retest reliability. The degree to which an instrument is stable, based on repeated administrations of the test to the same individuals over a specified time interval. (9)

theoretical sampling. In qualitative research, the process of data collection for generating theory by continuous analysis and recruitment of participants to add to themes. (21)

time-series design. (see *interrupted time-series design*)

tolerance. In multiple regression, a measure of collinearity among independent variables. Lower values of tolerance (<.2) indicate greater collinearity. (30)

transferability. In qualitative research, the extent to which findings can be generalized beyond the study. (21)

translational research. Clinical investigations with human subjects in which knowledge obtained from basic research is translated into diagnostic or therapeutic interventions that can be applied to treatment or prevention. (2)

treatment arm. Another term for independent groups in a clinical trial. (14)

trend. 1. The shape of a distribution of scores taken over time, reflecting the distribution's linearity or lack of linearity. (26) 2. In single-subject research, the direction of change in the target behavior within a phase or across phases. (18)

trend analysis. Using an analysis of variance, a test to assess trend within data taken over ordered intervals; can express data as linear, quadratic, or cubic, reflecting the number of changes in direction in the data over time. (26)

triangulation. The use of multiple methods to document and confirm observations related to a phenomenon. (21)

true negative. A test result that is negative for those who do not have the disease or condition of interest. (33)

true positive. A test result that is positive for those who do have the disease or condition of interest. (33)

truncation. Usually an * used to substitute for word endings that may have varied forms in a literature search. (6)

Tukey's honestly significant difference (HSD). A multiple comparison test for comparing multiple means following a significant analysis of variance. (26)

two standard deviation band method. A method of data analysis in single-subject research; involves calculating the mean and standard deviation of data points within the baseline phase and extending these values into the intervention phase. If two or more consecutive points in the intervention phase fall outside these bands, the change from baseline to intervention is considered significant. (18)

two-tailed test. A statistical test based on a nondirectional alternative hypothesis, in which critical values represent both positive and negative tails of a distribution. (22)

two-way analysis of variance. An analysis of variance with two independent variables. (25)

two-way design. An experimental or quasi-experimental study that involves two independent variables. (16)

Type I error. An incorrect decision to reject the null hypothesis, concluding that a relationship exists when in fact it does not. (23)

Type II error. An incorrect decision to not reject the null hypothesis, concluding that no relationship exists when in fact it does. (23)

unpaired *t*-test. A parametric test for comparing two means for independent samples; also called an independent *t*-test. (24)

unplanned comparisons. Multiple comparison tests that explore all possible comparisons following a significant analysis of variance. (26)

validity. 1. The degree to which an instrument measures what it is intended to measure. (10) 2. The degree to which a research design allows for reasonable interpretations from the data, based on control of bias and confounding (internal validity), appropriate operational definitions (construct validity), appropriate analysis procedures (statistical conclusion validity), and generalizability (external validity). (15)

variable. A characteristic that can be manipulated or observed and that can take on different values, either quantitatively or qualitatively. (3)

variance. A measure of variability in a distribution, equal to the square of the standard deviation. (22)

variance inflation factor (VIF). In multiple regression, a measure of collinearity, the inverse of tolerance. Higher values indicate greater collinearity. (30)

vector. In MANOVA, the combined mean of several dependent variables for each group. (31)

visual analog scale (VAS). An instrument used to quantify a subjective experience by marking a line between two anchors that represent extremes of the experience. A commonly used visual analog scale is a 10 cm line labeled with "no pain" as the left anchor, and "worst pain imaginable" as the right anchor. (11,12)

wait list control group. A control group composed of subjects for whom the experimental treatment is delayed, scheduled to receive the treatment following completion of the study. (14)

Wald statistic. Statistic used to assess significance of coefficients in a logistic regression. (31)

washout period. In a crossover design, that period of time between administration of the two treatments, allowing effects of the experimental treatment to dissipate. (16)

weighted kappa (κ_w). An estimate of percentage agreement, corrected for chance, based on weights reflecting levels of seriousness of disagreements. (32)

wildcard. Usually an * used in a literature search to substitute for several letters within a search term, to allow for alternate spellings. (6)

Wilcoxon signed-ranks test (*T*). A nonparametric statistical procedure, comparing two correlated samples (repeated measures); analogous to the paired *t*-test. (27)

Wilk's lambda (λ). Statistical test of significance in multivariate analysis of variance. (31)

withdrawal design. In single-subject research, a design that involves withdrawal of the intervention. (18)

within-groups variance. (see *error variance*)

within-subjects design (repeated measures design). A design in which subjects act as their own control. (16)

Yates' continuity correction. In the chi-square test, a correction factor applied when expected frequencies are too small, effectively reducing the chi-square statistic. (28)

z distribution. The standardized normal distribution, with a mean of 0 and a standard deviation of 1. (22)

Zelen design. (see *randomized consent design*)

z-score. The number of standard deviations that a given value is above or below the mean of the distribution; also called a standardized score. (22)

zero-order correlation. A bivariate correlation. (29)

■ Statistical Symbols and Abbreviations

Greek Letters

Symbol	Name	Description
α	*alpha*	1. Level of significance, denotes risk of Type I error; α_1 and α_2 represent one-tailed and two-tailed levels of significance (23) 2. Also used in Cronbach's alpha. (32)
α_{FW}		Familywise level of significance for a set of multiple comparisons. (26)
α_{PC}		Per comparison level of significance for individual comparisons when multiple comparisons are made. (26)
β	*beta*	1. Probability associated with Type II error. (23) 2. Coefficient in structural equation. (31 Supplement)
γ	*gamma*	Coefficient in structural equation. (31 Supplement)
ε	*epsilon*	Statistic for repeated measures ANOVA, used to adjust degrees of freedom to correct for unequal variances. (25)
η^2	*eta*	Eta-squared, effect size in one-way ANOVA. (25)
η_p^2		Partial eta-squared, effect size for two-way ANOVA. (25)
θ	*theta*	Effect size for proportions, used in sequential clinical trials. (16 Supplement)
κ	*kappa*	Chance-corrected measure of agreement. (32)
κ_w		Weighted kappa. (32 Supplement)
λ	*lambda*	1. A measure of association between categorical variables. (28) 2. Wilks' lambda, multivariate measure of effect. (31)
μ	*mu*	Population mean. (22)
ρ	*rho*	Population measure of correlation. (29)
σ	*sigma*	(lower case) population standard deviation. (22)
σ^2		Sigma-squared, population variance. (22)
$\sigma_{\bar{X}}$		Population standard error of the mean. (22)
Σ	*sigma*	(upper case) used to mean "the sum of." (22)
τ	*tau*	Kendall's tau. (29)
ϕ	*phi*	Phi coefficient measure of association. (28,29)
χ^2	*chi*	Chi-square test of significance for association between categorical variables. (28)
χ_r^2		Chi-square r, test statistic for the Friedman two-way ANOVA by ranks. (27)
ω^2	*omega*	Omega squared, effect size in ANOVA. (25)

Abbreviations

α	Constant (Y-intercept) in a regression equation. (30)
ANOVA	Analysis of variance. (25)
ANCOVA	Analysis of covariance. (30)
ARI	Absolute risk increase. (34)
ARR	Absolute risk reduction. (34)
b	Regression coefficient. (30)
c	Used to denote the number of comparisons in a set of comparisons. (26)
C	1. Contingency coefficient. (28) 2. Number of columns in a contingency table. (28)
CAT	1. Computer adaptive testing. (12) 2. Critically appraised topic. (36)
CER	Control event rate. (34)
CFA	Confirmatory factor analysis. (10,31)
CI	1. Confidence interval. (23) 2. Cumulative incidence. (34)
CV	Coefficient of variation. (22)
d	1. Difference score. (24) 2. Effect size index for the *t*-test, also Cohen's *d*. (24)
$\bar{d}$	Mean of a set of difference scores. (24)
df	Degrees of freedom. (23)
df_b	Degrees of freedom for between-groups source of variance in ANOVA. (25)
df_e	Degrees of freedom for error term (within subjects) in ANOVA. (25)
df_t	Total degrees of freedom. (25)
DOI	Digital object identifier, used to identify research publications. (6,38)
EER	Experimental event rate. (34)
EFA	Exploratory factor analysis. (10,31)
f	1. Frequency of scores. (22) 2. Effect size index for ANOVA. (25)
F	Test statistic for the ANOVA. (25)
H	Test statistic for the Kruskall-Wallis two-way ANOVA by ranks. (27)
H_0	Null hypothesis. (23)
H_1	Alternative hypothesis. (23)
HSD	Tukey's honestly significant difference multiple comparison test. (26)
I^2	Measure of heterogeneity in meta-analysis. (37)
ICC	1. Intraclass correlation coefficient. (32) 2. Item characteristic curve. (12 Supplement)
IQR	Interquartile range. (22)
IR	Incidence rate. (34)
IRT	Item response theory. (12)
ITS	Interrupted time series design. (17)
ITT	Intention-to-treat analysis. (15)
k	Number of groups, means, or predictor variables in an analysis. (25)

LR	Likelihood ratio, can be positive (LR+) or negative (LR–). (33)	
MANOVA	Multivariate analysis of variance. (31)	
MAR	Missing at random. (15)	
MCAR	Missing completely at random. (15)	
MCID	Minimal clinically important change. (10,32)	
MDC	Minimal detectable change. (9,32)	
MeSH	Medical subject headings. (6)	
MNAR	Missing not at random. (15)	
MS	Mean square. (25)	
MS_b	Between-groups mean square. (25)	
MS_e	Error mean square. (25)	
MTMM	Multitrait-multimethod matrix. (10)	
n	Number of subjects in a single sample or group. (22)	
N	Number of subjects in a total sample. (22)	
NNH	Number needed to harm. (34)	
NNT	Number needed to treat. (34)	
OR	Odds ratio. (31,34)	
p	Probability (23)	
P	1. Percentile. (22) 2. Prevalence. (33,34)	
PCA	Principal components analysis. (31)	
PCOR	Patient-centered outcomes research. (2)	
POEM	Patient-oriented evidence that matters. (2)	
PROM	Patient-reported outcome measures. (2)	
PCT	Pragmatic clinical trial (also *practical clinical trial*). (2,14)	
PICO	Elements of an evidence-based question: Population, Intervention, Comparison, Outcome. (3,5)	
PV	Predictive value, can be positive (PV+) or negative (PV–). (33)	
q	Studentized range statistic. (26)	
Q	1. Quartile. (22) 2. Cochrane's Q, a measure of heterogeneity in a meta-analysis. (37)	
r	1. Correlation coefficient. (29) 2. Range of ordered means in a multiple comparison test. (26)	
r^2	Coefficient of determination. (30)	
r_s	Spearman rank correlation coefficient. (29)	
$r_{XY\cdot Z}$	First order partial correlation. (29)	
r_{pb}	Point biserial correlation coefficient. (29)	
r_{rb}	Rank biserial correlation coefficient. (29)	
R	1. Multiple regression coefficient. (30) 2. Number of rows in a contingency table. (28) 3. Rank sum in a nonparametric test. (27)	
R^2	Multiple correlation coefficient squared. (30)	
RCT	Randomized controlled trial. (14)	

ROC	Receiver operating characteristic. (33)
RR	Relative risk. (34)
RRR	Relative risk reduction. (34)
s	Sample standard deviation. (22)
s^2	Sample variance. (22)
s_d	Standard deviation of a set of difference scores. (24)
$s_{\bar{d}}$	Standard error of the mean of a set of difference scores. (24)
$s_{\bar{X}}$	Standard error of the mean for a sample. (23)
$s_{\bar{X}_1 - \bar{X}_2}$	Standard error of the difference between means. (24)
SEE	Standard error of the estimate. (30)
SEM	1. Standard error of measurement. (9,32) 2. Structural equation modeling. (31)
SMD	Standardized mean difference. (24,37)
Sn	Sensitivity. (33)
SNK	Student-Newman-Keuls multiple comparison test. (26)
Sp	Specificity. (33)
SPC	Statistical process control. (18)
SRM	Standardized response mean. (32)
SS	Sum of squares. (22,25)
SS_b	Between-groups sum of squares. (25)
SS_e	Error sum of squares. (25)
SS_t	Total sum of squares. (25)
SSD	Single-subject design. (18)
t	Test statistic for comparison of two means. (24)
T	Test statistic for the Wilcoxon signed-ranks test. (27)
U	Test statistic for the Mann-Whitney U test. (27)
V	Cramer's V coefficient. (28)
$\bar{V}$	Mean vector in MANOVA. (31)
VAS	Visual analog scale. (12)
VIF	Variance inflation factor. (30)
x	Test statistic for the sign test and binomial test. (18,27)
X	1. Single score. (22) 2. Symbol for an independent variable in a regression equation. (30)
$\bar{X}$	Sample mean. (22)
Y	Symbol for a dependent variable in a regression equation. (30)
$\bar{Y}$	Mean for a sample of scores on variable Y. (30)
$\hat{Y}$	Predicted score in a regression equation (Y-hat). (30)
z	Standardized score. (22,23)

Index

Note: Page numbers followed by *f* refer to figures, those followed by *t* refer to tables. Numbers following *S* refer to online chapter supplements.

A-B-A-B design, 255, 256*f*
A-B-A-C design, 258
A-B-A design, 254, 255*f*
A-B design, 251, 251*f*, 254
Absolute effect, 534
Absolute reliability, 118, 492
Absolute risk (AR), 534
Absolute risk increase (ARI), 543
Absolute risk reduction (ARR), 541, 541*t*, 542, 542*f*
Abstracts, 290–91, 549, 602
Accessible population, 181
Accidental sample, 189
Active controls, 198–99
Active variable, 194
Adjusted means. *See* Analysis of covariance
Adjusted odds ratio (aOR), 460
Adjusted R Square, 444
Agreement, measures of, 494–96
   percent agreement, 494
   kappa, 494–97, 495*t*
   limits of, 499–501
Allocation concealment, 197–198, 584
Alpha (α),
   level of significance, 340–42
   Cronbach's alpha 122
Alphanumeric variable, 631
Alternate forms reliability, 122, 499–501
Alternating treatment design, 257–58
Alternative hypothesis (H_1), 338
AMSTAR–2, 591
Analysis of covariance (ANCOVA), 461–466, 463*t*
   adjusted means, 462–64, 464*f*
   covariate, 220, 462, 464, 465
   for confounding effects, 220
   homogeneity of slopes, 464
   intact groups, 465
   multiple covariates, 465
   null hypothesis, 462
   pretest-posttest adjustments, 465
   regression analysis, 462–65
   power and sample size, 464, S30–3
Analysis of variance (ANOVA), 365–82. *See also* Friedman ANOVA, Kruskal-Wallis ANOVA, MANOVA
   critical values table, 618*t*, *Appendix A Online*
   degrees of freedom, 368, 371, 375, 377, 378
   effect size, 369
   F statistic, 368–69, 371, 373, 377
   interaction effect, 371–73, 372*t*, 374*t*
   Intraclass correlation coefficient (ICC), 489
   main effect, 370–371, 371*f*

mixed designs, 378–81, 381*t*
null hypothesis, 366
   of regression, 444
   one-way, 365–70, 366*t*
   partitioning variance, 366–67, 367*f*, 370, 375
   power and sample size, 369, 369*b*, 373, 375, 378, 380, S25–2
   repeated measures, 373–78, 376*t*, 379*t*
   two-way, 370–73, 370*f*
Analytic epidemiology
   measures of risk, 533–39
   measures of treatment effect, 539–44
Anchor-based approach, 504–505
ANCOVA. *See* Analysis of covariance (ANCOVA)
ANOVA. *See* Analysis of variance (ANOVA)
Applied research, 11
Appraisal. *See* Critical appraisal
a priori tests. *See* Power
Arc sine transformation, 636
Area probability sampling, 188
Area under normal curve, 329*f*, 330, 331*f*, 614–16
Area under the curve (AUC), 521, 521*t*
Arm. *See* Treatment arm
Attribute variable, 194
Attrition
   bias, 584
   internal validity, 213, 222
Audit trail, 311
Authority, 54, 56*f*
Authorship, 599
Autocorrelation, 264
Autonomy, 90

Background question, 58
Backward inclusion, 452, 453
Bartlett's test of sphericity, 470*t*, 471
Basic research, 11, 19, 20*f*, 58, 201
Bayes' theorem, 515*b*
Belmont Report, 90
Bench research, 11
Beneficence, 90–91
Beta (β), 342, 637. *See also* Power
Beta weights, 448
Between-subjects design, 228
Bias
   ascertainment, 199
   attrition, 584
   case control study, 281–82
   Cochrane risk of bias tool, 584, 584*f*
   cohort study, 280
   detection, 199, 213, 584
   experimental, 217
   interviewer, 282

observation, 282
   performance, 199, 214, 584
   publication, 71, 345, 579
   reactive, 305
   recall, 282
   sampling, 185
   selection, 189, 213–214, 281–82, 584
Binomial test, 264, 264*t*, 613, S18–3*t*, S27–2*t*
Bland-Altman plot, 499–501, 500*f*, 501, 502*b*
Blinding, 199, 200, 201, 214, 215
Blocking variable, 219, 233
Block randomization, 195*t*, 196
Bonferroni correction, 384, 385*t*, S26–3
Boolean logic, 75–76, 77*f*
Box plot, 325–26, 325*f*

Canonical correlation, 480
Carryover effects, 120, 234
Case-control study, 12*f*, 13*t*, 280–82, 280*f*
   assessing methodological quality, 585
   case definition, 281, 281*b*
   confounding, 282
   interviewer bias, 282
   matching, 282
   observation bias, 282
   population-based/hospital-based study, 281
   recall bias, 282
   retrospective study, 280*f*
   selection bias, 281–82
   selection of cases and controls, 281
Case reports, 12*f*, 14*t*, 289–93, S20
   case series, 289
   epidemiologic reports, 292–93
   ethics, 292
   format, 290–292
   generalizability, 292
   purposes, 289–90
Case studies, 304–5
CAT. *See* Critically appraised topic
Causal modeling, 474
Cause-and-effect association, 273–74
   reverse causation, 277
Ceiling effect, 138
Celeration line, 263, S18–2
Censored observations, 482
Central tendency, 322–24
   and skewness, 323, 324*f*
   mean, 323, 324*f*
   median, 322–23, 324*f*
   mode, 322, 324*f*
Change, measuring, 136–38, 122–24, 501–6
   anchor-based approaches, 504
   distribution-based measures, 503

effect size, 503–4, 504t
global rating scale, 504–5, 505t
minimal clinically important difference (MCID), 136–38, 205–6, 501f, 503–6
minimal detectable change (MDC), 123–24, 123f, 136–38, 501–2, 501f
reliability, 122–24, 501
responsiveness, 501
validity, 136–38, 501
Change score, 122, 136
Changing criterion design, 259, S18–1
Chi-square, 415–27. *See also* McNemar test
  assumptions, 416
  chi-square statistic, 415–16
  contingency table, 419, 420f
  critical values table, 620t, *Appendix A Online*
  degrees of freedom, 416, 421, 424
  effect size, 423–24, 423t
  expected frequencies, 415, 416, 418, 420
  Fisher's exact test, 421
  goodness of fit, 416–19
  known distribution, 417–19, 418t
  McNemar test. *See* McNemar test
  null hypothesis, 415, 417–20, 424
  odds ratio, 425, 426b
  power and sample size, 423–424, 424b, S28
  standardized residuals, 419, 421
  testing proportions, 415–16
  tests of independence, 419–22, 422t
  uniform distribution, 416–17, 417t
  Yates' continuity correction, 421
CINAHL, 72–73, 72t, 579
Citation management applications, 85
Classical measurement theory, 115, 168
Classificatory scale, 109
Clinical practice guidelines (CPGs), 61, 575–76, 575t, 587, 590
Clinical prediction rules (CPR), 523–26
  diagnosis, 523–524, 524f
  intervention, 524
  prognosis, 524
  validation, 525–26, 526f
Clinical queries, 81, 82f
Clinical research
  defined, 2–3
  frameworks, 5–16
  types of research, 11–14, 12f, 13–14t
Clinical trials, 192–209
  active/attribute variable, 194
  allocation concealment, 197–98, 584
  blinding, 199, 200, 201, 214, 215
  block randomization, 195t, 196
  clinical trials registries, 193b
  cluster random assignment, 195t, 196–97
  control groups, 198–99
  defined, 192
  equipoise, 96b, 198b
  equivalence trial, 206

explanatory vs. pragmatic trial, 200–201, 201t
  non-inferiority trial, 205–6, 206f
  open-label trial, 199
  parallel group, 193
  phases of clinical trials, 19–21, 201–4
  PICO, 194
  placebo, 198, 198b
  pragmatic clinical trial (PCT), 200–201, 201t, 202b
  random assignment (allocation), 194–98, 195t
  randomized consent design, 195t, 197
  randomized controlled trial (RCT), 193, 193f, 200
  run-in period, 195t, 197
  stratified random assignment, 195t, 196
  superiority trial, 205, 206f
  wait list control group, 198
Closed-ended questions, 146
Cluster analysis, 477–78, 478f, 479f
Cluster random assignment, 195t, 196–97
Cluster sampling, 186t, 187–88, 188f
  multistage, 188, 188f
Cochrane Collaboration, 72t, 73, 576b, 579, 587, 588
Cochrane risk of bias tool, 584, 584f
Cochran's Q, 589
Code books, 633
Coding
  mixed methods research, 313–14
  qualitative research, 309
  regression analysis, 453–54
Coefficient of determination, 440
Coefficient of variation (CV), 328, 494
Cohen's f, 369, S25–2
Cohort effect, 287
Cohort studies, 12f, 13t, 278–80, 278f
  advantages/disadvantages, 279
  assessing methodological quality, 585
  bias, 280
  misclassification, 279–80
  prospective study, 280f
  retrospective study, 280f
  subject selection, 279
  types of, 278
Collinearity, 448–49, 448f
Common cause variation, 266
Common Rule, 90, S7
Communalities, 470t, 471
Comparative effectiveness research (CER), 19
Comparative studies, 35–36
Compensatory equalization, 215
Completer analysis, 223
Complex contrasts, 395
Complex hypothesis, 90
Computer adaptive test (CAT), 174
Concurrent validity, 129t, 131, 277, 278
Confidence intervals (CI), 336–338, 337f, 336f
  defined, 336
  diagnostic accuracy, 518–19

intraclass correlation coefficient (ICC), 489
  number needed to treat (NNT), 542
  paired *t*-test, 360
  relative risk, 535–36
  unpaired *t*-test, 357–60
Confidentiality, 93t, 97, 629
Confirmatory factor analysis (CFA), 134, 474, 475b
Conflict of interest (COI), 100
Confounding
  analysis of covariance (ANCOVA), 220
  case-control study, 282
  observational research, 275
  variable, 212, 538
Consecutive sampling, 189
CONSORT statement, 183, 184f, 600t, 601–2t
Constant comparison, 303
Constructs, 43–44, 108. 132, 133b, 159–73, 468–469, 473–478
  latent trait, 108, 469, 469f
Construct validity, 129f, 129t, 132–34, 215–17
  and content validity, 132
  convergence and discrimination, 133–34
  experimental bias, 217
  factor analysis, 134
  known groups method, 132
  methods of construct validation, 132
  multiple treatment interactions, 217
  multitrait-multimethod matrix (MTMM), 133–34
  Rasch analysis, 134
  subgroup differences, 216
  time frame, 216–17
  types of evidence, S10–2
Content analysis, 309
Content validity, 129–130, 129t, 129f
  universe of content, 130
  content validity index (CVI), 130, S10–1
Contingency coefficient (C), 423, 423t
Contingency table, 419
Continuity correction, 421
Continuous variable, 107
Contrast coefficient, 395
Control event rate (CER), 540, 541t
Control groups, 96, 198–99
  active controls, 198, 229
  inactive controls, 198
  placebo, 198, 229
  sham, 198
  wait list, 198
Convenience (accidental) sampling, 186t, 189
Conventional effect sizes
  d, 360
  η^2, 369
  f, 369
  f^2, 449
  r, 432
  R^2, 449
  w, 423

Convergent validity, 129t, 133
Correlation, 428–39
  assumptions, 429–30
  canonical, 480
  causation, and, 435–36, 436f
  comparison, and, 435
  correlation coefficient, 428–29
  critical values table, 619t, *Appendix A*
    Online
  curvilinear relationship, 430, 430f
  degrees of freedom, 432
  of dichotomies, 435, S29–2
  hypothesis testing, 429
  item-to-total, 497–99
  Kendall's tau-b, 434, 434t
  linear relationships, 429f, 430
  null hypothesis, 431
  outliers, 436–37, 436f
  null hypothesis, 431
  partial, 437–38, 438f
  Pearson correlation coefficient,
    431–32, 432t, 433b
  positive/negative, 428
  power and sample size, 432, S29–4
  range of test values, 437
  ranked data, 432–35
  scatter plot, 428, 429f
  Spearman rank correlation coefficient.
    See Spearman rank correlation
  zero-order, 438
COSMIN, 585
Covariate, 220, 440, 462, 464, 465
Cox proportional hazards model, 483
CPR. *See* Clinical prediction rules
Cramer's *V*, 423, 423t
Criterion referencing, 135
Criterion-related validity, 129t, 129f,
  130–31, 277, 278
  concurrent validity, 128t, 131
  predictive validity, 129t, 131–32
Critical appraisal, 557–73
  appraisal process, 558, 559t
  appraisal worksheets, S36–2
  are results meaningful?, 560–61
  are results relevant to patient?, 561–62
  core questions, 558–62
  critically appraised topic (CAT),
    568–71
  diagnostic accuracy studies, 564–65,
    564t
  evidence-based practice, and, 562f,
    561–562
  intervention studies, 562–64, 563t
  is the study valid?, 559–60
  levels of evidence, 557–58, 558t
  meta-analysis, 591
  prognosis studies, 565–67, 566t
  qualitative studies, 567–68, 567t
  systematic review, 591
Critically appraised topic (CAT), 568–71,
  570t
Critical region, 347, 347f
Critical value, 357
Cronbach's alpha, 497–99

Crossover design, 235, 235f, 259
  washout period, 235
Cross-sectional study, 276–78, 398
  accuracy of diagnostic test, 277, 278
  challenges, 277–78
  concurrent validity, 277, 278
  developmental research, 286–87
Crosstabulation, 494
C statistic, 265, S18–5
Cubic trend, 396
Cumulative incidence. *See* Incidence
Cumulative scales, 167–68
Cutoff scores, 161, 519–523

Data bases, 71–74, 72t, S6
Data cleaning, 633
Data collection, 630–32
Data management, 629–36
  confidentiality and security, 629
  data cleaning, 633
  data collection, 630–32
  data entry, 630, 633
  data modification/transformation,
    633–36
  listwise and pairwise deletion, 632
  missing data, 632
  monitoring subject participation, 629
  statistical programs, 629–30
  type of variable, 630–31
  variable names, 630
Data managing boards, 204b
Data modification, 633–36
Data transformation, 635–36
Declaration of Helsinki, 89–90, 96, 96b,
  198b
Deductive reasoning, 45–46
  deductive theories, 45–46
Degrees of freedom *(df)*, 354
Delphi survey, 142, S11–1
Dependent variable, 35, 36, 36f, 440
Descriptive research, 11, 12f, 14t, 32, 34,
  285–96
  case reports, 289–93
  descriptive survey, 12f, 288–89
  developmental research, 286–87, 287b
  epidemiology, 530–33
  historical research, 293–94
  normative studies, 287–88
Descriptive statistics, 318–32
  frequency distribution, 318–21
  graphs, 320–21, 320t
  measures of central tendency,
    322–24
  measures of variability, 324–28
  normal distribution, 322, 328–31
Design validity, 210–26. *See also* Validity
  construct validity, 215–17
  controlling subject variability, 218–20
  external validity, 217–18
  intention to treat (ITT), 222–23
  internal validity, 212–15
  missing data, 223–24
  non-compliance, 220–22
  overview, 211f, 211t

per-protocol analysis, 222
  statistical conclusion validity, 210–11
Detection bias, 199, 213, 584
Developmental research, 12f, 14t, 286–87
  cohort effect, 287
  natural history, 286
Diagnostic tests, 509–28
  clinical prediction rules (CPR), 523–26
  confidence intervals, 518–19
  critical appraisal of diagnostic studies,
    564–65, 564t, 585
  diagnostic accuracy, 511, 513
  gold standard, 510
  index test, 510
  likelihood ratios (LR), 516–17
  nomogram, 517–18, 518f
  positive and negative tests, 511
  predictive values (PV), 513
  pretest and posttest probabilities,
    514–19, 516f
  prevalence, 513
  QUADAS and QUADAS-2, 585
  ROC curves, 519–23, 522t
  ruling in and ruling out, 513–14, 514f
  sensitivity and specificity, 131b, 511,
    512t
Dichotomous variables, 106
Differences scores, 360, 499–501
Differential item functioning (DIF),
  173–74
Differential misclassification, 279
Direct costs, 553
Directional hypothesis, 38, 39
Discrete variable, 107
Discriminant analysis, 480–481, 481f
Discriminant validity, 129t, 133
Disease-oriented evidence (DOE), 24
Disproportional sampling, 186t, 188,
  S13–2
Disseminating research, 597–612
  authorship, 599, 599b
  choosing a journal, 597–99
  e-poster, 610
  journal impact factor, 597–8, 598b
  open access journals, 84, 598–99, 598b
  oral presentations, 607–8
  peer review, 605
  poster presentation, 608–9, 609f
  reporting guidelines, 599–600, 600t,
    602t, S38–1, S38–2
  standards for reporting, 599–600, 600t
  submitting the manuscript, 605–7
  supplementary materials, 605
  tracking metrics, 611
  types of submissions, 606, 610–11
Distribution, 318
  frequency, 318, 319t
  grouped frequency, 319–320
  normal, 328–31
  sampling, 335
  skewed, 322, 322f
Distribution-based approach, 503
Divergent validity, 133
Dose-response relationship, 272

Double-blind study, 199
Dummy variables, 453–54
Duncan's new multiple range test, 385t, S26–3
Dunnett's correctin, 285t, S26–3
Dunn's multiple comparison, 407, S27–1

Ecological validity, 218
EFA. *See* Exploratory factor analysis (EFA)
Effectiveness, 6, 19, 21–22. 26
Effect modification, 537–38, 528t
Effect size (ES), 343
  ANOVA, 369, 373, 378, 380
  chi-square, 423–24, 423t
  conventional values. *See* Conventional effect sizes
  effect size index, 503, 504t
  Friedman two-way ANOVA, 411
  Guyatt's responsiveness index, 504, 504t
  Kruskal-Wallis ANOVA, 407
  Mann-Whitney *U* test, 403–4
  meta-analysis, 587
  odds ratio, 536, S 34
  Pearson correlation coefficient, 432
  regression analysis, 449
  relative risk, 536, S34
  single-subject design, 267
  standardized response mean, 503–504, 504t
  t test, 361–63
  weighting, 587
  Wilcoxon signed-ranks test, 410
Efficacy, 6,18, 19, 26
Eigenvalue, 471
E-mail alerts, 85
Enablement theory, 49, S1
EndNote, 85
Endogenous variable, 476
Epidemiology, 11, 529–46
  absolute risk (AR), 534
  analytic, 533–544
  case reports, 292–93
  confounding, 538
  control event rate (CER), 540
  descriptive, 530–33
  disease frequency, 530–33
  effect modification, 537–38
  experimental event rate (EER), 540
  exposures, 533
  incidence, 532–33
  measures of risk, 533–39
  measures of treatment effect, 539–44, 541t
  number needed to harm (NNH), 542–44, 543b
  number needed to treat (NNT), 542, 542f, 543–44, 543b
  odds ratio (OR), 536, 537t
  power and sample size, 536, S34
  prevalence, 530–32
  relative risk (RR), 534–36, 540, 535t
  relative vs. absolute effects, 534

risk factors, 533
risk increase, 543
risk reduction, 540–42
vital statistics, 533
E-poster, 610
Epsilon, 377
Epub ahead of print, 84–85
Equipoise, 96b, 198b
Equivalence trial, 206
EQUATOR network, 558
Error variance, 351
Eta coefficient, 430, S29–3
Eta squared (η^2), 369
Ethical principles, 88–104
  autonomy, 90
  beneficence, 90–91
  case reports, 292
  Common Rule, 90, S7
  confidentiality, 93t, 97
  conflict of interest (COI), 100, 561, 599, 605
  fabrication, 99
  falsification, 99
  informed consent, 92–98
  institutional review board (IRB), 91–92, 92f
  justice, 91
  peer review, 100, 598b, 599, 603, 605
  plagiarism, 99–100
  replication, 32, 32b, 101
  research integrity, 98–102
  research misconduct, 98–100
  respect for persons, 90
  retractions, 101
Ethnography, 302
Event rate, 540
  control event rate (CER), 540, 541t
  experimental event rate (EER), 540, 541t
Evidence,
  absence of, 63b, 345b
  grading up or down, 65, 558t, 590, 591t
  levels of. *See* Levels of evidence
  misuse, 54, 55t
  overuse, 54, 55t
  quality of, 65
  reviews, 60
  underuse, 54, 55t
Evidence-based practice (EBP), 5–6, 22, 53–69
  acquire relevant literature, 59
  apply the evidence, 61–62
  appraise the literature, 61, 61t, 562f
  ask a clinical question, 58–59
  assess the EBP process, 62
  background question, 58
  barriers and facilitators to, 65, S5
  clinical decision-making, 53
  components of EBP, 56–57, 56f
  defined, 56
  EPB framework, 63f
  EBP process, 57–62
  foreground question, 58, 60t

implementation research, 25, 66
knowledge translation (KT), 66–67, 67b
misconceptions, 56
practice-based evidence (PBE), 22
qualitative research, 64–65, 298–99, 299f
ways of knowing, 54, 56f
Exclusion criteria, 181–82, 551, 560, 562, 565, 578, 580, 589, 603
Exempt review, 91
Exogenous variable, 476
Expedited review, 91
Experimental design, 11, 227–39
  design classifications, 227–28
  factorial design, 231–33
  mixed design, 236
  one-way, 228
  one-way repeated measures design, 233–36
  posttest-only control group design, 230–31
  pretest-posttest control group design, 228–30
  randomized block design, 233
  repeated measures design, 233–36, 228
  sequential clinical trials, 236–38, S16
  three-way factorial design, 233
  two-way factorial design, 232–33
  two-way repeated measures designs, 236
Experimental event rate (EER), 540, 541t
Experimental mortality, 213
Experimenter effects, 217
Explanatory research, 11, 12f, 13t, 34, 35–36, 200–201, 201t, 271
Exploding, in literature search, 78
Exploratory data analysis (EDA), 321b
Exploratory factor analysis (EFA), 134, 468–74, 469f, 470t
  Bartlett's test of sphericity, 470t, 471
  communalities, 470t, 471
  eigenvalue, 471
  extraction of factors, 471
  factor loadings, 471
  factor matrix, 470t, 471–73
  factor rotation, 472, 472f, 472b
  factor scores, 474
  Kaiser-Meyer-Olkin (KMO), 469
  latent traits, 469
  naming of factors, 470t, 473f
  principal axis factoring, 471
  rotated factor matrix, 470t, 473
  sample size, 474
Exploratory research. *See* Observational research
Exposures, 272, 529, 530, 532, 533, 534, 538
External validity, 217–18
Extraneous variable, 219, 220

Fabrication, 99
Face validity, 130
Factor, 34
  independent, 220, 236
  repeated, 220, 236

Factor analysis, 134, 135f, 468, 470–74, 470t. *See also* Exploratory and Confirmatory factor analysis
Factorial design, 231–33
  main effects, 232
  interaction effects, 232–33
  randomized block design, 233
Falsification, 99
False negative, 510
False positive, 510
Familywise error rate (α_{FW}), 383
Field notes, 305
Filters, in literature search, 80
First-order partial correlation, 438
Fisher's exact test, 421
Fisher's least significant difference (LSD), 385t, S26–3
Fixed effect, 419, 487
Floor effect, 138
Flow diagram, 184f, 221f
Focus group interviews, 307
Focusing, in literature search, 78
Follow-up study, 278. *See also* Cohort study
Foreground question, 58, 60t
Forest plot, 587–88, 588f
Forward inclusion, 452
Framingham Heart Study, 182b
Frequency distribution, 318–21, 320f
Friedman two-way ANOVA, 410–12, 412t
  critical values table, chi-square, 620, *Appendix A Online*
  degrees of freedom, 411
  effect size, 411
  multiple comparison, 411, S27–1
  null hypothesis, 411
F statistic. *See* Analysis of variance
Funnel plot, 589–90, 590f

Generalizability
  case reports, 292
  reliability, 119, 119b
  single-subject design, 267–68
Gold standard, 130, 510
Goodness of fit
  known distribution, 417–19
  structural equation modeling (SEM), 476–77
  uniform distribution, 416–17
Google Scholar, 73, 73b, S6
G*Power, 345, S23–34
GRADE system, 590, 591t
Grand mean, 367, 367f
Grand theory, 50
Graphs, 320–321, 320t
  box plot, 325–26, 325f, 326b
  histogram, 320
  line plot (frequency polygon), 321
  normal and skewed distribution, 322, 322f
  in presentations, 608
  stem and leaf plot, 321

Greenhouse-Geisser correction, 376t, 377
Grey literature, 70–71, 579, 580b
Grounded theory, 46, 303, 304f
Group centroid, 479
Grouped frequency distribution, 319–20, 320f
Guiding questions, 39, 144
Guttman scale, 167
Guyatt's responsiveness index (GRI), 504, 504t

Harmonic mean, 387, S26–2
Hawthorne effect, 217b
Hazard ratio (HR), 483
Health measurement scales, 159–77
  alternate forms, 164
  cumulative scales, 167–68
  cut-off scores, 161, 519–523
  item response theory (IRT), 168. *See also* Rasch analysis
  Likert scales, 162–64, S12–1
  numerical rating scale (NRS), 165–66, 166f
  Rasch analysis, 169–74
  short forms, 160
  subscales, 162
  summative scales, 161–67
  target population, 160
  unidimensionality, 160
  visual analog scale (VAS), 164–67, 164f, 165f, 167f
Henrietta Lacks, 89b
Heterogeneity, in meta-analysis, 589
Hierarchical regression, 453
HIPAA, 90
Histogram, 320, 320f
Historical controls, 246
Historical research, 12f, 14t, 293–94
History, in internal validity, 212
Homer-Lemeshow test, 459t, 460
Homogeneity of slopes, 464
Homogeneity of variance, 349, 353, 356, 368
  Levene's test, 356, 368
Hospital-based study, 281
Huynh-Feldt correction, 376t, 377
Hypotheses
  alternative, 338
  complex, 39
  deductive, 45
  directional/nondirectional, 38, 338–39
  null, 338–39
  research, 38
  simple, 39
  statistical, 38, 338
Hypothesis testing. *See also* Type I and Type II error
  alternative hypothesis (H_1), 338
  critical region, 347–48, 347f, 348f
  disproving the null, 339
  errors in, 340–345
  level of significance, 340–42
  null hypothesis (H_0), 338

one-tailed test, 348
power (*See* Power)
p value, 341
test statistic, 346
two-tailed test, 347
Hypothetical-deductive theory, 45–46

ICC. *See* Intraclass correlation coefficient (ICC)
ICF. *See* International Classification of Functioning, Disability and Health
Impact factor, 597
Implementation studies, 25–26, 66–67, 67b
Imputation, 223, 224
Inception cohort, 278
Incidence, 532–33
Inclusion criteria, 181–82, 551, 560, 562, 565, 578, 580, 585, 589, 592, 593, 603
Independent *t* test. *See* t-test
Independent variable, 34–35, 36, 36f
  independent factor, 220
  levels, 36
  repeated measure, 220
Index test, 510
Indirect costs, 554
Inductive reasoning, 46
Inferential statistics, 333–349
Informed consent, 92–98
  and usual care, 98
  confidentiality, 93t, 97, 629
  consent elements, 97–98
  control group, 96
  disclosure, 96
  elements, 93t
  equipoise, 96b
  information elements, 93–97
  informed consent form, 93f, 94–95f, 98
  lay language, 97
  placebo, 96b
  potential risks/benefits, 96–97
  surveys, 156–57
  usual care, 98
  "vulnerable" participants, 97–98
  withdrawing consent, 98
Institutional review board (IRB), 91–92, 92f, 156
Instrumentation effects, 213
Integrity. *See* Ethical principles
Intention to treat (ITT), 211, 222–23
Interaction effects, 232, 371, 390–92
Interlibrary loan, 84
Internal consistency, 122, 497–99, 498t
  Cronbach's alpha, 497
  item-to-total correlation, 497
Internal validity, 211t, 211f, 212–15, 584
  attrition, 212–213
  compensatory equivalization, 215
  compensatory rivalry, 215
  confounding variable, 212
  demoralization, 215
  diffusion or imitation of treatments, 214

history, 212
instrumentation, 213
maturation, 212
regression to the mean, 123, 213
ruling out the threats, 215
selection, 213–14
social threats, 214
testing effect, 213
International Classification of
Functioning, Disability and
Health (ICF), 6–8, 7*f*, *S1*
capacity and performance, 8
contextual factors, 7
Interprofessional research, 9–10
Interquartile range, 325
Inter-rater reliability, 121
Interrupted time series (ITS) design,
242–44
Interval recording, 253
Interval scale, 111–12
Interviewer bias, 282
Interviews, 142–43
face-to-face, 142
in qualitative research, 306–8
structured/unstructured, 142–43,
306–7
telephone, 143
Intraclass correlation coefficient (ICC),
486–90, 490*t*
ANOVA, 489
calculations, *S32–1*, *S32–2*
confidence intervals, 489
forms, 487
models, 487–88
Intra-rater reliability, 121
IRB. *See* Institutional review board (IRB)
I^2 statistic, 589
Item response theory (IRT), 168. *See also*
Rasch analysis
Item-to-total correlation, 497–99
ITS design. *See* Interrupted time series
(ITS) design
ITT. *See* Intention to treat (ITT)

Journal club, 571*b*
Journal impact factor (JIF), 597,
598*b*
Justice, 91

Kaiser-Meyer-Olkin (KMO) measure,
469, 470*t*
Kaplan-Meier estimate, 482
Kappa, 118, 494–96, 495*t*
weighted kappa, 456, *S32–3*
Kendall's tau-b, 434, 434*t*
Keywords, 74–76, 579, 602, 609
Knowing, ways of, 54, 56*f*
Knowledge translation (KT), 18,
66
Knowledge-to-action framework, 66,
67, 67*b*
Known distribution, chi-square, 417–19,
418*t*

Known groups method, 132
Kolmogorov-Smirnov test of normality,
349*b*, 643
Kruskal-Wallis ANOVA, 405–7, 406*t*
critical values table, chi-square, 620,
Appendix A Online
degrees of freedom, 407
effect size, 407
multiple comparison, 407, *S27–1*
null hypothesis, 405

Last observation carried forward
(LOCF), 224
Latent trait, 43,108, 168, 173, 469, 473,
475
Latin square, 235, 235*f*
Law, and theory, 50
Least squares method, 442
Level of significance, 340–42
Levels of evidence, 62–65, 64*t*, 557–58,
558*t*
qualitative research, 64–65
Levels of measurement, 109–14, 110*f*
interval scale, 111–12
nominal scale, 109–10
ordinal scale, 110–11
ratio scale, 112
Levene's test, 356, 368
Likelihood ratios (LR), 516–17
negative LR–, 517
positive LR+, 516
interpreting values, 517, 517*f*
Likert scales, 162–64, *S12–1*
Limits of agreement (LoA), 132,
499–501. *See also* Bland-Altman
plot
Linear regression. *See* Regression
Linear trend, 396
Line of best fit, 441, 442
Line plot, 320*f*, 321
Listwise deletion, 224, 632
Literature review, 33, 59, 86, 144.
See also Searching the literature
Logical positivism, 297
Logistic regression, 456–61, 459*t*
adjusted odds ratio (aOR), 460
classification table, 458, 459*t*
continuous variables, 460
Cox & Snell R Square, 458, 459*t*
Homer-Lemeshow test, 459*t*,
460
maximum likelihood estimation,
457
Nagelkerke R Square, 458, 459*t*
odds, 457–458, 458*b*
odds ratio, 457–58, 460
probabilities, 458*b*, *S30–2*
propensity scores, 461
sample size, 461, *S30–3*
Wald statistic, 459*t*, 460
Logit scores, 169, 171*f*, 172*t*,
173*t*
Log transformation, 635
Lonesome Doc, 84

Longitudinal studies, 274–76, 398
developmental research, 286
prospective study, 274–76
retrospective study, 276

Main effects, 232, 370, 371*f*, 390
Manifest variable, 476
Mann-Whitney *U* test, 403–5, 404*t*
critical values table, 613, *S27–2t*,
Appendix A Online
large samples, 403
null hypothesis, 403
MANOVA. *See* Multivariate analysis
of variance (MANOVA)
Marginal means, 370
Matching, 219, 282
Maturation, in internal validity, 212
Mauchly's test of sphericity, 376*t*, 377
Maximum likelihood estimation, 457
MCID. *See* Minimal clinically important
difference
McNemar test, 424–26, 425*t*
degrees of freedom, 424
effect size, 425
null hypothesis, 424
power and sample size, 426*b*, *S28*
MDC. *See* Minimal detectable change
Mean, 323, 324*f*
Mean square (MS), 327, 368
Measurement, 105–77
of change. *See* Change
classical measurement theory, 115,
168
indirect nature of, 107–8
levels of, 109–14, 110*f*
precision, 107
scales. *See* Health measurement scales
Measurement error, 115–17
random, 116, 116*f*, 128*f*
sources of, 116–17
systematic, 116, 116*f*, 128*f*
Mechanistic reasoning, 64
Median, 322–23, 324*f*, 402, 482
Medical subject headings (MeSH),
77, 80*t*
MEDLINE, 71–72, 72*t*, 579
Member checking, 311
Mendeley, 85
Merging, 313
MeSH. *See* Medical subject headings
Meta-analysis, 11, 12*f*, 61, 575*t*, 587–91,
S37–3. *See also* Systematic Reviews
advantages, 587
critical appraisal of, 591, 591*t*, *S37–2*
effect size, 587
forest plot, 587–88, 588*f*
funnel plot, 589–90, 590*f*
grading the evidence, 590, 591*t*
heterogeneity, 589
overview, 577*f*
sensitivity analysis, 589
standardized mean difference (SMD),
587
statistical heterogeneity, 589

Meta-theory, 50
Method error, 494, S32–4
Methodological studies, 11, 12f, 13t, 34, 124, 138–39
Middle-range theories, 49–50
Minimal clinically important difference (MCID), 136–38, 205–6, 501f, 503–6
    MCID proportion, 506
    non-inferiority margin, 205–6
Minimal detectable change (MDC), 123–24, 136–38, 137f, 501–2, 501f
    MDC proportion, 506
Minimum significant difference (MSD), 385–86
    Friedman two-way ANOVA, S27–1
    Kruskal-Wallis one-way ANOVA, S27–1
    Scheffé comparison, 390
    SNK test, 388–89
    Tukey's HSD, 386–87
Misclassification, 279–80
Missing data
    completer analysis, 223
    data imputation, 223–24
    design validity, 223–24
    identifying missing values, 632
    last observation carried forward, 224
    per-protocol analysis, 222
    surveys, 155
    "missingness," 223
Mixed methods research, 14t, 312–14. *See also* Qualitative Research
    coding and analysis, 313–14
    data collection, 313
    merging qualitative and quantitative data, 313–14, 314f
    sampling, 313
Mixed repeated measures design, 236
Mode, 322, 324f
Models, 44–45
Models of health and disability, 6, S1
Multicollinearity, *See* Collinearity
Multidimensional Health Locus of Control scale, 162–164, 163f, S12–1
Multi-factor design, 228
Multigroup pretest-posttest control group design, 229
Multiple baseline design, 255–57, S18–1
Multiple comparison tests, 369, 383–99, 385t, S26–3
    Bonferroni correction, 384t
    complex contrasts, 395, S26–3
    factorial designs, 390–92
    familywise error rate, 383
    minimum significant difference (MSD), 385
    planned, 394–98, S26–3
    post hoc, 384–90
    repeated measures, 392
    Scheffé comparison, 385t, 390, 391t
    simple effects, 391–92, 393t
    studentized range, q, 376, 387t, 613, *Appendix A Online*, S26–1t
    Student-Newman-Keuls (SNK) test, 385t, 387–89, 389t

trend analysis, 395–98, 396t, 397f
    unplanned, 384
    Tukey's honestly significant difference (HSD), 385t, 386–87
    Type I error rate, 383–84
Multiple imputation, 224
Multiple regression, 446–49
    adjusted R², 444
    beta weights, 448
    collinearity, 448–49, 448f
    hierarchical, 453
    null hypothesis, 446
    partial correlation, 448
    prediction accuracy, 446
    regression coefficients, 446, 448
    regression equation, 446
    stepwise, 449–53, 451t
    tolerance, 448
    variance inflation factor (VIF)_, 448
Multistage sampling, 188
Multitrait-multimethod matrix (MTMM), 133–34
Multivariate analysis, 468–85. *See also* Multiple regression and Logistic Regression
    cluster analysis, 477–78
    confirmatory factor analysis (CFA), 474
    defined, 468
    exploratory factor analysis (EFA), 468–74
    multivariate analysis of variance (MANOVA), 478–81
    structural equation modeling (SEM), 474–77
    survival analysis, 481–83
Multivariate analysis of variance (MANOVA), 478–81
    discriminant analysis, 480–81, 481f
    follow-up tests, 480–81
    purpose, 478
    test statistics, 479–80
    vectors, 479
My NCBI, 85

National Research Act, 90
Natural history, 286
Naturalistic inquiry, 302
Necessary exposure, 272b
Negative case analysis, 311
Negative likelihood ratio. *See* Likelihood ratios
Negative predictive value. *See* Predictive value
Newcastle-Ottawa Scale Quality Assessment Form (NOS), 585
Newman-Keuls test. *See* Student-Newman-Keuls test
NIH biosketch, 552, S35
NIH Roadmap, 17
NNH. *See* Number needed to harm (NNH)
NNT. *See* Number needed to treat (NNT)

N-of-1 trial, 12f, 259–60, 261b
Nominal scale, 109–10
Nomogram, 517, 518f, S33
Non-compliance, 220–22
Noncritical region, 347, 347f
Noncurrent multiple baseline design, 256, S18–1
Nondifferential misclassification, 279
Nondirectional hypothesis, 38
Nonequivalent group designs, 244–47
Nonequivalent posttest-only control group design, 246–47, 246f
Nonequivalent pretest-posttest control group design, 244–46
Non-inferiority trial, 205–6, 206f, 339b
    MCID, 205–206
    null and alternative hypotheses, 339b
    non-inferiority margin, 205–6, 339b
Nonlinear regression. *See* Polynomial regression
Nonoverlapping scores, in single-subject design, 267
Nonparametric tests, 113, 349, 400–414, 400t
    binomial test, 409, 409t, S27–2t
    Friedman two-way ANOVA, 410–12, 412t
    Kruskal-Wallis ANOVA, 405–7, 406t
    Mann-Whitney U test, 403–5, 404t, 405t, 613, S27–2t
    power-efficiency, 402, S27–3
    ranking scores, 402–3, 402t
    sample size, 402
    sign test, 407–9, 408t
    Wilcoxon signed-ranks test, 408t, 409–10, 410t, 613, S27–2t
Nonprobability sample, 151, 183, 186t, 188–90. *See also* Samples
Normal distribution, 328–31
    area under normal curve, 328–29, 329f, 330, 331f, 614–16
    normality tests, 349b
    standardized scores, 329–31, 330f, 331f
Normative research, 12f, 14t, 287–88
Norm-referenced test, 135–36
Null hypothesis (H_0), 38, 338
Number needed to harm (NNH), 542–44
Number needed to treat (NNT), 541t, 542, 542f, 543–44
Nuremburg Code, 88–89

Oblique rotation, 472b
Observational research, 11, 12f, 13t, 34, 36–8, 37f, 271–84
    case-control studies, 280–82, 280f
    causation, 273–74, 274b
    cohort studies, 278–80, 278f
    confounding, 275
    cross-sectional studies, 276–78
    hypotheses, 38–39
    longitudinal studies, 274–76
    Newcastle-Ottawa Scale of Quality Assessment (NOS), 585

prospective studies, 274–76, 275*f*
retrospective studies, 275*f*, 276
risk, 272, 533
Observation bias, 282
Odds, 457, 458*b*
Odds ratio (OR)
  adjusted odds ratio (aOR), 460
  case-control studies, 536, 537*t*
  chi-square, effect size, 421–22
  logistic regression, 458, 460
  McNemar test, effect size, 425
  power and sample size, 536, S30–3
Omega squared, 369
One-group pretest-posttest design, 241
One-tailed test, 348, 357*b*
One-way ANOVA, 365–70, 366*t*
  effect size, 369
  homogeneity of variance, 368
  partitioning the variance, 366–67, 367*f*
  power and sample size, 369, 369*b*
One-way design, 228
One-way pretest-posttest design, 241–42, 242*f*
One-way repeated measures design, 233–36
Open access journals, 84, 598–99, 598*b*
Open-ended questions, 145–46
Open Grey, 71
Open-label trial, 199
Operational definition, 36, 216
Operators, arithmetic, 633
Oral presentations, 607–8
Order effects, 235
Ordinal scale, 110–11
Orthogonal rotation, 472*b*
OT Search, 72*t*
Outcomes research, 23–25, S2
Outliers, 436–37, 436*f*
OVID, 73

Paired *t*-test. *See t*-test
Pairwise deletion, 224, 632
Paradigm shift, 5
Parallel forms reliability, 122
Parallel groups study, 193, 228
Parameters, 183, 318
Parametric statistics, 113, 348–49
Partial correlation, 437–38, 438*f*, 448
Partial eta squared, 373, 378
Participant observation, 305–6
Path analysis, 476
Path diagram, 476, 476*f*
Patient-Centered Outcomes Research Institute (PCORI), 24
Patient-centered outcomes research (PCOR), 24
Patient-oriented evidence that matters (POEM), 23–24
Patient-reported outcome measure (PROM), 24
Patient-reported outcome (PRO), 24
Pearson product-moment coefficient of correlation, 431–32. *See also* Correlation

PEDro, 72*t*, 73, 583–84, 583*t*
Peer review, 70, 100, 605
Percent agreement, 494
Percentiles, 325
Percent of nonoverlapping data (PND), 267
Per comparison error rate (α_{PC}), 383
Performance bias, 199, 214, 584
Per-protocol analysis, 222
person-item map, 169, 169*f*, 171*f*
Phases of clinical trials, 19–21, 20*f*, 201–204, 203*f*
Phi coefficient, 423, 423*t*, 435, S29–2
Physiotherapy Evidence Database. *See* PEDro
PICO, 34, 35*f*, 37*f*, 58, 59, 59*f*, 60*t*, 73, 75, 75*f*, 194
Pillai-Bartlett trace, 479
Pilot testing, 124, 145
Placebo, 96*b*, 198, 198*b*
Plagiarism, 99–100
Planned comparisons, 394–98
Point biserial correlation coefficient, 435, S29–2
Point estimate, 336
Polynomial regression, 454–56, 456*t*
Polytomous variables, 106
Population, 150, 180
  accessible, 181
  target, 160, 181
Population-based study, 281
Positive likelihood ratio. *See* Likelihood ratio
Positive predictive value. *See* Predictive value
Poster presentations, 608–9, 609*f*
Post hoc tests. *See* Multiple comparison tests
Posttest-only control group design, 230–31
Posttest probability, 515, 517–18, 518*f*, 519*b*
Power, 40, 102, 210, S24–34
  a priori sample size, 343–344
  beta (β), 342
  defined, 342
  determinants, 342
  effect size index, 343
  post hoc power analysis, 344
  underpowered trials, 102
Power-efficiency, nonparametric tests, 402
Practice-based evidence (PBE), 22
Practice effects, 234
Pragmatic clinical trial (PCT), 12*f*, 13*t*, 19, 21–22, 200–201, 201*t*, 202*b*
  pragmatic exploratory continuum indicator summary (PRECIS), 200, 202*b*
Precision, 107
Preclinical research, 11, 201
Predictive validity, 129*t*, 131–32

Predictive value (PV), 513
  negative PV–, 513
  positive PV+, 513
  and prevalence, 513
Presentations, 607–610
Pretest-posttest control group design, 228–30
Pretest probability, 515–16, 516*f*
Prevalence, 513, 530–32
Primary outcome, 25
Primary source, 71
Principal axis factoring, 471
Principal components analysis (PCA), 468, S31–1
Principal investigator (PI), 548–49
PRISMA, 581, 582*f*, S37–1
PRISMA-ScR, 592, S37–1
Privacy Rule, 90
Probability, 333–34, 341
Probability sampling, 150, 185–188, 186*t*
Prognosis studies, 565–67
  QUIPS, 585
Propensity score matching, 282
Propensity scores, 219, 461
Proportions, testing, 415–16
Proposal. *See* Research proposal
Proposition, 44
Prospective study, 274–76, 275*f*
  challenges, 275–76
  cohort study, 280*f*
PTNow Article Search, 72*t*
Publication bias, 71, 579
PubMed, 72, 74, 78, 85
  advanced search, 81*f*
  clinical queries, 81, 82*f*
  limits and filters, 78*f*, 80, 81*f*
  MeSH, 76*f*, 77, 80*f*
  My NCBI, 76*f*
  PMID, 79*f*
  send to, 78*f*
  tutorial, 76*f*
PubMed Central (PMC) repository, 72
Purposive sampling, 186*t*, 189–90, 308–9, 311, 313
p value, 341

Q-sort, 142, S11–2
QUADAS/QUADAS-2, 585
Quadratic trend, 396, 454
Quadruple Aim, 3*b*
Qualitative research, 11, 12*f*, 14*t*, 297–316
  audit trail, 311
  case study, 304–5
  coding, 309
  confirmability, 310*f*, 312
  content analysis, 309
  constant comparison, 303
  credibility, 310, 310*f*
  critical appraisal, 567–68, 567*t*
  data analysis and interpretation, 309–12
  data collection, 305–8
  dependability, 310*f*, 311

ethnography, 302
and EBP, 59, 298–99, 299f
field notes, 305, 311
grounded theory, 303, 304f
interviews, 306–8
levels of evidence, 64–65
member checking, 311
mixed methods, 312–14
negative case analysis, 311
observation, 305
participant observation, 305–6
phenomenology, 303–4
reflexivity, 312
research question, 299–302
sampling, 308–9
social constructivism, 3
sociocultural influences, 300–301
theoretical sampling, 309
and translational research, 299
transferability, 310f, 311
triangulation, 311
trustworthiness, 310–12
Quality improvement (QI), 26
Quartiles, 325
Quasi-experimental design, 12f, 13t, 214, 240–48, 242f, 243b
interrupted time series (ITS) design, 242–44
historical controls, 246
nonequivalent group design, 244–47, 246f
one-group pretest-posttest design, 241, 241f
repeated measures design, 241–42, 242f
Questionnaire, 142. *See also* Surveys
Questions. *See* Survey questions
QUIPS, 585
Quota sampling, 186t, 189

Random assignment (allocation), 194–98, 195t, 219
Random-digit dialing, 188
Random effect, 419, 487–88
Random error, 116, 116f
Randomized designs
between subjects, 228
block design, 233
consent design, 195t, 197
controlled trial (RCT), 12f, 13t, 18, 193, 193f, 200
crossover, 235–36, 235f
mixed, 236
one-way, 233–234
two-way, 236
Random numbers, 195–196, 196t, 621t, S13–1
Random sampling (selection), 185–87
Range, 324
Rank biserial correlation, 435, S29–2
Rasch analysis, 169–74, S12–2
computer adaptive test (CAT), 174
conversion scores, 172–73, 173t
differential item functioning (DIF), 173–74

fit statistics, 172–73
infit and outfit, 172, 172t
item and person separation, 170
item distribution, 170
logit scores, 169, 171f, 172t, 173t
mean square estimate, 172, 172t
person fit, 172
person-item map, 169, 169f, 171f
standardized residuals (ZSTD), 172, 172t
thresholds, 170
Rater reliability. *See* Reliability
Ratio scale, 112
RCT. *See* Randomized designs
Reactive bias, 305
Reactive effects, 213
Recall bias, 143, 282
Receiver operating characteristic curve. *See* ROC curve
Reciprocal transformation, 636
Recruitment, of participants, 182
in qualitative research, 308–309
Reference standard, 131, 510
Reflexivity, 312
RefWorks, 85
Regression analysis, 440–67. *See also* Multiple regression and Logistic regression
ANCOVA, 461–65
ANOVA, 444
coding, 453–54
coefficient, 442, 446
coefficient of determination, 440
constant, 442
dummy variables, 453–54
effect size, 449
explanation/cause and effect, 454
hierarchical regression, 453
least squares method, 442
line of best fit, 441–442, 442f, S30–1
logistic regression, 456–61
multiple regression, 446–49
null hypothesis, 444
polynomial (nonlinear) regression, 454–56, 456t
power and sample size, 449, 449b, S30–3
R^2, 444
regression line, 441, 442f
residuals, 445, 445f
simple linear regression, 440–46, 441f, 443t
standard error of estimate (SEE), 444
Regression to the mean (RTM), 123, 213
REGWF, REGWQ, 585t, S26–3
Relative effect, 534
Relative reliability, 118, 486
Relative risk (RR), 534–36, 535t, 540, 541t
power and sample size, 536, S34
Relative risk reduction (RRR), 540–41, 541t, 542, 542f
Reliability, 115–26, 486–501, 491b, absolute, 118, 492
agreement, measures of, 494–96

alternate (parallel) forms, 121–122, 499–501
carryover effects, 120
coefficient, 118
coefficient of variation (CV), 328, 494
generalizability theory, 119, 119b
internal consistency, 122, 497–99
inter-rater, 121, 488
intraclass correlation coefficient (ICC), 486–90
intra-rater, 121, 488
method error, 494, S32–4
methodological studies, 124
minimal detectable change (MDC), 123–24, 123f, 501–502
rater, 120–21
regression to the mean, 123
relative, 118, 486
split-half, 122
standard error of measurement (SEM), 118, 492–94
testing effect, 120
test-retest, 119–20, 492–494, 493t
validity, compared, 127–28
Repeated measures ANOVA, 373–78. *See also* Analysis of Variance
partitioning the variance, 375–77
power and sample size, 378, S25–2
sphericity, 377
two-factor designs, 378
Repeated measures design, 228, 233–36
crossover design, 235, 235f
mixed design, 236
one-way design, 233–36
time series design, 241–42
two-way designs, 236
within subjects, 228
Replication, 32, 101
single-subject design, 268
Reporting guidelines, 599–602, 600t, 601t, S38–1
Research
continuum, 11, 12f
definition, 2–3
evaluating. *See* Critical appraisal
hypotheses, 38–39
misconduct, 98–100
objectives, 38, 550
problem, 29–32, 550
process, 4–5
types of, 11–14, 12f, 13–14t, 34
ResearchGate, 85
Research proposal, 548–56
administrative support, 552–554
biosketch, 552, S35
budget, 549t, 553–54
components, 549–552, 549t
documentation of informed consent, 552
format, 554
funding, 555
statement of purpose, 549t, 550
submitting the proposal, 555
timeline, 551, 552t
writing the proposal, 554–55

Research question, 4, 29–41, 30f, 35f, 37f
  clinical experience, 30–31
  clinical theory, 31
  framing the question, 34–37
  good research questions, 39–40
  objectives and hypotheses, 38
  professional literature, 31
  research problem, 29–32
  research rationale, 32–33
  theory, 49
Research report 602–605. *See also*
    Disseminating research
Residuals, 172, 442, 444, 445
  standardized, 419, 445
Respect for persons, 90
Responsiveness, 136, 501. *See also* Change
Retractions, 101
Retrospective study, 275f, 276
  case-control study, 280f
  challenges, 276
  cohort study, 280f
  secondary analysis, 276b
Reverse causation, 277
Review of literature, 33, 59, 86, 144.
    See also Searching the literature
Risk
  absolute, 534
  analytic epidemiology, 533–39
  observational research, 272
  relative, 534–36, 540, 541t
Risk-benefit ratio, 91
Risk factor, 272, 533–34, 536, 538
Risk reduction, 540–42
ROC curve, 519–23, 522t
  area under the curve (AUC), 221
  cutoff scores, 519–523
  Youden index, 521
Rotated factor matrix, 470t, 472–73
Roy's largest characteristic root, 479
Run-in period, 195t, 197

Samples and sampling, 180–91
  accessible population, 181, 181f
  area probability sampling, 188
  cluster sampling, 186t, 187–88, 188f
  consecutive sampling, 189
  convenience (accidental) sampling,
    186t, 189
  disproportional sampling, 186t, 188,
    S13–2
  flow diagram, 183, 184f, 221f
  inclusion/exclusion criteria, 181–82
  mixed methods research, 313
  multistage sampling, 188, 188f
  nonprobability sampling, 186t, 188–90
  probability sampling, 185–88, 186t
  purposive sampling, 186t, 189–90,
    308–9, 313
  quota sampling, 186t, 189
  random-digit dialing, 188
  random sampling (selection), 183,
    185–86, 186t, S13–1
  sampling bias, 185
  sampling error, 183–85

selection criteria, 181–82
  snowball sampling, 186t, 190
  stratified random sampling, 186t, 187,
    187f
  systematic sampling, 186–87, 186t
  target population, 181, 181f
  theoretical sampling, 309
Sample size, 183, 343
  chi-square, 421, 424b, S28
  exploratory factor analysis (EFA), 474
  logistic regression, 461, S30–3
  McNemar test, 425, 426b, S28
  nonparametric tests, 402, S27–3
  one-way ANOVA, 369, 369b, S25–2
  Pearson correlation coefficient, 432,
    433b, S29–1
  power, and, 343
  a priori analysis, 343
  qualitative research, 308–9
  regression analysis, 449, 449b, S30–3
  relative risk/odds ratio, 536, S34
  repeated measures ANOVA, 378, S25–2
  surveys, 152
  two-way ANOVA, 373, 375b, S25–2
  t test, 360–363, 362b, 363b, S24–2
Sample variance, 327
Sampling bias, 185
Sampling distribution, 335
Sampling error, 151, 183–85, 334–35
Saturation, 303
Scales. *See* Health measurement scales
Scalogram analysis, 168
Scatter plot, 428, 429f
Scheffé comparison, 385t, 390, 391t, S26–3
  minimum significant difference, 390
Scientific method, 3–4
Scoping review, 11, 12f, 575t, 592–93,
    S37–6
SCOPUS, 579, S6
Screening accuracy, 131b
Searching the literature, 70–87. *See also*
    Literature review
  abstracts, 83–84
  automatic term mapping, 78
  Boolean logic, 75–76, 77f
  CINAHL, 72t, 72–73
  citation management applications, 85
  cited reference searching, 83
  clinical queries, 81, 82f
  Cochrane Database of Systematic
    Reviews, 72t, 73
  databases, 71–73, 72t, S6
  e-mail alerts, 85
  expanding search strategies, 83
  exploding, 78–79
  filters, 80
  focusing, 79
  full text, 84–85
  grey literature, 70–71, 579–80,
    580b
  interlibrary loan, 84
  journal and author searching, 83
  keyword searching, 74–76
  limits, 80

medical subject headings (MeSH), 77,
    79, 80t
MEDLINE, 71–72, 72t
meta-analysis. *See* Meta-analysis
My NCBI, 85
open access journals, 84
primary sources, 71
PubMed, 72, 72t, 74–82
reference lists, 83
refining the search, 80–83
related references, 83
saving searches, 85
scoping review, 575t, 592–93
search engines, 72t, 73, 73b
secondary sources, 71
sensitivity and specificity, 81
systematic review. *See* Systematic
    review
truncation, 75
wildcards, 75
Secondary analysis, 276b
Secondary outcome, 25
Secondary source, 71
Selection
  case-control study, 281–82
  cohort study, 279
  experimental design, 228
  internal validity, 213–14
  research question, 29
  sampling, 181–82
  surveys, 150–52
  systematic review, 578–79
Selection bias, 281–82, 584
Self-report, 143, 159, 160, 164
SEM. *See* Standard error of
    measurement; Structural equation
    modeling
Sensitivity, 131b, 511, 512t
  in literature search, 81
Sensitivity analysis, 589
Sequential clinical trials, 236–38, S16
Serial dependency, 264–65
Sham, 198
Shapiro-Wilk test of normality, 349b, 651
Sidak-Bonferroni procedure, 385t, S26–3
Significance, clinical vs. statistical,
    344–45, 345b
Sign test, 407–9, 408t
Simple effects, 391, 393t
Simple linear regression. *See* Linear
    regression
Simple random assignment, 195–96,
    195t
Simple random sampling, 185–86, 186t
Simpson's paradox, 539b
Single-blind study, 199
Single-factor design, 228
Single-subject design (SSD), 12f, 13t,
    249–70
  A-B-A-B design, 255, 256f
  A-B-A design, 254, 255f
  A-B design, 251, 251f, 254
  alternating treatment design, 257–58,
    258f

baseline data, 251–52, 252f, 256b
binomial test, 264, S18–3t
changing criterion design, 259, S18–1
C statistic, 265, S18–5
design phases, 250–53
effect size, 267
generalization, 267–68
level, 260–62, 262f
multiple baseline designs, 255–57, 257f, S18–1
multiple treatment design, 258–59
N-of-1 trial, 259–60, 261b
nonoverlapping scores, 267
replication of effects, 254, 268
serial dependency, 264–65
slope, 263
social validity, 268
split middle line, 263–64, 263f, S18–2
statistical process control (SPC), 265–67, 266f, S18–4
target behavior, 253–54
trend, 262–63, 262f
two standard deviation band method, 265. 265f
visual data analysis, 260–63
withdrawal designs, 254–55, 255f, 256f
Skewed distributions, 322, 322f, 323
SnNout, 514f
Snowball sampling, 186t, 190
Social threats, to internal validity, 214
Spearman rank correlation coefficient, 433–34, 434–35, 434t,
critical values table, 613, S29–1t, *Appendix A Online*
Special cause variation, 266
Specificity, 131, 511, 512t
in literature search, 81
Sphericity, 377
Bartlett's test, 470t, 471
Mauchly's test, 376t, 377
SPIDER, 59
Split-half reliability, 122
Split middle line, 263–64, 263f, S18–2
Split-plot ANOVA, 378
SPORTDiscus, 72t, S6
SpPin, 514f
Square root transformation, 635
Square transformation, 635
SRM. *See* Standardized response mean
Standard deviation, 327–28, 329f, S22
Standard error
of measurement (SEM), 118, 120, 492–94, 493t
of the difference between the means, 354
of difference scores, 360
of the estimate (SEE), 444
of the mean, 335, 335f
Standardized mean difference (SMD), 360, 587
Standardized normal curve, 329–30
Standardized residuals, 172, 419, 445
Standardized response mean (SRM), 503–4, 504t

Standardized scores, 329
Statistic, 183, 318
Statistical conclusion validity, 210–11, 211f, 211t
Statistical hypothesis, 38
Statistical hypothesis testing. *See* Hypothesis testing
Statistical inference, 333–50
confidence intervals, 336–38. *See also* Confidence intervals
hypothesis testing. *See* Hypothesis testing
nonparametric tests, 349
parametric statistics, 348–49
probability, 333–34
sampling error, 334–35
Statistical packages, 629–30, 630t
Statistical power. *See* Power
Statistical process control, S18–4. *See also* Single-subject designs
common cause and special cause variation, 266
control charts, 266
upper and lower control limits, 266, 266f
Statistical significance vs. clinical significance, 344–45
Statistical symbols, 654
Statistical tables, 613–21
area under normal curve, 614–16t
binomial test, 613, S18–3t, S27–2t, *Appendix A Online*
chi-square distribution, 620t
F statistic, 618t
Mann-Whitney U test, 613, S27–2t, *Appendix A Online*
Pearson correlations (r), 619t
Spearman's rank correlation coefficient, 613, S29–1, S29–1t, *Appendix A Online*
studentized range statistic, 613, S26–1t, *Appendix A Online*
table of random numbers, 621t
t test, 617t
Wilcoxon signed-ranks test, 613, S27–2t, *Appendix A Online*
Stem-and-leaf plot, 320f, 321
Stepwise multiple regression, 449–53, 451–52t. *See also* Multiple regression
forward or backward inclusion, 452–53
hierarchical regression, 453
step wise inclusion, 450
Stratified random assignment, 195t, 196
Stratified random sampling, 186t, 187, 187f
Structural equation modeling (SEM), 474–77
direct and indirect effects, 476, S31–2
endogenous variable, 476
exogenous variable, 476
goodness of fit, 476–77
interpretation of, 477
path diagram, 475–56, 476f

Studentized range, 386
critical values table, 613, S26–1, *Appendix A Online*
Student-Newman-Keuls (SNK) test, 385t, 387–89, 389t
comparison intervals, 387, 388f
critical values table, studentized range, 387, 613, S26–1t, *Appendix A Online*
minimum significant difference, 388
Subject-to-variables (STV) ratio, 474
Sufficient exposure, 274b
Summative scales, 161–67
Sum of squares (SS), 327, 327t, 367, 368, S25–1
Superiority trial, 205, 206f, 339b
Survey questions, *See also* Surveys
branching, 148
check-all-that-apply, 147
checklists, 147
closed-ended questions, 146
dichotomous questions, 146
double-barreled questions, 149
frequency and time measures, 149
multiple choice questions, 146
open-ended questions, 145–46
purposeful language, 148–49
rank-order questions, 148
sensitive questions, 149–50
writing good questions, 148–50
Surveys, 141–58
analysis of data, 154–55
bias, 143, 149
contacting respondents, 152–54
cover letter, 153–54, 153f
cross-tabulations, 155
demographics, 150
descriptive, 141, 288–289
ethical issues, 156–57
expert review, 145
hypothesis testing, 141, 144
incentives, 152
interviews, 142–43
missing data, 155
planning, 143–45
response rate, 151–52
sample size, 152, 152t
sampling error, 151
selecting a sample, 150–52
self-report, 143, 160
summarizing data, 155
type of questions. *See* Survey questions
Survival analysis, 481–83
censored observations, 482
Cox proportional hazards model, 483
hazard ratio (HR), 483
Kaplan-Meier estimate, 482
survival curve, 482f
Syllogism, 45, 46b
Synthesizing literature, 11, 574–96
See also Meta-analysis and Systematic Reviews
scoping review, 575t, 592–93
types of evidence synthesis, 575t

Systematic error, 116, 116f
Systematic review, 11, 12f, 60, 71, 575–87, 575t, S37–3
   AMSTAR-2, 591, S37–2
   Cochrane risk of bias tool, 584, 584f
   clinical practice guidelines, 590
   critical appraisal of, 591, S37–2
   data extraction, 580–81, S37–4
   data synthesis, 585, 586t
   methodological quality, 581–85
   overview, 577f
   PEDro scale, 583–84, 583t
   PRISMA flow diagram, 581, 582f, S37–1
   purpose, 575–76
   research question, 33, 576–77
   scoping review, 592–93
   screening references, 580
   search strategy, 579–80
   selection criteria, 578–79
   types of, 575t
Systematic sampling, 186–87, 186t

Table of random numbers, 186, 621
Target behavior, in single-subject design, 253
Target population, 160, 181
Testing effect, 120, 213
Test-retest reliability, 119–20. *See also* Reliability
Theoretical sampling, 309
Theory, 42–52
   characteristics, 47
   clinical, 31
   components, 43–44
   constructs, 43
   deductive, 45–46
   defined, 42
   development of, 45–46
   grand, 50
   grounded, 46, 303, 304f
   hypothetical-deductive, 45–46
   inductive, 46
   laws and, 50
   meta-, 50
   middle-range, 49–50
   models, 44
   practical applications, 48–49
   propositions, 44
   purposes, 42–43
   scope, 49–50
   testing, 46–47
   "tomato effect", 47b
Time series design, 241–44
   interrupted time series (ITS) design, 242–44
   one-group pretest-posttest design, 241
   repeated measures design, 241–42, 242f
Tolerance level, 448
Transformation of data, 445–46, 635–36, 635t, 636t
Translational research, 6, 10, 17–28, 20f
   basic research, 19, 20f
   defined, 6, 17
   effectiveness research, 21–22

implementation studies, 25–26
outcomes research, 23–25
qualitative research, 299
translation blocks, 19–21, 20f
translation continuum, 18–21
translation gap, 17–18
Treatment arms, 193
Tree plot, 587
Trend, in single-subject design, 262–63
Trend analysis, 369t, 397f, 395–98
Trial and error, 54, 56f
Triangulation, 311
Triple Aim, 3b
True negative, 510
True positive, 510
Truncation, 75
t-test, 351–64
   alternative hypothesis, 353
   confidence intervals, 357–358, 358b, 359–60
   critical values table, 617t, *Appendix A Online*
   degrees of freedom, 354, 360
   effect size, 360–63, 362f
   equal variances, 354–58
   error variance, 351
   homogeneity of variance, 353
   independent *t*-test. *See* unpaired
   misuse/inappropriate use, 363
   null hypothesis, 353, 360
   paired, 359–363, 361t
   power and sample size, 360–63, 362b, 363b, S24–2
   unequal variances, 358–59, S24–1
   unpaired, 353–59, 355t, 356f, 359t
Tukey's honestly significant difference (HSD), 385t, 386–87, 388t
   critical values table, studentized range, 387, 613, S26–1, *Appendix A Online*
   minimum significant difference, 386
Two-factor repeated measures design, 378
Two standard deviation band method, 265
Two-tailed test, 347, 357b
Two-way ANOVA, 370–73
   degrees of freedom, 371
   effect size, 373
   interaction, 371–373, 372t, 374t
   partitioning the variance, 370–71
   power and sample size, 373, 375b, S25–2
Two-way factorial design, 232–33, 370
Two-way repeated measures designs, 236
Type I error, 340–342, 340f
   error rate in multiple comparisons, 383–84
Type II error, 342–346, 340f

Uniform distribution, chi-square, 416–17, 417t
Unpaired *t*-test. *See t*-test

Unplanned comparisons, 384
U test. *See* Mann-Whitney *U* test

Validity, 127–40, 501–506
   ceiling effect, 138
   change, and, 136–38, 501–506, 501f
   concurrent, 129t, 131
   construct, 129f, 129t, 132–34, 215–17, 211f, 211t, S10–2
   content, 129–30, 129f, 129t, S10–1
   convergent, 129t, 133
   criterion-related, 129f, 129t, 130–31
   cross-sectional validity study, 277–78
   cultural validity, 160
   defined, 127
   diagnostic accuracy, of, 509–14
   discriminant, 129t, 133
   external, 217–18, 211f, 211t
   face, 130
   floor effect, 138
   internal, 212–215, 211f, 211t
   methodological studies, 138–39
   predictive, 129t, 131–32
   reliability, compared, 127–28
   social, 268
   statistical conclusion, 210–211, 211f, 211t
   strategies to maximize validity, 138–39
Variability, 324–28, 325t
   coefficient of variation (CV), 328
   interquartile range, 325
   percentiles, 325
   quartiles, 325
   range, 324
   standard deviation, 327–28, 329f, 327t
   standardized scores, 329, 329f
   variance, 326–27, 327t
Variables
   active and attribute, 194
   alphanumeric, 631
   blocking, 233
   categorical, 415, 419, 424, 453
   construct, 108
   continuous, 107
   dependent, 35, 440, 446, 457
   dichotomous, 106
   discrete, 107
   extraneous, 211, 214, 219, 220, 536
   grouping, 632
   independent, 34, 440, 449, 457
   latent, 43, 108, 168, 173, 469, 473, 475
   outcome, 440
   polytomous, 106
   response, 440
   string, 631
Variance, 117, 326–27, S22
   homogeneity of, 353, 368, 377
Variance inflation factor (VIF), 448
Varimax rotation, 472
VAS. *See* Visual analog scale
Vectors, 479
Venn diagram, 75, 77f

Visual analog scale (VAS), 147–48,
164–67, 164*f*, *165*t, 167*f*
anchors, 165
variations, 165–66
Vital statistics, 533

Wait list control group, 198
Wald statistic, 459*t*, 460
Washout period, 235, 235*f*
Web of Science, *S6*
Weighted kappa, 496, *S32–3*
Wilcoxon rank sum test, 400*t*, 404*t*

Wilcoxon signed-ranks test, 408*t*,
409–10, 613
critical values table, *S27–2t, Appendix A
Online*
degrees of freedom,
large samples, 410
null hypothesis, 410
power and sample size, 410, *S27–3*
Wildcard, 75
Wilk's lambda, 480
Withdrawal designs, 244, 254–55
Within-subject design, 228, 250

Writing
for dissemination, 606
in proposals, 554

Yates' continuity correction, 421
Youden index, 521

Zelen design, 197
zero-order correlation, 438
z-score, 329, 329*f*, 346
critical values table, 614–616*t*,
Appendix A Online